Neuroradiology THE REQUISITES

SERIES EDITOR   **James H. Thrall,** M.D.
Radiologist-in-Chief
Department of Radiology
Massachusetts General Hospital
Boston, Massachusetts

OTHER VOLUMES IN THE REQUISITES SERIES   Gastrointestinal Radiology
Pediatric Radiology
Nuclear Medicine
Cardiac Radiology
Genitourinary Radiology
Ultrasound
Thoracic Radiology
Mammography
Vascular and Interventional Musculoskeletal

Neuroradiology

THE REQUISITES

ROBERT I. GROSSMAN, M.D.

Louis Marx Professor and Chairman
Department of Radiology

Professor
Departments of Neurology, Neurosurgery,
and Physiology and Neuroscience
New York University School of Medicine
New York, New York

DAVID M. YOUSEM, M.D., M.B.A.

Director of Neuroradiology
Professor of Radiology
Johns Hopkins University School of Medicine
Baltimore, Maryland

Second Edition

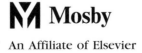

Mosby

An Affiliate of Elsevier

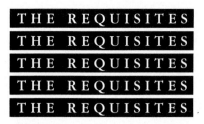

M Mosby
An Affiliate of Elsevier

The Curtis Center
Independence Square West
Philadelphia, Pennsylvania 19106

NEURORADIOLOGY: The Requisites   ISBN 0-323-00508-X

Library of Congress Cataloging in Publication Data
Grossman, Robert I.
    Neuroradiology : the requisites / Robert I. Grossman, David M. Yousem.—2nd ed.
      p. ; cm.
    Includes bibliographical references and index.
    ISBN 0-323-00508-X
     1. Nervous system—Radiography. I. Yousem, David M. II. Title.
    [DNLM: 1. Neuroradiography. 2. Central Nervous System Diseases—diagnosis. WL
141 G878 2003]
RC349.R3 G76 2003
616.8′04757—dc21
                        2002037859

Printed in the United States of America.

Last digit is the print number: 9 8 7 6 5 4 3 2 1

To Benjamin, David, and Elisabeth who supported me in peace and war, for better or worse—laissez les bons temps rouler.

R.I.G.

To Marilyn, Ilyssa, and Mitchell who have been supportive and understanding even when this book snatched precious family time
To the many students of neuroradiology who have inpsired us and who have been patient while we tried to write the best book possible
Live, learn, love, and leave a legacy.

D.M.Y.

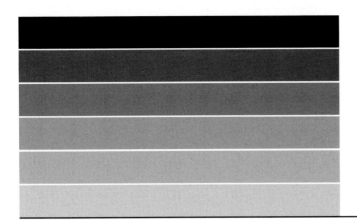

Foreword

The first edition of *Neuroradiology: The Requisites* has been one of the most successful books in the entire *Requisites* series. Drs. Grossman and Yousem produced a remarkable volume that captured both the philosophy of the series and their subject of neuroradiology extremely well. Readers found the first edition to be eminently readable and the subject was presented with a rare commodity for medical textbooks, humor! What better than to have an authoritative text that treats the reader to humor and encouragement.

In the nine years since the appearance of the first edition of *Neuroradiology: The Requisites*, much has happened in the field of neuroradiology. No, the anatomy, physiology and function of the nervous system have not changed. But, the level of understanding of each of these and the ability to translate that new knowledge and new understanding into the practice of neuroradiology has advanced the field dramatically. Drs. Grossman and Yousem have risen to the challenge of incorporating these advances into their book in a very efficient way for the reader. First, advances in technology, most importantly, CT and MRI are presented in the first chapter and subsequently the new imaging capabilities are addressed in a systematic way throughout the book. For example, in the discussion of magnetic resonance imaging techniques, sections have been added for functional magnetic resonance imaging, magnetization transfer imaging, MR spectroscopy, FLAIR and diffusion-weighted imaging among others. Application of these newer methods are woven into the remainder of the text.

I believe that anyone in the practice of medicine who deals with the nervous system will find the second edition of *Neuroradiology: The Requisites* to be an invaluable and entertaining approach to the subject. Residents on their first neuroradiology rotations face the unique problem of going from a minimal knowledge base of neuroradiology to a working knowledge in a very short period of time. *The Requisites* series was designed by intent to address this problem by making material efficiently accessible to the reader and reinforcing it with summary tables and boxes of the most important material.

The resident studying for the board exam faces the formidable task of covering the entire field of radiology. Again, the format of *The Requisites* makes this possible through the careful selection of material included in each text including this one. It is realistic to read each book in the series over the period of a few days during a subspecialty rotation or in board preparation.

For radiology practitioners, neurologists and neurosurgeons, *Neuroradiology: The Requisites* can actually serve as a useful reference book to help guide their understanding of imaging results and findings in their patients.

When *The Requisites* series was first established, it was our hypothesis and our hope that the format would make information readily accessible to the reader by eliminating extraneous material and covering those topics deemed most important to clinical practice by the respective authors. The success of the series over the past decade argues strongly in favor of the approach and format.

I have every confidence that the second edition of *Neuroradiology: The Requisites* will be equally well received and useful to its readers, as was the first edition. I again congratulate Drs. Grossman and Yousem for their outstanding text. They have truly brought to bear their authoritative knowledge and experience in neuroradiology for the benefit of the reader whether beginning resident or seasoned warrior.

James H. Thrall, M.D.

Radiologist-in-Chief
Massachusetts General Hospital
Professor of Radiology
Harvard Medical School
Boston, Massachusetts

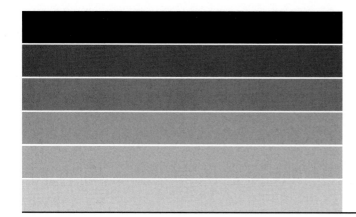

Preface to second edition

Neuroradiology has evolved considerably since our first edition was published in 1994 (thank the Lord—otherwise why would you cough up the big bucks for the second time around). We have attempted to capture this extended scope while at the same time tried to keep the same inimitable style that appeared to be successful in the first edition. As you can see, the size of the text has grown in keeping with the field. We believe that the vast majority of topics in the book are relevant to the practice and art of neuroradiology.

Our goal in writing a second edition was to produce a volume that was current with respect to neuroimaging including diagnosis, pathophysiology, and techniques. We have included diffusion, BOLD, magnetic resonance spectroscopy, perfusion imaging, etc. Some of this may not have migrated into the common practice but, if not, it is pretty close, and clearly important for the reader to understand. We are now in an era of genomics and proteinomics and molecular imaging; how do these relate to macroscopic imaging tools? Hard questions to be answered by a couple of small town doctors like us. There is considerable information here, more than our friend, the tire-kicking radiologist, may

need, but the board-taking resident or CAQee will be more than satisfied.

We still strove to write a book that you couldn't put down (literally and figuratively) that would be engaging to the reader. Frankly, adjusting the humor through the Clinton scandal years to the Gore-Bush non-election, to the era of terrorism and war was as difficult as describing Balo's concentric sclerosis. We hope that we have created a book that has the proper balance of irreverential humor, psy-ops, and scientific fact . . . or hearsay.

We have put our blood, sweat, and tears into this edition (our publisher guaranteed the last item). We hope that this book is as well-received as our first product. Please provide us with any suggestions, comments, criticisms, or corrections (be nice, we are very sensitive). DMY may be able to think about a third edition after his ulcer is healed. RIG has officially retired from writing Neuroradiology textbooks, although he still thinks about Neuroradiology.

Lastly, you the reader will be the ultimate arbiter of this book's success. Enjoy our baby!

Bob and Dave

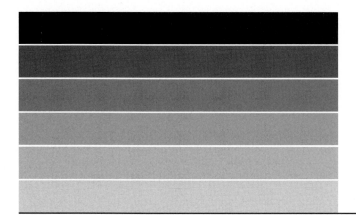

Acknowledgments

Whew! It is never over. This book has been a pustule on our rear for so long. I will never write a third edition—you can bet the estate on it. So yes David, you can be the first author of the third edition. You have been a splendid partner—doing more than your share of the work. We laughed and cried at the slings and arrows that were shot at us during the last two years. You have an exceptional work ethic and are an outstanding neuroradiologist—but your sense of humor still leaves much to be desired.

Let me start by acknowledging my past kismet. My career took a number of interesting turns. Leaving neurosurgery for radiology at the start of the CT era, training in neuroradiology at MGH with Ken Davis and the late Juan Taveras, coming to Penn and having MR dropped in my lap, and being able to build a magnificent section of Neuroradiologists including Scott Atlas (who is too much like this author), Linda Bagley, David Hackney, Robert Hurst, Laurie Loevner, and the junior author (David Yousem). I am extremely proud of about 100 fellows I helped train, many of whom hold prominent academic appointments throughout the world. Research fellows who have expanded my horizon include Jianping Dai, John Gomori, Vincent Dousset, Yulin Ge, Mark van Buchem, and Yukio Miki. Teaching and mentoring have been part of the rich and rewarding experience of academic life.

I was very fortunate to have the chance to assume the Chairmanship of Radiology at NYU in July 2001. Bob Glickman, the Dean, gave me this unique opportunity. I deeply respect him and am most grateful for all that he has done for me and Radiology. I inherited a wonderful department from Dr. Norman Chase (a neuroradiologist by training) who has been the perfect exchairman for me. Irv Kricheff first introduced me to NYU and has been a good friend and confidant. Eddie Knopp has now taken the torch and is lighting up the section.

When I landed at NYU I realized that the position required a team approach. I could not have recruited better mates. Bernie Birnbaum decamped with me to become a Vice Chair of Clinical Affairs. He is a magnificent individual in all respects and enables our department to thrive—*semper fi*. Andy Litt, Vice Chairman of Finance, is a most talented, industrious, and decent friend who has helped translate departmental dreams into reality. Nancy Genieser, Director of Radiology at Bellevue Hospital, has been at my side since the beginning. I deeply respect her intelligence and excellent advice. Alec Megibow, a gifted radiologist and Vice Chair for Education, is committed to our training program and has impacted the careers of countless radiologists. Vivian Lee, an exceptional radiologist/researcher and Vice Chair for Research, is propelling this vital aspect of our program to a leadership position in the world. Mike Harbeson, the splendid manager of our department, makes everyone's work better and easier.

There are a number of other individuals who deserve credit. Lois Mannon, research coordinator extraordinaire, has been the principal force that has managed to keep my research going throughout all of the chaos—you are too good. Oded Gonen, a friend, collaborator, and outstanding scientist, has impacted upon the understanding of disease and provided many new directions for my own research. Georgeann McGuinness provided invaluable editorial comments and introduced me to the martini which served me well through the tribulations of writing this book. One of my best recruits was Janice Ford-Benner. She is a fantastic Director of Corporate Relations and Continuing Medical Education and a special friend. Esther Roman, my secretary, and Sheilah

Rosen, my executive assistant, are immensely competent individuals who are committed to helping me maintain my sanity. They appreciate how much help I need and make me look competent.

Lastly to the countless friends, fellows, and loving family (Lisse—the best proof-reader and wife, David, Ben, Milton, Charlotte) who have enriched my existence. It has been a glorious marathon and I don't see the finish line.

Have a great life.

R.L.G.

"Writing the second edition of the book will be so much easier than the first. It'll be a breeze."

I wish that Bob and I could say that Liz Corra's prediction had come true. On the contrary, Bob and I have felt like we have weathered a tempest in concluding the second edition to this book. Liz had a baby or two and retired and so we have been through two new editors. These poor souls had to adjust to the demands that we made as authors as far as a tolerance for off color humor and a standard of excellence for the text and illustrations. Mosby became Harcourt became Saunders became Elsevier, corporate cultures changed, and electronic gremlins plagued the illustrations. We come to the end of this journey, bedraggled on the shore, wounded but still alive.

What have we accomplished? Bob and I have written a book again that we can be proud of. We read it and we laugh at the jokes, the alliterations, the analogies, the pithy sayings, the poems. It's a larger book with more depth than the first edition and it is more timely. It will stand the test of time. Hopefully it will garner the same level of satisfaction that the first edition achieved.

This is the acknowledgments section and so let's get to it. I thank Bob who has been a great partner in crime. He knew when to get angry and when to calm down during the upheavals that we went through to write the book. He remained passionate about what we were trying to achieve and provided me succor when I was devoid of energy to go on. He drove me, I drove him—this was harder to do than the first edition where we were a quarter of a mile away from each other instead of 200 miles away now. As many of you know, Bob has been my Svengali and I owe him thanks for excellent advice and friendship throughout my career in neuroradiology. He sometimes is more ambitious for me than I am for me. I appreciate the faith he puts in me.

The cast has changed since the first edition. While I want to continue to thank specific colleagues from my HUP days, Laurie Loevner, Bob Hurst, Joe Maldjian, Herb Goldberg, I now have a glorious cast of characters from Johns Hopkins who have "been there for me." Nafi Ay-

gun, Mike Kraut, Doris Lin, Marty Pomper, Deepak Takhtani, Bruce Wasserman, and Jim Zinreich now constitute my physician support system and because they are so good at what they do, I've been able to take the time to write this book. Without great neuroradiology fellows the work wouldn't get done and wouldn't be so much fun—I'm grateful to the 8 years of fellows that served during the making of this book. Thanks also to my former Chairmen, Stan Baum and Elias Zerhouni for modeling successful careers.

Two women in my life deserve extra bonuses of gratitude.

Melinda Hahn, as my administrative assistant, has made my life so much easier over the past 2 years. She is a pleasure to work with and honestly searches for ways to ease the stresses of my work life. I look forward to seeing her at her desk each day and it's cheering to know she's on my team. She's fun. Thanks Melinda. No more breaks.

Rena Geckle has run my research program for me for nearly a decade. I was fortunate that, living in Delaware, Rena was able to commute North or South to remain the caretaker of neuroradiology research at HUP and at Hopkins. Without Rena, I could never get a paper published or an IRB request approved. Being able to rely on her totally to keep all the various research projects afloat has been unbelievably reassuring. Plus Rena is a fantastic person who has a heart as big as Indiana. Thanks Rena.

Norm Beauchamp has been a very close buddy. Even though we now live coasts apart, I feel his presence still in the department here at Hopkins. Norm has outstanding leadership skills and helped me through some trying times that required his excellent counsel and friendship. Our families bonded and we connected in a very deep way. Norm has been through wars with me and I am a better person for that experience. Thanks buddy.

I'd also like to say thanks to research fellows that have been so productive and have done the hard work that I have been unable to perform with my role as Director of Neuroradiology at Hopkins. Over the years Mona Mohamed, Nina Browner, Kader Karli Oguz, and Aylin Tekes have put in very long hours crunching data, post-processing, and putting out manuscripts that have furthered the research mission. They are tireless workers who have bright futures ahead of them and for their work I thank them.

I also wish to thank some close friends at Hopkins. Mike Kraut shares many of the same values as me at work and has jumped on numerous grenades for me during the years I have been at Hopkins. He is a team player who believes in the institution and the values that we in the neuroradiology division strive towards. Buy some Cheetohs on me, Mike. Susan Bassett has been my closest bud outside of radiology. . . . a woman with a brilliant mind and a wonderful heart who has been inspirational in her dedication to quality research and nurturing junior faculty and students. Let's do lunch Susan!

Outside of work I have a cadre of wonderful friends from high school that I am still close with (Scott Glasser, Marty Pechter, Coos Hamburger, Jeff Mechanick, Steve Mandelberg, Bart Pachino, Todd Sarubin, Ronenn Roubenoff, Scott Markman). We meet each year at an undisclosed location and act like adolescents gossiping about friends, drinking booze, playing D&D, chucking the ball, and cutting each other up. It's rejuvenating. Thanks men. Stu Bobman—thanks for so many excellent contributions to our figures. Barry Zingler is my former roommate from college. He's a gastroenterologist in New Jersey and is a great doctor. He's hung in there with me. To Rob Evers, thanks for the friendship and MR support. To Laurie and John, fantastic friends, who make every return trip to Philadelphia a wonderful reunion. So glad we've stayed so close.

Of course, without family, nothing seems important. Mom, Dad, Sam, Penny—thanks for the support. To my life-partner Marilyn thanks for bringing up the kids, preparing the meals, keeping the house, providing emotional support to all of us, earning some dough, running the household, transporting the family, and maintaining the passion. I love you. To Lyss and Mit, I hope that someday you can think back on the breakfasts at Chestnut Ridge, the baseball practices, the soccer games where I ran around the field while training for my marathons, the Blast games, Marco island trips, Boca Raton trips, times in the pool together, the Chinese food dinners, the sleepovers, the birthday parties, the DVDs and videos brought home for dinner theater. If these stick in your memories, I hope that you'll view your Dad as someone who was there for you and loved you in a special way.

To all I recommend following the words of Stephen Covey "Live, learn, love and leave a legacy." Thank you.

D.M.Y.

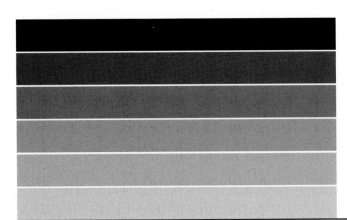

Contents

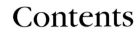

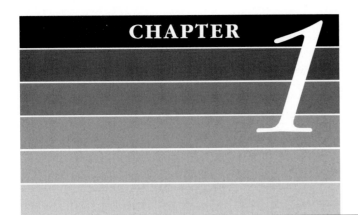

CHAPTER 1

Techniques in Neuroimaging

Central to the effective evaluation of an image is an understanding of the technical aspects of image production. This not only includes recently developed methodologies such as magnetic resonance (MR) and computed tomography (CT) but also the traditional techniques of angiography, myelography, ultrasound, nuclear scintigraphy, and plain film radiography. In some cases, individuals will limit their careers either to the more invasive aspect of neuroradiology (neurointerventionalists) or to the interpretive function (cross-sectional imagers). No matter which field one pursues it is necessary to have a rudimentary knowledge of the physics behind the modalities used. And who better to provide that rudimentary knowledge than two authors who have just that—a rudimentary knowledge of physics. Since the last edition of this book, the deficiencies in our "physical" fund of knowledge have expanded as newer techniques have developed. These imaging advances have been the motivating influence for updating *Neuroradiology: THE REQUISITES*. With these advances, our understanding of the pathophysiology of neurologic disease has improved dramatically. In essence we have moved from the low power of a light microscope to the high magnification detail of an electron microscope with faster scan times and better image resolution. We also have more techniques (e.g., functional MR, diffusion tensor imaging) to visualize brain physiology at our disposal. Let us start the journey. May the force be with you.

PLAIN FILMS

Skull radiographs have played an ever-decreasing role in neuroimaging since the advent of CT. Numerous studies have shown that abnormalities on skull radiographs in patients with trauma do not correlate well with intracranial abnormalities or neurologic deficits. Treatment is usually based on the intracranial effects of skull trauma, so CT and MR imaging are the more useful studies. For that reason the skull radiograph now has a virtually nonexistent role in the emergency department (ED) for the evaluation of closed and open head injuries, except to provide a map for identifying foreign bodies (e.g., a bullet), or to document child abuse. The present role of skull radiographs outside the ED appears to be very limited. Plain films may be useful in characterizing bone lesions in patients who have had ambiguous CT or bone scans, identifying lost sponges in the OR (never happens?), searching for radiopaque foreign bodies before MR, or localizing shunt tube disconnections. Most "plain films" we now interpret are the "scouts" from CT exams.

In a similar vein, plain radiographs of the paranasal sinuses have largely been supplanted by coronal CT, because plain films are notoriously inadequate for evaluating mucosal abnormalities. CT can also serve as a map for the endoscopic sinus surgeon. However, for patients in the ED or intensive care unit who are too unstable to be transported to a CT unit, plain radiographs of the sinus may be useful in determining the source of fever. One should understand, however, that the incidence of false-positive and false-negative findings for sinusitis by plain films is rather high.

Plain films are also occasionally used for the evaluation of facial trauma (Box 1-1) in those settings where CT is unavailable in the ED (Taliban medical centers, MASH units in Kuwait and backwater academic institutions like ours).

Although these studies may identify gross fractures, multiplanar CT scanning often is required for surgical planning and for true assessment of deep facial trauma. This is particularly true if one is considering sphenoid sinus, skull base, or temporal bone fractures where plain films are even less accurate.

With plain radiography the x-ray beam serves as the source of photon energy and the film is the "detector." The x-ray beam is generated when electrons produced

in the cathode of an x-ray tube hit the anode (usually tungsten alloy) target. The electron current is measured in milliamperes (mA) and the potential difference across the x-ray tube is the peak kilovoltage (kVp). Increasing the kVp increases the energy of the electrons flowing towards the anode and therefore increases the amount and energy of x-rays produced. The time that the x-ray tube is in operation is multiplied by the mA to calculate the mAs (milliampere-seconds). Lowering the kVp increases image contrast, but penetration of the photon beam decreases. Increasing the mAs yields greater exposure at the cost of higher current and heat load on the x-ray tube. This has not changed since Roentgen.

Contrast in plain radiography is based on the differential attenuation of the x-ray beam by various tissues. As the density, atomic number, and electrons per gram of a tissue increase, the degree of attenuation of an x-ray beam increases. The greater the attenuation of photons of an x-ray beam, the lighter the image on the film. Thus, metal and bone have a greater degree of attenuation of the x-ray beam than air or soft tissue. Metal and bone will look white on an x-ray film; air is black. By virtue of lower density, fat also has a lesser degree of x-ray attenuation (Fig. 1-1). So a fat Oprah attenuates less than a muscular Oprah.

Digital radiography has also invaded the workspace. This allows collection and storage of data on digital detectors and computers rather than merely relying on hard copy film for plain film studies. This has led to a debate between hard and soft copy as it relates to expense versus ease of use versus storage needs, and so on. Some manufacturers have switched to silicon flat panel detectors, with cesium iodide scintillators to improve image quality, decrease radiation dose, and allow long-term storage of data. The x-ray photons are converted to light by the cesium scintillator, which in turn produces an electrical charge, which is transformed into a digital readout on an electronic processor. Digital images may be read on film, computer monitors, or even video screens. Thus the innovators have taken a relatively simple technology and made it as complex as rocket science. The trend has been from low cost–low tech to high cost–high tech methodology with constant software upgrades. Besides freeing film librarians for longer coffee breaks this has lined the pockets of equipment manufacturers and saddled the departments with extra high cost propellor heads in information technology. Digital radiography has largely been implemented in such plain-film bastions as the intensive care units (ICU) and mammography units (where the debate between hard versus soft also rages). As these areas are often services that are "in the red" to begin with, the negative margin only increases. Technology marches on. Profit declines.

Subtraction angiography is based on the principle that a baseline film of an area of anatomy without vascular opacification can be subtracted from a film of the same

---

Box 1-1 Current *Alleged* Utility of Plain Films

Rule out foreign body (before magnetic resonance scan)
Skull fractures
Acute sinusitis screen
Rule out opaque salivary gland calculi
Characterize bony lesions
Rule out epiglottis vs croup in emergency room
Cervical spine fractures
Flexion-extension views for instability
Spondylolysis
Facial trauma: gross fractures
Find needle in haystack

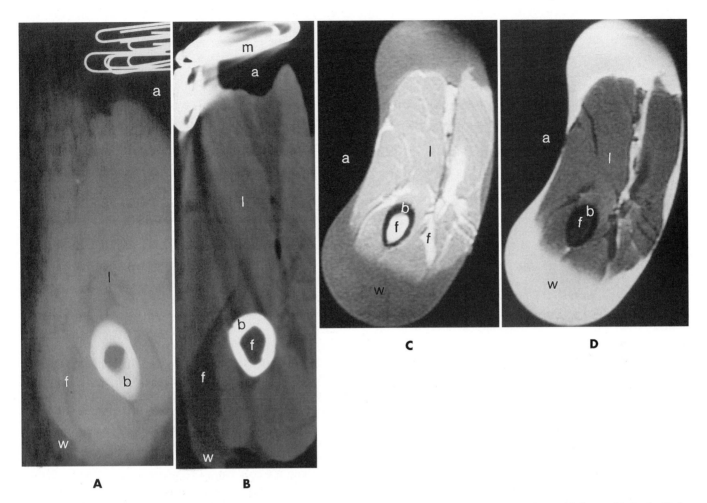

Fig. 1-1 Multimodality imaging of different tissues. **A,** Plain film of last night's entree reveals water *(w)*, air *(a)*, bone *(b)*, lamb *(l)*, fat *(f)*, and a paper clip (metal *[1]*) (yum!). **B,** CT performed with standard algorithm and filmed at soft-tissue settings shows good differentiation of bone *(b)*, metal *(m)*, lamb *(l)*, air *(a)*, and fat *(f)*. Note that water and lamb have similar densities at this window setting. **C,** T1WI shows high intensity fat *(f)*, low intensity water *(w)*, and intermediate intensity lamb muscle *(l)*. Air *(a)* and bone *(b)* are black. Unfortunately, the paper clips flew into the bore of the scanner before they could be imaged. **D,** Items on T2WI include intermediate intensity fat *(f)* and lamb muscle *(l)*, bright water *(w)*, black air *(a)*, and bone *(b)*. Paper clips are still stuck in the scanner.

area with vascular opacification, yielding an image of the vascular structures alone. The administration of iodinated contrast allows one to opacify the blood vessels because of the differential attenuation of the x-ray beam by iodine compared with the skull and nonopacified portions of the brain, head, and neck. Taking a "negative image" of the scout film and manually applying that to one where the vessels are opacified, yields a composite vessel-only study. Thankfully, the late 20th century brought computer technology to the art of subtraction imaging so that the days of "lining up the subs" and putting them through the processor are now over.

COMPUTED TOMOGRAPHY

Parameters and Units

Nobel prize winner Sir Godfrey Hounsfield developed CT for clinical use between 1972 and 1973. The first

company to introduce a CT scanner was EMI (English Musical Instruments), the same company the Beatles used for distributing their music on the Apple label. The music of the Beatles will, hopefully, survive the generations and corporate mergers—"all you need is love."

The principles of differential x-ray beam attenuation apply to CT, only CT uses a highly collimated x-ray beam. The photons that pass through the patient are collected by CT detectors, which show a differential rate of intensity on a gray scale depending on the degree of absorption along the narrow x-ray beam. The CT scanner's x-ray beam is rotated over many different angles so as to get differential absorption patterns across various rays through a single slab of a patient's body. By a mathematical analysis known as projection reconstruction, one is then able to obtain an absorption value for each point (pixel) within a CT slice. To understand the concept of a pixel, one must understand how pixel size relates to the matrix and field of view (FOV).

The matrix refers to the number of imaging partitions in the x-y plane of a slice, assuming an axial slice is in the Z plane. The in-plane pixel size is determined by dividing FOV by the matrix dimensions. The FOV is the linear dimension of the space to be imaged. The machine operator can select both the FOV and the matrix size. The matrix sizes of the CT scanners have increased several fold since the original 80×80 matrix of the EMI scanner in 1972. At present, matrices on the order of 128×128 to 512×512 are used. As an example, a 20-cm FOV scanned with a 512×512 matrix would yield pixels that are 0.39 mm (200 mm/512) by 0.39 mm. The final dimension one must know in CT imaging is the slice thickness. At present, CT slice thicknesses can be less than 1 mm thick. The three-dimensional imaging unit is called a voxel; in the example just given, the voxel size would be $1.0 \times 0.39 \times 0.39$ mm^3. For an 18-cm FOV with a 256×256 matrix and 8 mm slice thickness, the voxel size would be (180 mm/256) $\times$ (180 mm/256) $\times$ 8 mm. For high-resolution imaging, as desired in the temporal bone or orbits, a large matrix and a small FOV are used with slice thicknesses of 0.5 mm.

The scale for CT absorption generally ranges from $+1000$ to -1000, with zero allocated to water and -1000 to air (Table 1-1). The units are termed Hounsfield units (HU) named to honor the discoverer of the technique (just as the term "neuroradiology" has been coined by our profession to honor the success of our book "*Neuroradiology: THE REQUISITES*"). White matter and gray matter are in the 30 to 50 HU range. Hematomas tend to range from 50 to 80 HU, and calcification is generally 150 HU or greater. These values vary by approximately 10 to 25 HU according to the particular CT machine that is used. Dense bone and metal are the materials at the highest HU range. High protein concentrations equate with higher HU values (clotted blood, tenacious sinus secretions, the lens of the eye). At values less than zero one finds the structures that show less CT attenuation than water. Fat is usually in the -40 to -100 HU range. In human beings, the structures with less CT attenuation than fat are relatively limited to air-containing materials (lungs, sinuses, airheads?).

Evolution of CT Scanners

CT technology has evolved over several generations, each one designed to reduce scan time and increase image quality. The first-generation CT scanner had a thin x-ray beam and one detector. The second-generation scanners used a fan-shaped beam and multiple detectors. The arc of scanner gantry motion improved from 1-degree increments to as much as 30-degree differences. Third-generation scanners used an even wider fan-shaped beam and 10 times as many detectors as the second-generation scanner. The gantry rotated 360 degrees and moved continuously. Fourth-generation scanners use circumferential detectors so that only the x-ray tube moves in a 360-degree arc.

Most CT scanner manufacturers now use "slip ring technology," which allows continuous data acquisition and gantry rotation throughout the scanning procedure as the table moves without stopping and starting for each slice. This procedure, called spiral scanning, has allowed scan times per slice to be reduced to 1 second or less. The increased heat capacity of the newer x-ray tubes and the increasing sensitivity of the CT detectors have allowed more rapid image acquisition and more slices before x-ray tube heating becomes prohibitive. Other advances in CT collimation have allowed thinner and thinner slice profiles to be obtained. At present, 0.5 mm thick sections are often used for evaluation of fine anatomic structures such as the ossicles in the temporal bone or for CT angiography studies. Because the beam is so well collimated, x-ray exposure to the patient is limited to the area of scanning, and if overlapping sections are not used, the overall dose to the patient is less than 3 rad to the imaged volume. Of course, one cannot help but get "scatter radiation," which may affect radiosensitive organs such as the thyroid glands or gonads (both of which are hypometabolic in RIG). Helical (spiral) scanning has allowed excellent quality CT angiography studies to be performed, thus enabling CT to compete with ultrasound and MR angiography for the evaluation of neck and intracranial vessels.

One of the terms used to define the parameters for helical scanning is "pitch," which is defined as the table speed times the tube rotation time divided by the slice width. As an example, if a scanner has a table speed of 5 mm/sec and you scan for 0.8 seconds and have a slice thickness of 3 mm your pitch would be $5 \times 0.8/3 = 1.33$ pitch. In the past the pitch floated between 0.75 and 1.50, but as table speeds have increased and slice thicknesses reduced, pitches of 2.0–10.0 are not uncommon. Fast table speed is desirable to cover more anatomy in a scan, however, spatial resolution decreases with higher pitch

Table 1-1 HU of central nervous system structures on CT	
Structure	**HU**
Acute blood	56 to 76
Air	-1000
Bone	1000
Calcification	140–200
Cerebrospinal fluid	0
Fat	-30 to -100
Gray matter (caudate head)	32 to 41
White matter (centrum semiovale)	23 to 34

(like Nolan Ryan's fastball—the faster it moves the more the ball blurs—from a hitter's standpoint).

Another advantage to helical scanning is that once you have a volume of tissue scanned, you can slice it in as many thin sections or in as many planes as you wish. In general, the best image quality is produced when images are reconstructed using at least half the collimator setting. You can play with overlapping images and thinner slice reconstructions for CT angiography studies.

The latest refinement in CT technology is the multidetector system. In this scenario, instead of 1 mm × 20 mm detector channels you have 1 mm × 1.25 mm channels. The key to optimizing scanning is deciding which detectors to turn on when. Image thickness is selected by changing collimation, detector configuration, and reconstruction algorithm. In practical terms, with one rotation of the gantry, one is able to perform interweaving helices producing multiple (one to eight to sixteen . . . and beyond) slices instead of one per rotation. The speed of data acquisition and patient throughput can be accelerated in this way, or, alternatively, thinner slices and higher resolution can be achieved. The evolution of CT has thus progressed from 0.5 image per second (single slice with 1 second of scanning and 1 second of table movement), through 2 images per second (helical imaging with 2 images in 1 second as the table moves), to 16 images per second (multidetector mode with 16 images in 1 second as the table moves). Whether one wants to use single step and shoot techniques with four nonoverlapping slices with each rotation or perform overlapping helices depends on the indications and the need for resolution versus speed. Table speeds of 15 to 30 mm per rotation to perform four 5-mm slices have been advocated for brain images. At 2 seconds per rotation, a 25-cm brain study could take as little as 18 seconds to perform at high-speed helical mode. The heat load on the x-ray tube is, if anything, decreased with helical and multidetector scanning. The ability to acquire eight slices per second, a pitch of eight (80 mm per second) with scanner rotation speeds of 0.5 seconds would translate to performing a brain study in less than 5 seconds. Think of the potential in increasing your daily relative value units (RVUs).

CT Perfusion

Xenon 133 CT is a method for evaluating cerebral perfusion. The xenon is inhaled in combination with oxygen, and CT scans are performed to determine cerebral blood flow at multiple locations in the brain. Brain xenon concentration is related to the concentration of xenon absorbed in the bloodstream, the brain blood flow, and the time of exposure to xenon. Decreased flow has been documented in patients with meningitis, vasospasm, head trauma, sickle cell disease, and stroke. Side effects of xenon inhalation may include sedation, bronchospasm, and respiratory depression.

Iodine-based CT perfusion has also been introduced recently. A large rapid bolus of contrast is infused during continuous rapid scanning of a single slice and the wash-in and wash-out of the bolus can be analyzed by a computer to generate semi-quantitative images of brain perfusion. Commonly measured parameters are mean transit time (MTT), cerebral blood volume (CBV), and/or cerebral blood flow (CBF = CBV/MTT). On CT perfusion images, the differential density between normal brain and hypoperfused brain can be accentuated through computer manipulation to demonstrate areas of ischemia in the brain. The main disadvantages to this technique are the large bore catheter required (14 to 16 gauge), the rapid injection rate (5–10 cc per second), patient discomfort (one should use nonionic contrast to reduce the "barf" factor), the single slice acquisitions that limit the region of study (though we predict we will be seeing multislice CT perfusion by the time you read this page), and the reluctance of clinicians to give iodinated contrast to patients with strokes. To that end, MR still has an advantage in that only milliosmoles are delivered with gadolinium injections (see discussion of MR).

CT perfusion cerebral blood flow maps are noted to be more sensitive to ischemia than blood volume or time to peak maps. Infarctions may occur in most patients in areas of the brain with CBF values ≤30% of normal tissue and in 50% of patients where the CBF of affected tissue is 30% to 50% that of normal tissue.

CT technology has really taken off in the last 5 years and the sanctity of MR as the premiere means for evaluating intracranial pathology now rests more in the elimination of radiation exposure and increased soft-tissue contrast than in image resolution and functionality.

Algorithms, Windows, and Contrast Agents

Different reconstruction algorithms, or kernels, can be used to highlight a particular tissue with CT. Thus, bone disease may be best visualized with a bone, edge, or detail algorithm used to accentuate the interface between the bone and the soft tissue (Box 1-2). Alterna-

---

Box 1-2 Uses of Bone Algorithms in CT Scanning

Fracture identification
Temporal bone trauma, inflammatory disease
Sinusitis for bony anatomy of ostiomeatal complex (OMC)
Skull base lesions
Degenerative spine disease
Odontogenic disease

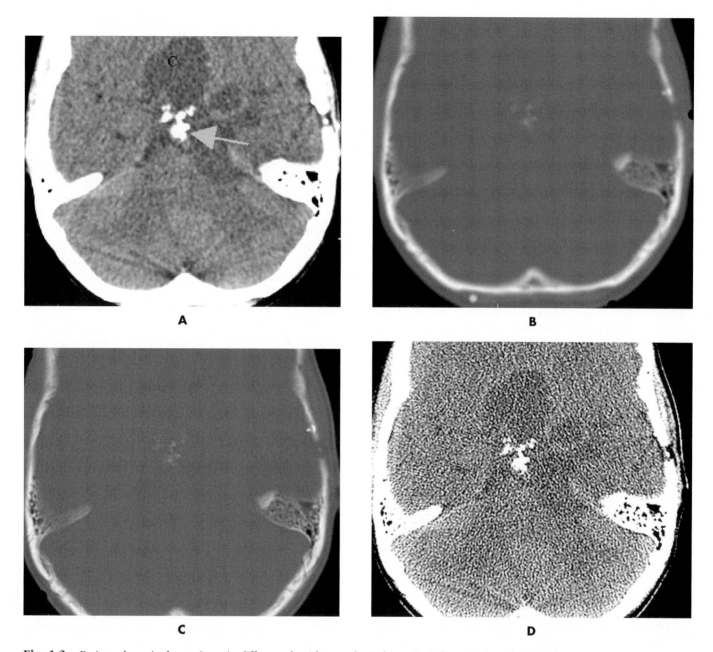

Fig. 1-2   Brain and craniopharyngioma in different algorithms and windows. **A,** Soft-tissue algorithm filmed in soft-tissue window settings: you can see the brain, the cystic portion of the mass (c) and the calcifications *(arrow)*. **B,** Soft-tissue algorithm, bone window allows one to see that the calcification and bone are of the same density, but one loses the soft tissue resolution to distinguish cystic fluid from brain. Note also shunt tubing in subcutaneous tissue right occiput and evidence of craniotomy on left with small clip. **C,** Bone algorithm, bone window: Note how much crisper the calcification and the bony walls appear in this imaging kernel. Now the clip on the left is well seen and even edges of the bone are sharper than in B. **D,** Bone algorithm, soft-tissue window: The noise of this image is not due to the scanning parameters but the combination of the bone algorithm and soft-tissue windows. The best combinations are, naturally, bone algorithm, bone window and soft-tissue algorithm, soft-tissue window.

tively, the algorithm for data reconstruction can be set to highlight differences in soft-tissue attenuation of structures (Fig. 1-2). If you save the raw data from a scan, any number of algorithms can be used retrospectively to analyze (target) the tissues studied. With helical scanning, this can also be translated into high quality oblique or multiplanar reconstructions. The problem is that saving the raw data eats up disk space and is time intensive for technologists. Raw data are like sushi; they can't be saved for very long before they stink.

The images from a given algorithm may be displayed with different window widths and levels to photograph the pictures in a manner that accentuates differences in CT attenuation between structures. Window widths refer to the HU range selected for gray-scale display, whereas the window level refers to the center point about which the range is displayed. By using small window widths (80 to 400 HU) and center levels (20 to 80 HU) you can highlight subtle soft tissue differences. To visualize tissues with wide variations in CT attenuation, as in bone versus air, a larger width (2000 to 3000 HU) and level (300 to 600 HU) are used.

Contrast enhancement is often used in cranial CT to opacify blood vessels and to detect areas of abnormal blood-brain barrier breakdown, where iodinated contrast will seep into the parenchyma. One hundred milliliters of intravenous iodinated contrast at a concentration of 240 mg/mL delivered by rapid bolus gives excellent vascular opacification. The factors that determine contrast enhancement of a lesion include (1) the volume and delivery of the contrast to the intravascular system, (2) the size of the intravascular space, (3) lesion vascularity, (4) permeability of lesion blood vessels, and (5) size of extravascular intralesional space. The blood-brain barrier is discussed more fully in Chapter 2.

Occasionally, intrathecal contrast is administered through a lumbar, cervical, cisternal, or ventricular approach to visualize *intracranial* pathology. Approximately 3 mL of nonionic contrast material (iodine, 180 mg/mL) can be administered through the cisternal or ventricular approach without risk of deleterious effects (seizures, headache, nausea, vomiting, and neuralgia). Myelographic doses will be discussed later.

Current Role of CT in Neuroimaging

What is the role of CT in neuroimaging (Box 1-3)? It remains the quickest, most efficient screening technique

---

Box 1-3 Most Effective Uses of CT in Neuroradiology

Ruling out subarachnoid hemorrahage
Acute head trauma
Fractures of orbit, temporal bone, face, skull
Sinusitis
Salivary gland calculous disease
Subtle bony irregularities
Detection of calcification in lesions
Odontogenic lesions
Degenerative disease
CT angiography
CT perfusion
Bony spinal stenosis
When MR is contraindicated or unavailable
Immediate postoperative evaluation
Temporal bone (external, middle, inner ear) disease

---

in patients with head trauma. It is the most sensitive imaging study for the detection of subarachnoid hemorrhage and is the study of choice for initial evaluation of patients with signs and symptoms suggestive of subarachnoid hemorrhage. The sensitivity of CT for calcification is critical in increasing diagnostic specificity, particularly for central nervous system (CNS) tumors (e.g., craniopharyngioma, oligodendroglioma, neurocytoma, retinoblastoma, meningioma), metabolic disorders (e.g., parathyroid imbalances), and congenital lesions (e.g., TORCH infections, tuberous sclerosis). In the head and neck, chondroid and osseous lesions are well depicted on CT and may be confusing in their appearances on magnetic resonance imaging. CT is the best study for bony (non–marrow-replacing) lesions and is indispensable in evaluating the temporal bone in general and the skull, face, and spine for fractures. It is critical for defining the intricate anatomy of the paranasal sinuses. In the spine, CT still holds its own in the evaluation of cervical and lumbar bony spinal stenosis, trauma, and postoperative studies where the hardware precludes adequate MR definition. MR may have invaded CT's space, but it will not replace it completely.

Since the last edition of this book, CT has made substantive inroads through CT angiography of neck and intracranial vessels, CT perfusion to acutely detect ischemic brain, multiplanar reconstructions, and virtual endoscopy. At the same time speeds, resolution, and dose efficiency has improved. Using CT angiography (CTA) to define necks of aneurysms, atherosclerotic disease, or occluded vessels in the ED (where CT has a more captive audience), has created newfound growth in CT usage for neuroradiology.

MAGNETIC RESONANCE IMAGING

Summarizing the principles of magnetic resonance (MR) imaging in just a few pages does a disservice to the complexity and elegance of the technique, but is about all we can muster given the constraints our editors have placed on the length of this tome. Fortunately, the anatomy that has been demonstrated with MR is well integrated into the knowledge that has been achieved through CT. However, the contrast mechanisms for the two studies are completely different. CT relies on differential attenuation of an x-ray beam, whereas MR relies on a complex interplay of the response of tissues to applied magnetic fields.

Magnets

The two main types of magnets used in clinical imaging are permanent magnets and superconducting magnets. Permanent magnets can be thought of as two bar magnets that generate a uniform magnetic field between them. Typically, the magnets are composed of metallic alloys, with iron used as the material that outlines the two magnets and conducts the magnetic field from one bar to the next. Permanent magnets, as the name implies, do not require continual energy to maintain the magnetic field. With a patient lying between the two permanent magnets, the magnetic field is oriented perpendicular to the axis of the supine body.

Superconducting magnets require no additional energy input once they have been "magnetized," mainly because they are encased in a liquid helium shell that prevents dissipation of the energy. The helium keeps the magnet cold enough to maintain its superconductance (i.e., zero resistance). An outer insulating layer of supercoolant liquid nitrogen is often used to keep the helium cold. The nitrogen requires constant replenishment. The coils of superconducting material that produce the magnetic field in a superconducting magnet are generally made of niobium-titanium wire. The static magnetic field of a superconducting magnet is oriented parallel to the axis of the supine patient body.

Because of their heavy weight from the iron yoke that surrounds and connects them and the weight of the magnets themselves, the maximum field strength of the permanent magnet scanner is relatively low, usually 0.5 tesla. A tesla (T) is a unit of magnetic field strength and is equivalent to 10,000 gauss (G). By comparison, the earth's magnetic field is approximately 0.5 G. Aren't you impressed now with "low-field strength" (0.15 to 0.5 T) magnets? They are much stronger than Mother Earth! Most nonopen superconducting magnets in clinical use range from 1.0 to 3.0 T systems, but scanners with field strengths up to 8.0 T are available and can blow your ears off with the noise they generate. Open magnets range from 0.1–1.0 T in strength.

Gradient Coils

The concept of gradient coils is important to understanding MR. To localize a point in space, the magnetic field at that point must be unique. The way to alter the magnetic field (which is uniform in strength) within the bore is to pass current through gradient coils, which create an organized continuous gradation. That is, for a z gradient, there is an orderly increase in field strength of the main magnet from one end to the other. Each coordinate axis has a series of gradient coils, which are essentially loops or half-loops of wire that carry current. By winding different-shaped coils around a cylinder, one is able to achieve an x-, y-, or z-oriented magnetic gradient field. Therefore, at any point in the x-, y-, and z-planes a unique magnetic vector will be present in the scanner. A proton in that location in the scanner will precess with a unique frequency that is proportional to

the magnetic field it "feels." By tuning to a particular frequency you can localize that point and judge the amplitude of its signal. This is one way that spatial localization is achieved with MR. Turning the imaging gradient coils off and on is what gives MR its characteristic loud noise (like an M-16 in a Tora Bora cave).

Obviously the homogeneity (uniformity of magnetic field strength across an FOV) of a magnetic field affects the image quality. Other coils (called shim coils) are used to correct any unwanted localized inhomogeneities to the main magnetic field. Much emphasis in recent years has therefore been placed on those gradient shim coils that allow better homogeneity to the applied magnetic field. These shim coils should not be confused with the three gradient coils used to localize a particular region of interest within an x-y-z coordinate system.

The MR manufacturers are in a never-ending battle to upstage each other with the strength of their gradient packages. What this translates to for the physician is shorter times to echo (TEs), smaller FOVs, faster scanning, and higher resolution. We encourage these battles with our demands for image quality, but pay through one of our apertures for the cost.

Radiofrequency Receiver Coils

Radiofrequency receiver coils are used to receive magnetic signals from the region of interest within the body. In most cases, except for the head and whole body coils, which transmit signal, the surface coils are limited to receiving signal from the imaged volume after the body coil stimulates it. Innovations in surface coil technology have led to the creation of more specialized coils including those used for the spine, temporomandibular joint, shoulder, knee, and even rectal and intravaginal coils (yikes). The smaller the surface coil, the higher the signal to noise ratio (SNR) but the smaller the sensitive volume. One is therefore forced to strike a compromise between sensitivity profile (coverage), SNR, and resolution. If the coil is too small, one obtains excellent resolution and SNR but insufficient coverage. If the coil is too large, one obtains adequate coverage but insufficient SNR to support the resolution one desires. This has led to the concept of phased-array coil (multicoil) systems in which signal is obtained from several small coils simultaneously to scan a large volume (Fig. 1-3). For example, a multicoil spine system may use a linear array of four coils, each approximately 6 inches in size, ample to cover from C1—L2. The four coils are electrically isolated from one another (with low-input impedance preamplifiers and overlapping fields) and are each connected to a separate MR receiver, preamplifier, and digitizer. Each coil has limited coverage but very high resolution. The four separate images are then combined (by sophisticated computers) to form one

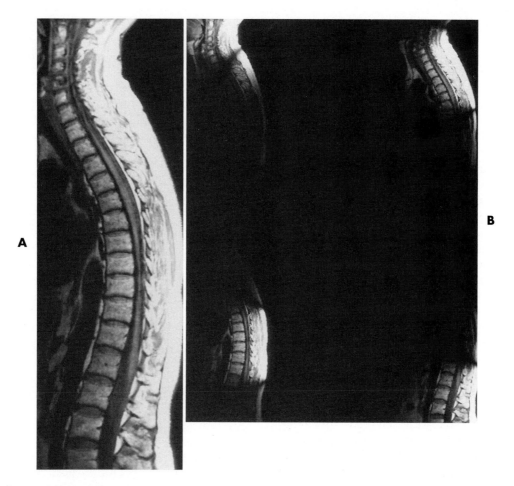

Fig. 1-3   Phased-array multicoil image of the spine. **A,** Composite image of the spine from four separate coils. Note the 48-cm FOV covers from C2–L3 with high SNR. **B,** Individual images from each of the four coils connected in an array can be demonstrated by evaluating each coil separately. The computer does the rest, cleaning up the overlap and smoothing the image. And voila, Fig. 1-3, A; c'est magnifique!

composite image that has maximal coverage, SNR, and resolution.

Larmor Frequency

Most of MR consists of proton imaging of the hydrogen nucleus because it is very abundant within human tissue. The hydrogen nucleus precesses in a magnetic field at its own resonant frequency, called the Larmor frequency. The Larmor frequency of the hydrogen nucleus is linearly related to field strength by the following equation:

Precessional (or Larmor) Frequency
$$= \text{Field Strength} \times \text{Gyromagnetic Ratio}$$

The gyromagnetic ratio of each nucleus is unique and does not vary in different field strength magnets. At 1 T the Larmor frequency for hydrogen is 42.6 MHz, whereas at 1.5 T the Larmor frequency is roughly 63.86 MHz. To stimulate the hydrogen nuclei, a radio frequency (RF) pulse must be tuned to the Larmor frequency of the hydrogen nucleus (its resonant frequency). As the hydrogen nucleus is put into a magnetic field with a gradient of magnetism, the location of a particular hydrogen nucleus can be determined by its resonant frequency within that gradient. Again, the frequency varies slightly, depending on where in the field the nucleus resides. The ability to localize protons by variations in their Larmor frequency as a response to a graded magnetic field allows the spatial characterization that distinguishes MR imaging from nuclear magnetic resonance (NMR), or chemical spectroscopy.

Relaxation Times

When a sample containing hydrogen nuclei is placed in a magnet, its magnetization aligns along the direction of the magnetic field (z direction). After stimulation of the hydrogen nuclei by applying a 90-degree RF pulse at the Larmor frequency of its nucleus, the magnetization vector rotates from the z-axis to the transverse x-y plane, where the protons precess at the Larmor frequency. According to Faraday's law of induction, the precessing magnetization creates voltage in a properly oriented receiver coil (the same coil that is used to apply the RF pulse when the head or body coils are used). One can vary the angle at which the vector is tipped from the z-axis by varying the amplitude and duration of the RF pulse. The hydrogen nuclei then relax by two mechanisms. The first is termed T1 or spin lattice relaxation. As the nucleus relaxes back to equilibrium after being excited by an RF pulse, there is an exponential increase in the amplitude of the z-direction magnetization until there is complete return of the magnetization towards its baseline position. T1 is defined as the time it takes for the hydrogen nucleus to recover 63% of its longitudinal (Z axis) magnetization. At the same time, the transverse magnetization in the x-y plane also decays towards zero in an exponential fashion. This exponential decay is characterized by a time constant that is termed T2, or spin-spin relaxation time. The signal created in a proton's decay is called a free induction decay (FID). In spin-echo imaging, rather than detecting the FID, a 180-degree RF pulse is given at some time (half the time to echo [TE]) after the initial 90-degree RF pulse. This rephases the spins after another $\frac{1}{2}$ TE and when all the spins are coherent produces the so-called "spin echo." Thus, the TE is the time from the 90-degree pulse to the echo. The analogy is to a race where the slow and fast runners start together (in phase), but very soon thereafter the fast runners pull ahead of the slow runners. At a certain time ($\frac{1}{2}$ TE) in the race the runners are told to turn around and head back to the starting line (180 degrees pulse). All the runners should return across the starting line at the same time (spin echo) if they have kept up their original pace.

Because T1 and T2 relaxation mechanisms are independent of each other by and large, one can completely lose signal in the x-y axis without having completely returned all the magnetization to the z axis. The T2 or transverse (spin-spin) relaxation is due to dephasing caused by the adjacent hydrogen nuclei, which are not totally in concert with each other. T2 is defined as the time for 63% of the transverse magnetization signal to be lost owing to this natural dephasing process. By and large, T2 values in the CNS are shorter than T1 values. The T1 and T2 values of some normal tissues seen in the CNS are listed in Table 1-2.

The overriding concept of T2 relaxation is that of phase dispersion or incoherence caused by local field inhomogeneity. However, phase dispersion may be due to three factors: (1) the magnetic environment of the hydrogen protons (true T2), (2) the heterogeneity in the main magnet itself (extrinsic variations caused by magnetic field imperfections and other inhomogeneities produce phase dispersion characterized by the time con-

Table 1-2   Representative T1 and T2 relaxation times of CNS structures at 1.5 T

Structure	T1 (msec)	T2 (msec)
Gray matter	980-1040	64-71
White matter	740-770	64-70
CSF	>2000	>300
Muscle (at 1.0 T)	600	40
Fat (at 1.0 T)	180	90

From Berger RK, Rimm AA, Rischer ME, et al: T1 and T2 measurements on a 1.5-T commercial MR image. *Radiology* 171:273-279, 1989. Data for 1.0 T from Bushong SC: *Magnetic resonance imaging; physical and biological principles*, St Louis, 1988, Mosby.

stant T2'), and (3) the paramagnetic substance-induced field inhomogeneities (blood or iron) known as T2". Now you can understand that various tissues within the human body have varying magnetic susceptibilities (affinities to be magnetized), which result in different local field strengths and which cause phase dispersion as the patient's body is placed in the "uniform" magnetic field. To reiterate, consider three components: T2 from spin-spin relaxation, T2' caused by main field inhomogeneity, and T2" from susceptibility effects. The reciprocal of these relaxation times (relaxation rates), when summed, can be related by this equation:

$$1\backslash T2^* = 1/T2 + 1\backslash T2' + 1\backslash T2''.$$

The reason these three factors are worth emphasizing becomes clear in a discussion of the differences between spin echo and gradient echo pulse sequences. (Now you know why President Bush went into politics and not physics.)

Pulse Sequences

Conventional spin-echo imaging

Different pulse sequences have been developed that emphasize T1 and/or T2 relaxation effects. T1-weighted images (T1WI) are used for tissue discrimination and in conjunction with the gadolinium contrast agents because enhancing lesions become bright on T1WI. T2-weighted images (T2WI) are very sensitive to the presence of increased water and can visualize edema to great advantage. T2WI are also most sensitive to differences in susceptibility between tissues. Usually both T1WI and T2WI are used in routine brain, spine, and neck imaging. The combination of signal intensities on the two sequences often allows some tissue specificity. However, as you can imagine, the combinations of bright or dark on these two images are limited, which is why MR specificity is also limited. Proton density–weighted images (PDWI) are variably used and are occasionally helpful from the standpoint of diagnostic specificity. Proton density weighted scans display contrast based on available mobile hydrogen proton concentrations.

The most common pulse sequence currently used is the spin-echo pulse sequence. This consists of a 90-degree pulse that flips the longitudinal magnetization from the z-axis to the x-y axis. This is followed by a 180-degree pulse, which rephases the protons that are dephased because of magnetic field distortions (T2). T2' and T2" can be rephased by the spin-echo technique, but gradient echo scanning (see following paragraph) unmasks these contributions to total transverse relaxation.

By varying the repetition time (TR), which is the time between 90-degree pulses, and the echo time (TE), one can obtain T1WI and T2WI. In general, a short-TR (<1000 milliseconds), short-TE (<45 milliseconds) scan is T1-weighted. A long-TR (>2000 milliseconds), short-TE (<45 milliseconds) scan is weighted towards proton density. A long-TR (>2000 milliseconds), long-TE (>60 milliseconds) scan is weighted towards T2 information. The terms short and long here are relative. The intensity of a voxel in a spin-echo sequence is determined by both tissue intrinsic and scanner extrinsic factors (Boxes 1-4 and 1-5).

Another factor in scanning is the inversion time TI, the length of time before the 90-degree pulse that a 180-degree inversion pulse is placed. This parameter can be set to various values to generate contrast and/or to null the signal of a specific tissue in the brain, spine, or head and neck. The most frequent uses in neuroradiology are in suppressing fat in the orbits, neck, or bone marrow (short tau inversion image recovery [STIR]), or in suppressing cerebrospinal fluid (CSF) signal in the brain (fluid-attenuated inversion recovery [FLAIR]). One can use this technique in a T1-weighted or T2-weighted sequence. The values of the TI vary with TR, field strength, and tissue to be suppressed. Use a TI of 16 to suppress your teenagers' raging hormones.

Box 1-4 Intrinsic Contrast Factors of Tissue

T1
T2
Proton density
Blood-brain barrier
Velocity of movement
Viscosity
Diamagnetic and ferromagnetic disturbances to
   magnetic field
Magnetization transfer
Diffusion coefficient

Box 1-5 Extrinsic Factors for Contrast Manipulation

TR
TE
Flip angle
Saturation pulses
Velocity-encoding schemes
Spoiler gradients
Gradient moment nulling
FSE design
Contrast administration

Gradient echo imaging

In gradient echo scanning the magnetization vector of the protons also is tipped off the z-axis to the x-y coordinate system (usually less than 90 degrees). As opposed to the 180-degree *spin-echo* pulse, a rephasing gradient pulse follows the initial flip-angle magnetization. Therefore, the gradient echo scans can be devised to be more susceptible to magnetic field inhomogeneities, because of the lack of 180-degree rephasing pulse (Table 1-3). Blood products, iron, calcium, and manganese deposition are seen more readily with gradient echo scanning. These scans are part of routine trauma or stroke protocols searching for blood or in cases where calcified le-

---

Table 1-3 Utility of gradient echo scanning

Feature	Advantage	Clinical use
Shorter TR	Faster	Uncooperative patient, rapid localizer scans
Can be used without 180-degree pulse	Higher susceptibility sensitivity	Better for looking for blood products, calcification
Can be used with 180-degree pulse	"Echoplanar scanning"	Fast imaging, functional studies
Flow-related enhancement	Bright blood	Basis of time-of-flight MR angiography, CSF flow imaging
Less gradient stress	Thinner slices	Cervical spine, sella, temporal bone, MR angiography, 3DFT images
Shorter TE	More slices	Thin section T1WI-SPGR

CSF, Cerebrospinal fluid; 3DFT, three-dimensional Fourier transform.

sions are suspected. Remember that CT is the study of choice, however, for the detection of calcification. MR rates only a B−. When gradient echoes are applied, the most important factors to create T1 or T2 weighting are the value of the angle of nutation or "flip angle," the TR, and the TE. At low flip angles, more T2 weighting is achieved. The lower the flip angle (5 to 10 degrees) and the longer the TE (>40 milliseconds), the greater the susceptibility sensitivity. The cost of extending the TEs to achieve higher susceptibility sensitivity is a reduction in slices available and in signal. To get through the brain, longer scan times are needed. However, gradient echo imaging generally is more rapid than conventional spin-echo imaging and also allows one to obtain bright blood from flow-related enhancement, which is used for magnetic resonance angiography (MRA). Three-dimensional gradient echo scanning is also possible and allows very thin slices while maintaining high SNR. The three-dimensional data set may be manipulated into multiplanar reconstructions with relative ease.

At larger flip angles (45 to 60 degrees), and a shorter TR, a more T1-weighted or proton density–weighted gradient echo image is achieved. However, other factors such as spoiler gradients or steady-state free precession factors can cause T1 weighting or T2 weighting within a gradient echo scan. Spoiler gradients generally reduce T2 contribution to the signal by eliminating or spoiling the residual transverse magnetization after a gradient echo pulse. With steady-state free precession scanning, T2 information is highlighted by shortening the TR to a sufficient degree that there continues to be transverse relaxation, which, although incomplete, provides the contrast. This allows T2WI to be performed with short TRs, shortening scan time. This technique, also called FISP, does suffer artifacts due to magnetic field inhomogeneities.

Fast spin echo

To achieve more rapid T2WI, fast spin echo (FSE) scans are usually used. The FSE method produces spin density and T2-like images in scan times that can be up to 64 or more times faster than conventional spin-echo images. The trick is that in conventional spin-echo imaging one phase encoding step is acquired per TR, whereas with FSE multiple phase encoding steps are acquired during the same TR interval (nowadays anywhere from 2 to 256 steps). The echo train length is the number of echoes (phase encoding steps) per TR and essentially determines how much faster the FSE will be than the conventional spin echo.

If you imagine that a TV image is based on multiple raster lines across a tube, an MR image is filled with lines in "K-space." Conventional spin echo scanning determines one raster line per TR. Fast spin echo can determine "n" lines of k-space where n is the echo train length. Contrast is weighted toward the time to echo of the 180 degree pulse at the center of k-space. The echo train length also determines the number of slices per TR available. As the echo train length is increased, the contribution of T2 differences increases. The time between successive echoes within the echo train is termed the echo spacing.

To reemphasize, in FSE each echo is acquired with a different phase-encoding gradient. This is different from the traditional spin-echo experiment where one line of k-space (the data coordinate system from which a magnetic resonance image is calculated by Fourier transformation) is acquired per TR. Another important difference is that all the echoes acquired during an echo train contribute to the image signal, so the TE really represents an "effective" TE and not a true TE. The middle lines of k-space (low spatial frequencies) provide the greatest contrast and have the most signal. The outer lines of k-space (high spatial frequencies) add much less to the image with respect to signal-to-noise ratio and contrast but are used for fine-detail information. Thus the lower amplitudes of the phase-encoding gradient generate the highest signal and occur at the effective TE. This makes sense because the data from the effective echo are placed in the middle of k-space.

As an aside, one can use partial k-space sampling to speed up the scan times. This technique is being used frequently for fast-enhanced MRA where time is critical to prevent venous contamination of the MR arteriogram.

Echo Planar Imaging (EPI)

EPI is similar to FSE in its utilization of numerous echoes within a TR to fill k-space, however, instead of a train of 180-degrees RF pulses (FSE), in EPI we have a faster train of gradient echo pulses. The method uses a series of rapidly oscillating gradient reversals to encode spatial information. The k-space is filled much more efficiently in EPI; usually the whole of k-space (a whole slice) is filled in one TR. Its sensitivity to susceptibility effect leads to marked artifacts at the air-bone interfaces with tissue, producing geometric distortions. EPI is used to produce motion free images for diffusion and perfusion and functional MR scans. EPI imaging is also useful in uncooperative patients, fetal scanning, and pediatric imaging. The images are not nearly of as good quality as spin echo or FSE images if the patient is cooperative.

Fluid Attenuation Inversion Recovery (FLAIR)

FLAIR stands for fluid attenuation inversion recovery and its concept is simple: obtain T2-weighted contrast while keeping the CSF dark. You can null the intensity of CSF by setting the TI at 0.69 times the T1 relaxation time of pure water (around 2 seconds at 1.5 Tesla scanning). This changes the dynamic range of the image so that even subtle areas of T2 relaxation abnormality can be detected, particularly at the borders with CSF. Previously the proton density weighted scan provided this contrast. However, FLAIR provides a better contrast range with more conspicuous delineation of pathology. Suddenly, even a professor emeritus can identify vasogenic and cytotoxic edema opposite the dark CSF background. This technique has been particularly effective to identify periventricular ischemic foci and multiple sclerosis plaques and to differentiate perivascular spaces (dark) from ischemic zones (bright).

FLAIR has also been advocated for extending the realm of MR to identification of subarachnoid disease. Blood and pus in the subarachnoid space can cause the normally dark signal of CSF on FLAIR imaging to turn bright. Even carcinomatous meningitis may "brighten" the FLAIR CSF. FLAIR and the CSF is like my child's description of a day in school; nonspecific and of questionable sensitivity at this time. The pitfalls of hanging your hat on the bright CSF sign include cisternal CSF flow artifacts and some anesthetic techniques that use 100% O_2. The O_2 causes a reduction in the T1 of CSF and leads to high signal on FLAIR scans. Oxygen, not the anesthetic, is the purported culprit. The sensitivity to meningeal and subarachnoid pathology may be increased with gadolinium-enhanced FLAIR scanning. This technique appears to be more sensitive than enhanced T1-weighted scanning for carcinomatosis and subarachnoid seeding. Some have also advocated using gadolinium-enhanced FLAIR scanning for parenchymal masses.

Pitfalls with FLAIR are limited to reduced visibility of cystic lacunae in the deep gray matter and posterior fossa structures, old ischemic foci that are vacuolated and hence have CSF intensity, and the presence of flow-related high signal intensity and incomplete CSF suppression in the posterior fossa. It should be noted that FLAIR scans are generally performed as a fast/turbo spin echo (FSE) technique and therefore have the limited susceptibility sensitivity for hemorrhage that plagues other FSE techniques. Another recent study has reported that posterior fossa abnormalities are not as conspicuous on FLAIR scans as supratentorial ones. Consult the FSE T2WI for posterior fossa lesions. (You have been warned.) At present, FLAIR imaging has not been implemented in the spine, owing to the issues of CSF pulsation. So, do not toss the vanilla T2-weighted scans yet!

For an example of how all these pulse sequences look at the same section of imaging, see Figure 1-4.

MR Angiography

MR angiography (MRA) capitalizes on creating intensity differences between flowing (or intravascular) tissue and stationary tissue. By suppressing background stationary tissue and focusing only on the high-signal flowing blood, one can obtain a data set that depicts only vascular structures. If used with contiguous sections or three-dimensional volumetric acquisitions, one can produce very thin section MR angiograms that can be rotated in space to visualize the intracranial circulation, cervical vessels, and/or origins of the vessels from the aorta (Fig. 1-5). Suddenly MR is capable of detecting atherosclerotic narrowing or intracranial aneurysms in three-dimensional space.

Two main types of MRA pulse sequences have been developed (see Table 1-4). The first, time-of-flight (TOF) imaging, capitalizes on the difference in longitudinal magnetization between nonsaturated spins (with high signal) moving into the imaging slice and stationary ones within the slice that have been saturated (low-signal) by the RF pulses creating the image. This effect, termed flow-related enhancement, explains why inflowing blood on gradient echo images is bright. The source images may then be processed with any number of different postprocessing algorithms, the most commonly used is the maximal intensity pixel (MIP) method, which projects only the brightest pixels (flowing blood) in the image for display. The MIP images can be projected in any plane to provide multiple views of the vascular anatomy.

Phase contrast (PC) imaging is the second MRA technique. PC MRA capitalizes on the change in transverse magnetization (phase shifts) that occurs when flowing protons encounter changes in gradient strength, which are produced by bipolar gradient pulses. By applying a bipolar "flow-encoding" gradient pulse to the tissue between the initial excitation and readout pulse, a phase shift is induced in moving spins but not in stationary tissue. Two acquisitions are performed, with flow-encoding pulses of opposite polarity. Then, by complex subtraction of the two acquisitions, stationary protons creating the background are snuffed out and phase shifts of flowing spins are additive. Because this subtraction completely nulls background signal, the background suppression of PC is superior to TOF MRA, and unlike TOF imaging, where bright fat or bright subacute thrombus may superimpose on the MIP projection, these stationary tissues are well suppressed with PC. PC MRA also allows one to obtain velocity information, not easily obtainable with TOF MRA. By adjusting the flow-encoding gradients to the range of velocities in which one is interested, one can obtain a PC image of slow-flow venous

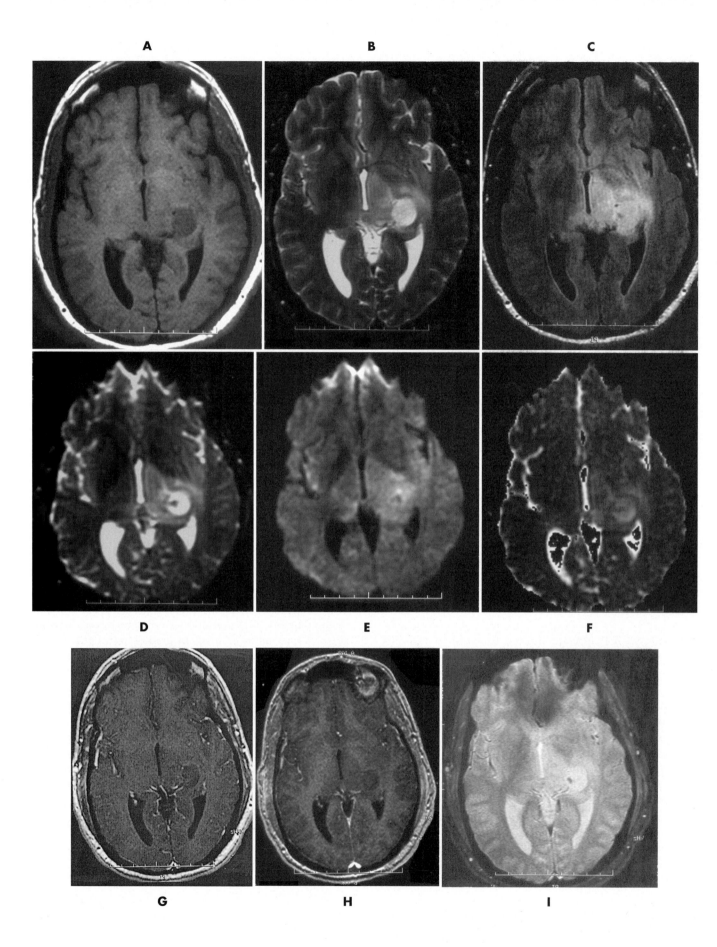

A　　　　　　　　　B　　　　　　　　　C

D　　　　　　　　　E　　　　　　　　　F

G　　　　　　　　　H　　　　　　　　　I

Table 1-4   Comparison of MRA techniques

Technique	Advantages	Disadvantages
2DFT TOF	Sensitive to slow flow	Thick slices
	Fast	Poor background suppression of fat, hemorrhage
	Less in-plane saturation	Insensitive to in-plane flow
	Good for venous studies	Gradient moment nulling used leading to longer TEs, more dephasing
		Overestimates stenoses from dephasing
3DFT TOF	Thin slices possible	Patient motion artifacts
	Reasonably fast	Poor background suppression of fat, hemorrhage
	Short TEs possible, so less dephasing	Less sensitive to slow flow because of saturation effects
	High SNR from slab	
2DFT PC	Fast	Thick slices leading to intravoxel dephasing
	Can direction- and velocity-encode for slow flow	No multiplanar reconstructions
	Excellent background suppression	
	Intensity related to velocity	
3DFT PC	Thin slices so less intravoxel dephasing	Requires postprocessing
	Can direction- and velocity-encode for slow flow	Patient motion artifacts
	Excellent background suppression	Worse dephasing with turbulence
	Improved SNR from slab	Longer scan time
Enhanced 3DTOF	Less artifact	Slightly invasive
	Can see arch vessel	Need sophisticated software (or timely fellow), gradients to avoid venous contamination
	Longer field of view	
	No saturation	Slab is not wide
	Improved estimation of stenosis	One time only

blood or very fast-flow central arterial blood. One can also perform directional encoding in PC MRA so that, for example, right-to-left flowing blood is bright, but left-to-right flowing blood is dark. Heady stuff, and the physics behind all these sequences is mind boggling (Stephen Hawking, move over).

PC and TOF sequences can be performed in a three-dimensional Fourier transform (3DFT) or two-dimensional Fourier transform (2DFT) mode. With 3DFT one is able to excite a slab of tissue and partition it into thinner sections (1 mm) than 2DFT images (2 to 3 mm). The advantage of 3DFT imaging is (1) improved signal-to-noise ratio (SNR) in a thick slab excitation and (2) thinner sections leading to less saturation of spins, thereby maintaining bright signal in a vessel. The drawbacks of 3DFT scanning are that the TE is slightly longer, which may lead to greater dephasing, scan times are slightly longer, and the technique is slightly less sensitive to slow flow because of saturation within the volume.

At the time of the last edition of this volume, most centers used 2DFT or 3DFT TOF MRA to evaluate the carotid bifurcation and 3DFT TOF or PC MRA (less commonly) to evaluate the intracranial circulation. Increasingly, those of us with less cost consciousness and more time constraints have opted to go to gadolinium-enhanced MRA to evaluate the neck vessels. Believe it or not, the body guys have really driven this business, having shown neuroradiologists the way with stellar examples of enhanced MRAs of the renal arteries and peripheral vessels. The key to great quality enhanced three-dimensional TOF carotid MRAs is the timing of the bolus injection and the tightness of the bolus. It is best to use an injector (2 cc of gadolinium/sec will suffice for a total of 40 cc). Some centers use "SmartPrep" (we use "dumb fellows") or a test bolus to optimize the start of the scans (thereby reducing venous contamination of the MR arteriogram) when the bolus arrives in the vessels. However, if your gradient hardware package allows

Fig. 1-4   Appearance of the various pulse sequences, same slice through a thalamic neoplasm. **A,** T1WI: dark CSF, bright fat, dark lesion. **B,** T2WI: bright CSF, dark (suppressed) fat, bright lesion. **C,** FLAIR: dark CSF, bright fat, bright lesion. **D,** B0 DWI: bright CSF, bright fat, bright lesion. **E,** Composite DWI: dark CSF, bright fat, bright lesion (vasogenic edema). **F,** ADC map: bright CSF, bright vasogenic edema (contrast with Fig. 1-5). **G,** Postgadolinium conventional T1WI: dark CSF, bright fat, dark lesion with enhancing portion. **H,** Postgadolinium spoiled gradient echo T1WI: dark CSF, bright fat, dark lesion with enhancing portion, better gray-white contrast than **G. I,** Gradient echo T2WI: bright CSF, dark fat, bright lesion with increased susceptibility sensitivity.

you to obtain MRAs in less than 12 seconds per MRA series, you should have at least one series where the arteries alone show contrast. What you do is repetitively scan at the same location up to five times in a row after injecting the contrast. Although your initial scans may not have any contrast visible (seen as bright signal on your three-dimensional TOF MRA) and your last scans may merely show venous flow, one or more of the middle sets will have gadolinium in the arteries (because the circulation time in most individuals runs from 10 to 25 seconds). However, gadolinium-enhanced MRA is a one shot deal—it is hard to go back and try it again. The advantages to this technique are (1) it is quick so that 5 sets of 12 seconds each yields a scan time of under 2 minutes, (2) it is performed coronally with a large FOV so you can see the origins of the arteries from the aorta to the intracranial vessels, (3) it shows tight narrowing better than two-dimensional TOF, (4) it shows slow flow better than unenhanced three-dimensional TOF, (5) it is unencumbered by flow artifacts, and (6) when performed well it looks beautiful (Fig. 1-5).

Spin-echo scans should always accompany an MRA sequence to evaluate for thrombosed or dissected vessels. What is bright on an MRA may be fat, hematoma, high protein, or cholesterin, not necessarily flow, so it is best to perform T_1-weighted spin-echo scans with every MRA.

Nonetheless, conventional angiography should continue to be considered the gold standard of vascular imaging. Catheters are not obsolete yet!

Diffusion-Weighted Imaging (DWI)

Trying to explain DWI (diffusion-weighted imaging) may be as difficult as DWI (driving while under the influence). We recommend the former but not the latter. Let us just say that the concept of DWI is to assess the local environment of the cell to determine the ease of water diffusion. As dilettantes in physiology we offer the following supercilious explanation. As cells swell (as in cytotoxic edema) the ability of water protons to diffuse extracellularly is restricted. Think of yourself in your chair reading this passage. You are probably antsy, twisting in your seat, getting anxious about all this physics. You move around a lot in your chair nervously and randomly. Now imagine that you have just gained 50 pounds and 4 inches to your waistline. Probably, you would not have as much room to move in your chair, eh? Your ability to move randomly would be restricted sort of like a swollen apoptotic cell. This restriction of diffusibility corresponds to high signal intensity on DWI images and a reduction in the apparent diffusion coefficient (ADC) of local water. The ADC is a quantity corresponding to a matrix of tensor vectors in various directions. The mechanism for the increased intracellular water is be-

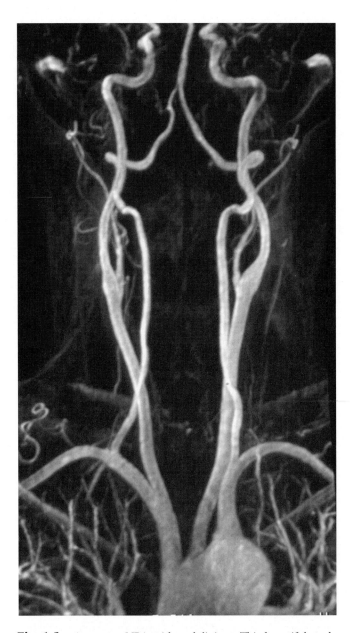

Fig. 1-5 Awesome MRA with gadolinium. This beautiful study was done by our chief technician in just 23 seconds. Contrast was administered via a power injector at a rate of 3 cc per second. Note how well the origins of the carotid and vertebral vessels from the arch were visualized and how large the display field of view is. The bifurcations of the carotids and proximal intracranial circulation are nicely demonstrated all at once. (Compliments of Rob Evers, RT)

lieved to be due to the failure of the sodium-potassium pump at the cell membrane. Other explanations have also been offered but we do not want to confuse ourselves.

Now let us think on a more global scale. Let us say you are in your chair in a row reading this chapter with everyone else in class, everyone individually twitching with ants in their pants. Suddenly, the fire alarm goes off. There is a scramble for the exits, but the aisles and rows of chairs presents a natural flow of people in the room. That is, though individually you can twitch away, as a unit there is nonrandomness in the movement of the group. This is the concept behind diffusion tensor tractopathy or white matter mapping. There is some organization to the white matter societal movement that can be characterized by the asymmetry, because the water protons cannot diffuse equally in all directions. This is termed diffusion anisotropy. Diffusion tensor imaging is a means to map white matter tracts and obtain three-dimensional ADC values. To perform this study, diffusion gradients are placed in at least six directions and calculations of the tensor in three-dimensional space are performed. From these studies, one can determine white matter directionality and, in some cases, diagnose abnormalities in the white matter.

When one performs DWI studies there are a few relevant parameters: (1) the direction the DWI gradients are applied; one can look for diffusion contrast in one or all three x, y, and z directions, (2) the b value in sec/mm^2 as a reflection of gradient strength.

The importance of understanding DWI is that it can show cerebral ischemia within minutes of irreversible damage. DWI is the most sensitive way of detecting acute infarction, and can be used to distinguish new (low ADC) from old (high ADC) strokes (Fig. 1-6). Transient ischemic attacks usually do not show DWI abnormality whereas completed infarcts do, eliminating the confusion as to the reversibility of patients' deficits. By the same token, one must understand that not all bright areas on DWI are due to strokes; T2 "shine-through," areas of high intensity on T2-weighted scans, may lead to bright signal on DWI scans yet the ADC may not be reduced. This is because DWI scans are intrinsically T2-weighted scans. To eliminate the T2 effect, we take a scan with a b value of 0 (diffusion gradients off) and a scan with the b value in the over 800 range (diffusion gradients on) and divide the latter by the former (giving the exponential image). This is one of several means for eliminating the T2 effect and just seeing the ADC effect. Absolute ADC imaging is being implemented as a commercial product by most manufacturers. This will allow the distinction between T2 shine-through brightness on diffusion-weighted images from true ADC decreases in a qualitative way. Quantitation of ADC values can be made from region of interest measures. The term "trace images" refers to the sum of the true ADC maps in each direction (x, y, and z).

By these means, DWI can also distinguish between cytotoxic (low ADC) and vasogenic (high ADC) edema, but beware because both may appear bright on the DWI image. Check those ADC values. DWI scans, because they are gradient echo scans, also tend to be somewhat more sensitive to the presence of hemorrhage than fast spin echo scans.

Perfusion Scanning

Diffusion-weighted scanning is often combined with perfusion scanning, which allows the evaluation of relative cerebral blood flow (CBF), cerebral blood volume (CBV), mean transit times, and times to peak perfusion. These techniques usually require high volume gadolinium bolus injections in which the rate at which the gadolinium circulates through the brain is determined. The technique uses rapid echo planar imaging of the brain with a power injector bolus of a gadolinium agent at a rate of 3 to 5 cc per second. Multiple scans at the same locations are performed as the concentrated gadolinium enters the brain (appearing dark in signal on a gradient echo T2-weighted scan). Graphically, one can see the subsequent decrease from baseline of the signal intensity of the gray and white matter as the gadolinium enters the capillary bed that perfuses the tissue (Fig. 1-6). With a rapid bolus T2-weighted scan, highly concentrated gadolinium leads to signal decrease. As the first pass of gadolinium leaves the capillary bed, the signal intensity of the adjacent brain rises. Plotting the inflow curve will allow the subsequent analysis of blood flow parameters. It is easy enough just from the raw data with intensity on the y-axis and the time on the x-axis to compute the time to peak gadolinium effect and the mean transit time.

Alternatively, there are techniques to tag the blood without administering a contrast agent—spin tagging or arterial spin labeling (ASL). These differ from the "first-pass gad" techniques which are one-time deals where you lose the ability to repetitively sample due to the recirculation of the gadolinium. The arterial spin labeling techniques are much more sophisticated and hence less widely available. However, they allow accurate evaluation of absolute cerebral blood flow and can be used repetitively in the same patient. ASL allows real-time monitoring of therapeutic measures that influence cerebral blood flow in a single setting. Essentially, ASL techniques label the inflowing blood with a saturation pulse instead of gadolinium and make images of CBF by subtracting images recorded with and without the saturation pulse. The drawbacks of ASL are in low signal to noise and susceptibility artifacts.

Functional Magnetic Resonance Imaging (fMRI)

fMRI is still struggling to find its role in routine clinical imaging. The blood oxygen level-dependent (BOLD) contrast method is the basis for most fMRI studies performed at present. This technique relies on the T2* effect of deoxyhemoglobin in the tissue. Essentially, when the brain is activated by a task, there is conversion of

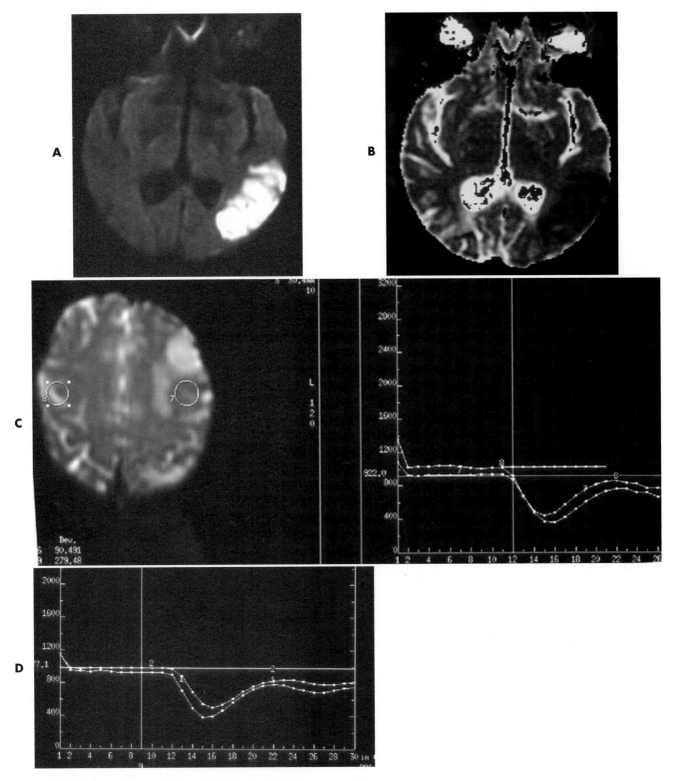

Fig. 1-6   DWI, ADC, and PWI in a CVA. **A,** DWI scan shows the wedged shape bright stroke in the left MCA distribution. **B,** ADC map is dark in that area, implying restricted diffusion. **C,** PWI graph shows a delay in decrease in signal intensity and the amplitude of the diminution is less on the affected side. **D,** Another stroke showing delay in downturn and reduced amplitude (line 2) compared to normal side (line 1).

oxyhemoglobin to deoxyhemoglobin and utilization of glucose. Although this may lead one to believe that the local brain tissue will therefore have lower signal intensity on a T2-weighted scan (due to the T2 shortening effects of deoxyhemoglobin), the exact opposite is seen. How is this possible, you ask? Well the brain is so good at perfusion that it actually increases blood flow to the functioning tissue leading to a wash-out of deoxyhemoglobin and an abundance of diamagnetic oxyhemoglobin. Thus, the intensity increases. Hence, the BOLD effect.

Initially most fMRI studies were performed with a block design of 15 to 40 seconds of a task alternating with 15 to 40 seconds of rest. The intensity of the tissue between the two periods was evaluated with very sophisticated mathematical analysis that belie our early algebraic limitations. (Calculus to us means a salivary gland stone.) Nowadays there has been a movement to "single trial analysis" where a single event is analyzed for the slopes of the curve of signal intensity and for its localization. This eliminates the worry of accommodation or fatigue as a subject performs the task.

Clinical fMRI studies have focused on the ability to localize the motor strip, speech areas, and memory centers in patients who are undergoing frontotemporal resections of adjacent tumors. The information is useful from the standpoint of operative approach and preoperative counseling of patients. On the research side, the possibilities are endless as we try to map and understand cortical function in humans (Fig. 1-7). "The brain, boss, the brain."

Scan Times

Scan times (Box 1-6) for 2DFT imaging are traditionally determined by the following equation:

Scan time = No. of Excitations
$$\times \text{ TR} \times \text{No. of Phase Encodings}$$

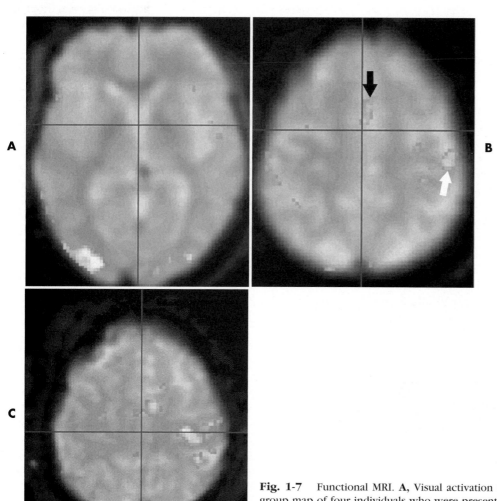

Fig. 1-7 Functional MRI. **A,** Visual activation in the occipital lobe is seen on this group map of four individuals who were presented with a colored visual cue. **B,** Motor activation in the primary motor strip *(white arrow)* and the supplementary motor area *(black arrow)* can be seen on this group map. Note that bilateral activation even with unilateral motor activity is to be expected. **C,** An individual subject's motor map shows greater variation in activation.

Box 1-6 Factors Relating to Scan Time

TR
Phase-encoding steps
Number of excitations
Number of acquisitions
Echo train length (FSE schemes)
Interleaving

Factors relating to number of slices per scan

TR
TE
Saturation pulses, gradient moment nulling
Echo train length, echo spacing

Box 1-8 Techniques to Increase SNR

Increase excitations
Decrease TE
Use surface coils
Increase FOV
Decrease matrix size
Sample full echo
Reduce bandwidth
Thicken slices
Increase field strength

For a TR of 600 milliseconds, 2 excitations, and 256 × 256 matrix (phase encodings × frequency encodings matrix), the scan time would be 0.6 second × 2 × 256, or 307 seconds. Increasing the matrix size increases resolution but decreases the SNR as smaller pixels are created. Increasing the number of phase-encoding steps increases the scan time. Increasing the number of excitations (or averages) increases the SNR but also increases scan times. In MR a constant battle is waged between increasing resolution, increasing SNR, increasing the number of slices, changing contrast, and decreasing the slice thickness, versus the almighty scan time (Boxes 1-7 and 1-8).

How do these factors interrelate? Doubling the Number of EXcitations (NEX) (averages or NEX) causes a twofold increase in scan time but only an increase of the square root of 2 (1.42) in SNR, so there is an unequal trade-off in scan time to SNR. If slice thickness (or voxel size) is doubled, SNR doubles, so these are linearly related. If the FOV is doubled, the voxel size is quadrupled (doubled in two dimensions of the matrix, yielding poorer resolution) and SNR doubles. If one dimension of the matrix is doubled (going from 128 phase encodings to 256 phase encodings) but the other dimension is kept constant, SNR decreases by two, because voxel size is halved (and resolution doubled), but SNR in-

creases by the square root of two because acquisition time is doubled (as with NEX). The net effect is a decrease in SNR by 0.71.

The receiver bandwidth is another factor involved in SNR. The receiver bandwidth refers to the range of frequencies that are sampled in the frequency-encoded dimension. The higher the bandwidth the shorter the read-out time and susceptibility and chemical shift artifacts are reduced. The greater the range of frequencies sampled, the less SNR is obtainable at any one frequency. Therefore as bandwidth is increased, SNR decreases. It does so by a factor of the square root of the reciprocal of bandwidth. The trade-off for reducing the bandwidth to obtain higher SNR is decreased resolution. Finally, increasing field strength increases SNR by a complex mechanism.

Because of the implications of these parameters on scan time, there has been a strong push to create pulse sequences that reduce scan times while maintaining SNR. More and more rapid scanning techniques have been developed and include preparation pulses applied to tissue before actual imaging to achieve faster scan times and more T1WI. These sequences allow scan times in the range of fractions of seconds.

Box 1-7   Dependence of SNR on Imaging Parameters

$\sqrt{\text{Number of excitation averages}}$
$\sqrt{\text{Frequency-encoding steps}}$
$\sqrt{\text{Phase-encoding steps}}$
$\sqrt{1/\text{bandwidth}}$
Pixel area
Slice thickness

Contrast Agents

Gadolinium is a paramagnetic agent that is responsible for T1 shortening on MR images. Because shortening of T1 leads to higher signal intensity on a T1WI, areas of gadolinium accumulation appear bright or "enhanced." Actually gadolinium shortens both T2 and T1 because of its paramagnetic effect on adjacent hydrogen protons; however, the T1 shortening effect is dominant after the first pass (see perfusion scanning). The same percentage shortening of T1 is manifested to a greater extent than that of T2 because T1 values are much larger in the CNS than T2 values. This causes high signal intensity on T1WI after administration of gadolinium in areas of blood-brain barrier absence or breakdown. The standard dose of gadolinium currently recommended is 0.1 mmol/kg. Utilization of higher doses (0.3 mmol/kg) of gadolinium has largely been stymied in this medical care market because of the added expense and often little reward except in cases of enhanced MRA and for perfusion studies. Allowing a delay after contrast administration or applying a magnetization transfer suppression pulse to the sequence may afford the same added lesion conspicuity as doubling or tripling the gadolinium dose. Various iron-containing contrast agents have been proposed to be used in conjunction with T2WI. They generally shorten T2 as a result of paramagnetic effects and cause decreased signal intensity on long-TR images. These are under investigation in studies looking at the lymph nodes where uptake of small T2 shortening particles implies a normally functioning (nonneoplastic) lymph node. We also use the T2 shortening effects of gadolinium agents to perform first pass bolus perfusion scans. As the gadolinium flows in the arteries, its T2 shortening characteristics cause the adjacent brain tissue to have reduced signal on $T2^*$ studies. This is as simple as black and white. No perfusion—less T2 shortening, brighter brain. Good perfusion—more T2 shortening, darker brain.

Magnetization transfer imaging

Magnetization transfer (MT) imaging manipulates the differences in relaxation of three pools of protons in a given magnetic resonance experiment. There are (1) freely mobile unbound (water) protons, to which MR imaging is highly sensitive; (2) immobile restricted motion protons, which are invisible to MR; and (3) boundary layer protons through which exchange of MT occurs. Simplistically, one is able to determine the contribution of MT from the immobile proton pool (consisting of protons from cell membranes, macromolecules, and lipid bilayers) by observing the change in the MR signal when these protons are suppressed from when they are not suppressed. By applying a suppressor pulse with a large amplitude far away from the water and fat frequency into the macromolecular pool (which has broad resonance frequency) one can saturate the magnetization of these compounds. These saturated protons then exchange their magnetization with water. Scans with and without the suppression pulse may then be analyzed quantitatively or qualitatively to assess a contribution of the macromolecular pool to the signal intensity of a given structure or lesion.

The clinical applications of MT can be separated into three categories: (1) utilization of MT as a means of suppressing background tissue (used in magnetic resonance angiography and postgadolinium T1-weighted scans), (2) utilization of MT pulses to affect contrast on unenhanced scans, and (3) use of MT to assess the biochem-ical macromolecular composition of a lesion. Most frequently, MT is used to suppress background tissue in MR angiography. TOF MRA suffers from more background signal than that of PC MRA. Applying an MT pulse decreases the background intensity of normal brain for TOF MRA images. Using MT subtraction, the background signal intensity of the brain could be decreased anywhere from 15% to 30%, which allows greater visualization of vessels through the maximum intensity projection (MIP) algorithm. Improved distal blood vessel visualization and accurate representation of the caliber of proximal vessels are obtainable with suppression with MT. This technique can be coupled with varying the flip angle through a three-dimensional TOF MRA slab (RAMP/TONE pulse) to obtain the benefits of low and high flip angles and MT.

Recent studies have used MT in combination with postgadolinium spin-echo imaging. Again, the theory behind these studies consists of improved background suppression in the evaluation of enhancing lesions of the brain. Because the white matter of the brain has a greater degree of suppression with MT than gray matter structures, gray matter structures along the central sulcus, the basal ganglia, and substantia nigra are more intense than the white matter, which has been suppressed to a greater degree. This provides better conspicuity of enhancing lesions in the white matter. Particularly, if MT imaging is combined with high doses of gadolinium, one may be able to detect the parenchymal, intravascular, and meningeal enhancement associated with the various stages of infarct. The problem is that sometimes things look bright even without gadolinium on MT images, so you need to do both pre and postcontrast scans. Remember, time is money in practice.

MT T1 spin-echo images show a 37% reduction to background signal intensity and provide a twofold improvement in the contrast-to-noise of enhancing brain lesions (including metastases) over T1-weighted postgadolinium spin-echo images. A single-dose postgadolinium scan used with MT may be equivalent to a triple-dose postgadolinium scan without MT applied. Save money. Do MT. Eat more chikn.

In FSE imaging it is thought that the repetitive 180-degree pulses cause an effect that is similar to MT by having sinc pulses placed at a point removed from the center frequency of water. Therefore, for any given TR and TE an FSE image should have a greater degree of MT effect than that of a conventional spin-echo scan. This causes a more T2-weighted appearance on long TR, long TE scans, which has been noted on comparison of fast and conventional spin-echo imaging. The white matter on an FSE long-TR long-TE sequence tends to be darker than that in a conventional spin-echo long-TR long-TE sequence. Some authors have proposed that this causes an increased sensitivity to white matter abnormalities such as demyelinating lesions. If T1WI with FSE are used (echo train length [ETL = 4]) you can gain MT suppression for your postcontrast scans while you also decrease scan times. Now that is using your noggin!

MT can provide a window into the biochemical nature of a lesion. Some multiple sclerosis (MS) gurus have demonstrated that demyelinating and edematous plaques may be differentiated on the basis of their MT. The breakdown of the myelin protein in demyelinating lesions causes a greater reduction in MT than that of lesions where the myelin is intact (though edematous). In both of these situations, the MT ratio (calculated as 1−the intensity before divided by the intensity after the application of the suppressor-pulse) is less than that of normal white matter. Furthermore, even normal appearing white matter on T2 weighted and postgadolinium scans may demonstrate abnormal MT. This suggests that multiple sclerosis is a diffuse disease, which has alterations at a biochemical level that may be invisible to standard MR imaging.

Other researchers have shown that the MT in strokes decreases progressively from the acute setting to the chronic setting. Although this may represent cell membrane loss and/or global cortical tissue loss effect, it may also represent the influence of edema and encephalomalacia on the lesions. Exciting stuff, but there is more . . . .

MR spectroscopy (MRS)

MR spectroscopy has also moved from the realm of a research technique to clinical use during the years that we have been garnering large royalties from the first edition of this book. MR spectroscopy attempts to interrogate the chemical environment of the brain noninvasively. Initially the sample (voxel) of the brain that one was able to investigate had to be large (3 cm × 3 cm × 3 cm) and singular for SNR and speed reasons. At present "chemical shift imaging" (CSI) or MR spectroscopic imaging (MRSI) has evolved to the point where one can obtain 32 × 32 matrix scans in multiple 5-mm thick slices of brain using proton MRS. Metabolite maps are able to be generated and used to determine pathology. Many practices are still just employing single voxel MRS; MRSI is usually relegated to academic-based practices because of time limitations and postprocessing requirements.

Two flavors of MRS dominate: phosphorus and proton spectroscopy (Fig. 1-8). Right now proton is the flavor du jour, but initially the energetics of the brain were explored with phosphorus MRS. As one would imagine, by evaluating the relative states of inorganic phosphate, phosphomonoesters, phosphodiesters, ATP, and ADP one could determine the bioenergetic state of the tissue as well as measure other parameters such as pH. In so doing, one could differentiate ischemic tissue, where glycolysis was dominant, from healthy tissue, where the Krebs cycle was being used. Deposition of inorganic phosphorus also belied dead tissue. Phosphorous MRS is rarely used these days because it requires large volumes to be sampled, owing to the relative scarcity of the element and low SNR.

Now hydrogen is all over the place—hard to avoid hydrogen in our houses. Hydrogen or proton spectroscopy seems much more versatile than phosphorous. The proton MR spectrum is characterized by at least three peaks representing the compounds creatine and phosphocreatine (Cr), which is associated with cellular energy metabolism, choline (Cho), associated with cell membrane synthesis, and N-acetyl aspartate (NAA), which is considered to be a marker of neuronal integrity. Lactate is not detectable in the normal spectrum but may be seen with inflammation, infarction, and some neoplasms. MR spectra are acquired using primarily one of two volume localization techniques, point resolved spectroscopy (PRESS), and stimulated echo acquisition mode (STEAM). The techniques can be used at different TEs; long-TEs (>200 msec) or short TEs (<35 msec). With short TEs one has better SNR and can better identify myoinositol, lipids, glutamate, glutamine, gamma aminobutyric acid (GABA), and other amino acids. With CSI, (usually done at long TE), one can make whole brain maps of the more abundant compounds of NAA, Cho, or Cr. It turns out that although NAA is shown to be depleted very commonly in most diseases that destroy or replace neurons, Cho can be used to suggest increased cellular turnover as in neoplasms. Cr is a relatively constant compound in the brain. With demyelinating disorders, you may see reductions in NAA peaks reflecting axonal damage and/or elevations in the Cho, myoinositol, glutamine, and glutamate levels. Myoinositol has also been implicated as a marker for Alzheimer disease. Alanine is said to be elevated with meningiomas. NAA is markedly elevated in Canavan disease—one of the few conditions to show elevated NAA. Lipid peaks are often found in metastases and acute multiple sclerosis plaques.

Proton MRS can also determine "energetics" through the demonstration of lactate doublet peaks. This again is a marker for anaerobic metabolism and hence is elevated in stroke and in recent seizures. High grade or necrotic neoplasms often show elevated lactate doublets.

The clinical uses of MRS remain relegated to assessing seizure foci, trying to predict neoplasms from other causes of abnormal brain signals, distinguishing radiation necrosis from recurrent neoplasms, defining white matter diseases and their extent, assessing metabolic abnormalities, and characterizing masses in the brain.

We have included a table with various MRS identifiable compounds and their associations with disease states (Table 1-5)

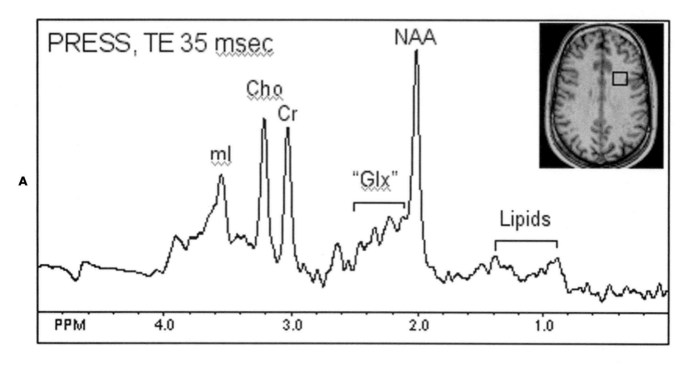

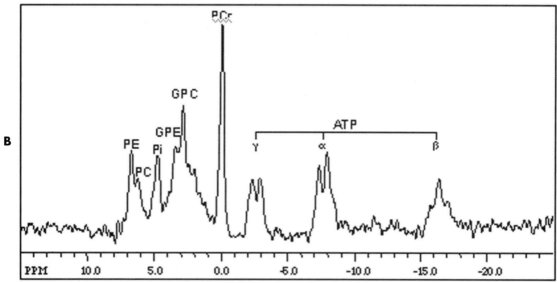

Fig. 1-8   Spectra from the brain. **A,** The proton MRS plot shows the dominant N-acetyl aspartate (NAA) peak with creatine and phosphocreatine (Cr) and choline containing compounds (Cho) at 2.0, 3.0, and 3.2 ppms, respectively. Also seen are lipid peaks between 1.0 and 1.5 ppm, glutamine and glutamate residues (61x) at 2.3 ppm, and myoinositol (MI). **B,** The phosphorous spectrum demonstrates peaks from ATP, phosphocreatine (PCr), phosphomonoesters (PE, PC), phosphodiesters (GPE, GPC), and inorganic phosphate (Pi). (Compliments of Peter Barker, D.Phil.)

Role of MR in Neuroimaging

MR is the initial study of choice to evaluate most brain and spine lesions. However, we will reiterate some caveats:

1. MR is less sensitive to subarachnoid hemorrhage even given the purported increased sensitivity of FLAIR. Thus, the typical ED patient who has a severe headache, sudden mental status change, or neurologic event, where bleeding from an aneurysm is a possible cause, must be studied by CT first before proceeding with MR.

2. MR is less sensitive than CT for the detection of calcification. Therefore, some lesions that have signature appearances of calcification (whorls as in chondrosarcoma, eggshell as in craniopharyngiomas, periventricular as in tuberous sclerosis,

Table 1-5 Various MRS indentifiable compounds and their associations with disease states

	mI	Cho	Cr	Glx	NAA	Lac	Lipid	Alanine
Brain tumors								
Low grade	+	+			−			
High grade	+ +	+ + +			− − −	+	+	
Necrotic/treated		−	−		− − −	+?	+	
Meningioma		+	− −		− −			+?
Seizure foci		+?			−	+*		
Mitochondrial disorders					−	+?		
Stroke								
Acute					−	+		
Chronic		+/−	−		− − −	+?	+?	
HIE (birth asphyxia, near drowning, CO poisoning)					−	+		
Demyelinating diseases								
Acute	+ +	+ +			−		+	
Chronic		−	−		−			
Miscellaneous								
ALS					−			
Alzheimer's	+	+?			−			
Canavan disease					+ +			
Creatine deficiency (GAMT)			− − −					
Cysts/CSE	−	−	−	−	−	+?		
Hemorrhage**								
Hepatic encephalopathy	−	−		+				
HIV encephalopathy	+	+			−			
Infection/inflammation					−	+?		
Trauma					−			

blank or ? - not a consistent observation

*ictal or early post-ictal

**very broad lines due to paramagnetic blood products

+increased

−decreased

(Compliments of Peter Barker, D.Phil.)

gyriform as in Sturge-Weber syndrome, punctate in the basal ganglia as in calcium-phosphorus dysmetabolism, serpiginous within arteriovenous malformations) may be nondetectable with MR. If the calcification is complexed to iron, MR may be more sensitive than CT for its presence, but calcium alone is weakly paramagnetic and hard to see on spin-echo MR.

3. MR is also relatively insensitive to bony cortical abnormalities. Although MR can detect the fat in bone marrow easily (and therefore is good for intramedullary bone lesions), the cortex of bone appears as a signal void on MR. Therefore, subtle fractures and even some minimally displaced ones can be overlooked with MR. Displaced shards of bone or foreign matter may not be picked up by MR; again, this justifies the use of CT over MR in the acute traumatic setting.

4. MR cannot be performed in patients who have pacemakers, non–MR-compatible vascular clips, pain stimulator implants, metallic implants or foreign bodies in the eyes, and severe claustrophobia. Because the risks to fetuses are unknown at this time, MR should not be performed on an elective basis in early term pregnant women. As an aside, for the evaluation of intraorbital foreign bodies, two anteroposterior (AP) plain films with different film cassettes will suffice. Particles that would be missed by plain films most likely would not penetrate the sclera.

5. Certain metallic artifacts may preclude adequate evaluation of some regions of the body including braces on the teeth, fixation hardware in the spine, and La Cage Aux Folles mascara.

ANGIOGRAPHY

Cerebral angiography is usually performed by the transfemoral artery technique. This requires the insertion of a needle into the common femoral or deep femoral artery and the threading of a wire and a catheter into the vessel via the Seldinger technique. Care should be taken not to force a wire subintimally into a vessel; if any resistance is met passing the wire, stop and analyze where you are. Gentle is the watchword. Carotid angiography is associated with an overall complication rate of 5% (groin hematomas, minor allergic reactions to contrast agents, femoral artery thromboses and/or arteriovenous fistulae, and retroperitoneal hematomas), including a permanent stroke rate of 0.5% to 1.0%.

Catheter Selection

The philosophy of "smaller, softer, safer" has dominated the catheter and wire technology used for cerebral angiography. At present, 5F (1F = 0.33 mm, so 5F = 1.66 mm or 0.066 inch) polyethylene catheters are relatively standard for most institutions that perform cerebral angiography and selective internal carotid artery catheterization. Catheter selection for any given patient is based on the anatomy of the takeoffs of the common carotid, innominate, and subclavian arteries from the aortic arch; the anatomic variations from person to person; the patient's age; and the vessel desired to be catheterized. This selection is not without a degree of subjectivity. In a young patient (<40 years old) you are likely to be able to catheterize all the necessary blood vessels for an aneurysm study with a simple hockey stick-shaped catheter (Fig. 1-9).

Catheters are usually described in terms of three curves. The tertiary curve is its most proximal one and is usually used to seat the catheter against the wall of the ascending aorta. The secondary curve points the catheter tip upward towards the supraaortic vessel origins. The primary curve is in the opposite direction of the tertiary curve and is the most distal. It is ideally shaped to the angle and curvature of the vessel's origin from the aorta.

Guide wires are used to pass the catheters through the groin or into a selected vessel. They are usually made of stainless steel with a flexible, tapered tip. Using a 5F catheter, one can use a 0.038-inch guide wire or, preferably, a "softer, smaller, safer" 0.035-inch wire. Wires also run in various stages of stiffness, with the Bentson wire the most floppy and a rigid Newton (Mandril) LT (long taper) wire on the stiffer side. To achieve "purchase" (enough rigidity and stability of a wire or catheter to prevent its movement in more tortuous blood vessels), the stiffer wires may need to be used. Highly slippery Terumo glide/guide wires are increasingly used with torque control devices to help guide catheters.

Technique

Once the catheter is in the carotid circulation, it is critical to avoid jerky motions for fear of injuring the vessel and setting up a nidus for thrombi. Double flushing of the catheter with heparinized saline solution to prevent propagation or development of catheter-induced emboli is the norm. Selective catheterization of smaller branches is weighed against the potential risk or discomfort to the patient.

Obviously, the amount of injection varies according to the size of the blood vessels (Table 1-6). Injection rates should be adjusted for children because their vessels are much smaller than those of adults. In addition, one should adjust the rate according to what one wishes to visualize. If a purely arterial view is required, one should decrease the total injection while maintaining the rate of injection. When one increases the total injection volumes, the time that the vessel is in contact with the contrast increases.

The explosive development of interventional neuroradiology has required smaller and more flexible catheters. Some of these catheters have tiny balloons at the end of their tips that can be used to flow-direct the catheter into ever-smaller branches of the carotid or vertebrobasilar system. These tiny (3F) catheters are generally introduced through a coaxial system using a 5F to 7F introducer catheter. Embolic agents may then be introduced into the vasculature from a site localized to the vascular abnormality without endangering normal vessels. Short-term occlusion of small vessels (as in an arteriovenous malformation [AVM] nidus or meningioma) can be achieved by embolizing with agents such as absorbable gelatin sponge or polyvinyl alcohol. Detachable balloons, metallic coils, and cyanoacrylates can be used for long-term occlusion of larger vessels (e.g., aneurysms, fistulas, or preoperative carotid occlusion). Stents are also now used in treatment of extracranial vascular stenoses, often coupled with balloon angioplasty.

Contrast Agents

Nonionic contrast agents are nearly exclusively used in the CNS, particularly in patients who have a lowered seizure threshold. In patients who are at risk of vasospasm, seizures, subarachnoid hemorrhage, ischemia, vasculitic reaction, and neoplasm, nonionic contrast agents are standard fare (Box 1-9). There has been considerable debate within the literature as to whether the nonionic agents have a higher degree of thrombotic complications because of clot formation within the syringe and/or the catheter. The ionic contrast agents appear to have an anticoagulant effect that is not found with the nonionic contrast agents. Thus, it is important to flush regularly with heparinized saline solution and to be wary of clot formation within syringes in contact with the nonionic contrast agent. The longer the blood vessel is in contact with iodinated contrast, the more likely it is that seizures and other vasculopathic complications will occur. These complications are rare with the nonionic con-

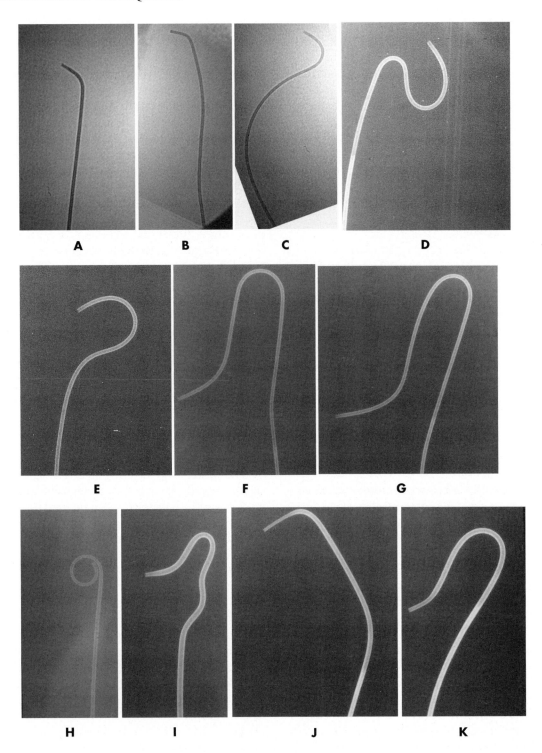

Fig. 1-9   Catheters. Radiographs of commonly used catheters. **A,** At our institution the most commonly used intracranial catheters that do not need to be formed are the hockeystick 1 (Berenstein) catheter **(A)**, the JB-1 **(B)**, and JB-2 **(C)** catheters. The next most frequently used catheters are the HN4 (Mani) **(D)**, and HN5 **(E)** catheters. When the arteries are particularly tough to selectively catheterize, you may need a Simmons 2 **(F)** or Simmons 3 **(G)** catheter. These are usually formed in the subclavian artery or ascending aorta. For arch injections, use a pigtail catheter **(H)** so that the tip does not get embedded in an atherosclerotic plaque. For spinal arteriograms either a Mikaelsson **(I)** or 5 Fr Cobra glide catheter **(J)** is typically selected. For axillary arteriograms, try a Hinck catheter **(K).**

Table 1-6 Representative injection rates for vessels

Vessel	Rate (mL/sec)	Total contrast given (mL)
Common carotid artery	7	11
Internal carotid artery	6	8
External carotid artery	3	5
Vertebral artery	5	8
Subclavian artery	10	15
Aortic arch	22	45
Intercostal artery	1-2	2-4

From Yousem DM, Trinh BC: AJNR 22:1838-1840, 2001.

trast agents now in use, but injection rates and durations should be kept to the minimum necessary to visualize the relevant anatomy completely.

According to the literature on nonionic contrast agents, the incidence of significant cardiovascular events with an agent such as iohexol is 0.3%. Fatalities associated with contrast agents occur in 1 in 20,000 to 40,000 doses. According to Caro and co-workers (see Selected Readings), reviewing safety studies from 1980 to 1990, the risk of death from high-osmolar (ionic) agents was 0.9 per 100,000 uses and the risk of severe reactions was 157 per 100,000 uses. There was no reduction in the risk of death with low-osmolar (nonionic) agents, but the number of severe reactions was as low as 126 per 100,000 uses. Treatment of contrast reactions is outlined in the Appendix taken from American College of Radiology guidelines.

These agents should be treated as drugs, with a physician or nurse on hand to administer the contrast and to monitor the patient thereafter. These rates of complications are intrinsic to the use of iodinated contrast media and not specific to contrast arteriography. In fact, in most studies, arterial injection of contrast led to fewer complications than intravenous injections.

Iodinated contrast agents are potentially nephrotoxic (Box 1-10). Decreases in creatinine clearance are rou-

tinely seen after administration of iodine agents. In the short term at least, the effect on creatinine clearance appears to be less with nonionic agents than with ionic compounds. The potential for severe renal damage is greatest in patients who have predisposing illnesses for renal impairment.

Transient ischemic attacks and cerebral infarctions in high-risk patients during cerebral intraarterial angiography, according to the package insert for iohexol, occur in 1.6% of cases. Groin hematomas occur in about 10% to 15% of cases in most major series, but most only require a muscular resident or fellow applying adequate compression to treat. Intimal tears or dissections of catheterized vessels occur in fewer than 1% of cases. Transient global amnesia has been reported with both ionic and nonionic iodinated agents. This entity is usually self-limited but can be very frightening because the patient suddenly loses short-term memory and becomes disoriented in the middle of arteriography. The problem usually resolves after a few hours, but in the meantime, the neuroradiologist sweats bullets. The cause is thought to be limbic ischemia. Vertebral artery injections seem to elicit the syndrome more commonly.

Spinal arteriograms are associated with a 2.2% risk of neurologic complications resulting from cord ischemia. Limited flow injections, often performed by hand, are commonly used, and the catheter should never be allowed to occlude flow to the cord. Repetitive injections are avoided. To perform a search for a spinal vascular malformation, one must perform selective right-sided and left-sided catheterizations of the intercostal arteries, lumbar arteries, iliac arteries, vertebral arteries, subclavian arteries (to opacify thyrocervical, costocervical, and ascending cervical branches), the distal aorta (to see median sacral branches), and external carotid arteries. This is often a laborious task with the technologists and nurses ticking off a ledger that specifies each of the over 40 vessels catheterized. The nice part about spinal an-

Box 1-9 Indications for Use of Low-Osmolar (Nonionic) Contrast Agents

Previous adverse reaction to high-osmolar agent
History of asthma
Cardiac abnormalities: arrhythmia, congestive heart failure, unstable angina, recent myocardial infarction, pulmonary hypertension
Generalized severe debilitation
By patient request

Box 1-10 Predisposing Factors to Nephrotoxicity from Iodinated Contrast

Multiple myeloma or other paraproteinemias where precipitation of proteins in tubules can cause acute renal failure
Severe diabetes
Dehydration
Recent aminoglycoside exposure
Anuria
Hepatorenal syndrome
Serum creatinine >3 mg/dL
Metformin (glucophage) usage

giograms is that, because of all these selective catheterizations, once you have done one thoroughly, you are well trained for life. Of course the reimbursement will probably only be about $3.49. On the other hand, if you screw up and you infarct the cord, the settlement will be about $3.49 billion dollars. Oh the lack of justice in it all.

MYELOGRAPHY

Is myelography becoming obsolete? Perhaps. In centers where MR has become dominant, myelography has taken it on the chin. Only patients with pacemakers, claustrophobia, and postop metallic hardware (thank the lord for pedicle screws!) keep our myelography census high enough that we can train neuroradiology subspecialists in the waning art of myelography.

Myelography has played a smaller role in neuroimaging because of the greater safety and noninvasiveness of MR for imaging the spine for degenerative disease. The role of myelography with CT has been relegated to imaging the spine in patients who are unable to undergo MR or for confirmation of equivocal MR findings, particularly in the cervical spine. Occasionally, neurosurgeons order myelograms to visualize nerve roots in a direct coronal plane to assess better the degree of compression seen on MR. Other spine surgeons prefer myelography and CT because of the distinct appearance of osteophytic disease or because of their familiarity with the technique. A good CT-myelogram study of the cervical spine cord still is a thing of beauty and the gold standard for degenerative disease.

We include here a section on myelographic techniques because professors long in the tooth are still around to examine at the boards. We are sure most of the pneumoencephalographers have abandoned that technique by now.

Lumbar Myelographic Technique (Fig. 1-10)

Performing lumbar myelography is relatively simple. The patient is informed of the risks of bleeding, infection, pain, seizures, contrast dye reactions, and, most commonly, severe headaches after the study, and consent is obtained. Patients who have been taking medications that lower the seizure threshold (Box 1-11) should have these medications stopped at least 24 to 48 hours before the study. The patient is placed in a prone position on the examining table and the back is sterilized from the L1 to L3 levels. Initial plain films or fluoroscopy are done to map out strategy for placement of the spinal needle and to identify bony abnormalities or normal variations such as transitional vertebrae or rib-bearing lumbar bodies.

Two approaches to inserting the needle can be used. With the patient left in a prone position, the needle is inserted from a position 2 to 3 cm off midline at the L2-L3 level. The needle is angled (depending on the thickness of the patient's back) to course under the ipsilateral lamina into the thecal sac. Alternatively, the patient may be placed on a bolster or rotated on the scan table so that the needle direction is straight down in an obliquely positioned patient. This allows visualization of a boneless "bull's eye" into the spinal canal under the lamina. Because the spinous processes overlap in the prone position and the needle tip invariably ends up at the disk level, midline insertion of the needle between spinous processes is a less than ideal approach. The disk level is usually the area most stenotic in patients with degenerative spine disease.

Often the patient and the neuroradiologist feel a "pop" as the posterior ligaments of the spinal canal are crossed and a second pop at the entry point into the thecal sac. To the person on the hub side of the needle one of the most gratifying sensations in neuroradiology is "the pop" that tells you the needle is intrathecal. It is almost anticlimactic to pull the stylet and see clear cerebrospinal fluid (CSF) flow out the hub; you know before then that you have done the puncture correctly. Once the needle is within the thecal sac, CSF is removed for laboratory examination (in the appropriate setting) unless the examination is being performed to evaluate for the possibility of cord compression, where there is at least a theoretic risk of herniation caused by the negative pressure transmitted by the open-ended needle.

In general, a 3.06-g limit of iodinated contrast medium instilled intrathecally in the lumbar or cervical region is followed. Thus, one is able to administer 10 mL of contrast material with a 300 mg/mL concentration or approximately 12 mL at a 240 mg/mL concentration. These are the usual doses used for lumbar puncture myelography. In children, manufacturers recommend no more than 2.94 g of iodine intrathecally and a concentration no greater than 210 mg/mL. The contrast is instilled with intermittent fluoroscopy to determine the correct amount of contrast to be administered. Patients with small thecal sacs require less than those with capacious sacs. If one is performing a cervical myelogram through a lumbar puncture approach, the maximum contrast load should be given and an attempt should be made to keep the contrast collected as a "bolus" for passage to the cervical region.

AP, lateral, and oblique films are obtained in the lumbar region to detect nerve root compression and extradural impressions. These are obtained in the prone position. Standing views may be helpful to accentuate gravity-induced disk protrusions. Because the conus

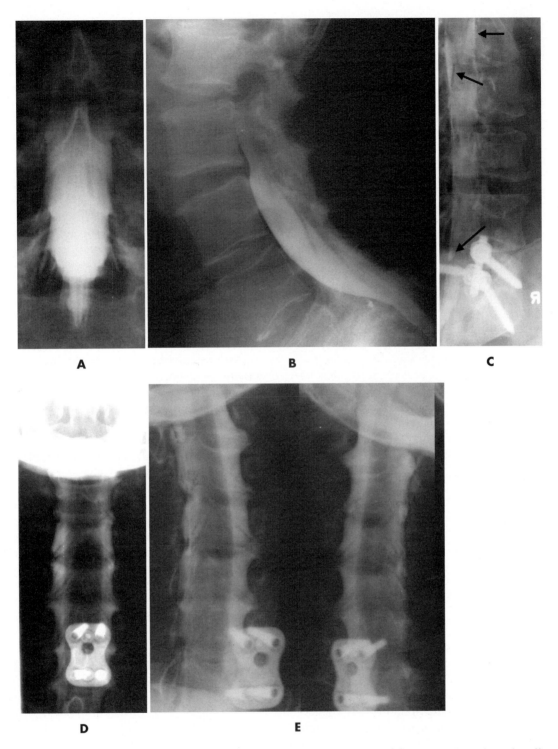

A   **B**   **C**

D   **E**

Fig. 1-10   Myelography. Lumbar myelography requires AP (**A**), Lateral (**B**), and oblique (**C**), views to best show the effects of disks on nerve roots and the thecal sac. Posterior impressions are usually from facet joint disease, anterior ones from disks or osteophytes. This patient has grade II spondylolisthesis at L5–S1 as seen on the lateral view. Skip ahead to Chapter 16 for the definition of this six-syllable word. **C**, Subdural injections are identified when focal collections of contrast accumulate and do not flow appropriately in the subarachnoid space. They are hard to readily identify when one has a mixed subarachnoid-subdural injection as in this case, when your fluoroscopy is from Roentgen's era, or you are dealing with a very obese patient. **D**, Cervical myelograms look best when a C1–C2 puncture has been performed and the contrast is locally collected. With instillation from a lumbar approach the contrast may be diluted as it is passed superiorly to the neck. Hence, the use of 10 mL of 300 mg/mL concentration of iodine dye is recommended. The AP view on the cervical study (**D**) usually shows nerve root truncation or compression the best, but the oblique views (**E**) are also helpful.

medullaris generally lies in the posterior half of the thecal sac, supine conus views are obtained, although in a well-filled thecal sac prone views are adequate. The myelographic and clinical findings direct the postmyelogram CT examination. CT sections angled through the disks are obtained. Contiguous straight transaxial sections allow high-quality sagittal and coronal reconstructed images that ideally visualize nerve root and thecal sac compression. 3D reconstructions should be produced. CT detects the lateral herniations that are invisible to myelography because they occur beyond the confines of the thecal sac.

Cervical Myelographic Technique

Cervical or thoracic myelography can be performed through a lumbar or cervical approach. Because of their ease of performance, reduced patient anxiety, and lower complication rate, lumbar approaches are more common today. The contrast is inserted in the lumbar region of the spine and maintained as a bolus as the patient is tilted downward, allowing the flow of contrast to the cervical region. The patient's head is maintained in a hyperextended fashion to prevent contrast from entering the intracranial space. In patients with kyphosis or scoliosis, the patient may be placed in an oblique or prone position to help the contrast medium flow to the neck. Once contrast streams into the cervical region, the patient's position is flattened and the contrast pools in the natural lordosis of the cervical spine.

If the cervical approach is preferred, the needle is inserted just anterior to the spinal lamina line at the C1–C2 level from a lateral puncture site with cross-table lateral and AP fluoroscopy. The patient is positioned in a prone, face-down position with verification that the patient is in a true lateral position to the lateral fluoroscopic tube by making sure the mandibular condyles and necks superimpose. The needle is inched forward from just anterior to the spinal lamina line, with lateral fluoroscopy to ensure that one is not proceeding too far anteriorly

where the spinal cord could be punctured. Usually, one need not go farther anteriorly than the posterior third of the spinal canal. On AP fluoroscopy the tip of the needle, when properly positioned, should be medial to the lateral margin of the dens. Although puncturing the spinal cord elicits an immediate dramatic reaction by the patient and physician (usually lightning shots in the legs for the former, and checks of malpractice premiums for the latter), permanent injury to the cord is extremely rare unless one injects contrast into the cord itself. Low-dose contrast can be instilled into the thecal sac for a cervical examination. AP, lateral, and oblique views (the latter can be obtained by having the patient perform Schwartzeneger-esque one-arm push-ups) are obtained in the cervical region. CT scans are obtained with 1.0 to 3.0 mm thick sections through suspicious levels, angled to the disks or straight transaxial for optimal reconstructed images.

Postprocedure Orders

Postmyelography orders should include restriction of activity for 24 hours with no heavy lifting or bending, vigorous rehydration, elevation of the head to limit contrast flowing intracranially, and resumption of restricted medications after 24 hours. The patient should be warned about the severity and duration of postspinal tap headaches, which can be incapacitating to some persons. Epidural blood patches for CSF leaks are very effective at relieving those headaches.

ULTRASOUND

In skilled hands, ultrasound (Box 1-12) can be a useful technique for evaluating disorders of the CNS. The acoustic barrier of the skull and vertebrae prevents routine evaluation of the adult patient; however, one can use the anterior and posterior fontanelles in infants as an effective window into the brain. In addition, intraoperative ultrasound may be useful for localizing lesions in the brain or spine once the overlying bones have been removed.

Portable real-time ultrasound can be used effectively in the operating room or the neonatal nursery. Ultrasound studies the ability of structures to transmit or impede sonic waves transmitted from a transducer. The transducer also serves as the receiver, detecting the sound waves that have bounced off structures back to the surface. The concept is identical to that of sonar, used by surface ships to detect submarines, fish, and ocean-bottom irregularities. The benefit of no ionizing radiation is of particular value in studying infants and in the operating room, where the personnel are at no risk from the procedure. In general, one uses high-frequency (5.0 to 10.0 MHz) transducers for shallow imaging, with the probe covered with coupling gel in a sterile glove.

In infants or in utero, one can readily detect regions of intraparenchymal and/or intraventricular hemorrhage as areas of increased echogenicity compared with hypoechoic brain or anechoic CSF. Such congenital anomalies as Dandy-Walker cysts, agenesis of the corpus callosum, lipomas, and holoprosencephaly can also be detected. Extraaxial collections, hydrocephalus, and cystic encephalomalacia may also be seen. In utero ultrasound has been used to detect anencephaly, hydrocephalus, and neural tube defects in the spinal canal (myelomeningoceles and spina bifida) in patients with elevated α-fetoprotein levels.

In adults at surgery, gliomas are usually hyperechoic to normal brain tissue. Necrosis is seen as an area of increased echogenicity. Ultrasound's role in determining the optimal site for biopsy intraoperatively has been well established for the brain and the spine. The needle used for a biopsy can be tracked in real time as it enters a lesion. Syringes in the cord can be seen as anechoic areas with increased transmission.

Sonography of the carotid bifurcation is an excellent screening test for significant stenoses and plaques. Combining the visual inspection of the vessel with frequency analysis and spectral patterns reflecting flow velocity, one has two means for detecting arterial narrowing (Fig. 1-11). The days when ultrasound was belittled as looking like menacing cloud formations on a dark screen are over; color-flow Doppler ultrasound of the arteries can give information about flow direction, velocity, turbulence, and patency.

Recent studies have suggested that peak systolic velocities over 200 cm/sec on power Doppler studies are the best sonographic indicator of stenoses of the internal carotid artery that are greater than 70%. This is critical to know because 70% is the criterion most cited for recommending surgery over medical therapy for carotid atherosclerotic disease.

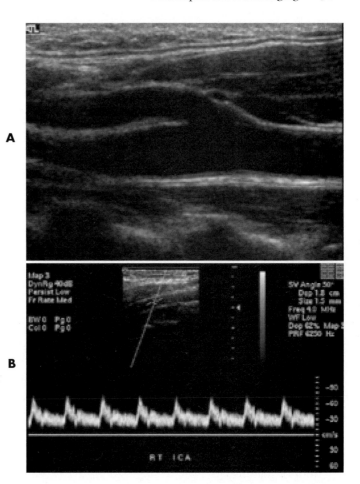

Fig. 1-11   Sonography. **A,** Carotid ultrasound examination shows a beautifully pristine carotid bifurcation with internal carotid artery lying posterior and external carotid anterior. **B,** The Doppler study shows a peak systolic rate of approximately 80 cm/sec, well within the normal limits. We get worried when peak velocities exceed 200 cm/sec.

Ultrasound is also used extensively by ophthalmologists. Because the globe is filled with fluid, it serves as an excellent transmitter of sound waves. Retinal lesions or, for that matter, most intraocular masses can be readily evaluated with ocular sonography. The technique can be used in combination with color-flow Doppler ultrasound to evaluate the direction of flow in the superior ophthalmic vein, to suggest the diagnosis of cavernous-carotid fistulas (where the flow is reversed).

Transcranial Doppler studies are used to evaluate velocities of intracranial vessels. These will be increased in patients with vasospasm, usually in the setting of subarachnoid hemorrhage. Occasionally, occluded vessels will also be identified.

NUCLEAR MEDICINE

The theory behind nuclear medicine is to instill radioactive substances into the body and then detect the emissions of these agents with crystal scintillation devices (gamma cameras). The amplitude of the gamma-emissions by the radiotracer is reflected in the intensity on the scintillation device. The nuclear agent used most frequently in planar brain scanning is technetium, which is a gamma ray emitter of 140 keV photons and has a half-life of 6 hours. Use of nuclear medicine technetium pertechnetate scanning is limited to studies on brain death. Because no flow enters the brain with brain death, no accumulation of the tracer in the brain is seen, yielding a "cold study." Areas of blood-brain barrier breakdown may demonstrate radiotracer activity; otherwise, on a normal scan the uptake is only in vascular (usually venous) structures.

In patients suspected of having communicating hydrocephalus an indium 111-diethylenepentaacetic acid study is sometimes ordered. This agent emits gamma rays at 173 keV and has a half-life of 2.8 days. The agent is instilled in the CSF through a lumbar puncture. The normal circulation of the CSF should produce radiotracer uptake in the basal cisterns by 2 to 4 hours after instillation. By 24 hours tracer should be seen over the vertex. In cases of communicating hydrocephalus and normal-pressure hydrocephalus, reflux of the tracer into the ventricles is seen with lack of tracer accumulation over the convexities. Patients who demonstrate this scintigraphic appearance may have a better response to shunting than patients with equivocal indium studies.

Indium may also be used to detect sinonasal CSF leaks. Multiple pledgets are inserted in the nose or ears before instillation of the radiotracer in the lumbar thecal sac. Twenty-four hours later the detection of elevated counts in specific pledgets can grossly localize or verify the site of active CSF leak.

Positron emission tomography (PET) uses positron-emitting isotopes of chemical elements produced in a cyclotron. A positron is a positively charged antimatter equivalent of an electron that is emitted by the isotope that combines with negatively charged electrons to produce gamma-radiation, which can be detected by scintillation cameras on opposite sides of the patient. Is that a lot in one sentence? You bet! The typical agents used for PET studies are fluorine 18-labeled deoxyglucose (FDG), carbon 11-labeled deoxyglucose, or methionine. These agents are used to determine glucose utilization or blood flow in the brain. The most frequent intracranial clinical indication for these studies is differentiation of tumor from radiation necrosis. FDG PET combined with CT scanners is now also being used to identify head and neck cancers before and after treatment. The metabolic rate of a neoplasm can be determined by ^{18}F-deoxyglucose. Dopamine analogues have been used with radioactive fluorine or carbon to analyze activity in patients with Parkinson disease (the activity is decreased in the putamen), Alzheimer disease (temporal lobe and hippocampal activity is markedly depressed, but putamen activity is normal), and neu-

ropsychiatric disorders. Effectiveness of drug treatment in neuropsychiatric disorders can be assessed with PET. The relatively poor resolution, need for a cyclotron in many instances, high cost, and decreased availability in the community of PET scanning is its chief downfall at this time.

Single-photon emission computed tomography (SPECT) uses iodinated radiotracers (iodine 123-labeled iodo-amphetamine) or technetium 99m agents as cerebral perfusion and extraction agents. These agents are relatively stable and an on-site cyclotron is not required, making the technique easier and cheaper than PET. The agents are used to study blood flow and cerebral metabolism. These agents have been used to study stroke, epilepsy, and dementia. Subclinical ischemic areas may be detected by SPECT studies at an earlier stage than CT. Perfusion defects in Alzheimer's disease have been demonstrated in parietal association areas with ^{123}I-SPECT, but spatial resolution tends to be lower than PET.

SEDATION

We tend to use oral diazepam or alprazolam to help our adult patients make it through CT and MRI scans and the occasional myelogram. During angiography, a cocktail of midazolam (Versed) and/or pentobarbital (Nembutal) seems to do the trick to reduce anxiety and allow a comfortable study. In children under 5 years of age, chloral hydrate at doses between 60 and 100 mg/kg seems to adequately sedate the subject for the time needed to do the cross-sectional imaging study with very little risk of complications. If intravenous sedation is required, we rely on pentobarbital and fentanyl. Others are advocating ketamine hydrochloride (Ketalar) intravenous or intramuscular sedation in children younger than 11 years old for interventional radiologic procedures. The short induction time, rapid recovery, and minimal respiratory depression are cited as advantages of this sedative.

The Ideal World

In our ideal neuroradiology section (located on I-95 between Manhattan and East Baltimore), CT would be located in the ED trauma bay for acute scanning of patients with head injuries. For nearly all outpatient neurologic imaging procedures of the brain and spine MR would be performed. Tissue specific diagnoses would be made with the aid of high resolution echoplanar sequences, instantaneous spectroscopy, molecular imaging and perfusional analysis. Preoperative planning would include fMRI localization and three-dimensional imaging with interactive image guidance. After MR, some patients would be referred for CT to detect calcification and to characterize skull lesions. Skull base and neck cases could be equally distributed between CT (inflammatory sinus, temporal bone, and salivary gland calculous disease) and MR (aerodigestive system malignancies and nonmucosal neck masses). Myelography would be performed only in conjunction with CT and only in non–MR-compatible patients or for clarification of degenerative spondylitic abnormalities seen on MR. Ultrasound would be used for prenatal screening for CNS anomalies, and neonatal cranial examinations for complications of prematurity (intraventricular hemorrhage and germinal matrix bleeds) and delivery. Although angiography would be the authoritative method for evaluating vascular lesions of the brain (aneurysms and AVMs) and neck (carotid bifurcations and dissections of neck vessels), most cases could be handled with CTA, MRA, and color-flow Doppler ultrasound (performed by radiologists not vascular surgeons). Clinical nuclear medicine studies would be confined to indium studies for CSF leakage and for predicting response to shunting in patients with communicating hydrocephalus. PET and SPECT studies would be highly sensitive, specific, and reimbursed. These techniques would help us better understand metabolism, mental illness, physiology, and tumor recurrence.

PET would help build our molecular imaging program that would be predominantly MR/MRSI based. We would read all these cases from our summer homes in the islands over high speed Internet lines. Of course, in this ideal world everyone would have fee for service insurance, and the choice of the finest doctors who write textbooks. Yes, there is a Santa Claus, Virginia!

> To maintain the state-of-the-art
> Would take a CFO's part
> He'd charge for injections
> And multi-projections
> And rip out the HMO's heart

> There is a department with fame
> That has the best equipment in name
> But the staff continue to whine
> The residents still read like they're blind
> Things change but human nature remains the same

APPENDIX
American College of Radiology Guidelines on Management of Contrast Reactions

Urticaria
Treatment
1. Discontinue injection.
2. No treatment needed in most cases.
3. H_1-receptor blocker: Diphenhydramine (Benadryl), 25 to 50 mg PO/IM/IV, or hydroxyzine (Vistaril), 25 to 50 mg.

H_2-receptor blocker may be added: Cimetidine (Tagamet) 300 mg PO or IV slowly, diluted in 10 mL D5W solution; or ranitidine (Zantac), 50 mg PO or IV slowly, diluted in 10 mL D5W solution.

If severe or widely disseminated, use α-agonist (arteriolar and venous constriction): epinephrine (1:1000), 0.1 to 0.3 mL SC (if no cardiac contraindication).

Facial/laryngeal edema
Treatment
1. α-Agonist (arteriolar and venous constriction): Epinephrine (1:1000), 0.1 to 0.3 mL SC or, if SC route fails or if peripheral vascular collapse, then 1.0, 1:10,000 slowly IV. May repeat up to maximum of 1.0 mg.
2. O_2, 2, to 6 L/min.

If not responsive to therapy or for obvious laryngeal edema (acute)
1. Call anesthesiologist/CODE team.
2. Consider intubation.

Bronchospasm
Treatment
1. O_2, 6 to 10 L/min; monitor ECG; O_2 saturation (pulse oximeter); blood pressure.
2. Epinephrine (1:1000), 0.1 to 0.3 mL SC or β-agonist inhalers (bronchiolar dilators, i.e., metaproterenol [Alupent], terbutaline [Brethaire], or albuterol [Proventil]). If SC route fails or if peripheral vascular collapse, then 1.0 (1:10,000) slowly IV. May repeat 3 times prn to maximum of 1.0 mg.

Alternative treatment
1. Aminophylline, 6.0 mg/kg IV in D5W over 10 to 20 min (loading dose), then 0.4 to 1.0 mg/kg/hr prn, or terbutaline, 0.25 to 0.5 mg IM or SC.
2. Call CODE for severe bronchospasm (or if O_2 saturation < 88%).

Hypotension with tachycardia
Treatment
1. Legs up; Trendelenburg position; monitor blood pressure; also ECG, pulse oximetry.
2. O_2, 6 to 10 L/min.
3. Rapid administration of large volumes of isotonic Ringer's lactated solution (Ringer's lactate > normal saline > D5W).

If poorly responsive, administer epinephrine 1.0 mL (1:10,000) slowly IV. May repeat prn up to maximum of 1.0 mg. If still poorly responsive, transfer to ICU for further management.

Hypotension with bradycardia: vagal reaction
1. Legs up; Trendelenburg position; secure airway; monitor vital signs; give O_2 (6–10 L/min).
2. Give atropine 0.6 to 1.0 mg IV slowly.
3. Secure IV access; push fluid replenishment IV (Ringer's lactate > normal saline > D5W).
4. Repeat atropine up to 2.0 mg total dose.

Hypertension, severe

1. Monitor blood pressure; also place ECG, pulse oximeter.
2. Nitroglycerin 0.4 mg tablet SL (may repeat × 3).
3. Sodium nitroprusside: Arterial line; infusion pump necessary to titrate.
4. Transfer to ICU.
5. For pheochromocytoma, phentolamine, 5.0 mg (1.0 mg in children) IV.

Seizures/convulsions

1. O$_2$, 6 to 10 L/min.
2. Consider diazepam (Valium), 5.0 mg or midazolam (Versed), 2.5 mg IV.
3. If longer effect needed, obtain consultation; consider phenytoin (Dilantin) infusion, 15 to 18 mg/kg at 50 mg/min.
4. Careful monitoring of vital signs required.

Pulmonary edema

1. Elevate torso; apply rotating tourniquets (venous compression).
2. O$_2$, 6 to 10 L/min.
3. Diuretics: Furosemide (Lasix), 40 mg IV slowly.
4. Consider morphine.
5. Corticosteroids optional.

Premedication regimens:
Prednisone 50 mg by mouth 13, 7,
and 1 hours before the procedure
50 mg diphenhydramine IV, IM, PO
1 hour before contrastadministered
or
Methylprednisolone 32 mg by mouth 12
and 2 hours before contrast administration
or
200 mg hydrocortisone intravenously 7
and 1 hour before contrast administration.

Pediatric sedation:
Chloral hydrate 80 to 100 mg/kg PO up to 2 g maximum
Pentobarbital (Nembutal) 2 to 4 mg/kg IV up to 150 mg
Fentanyl (Sublimase) 0.5 to 1.0 mcg/kg IV
Lorazepam (Ativan) 0.05 to 0.1 mg/kg up to 2 mg

SELECTED READINGS

Achten E, Jackson GD, Cameron JA, Abbott DF, Stella DL, Fabinyi GC: Presurgical evaluation of the motor hand area with functional MR imaging in patients with tumors and dysplastic lesions, *Radiology* 210:529-538, 1999.

Bakshi R, Kamran S, Kinkel PR, et al: Fluid-attenuated inversion-recovery MR imaging in acute and subacute cerebral intraventricular hemorrhage, *Am J Neuroradiol* 20:629-636, 1999.

Beauchamp NJJ, Barker PB, Wang PY, vanZijl PC: Imaging of acute cerebral ischemia, *Radiology* 212:307-324, 1999.

Bradley WG Jr: Pathophysiologic correlates of signal alterations. In Brant-Zawadzki M, editor: *Magnetic resonance in the central nervous system,* New York, 1986, Raven Press.

Bradley WG Jr, Tsuruda JS: MR sequence parameter optimization: an algorithmic approach, *AJR* 149:815-823, 1987.

Breger RK, Rimm AA, Fischer ME, et al: T1 and T2 measurements on a 1.5-T commercial MR imager, *Radiology* 171: 273-276, 1989.

Breger RK, Wehrli FW, Charles HC, et al: Reproducibility of relaxation and spin density parameters in phantoms and the human brain measured by MR imaging at 1.5T, *Magn Reson Med* 3:649-662, 1986.

Bushong SC: *Magnetic resonance imaging: physical and biological principles,* St Louis, 1988, Mosby-Year Book.

Caro JJ, Trindade E, McGregor M: The risks of death and of severe nonfatal reactions with high- vs low-osmolality contrast media: a metaanalysis, *AJR* 156:825-832, 1991.

Cenic A, Nabavi DG, Craen RA, Gelb AW, Lee TY: Dynamic CT measurement of cerebral blood flow: a validation study, *AJNR* 20:63-73,1999.

Forbes G, Nichols DA, Jack CR Jr, et al: Complications of spinal cord arteriography: prospective assessment of risk for diagnostic procedure, *Radiology* 169:479-484, 1988.

Fullerton GD: Physiologic basis of magnetic relaxation. In Stark DD, Bradley WG Jr, editors: *Magnetic resonance imaging,* ed 2, St Louis, 1992, Mosby-Year Book.

Giang DW, Kido DK: Transient global amnesia associated with cerebral angiography performed with use of iopamidol, *Radiology* 172:195-196, 1989.

Hans P, Grant AJ, Laitt RD, Ramsden RT, Kassner A, Jackson A, Comparison of three-dimensional visualization techniques for depicting the scala vestibuli and scala tympani of the cochlea by using high-resolution MR imaging. *AJNR* 20: 1197-1206, 1999.

Hara Y, Nakamura M, Tamaki N: A new sonographic technique for assessing carotid artery disease: extended-field-of-view imaging [see comments], *AJNR* 20:267-270, 1999.

Johnson BA, Schellhas KP, Pollei SR, Epidurography and therapeutic epidural injections: technical considerations and experience with 5334 cases [see comments], *AJNR* 20:697-705,1999.

Lantz EJ, Forbes GS, Brown ML, et al: Radiology of cerebrospinal fluid rhinorrhea, *AJNR* 1:391-398, 1980.

Manelfe C, Cellerier P, Sobel D, et al: Cerebrospinal fluid rhinorrhea: evaluation with metrizamide cisternography, *AJNR* 3:25-30, 1982.

Melhem ER, Caruthers SD, Faddoul SG, Tello R, Jara H: Use of three-dimensional MR angiography for tracking a contrast bolus in the carotid artery [see comments], *AJNR* 20:263-266, 1999.

Otto PM, Otto RA, Virapongse C, et al: Screening test for detection of metallic foreign objects in the orbit before magnetic resonance imaging, *Invest Radiol* 27:308-311, 1992.

Pike GB, de Stefano N, Narayanan S, Francis GS, Antel JP, Arnold DL: Combined magnetization transfer and proton spectroscopic imaging in the assessment of pathologic brain lesions in multiple sclerosis, *AJNR* 20:829-837, 1999.

Schaefer PW, Grant PE, Gonzalez RG: Diffusion-weighted MR imaging of the brain, *Radiology* 217:331-345, 2000.

Schmalbrock P, Chakeres DW, Monroe JW, Saraswat A, Miles BA, Welling DB: Assessment of internal auditory canal tumors: a comparison of contrast-enhanced T1-weighted and steady-state T2-weighted gradient-echo MR imaging, *AJNR* 20:1207-1213, 1999.

Shetty PG, Shroff MM, Sahani DV, Kirtane MV: Evaluation of high-resolution CT and MR cisternography in the diagnosis of cerebrospinal fluid fistula, *AJNR* 19:633-639, 1998.

Strother CM: The rapidly expanding role of MR imaging techniques in the endovascular treatment of CNS diseases [editorial; comment], *AJNR* 20:4-5, 1999.

Sunshine JL, Tarr RW, Lanzieri CF, Landis DM, Selman WR, Lewin JS: Hyperacute stroke: ultrafast MR imaging to triage patients prior to therapy, *Radiology* 212:325-332, 1999.

Sutherland GR, Kaibara T, Louw D, Hoult DI, Tomanek B, Saunders J: A mobile high-field magnetic resonance system for neurosurgery, *J Neurosurg* 91:804-813, 1999.

Thompson MR, Venkatesan R, Kuppusamy K, et al: Increased-contrast, high-spatial-resolution, diffusion-weighted, spin-echo, echo-planar imaging, *Radiology* 210:253-259, 1999.

Tonami H, Ogawa Y, Matoba M, et al: MR sialography in patients with Sjögren syndrome [see comments], *AJNR* 19:1199-1203, 1998.

Tsuchiya K, Inaoka S, Mizutani Y, Hachiya J: Echo-planar perfusion MR of moyamoya disease, *AJNR* 19:211-216, 1998.

Tsuchiya K, Yamakami N, Hachiya J, Kassai Y: MR cisternography using a three-dimensional half-fourier single-shot fast spin-echo sequence, *European Radiology* 8:424-426, 1998.

Ulug AM, Moore DF, Bojko AS, Zimmerman RD: Clinical use of diffusion-tensor imaging for diseases causing neuronal and axonal damage, *AJNR* 20:1044-1048, 1999.

Yamada N, Imakita S, Sakuma T: Value of diffusion-weighted imaging and apparent diffusion coefficient in recent cerebral infarctions: a correlative study with contrast-enhanced T1-weighted imaging, *AJNR* 20:193-198, 1999.

Yamamoto Y, Kunishio K, Sunami N, et al: Identification of CSF fistulas by radionuclide counting, *AJNR* 11:823-826, 1990.

Cranial Anatomy

Nothing is more fascinating and has more layers of potential knowledge than the anatomy of the central nervous system (CNS). Like the microcircuits of a computer, each portion of the CNS interconnects to another. Although we will deal with the development of the brain in Chapter 9, we will address only the pertinent aspects of normal anatomy in this chapter. We stress the concept of "pertinent" in part because we are impertinent kind of guys and also because a treatise on human anatomy is about as exciting to the readers (and authors) as half-time entertainment at the curling tournament. Our approach in this chapter is to introduce the basic morphologic building blocks of the CNS in the first section, followed by the functional units in the latter section. (Function follows form.) Functional magnetic resonance (MRI) and the emphasis on radiologic-clinical-pathologic correlation demands that functional anatomy be emphasized.

TOPOGRAPHIC ANATOMY

Cerebral Hemispheres

There are four lobes of the cerebral hemisphere: the frontal, parietal, occipital, and temporal lobes. The frontal lobe is separated from the parietal lobe by the central (Rolandic) sulcus, the parietal lobe is separated from the occipital lobe by the parietooccipital sulcus, and the temporal lobe is separated from the frontal and parietal lobes by the sylvian (lateral) fissure.

The main named areas of the frontal lobe are the precentral gyrus (the primary motor strip of the cerebral

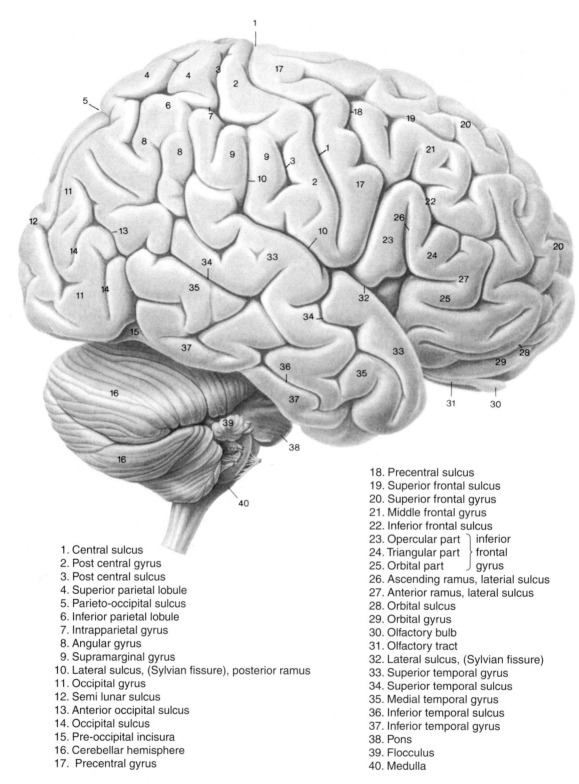

Fig. 2-1   Surface anatomy of the brain from a lateral view. Gyri are labeled in this figure. (From Nieuwenhuys R, Voogd J, van Huijen C: *The human central nervous system: a synopsis and atlas,* rev ed 1, Berlin, Springer-Verlag, 1988.)

1. Central sulcus
2. Post central gyrus
3. Post central sulcus
4. Superior parietal lobule
5. Parieto-occipital sulcus
6. Inferior parietal lobule
7. Intrapparietal gyrus
8. Angular gyrus
9. Supramarginal gyrus
10. Lateral sulcus, (Sylvian fissure), posterior ramus
11. Occipital gyrus
12. Semi lunar sulcus
13. Anterior occipital sulcus
14. Occipital sulcus
15. Pre-occipital incisura
16. Cerebellar hemisphere
17. Precentral gyrus
18. Precentral sulcus
19. Superior frontal sulcus
20. Superior frontal gyrus
21. Middle frontal gyrus
22. Inferior frontal sulcus
23. Opercular part ⎤ inferior
24. Triangular part ⎬ frontal
25. Orbital part ⎦ gyrus
26. Ascending ramus, lateral sulcus
27. Anterior ramus, lateral sulcus
28. Orbital sulcus
29. Orbital gyrus
30. Olfactory bulb
31. Olfactory tract
32. Lateral sulcus, (Sylvian fissure)
33. Superior temporal gyrus
34. Superior temporal sulcus
35. Medial temporal gyrus
36. Inferior temporal sulcus
37. Inferior temporal gyrus
38. Pons
39. Flocculus
40. Medulla

cortex) and the three frontal gyri anterior to the motor strip: the superior, middle, and inferior frontal gyri (Fig. 2-1). On the medial surface one finds the cingulate gyrus just superior to and bounding the corpus callosum, and

the gyrus rectus extending along the medial basal surface of the anterior cranial fossa (Fig. 2-2).

The parietal lobe contains the postcentral gyrus (the center for somatic sensation), the supramarginal gyrus

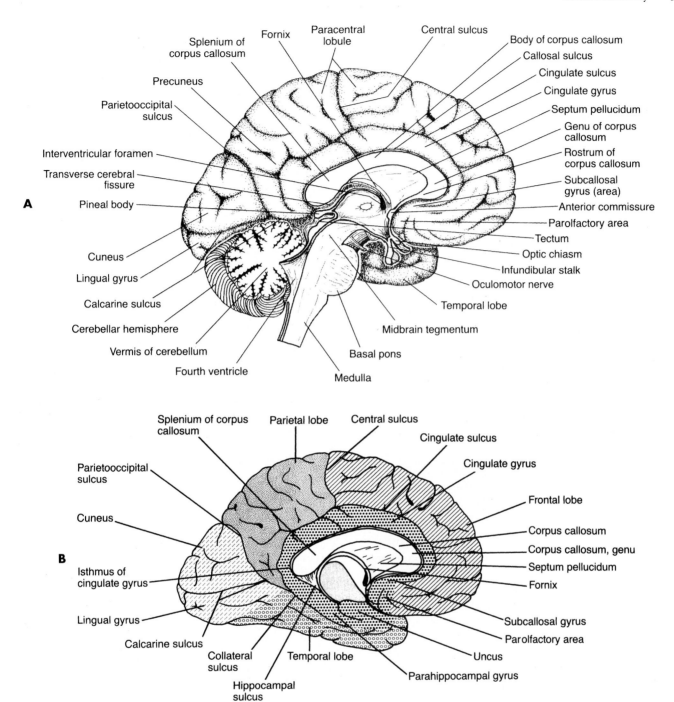

Fig. 2-2   Medial surface of brain. **A,** Midsagittal view of the brain. **B,** Midsagittal view of the left cerebral hemisphere illustrating the major cortical lobes. Frontal lobe, (*diagonal lines*); parietal lobe, (*stippled area*); occipital lobe, (*dashed lines*); temporal lobe, (*open circles*); and limbic lobe, (*filled circles*). (From Burt AM: *Textbook of neuroanatomy.* Philadelphia, WB Saunders, 1993, pp. 159, 160.)

just above the temporal lobe, and the angular gyrus near the apex of the temporal lobe (see Fig. 2-1). Two superficial gyri of note are the superior and inferior parietal lobules, which are separated by an interparietal sulcus. On its medial side the precuneate gyrus is present in front of the parietooccipital fissure, with the cuneate gyrus posteriorly in the occipital lobe (see Fig. 2-2).

The temporal lobe contains the brain-functioning elements of speech, memory, and hearing. Superior (auditory), middle, and inferior temporal gyri are seen on the superficial aspect of the brain (see Fig. 2-1). Deep to the sylvian fissure is the insula, or isle of Reil (southwest of the Isle of Kent and north of the Isle of Wight), which is bounded laterally by the opercular regions. The frontal

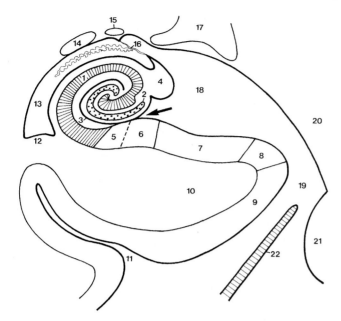

Fig. 2-3 Hippocampal anatomy. *Arrow* indicates the hippocampal sulcus (superficial part). *1,* cornu Ammonis (Ammon's horn); *2,* gyrus dentatus; *3,* hippocampal sulcus (deep or vestigial part); *4,* fimbria; *5,* prosubiculum; *6,* subiculum proper; *7,* presubiculum; *8,* parasubiculum; *9,* entorhinal area; *10,* parahippocampal gyrus; *11,* collateral sulcus; *12,* collateral eminence; *13,* temporal (inferior) horn of the lateral ventricle; *14,* tail of the caudate nucleus; *15,* stria terminalis; *16,* choroid fissure and choroid plexuses; *17,* lateral geniculate body; *18,* lateral part of the transverse fissure (wing of ambient cistern); *19,* ambient cistern; *20,* mesencephalon; *21,* pons; *22,* tentorium cerebelli. (Modified after Williams, 1995. From Duvernoy HM: *The Human Hippocampus.* New York, Springer-Verlag, 1998, p. 18. Used with permission.)

operculum (superior to the sylvian fissure and in the frontal lobe) contains portions of the motor speech area. The inferior part of the insula near the sylvian fissure is called the limen of the insula. The inferior and medial surface of the temporal lobe reveals the parahippocampal gyrus with the hippocampus just superior to it (Fig. 2-3). Anteriorly, the almond–shaped amygdala dominates. If you walked along the cortex of the parahippocampal-hippocampal region of the inferomedial temporal lobe, you would get dizzy because it simulates a spiral staircase. But if you started at the right collateral sulcus (in the coronal plane) just inferior to the parahippocampus and traveled northward, you would first hit the entorhinal cortex, then turn at the parasubiculum, pass along the subiculum proper, and continue laterally to the presubiculum. All of these represent parahippocampal structures. You would then curl in a spiral into the hippocampus' cornu ammonis and dentate gyrus with the fimbria found superomedially and the alveus on top of the cornu ammonis. The cornu itself has four zones of granular cells. CA1 (Sommer sector) is lateral, CA2 (dorsal resistant zone) is superior, CA3 (resistant Spielmeyer sector) is superomedial, and CA4 (end folium).

CA1 is also called the vulnerable sector because it is the most sensitive area of the brain (with the globus pallidus) to anoxia. CA3 is resistant to anoxic damage. Sclerosis of CA1 is the etiology of mesial temporal sclerosis or hippocampal atrophy and has been linked to febrile seizures.

The occipital lobe is the lobe most commonly associated with visual function. At its apex is the calcarine sulcus, with the cuneate gyrus just above it (posteroinferior to the parietooccipital fissure) and the calcarine gyrus just below it (see Figs. 2-1 and 2-2).

The diencephalon contains the thalamus and hypothalamus. The diencephalic syndrome refers to visual changes, euphoria, increased appetite, emaciation, amnesia, with alertness, usually caused by a hypothalamic astrocytoma (or adolescence). The thalamus has many nuclei, the most important of which are the medial and lateral geniculate nuclei associated with auditory and visual functions, respectively (see the following sections). The thalamus is found on either side of the third ventricle and connects across the midline by the massa intermedia. Its other functions include motor relays, limbic outputs, and coordinations of movement. Portions of the thalamus also subserve pain. The hypothalamus is located at the floor of the third ventricle, above the optic chiasm and suprasellar cistern. The hypothalamus is connected to the posterior pituitary via the infundibulum, or stalk, through which hormonal information to the pituitary gland is transmitted. The hypothalamus is critical to the autonomic functions of the body.

Brain Stem

The mesencephalon differentiates into the midbrain. The midbrain is the site of origin of the third and fourth cranial nerves. Additionally, the midbrain contains the red nucleus, substantia nigra, and cerebral aqueduct, or aqueduct of Sylvius (Fig. 2-4). White matter tracts conducting the motor and sensory commands pass through the midbrain. The midbrain is also separated into the tegmentum and tectum, which refer to portions of the midbrain anterior and posterior to the cerebral aqueduct, respectively. The tectum, or roof, consists of the quadrigeminal plate (corpora quadrigemina), which houses the superior and inferior colliculi. The tegmentum contains the fiber tracts, red nuclei, third and fourth cranial nerve nuclei, and periaqueductal gray matter. The substantia nigra is the anterior border of the tegmentum. Anterior to the tegmentum are the cerebral peduncles.

The metencephalon develops into the pons and cerebellum (see following section). The pons contains the nuclei for cranial nerves V, VI, VII, and VIII (Fig. 2-5, Fig. 2-6). Pontine white matter tracts transmit sensory and motor fibers to the face and body (see Fig. 2-5). The pons also houses major connections of the reticular activating system for vital functions (like keeping you awake

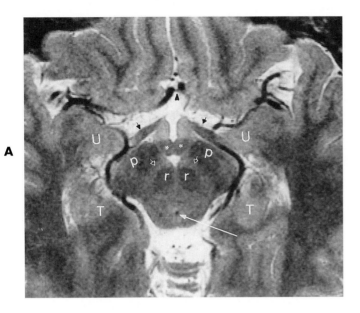

A

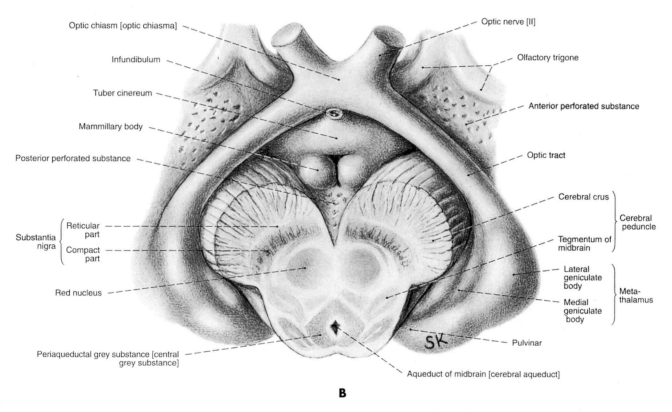

Optic chiasm [optic chiasma]

Infundibulum

Tuber cinereum

Mammillary body

Posterior perforated substance

Substantia nigra { Reticular part / Compact part }

Red nucleus

Periaqueductal grey substance [central grey substance]

Optic nerve [II]

Olfactory trigone

Anterior perforated substance

Optic tract

Cerebral crus } Cerebral peduncle

Tegmentum of midbrain

Lateral geniculate body } Meta-thalamus

Medial geniculate body

Pulvinar

Aqueduct of midbrain [cerebral aqueduct]

B

Fig. 2-4   Midbrain anatomy. **A,** Axial T2WI demonstrates the mamillary bodies *(asterisks)*, the optic tracts *(short arrows)*, the cerebral peduncles *(p)*, the red nuclei *(r)*, and the cerebral aqueduct *(long arrow)*. The posterior cerebral arteries course around the midbrain and show flow voids. Other structures identified include uncus *(U)*, anterior communicating artery *(arrowhead)*, and substantia nigra *(open white arrow)*. One of the authors is having a fantasy thought *(T)*. **B,** Midbrain anatomy diagram. Note the intimate relationship of the optic chiasm and postchiasmal tracts with the midbrain.

Illustration continued on following page

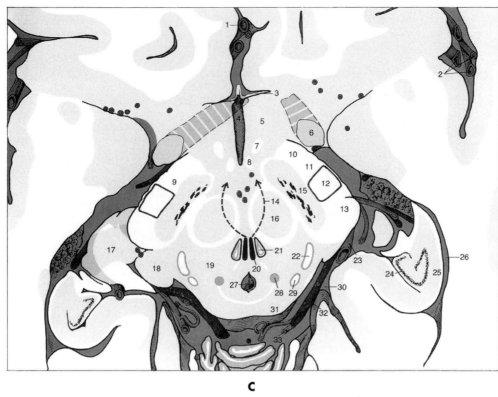

1 Anterior cerebral artery
2 Insular arteries
3 Lamina terminalis
4 Third ventricle
5 Hypothalamus
6 Optic tract
7 Fornix
8 Mamillothalamic tract
9 Base of cerebral peduncle
   (crus cerebri)
10 Frontopontine tract
11 Corticonuclear tract
12 Corticospinal tract
13 Occipitotemporopontine
   tract
14 Oculomotor nerve
   (within the slice)
15 Substantia nigra
16 Red nucleus
17 Lateral geniculate body
18 Medial geniculate body
19 Reticular formation
20 Oculomotor nucleus
21 Medial longitudinal
   fasciculus
22 Medial lemniscus
23 Posterior cerebral artery
24 Dentate gyrus
25 Hippocampus
26 Temporal (inferior) horn
   lateral ventricle
27 Aqueduct
28 Mesencephalic neuleus
   trigeminal nerve
29 Spinothalamic tract
30 Ambient cistern
31 Superior colliculus
32 Basal vein (of Rosenthal)
33 Lateral posterior
   choroidal artery

C

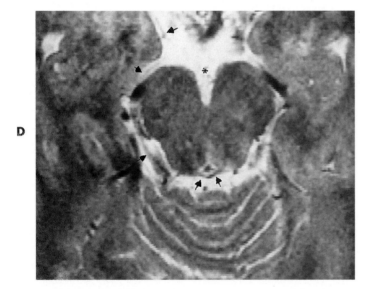

D

Fig. 2-4 *Continued.* **C,** Upper midbrain level showing nuclei and tracts at the superior colliculus. **D,** Axial T2WI demonstrates the course of cranial nerve IV around the cerebral aqueduct *(black arrows).* Cranial nerve III emanates from the interpeduncular cistern *(asterisk).*

Illustration continued on following page

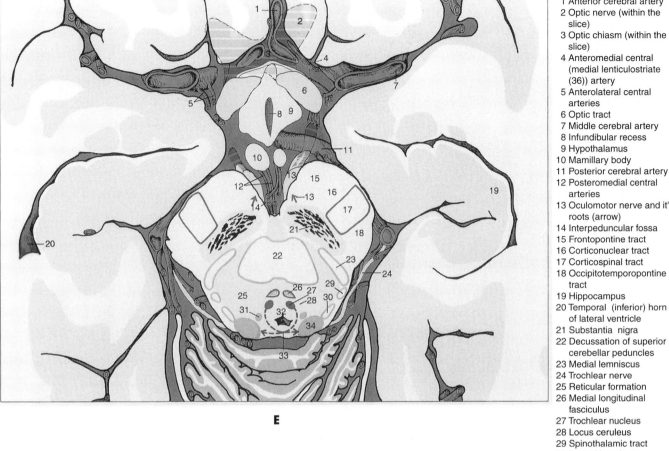

1 Anterior cerebral artery
2 Optic nerve (within the slice)
3 Optic chiasm (within the slice)
4 Anteromedial central (medial lenticulostriate (36)) artery
5 Anterolateral central arteries
6 Optic tract
7 Middle cerebral artery
8 Infundibular recess
9 Hypothalamus
10 Mamillary body
11 Posterior cerebral artery
12 Posteromedial central arteries
13 Oculomotor nerve and it's roots (arrow)
14 Interpeduncular fossa
15 Frontopontine tract
16 Corticonuclear tract
17 Corticospinal tract
18 Occipitotemporopontine tract
19 Hippocampus
20 Temporal (inferior) horn of lateral ventricle
21 Substantia nigra
22 Decussation of superior cerebellar peduncles
23 Medial lemniscus
24 Trochlear nerve
25 Reticular formation
26 Medial longitudinal fasciculus
27 Trochlear nucleus
28 Locus ceruleus
29 Spinothalamic tract
30 Lateral lemniscus
31 Mesencephalic nucleus of trigeminal nerve
32 Aqueduct
33 Decussation of trochlear nerves (within the slice)
34 Inferior colliculus

E

Fig. 2-4 *Continued.* **E,** Inferior midbrain structures are identified in this axial diagram. (B from Putz R, Pabst R [eds]: *Sobotta atlas of human anatomy,* ed 13, Philadelphia, Lippincott Williams & Wilkins, 1996, p. 296; C and E from Kretschmann H-J, Weinrich W: *Cranial neuroimaging and clinical neuroanatomy: magnetic resonance imaging and computed tomography,* rev ed 2, New York, Thieme, 1993, pp. 145, 143, respectively.)

through this chapter). One identifies the pons on the sagittal scan by its "pregnant belly."

The myelencephalon becomes the medulla. The medulla contains the nuclei for cranial nerves IX, X, XI, and XII. Again, the sensory and motor tracts to and from the face and brain are transmitted through the medulla. Other named portions of the medulla include the pyramids, an anterior paramedian collection of fibers transmitting motor function, and the olivary nucleus in the mid-medulla (Fig. 2-7).

Cerebellum

The cerebellum is located in the infratentorial space posterior to the brain stem. The anatomy of the cerebellum is complex, with many named areas. For sim-

plicity's sake, most people separate the cerebellum into the superior and inferior vermis and reserve the term cerebellar hemispheres for the rest of the lateral and central portions of the cerebellum. For those interested in details, the superior vermis has a central lobule and lingula visible anteriorly, and the inferior vermis has a nodulus, uvula, pyramid, and tuber on its inferior surface (Fig. 2-8). The superior surface provides a view of the culmen, declive, and folium of the superior vermis. Superolaterally, there is a bump called the flocculus, which may extend toward the cerebellopontine angle cistern. This is a potential "pseudotumor," often misidentified as an acoustic schwannoma by less erudite, misguided persons. The tonsils are located inferolaterally and are the structures that herniate downward through the foramen magnum in Chiari malformations.

Text continued on page 49

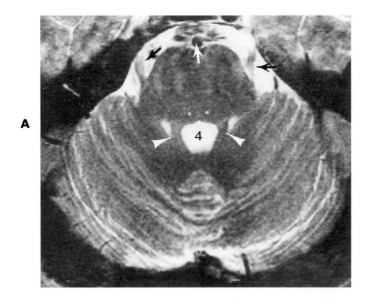

A

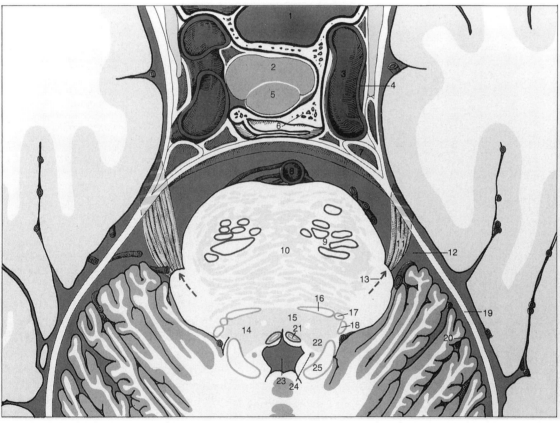

B

1 Sphenoid sinus
2 Adenohypophysis
3 Internal carotid artery
4 Cavernous sinus
5 Neurohypophysis
6 Dorsum sellae
7 Superior petrosal sinus
8 Basilar artery
9 Corticospinal tract
10 Nuclei pontis
11 Trigeminal nerve
12 Cerebellopontine (angle cistern (519)
13 Trigeminal nerve (within the slice)
14 Reticular formation (PPRF)
15 Paramedian pontine reticular formation
16 Medial lemniscus
17 Spinothalamic tract
18 Lateral lemniscus
19 Tentorium cerebelli
20 Primary fissure
21 Medial longitudinal fasciculus
22 Locus ceruleus
23 Fourth ventricle
24 Mesencephalic nucleus trigeminal nerve
25 Superior cerebellar peduncle

Fig. 2-5   Pontine anatomy. **A,** Axial T2WI shows cranial nerve V exiting the pons *(black arrows)*. Note the superior cerebellar peduncles *(arrowheads)*, fourth ventricle *(4)*, medial longitudinal fasciculus (MLF) *(asterisk)*, and basilar artery *(white arrow)*. **B,** Pontine anatomy at the level of the superior cerebellar peduncle (25) shows several descending and ascending tracts.

Illustration continued on following page

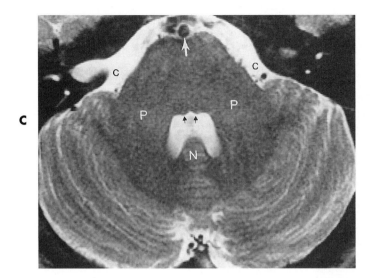

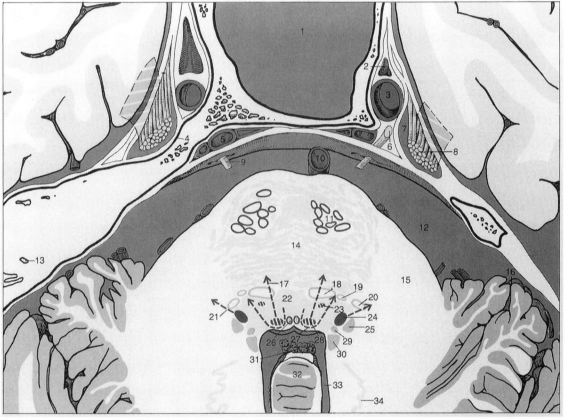

D

1 Sphenoid sinus
2 Cavernous sinus
3 Internal carotid artery
4 Trigeminal impression
5 Inferior petrosal sinus
6 Abducens nerve
7 Opening of trigeminal cistern
8 Triangular part of trigeminal nerve
9 Abducens nerve near opening of dura mater
10 Basilar artery
11 Corticospinal tract
12 Cerebellopontine (angle) cistern (519)
13 Anterior semicircular canal
14 Nuclei pontis
15 Middle cerebellar peduncle
16 Primary fissure
17 Abducens nerve (within the slice)
18 Medial lemniscus
19 Spinothalamic tract
20 Lateral lemniscus
21 Portio minor of trigeminal nerve (within the slice)
22 Reticular formation
23 Facial nucleus (in the caudal part of the slice)
24 Motor nucleus of trigeminal nerve
25 Main sensory (pontine) necleus of trigeminal nerve
26 Medial longitudinal fasciculus
27 Genu of facial nerve
28 Abducens nucleus (within the slice)
29 Mesencephalic nucleus of trigeminal nerve
30 Superior vestibular nucleus
31 Choroid plexus in fourth ventricle
32 Nodule of vermis
33 Posterior recess of fourth ventricle
34 Dentate nucleus

Fig. 2-5 *Continued.* **C,** Facial colliculi *(arrows)* are clearly seen on this axial T2WI. The middle cerebellar peduncle *(P)* is the dominant structure leading to the cerebellum. Also shown are the basilar artery *(white arrow),* cerebellar pontine angle cistern *(C),* and nodulus *(N).* **D,** A₄ the factial colliculus (27) one finds numerous cranial nerve nuclei and traversing lemnisci. (B and D from Kretschmann H-J, Weinrich W: *Cranial neuroimaging and clinical neuroanatomy: magnetic resonance imaging and computed tomography,* rev ed 2, New York, Thieme, 1993, pp. 139, 137, respectively.)

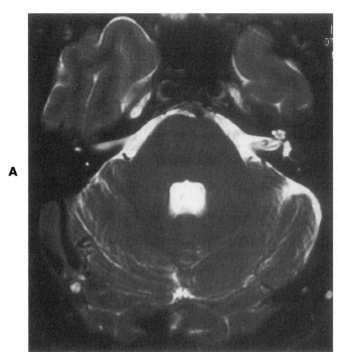

1 Sphenoid sinus
2 Internal carotid artery
3 Trigeminal (semilunar Gasserian) ganglion
4 Trigeminal nerve
5 Cochlea
6 Basilar artery
7 Abducens nerve
8 Greater petriosal nerve
9 Internal acoustic (auditory) meatus
10 Nuclei pontis
11 Corticospinal tract
12 Facial nerve and
13 Abducens nerve (within the slice)
14 Facial nerve (within the slice)
15 Vestibulocochlear nerve
16 Cerebellopontine (angle) cistern (519)
17 Medial lemniscus
18 Spinothalamic tract
19 Dorsal nucleus of corpus trapezoideum
20 Reticular formation
21 Facial nucleus
22 Pars oralis of spinal nucleus of trigeminal nerve
23 Flocculus
24 Middle cerebellar peduncle
25 Medial longitudinal fasciculus
26 Vestibular nuclei
27 Inferior cerebellar peduncle
28 Anterior inferior cerebellar artery (AICA)
29 Fourth ventricle
30 Nodule of vermis
31 Posterior recess of fourth ventricle
32 Dentate nucleus

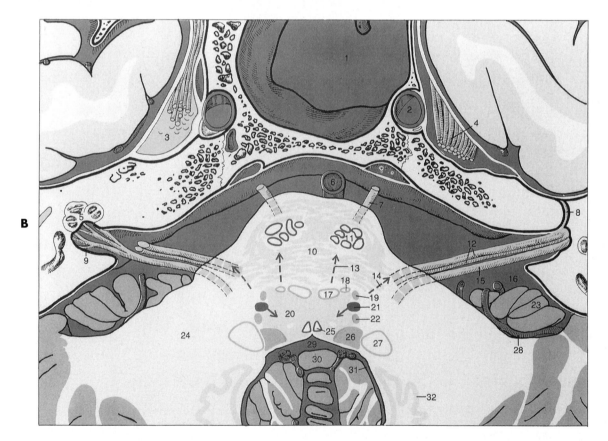

Fig. 2-6   Lower pons. **A,** T2 of IACS showing nerves. **B,** Sphenoid sinus with the adjoining trigeminal ganglion *(left)* and the trigeminal nerve *(right).* The cross section through the caudal pons portion reveals the middle peduncles of the cerebellum. The seventh and eighth cranial nerves enter the internal acoustic meatus. (B from Kretschmann H-J, Weinrich W: *Cranial neuroimaging and clinical neuroanatomy: magnetic resonance imaging and computed tomography,* rev ed 2, New York, Thieme, 1993, p. 135.)

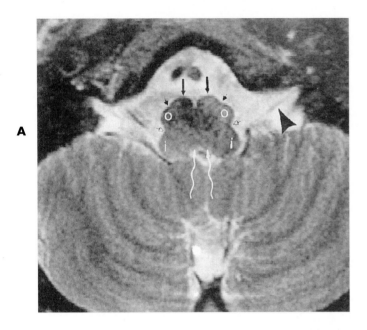

A

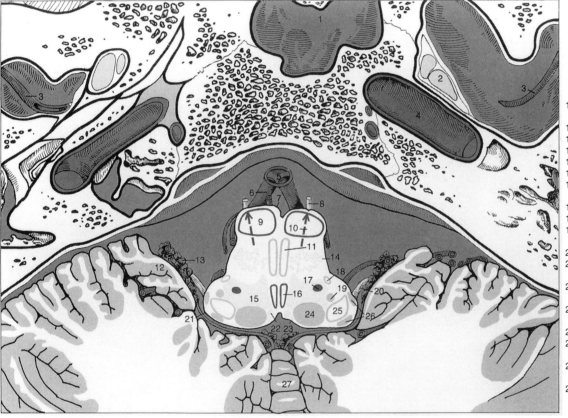

1 Sphenoid sinus
2 Mandibular nerve
3 Middle meningeal artery
4 Internal carotid artery
5 Basilar artery
6 Vertebral artery
7 Pyramid
8 Abducens nerve
9 Corticospinal tract
10 Abducens nerve (within
   the slice)
11 Medial lemniscus
12 Flocculus
13 Choroid plexus
14 Inferior olivary nucleus
15 Reticular formation
16 Medial longitudinal
   fasciculus
17 Nucleus ambiguus
18 Sinothalamic tract
19 Pars oralis of spinal
   nucleus of trigemi nerve
20 Vestibular nuclei
21 Lateral aperture (of
   Luschka)
22 Nucleus preposilus
   hypoglossi
23 Floor of rhomboid fossa
   and fourth ventricl
24 vestibular nuclei
25 Inferior cerebellar
   peduncle
26 Dorsal and ventral
   cochlear nuclei
27 Uvula of vermis

B

Fig. 2-7   Medulla anatomy. **A,** Axial T2WI shows the preolivary sulcus *(short arrows),* the olivary sulcus *(open arrows),* pyramidal tract *(long black arrows)* and the inferior cerebellar peduncle *(i),* hypoglossal nuclei *(squiggly arrows),* and nerve complex (cranial nerves IX and X) *(arrowhead).* The olive *(o),* "which is stirred and not shaken," is well demonstrated. **B,** The segment reveals the junction of the vertebral arteries to the basilar artery. The roots of the abducens nerve arise at the border between the medulla oblongata and pons. The upper part of the inferior olivary nucleus is positioned in the medulla oblongata.

Illustration continued on following page

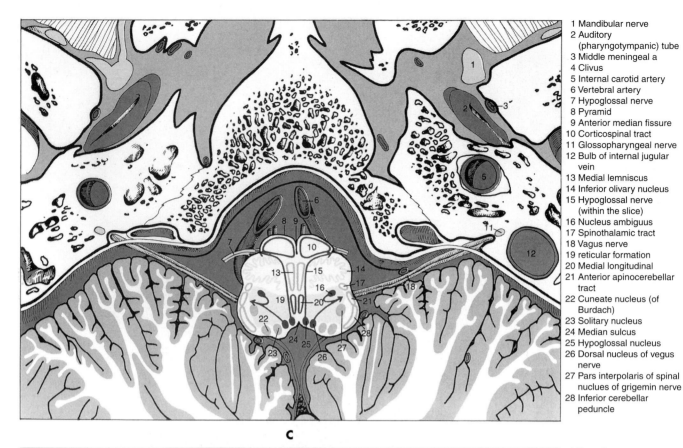

1 Mandibular nerve
2 Auditory (pharyngotympanic) tube
3 Middle meningeal a
4 Clivus
5 Internal carotid artery
6 Vertebral artery
7 Hypoglossal nerve
8 Pyramid
9 Anterior median fissure
10 Corticospinal tract
11 Glossopharyngeal nerve
12 Bulb of internal jugular vein
13 Medial lemniscus
14 Inferior olivary nucleus
15 Hypoglossal nerve (within the slice)
16 Nucleus ambiguus
17 Spinothalamic tract
18 Vagus nerve
19 reticular formation
20 Medial longitudinal
21 Anterior apinocerebellar tract
22 Cuneate nucleus (of Burdach)
23 Solitary nucleus
24 Median sulcus
25 Hypoglossal nucleus
26 Dorsal nucleus of vegus nerve
27 Pars interpolaris of spinal nuclues of grigemin nerve
28 Inferior cerebellar peduncle

C

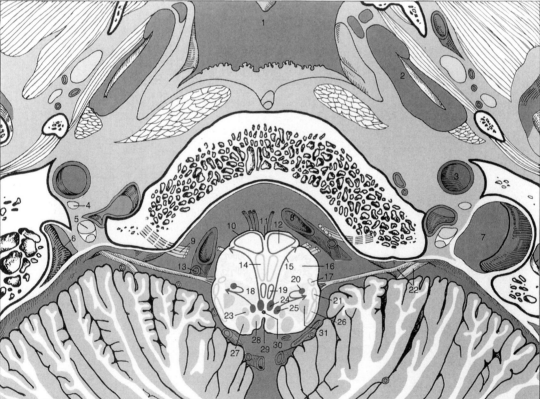

1 Nasopharynx
2 Cartilage of auditory tube
3 Internal carotid artery
4 Glossopharyngeal nerve
5 Vagus nerve
6 Internal jugular vein (var.)
7 Bulb of internal jugular vein
8 Vertebral artery
9 Hypoglossal nerve
10 Pyramid
11 Anterior median fissure
12 Corticospinal tract
13 Posterior inferior cerebellar artery (PICA)
14 Medial lemniscus
15 Hypoglossal nerve (within the slice)
16 Inferior olivary nucleus
17 Spinothalamic tract
18 Reticular formation
19 Medial longitudinal fasciculus
20 Nucleus ambiguus
21 Anterior spinocerebellar tract
22 Cranial and spinal roots of accessor nerve
23 Solitary nucleus
24 Hypoglossal nucleus
25 Dorsal nucleus of vagus nerve
26 Posterior spinocerebellar tract
27 Cuneate nucleus (of Burdach)
28 Gracile nucleus (of Goll)
29 Obex
30 Central canal
31 Pars caudalis of spinal nucleus of trigeminal nerve

D

Fig. 2-7 *Continued.* **C,** The mandibular nerve lies just below the foramen ovale. The roots of the vagus nerves branch off the medulla oblongata. **D,** The sectioning plane cuts through the cartilaginous part of the auditory tube, the caudal part of the inferior olivary nucleus and the origin of the posterior inferior cerebellar artery (PICA) from the vertebral artery. Both internal jugular veins are asymmetrical. The right side shows the jugular foramen to be extended with an enlarged bulb of the internal jugular vein (variability).

Illustration continued on following page

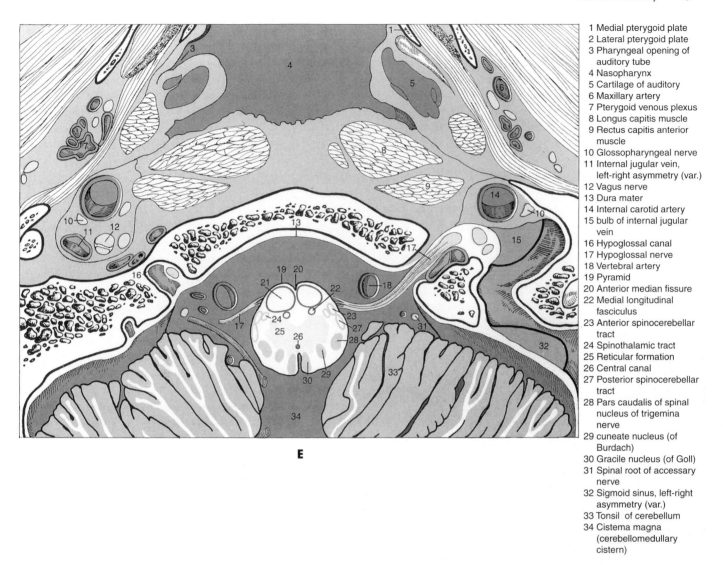

1 Medial pterygoid plate
2 Lateral pterygoid plate
3 Pharyngeal opening of
   auditory tube
4 Nasopharynx
5 Cartilage of auditory
6 Maxillary artery
7 Pterygoid venous plexus
8 Longus capitis muscle
9 Rectus capitis anterior
   muscle
10 Glossopharyngeal nerve
11 Internal jugular vein,
   left-right asymmetry (var.)
12 Vagus nerve
13 Dura mater
14 Internal carotid artery
15 bulb of internal jugular
   vein
16 Hypoglossal canal
17 Hypoglossal nerve
18 Vertebral artery
19 Pyramid
20 Anterior median fissure
22 Medial longitudinal
   fasciculus
23 Anterior spinocerebellar
   tract
24 Spinothalamic tract
25 Reticular formation
26 Central canal
27 Posterior spinocerebellar
   tract
28 Pars caudalis of spinal
   nucleus of trigemina
   nerve
29 cuneate nucleus (of
   Burdach)
30 Gracile nucleus (of Goll)
31 Spinal root of accessary
   nerve
32 Sigmoid sinus, left-right
   asymmetry (var.)
33 Tonsil of cerebellum
34 Cistema magna
   (cerebellomedullary
   cistern)

Fig. 2-7   *Continued.* **E,** The caudal portion of the medulla oblongata, the rootlets of the hypoglossal nerves, and the hypoglossal canal are included. (B–E from Kretschmann H-J, Weinrich W: *Cranial neuroimaging and clinical neuroanatomy: magnetic resonance imaging and computed tomography,* rev ed 2, New York, Thieme, 1993, pp. 133, 131, 129, 127, respectively.)

Gray matter masses in the cerebellum include the fastigial, globose, emboliform, and dentate nuclei; the dentate nuclei are seen well on T1WI whereas the fastigial, globose, and emboliform nuclei cannot be discerned. The dentate nuclei are situated laterally in the white matter of the cerebellum, and can be seen on CT because they may calcify in later life.

Three major white matter tracts connect the cerebellum to the brain stem (Fig. 2-9). The superior cerebellar peduncle (brachium conjunctivum) connects midbrain structures to the cerebellum, the middle cerebellar peduncle connects the pons to the cerebellum, and the inferior cerebellar peduncle (restiform body) connects the medulla to the cerebellum.

The functional divisions of the cerebellum are discussed in the following section. The flocculonodular lobe, fastigial nucleus, and uvula of the inferior vermis receive input from vestibular nerves and are thought to be involved primarily with maintaining equilibrium. Lesions of this part of the cerebellum, the archicerebellum, cause wide-based gait and dysequilibrium.

The superior vermis, most of the inferior vermis, and globose and emboliform nuclei receive spinocerebellar sensory information. Muscle tone information, postural tone, and coordination of locomotion appear to be influenced by these sites and by their effect on brain stem fibers, the red nuclei, and vestibular nuclei. The hemispheric portions of the cerebellum receive information from the pons and help to control coordination of voluntary movements. Abnormalities of the hemisphere (or the neocerebellum) include dysmetria, dysdiadochokinesis, intention tremors, nystagmus, and jⁿeᵣₖy ataxia.

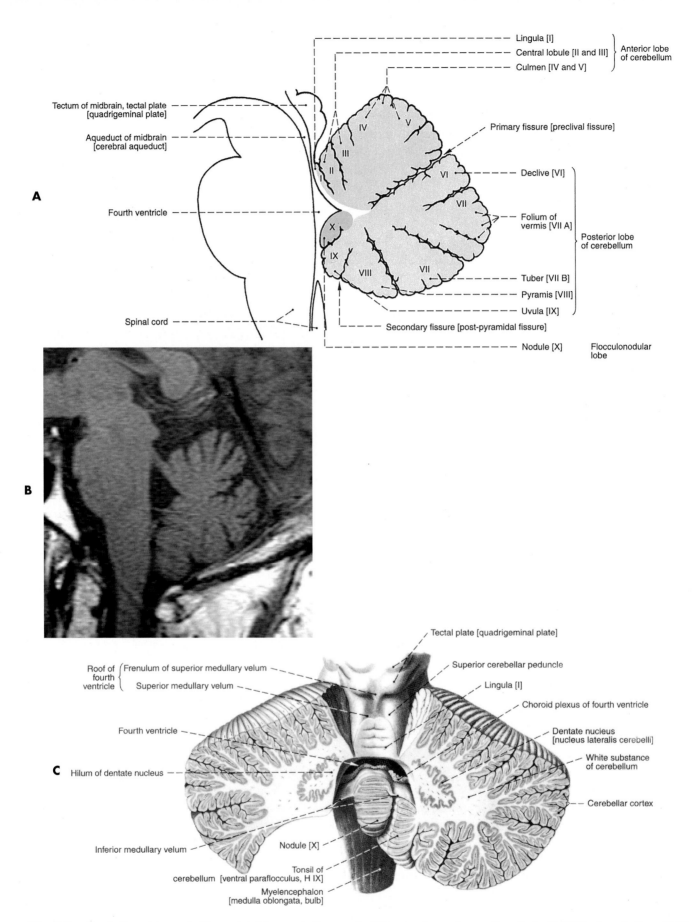

Fig. 2-8   Cerebellar anatomy. **A,** The parts of the cerebellar vermis. Diagram of a median section. **B,** Sagittal MR of cerebellum. **C,** Diagram of the cerebellar lobes and their lobules. (A and C from Putz R, Pabst R [eds]: *Sobotta atlas of human anatomy,* ed 13, Philadelphia, Lippincott Williams & Wilkins, 1996, pp. 292, 293.)

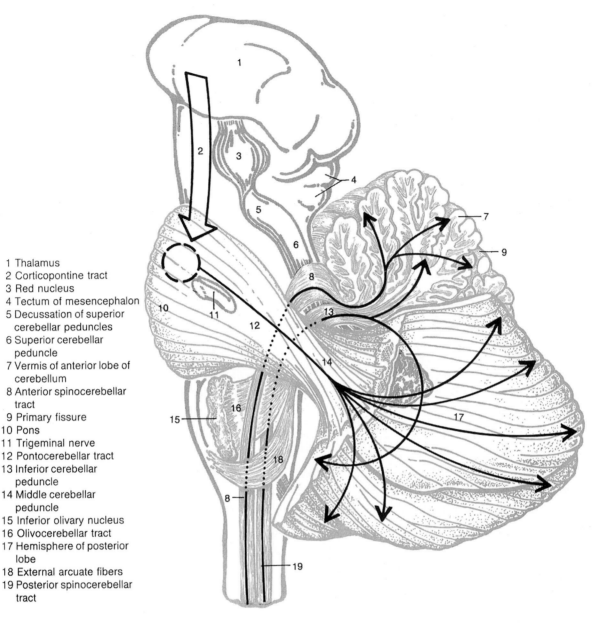

1 Thalamus
2 Corticopontine tract
3 Red nucleus
4 Tectum of mesencephalon
5 Decussation of superior
  cerebellar peduncles
6 Superior cerebellar
  peduncle
7 Vermis of anterior lobe of
  cerebellum
8 Anterior spinocerebellar
  tract
9 Primary fissure
10 Pons
11 Trigeminal nerve
12 Pontocerebellar tract
13 Inferior cerebellar
   peduncle
14 Middle cerebellar
   peduncle
15 Inferior olivary nucleus
16 Olivocerebellar tract
17 Hemisphere of posterior
   lobe
18 External arcuate fibers
19 Posterior spinocerebellar
   tract

Fig. 2-9 Cerebellar pathways. **A,** The afferent systems of the cerebellum (lateral view). The left half of the anterior lobe of the cerebellum was removed. The archeocerebellum was separated and removed caudally from the middle cerebellar peduncle.

Illustration continued on following page

Corpus Callosum

The medial surface of the brain in the midline is dominated by the corpus callosum. This is the large white matter tract that spans the two hemispheres. Its named parts include the rostrum (its tapered anteroinferior portion just above the anterior commissure), the genu (the anterior wide sweep over the third ventricle), the body or trunk (the superiormost aspect), and the splenium (the posteriormost aspect) (see Fig. 2-2). Embryologically, the genu and body form first, then comes the splenium, and finally the rostrum. This is useful in understanding partial agenesis of the corpus callosum.

Other white matter tracts that cross the midline include the anterior commissure, located at the inferior aspect of the corpus callosum just above the lamina terminalis, and the posterior commissure, just anterior to the pineal gland near the habenula. The anterior commissure transmits tracts from the amygdala and temporal lobe to the contralateral side. The habenula and hippocampal commissures cross-connect the two hemispheres and thalami.

"If you are not a good kisser"
Said a madame to her monsieur,
"The info from my amygdala
Will not pass thru my habenula
And you can never cross my commissure"

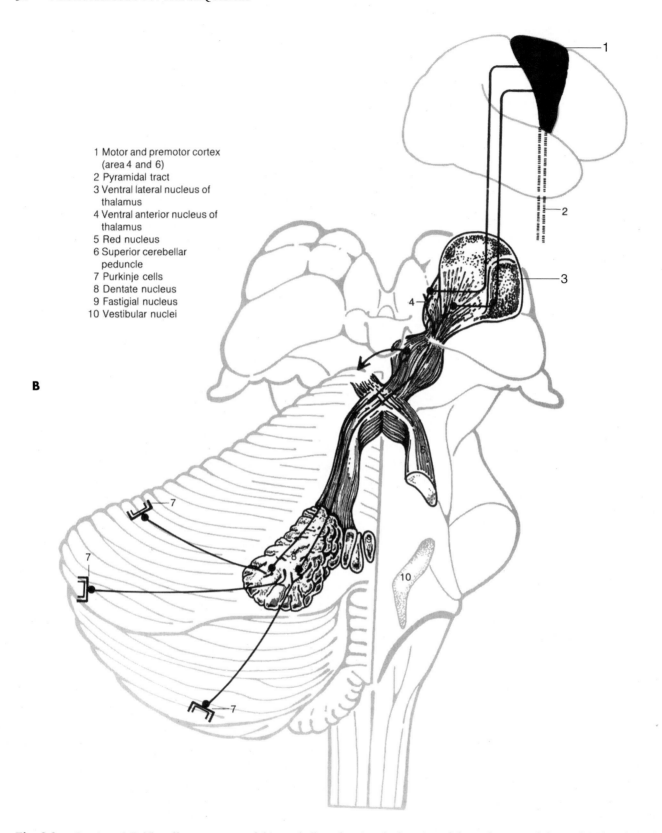

1 Motor and premotor cortex
  (area 4 and 6)
2 Pyramidal tract
3 Ventral lateral nucleus of
  thalamus
4 Ventral anterior nucleus of
  thalamus
5 Red nucleus
6 Superior cerebellar
  peduncle
7 Purkinje cells
8 Dentate nucleus
9 Fastigial nucleus
10 Vestibular nuclei

B

Fig. 2-9 *Continued.* **B,** The efferent systems of the cerebellum showing the location of the pathways and the nuclei (dorsal view). The cerebellum was dissected in the median plane and the right half was removed with the exception of the superior cerebellar peduncle. (From Kretschmann H-J, Weinrich W: *Cranial neuroimaging and clinical neuroanatomy: magnetic resonance imaging and computed tomography,* rev ed 2, Thieme, 1993, pp. 326, 327, respectively.)

There once was a sad man from Tojo
Who noted his function was no go
His hippocampi were small
The pineal gland tall
But Viagra restored his Mojo

Deep Gray Nuclei

The basal ganglia are known by a number of names in the neuroanatomic literature. These gray matter structures lie between the insula and midline. The globus pallidus is the medial gray matter structure identified just lateral to the genu of the internal capsule (Fig. 2-10). Superficial to it lies the putamen. The caudate nucleus head indents the frontal horns of the lateral ventricle and is anterior to the globus pallidus; however, the body of the caudate courses over the globus pallidus, paralleling the lateral ventricle and ending in a tail of tissue near the amygdala.

Additional terms used referring to the various portions of the basal ganglia include the corpus striatum (all three structures and the amygdala) and the lentiform or lenticular nuclei (the globus pallidus and putamen).

The basal ganglia receive fibers from the sensorimotor cortex, thalamus, and substantia nigra, as well as from each other. Efferents go to the same locations and to the hypothalamus. The main function of the basal ganglia appears to be coordination of smooth movement. Who is smoother Michael Jordan or Bill Clinton? In this case, we are referring to motor rather than Mojo regions so we will pick Michael's deep gray nuclei from the base line and basal ganglia.

The other deep gray matter structures of interest in the supratentorial space are the thalami, which sit on either side of the third ventricle. The thalamus is subdivided into many different nuclei by white matter striae. As will be discussed, the medial and lateral geniculate nuclei, located along the posterior aspect of the thalamus, are the most significant nuclei within the thalamic deep gray structures, because they serve as relay stations for visual and auditory function. The pulvinar is the posterior expansion of the thalamus. Behind the pulvinar are the wings of the ambient cistern. The massa intermedia connects the thalami across the third ventricle.

In the infratentorial space, the dentate nucleus, the largest deep gray matter structure, has connections to the red nuclei and to the thalami. The deep gray matter structures are most important in coordinative movements of the limbs and the trunk. Other central nuclei within the cerebellum include the emboliform nucleus, globose nucleus, and the fastigial nucleus. As we frequently say, repetition is the mother of all learning techniques.

Ventricular System

The normal volume of cerebrospinal fluid (CSF) in the entire CNS is approximately 150 mL, with 75 mL distributed around the spinal cord, 25 mL within the ventricular system, and 50 mL surrounding the cortical sulci and in the cisterns at the base of the brain. In elderly persons, the intracranial CSF volume increases from 75 mL to a mean of approximately 150 mL in women and 190 mL in men (a statistically significant difference), a further indication of women's phylogenetic superiority over men—less water, more brains. The normal production of CSF has been estimated to be approximately 450 mL/day, thereby replenishing the amount of CSF two to three times a day. As one might expect, the reabsorption of CSF is critical in this instance, and the arachnoid villi are the major sites where CSF is resorbed into the intravascular system from the extracellular fluid.

The flow of CSF runs from the choroid plexi in the floor of the lateral ventricles via the foramina of Monro, to the third ventricle, out the cerebral aqueduct of Sylvius, and into the fourth ventricle (Fig. 2-11). Each ventricle's choroid plexus contributes to CSF production. After leaving the foramina of Magendie (medially) and Luschka (laterally) of the fourth ventricle, CSF flows into the cisterns of the brain and the cervical subarachnoid space and then down the intrathecal spinal compartment. The CSF ultimately percolates back up over the convexities of the hemispheres, where it is resorbed by the arachnoid villi into the intravascular space.

There are several named cisterns around the brain. The names, locations, and the structures traversing these cisterns are summarized in Table 2-1.

Physiologic Calcifications

The pineal gland calcifies with age. A small percentage (2% of children less than 8 years old and 10% of adolescents) of children show calcification of the pineal gland. By 30 years of age, most people have calcified pineal glands. Anterior to the pineal gland, one often sees the habenular commissure as a calcified curvilinear structure.

The choroid plexus is calcified in about 5% of children by age 15, and most adults by age 40.

The dura of the falx and/or tentorium is virtually never calcified in children and should be viewed as suspicious for basal cell nevus syndrome in that setting. The dura shows higher rates of calcification in patients who have had shunts placed or have been irradiated.

Basal ganglia calcification is also rarely observed in individuals less than 30 years of age and should provoke

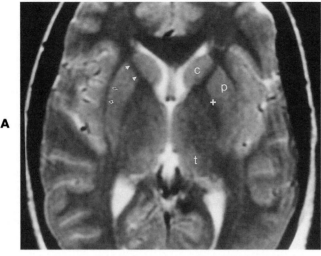

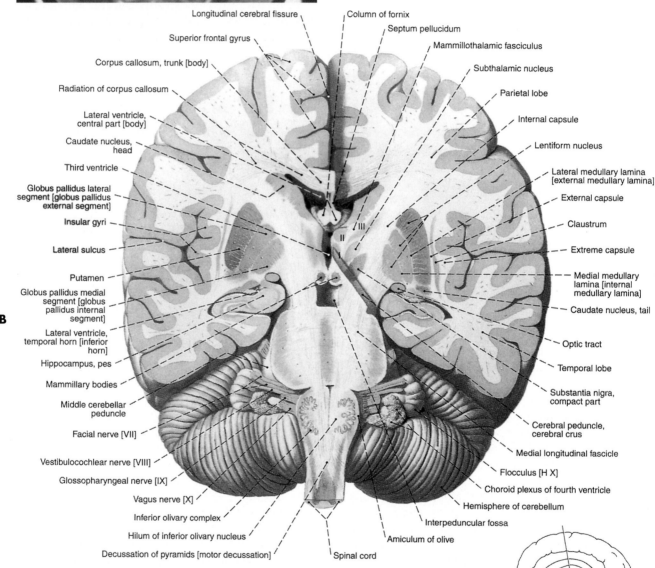

Longitudinal cerebral fissure
Column of fornix
Septum pellucidum
Superior frontal gyrus
Mammillothalamic fasciculus
Corpus callosum, trunk [body]
Subthalamic nucleus
Radiation of corpus callosum
Parietal lobe
Lateral ventricle, central part [body]
Internal capsule
Caudate nucleus, head
Lentiform nucleus
Third ventricle
Lateral medullary lamina [external medullary lamina]
Globus pallidus lateral segment [globus pallidus external segment]
External capsule
Insular gyri
Claustrum
Lateral sulcus
Extreme capsule
Putamen
Medial medullary lamina [internal medullary lamina]
Globus pallidus medial segment [globus pallidus internal segment]
Caudate nucleus, tail
Lateral ventricle, temporal horn [inferior horn]
Optic tract
Hippocampus, pes
Temporal lobe
Mammillary bodies
Substantia nigra, compact part
Middle cerebellar peduncle
Cerebral peduncle, cerebral crus
Facial nerve [VII]
Medial longitudinal fascicle
Vestibulocochlear nerve [VIII]
Flocculus [H X]
Glossopharyngeal nerve [IX]
Choroid plexus of fourth ventricle
Vagus nerve [X]
Hemisphere of cerebellum
Inferior olivary complex
Interpeduncular fossa
Hilum of inferior olivary nucleus
Amiculum of olive
Decussation of pyramids [motor decussation]
Spinal cord

Fig. 2-10 Basal ganglionic anatomy. **A,** This T2WI nicely distinguishes the head of the caudate *(c)*, the dark iron-containing globus pallidus *(1)*, the more lateral putamen *(p)*, and portions of the thalamus *(t)*. The low intensity of the internal capsule *(small arrows)* and the external capsule *(small open arrows)* is shown on the right side. **B,** Coronal section through basal ganglia shows relationship to ventricular system, internal capsule, and brain stem. (citation to come)

Illustration continued on following page

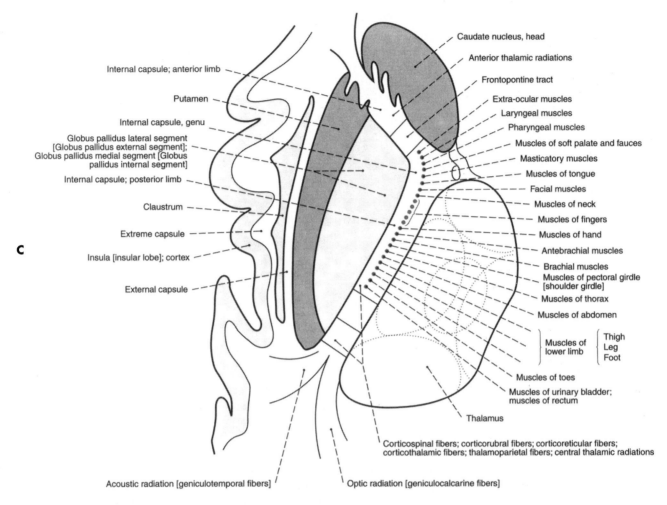

Fig. 2-10 *Continued.* **C,** Functional organization of the internal capsule. (From Putz R, Pabst R [eds]: *Sobotta atlas of human anatomy,* ed 13, Philadelphia, Lippincott Williams & Wilkins, 1996, p. 323.)

a search for metabolic disorders or a past history of perinatal infections if seen in youngsters (See the Appendix for causes of basal ganglia calcification).

FUNCTIONAL ANATOMY

Understanding the functional anatomy requires a little bit of the cartographer in each of us. After having assimilated the destinations and points of departure, one should talk about the entire routes of neuronal travel. For functional anatomy, we can now use functional magnetic resonance imaging (fMRI) to identify the sites of cortical activation (the points of departure and destinations). We have just started using diffusion tensor imaging to perform white matter tracking. This allows us to see the white matter highways between the two gray matter sites and the various routes to getting there. Directionality of these white matter tracts can also be inferred now. In some cases the maze may seem a bit like

New York's thruway system, with exit and entrance ramps coming at you from all directions and no clue as to why the designers planned it that way. We will leave the "whys" to the Great Architect in the sky . . . or to Hillary Rodham Clinton the New York State's senator who is now responsible for funding that highway system . . . and its path back to the White House.

Brodmann Areas

The functional units of the cerebral hemispheres have been separated into what are called Brodmann areas. These numbered areas correspond to different gyri that subserve various functions. The Brodmann areas are the currency with which functional MRI scientists transact business and are therefore important to learn. In addition, knowing which gyri are responsible for which properties can be critical to predicting deficits in patients with strokes. This knowledge will also direct YOUR attention as the reader of images with a given clinical his-

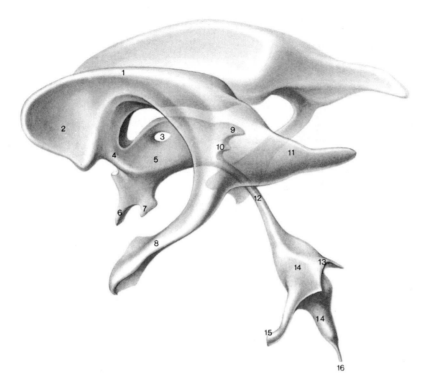

1 Lateral ventricle, body
2 Lateral ventricle, frontal horn
3 Massa Intermedia
4 Foramen of Monro
5 Third ventricle
6 Optic recess, third ventricle
7 Infundibular recess, third ventricle
8 Temporal horn, lateral ventricle
9 Suprapineal recess, third ventricle
10 Pineal recess, third ventricle
12 Aqueduct of sylvius
13 Fastigium
14 Fourth ventricle
15 Lateral recess, Foramen
    Luschka, fourth ventricle
16 Central canal

Fig. 2-11 Ventricular system of the brain. Three-dimensional diagram of the ventricular system of the brain is labeled. (From Nieuwen-huys R, Voogd J, van Huijen C: *The human central nervous system: a synopsis and atlas,* rev ed 3, Berlin, Springer-Verlag, 1988.)

tory to a specific site where subtle pathology may reside. Neuroradiologists often receive requisitions for studies in which only the patient's symptoms or neurologic signs are given (if they are lucky!!!). Thus, you may need to trace the pathway for that particular symptom or sign and localize the lesion better. It is only by knowing the pathway that might account for the patient's symptom that you develop a well-trained eye for detecting disease. You see what you know.

Although this is by no means an exhaustive review, Table 2-2 will help you define structure and function in Brodmann's terms.

Table 2-1 Cisterns of the brain

Name	Location	Structures traversing cistern
Cisterna magna	Posteroinferior to 4th ventricle	None important
Circummedullary cistern	Around medulla	Posterior inferior cerebellar artery
Superior cerebellar cistern	Above cerebellum	Basal vein of Rosenthal, vein of Galen
Prepontine cistern	Anterior to pons	Basilar artery, cranial nerves V and VI
Cerebellopontine angle cistern	Between pons and porus acousticus	Anterior inferior cerebellar artery, cranial nerves VII and VIII
Interpeduncular cistern	Between cerebral peduncles anterior to midbrain	Cranial nerve III
Ambient (crural) cistern	Around midbrain	Cranial nerve IV
Quadrigeminal plate cistern	Behind midbrain	None important
Suprasellar cistern	Above pituitary	Optic chiasm, cranial nerves III, IV, carotid arteries, pituitary stalk
Retropulvinar cistern (wings of ambient cistern)	Behind thalamus	Posterolateral choroidal artery
Cistern of lamina terminalis	Anterior to lamina terminalis, anterior commissure	ACA
Cistern of velum interpositum	Above 3rd ventricle	Internal cerebral vein, vein of Galen
Cistern of the ACA	Above corpus callosum	ACA

ACA, Anterior cerebral artery.

Table 2-2 Functional Anatomy by Brodmann Areas

Brodmann area # (alias)	Location	Function
1 (S1)	Post-central gyrus, paracentral lobule, parietal lobe	Primary somatosensory, rapidly adapting skin sensors, position sense
2	As above, posterior to 1	As above, proprioception from joints
3 (a = motor, b = sensory)	As above, anterior to 1	As above, fine tactile receptors in b, stretch receptors in a
4 (M1)	Precentral gyrus, frontal lobe	Primary motor
5 (S2)	Superior parietal lobule, posterior to 2	Somatosensory association area, gross sensory areas
6 (SMA, premotor)	Superior and middle frontal gyrus, anterior to 4, has lateral and medial surface parts	Premotor area, supplemental motor area, word retrieval, hand movement, stuttering, programming movements
7	Superior parietal lobule, posterior to 5, some of pre-runers	Counting, mathematics, somatosensory association, mental rotation
8 (premotor)	Anterior superomedial frontal gyrus, superior frontal gyrus	Frontal eye fields, mental state assessment, spatial attention and orientation
9	Orbitofrontal, prefrontal, frontal gyri	Emotions, pain, motor association, intelligence
10	As above, anterior and inferior to 9 Frontopolar region	Emotions, pain, higher intelligence, motor association
11	Gyrus rectus, inferior pole frontal lobe, orbital gyri	Emotions, pain, olfaction, intelligence
12	Superior to 11, below 10 inferior frontal lobe, prefrontal	As above
13	Lost in adolescence	
14	Lost in adolescence	
15	Lost in adolescence	
16	Lost in adolescence	
17 (V1—striate cortex)	Calcarine fissure region, posterior pole, medially	Primary viscal cortex, chromatic, luminence
18 (V2—extra-circumstriate, parastriate)	Anterolateral to 17, both superior and inferior, lingual gyrus regions, lateral occipital gyrus	Visual association area, faces
19 (V3, V4, V5, VP peristriate)	Anterolateral to 18, both superior and inferior, cuneus, lingual, superior occipital gyrus	Visual fields, color, motion
20	Inferior temporal gyrus	Visual association
21 (Wernicke)	Middle temporal gyrus, lateral surface only	Higher order audition, visual association
22 (Wernicke)	Posterior-superior temporal gyrus, lateral aspect	Speech reception, auditory association
23	Posterior cingulate, medial surface	Emotions, facial familiarity
24	Anterior cingulate	Emotions, pain, itch, bimanual coordination
25	Lamina terminalis region, medial perforating substance	? Olfaction
26	Posterior commisure region	
27	Superomedial temporal lobe	
28 (entorhinal)	Medial surface anterior-inferior temporal lobe, hippocampus, entorhinal cortex	Gender classification, memories, emotions, olfaction, limbic
29	Posterior cingulate, region, posterior induseum griseum	
30	As above	Visual attention
31	Pre-cuneus, posterior cingulate	Emotions, pitch of music, familiar faces
32	Anterior to cingulate, callosomarginal region, anterior internal frontal	Pain
33	Induseum griseum, anterior cingulate	Emotions
34	Medial temporal lobe, amygdala, entorhinal	Olfaction, limbic, sadness on left, happiness on right
35	Inferior temporal lobe, medial aspect, parahippocampus, perihinal	Limbic, olfaction
36	Posteroinferior temporal lobe, medial aspect, parahippocampus, fusiform gyrus	Gender classification, memories, emotions, face, information for memories
37, middle temporal visual (area = MT/V5 with 19)	Posterior to 36, extends from medial to lateral inferior temporal lobe, fusiform gyrus	Visual motion, speech, visual association, spatial recognition, naming objects
38	Anteromedial tip of temporal lobe, temporopolar	Emotions, pain

Table continued on following page

Table 2-2   Functional Anatomy by Broadmann Areas *(continued)*

Brodmann area # (alias)	Location	Function
39 (extrastriate cortex)	Angular gyrus of inferior parietal lobe	Face recognition, spatial attention, visual association, making analogies
40	Supramarginal gyrus in inferior parietal lobule	Sensory analysis, pain
41 (A1-Wernicke) (STG-Heschl's gyrus = transverse temporal gyrus)	Superior-most temporal gyrus, lateral aspect, anterior transverse gyrus	Primary auditory
42 (A2-Wernicke)	Just inferior to 41, superior temporal gyrus	Auditory association, speech recognition
43	Frontal opercular region, postcentral gyrus	Language perception
44 (Broca's)	Inferior frontal gyrus, opercular region lateral aspect	Broca's speech expression, motor toe and finger
45 (Broca's)	Anterior to 44, inferior frontal, lateral aspect, "triangular" gyrus	Broca's motor speech (posteriorly), tongue movement, upper extremity motor, some perception of speech seen anteriorly
46	Anterior to 45, inferior frontal–dorsolateral prefrontal cortex, middle frontal gyrus	Emotions, memory, visual cues
47	Lateral orbitofrontal	Emotions, familiarity, memory, olfaction, verb generation

Legend:
- Frontal eye fields
- Somatosensory
- Motor
- ??
- Broca's
- Audition
- Wernicke's
- Cognition
- Emotion
- Vision
- Visual-parietal
- Visual-temporal
- Olfaction

(With permission from Mark Dubin, Boulder, Colorado)

Talairach and Tourneaux Space

The output of fMRI images is often transposed onto a standard space that every neuroscientist can use to determine the location of gyri. This means that people's brains become warped—to a standard space defined by Madame Talairach, the wife of a 20th century neuroanatomist. Hers has become the standard by which all brains are judged. If we knew the volume of cheap French wines that she imbibed over her lifetime, we might not rush to use her brain as our standard in neurophysiology. The use of Talairach space also allows "summing of data" of many brains to one agreed upon standard.

The anterior commissure to posterior commissure (AC-PC) line is frequently used to select axial sections in a reproducible fashion and is also the basis for "Talairach space." The Talairach coordinates in X (right to left), Y (anterior to posterior), and Z (superior to inferior) axes are used in functional MRI to identify the location of gyri. A spot that has a negative X location is to the right, positive X is to the left, positive Y is anterior to the midpoint of the AC-PC line, negative Y is posterior to the midpoint of the AC-PC line, negative Z is below the plane of the AC-PC line and positive Z is above the AC-PC line.

Motor System

"If I could only lay my hands on him!" What brain connections will this simple task require?

The primary origin of the stimulus for motor function is the precentral gyrus of the frontal lobe, which receives input from many sensory areas (Fig. 2-12) (Table 2-3). Stimulation of the motor area of one precentral gyrus

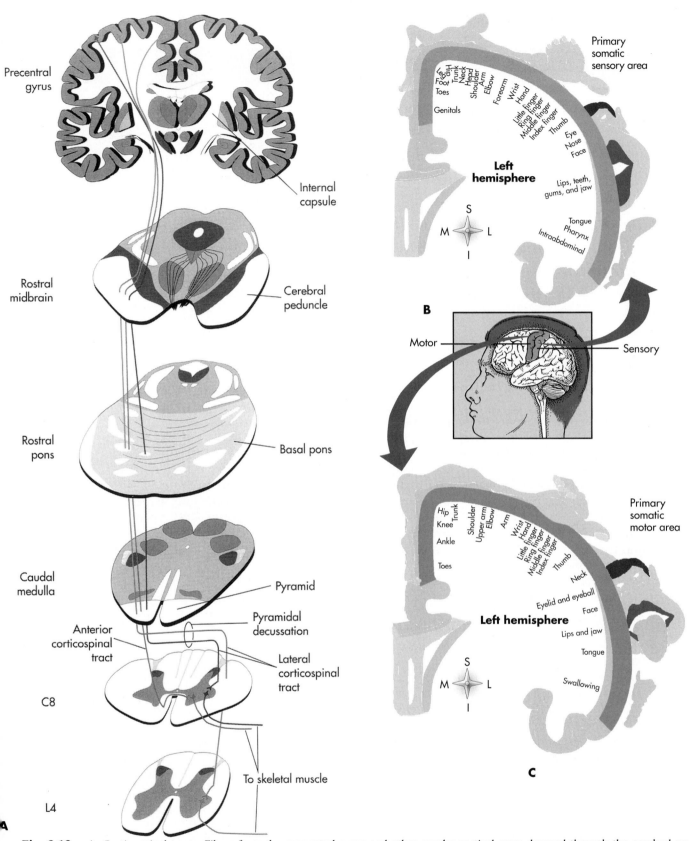

Fig. 2-12   **A,** Corticospinal tracts. Fibers from the precentral gyrus and other nearby cortical areas descend through the cerebral peduncles, pons, and medullary pyramids; most cross in the pyramidal decussation to form the lateral corticospinal tract. Those that do not cross in the pyramidal decussation form the anterior corticospinal tract; most of these fibers cross in the anterior white commissure before ending in the spinal gray matter. Most corticospinal fibers do not synapse directly on the motor neurons. They are drawn that way here for simplicity. Primary somatic sensory **(B)** and motor **(C)** areas of the cortex. The body parts illustrated here show which parts of the body are "mapped" to correlates in each cortical area. The exaggerated face indicates that more cortical area is devoted to processing information to/from the many receptors and motor units than for the leg or arm, for example. (A from Nolte J: *The human brain: an introduction to its functional anatomy,* ed 4, St. Louis, Mosby, 1999, p. 249. B and C from Thibodeau GA, Patton KT: *Anatomy and physiology,* ed 4, St. Louis, Mosby, 1999, p. 394.)

Table 2-3   Motor pathways

Pathway	Course	Function
Lateral corticospinal tract	Primary motor cortex to corona radiata to posterior limb of internal capsule to cerebral peduncle to central pontine region to medulla through pyramidal decussation to posterolateral white matter of cord	Motor to contralateral extremities
Anterior corticospinal tract	Primary motor cortex to corona radiata to posterior limb of internal capsule to cerebral peduncle to central pontine region to medulla to anterior funiculus and anterior column of spinal cord	Motor to ipsilateral muscles
Rubrospinal tract	Red nucleus to decussation in ventral tegmentum of the midbrain through the lateral funiculus of the spinal cord to the posterolateral white matter of cord (with lateral corticospinal tract)	Motor control of contralateral limbs
Reticulospinal tract	Pons and medulla to ipsilateral anterior column of cord	Automatic movement of axial and limb muscles (walking, stretching, orienting behaviors)
Vestibulospinal tract	Vestibular nuclei to ipsilateral anterior columns in cord	Balance, postural adjustments, and head and neck coordination

causes contraction of muscles on the opposite side of the body. The motor cortex, like the sensory area, is arranged such that the lower extremity is located superomedially along the paracentral lobule in the midline, whereas the upper extremity is located inferolaterally. The cells innervating the hip are at the top of the precentral sulcus; the leg is draped over medially along the interhemispheric fissure. The face (especially the tongue and mouth) has an inordinately large area of motor and sensory representation along the inferiormost aspect of the precentral motor strip on the surface of the brain, just above the sylvian fissure. This picture of the homunculus, with leg hanging over the vertex and with an enormous mouth and tongue, reminds a baby boomer of Mick Jagger (Chris Rock for the X generation, Maria Bartiromo for the $$$ generation), with mouth open, jabbering away. The motor contribution to speech is located at the inferior frontal gyrus (frontal operculum regions). In politicians, one often finds this gyrus to be hypertrophied despite severe generalized cerebral atrophy elsewhere.

Sometimes finding the central sulcus can be a bear (Fig. 2-13). This is necessary for discriminating motor from sensory areas particularly when surgery to resect a peri-Rolandic tumor is contemplated. Retaining motor function is desired. Consult Box 2-1 for some clues on how to identify the central sulcus.

From the motor cortex of the frontal lobe, the white matter fibers pass into the corticospinal tract, which extends through the white matter of the centrum semiovale to the posterior limb of the internal capsule. From the posterior portion of the posterior limb of the inter-

nal capsule, the corticospinal tract continues through the central portion of the cerebral peduncle in the anterior portion of the midbrain. These fibers continue in the anterior portion of the pons to the pyramids of the medulla, where most of them decussate (in the pyramidal decussation) and proceed inferiorly in the lateral corticospinal tract of the spinal cord. Fifteen percent of fibers do not decussate in the medulla. (Does not decussate sound like something you would like to do to your foul-mouthed teenager?). These fibers pass into the anterior funiculus along the anterior median fissure of the spinal cord as the anterior corticospinal tract. The fibers of the pyramidal tract, which include both the lateral and anterior corticospinal tract, synapse with the anterior horn cell spinal cord nuclei.

Motor supply to the face travels from the cortex, through the corona radiata, into the genu of the internal capsule, via the corticobulbar tract. The corticobulbar fibers are located more anteromedially in the cerebral peduncles and have connections to the brain stem nuclei as they descend. Most of the connections to the various cranial nerve nuclei are contralateral to the cortical bulbar tract; however, some ipsilateral fibers are present as well.

The pyramidal tract is responsible for voluntary movement and contains the corticospinal and corticobulbar fibers. The extrapyramidal system includes the corpus striatum, which receives fibers from the cerebral cortex, the thalamus, and the substantia nigra, with connections to the caudate nucleus and putamen. These fibers originate from the cerebral cortex but pass through the internal and external capsule to reach the basal ganglia.

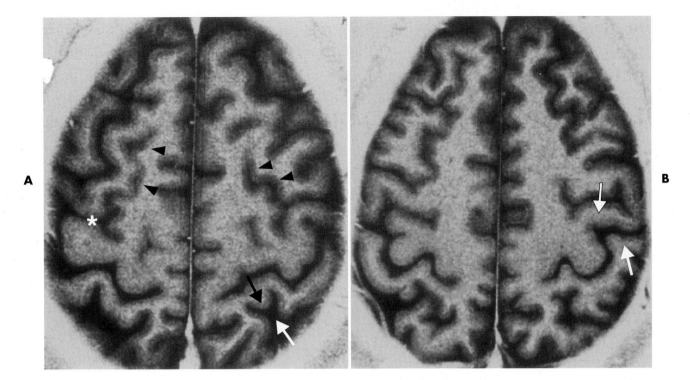

Fig. 2-13   Central sulcus. **A,** Note the shape of the medial end of the postcentral sulcus, the bifid y *(black arrows)* and how the superior frontal sulcus *(arrowheads)* terminates in the precentral sulcus *(asterisk)*. **B,** The central sulcus is the next sulcus posterior to the precentral sulcus. Note that precentral gyrus' cortical gray matter *(open arrow)* thickness is greater than that of the postcentral gyrus *(white arrow)* cortical thickness. Usually PRE/POST thickness ≥1.5.

The dentate nuclei, found in the cerebellar hemispheres, also send tracts to the thalamus and motor areas of the frontal cortex. The red nucleus of the midbrain receives fibers from the cortical motor area and transmits fibers via the rubrospinal tract to the spinal cord, which also regulates motion.

Abnormalities of the pyramidal system mainly produce weakness, paralysis, or spasticity of voluntary motor function. Extrapyramidal system abnormalities often produce involuntary movement disorders including tremors, choreiform, (jerking) movements, athetoid (slow sinuous) movements, hemiballismic (flailing) motions, and muscular rigidity (pyramid, paralysis; extrapyramidal, extremity excesses).

Sensory System (Fig. 2-14)

Supposedly, humans get the greatest degree of satisfaction from their sense of touch. Certainly, a good back scratch can satiate many a need, but the sense of touch goes beyond merely a light touch on the back. It also includes pain (an inadvertent scratch by the nails), vibration (add a pulsating massager), and position sense (lying on one's stomach).

The sensory system of the CNS is separated into fibers that transmit the sensations of pain and temperature, position, vibration, and general fine touch (Table 2-4). From the body, pain and temperature primary neuron fibers are transmitted by peripheral nerve fibers. The pain and temperature sensations are transmitted to the dorsal root

---

Box 2-1   Localization of the Central Sulcus (see Fig. 2-13)

1. The central sulcus enters the paracentral lobule anterior to the marginal ramus of the cingulate sulcus.
2. The medial end of the post central sulcus is shaped like a bifid "y" and the bifid ends enclose the marginal ramus of the cingulate sulcus.
3. The superior frontal sulcus terminates in the precentral sulcus and the central sulcus is the next sulcus posterior to the precentral sulcus.
4. The interparietal sulcus intersects the postcentral sulcus.
5. The knob representing the hand motor area is in the precentral gyrus.
6. The precentral gyrus' cortical gray matter thickness is greater than that of the postcentral gyrus thickness. Usually PRE/POST thickness ratio is about 1.5/1.
7. The peri-Rolandic cortex is more hypointense than surrounding cortex on FLAIR.

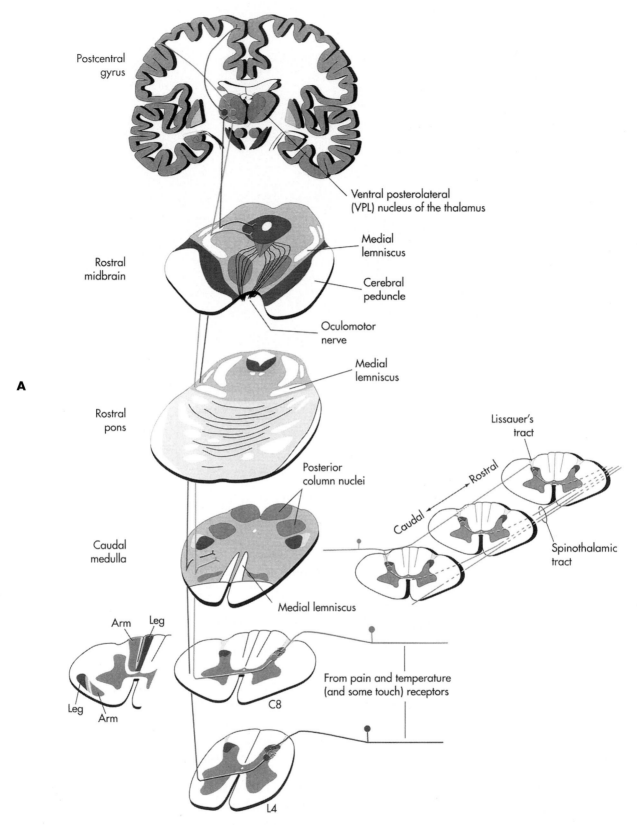

Fig. 2-14 The sensory pathways of the body. **A,** Spinothalamic tract. Pain, temperature, and some touch and pressure afferents end in the posterior horn. Second- or higher-order fibers cross the midline, form the spinothalamic tract, and ascend to the ventral posterolateral *(VPL)* nucleus of the thalamus (and also to other thalamic nuclei not indicated in this figure). Thalamic cells then project to the somatosensory cortex of the postcentral gyrus and to other cortical areas (also not indicated in this figure). Along their course through the brain stem, spinothalamic fibers give off many collaterals to the reticular formation. The inset to the left shows the lamination of fibers in the posterior columns and the spinothalamic tract, in a leg-lower trunk-upper trunk-arm sequence. The inset to the right shows the longitudinal formation of the spinothalamic tract. Primary afferents ascend several segments in Lissauer's tract before all their branches terminate; fibers crossing to join the spinothalamic tract do so with a rostral inclination. As a result, a cordotomy incision at any given level

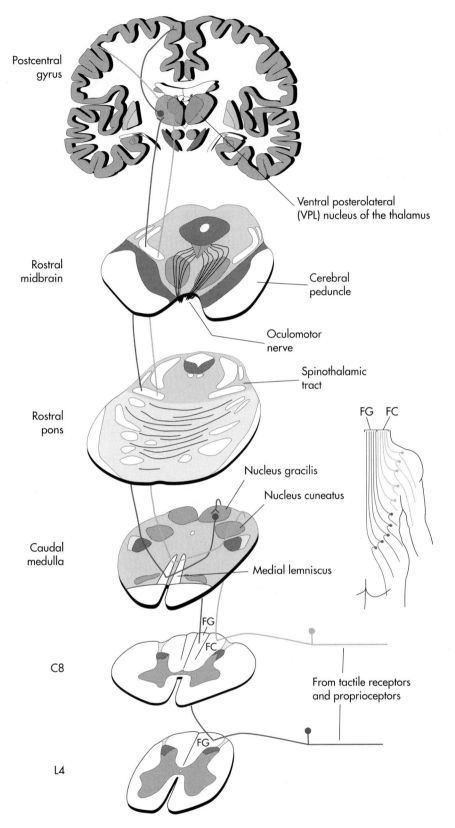

Postcentral gyrus

Ventral posterolateral (VPL) nucleus of the thalamus

Rostral midbrain

Cerebral peduncle

Oculomotor nerve

Spinothalamic tract

B

Rostral pons

FG   FC

Nucleus gracilis

Nucleus cuneatus

Caudal medulla

Medial lemniscus

FG

FC

C8

From tactile receptors and proprioceptors

FG

L4

will spare most of the information entering the contralateral side of the spinal cord at that level, and to be effective the incision must be made several segments rostral to the highest dermatomal level of pain. **B,** Posterior column-medial meniscus pathway. Primary afferents carrying tactile and proprioceptive information synapse in the posterior column nuclei of the ipsilateral medulla. The axons of second-order cells then cross the midline, form the medial lemniscus, and ascend to the ventral posterolateral nucleus of the thalamus. Third-order fibers then project to the somatosensory cortex of the postcentral gyrus. A somatotopic arrangement of fibers is present at all levels. The beginning of this somatotopic arrangement, as a lamination of fibers in the posterior columns, is indicated in the inset to the right. (From Nolte J: *The human brain: an introduction to its functional anatomy,* ed 4, St. Louis, Mosby, 1999, pp. 244, 245.)

Table 2-4 Sensory tracts

Tract	Course	Function
Medial lemniscus	From posterior white matter of cord to dorsal nuclei of medulla, through decussation, to medial lemniscus to thalamus to anterior limb of internal capsule to primary sensory cortex	Touch and limb position sense
Spinothalamic tract	Dorsal horn of cord to spinal decussation to anterolateral spinal tract to reticular formation of pons, medulla, thalamus	Pain and temperature
Lateral lemniscus	From auditory fibers in caudal pons, crossed and uncrossed, to inferior colliculus, to medial geniculate of thalamus to primary auditory cortex	Auditory

ganglia of the spinal cord, where fibers may ascend or descend for one or two spinal segments before terminating in the region of the substantia gelatinosa of the dorsal horn. From the secondary neurons of the nucleus proprius of the dorsal horn, the fibers cross the midline in the anterior white commissures of the spinal cord and ascend in the lateral spinothalamic tract. The lateral spinothalamic tract is identified in the lateral midportion of the medulla and centrally in the pons where it is renamed the spinal lemniscus (see Fig. 2-14A). The spinal lemniscus proceeds through the anterolateral portion of the dorsal pons and along the lateral aspect of the midbrain. From there the fibers synapse with tertiary neurons in the ventral posterolateral thalamic nucleus and then terminate in the somesthetic area of the parietal lobe in the postcentral sulcus region.

Pain and temperature sensation from the face is transmitted via the primary neuron axons of cranial nerve V, with the nuclei identified in the trigeminal ganglion (Fig. 2-15A). The axons from the trigeminal ganglion descend in the spinal trigeminal tract. The fibers terminate in the secondary neuron nucleus of the trigeminal spinal tract, which extends from the lower medulla to the C3 level of the spinal cord. At this point the pain and temperature fibers cross the midline to the contralateral side and ascend as the trigeminothalamic tract, which passes medial to the lateral spinothalamic tract but terminates also in the ventral posterior (lateral) thalamic nucleus. From there tertiary neuron fibers pass to the somesthetic area of the cerebral cortex.

Light touch and pressure from the body are transmitted in the ipsilateral posterior column of the spinal cord and contralateral anterior column (see Fig. 2-14B). The ascending branches may travel up to six to eight segments of the spinal cord before crossing to the contralateral side. Once again, a synapse is present in the nucleus proprius of the dorsal horn. From there, the white matter tracts form the anterior spinothalamic tracts, also included as part of the spinal lemniscus. These axons also terminate in the ventral posterior (lateral) thalamic nucleus passing through the anterior portion of the internal capsule and the centrum semiovale to the somesthetic cortex. The spinal lemniscus lies lateral to the medial lemniscus in the posterior pons.

The pathway for light touch of the face is identical to that of the pain and temperature. However, termination of these cranial nerve V fibers occurs in a more superior portion of the nucleus of the trigeminal spinal tract. In addition, these fibers may bifurcate on entering the pons and synapse with the chief sensory nucleus of V within the pons.

The body's sense of proprioception, fine touch, and vibration is transmitted via proprioceptors, which bifurcate in the posterior columns of the spinal cord. A portion of the fibers descend and make up the afferent loop of fiber reflex arcs; however, the ascending portion passes superiorly in the fasciculus gracilis and the fasciculus cuneatus, which terminate in their respective nuclei in the medulla. These fibers ascend ipsilaterally only. From the nucleus gracilis and nucleus cuneatus the axons cross the midline of the medulla and continue superiorly as the medial lemniscus found in the posterior portion of the medulla and pons before terminating in the ventral posterolateral (VPL). From the VPL, the path is through the internal capsule to get to the primary somatosensory cortex nucleus of the thalamus.

Fine tactile fibers from the face terminate in the chief sensory nucleus or the mesencephalic nucleus of cranial nerve V (see Fig. 2-15B). The fibers going to the chief sensory nucleus of cranial nerve V then cross the midline and ascend as the trigeminothalamic tract (ventral trigeminal lemniscus), whereas the fibers going to the mesencephalic nucleus of nerve V ascend ipsilaterally in the dorsal trigeminal lemniscus. From the mesencephalic nucleus in the midbrain, however, these fibers cross the midline at the red nucleus level and ascend to the ventral posteromedial thalamic nucleus. The pathways from both the body and face terminate in the somesthetic area of the cerebral cortex after passing through the posterior limb of the internal capsule.

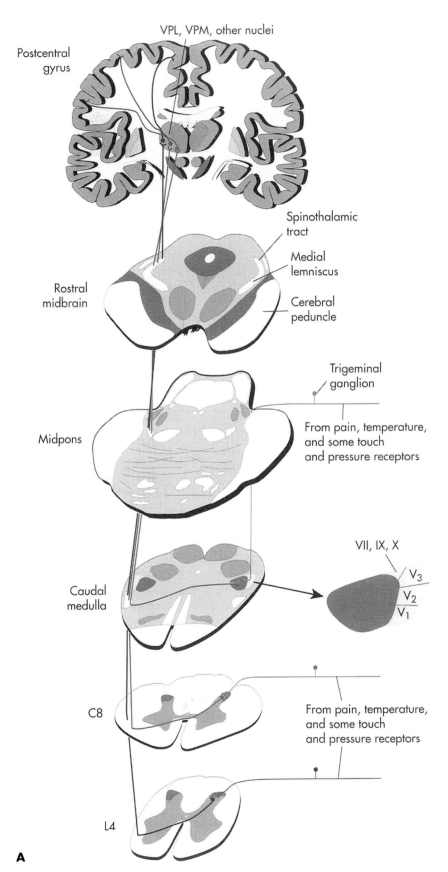

Fig. 2-15 Ascending trigeminal pathways from the spinal nucleus. **A,** The insert near the caudal medulla section indicates the arrangement within the spinal trigeminal tract of fibers from the three subdivisions of the trigeminal nerve, as well as those from cranial nerves VII, IX, and X that innervate the outer ear. Ascending trigeminal pathways from the spinal nucleus. The inset near the caudal medulla section indicates the arrangement within the spinal trigeminal tract of fibers from the three subdivisions of the trigeminal nerve, as well as those from cranial nerves VII, IX, and X that innervate the outer ear. (Trigeminal pain information, like pain information from the body, also projects to other parts of the thalamus and cortex not indicated in this figure.)

Illustration continued on following page

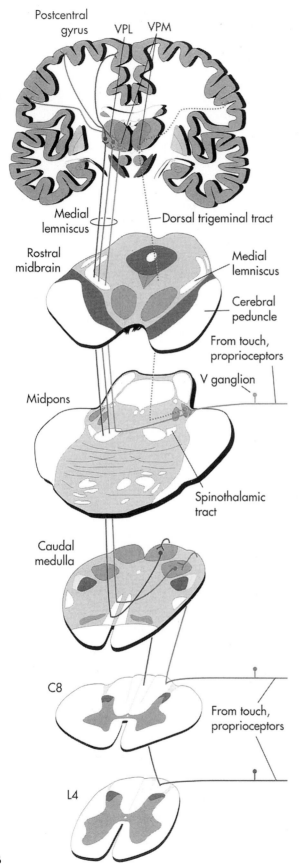

B

For those of you who have become lost with this verbose description, look at the figures instead. That is why you are a radiologist—you prefer the pictures! Clearly, a picture is worth a thousand words.

Visual Pathway

Next to taste (wine, coffee, and Krispy Kremes), vision (films, journals, stock market trends, paychecks) is the radiologist's favorite sense. Although taste ultimately is transmitted to the limbic system where it gets mixed up with all those crazy emotions (see discussion later in this section), vision remains blessedly cerebral and intellectual. Its circuitry, although extensive, is well organized. These are the circuits that select for radiologists in a Darwinian sense.

The image received by the rods and cones of the retina is passed to secondary sensory ganglion cells of the retina and is then transmitted along the second cranial nerve—the optic nerve. The optic nerve ascends obliquely through the optic canal to join fibers from the contralateral optic nerve at the optic chiasm (Fig. 2-16). The temporal retina fibers (nasal field) remain uncrossed and pass to the ipsilateral optic tract. The fibers from the nasal retina (temporal fields) decussate to join the nondecussating nasal field fibers from the opposite optic nerve continuing in the postchiasmal optic tract. However, before they cross, some of the inferonasal retinal fibers loop for a short distance up into the contralateral optic nerve in what is termed Wilbrand's knee. This accounts for the signs of the "junctional syndrome" found in a lesion that compresses one optic nerve and the looping contralateral Wilbrand's fibers. This results in a central scotoma in the ipsilateral eye and a superotemporal visual defect in the contralateral eye. Ninety percent of the fibers in the chiasm are from the macula of the retina; the crossing fibers lie superiorly and posteriorly in the chiasm. The optic tract encircles the anterior portion of the midbrain before terminating in the lateral geniculate body of the thalamus. The lateral geniculate body is located in the posterolateral portion of the thalamus within the pulvinar nucleus. A few fibers ascend to the Edinger-Westphal nucleus (cranial nerve III) in the pretectal portion of the midbrain as part of the pupillary reflex, and some connect to the superior colliculus for tracking ability. From the lateral geniculate nucleus, tertiary neuronal fibers pass in the geniculocalcarine tract (optic radiations), course through portions of the posterior limb of the internal capsule and around the lateral ventricle, and

Fig. 2-15 *Continued.* **B,** Ascending trigeminal pathways from the main sensory nucleus. (A, B from Nolte J: *The human brain: an introduction to its functional anatomy,* ed 4. St. Louis, Mosby, 1999, pp. 308, 306, respectively.)

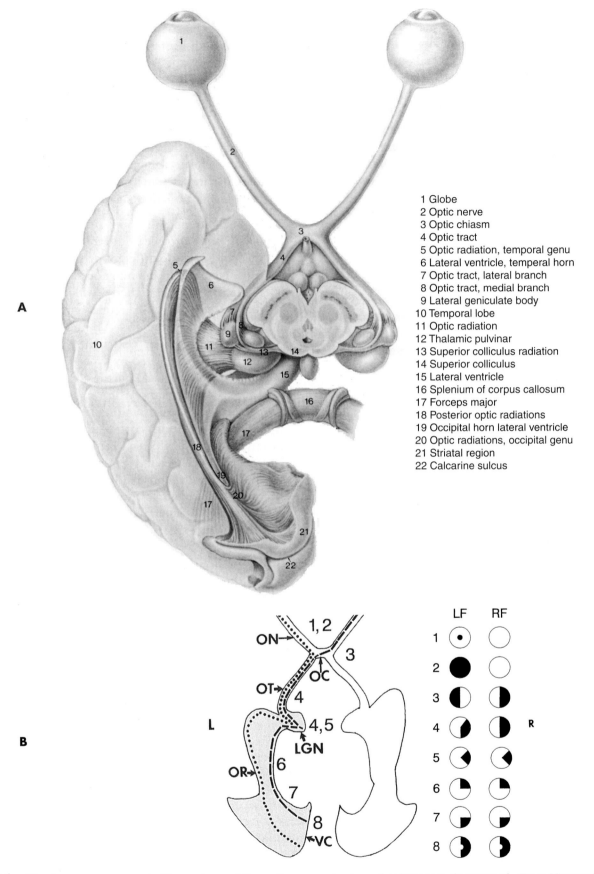

1 Globe
2 Optic nerve
3 Optic chiasm
4 Optic tract
5 Optic radiation, temporal genu
6 Lateral ventricle, temperal horn
7 Optic tract, lateral branch
8 Optic tract, medial branch
9 Lateral geniculate body
10 Temporal lobe
11 Optic radiation
12 Thalamic pulvinar
13 Superior colliculus radiation
14 Superior colliculus
15 Lateral ventricle
16 Splenium of corpus callosum
17 Forceps major
18 Posterior optic radiations
19 Occipital horn lateral ventricle
20 Optic radiations, occipital genu
21 Striatal region
22 Calcarine sulcus

Fig. 2-16 Visual system anatomy. **A,** The anatomy of the optic nerves, tracts, and radiations is diagrammed. (From Nieuwenhuys R, Voogd J, van Huijen C: *The human central nervous system: a synopsis and atlas,* rev ed 3, Berlin, 1988, Springer-Verlag.) **B,** Optic chiasm: correlation of lesion site and field defect. Note the most ventral nasal fibers (mostly from inferior nasal retina) temporarily travel within the fellow optic nerve in Wilbrands' knee.

terminate in the visual calcarine cortex in the medial occipital lobe. The superior optic radiations (inferior visual fields) pass through the parietal lobe on their way to the superior visual cortex of the occipital lobe. The inferior optic radiations (superior visual fields) are called Meyers loop fibers. They pass over the anteroinferior aspect of the lateral ventricle (around the temporal horn) into the temporal lobe to terminate in the inferior visual cortex just below the calcarine sulcus. An optic radiation lesion is localized depending on whether there are signs of neglect or sensory loss (superior radiation–parietal lobe lesion) or dysphasia and memory loss (Meyers loop temporal lobe lesion).

Thus, lesions in the optic nerve cause blindness of the ipsilateral eye. Lesions in the midline at the level of the optic chiasm will cause a bitemporal hemianopsia. Lesions compressing the lateral edge of the optic chiasm cause a nasal hemianopsia of the ipsilateral eye. Lesions of the optic tract extending to the lateral geniculate, and primary lesions of the lateral geniculate nucleus cause a contralateral homonymous hemianopsia. Lesions of the geniculocalcarine tract or visual cortex cause a contralateral homonymous hemianopsia (see Fig. 2-16B).

Sparing of macular vision with cortical strokes is common, and one of four explanations is possible: (1) localization of macular fibers to the watershed area of middle and posterior cerebral artery supply, allowing for dual vascular supply to be present; (2) a very large cortical area devoted to central vision, meaning that small strokes will not affect all fibers; (3) some decussation of macular fibers, so that they are bilaterally represented, and (4) testing artifact due to poor central fixation by the subject.

Auditory System (Fig. 2-17)

What goes on in your head when your cell phone chirps? Sound is transmitted through the external ear via vibrations of the tympanic membrane to the middle ear ossicles. It is transmitted to the hair cells of the organ of Corti in the cochlea. The cochlear division of the eighth cranial nerve runs in the anterior inferior portion of the internal auditory canal. From the canal, the nerve enters the brain stem at the junction between the pons and the medulla. The fibers end in the dorsal and ventral cochlear nuclei, which are identified in the upper part of the medulla along its dorsal surface. After this primary synapse the secondary nerves for hearing may cross the midline at the level of the pons and ascend in the lateral lemniscus in what is termed the trapezoid body. A synapse may occur in the trapezoid body, but other fibers may synapse in the superior olivary nucleus (whose function is thought to be involved in the sound localization of an olive dropped into a Martini). Some fibers may remain on the ipsilateral side and synapse in the ipsilateral superior olivary nucleus to ascend in the ipsilateral lateral lemniscus. The tertiary neurons of the lateral lemniscus pass through the ventral portion of the pons and midportion of the midbrain before synapsing at the inferior colliculus (thought to be instrumental in frequency discrimination). From the inferior colliculus, the fourth-order fibers pass to the medial geniculate nucleus of the thalamus. It should be noted, however, fibers may bypass each of these nuclei to get to the next level in the auditory pathway.

Fibers from the medial geniculate course in the posterior limb of the internal capsule as the auditory radiations and terminate in the anterosuperior transverse temporal gyri superior temporal gyrus. The auditory association cortex is also located in the temporal lobe. Unilateral lesions in the auditory cortex do not induce complete deafness in the contralateral ear, but there is a decrease in auditory acuity because of crossing fibers in the lateral lemniscus and crossed connections between the nuclei of the lateral lemniscus and the inferior colliculi. Most causes of unilateral hearing loss are at the level of the inner and middle ear.

Limbic System

The limbic system anatomy is enough to lead you to think that its primary purpose is to make you nuts. The main components of the limbic system include the fornix, the mamillary bodies, the hippocampus, the amygdala, and the anterior nucleus of the thalamus. The limbic system controls the emotional responses to visceral stimuli. In addition, portions of memory function are contained within the limbic system.

The olfactory and gustatory systems tie into the limbic system (Fig. 2-18). The olfactory bulb receives nerve fibers located in the upper nasal cavity, the ciliary nerves. The olfactory bulbs feed into the olfactory tracts lying just under the gyrus rectus region in the olfactory sulcus of the frontal lobes. The olfactory tracts penetrate the brain just under the lamina terminalis and send nerve fibers to the septal nuclei, the parahippocampus, the uncus, and the amygdala.

The amygdala is a primary work station for emotions. In addition to input from the olfactory system, it receives fibers from the thalami and the hypothalamus. Efferent fibers are sent from the amygdala to the temporal and frontal lobes, the thalamus, the hypothalamus, and the reticular formation in the brain stem. Lesions of the amygdala and other portions of the limbic system may cause anhedonia with a lack of emotional response to what are normally pleasurable stimuli (is she playing possum or hard to get? Or is she Anne Hedonic).

The fornices are white matter tracts lying medially beneath the corpus callosum and are the major white matter relays from one hippocampus to the other and on to

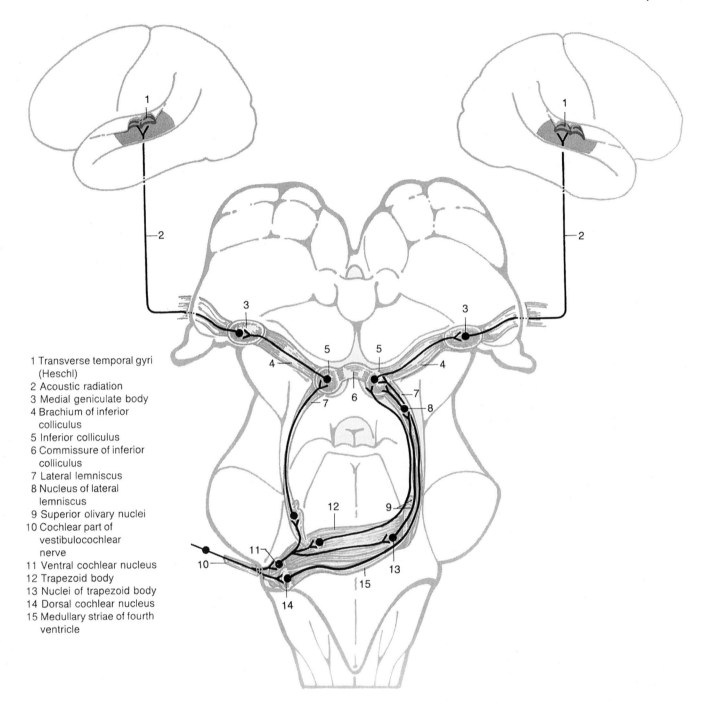

1 Transverse temporal gyri (Heschl)
2 Acoustic radiation
3 Medial geniculate body
4 Brachium of inferior colliculus
5 Inferior colliculus
6 Commissure of inferior colliculus
7 Lateral lemniscus
8 Nucleus of lateral lemniscus
9 Superior olivary nuclei
10 Cochlear part of vestibulocochlear nerve
11 Ventral cochlear nucleus
12 Trapezoid body
13 Nuclei of trapezoid body
14 Dorsal cochlear nucleus
15 Medullary striae of fourth ventricle

Fig. 2-17   The auditory system in the brain stem and diencephalon (dorsal view) and in the cerebrum (lateral view). (From Kretschmann H-J, Weinrich W: *Cranial neuroimaging and clinical neuroanatomy: magnetic resonance imaging and computed tomography,* rev ed 2, New York, Thieme, 1993, p. 284.)

the hypothalamus. The fornical columns invaginate into the lateral and third ventricles as they sweep anteroinferiorly to end in the mamillary bodies. The anterior portions of the fornices parallel the corpus callosum but are more inferiorly and centrally located.

The hippocampal formation includes the hippocampus (located in the temporal lobe above the parahippocampus), the indusium griseum (a fine gray matter tract situated between the corpus callosum and cingulate gyrus connecting septal nuclei to parahippocampal gyri), and the dentate gyrus (just above the parahippocampal gyrus). The hippocampus is found along the medial temporal lobe adjacent to the inferior temporal horn of the lateral ventricle and the choroidal fissure. (See temporal lobe anatomy earlier.)

The hippocampus receives afferents from the indu-

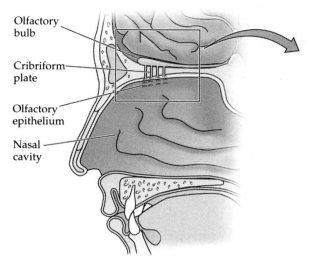

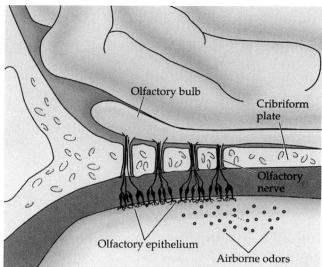

A

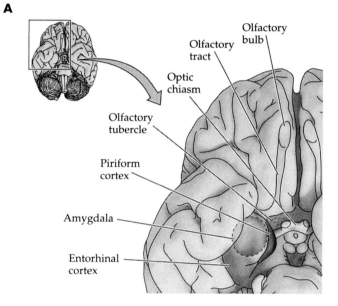

B

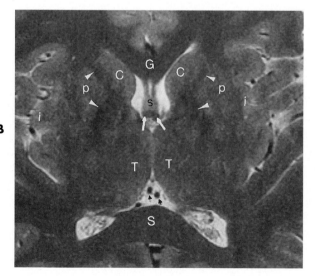

Fig. 2-18   Olfactory system. **A,** Organization of the human olfactory system. Peripheral and central components of the olfactory pathway. Enlargement of region showing the relationship between the olfactory epithelium, containing the olfactory receptor neurons, and the olfactory bulb (the central target of olfactory receptor neurons). Central components of the olfactory system. (From Dale Purves et al [eds]: *Sinauer neuroscience,* ed 2, Sunderland, MA, Sinauer Associates, 2001, p. 318.) **B,** Axial T2WI delineates the columns of the fornices *(arrows),* the caudate nucleus *(C),* the thalami *(T),* septum pellucidum *(small black s),* putamen *(p),* insular cortex *(i),* and the internal capsule *(arrowheads).* Genu *(G)* and splenium *(white S)* of the corpus callosum are the white matter tracts seen in front of and behind the lateral ventricular system.

sium griseum. The hippocampus also receives input from the parahippocampal gyrus. The hippocampus is involved primarily with visceral responses to emotions (with the hypothalamus) and memory, with less input into olfaction.

When both temporal lobes are removed, a syndrome characterized by increased appetite and sexual activity with decreased aggressiveness has been described and is known as the Klüver-Bucy syndrome. Before the reader makes an elective appointment with his or her neurosurgeon for bilateral temporal lobectomies for a spouse, remember the other important functions in the temporal lobe (speech, hearing, and memory). In summary, the limbic system controls such aggressive emotions as fear and anger, as well as the emotions associated with sexual behavior and olfactory stimulation. Many of the responses to stimuli in the limbic system result in autonomic nervous system action controlled through the hypothalamus.

Taste (Fig. 2-19)

Taste from the anterior two thirds of the tongue is transmitted by the chorda tympani, a branch of cranial nerve VII that runs with fibers from the third division of cranial nerve V as the lingual nerve. From the chorda tympani, the fibers run through the otic and geniculate ganglia to end at the cell bodies in the nucleus solitarius. The taste papillae of the posterior third of the tongue are supplied by cranial nerve IX. These fibers course through the petrosal ganglion of cranial nerve IX to reach the cell bodies in the nucleus solitarius. Some bitter taste fibers may be supplied via the vagus nerve's nodose ganglion from the epiglottis. This may be the source of laryngospasm from some food items.

From the nucleus solitarius, projections are made to the pons, both ventromedial nuclei of the thalamus, hypothalamus, and amygdala. These limbic structures monitor the visceral (nausea, vomiting, sweating, flushing, salivation) and emotional responses (elation, disgust, satiation) to certain foods, like jalapeños. From the thalamus, fibers track up to both sides of the sensory cortex, where the tongue occupies a huge proportion of the homunculus projection of the body on the brain surface.

Speech

Obviously, speech ties into the motor and auditory pathways described previously. Nonetheless, a brief description of the speech pathway is warranted because of its critical role in humans. If silence were golden, academic radiologists would not be able to travel on university budgets.

Speech requires coordination between the left hemisphere's temporoparietal areas assigned to the sensation of speech and the inferior frontal gyrus (Broca's area) assigned to motor function. Portions of the arcuate fasciculus connect these two areas. In a few persons (usually left-handed), speech may be localized to the right hemisphere. Portions of the superior and middle temporal gyri and the inferior parietal lobule control ideational language. The auditory association cortex of the superior temporal gyrus (Wernicke's area) handles receptive understanding of speech. Some people, it seems, choose to ignore their Wernicke's input to concentrate on Broca's output. If the inferior frontal gyrus is injured, coordination of intelligible expressive speech is lost (motor aphasia). Receptive aphasia develops with lesions in Wernicke's area, and conductive aphasia (disturbance in speech in response to verbal command but not spontaneously [ideomotor dyspraxia]) occurs with arcuate fasciculus lesions. This is a very complex subject summarized by a dysphasic neuroradiologist. For a greater understanding, do a neurology residency.

CRANIAL NERVES

How many medical students over the years have recited one of the classic mnemonics for the cranial nerves: On old Olympus' towering tops, a Finn and German viewed some hops (olfactory, optic, oculomotor, trochlear, trigeminal, abducens, facial, acoustic, glossopharyngeal, vagus, spinal accessory, and hypoglossal nerves)? The phrase remains imprinted forever, but here is a refresher on the anatomy.

The cranial nerves can be organized in groups of four. Cranial nerves I through IV arise from the midbrain (oculomotor and trochlear) or above (olfactory and optic nerves). Cranial nerves V through VIII arise from the pons. The last four cranial nerves arise from the medulla. Fortunately, the numbering of the cranial nerves was established by someone with an eye for the future and simplicity; as the nerve number goes up, its site of entry or exit from the brain stem goes down (Fig. 2-20).

Olfactory Nerve

The first cranial nerve, the olfactory nerve (see Fig. 2-18A), consists of primary afferent neurosensory cells in the roof of both nasal cavities. The cells have efferent axons that pass through the cribriform plate to synapse on secondary sensory neurons in the olfactory bulb situated along the medial and inferior portions of the anterior cranial fossa. The central connections to the brain from the olfactory bulbs and tracts enter the inferior frontal regions via the medial and lateral olfactory striae. Neuronal pathways pass to the subcallosal medial frontal lobe (via medial olfactory stria) and the inferomedial temporal lobes (via lateral olfactory stria). Specifically, the gyrus

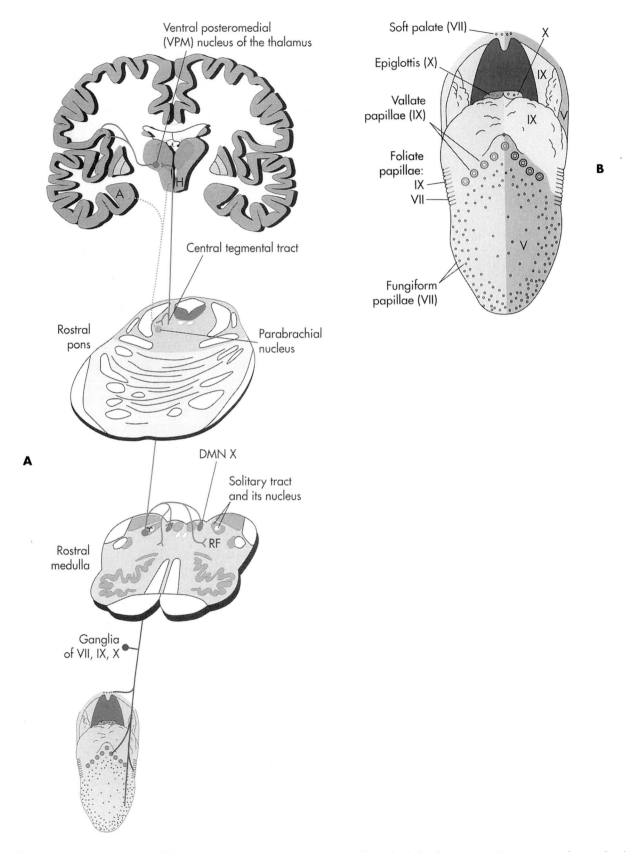

Fig. 2-19 Taste pathways in the CNS. **A,** Second-order neurons feed into reflexes both by direct projections (e.g., to the nearby dorsal motor nucleus of the vagus) and by connections with the reticular formation. The projection from the parabrachial nucleus to the hypothalamus and amygdala is dashed because its existence in primates has not been demonstrated conclusively. **B,** Distribution and innervation of taste buds and innervation of the lingual epithelium. The trigeminal nerve (V) subserves general sensation from the anterior two thirds of the tongue, and the glossopharyngeal nerve (IX) has a similar function with taste for the posterior third of the tongue. Taste is controlled anteriorly by the chorda tympani of the facial nerve (VII). (A, B from Nolte J: *The human brain: an introduction to its functional anatomy,* ed 4, St. Louis, Mosby, 1999, pp. 324, 320, respectively.)

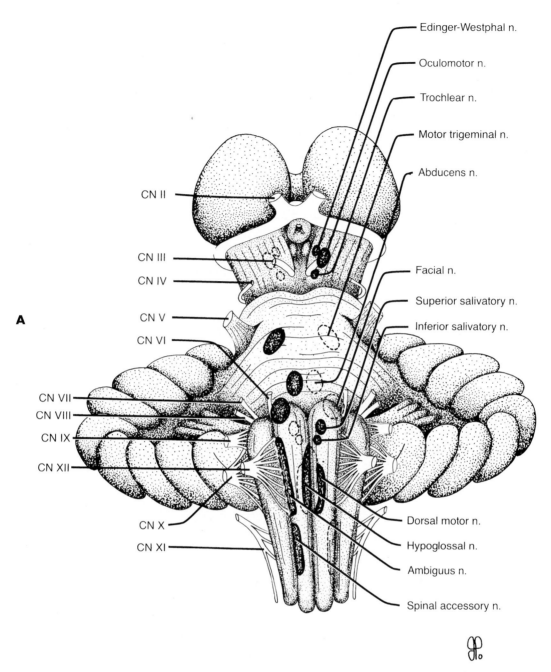

CN II

CN III

CN IV

A   CN V

CN VI

CN VII

CN VIII

CN IX

CN XII

CN X

CN XI

Edinger-Westphal n.

Oculomotor n.

Trochlear n.

Motor trigeminal n.

Abducens n.

Facial n.

Superior salivatory n.

Inferior salivatory n.

Dorsal motor n.

Hypoglossal n.

Ambiguus n.

Spinal accessory n.

Fig. 2-20   Cranial nerve anatomy. **A,** Cranial nerve nuclei locations 1-brain stem.

Illustration continued on following page

semilunaris and gyrus ambiens (forming the prepiriform cortex), the entorhinal-parahippocampal cortex (forming the inferomedial margin of the temporal lobe anterior to the amygdala), and the amygdala receive afferents via the lateral stria. The anterior paraterminal gyrus of the frontal lobe and the lamina terminalis appear to receive fibers from the medial stria. The tertiary pathways from these olfactory projections are located in the (1) orbitofrontal cortex (responding to odor stimulation in monkeys), (2) the hypothalamus via the septum pellucidum, (3) the hippocampus, and (4) the limbic system.

The limbic responses to olfaction are derived through connections from the olfactory area to the hypothalamus, habenular nucleus, reticular formation, and cranial nerves controlling salivation, nausea, and gastrointestinal motility. A rose by any other name would smell so sweet (hence the separation of olfaction from speech).

Optic Nerve (CN II)

The visual pathway has been described previously (see Fig. 2-16).

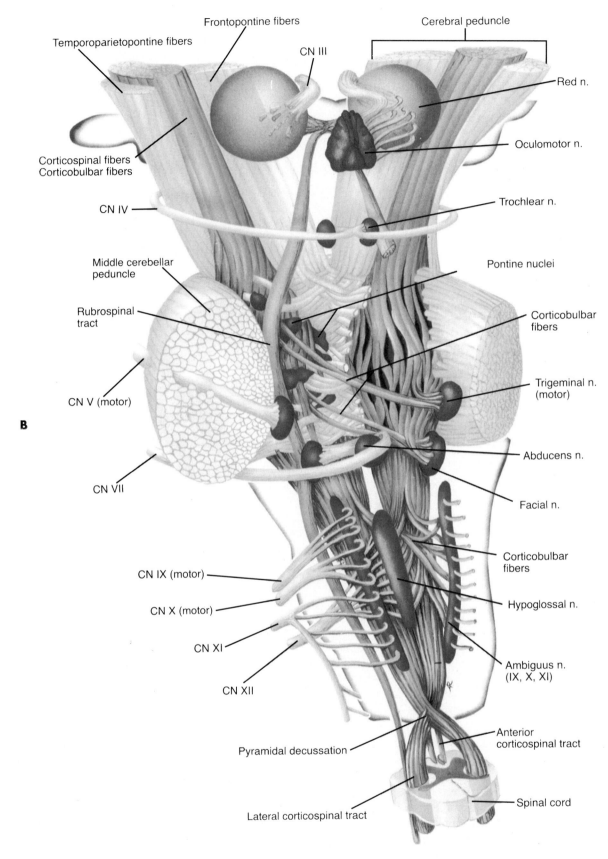

Fig. 2-20 *Continued.* **B,** Descending tracts from cranial nerves and motor nuclei. (From Hendelman WJ: *Student's atlas of neuroanatomy.* Philadelphia, WB Saunders, 1994, pp. 59, 119.)

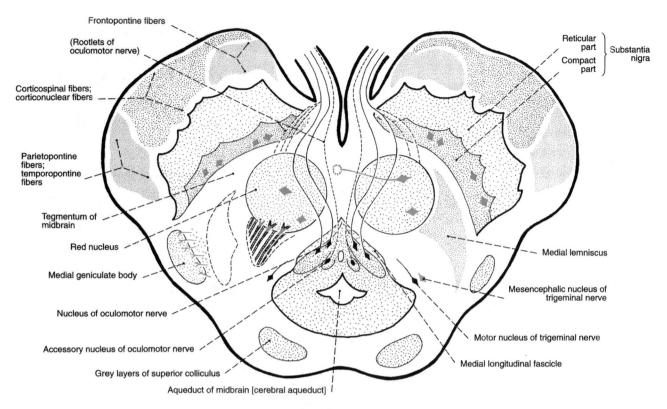

Fig. 2-21   Nuclei and fibers tracts of midbrain. Schematic cross-section at the level of the superior colliculi. Note location of oculomotor nucleus and tracts leaving via interpeduncular cistern. (From Putz R, Pabst R [eds]: *Sobotta atlas of human anatomy,* ed 13, Philadelphia, Lippincott Williams & Wilkins, 1996, p. 301.)

Oculomotor Nerve (CN III)

The nucleus of the oculomotor nerve is identified in the midbrain just posterior to the red nucleus and anterior to the superior aspect of the cerebral aqueduct (Fig. 2-21 and see Fig. 2-4). The oculomotor nuclei are paramedian structures that transmit the oculomotor nerve as it courses around and through the red nucleus, with its exit from the midbrain in the interpeduncular cistern. The oculomotor nerve then proceeds anteroinferiorly between the posterior cerebral and superior cerebellar arteries and lateral to the posterior communicating artery (PCOM). This close approximation to the PCOM accounts for the third nerve palsy often seen with PCOM aneurysms. It then enters the cavernous sinus lying in the superolateral portion of the cavernous sinus just above and lateral to the carotid artery. The oculomotor nerve enters the orbit through the superior orbital fissure. The parasympathetic nucleus of the oculomotor nerve, the Edinger-Westphal nucleus, controls the pupillary muscles of the eye for constriction and dilation. The motor portion of the cranial nerve III supplies the extraocular muscles except for the lateral rectus and superior oblique muscles (see following paragraph). The voluntary portion of the levator palpebrae muscle is also supplied by the oculomotor nerve, accounting for the ptosis seen in third nerve palsies. The sympathetic system supplies Müller's muscle (superior tarsus portion of levator palpebrae), which is why one gets a ptosis with Horner syndrome (ptosis, anhidrosis, miosis, and enophthalmos).

Trochlear Nerve (CN IV)

Cranial nerve IV, the trochlear nerve, has a nucleus in the midbrain in a location just below the nucleus of cranial nerve III, anterior to the aqueduct (see Fig. 2-6). Cranial nerves III, IV, and VI interconnect via the medial longitudinal fasciculus (MLF) to coordinate conjugate extraocular muscle movements. The MLF is located anterior to these three cranial nerve nuclei. The MLF is analogous to the long-distance telephone system, receiving connections from many sites, including the nuclei of nerves III, IV, VI, VII, XI, and XII; the vestibular system; and the spine.

Cranial nerve IV is unique in that it is the only one where the nerve exits the posterior portion of the brain stem and it is also the only one that crosses completely (the optic nerve has portions that cross). The fibers of the trochlear nerve decussate just below the inferior colliculi in a small area posterior to the cerebral aqueduct (Fig. 2-22). After leaving the brain stem, the cranial nerve

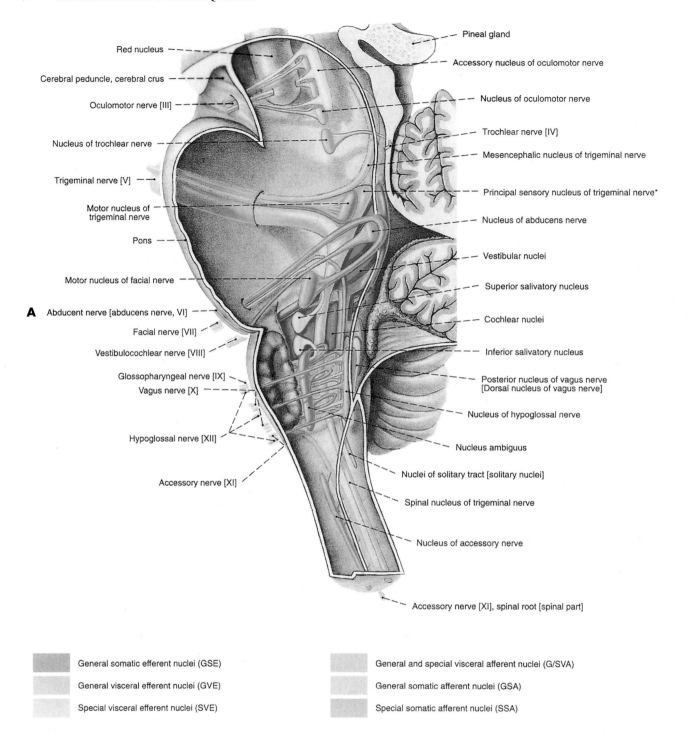

Red nucleus

Cerebral peduncle, cerebral crus

Oculomotor nerve [III]

Nucleus of trochlear nerve

Trigeminal nerve [V]

Motor nucleus of trigeminal nerve

Pons

Motor nucleus of facial nerve

A Abducent nerve [abducens nerve, VI]

Facial nerve [VII]

Vestibulocochlear nerve [VIII]

Glossopharyngeal nerve [IX]

Vagus nerve [X]

Hypoglossal nerve [XII]

Accessory nerve [XI]

Pineal gland

Accessory nucleus of oculomotor nerve

Nucleus of oculomotor nerve

Trochlear nerve [IV]

Mesencephalic nucleus of trigeminal nerve

Principal sensory nucleus of trigeminal nerve*

Nucleus of abducens nerve

Vestibular nuclei

Superior salivatory nucleus

Cochlear nuclei

Inferior salivatory nucleus

Posterior nucleus of vagus nerve [Dorsal nucleus of vagus nerve]

Nucleus of hypoglossal nerve

Nucleus ambiguus

Nuclei of solitary tract [solitary nuclei]

Spinal nucleus of trigeminal nerve

Nucleus of accessory nerve

Accessory nerve [XI], spinal root [spinal part]

General somatic efferent nuclei (GSE)

General visceral efferent nuclei (GVE)

Special visceral efferent nuclei (SVE)

General and special visceral afferent nuclei (G/SVA)

General somatic afferent nuclei (GSA)

Special somatic afferent nuclei (SSA)

Fig. 2-22 Cranial nerve brain stem origins. **A,** Trochlear nerve nucleus arises in brain stem and nerve leaves posteriorly. It loops around midbrain. Note also motor loop of facial nerve looping around the abducens nucleus. (From Sobotta, Philadelphia, Lippincott Williams & Wilkins, 2001, p. 301, Fig. 5-17.)

Illustration continued on following page

IV fibers course anteroinferiorly around the midbrain below the tentorium to enter the cavernous sinus lying just below the cranial nerve III fiber tracts. The trochlear nerve, together with the oculomotor nerve and cranial nerve VI, enters the orbit through the superior orbital fissure. The trochlear nerve supplies the superior oblique muscle.

Trigeminal Nerve (CN V)

The nuclei of cranial nerve V have been described previously in discussions of tactile sense and motor function of the face (see previous sections). Cranial nerve V exits the lateral aspect of the pons and courses anteri-

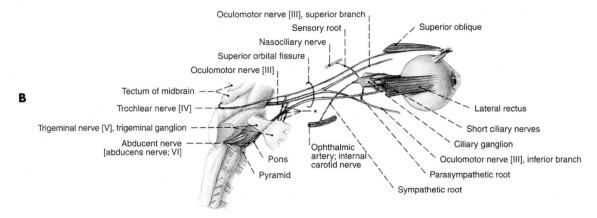

Fig. 2-22 *Continued.* **B,** Branches of cranial nerves to oculomotor muscles are seen. (From Putz R, Pabst R [eds]: *Sobotta atlas of human anatomy,* ed 13, Philadelphia, Lippincott Williams & Wilkins, 1996, p. 271.) or **B,** figure 51, p. 125 Hendelman 1994 edition.

orly to synapse in Meckel's cave (see Fig. 2-5, Fig. 2-23). The ganglion in Meckel's cave is known as the gasserian or semilunar ganglion. From the gasserian ganglion cranial nerve V trifurcates. Its first division is the ophthalmic nerve, which branches out to the tentorium and then runs anteriorly into the inferior portion of the cavernous sinus, enters the superior orbital fissure, and provides sensory afferents to the upper portion of the face, the eye, the lacrimal gland, and the nose.

The second division of cranial nerve V enters the foramen rotundum and courses anteriorly to the pterygopalatine fossa; from there it supplies sensory innervation throughout the maxillofacial region below the orbits (see description in Chapter 14). It has a meningeal branch to the middle cranial fossa. The maxillary nerve enters the inferior orbital fissure, passing through the infraorbital groove to supply the inferior eyelid, upper lip, and nose. The upper teeth and gingiva are supplied by alveolar nerves, which have branches arising from the zygomatic nerve off the maxillary nerve in the pterygopalatine fossa (Fig. 2-24).

The third division of the trigeminal nerve, the mandibular division, supplies motor function to the muscles of mastication. In addition, sensory fibers contributing to the lower portion of the face, ear, temporomandibular joint, temple, and tympanic membrane are transmitted through the mandibular division of cranial nerve V. The mandibular nerve passes through the foramen ovale as it exits through the skull base. A meningeal branch returns through the foramen spinosum with the middle meningeal artery. In addition to the masseter, temporalis, and both pterygoid muscles, the mandibular nerve supplies motor function to the tensor tympani, tensor veli palatini, anterior belly of the digastric muscle, and mylohyoid muscle. The posterior branch of the mandibular nerve divides into auriculotemporal, lingual, and inferior alveolar nerves. The lingual nerve contains general sensory fibers and taste fibers from the chorda tympani (fa-

cial nerve) arising from the anterior two thirds of the tongue. The inferior alveolar nerve enters the mandible through the mandibular (inferior alveolar) canal, giving off motor supply to the mylohyoid muscle and anterior digastric muscle. Its sensory fibers supply the gingiva and teeth of the mandible. What a mouthful!

Abducens Nerve (CN VI)

Cranial nerve VI, the abducens nerve, has its nucleus in the middle of the pons near the floor of the fourth ventricle (see Figs. 2-5, 2-6, 2-22A). The facial nerve encircles this nucleus and makes a tiny bump on the anterior margin of the fourth ventricle (facial colliculus). The abducens nerve courses from the nucleus anteriorly, leaving the brain stem at the junction of the pons and the pyramids of the medulla. Cranial nerve VI courses through Dorello's canal before entering the cavernous sinus, where it lies lateral to the carotid artery (see description of CN VI in Chapter 11). In this location, it is the nerve closest to the artery and therefore most sensitive to cavernous carotid artery disease. The nerve then enters the superior orbital fissure and innervates the lateral rectus muscle.

Facial Nerve (CN VII)

The facial nerve has its motor nucleus in the midpons, situated anterolateral to that of the abducens nucleus (see Figs. 2-6, 2-22A). From the motor nucleus of the facial nerve the fibers course initially posteriorly to encircle the abducens nucleus (facial colliculus) before turning back anteriorly to join fibers from the superior salivatory nucleus and the nucleus solitarius of cranial nerve VII, to be joined by the spinal tract of cranial nerve V. The nucleus solitarius receives taste afferents from VII (anterior tongue), IX (posterior tongue), and X (epiglottis). Nerve VII leaves the pons further lateral than the abducens nerve and crosses the cerebellopontine angle cis-

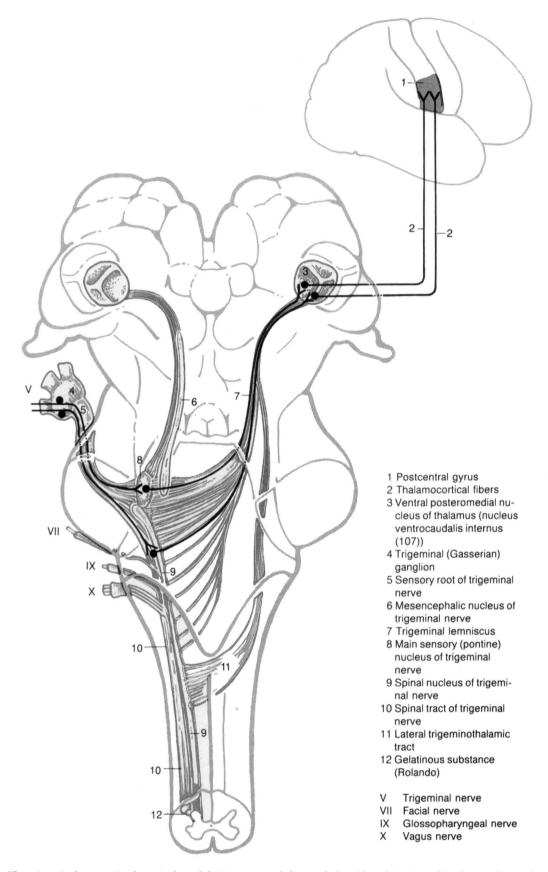

1 Postcentral gyrus
2 Thalamocortical fibers
3 Ventral posteromedial nucleus of thalamus (nucleus ventrocaudalis internus (107))
4 Trigeminal (Gasserian) ganglion
5 Sensory root of trigeminal nerve
6 Mesencephalic nucleus of trigeminal nerve
7 Trigeminal lemniscus
8 Main sensory (pontine) nucleus of trigeminal nerve
9 Spinal nucleus of trigeminal nerve
10 Spinal tract of trigeminal nerve
11 Lateral trigeminothalamic tract
12 Gelatinous substance (Rolando)

V   Trigeminal nerve
VII Facial nerve
IX Glossopharyngeal nerve
X   Vagus nerve

Fig. 2-23   The trigeminal system in the spinal cord, brain stem, and diencephalon (dorsal view) and in the cerebrum (lateral view). Roman numerals indicate the cranial nerves. (From Kretschmann H-J, Weinrich W: *Cranial neuroimaging and clinical neuro-anatomy: magnetic resonance imaging and computed tomography,* rev ed 2, New York, Thieme, 1993, p. 267.)

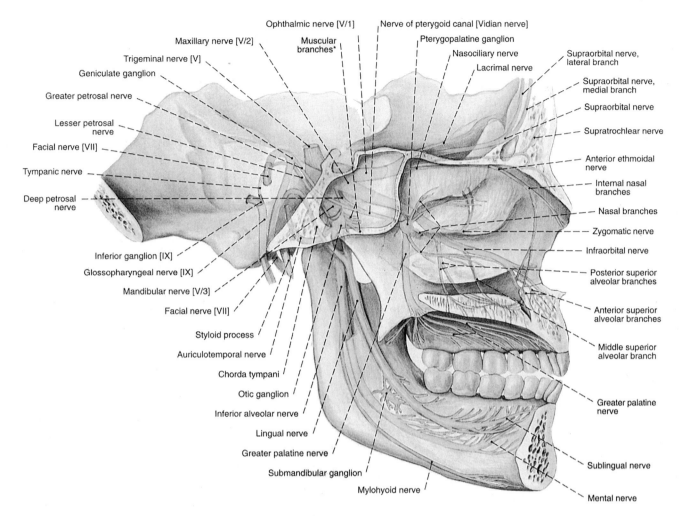

Fig. 2-24   The nerves of the face, the trigeminal, facial, glossopharyngeal nerves and their branches. *Asterisk* indicates muscles of mastication. (From Putz R, Pabst R [eds]: *Sobotta atlas of human anatomy,* ed 13, Philadelphia, Lippincott Williams & Wilkins, 1996, p. 78.)

tern to enter the internal auditory canal. The seventh nerve has a larger motor component and a smaller sensory portion termed the nervus intermedius. The nervus intermedius contains fibers for taste and has parasympathetic fibers as well. The nervus intermedius lies between (intermediate) the motor component of CN VII and CN VIII in the internal auditory canal. The cranial nerve VII fibers run in the anterior superior portion of the internal auditory canal and the sensory fibers have their first synapse at the geniculate ganglion located along the anterior surface of the petrous bone at the level of the middle ear ossicles. From the geniculate ganglion, these fibers leave as the greater superficial petrosal nerve, which transmits fibers to the lacrimal apparatus. Cranial nerve VII then turns inferiorly, branching off a nerve to the stapedius muscle and, in the lower mastoid portion of the temporal bone, transmits the chorda tympani branch of the facial nerve. This joins the lingual branch of the mandibular nerve and provides taste sensation to the anterior two thirds of the tongue. On leaving the

mastoid portion of the temporal bone through the stylomastoid foramen, the nerve passes laterally around the retromandibular vein in the parotid gland, coursing superficially through the masticator space to innervate the muscles of facial expression.

Vestibulocochlear (Acoustic) Nerve (CN VIII)

Cranial nerve VIII has been described in a previous section. The nuclei of cranial nerve VIII are located in the superior aspect of the medulla along the base of the inferior cerebellar peduncle (see Figs. 2-6 and 2-7). The cochlear and vestibular nuclei are situated adjacent to each other, with the vestibular nuclei located more medially. The nerves exit the pontomedullary junction posterior to the inferior olivary nucleus. The cochlear division of the vestibulocochlear nerve runs in the anteroinferior portion of the internal auditory canal whereas the vestibular branches run in the superior and inferior posterior portions of the internal auditory canal. The nerves end within the cochlea and the semicircular canals.

Glossopharyngeal Nerve (CN IX)

Cranial nerve IX has its nucleus in the medulla just posterior to the inferior olivary nucleus (see Fig. 2-7). The nuclei of the glossopharyngeal nerve include the nucleus ambiguus (for motor function), the inferior salivatory nucleus (for salivation), and nucleus of the tractus solitarius (for taste). The vagus and glossopharyngeal nerves share the nucleus ambiguus and the dorsal vagal nuclei (touch, pain, and temperature to tongue) as sites of origin. The fibers from cranial nerve IX pass through the olivary sulcus to enter the pars nervosa of the jugular foramen. The nerves pass through the jugular foramen, perforate the superior constrictor muscles, and innervate the pharynx and stylopharyngeus muscles. Taste and general somatic sensation to the posterior third of the tongue and part of the soft palate are supplied by nerve IX. Meningeal branches to the posterior fossa, tympanic branches (Jacobson's nerve, responsible for glomus tumors), and carotid body fibers are transmitted through cranial nerve IX. The otic ganglion, which receives the lesser petrosal nerve from tympanic branches of the glossopharyngeal nerve, has secretomotor fibers for the parotid gland from CN VII and may communicate with the chorda tympani and vidian nerve (see Fig. 2-24).

Vagus Nerve (CN X)

The vagus nerve (cranial nerve X) has three parent nuclei within the medulla (see Fig. 2-7). The nucleus ambiguus gives rise to motor fibers to the larynx and pharynx. The dorsal nucleus of the vagus nerve is identified just anterior to the fourth ventricle in its inferior aspect. It receives sensory information and transmits motor information to and from the cardiovascular, pulmonary, and gastrointestinal tracts. The nucleus solitarius receives CN X taste afferents from the epiglottis and valleculae (see Fig. 2-22). The vagus nerve exits the medulla through the olivary sulcus and enters the pars vascularis of the jugular foramen. It receives efferents from the cranial root of the spinal accessory nerve, which provide innervation to the recurrent laryngeal nerves. The main trunks of the vagus nerve then run in the carotid sheath with the internal carotid arteries and internal jugular veins. Recurrent laryngeal nerves loop under the aorta on the left side and subclavian arteries on the right, and travel in the tracheoesophageal grooves, before supplying all the laryngeal muscles except the cricothyroids (supplied by the superior laryngeal nerve, also a branch of the vagus).

Spinal Accessory Nerve (CN XI)

The spinal accessory nerve receives fibers from the first three cervical spinal levels as well as the motor cortex. The nerves ascend as the ansa cervicalis (running along the carotid sheath) and course with cranial nerve X out the postolivary sulcus into the jugular foramen's pars vasculosa along with the internal jugular vein. The spinal accessory nerve's motor nucleus is in the lower medulla and upper cervical spinal cord (see Fig. 2-7), and it supplies branches to the sternocleidomastoid muscle and trapezius muscle. The ansa cervicalis (C1-C3) fibers innervate the infrahyoid strap muscles.

Hypoglossal Nerve (CN XII)

The hypoglossal nerve has its nucleus along the paramedian area of the anterior wall of the fourth ventricle in the medulla (see Fig. 2-7). The nerve fibers course anteriorly to exit the medulla in the preolivary sulcus. From there, the nerve courses through the hypoglossal canal. It supplies the intrinsic muscles of the tongue as well as the genioglossus, styloglossus, and hyoglossus muscles. Ansa cervicalis branches run with the hypoglossal nerve to supply the anterior strap muscles.

A picture is worth a thousand words. You have just read nearly that many on the cranial nerves, now study the pictures.

VASCULAR ANATOMY

At a grand rounds lecture it was opined that knowledge of the vascular anatomy of the brain, particularly the venous anatomy of the posterior fossa, is better correlated with a neuroradiologist's age than his or her abilities. There was a nasty, disdainful response from the elder statesmen in the department after that gaffe. Nonetheless, the advent of cross-sectional imaging modalities has relegated conventional angiography to the role of delineating vascular lesions including aneurysms, vasculitis, and arteriovenous malformations, not detection or localization of masses as in yesteryear. Now, even magnetic resonance angiography and CT angiography are largely replacing diagnostic angiography. It is a bit of a shame; some of the most satisfying adventures in neuroradiology have come from the end of a catheter. In the not too distant future people will talk about the old geezers (us) who used to diagnose aneurysms with catheter angiography. There will be revenge.

The common carotid artery bifurcates into an external and internal carotid artery approximately at the level of the third or fourth cervical vertebral body in most persons. The angle of the mandible is another good marker

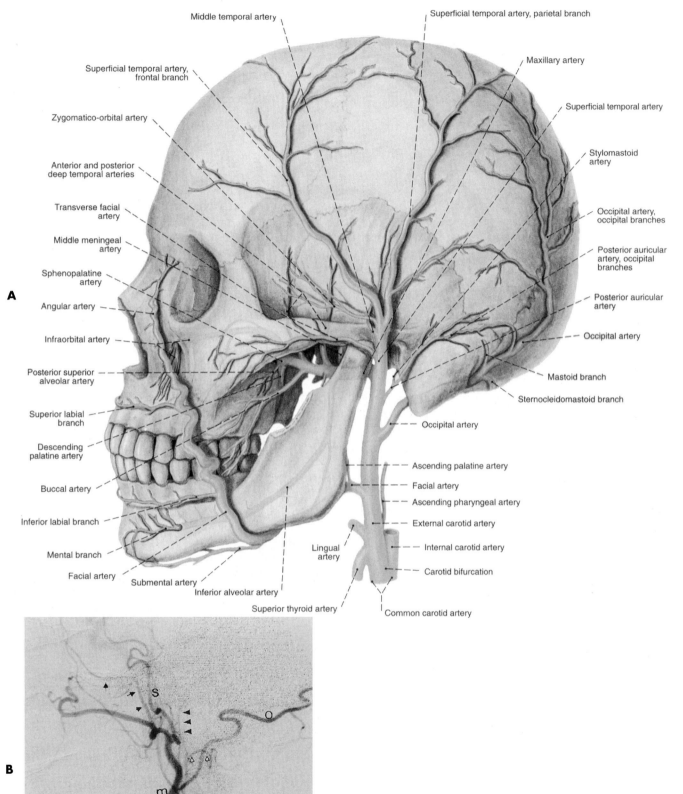

Middle temporal artery

Superficial temporal artery, parietal branch

Superficial temporal artery, frontal branch

Maxillary artery

Zygomatico-orbital artery

Superficial temporal artery

Anterior and posterior deep temporal arteries

Stylomastoid artery

Transverse facial artery

Occipital artery, occipital branches

Middle meningeal artery

Posterior auricular artery, occipital branches

Sphenopalatine artery

Posterior auricular artery

Angular artery

Occipital artery

Infraorbital artery

Posterior superior alveolar artery

Mastoid branch

Sternocleidomastoid branch

Superior labial branch

Occipital artery

Descending palatine artery

Ascending palatine artery

Facial artery

Buccal artery

Ascending pharyngeal artery

Inferior labial branch

External carotid artery

Internal carotid artery

Mental branch

Lingual artery

Carotid bifurcation

Facial artery

Submental artery

Inferior alveolar artery

Superior thyroid artery

Common carotid artery

A

B

Fig. 2-25 ECA anatomy. **A,** The external carotid artery and its branches, lateral aspect (60%). (From Putz R, Pabst R [eds]: *Sobotta atlas of human anatomy,* ed 13, Philadelphia, Lippincott Williams & Wilkins, 1996, p. 76.) **B,** External carotid artery circulation. Lateral view of a common carotid injection with preferential filling of the external system shows lingual *(l),* facial *(f),* ascending pharyngeal *(arrowheads),* internal maxillary *(m),* occipital *(o),* and superficial temporal *(s)* branches. The middle meningeal artery *(arrows)* is seen and the posterior auricular artery *(open arrows)* is superimposed on the occipital artery.

for the carotid bifurcation. Above this level it becomes harder and harder for the surgeon performing a carotid endarterectomy (CEA) to get control of the vessel. The external carotid artery courses anteromedial to the internal carotid artery from the bifurcation. However, the internal carotid artery crosses medial to the external carotid artery at approximately the C1–2 level as it turns to enter the skull.

External Carotid Branches

The branches of the external carotid artery can be remembered by the mnemonic, "She always likes friends over Papa, Sister, and Mamma." With this memory aid, you can remember the external carotid artery branches of superior thyroidal, ascending pharyngeal, lingual, facial, occipital, posterior auricular, superficial temporal, and maxillary arteries (Fig. 2-25). Knowing the branches of the external carotid artery is important for understanding the vascular supply to head and neck and skull base tumors such as glomus tumors, angiofibromas, and meningiomas. Anterior and middle cranial fossa meningiomas by and large are supplied by the anterior and posterior divisions of the middle meningeal artery, a branch of the internal maxillary artery. The ascending pharyngeal artery is the artery that is typically implicated in supply of glomus jugulare, glomus tympanicum, carotid body tumors, and juvenile angiofibromas.

The superior thyroidal artery emerges off the anterior aspect of the external carotid artery and supplies the rostral aspect of the thyroid gland. It runs with the external laryngeal nerve (a branch of the vagus' superior laryngeal nerve, which supplies the cricothyroideus muscle) and gives limited blood supply to the larynx. The thyroid gland also receives blood supply from inferior thyroidal vessels from the subclavian artery's thyrocervical trunk.

The ascending pharyngeal artery has three divisions. Whereas its anterior (pharyngeal) branch supplies the posterolateral pharyngeal wall and palatine tonsil, the middle (neuromeningeal) and posterior branches have extensive supply to the jugular foramen region, supplying the vasa nervorum of cranial nerves IX, X, and XI.

The lingual artery arises anteriorly off the external carotid artery and has a characteristic hook in it. It supplies the tongue and pharynx, eventually entering the sublingual space and coursing along to supply the mandible and submandibular gland.

The facial artery also supplies the region around the mandible, submandibular gland, and maxilla before anastomosing with distal branches of the internal maxillary artery to supply the remainder of the anterior lower facial region. It has labial artery branches for the upper and lower lips, a lateral nasal branch to the nose, and a terminal angular artery at the medial canthus of the eye.

Its nasal and orbital ramifications anastomose with ophthalmic branches to the same region.

The occipital artery arises posteriorly off the external carotid artery and branches off to the sternocleidomastoid muscle, posterior belly of the digastric muscle, the back of the head, and the meninges. The stylomastoid branch of the occipital artery may supply skull base lesions such as glomus tumors.

The posterior auricular artery supplies the back of the ear and has meningeal anastomoses to the posterior fossa.

The superficial temporal branch supplies the parotid gland, masseter, buccinator muscles, lateral part of the scalp, and the anterior scalp and cheek. Anterior branches anastomose with ophthalmic artery branches whereas posterior branches join posterior auricular and occipital artery supply.

Branches of the internal maxillary artery are significant for supplying collateral circulation to the distal internal carotid artery when internal carotid artery thrombosis occurs. The middle meningeal artery may anastomose with ethmoidal branches of the ophthalmic artery, or collateral circulation may be achieved by way of the meningolacrimal artery to the ophthalmic artery (see Chapter 10). On the lateral arteriogram the middle meningeal artery can be distinguished from the superficial temporal artery by (1) its less sinuous appearance, (2) its entrance at the foramen spinosum, (3) its origin from the internal maxillary artery, (4) its persistence within the confines of the skull, and (5) its characteristic course and divisions running anteriorly and posteriorly. Other internal maxillary artery branches besides the middle meningeal artery such as the ethmoidal, temporal, lacrimal, palpebral, or muscular branches may also anastomose to the ophthalmic artery. The artery of the foramen rotundum from the maxillary artery may anastomose with branches of the inferolateral trunk of the cavernous segment of the internal carotid artery. The vidian artery may also anastomose to the cavernous carotid artery. Additional external carotid–internal carotid artery vascular anastomoses include the branches of the ascending pharyngeal artery to the internal carotid artery via petrous and carotid artery branches. The occipital artery may anastomose to the internal carotid via the stylomastoid artery.

External carotid system anastomoses to the vertebral artery may occur via the occipital artery, ascending pharyngeal artery, or posterior auricular artery. The occipital artery supplies the scalp and occipital musculature. It sends meningeal branches to the foramen magnum, the jugular foramen, the hypoglossal canal, and the mastoid canal.

Several anastomotic channels that are present in fetal life and connect carotid and vertebral circulations usually regress in utero but can remain patent in rare instances (Fig. 2-26). The persistent trigeminal artery is a

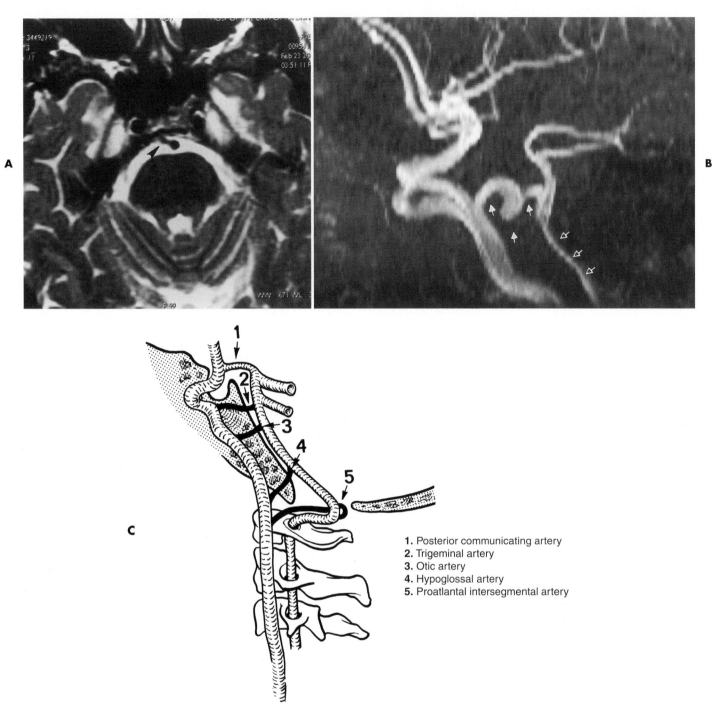

Fig. 2-26 Persistent fetal connections. **A,** Axial T2WI demonstrating a persistent trigeminal artery *(arrowhead)* exiting the basilar artery and heading into the cavernous sinus. **B,** MRA shows the persistent trigeminal artery *(arrows).* The hypoplastic basilar artery is also visualized *(open arrows).* **C,** Anatomic diagram depicts the embryonic carotid-basilar and carotid-vertebral anastomoses. The anterior communicating artery is the only vessel that normally persists; the other four, shown in black, usually regress completely. (From Osborne AG: *Diagnostic cerebral angiography,* ed 2, Philadelphia, Lippincott, Williams & Wilkins 1998, p. 69, Fig 3-14.)

vessel that connects the cavernous carotid artery to the upper basilar artery in 0.1% to 0.2% of people. This normal variant may be associated with hypoplasia of the vertebrobasilar system below the anastomosis. The persistent otic and hypoglossal arteries are found more inferiorly (and much more rarely) connecting the petrous (otic) and cervical (hypoglossal) internal carotid artery to the lower basilar artery. A persistent proatlantal artery is found at the C2 level and connects the cervical carotid to the vertebral artery (Table 2-5).

Table 2-5   Persistent vascular connections

Persistent artery	Origin	Feeds	Location	Coexistent findings
Trigeminal	Cavernous carotid	Top of basilar	Suprasellar cistern	Aneurysms
Otic	Petrous carotid	Mid basilar	Internal auditory canal	
Hypoglossal	High cervical internal carotid at skull base	Intracranial vertebrobasilar circulation	Hypoglossal canal	
Proatlantal type 1	Low internal carotid	Cranial and cervical Vertebrobasilar circulation	C2 level	
Proatlantal type 2	External carotid	Cranial and cervical Vertebrobasilar circulation	C2 level	Hypoplastic vertebral arteries

Intracranial Circulation

The intracranial circulation is supplied by paired internal carotid arteries and paired vertebral arteries, the latter of which join to form the basilar artery. (Everything good comes in pairs!) Because of the collateral network inherent in the circle of Willis, where the carotid and vertebrobasilar systems are connected, the brain possesses a redundant defense against major-vessel occlusive disease. Such is not the case with the branches distal to the circle of Willis, where collateral circulation is less easily supplied. Therefore, it is important to understand the vascular anatomy and arterial supply to localize vasculopathy.

The internal carotid arteries have cervical (C1), petrous (C2), lacerum (C3), and cavernous portions (C4) before they pierce the dura to enter the intracranial space. The clinoid segment (C5), ophthalmic segment (C6), and communicating segment (C7) follow the cavernous segment (C4). On routine angiography in a normal patient, you do not see branches in the cervical or petrous portions of the internal carotid artery. Occasionally, the ophthalmic artery may arise below the dura from the intracavernous carotid artery, and rarely one may be able to see hypophyseal branches from the cavernous carotid artery. When carotid occlusive disease or vascular masses are present, the small branches from the petrous carotid artery (the tympanic arteries, vidian artery, and caroticotympanic branch) may be enlarged and visible on lateral carotid injections. The cavernous carotid branches include the (1) lateral mainstem artery (inferolateral trunk), (2) meningohypophyseal arteries, and (3) capsular sellar branches of McConnell. The tentorial artery off the meningohypophyseal trunk of the cavernous carotid artery is given the eponym the artery of Bernasconi-Casanari (see Fig. 3-9). This is a classic question asked at the board examinations. Remember it.

In 80% to 90% of cases, the ophthalmic artery arises intradurally, just below the anterior clinoid process. Branches of the ophthalmic artery anastomose with those from the maxillary artery, providing a rich network for collateral supply in the event of proximal carotid artery occlusion. The ophthalmic artery supplies the orbit, the globe, the frontal scalp region, the frontal and ethmoidal sinuses, and the upper part of the nose. It has anastomoses with facial and internal maxillary artery branches.

The next branch of the internal carotid artery distal to the ophthalmic artery is the posterior communicating artery (PCOM) (Fig. 2-27). It connects the anterior carotid circulation with the posterior vertebrobasilar artery circulation. Occasionally, the connection to the basilar artery is absent and the PCOM directly feeds the posterior cerebral artery on that side (a fetal PCA). The PCOM supplies parts of the thalamus, hypothalamus, optic chiasm, and mamillary bodies. Its named branches are the anterior thalamoperforate vessels. They supply parts of the thalamus, internal capsule, and optic tracts. Posterior thalamoperforate arteries, the artery of Persheron, and thalamogeniculate branches arise from the proximal posterior cerebral artery (the P1 segment), but the PCOM may give minimal supply to these areas.

The anterior choroidal artery is the next branch of the supraclinoid intradural carotid artery. The anterior choroidal artery courses through the ambient cistern before entering the choroid plexus of the temporal horn via the choroidal fissure at the plexal point. The anterior choroidal artery supplies (and follows) portions of the optic tract, medial temporal lobe, uncus, amygdala, hippocampus, anterior limb of the internal capsule, choroid plexus of the lateral ventricle, inferior globus pallidus,

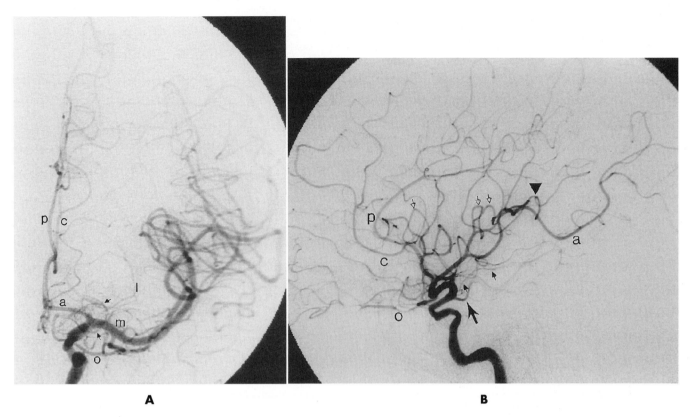

A   **B**

Fig. 2-27   Internal carotid artery anatomy (digital subtraction arteriogram). **A,** AP view of an internal carotid artery injection shows filling of ACA and MCA branches. Minimal PCOM filling is seen *(arrows)*. The M-1 *(m)* and A-1 *(a)* segments are labeled. Note that the pericallosal artery *(p)* remains closer to the midline than callosal-marginal *(c)* branches. Lenticulostriate branches *(l)* and the ophthalmic artery *(o)* can also be made out. **B,** Lateral view again demonstrates partial filling of the PCOM *(large arrow)* and good opacification of the pericallosal *(p)* and callosal-marginal *(c)* branches. The ophthalmic artery *(o)*, anterior choroidal artery *(small arrows)*, sylvian loops of the insula *(open arrows)*, sylvian point *(large arrowhead)*, and angular branch *(a)* of the MCA can be identified.

caudate nucleus, cerebral peduncles, and midbrain. That is a lot of territory for a relatively small artery seen at angiography.

Anterior Cerebral Artery System

The internal carotid artery terminates at a bifurcation into the anterior and middle cerebral arteries. The first, horizontal portion of the anterior cerebral artery (ACA) is termed the A-1 segment, and as it turns superiorly along the genu of the corpus callosum it forms the A-2 segment. This then bifurcates into pericallosal and callosomarginal arteries. The ipsilateral A-1 and contralateral A-1 ACAs are connected via the anterior communicating artery (ACOM). The A-1 segment gives off medial lenticulostriate arteries to the basal ganglia and anterior limb of the internal capsule. Infarctions in the medial lenticulostriate distribution affect motor function of the face and arm. One named branch, the recurrent artery of Heubner, supplies the head of the caudate and anteroinferior internal capsule. The ACOM also gives off small perforating vessels.

Distal branches of the ACA supply the olfactory bulbs and tracts, the corpus callosum, and the medial aspects

of the frontal and parietal lobes (Fig. 2-28). Therefore ACA infarctions affect olfaction, thought processes (the medial inferior frontal lobe), motor function of the leg (precentral gyrus medially), sensation to the leg (postcentral gyrus medially), memory, and emotion (the cingulate gyrus).

A series of internal frontal and internal parietal arteries arise from the callosomarginal artery after it gives off anteroinferior orbitofrontal and frontopolar branches. The terminations of the pericallosal artery and the callosomarginal artery are the splenial and cuneal arteries, respectively.

In the days of the radiologic giants (before CT or MR), the ACA on the frontal projection was used to identify the location of intraparenchymal masses. It is hard to believe that suprasellar extension of pituitary adenomas used to be diagnosed by superior displacement of the A-1 segment of the ACA on angiograms. However, the giants were able to derive even more information from the course of the ACA and its relationship to the falx. Because the falx cerebri extends inferiorly and has a tough, inflexible, long posteriormost portion, the ACA is not as mobile posteriorly as anteriorly. The so-called round shift is caused by a frontal mass, and the ACA is

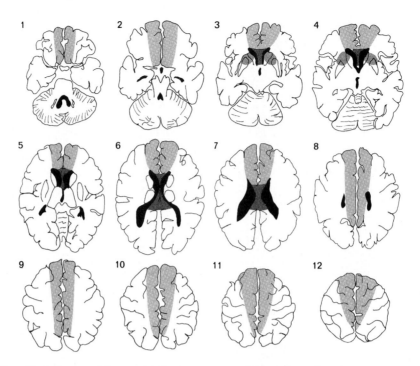

Fig. 2-28 ACA distribution. Shaded areas of these axial diagrams, arranged in sequence from base to vertex, outline the territory of the ACA including the medial lenticulostriate (*medium shading*), callosal (*dark shading*), and hemispheric branches (*light shading*). (From Latchaw RE: *MR and CT imaging of the head, neck, and spine,* ed 2, St. Louis, Mosby, 1991.)

seen to bend freely and smoothly in an arc anteriorly, returning to the midline posteriorly as it becomes confined by the posterior falx (Fig. 2-29). A "square shift" of the ACA denotes a posterior mass, be it temporal, posterior frontal, or anterior parietal. The ACA branches start out across the midline anteriorly, then return sharply to the midline posterior to the mass. A "proximal shift" is seen with low frontal and anterior temporal masses. The inferoanterior portion of the ACA, before its course around the genu of the corpus callosum, is shifted across the midline. It gradually returns to midline as it proceeds more distally. Finally, a "distal shift" implies parietal, posterior temporal, or occipital lobe lesions. The anterior ACA tributaries are in the midline, but the posterior course is shifted gradually across midline, confined by the tough posterior falx. The shift is usually rather contained and the return to midline abrupt.

Middle Cerebral Artery System

The horizontal portion of the middle cerebral artery (MCA) is termed its M-1 segment, and it too gives off (lateral) lenticulostriate arteries that supply the globus pallidus, putamen, and internal capsule. Lateral lenticulostriate infarctions cause internal capsule damage typically resulting in hemiparesis and sensory deficits on the contralateral side of the body. Speech may be affected because the medial temporal lobes are affected. Vision may be affected because of involvement of the optic ra-

diations as they sweep from the lateral geniculate to Meyer's loop in the temporal lobes.

The M-2 segment refers to the sylvian segment of the MCA after it trifurcates into an anterior division, posterior division, and the anterior temporal artery. The distal branches of the MCA course lateral to the insula, and then loop around the frontal operculum to form the "candelabra" effect of the sylvian triangle on the lateral surface of the cortex (M-3 segment). The last branch of the sylvian vessels of the MCA is the angular artery supplying the angular gyrus just beyond the sylvian fissure. Other branches supply frontal and parietal lobes. Anterior and inferior temporal branches supply the vast majority of the temporal lobe (Fig. 2-30).

MCA infarctions may affect motor and sensory function of the face, arm, and trunk (lateral precentral and postcentral gyri), speech (inferior lateral frontotemporal gyri), thought processes (anteroinferolateral frontal lobes), hearing (superior temporal gyri), memory and naming of objects (temporal lobe), and taste (insular cortex).

It is important to understand that the circle of Willis may be congenitally incomplete or narrowed in many cases. The intact ring from distal internal carotid artery to A-1 ipsilateral ACA, to ACOM, to contralateral A-1, to contralateral distal internal carotid artery, to contralateral PCOM, to contralateral P-1 segment of the posterior cerebral artery (PCA), to basilar artery, to ipsilateral P-1 PCA, to ipsilateral PCOM, back to ipsilateral internal carotid artery is most frequently broken by a hypoplastic or absent A-1 segment (Fig. 2-31). Fetal origin of the

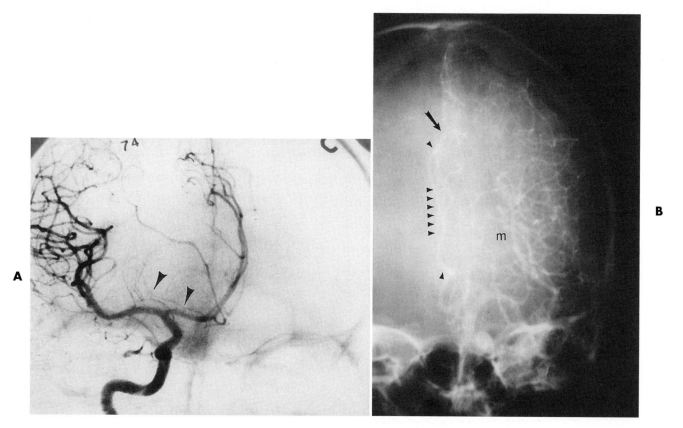

Fig. 2-29 ACA shifts. **A,** Round shift. This right internal carotid artery arteriogram demonstrates a round shift of the ACA caused by medial basal ganglionic hemorrhage. Note that the artery of Heubner *(arrowheads)* is displaced laterally. **B,** Square shift. This unsubtracted (yuk!) arteriogram from the old geezer's collection shows a square shift *(black arrowheads).* Notice that the distal ACA goes back under the falx *(arrow).* The MCA *(m)* is shifted medially. What is the etiology? Answer (read backwards): tfel no amotameh larudbus gib (note that the MCA branches do not go as far laterally as the inner table of the skull). Can you image diagnosing slarudbus this way?

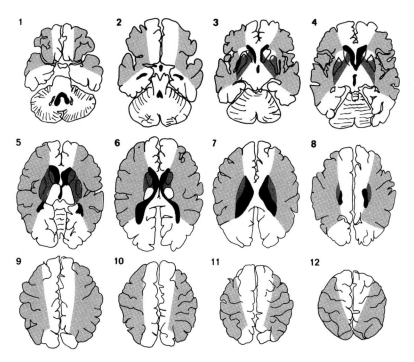

Fig. 2-30 MCA distribution. This diagram of the axial sections, arranged in sequence from base to vertex, outlines the MCA distribution with the lateral lenticulostriate *(medium shading)* and hemispheric branches *(light shading).* (From Latchaw RE: *MR and CT imaging of the head, neck, and spine,* ed 2, St Louis, Mosby, 1991.)

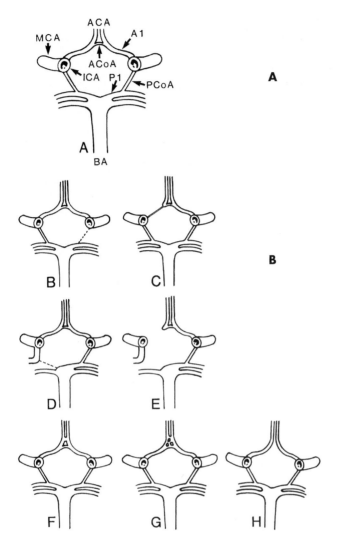

Fig. 2-31 COW. **A,** Arterial circle of Willis. **B,** Anatomic diagrams depict the circle of Willis *(a)* and its common variations *(b-h)*. *A:* A "complete" circle of Willis is present. Here all components are present and none are hypoplastic. This configuration is seen in less than half of all cases. *B:* Hypoplasia (right) or absence (left) of one or both posterior communicating arteries (PCoAs) is the most common circle of Willis variant, seen in 25% to 33% of cases. *C:* Hypoplasia or absence of the horizontal (A1) anterior cerebral artery segment is seen in approximately 10% to 20% of cases. Here the right A1 segment is absent. *D:* Fetal origin of the posterior cerebral artery (PCA) with hypoplasia of the precommunicating (P1) PCA segment, seen in 15% to 25% of cases. *E:* If both a fetal PCA and an absent A1 occur together, the internal carotid artery (ICA) is anatomically isolated with severely restricted potential collateral blood flow. Here the right ICA terminates in an MCA and fetal-type PCA. *F:* Multichannel (two or more) anterior communicating artery segments, seen in 10% to 15% of cases. Here the duplicated ACoAs are complete and both extend across the entire ACoA. *G:* In a fenestrated ACoA, the ACoA has a more plexiform appearance. *H:* Absence of an ACoA is shown. ACA, distal anterior communicating artery segments; A1, horizontal ACA segment; P1, horizontal (precommunciating) PCA segment. (From Osborne AG: *Diagnostic cerebral angiography,* ed 2, Philadelphia, Lippincott Williams & Wilkins, 1999, p. 113.)

PCA where the PCOM feeds the PCA without communication with the basilar artery is also a common variant, as is hypoplasia of the PCOMs. Fenestrated (multichanneled) ACOMs are also seen.

Vertebral Arteries

The vertebral arteries arise from the subclavian arteries and course superiorly between the longus colli and scalene muscles (V-1) before entering the vertebral canal. The artery enters at the C6 transverse foramen in 95% of cases and continues upward in the foramina of the vertebrae (V-2) before exiting at the C1-2 level. The left is bigger than the right in 75% of cases and therefore should be the first choice of vertebral arteries if you are on a search for a posterior fossa aneurysm or for basilar artery stenosis. Branches of the vertebral artery include muscular arteries to the neck, occipital, segmental spinal arteries, and the anterior spinal artery, which supplies most of the spinal cord. Posterior meningeal branches are found as the vessel travels from the atlas to pierce the dura (V-3), entering the intracranial compartment via the foramen magnum. The first branch of the vertebral artery in the intracranial compartment (V-4) is the posterior inferior cerebellar artery (PICA). This vessel loops around the medulla and tonsil while supplying the posterolateral medulla, the inferior vermis, the choroid plexus of the fourth ventricle, and the inferior aspect of the cerebellum. The inferior vermian artery and tonsillohemispheric arteries are the terminating branches of the PICA. The size of the PICA is inversely proportional to the size of the anterior inferior cerebellar artery (AICA).

PICA infarcts can induce the lateral medullary (Wallenberg) syndrome. This causes loss of pain and temperature of the body on the contralateral side (lateral spinothalamic tract) and face on the ipsilateral side (descending trigeminothalamic tract), ataxia (cerebellar connections), ipsilateral swallowing and taste disorders (ninth cranial nerve), hoarseness (tenth cranial nerve), vertigo and nystagmus (eighth nerve), and ipsilateral Horner syndrome.

Basilar Artery Branches

The two vertebral arteries join to form the basilar artery at the pontomedullary level. The basilar artery has many tiny branches to the pons and medulla that are never seen at angiography. The first major branch seen from the basilar artery is the AICA (Fig. 2-32). This vessel runs toward the cerebellopontine angle and may loop into the internal auditory canal, where it gives off labyrinthine branches to the inner ear before supplying the anteroinferior part of the cerebellum. Medullary and pontine branches also arise from the AICA.

The superior cerebellar artery is the last infratentorial branch off the basilar artery. The lateral marginal and

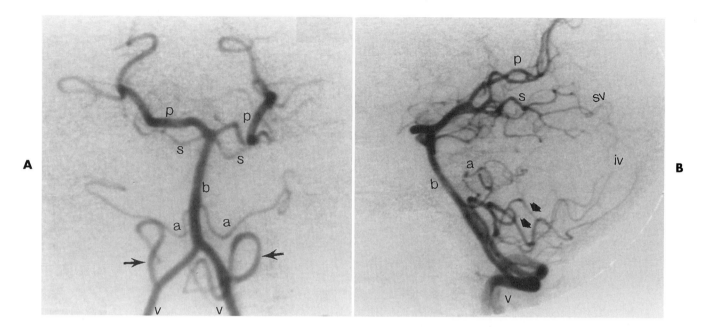

Fig. 2-32   Vertebrobasilar artery circulation. **A,** Vertebral artery arteriogram depicts the vertebral arteries *(v)*, the PICAs *(arrows)*, the AICAs *(a)*, the superior cerebellar arteries *(s)* and PCAs *(p)* on this anteroposterior view. **B,** Lateral view shows the same vascular anatomy. Basilar artery *(b)*, superior vermian *(sv)* branch of superior cerebellar artery, and inferior vermian *(iv)* branch of PICA are shown.

hemispheric branches supply the upper part of the cerebellum before the vessel terminates in the superior vermian artery. Other fine branches help supply the pons, the superior cerebellar peduncle, and the inferior colliculus. The superior vermian vessel anastomoses with the inferior vermian artery of the PICA.

The basilar artery terminates in the two PCAs and a few small perforating vessels from its vertical dome. Midbrain perforating arteries arise from the basilar artery and proximal PCAs. Infarctions of these perforating vessels can affect cranial nerves III and IV, causing oculomotor deficits; the cerebral peduncles, affecting motor strength; the medial lemniscus, altering sensation; the red nucleus and substantia nigra, affecting coordination and motor control; and the reticular activating substance, affecting the level of consciousness.

The PCAs join the anterior circulation via the PCOMs. The PCAs also have small premamillary, posterior thalamoperforate, and thalamogeniculate branches supplying the hypothalamus, midbrain, and inferior thalami. Infarctions of these vessels may affect memory and emotion (anterior thalamus), endocrine function (hypothalamus), language (pulvinar), pain sensation (thalami), sight (lateral geniculate), and motor control (subthalamic nuclei).

The next branches of the PCA are the medial and lateral posterior choroidal arteries that supply the trigone region of the lateral ventricles. Medial posterior choroidal arteries pass around the midbrain and course medially toward the pineal gland. They supply the tectum, the choroid plexus of the third ventricle, and the thalami. The lateral posterior choroidal arteries run behind the pulvinar into the choroidal fissure and supply the

choroid of the lateral and third ventricles, the posterior thalamus, and the fornix (see Fig. 2-32).

The PCA continues, branching off anterior and posterior temporal arteries and a posterior pericallosal artery before terminating into parietooccipital branches and calcarine arteries to the occipital lobe. PCA infarctions affect vision most commonly (occipital lobes) but also affect memory (posteroinferior temporal lobe), smell (hippocampal region), and emotion posterior fornix (Fig. 2-33).

Venous Anatomy

By the superficial manner in which the venous drainage of the brain is covered here, you can tell that this is the new (CT-MR) generation. No apologies are rendered; hop in your DeLorean and go "back to the future" for more venous anatomy teachings. However, at least a working knowledge of this anatomy is important when you are confronted by vascular malformations and sinus occlusions. In the right hands, venous anatomy is also useful for localization of lesions on angiograms.

Superficial Drainage

The superficial drainage of the brain is remarkable for the superficial vein of Labbé (draining from the sylvian fissure laterally), which drains into the transverse sinus, and the superior superficial vein of Trolard (draining from the sylvian fissure to the top), which empties into the superior sagittal sinus (Fig. 2-34). Superior cerebral veins also empty directly into the superior sagittal sinus.

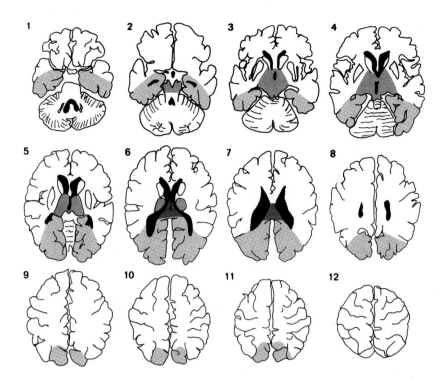

Fig. 2-33 PCA distribution. Axial diagrams arranged in sequence from base to vertex outline supply from the PCA, the thalamic and midbrain perforators (*medium shading*), callosal (*dark shading*), and hemispheric branches (*light shading*). (From Latchaw RE: *MR and CT imaging of the head, neck, and spine,* ed 2, St. Louis, Mosby, 1991.)

A

Superficial veins of cortical regions and their sinuses:
  1 Superior (superficial) cerebral veins
  2 Superior sagittal sinus
  3 Superficial middle cerebral vein (of Sylvius)
  4 Cavernous sinus
  5 Inferior petrosal sinus

Deep veins of central and nuclear regioins and their sinuses:
  6 Anterior vein of septum
  7 Superior thalamostriate
  8 Venous angle
  9 Internal cerebral vein
  10 Great cerebral vein (of Galen)
  11 Inferior sagittal sinus
  12 Basal vein (of Rosenthal)
  13 Straight sinus
  14 Confluence of sinuses
  15 Transverse sinus
  16 Sigmoid sinus
  17 Internal jugular vein

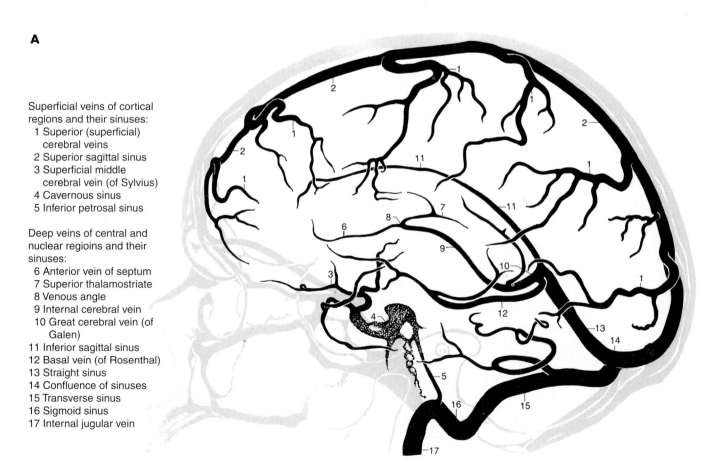

Fig. 2-34 Venous anatomy. **A,** Lateral view of the head illustrating the cerebral veins and sinuses. The sequence of the numbers takes into account both the areas drained by the veins and the direction of blood flow.

Illustration continued on following page

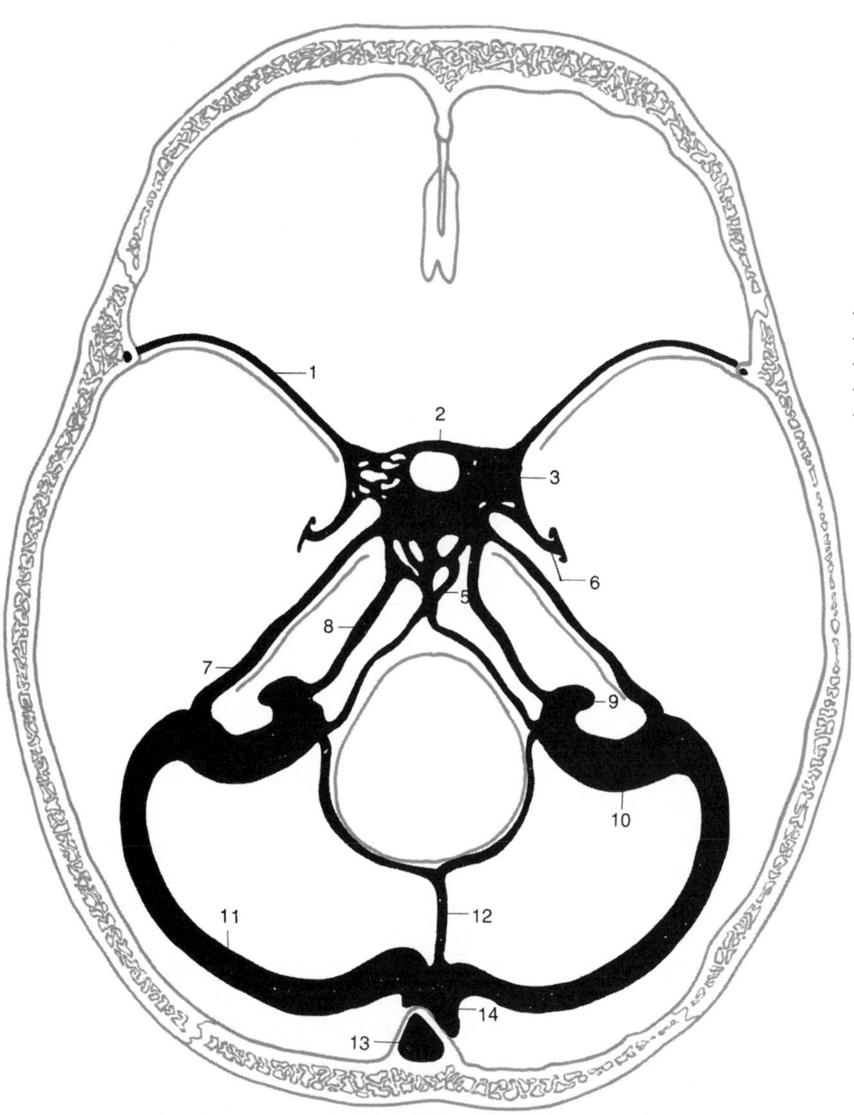

1 Sphenoparietal sinus
2 Anterior intercavernous sinus
3 Cavernous sinus
4 Posterior intercavernous sinus
5 Basilar plexus
6 Venous plexus of foramen ovale
7 Superior petrosal sinus
8 Inferior petrosal sinus
9 Internal jugular vein (running caudally)
10 Sigmoid sinus
11 Transverse sinus
12 Occipital sinus
13 Superior sagittal sinus
14 Confluence of sinuses

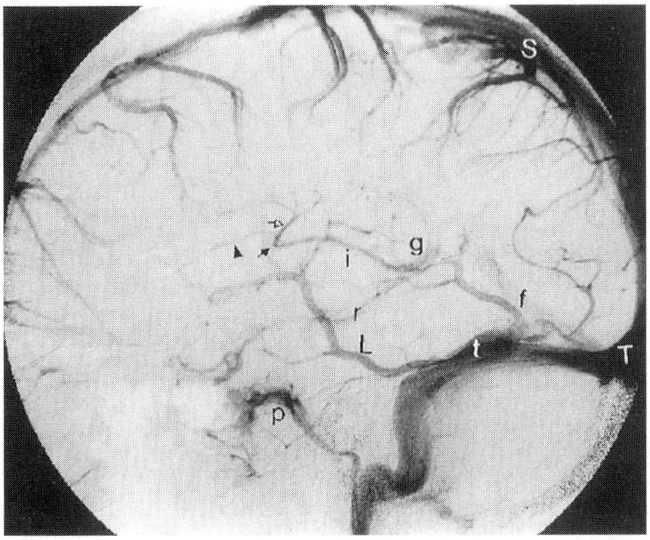

Fig. 2-34 *Continued.* **B,** The basal sinuses. **C,** Deep venous anatomy on angiography. This lateral view shows the internal cerebral vein *(i),* vein of Galen *(g),* straight sinus, torcular *(white T),* and superior sagittal sinus *(S).* The venous angle *(small black arrow)* is formed by the thalamostriate vein *(open black arrow)* and the internal cerebral vein, which is also the drainage site of the septal vein *(arrowhead).* The vein of Labbé *(L)* is superimposed and can be seen draining to the transverse *(white t)* sinus. Faintly seen are the basal vein of Rosenthal *(r)* and inferior petrosal sinus *(p).* (A and B from Kretschmann H-J, Weinrich W: *Cranial neuroimaging and clinical neuroanatomy: magnetic resonance imaging and computed tomography,* rev ed 2, New York, Thieme, 1993, pp. 214, 215.)

The superficial middle cerebral vein drains from the sylvian fissure into the cavernous sinus. The vein of Labbé may arise from the posterior extent of the superficial middle cerebral vein.

Deep Supratentorial Drainage

The deep venous drainage of the supratentorial space centers on the internal cerebral vein and the vein of Galen. Medullary veins radiate downward from the superficial white matter to drain to the subependymal and thalamostriate veins. Choroidal, caudate, terminal, lateral, atrial, and ventricular veins drain to the medial subependymal septal vein and the lateral subependymal thalamostriate vein. The septal vein courses around the anteromedial aspect of the lateral ventricle before passing behind the foramen of Monro to join the internal cerebral vein at the "true venous angle" (see Fig. 2-34). If the septal vein joins the internal cerebral vein further posteriorly than the demarcation of the foramen of Monro, the junction is called the "false venous angle." Thus, the internal cerebral veins usually begin at the foramina of Monro and run on either side of the roof of the third ventricle (velum interpositum). The internal cerebral veins unite to form the great vein of Galen. The vein of Galen drains to the straight sinus. The internal cerebral veins are a marker for midline shift, behind the foramen of Monro. They should not deviate more than 2 mm from the midline.

Deep Infratentorial Drainage

The anatomy of posterior fossa venous drainage is more complex. Superior vermian, posterior pericallosal, mesencephalic, and internal occipital veins drain into the vein of Galen at the tentorial hiatus. This vein also receives drainage from the basal vein of Rosenthal, which in turn receives venous supply from the insular lateral mesencephalic veins, and deep middle cerebral and anterior cerebral veins in the supratentorial space (Fig. 2-35). The vein of Galen and the inferior sagittal sinus drain to the straight sinus, which in turn drains into the torcular herophili. The torcular is the common dumping ground (toilet) of the venous system. It also receives the drainage from the superior sagittal sinus.

From the torcular, blood flows to the transverse sinus, which receives drainage from the superior petrosal sinus, diploic veins, and lateral cerebellar veins. It courses laterally in the leaves of the tentorium and continues as the sigmoid sinus, which also drains the occipital sinus. The sigmoid sinus terminates as the internal jugular vein. The inferior vermian veins and superior hemispheric veins drain into the straight sinus. The transverse sinus receives blood from the inferior and superior hemispheric venous system. The deep middle cerebral vein courses deep in the sylvian fissure, and it meets with the anterior cerebral vein (which runs with the corresponding artery) to form the basal vein of Rosenthal arising along the brain stem. The basal vein of Rosenthal receives blood from the anterior pontomesencephalic vein in front of the brain stem, the lateral mesencephalic veins, and the precentral cerebellar vein (just anterior to the superior vermis behind the fourth ventricle).

Anterior venous drainage centers on the cavernous sinuses (see Fig. 2-34). These venous channels receive blood from superior and inferior ophthalmic veins, the sphenoparietal sinus, and the superficial middle cerebral vein. The cavernous sinus communicates via (1) an extensive network across midline to the opposite cavernous sinus via the intercavernous sinus, (2) posteriorly via the superior petrosal sinus to the transverse sinuses just before the latter dive inferiorly to the sigmoid sinus, and (3) inferiorly into the inferior petrosal sinuses, which subsequently drain directly to the jugular bulbs. The inferior petrosal sinus also drains the internal auditory canal venous system.

Arachnoid granulations often arise in the transverse and sigmoid venous sinuses and can simulate clots or other lesions. They look like filling defects on angiography, MRA, and CT in or partially outside the sinus with CSF density. They have CSF intensity on MR with fibrous septa or vessels appearing as dark signal within them. They occur in approximately 1% of patients. Learn to ignore them. They may also look like little lytic lesions in the calvarium usually close to the torcular or inion.

Blood-Brain Barrier

It is probably appropriate after a vascular anatomy section to emphasize the role of the blood-brain barrier (BBB) in neuroimaging and in CNS pathology. The anatomy of the BBB is based on the microanatomy of the capillary endothelial cells. There are tight junctions between normal endothelial cells without gaps or channels. Very little pinocytic activity of these cells occurs under normal conditions. The astrocytic foot processes of endothelial cells cover the basement membrane. The basement membrane maintains the tubular conformation of the capillary and holds the endothelial cells together. In only a few regions in the brain do channels exist so that direct communication is present between the capillary and extracellular fluid or neurons. Such sites play a role in the feedback mechanism for hormonal homeostasis and as a port of entry into the brain for certain pathogens. They include the choroid plexus of the ventricles, the pineal gland, pituitary gland, median eminence, subcommissural organ, subfornical organ, area postrema, and organum vasculosum of the lamina terminalis.

After injection of contrast, increased attenuation is noted immediately in the vessels of the brain and struc-

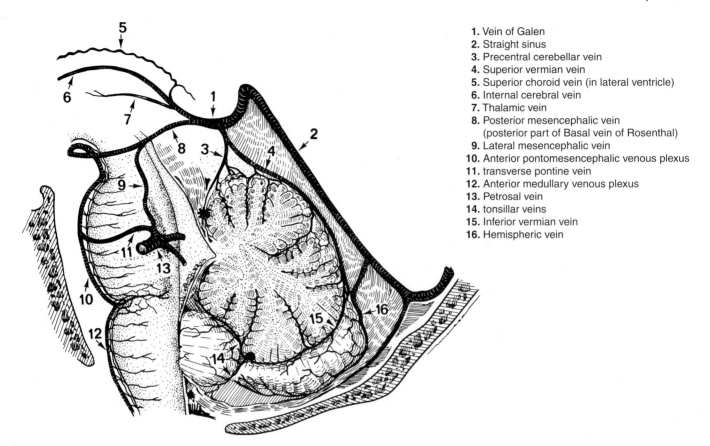

1. Vein of Galen
2. Straight sinus
3. Precentral cerebellar vein
4. Superior vermian vein
5. Superior choroid vein (in lateral ventricle)
6. Internal cerebral vein
7. Thalamic vein
8. Posterior mesencephalic vein
   (posterior part of Basal vein of Rosenthal)
9. Lateral mesencephalic vein
10. Anterior pontomesencephalic venous plexus
11. transverse pontine vein
12. Anterior medullary venous plexus
13. Petrosal vein
14. tonsillar veins
15. Inferior vermian vein
16. Hemispheric vein

Fig. 2-35   Anatomic drawing depicts the major posterior fossa veins as seen from the lateral view. The black star represents the colliculocentral point, an angiographic landmark that should be about halfway between the tuberculum sellae and the torcular herophili. *1,* vein of Galen; *2,* straight sinus; *3,* precentral cerebellar vein; *4,* superior vermian vein; *5,* superior choroid vein (in lateral ventricle); *6,* internal cerebral vein; *7,* thalamic vein; *8,* posterior mesencephalic vein; *9,* lateral mesencephalic vein; *10,* anterior pontomesencephalic venous plexus; *11,* transverse pontine vein; *12,* anterior medullary venous plexus; *13,* petrosal vein; *14,* tonsillar veins; *15,* inferior vermian veins; *16,* hemispheric vein. (From Osborne AG: *Diagnostic cerebral angiography,* ed 2, Philadelphia, Lippincott William & Wilkins, 1998, p. 234.)

tures without a BBB. Slightly increased density is also demonstrated in the cerebral parenchyma (gray matter denser than white matter) because of the cerebral blood volume (4% to 5% of total brain volume). The normal cerebral parenchymal enhancement is minimal.

Alterations of the BBB are the major component producing parenchymal enhancement. Any alteration of the BBB from factors such as inflammation, infection, neoplasm, and trauma can produce intraparenchymal enhancement. The alteration is usually in the form of unlocking of the tight junctions, increased pinocytosis of contrast agents, vascular endothelial fenestration (formation of transendothelial channels), or increased permeability of the endothelial membrane. Furthermore, in many neoplastic conditions the BBB is not competent and contrast material is distributed into the extravascular spaces. A minority of enhancement is due to increased blood volume in certain neoplastic lesions. This has recently been demonstrated by perfusion weighted MR studies of high grade neoplasm. Lack of angiographic

vascularity has little bearing on contrast enhancement. Angiogenesis at a microvascular level may also be an important factor in enhancement.

Miscellaneous   The skull base foramina, their contents, and common disorders associated with each site are summarized in Table 2-6 and depicted in Fig. 2-36.

A word on neurotransmitters: Excitatory amino acid neurotransmitters are glutamate and aspartate whereas gamma amino butyric acid (GABA), glycine, and taurine are inhibitory. Excessive accumulation of intracellular calcium can lead to neuronal death and injury and may be mediated by the NMDA (*N*-methyl D-aspartate) ionotropic receptors on the postsynaptic membrane for glutamate. The NMDA receptors activate the channels that allow the influx of the extra-cellular calcium. Overstimulation of NMDA receptors leads to calcium overload and cell death. Opening of the sodium-calcium channels causes membrane depolarization, which activates voltage dependent calcium channels, which further in-

Table 2-6   Skull base foramina and contents (see Fig. 2-29)

Skull base foramen	Contents	Disease
Cribriform plate	Olfactory nerves, anterior ethmoidal artery	Esthesioneuroblastoma
Optic canal	Optic nerve, ophthalmic artery	Optic nerve gliomas, meningiomas
Superior orbital fissure	Oculomotor, trochlear, abducens, and ophthalamic (V-1) nerves, ophthalmic veins, sympathetic nerve plexus, orbital branch of middle meningeal artery, recurrent branch of lacrimal artery	
Foramen rotundum	Maxillary (V-2) nerve	Schwannomas, meningiomas, PNS
Foramen ovale	Mandibular (V-3) nerve, accessory meningeal artery, emissary veins	Schwannomas, meningiomas, PNS
Stylomastoid foramen	Facial nerve, stylomastoid artery	PNS, Bell's palsy, schwannoma
Internal auditory canal	Facial and vestibulocochlear nerves, labyrinthine artery (branch of AICA)	Schwannomas, meningiomas, epidermoids, arachnoid cysts
Jugular foramen, pars nervosa	Glossopharyngeal nerve, inferior petrosal sinus	Schwannomas, meningiomas, PNS
Jugular foramen, pars vascularis	Vagus, spinal accessory nerves, internal jugular vein, ascending pharyngeal and occipital artery branches	Glomus tumors, schwannomas, meningiomas, PNS, metastases
Hypoglossal canal	Hypoglossal nerve, meningeal branch of ascending pharyngeal artery, emissary vein	Schwannomas
Foramen magnum	Spinal cord, vertebral arteries, spinal arteries and nerves	Meningiomas, chordomas, schwannomas
Foramen spinosum	Middle meningeal artery, meningeal branch of V-3	
Foramen lacerum	Carotid artery lies on top of it, greater petrosal nerve, vidian nerve pass above it	PNS
Incisive canal/nasopalatine canal	Nasopalatine nerve, palatine arteries	Cysts
Greater palatine canal	Greater palatine nerve, palatine vessels	PNS
Lesser palatine canal	Lesser palatine nerve and artery	PNS
Carotid canal	Internal carotid artery, sympathetic plexus	Aneurysms
Foramen of Vesalius	Emissary veins	
Petrosal	Lesser petrosal nerve	
Foramen cecum	Emissary vein	
Vestibular aqueduct	Endolymphatic duct, meningeal branch of occipital artery	Meniere's disease, congenital stenosis or patulousness
Condylar canal	Emissary vein, meningeal branch of occipital artery	
Mastoid foramen	Emissary vein, meningeal branch of occipital artery	
Palatovaginal canal	Pharyngeal branches of pterygopalatine ganglion and maxillary artery	PNS
Cochlear aqueduct	Perilymphatic duct, emissary vein	Congenital stenosis or patulousness
Inferior orbital fissure	Maxillary nerve, zygomatic nerve, orbital branches of pterygopalatine ganglion, infraorbital vessels, inferior ophthalmic veins	PNS, schwannomas
Infraorbital foramen	Infraorbital nerve and vessels	Blow-out fractures
Mental foramen	Mental nerves and vessels	Squamous cell carcinoma
Mandibular foramen	Inferior alveolar nerve and vessels	Schwannomas, squamous cell carcinoma
Pterygomaxillary fissure	Maxillary artery, maxillary nerve, sphenopalatine veins	Juvenile angiofibromas
Vidian canal	Vidian nerve and artery	PNS

PNS, Perineural spread of cancer.

creases intracellular calcium levels. Causes of excessive glutamate accumulation are separated into those that cause increased release of glutamate into the extracellular space, decreased glutamate uptake from the synap-tic space, or spillage from an injured neuron. Trauma can cause spillage of glutamate from transected neurons. Parenchymal loss in age-associated dementia is thought to be related to glutamate cytotoxic injury. This may also

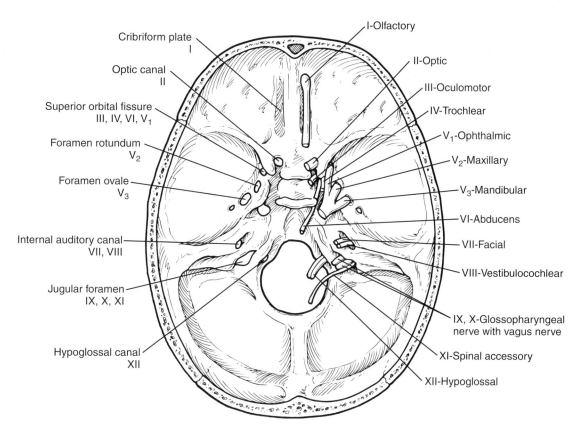

Fig. 2-36 Skull base foramina. This diagram illustrates the exits of the cranial nerve through the skull base foramina.

occur with mesial temporal sclerosis. Ischemia due to abnormal release of glutamate from storage sites can lead to excessive glutamate accumulation and the resultant injury impairs reuptake by the glutamate transporters. To protect against the toxic affects of glutamte, sodium channel blockers can be used to decrease glutamate release. Voltage dependent channel blockers can also decrease glutamate release.

"You're not a man" is an anagram of "Neuroanatomy," and "You're not a woman" is an anagram of "Wo, neuroanatomy!" Now that you have learned it, you are men and women of neuroradiology. See you next chapter.

SUGGESTED READINGS

Alsop DC, Detre JA, D'Esposito M, et al: Functional activation during an auditory comprehension task in patients with temporal lobe lesions, *Neuroimage* 4:55-59, 1996.

Barkovich AJ: MR of the normal neonatal brain: assessment of deep structures, *AJNR* 19:1397-1403, 1998.

Carpenter MB, Sutin J: *Human neuroanatomy,* ed 8, Baltimore, 1983, Williams & Wilkins.

Chong VF, Fan YF: Radiology of the jugular foramen, *Clin Radiol* 53:405-416, 1998.

Davatzikos C, Vaillant M, Resnick SM, et al: A computerized approach for morphological analysis of the corpus callosum, *J Comput Assist Tomogr* 20:88-97, 1996.

Frackowiak RS, Zeki S, Poline JB, Friston KJ: A critique of a new analysis proposed for functional neuroimaging [see comments], *Eur J Neurosci* 8:2229-2231, 1996.

Friston KJ, Frith CD, Fletcher P, et al: Functional topography: multidimensional scaling and functional connectivity in the brain, *Cerebral Cortex* 6:156-164, 1996.

Gilissen E, Zilles K: The calcarine sulcus as an estimate of the total volume of human striate cortex: a morphometric study of reliability and intersubject variability, *J Hirnforschung* 37:57-66, 1996.

Hayman LA, Fuller GN, Cavazos JE, et al: The hippocampus: normal anatomy and pathology, *AJR* 171:1139-1146, 1998.

Hayman LA: *Clinical brain imaging: normal structure and functional anatomy,* St Louis, 1992, Mosby.

Insausti R, Tunon T, Sobreviela T, et al: The human entorhinal cortex: a cytoarchitectonic analysis, *J Comparative Neurol* 355:171-198, 1995.

Kier EL, Fulbright RK, Bronen RA: Limbic lobe embryology and anatomy: dissection and MR of the medial surface of the fetal cerebral hemisphere, *AJNR* 16:1847-1853, 1995.

Lanziere CF: MR imaging of the cranial nerves, *AJR* 154:1263-1278, 1990.

Latchaw RE: *MR and CT imaging of the head, neck, and spine,* ed 2, St. Louis, 1991, Mosby.

Murphy DG, DeCarli C, McIntosh AR, et al: Sex differences in human brain morphometry and metabolism: an in vivo quantitative magnetic resonance imaging and positron emission tomography study on the effect of aging, *Arch Gen Psychiatr* 53:585-594, 1996.

Netter FH: *CIBA collection of medical illustrations,* 1993, CIBA-GEIGY Corporation.

Nieuwenhuys R, Voogd J, van Huijzen C: *The human central nervous system,* ed 3, Berlin, 1988, Springer-Verlag.

Price CJ, Wise RJ, Warburton EA, et al: Hearing and saying. The functional neuro-anatomy of auditory word processing, *Brain* 119:919-931, 1996.

Royet JP, Koenig O, Gregoire MC, et al: Functional anatomy of perceptual and semantic processing for odors. *J Cogn Neurosci* 11:94-109, 1999.

Schlaepfer TE, Harris GJ, Tien AY, et al: Structural differences in the cerebral cortex of healthy female and male subjects: a magnetic resonance imaging study, *Psychiatr Res* 61:129-135, 1995.

Soares JC, Mann JJ: The functional neuroanatomy of mood disorders, *J Psychiatr Res* 31:393-432, 1997.

Stock KW, Wetzel S, Kirsch E, et al: Anatomic evaluation of the circle of Willis: MR angiography versus intraarterial digital subtraction angiography, *AJNR* 17:1495-1499, 1996.

Waldemar G: Functional brain imaging with SPECT in normal aging and dementia. Methodological, pathophysiological, and diagnostic aspects. *Cerebrovascular & Brain Metabolism Reviews* 7:89-130, 1995.

Wilson-Pauwels L, Akesson EJ, Stewart PA: *Cranial nerves,* Toronto, 1988, BC Decker.

Neoplasms of the Brain

In the first edition of this textbook, we described the appearances of neoplasms of the central nervous system (CNS) as the artistic masterpieces of neuroradiology. The analogies we used apparently lacked universal appeal (the reviewer from *Radiology* wrote ". . . the fact that I found these references more confusing than helpful is simply an admission of my artistic naiveté"). Despite our lofty intention of raising neuroradiology to an art form, we have been forced to rethink our approach to brain tumors. Perhaps they do not constitute the beauty of the art gallery—maybe they are more like the offerings of a Lancaster-style smorgasbord. Perhaps that analogy is more universally appealing. So join us on this stroll down the banquet hall as we sample from the wide array of tumors offered. Predicting the pathology of a tumor affords the neuroradiologist an opportunity to truly shine and leave the reading room with a good taste in his/her mouth.

We will be basing our analysis in part on the latest World Health Organization (WHO) classification of tu-mors. Members of the International Society of Neuropathology, International Academy of Pathology, and Preuss Foundation for Brain Tumor Research met in Lyon France for several bottles of wine and a lengthy discussion of whether to spell the word "tumor" or "tumour." On the last day they concocted a classification of brain tumors that we will share with you in this book. WHO let the tumours out? WHO? WHO? WHO? WHO?

The first taste is the most critical. The essential distinction that a neuroradiologist must make is whether a lesion is intraaxial (intraparenchymal) or extraaxial (outside the brain substance; i.e., meningeal, dural, epidural, or intraventricular). Think of tasting a new food blindfolded. Probably the first distinction you would make is whether the food is a fruit, meat, or a vegetable. This distinction has been made easier by the multiplanar capabilities of magnetic resonance (MR) imaging. The quintessential and most common *extraaxial* mass is the meningioma, a readily treatable and diagnosable lesion. The meningioma is not only extraaxial but also *intradural*. Extraaxial intradural lesions buckle the white matter, expand the ipsilateral subarachnoid space, and sometimes cause reactive bony changes. On MR scans you can visualize the dural margin and determine that the lesion is extraaxial. The prototypical *extradural* (epidural) extraaxial mass, a bone metastasis, displaces the dura inward (is superficial to the dural coverings) but otherwise may have the same contour as an intradural extraaxial mass (Fig. 3-1 A and B).

When you are confronted with a solitary *intraaxial* mass in an adult, the odds are nearly even that the lesion is either a solitary metastasis or a primary brain tumor. Fifty percent of metastases to the brain are solitary, so the lack of multiplicity should not dissuade you from considering a metastasis in the setting of a single intraaxial lesion. You can classify a lesion as intraaxial if (1) it expands the cortex of the brain; (2) there is no ex-

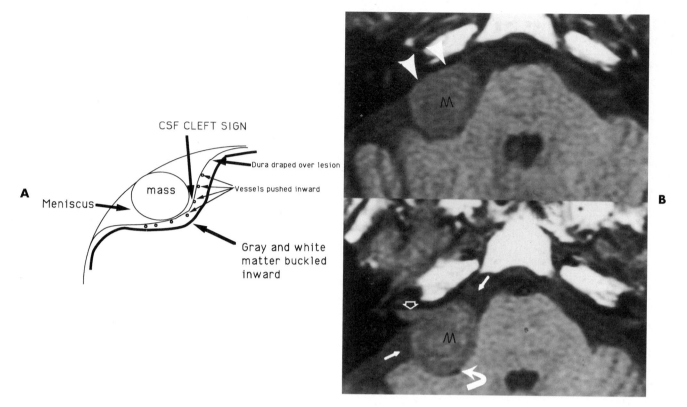

Fig. 3-1 Extra-axial lesion signs. **A,** A skull-based extradural mass is depicted diagrammatically, producing a meniscus sign, displacement of the subarachnoid veins inward, and buckling of the gray-white interface. Dura may be seen stretched over the mass. **B,** Extra-axial mass. The classic extra-axial mass (M) expands the subarachnoid space at its borders *(straight arrows)*, has a dural base *(arrowheads)*, and displaces blood vessels in the subarachnoid space medially *(curved arrow)*. This was a vestibular schwannoma, but on the top image it could just as easily be a meningioma with that dural base. Notice the extension into the internal auditory canal on the lower image *(open arrow)*.

pansion of the subarachnoid space; (3) the lesion spreads across well-defined boundaries; and (4) the hypointense dura and pial blood vessels are peripheral to the mass.

Occasionally, the distinction between intraaxial and extraaxial lesions may be blurred, because some extraaxial lesions may aggressively invade the underlying brain (aggressive meningiomas, dural metastases). Conversely, an intraaxial lesion may invade the meninges. Although the latter is somewhat atypical, it has been described in neoplasms such as lymphoma, glioblastoma multiforme, and parenchymal metastases.

If you err initially in your gustatory analysis, all other ruminations will be flawed. It is understandable that you will occasionally run across a soy burger or ballpark frank that you will not know whether the food is an animal, vegetable, or mineral (and for the ballpark frank we may never know). Sometimes, as with the low quality (nonkosher) hot dog, you may obtain a biopsy and it comes back vegetable filling or rodent hair—clearly a case of sampling error, which also occurs with some brain tumors that are of mixed grade. You must stand your ground then and insist that the lesion in question is a wienie. In a similar fashion you must localize a lesion as intraaxial or extraaxial so your differential diag-

nosis will be relevant. Once you have made that decision, you must appreciate its other qualities; its shape (margination), its consistency (solid, hemorrhagic, calcified, fatty, cystic), its colors (density), its aftertaste (enhancement). These are the secondary features in intraaxial and extraaxial lesions that allow you to arrive at the specific delicious diagnosis. If you get the right diagnosis you are cooking with gas, and then YOU will be the hot dog!

EXTRAAXIAL TUMORS

Tumors of the Meninges

Meningiomas
Meningiomas constitute the most common extraaxial neoplasm of the brain (Box 3-1). These tumors can be likened to cooked eggs. Although the shape of this lesion often looks like an egg cooked over easy, what with a central mass (the yolk of the egg) and a trailing dural based edge (the whites of the egg at the periphery), occasionally, they may be appear wholly ovoid like a hardboiled egg. That said, meningiomas can also grow into

Box 3-1 WHO Classification of Tumors of the Meninges

TUMORS OF MENINGOTHELIAL CELLS

Meningioma
Meningothelial
Fibrous (fibroblastic)
Transitional (mixed)
Psammomatous
Angiomatous
Microcystic
Secretory
Lymphoplasmacyte-rich
Metaplastic
Clear cell
Chordoid
Atypical
Papillary
Rhabdoid
Anaplastic meningioma

MESENCHYMAL, NON-MENINGOTHELIAL TUMORS

Lipoma
Angiolipoma
Hibernoma
Liposarcoma
Solitary fibrous tumor
Fibrosarcoma
Malignant fibrous histiocytoma
Leiomyoma
Leiomyosarcoma
Rhabdomyoma
Rhabdomyosarcoma
Chondroma
Chondrosarcoma
Osteoma
Osteosarcoma
Osteochondroma
Hemangioma
Epithelioid hemangioendothelioma
Hemangiopericytoma
Angiosarcoma
Kaposi Sarcoma

PRIMARY MELANOCYTIC LESIONS

Diffuse melanocytosis
Melanocytoma
Malignant melanoma
Meningeal melanocytosis

TUMORS OF UNCERTAIN HISTIOGENESIS

Hemangioblastoma

---

neoplasms in men and in adults of all age groups. The most common locations for meningioma (in descending order) are the parasagittal dura, convexities, sphenoid wing, cerebellopontine angle cistern, olfactory groove, and planum sphenoidale. Ninety percent occur supratentorially. One percent of meningiomas occur outside the CNS, presumably from embryologic arachnoid rests. The most common sites for these "extradural" meningiomas are the sinonasal cavity, parotid gland, and skin (Hey this is supposed to be a brain chapter!). Because meningiomas arise from arachnoid cap cells, they can occur anywhere that arachnoid exists.

On unenhanced CT scans, approximately 60% of meningiomas are slightly hyperdense compared with normal brain tissue (Fig. 3-2). You may see calcification within meningiomas in approximately 20% of cases. Rarely, cystic, osteoblastic, chondromatous, or fatty degeneration of meningiomas occurs (Fig. 3-3). The specific histologic subtypes of meningioma—transitional, fibroblastic, and syncytial—cannot be readily distinguished on imaging.

MR is superior to CT in detecting the full extent of meningiomas, sinus invasion and/or thrombosis, vascularity, intracranial edema, and intraosseous extension. The typical MR signal intensity characteristics of meningiomas consist of isointensity to slight hypointensity relative to gray matter on the T1-weighted image (T1WI) and isointensity to hyperintensity relative to gray matter on the T2-weighted image (T2WI). The "cleft sign" has been described in MR to identify extraaxial intradural lesions such as meningiomas. The cleft usually contains

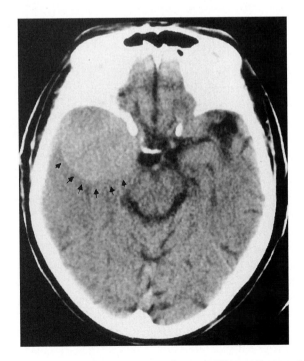

Fig. 3-2 Meningioma. Axial unenhanced CT scan shows a hyperdense *(arrows)* extraaxial mass in the middle cranial fossa.

---

the bone or through the dura on occasion. This lesion commonly affects middle-aged women (women . . . eggs—good analogy). However, because of its incidence, it represents a significant proportion of the extraaxial

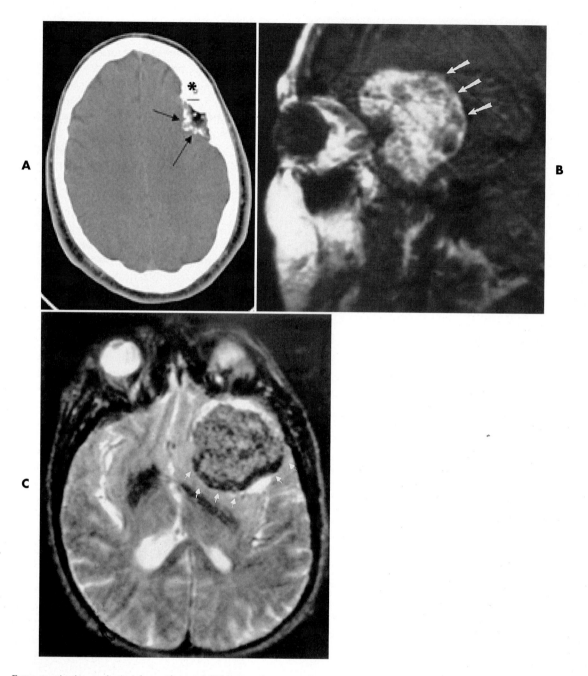

Fig. 3-3 Fatty meningioma. **A,** Axial unenhanced CT image shows an extraaxial fat-containing mass (low density centrally), which represents fatty degeneration of a meningioma. The lesion also has calcification *(arrows)* along its medial border The bone is thickened superficially *(asterisk)* which also suggests the correct diagnosis. **B,** Sagittal T1WI shows a high signal intensity extraaxial mass *(arrows)* in the left frontotemporal region on an unenhanced scan. **C,** On T2WI this scan demonstrates a chemical shift artifact *(arrows)* identifying its fatty composition. The lesion has a bright anterior and dark posterior border because of the frequency shift from fat.

one or more of the following: (1) cerebrospinal fluid (CSF) between the lesion and the underlying brain parenchyma, (2) hypointense dura (made of fibrous tissue), and (3) marginal blood vessels trapped between the lesion and the brain. Just as the yolk of an egg may have a vascular connection, one may see vascular flow voids on MR within and around a meningioma. Avid en-

hancement after contrast is also seen (Fig. 3-4), but occasionally, meningiomas may have necrotic centers or calcified portions, which may not enhance. With MR you may be able to identify the "dural tail"; enhancement of the dura trailing off away from the lesion in crescentic fashion, which is typical of meningiomas and has been exhibited in up to 72% of cases (Fig. 3-5). There has been

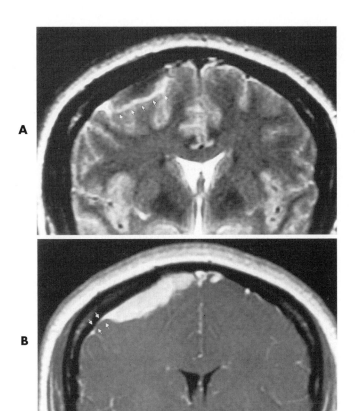

Fig. 3-4 Parasagittal meningioma. **A,** This meningioma is really dark on T2WI but the adjacent bright CSF demonstrates its extraaxial location nicely (CSF cleft sign designated by arrows). **B,** Add a dural tail *(arrows)* and strong enhancement and you should be dictating this case as a meningioma.

a debate in the radiologic literature as to whether the dural tail always represents neoplastic infiltration of the meninges by the meningioma or, alternatively, a reactive fibrovascular proliferation of the underlying meninges. In the typical situation where a differential diagnosis of acoustic schwannoma, meningioma, or fifth-nerve schwannoma is debated, the dural tail may be a useful sign to suggest meningioma rather than other diagnoses (Table 3-1). The dural tail is not usually seen with schwannomas, although dural metastases may demonstrate a similar finding.

Meningiomas may encase and narrow adjacent vessels. This finding helps in the sella region, because pituitary adenomas, the other culprit in this location, virtually never narrow the cavernous carotid artery.

The degree of parenchymal edema is variable in meningiomas. Although it is true that larger meningiomas tend to have a greater degree of parenchymal edema, there are exceptions where smaller meningiomas incite a large amount of white matter edema. The degree of edema seems to correlate with location, because menin-

giomas adjacent to the cerebral cortex tend to incite greater edema than those along the basal cisterns or planum. Edema associated with meningiomas may be caused by compressive ischemia, venous stasis, aggressive growth, or parasitization of pial vessels. Venous sinus occlusion or venous thrombosis can also cause intraparenchymal edema from a meningioma. So, though we usually think of eggs and meningiomas as benign entities, you still have to watch your cholesterol because over the long term, these both may become bad for you.

Intraosseous meningiomas may appear as expansions of the inner and outer tables of the calvarium or may even extend into the scalp soft tissues (Fig. 3-6). No dural component may be present at all. This type of meningioma strongly resembles a blastic osseous metastasis. Intraventricular meningiomas typically occur around the choroid plexus (80%) in the trigone of the lateral ventricle and have a distinct propensity for the left lateral ventricle (Fig. 3-7). Only 15% of intraventricular meningiomas occur in the third ventricle, and 5% occur in the fourth ventricle. Intraventricular meningiomas calcify in 45% to 68% of cases, and their frequency is higher in children. Multiple meningiomas are associated with neurofibromatosis type 2.

Bony changes associated with meningiomas may be hyperostotic or osteolytic, and occur in 20% to 46% of cases. Hyperostosis is particularly common when the tumor is at the skull base or anterior cranial fossa, and here it may resemble fibrous dysplasia or Paget disease. The presence of bony reaction may be a helpful feature to distinguish meningiomas from other extraaxial masses, particularly schwannomas, which do not elicit a bony reaction. Bony changes, according to the neuropathology literature, may be due to actual tumor infiltration of the

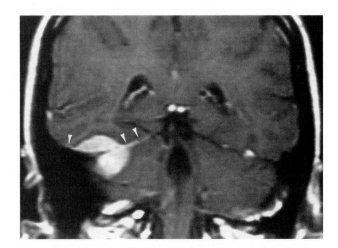

Fig. 3-5 Another piece of tail in a meningioma. Coronal enhanced T1WI of this tentorial meningioma shows enhancing tails *(arrowheads)* coursing medially and laterally from the main portion of the tumor. Note that tumor extends to either side of the tentorium.

Table 3-1 Differential diagnosis of meningioma versus schwannoma

Feature	Meningioma	Schwannoma
Dural tail	Frequent	Extremely rare
Bony reaction	Osteolysis or hyperostosis	Rare
Angle made with dura	Obtuse	Acute
Calcification	20%	Extremely rare
Cyst/necrosis formation	Rare	Up to 10%
Enhancement	Uniform	Inhomogeneous in 32%
Extension into the internal auditory canal	Rare	80%
MRS	Alanine	Taurine, GABA
Precontrast CT attenuation	Hyperdense	Isodense
Hemorrhage	Rare	Somewhat more common

marrow space with osteoblastic metaplasia or merely due to the involved dura inciting hypervascularity of the periosteum and subsequent benign osteogenesis (Fig. 3-8). Therefore if the hyperostosis is along the inner table only, you cannot say whether it is due to neoplastic invasion or reactive changes. If the outer table is transgressed, tumor is most likely.

Meningiomas are one of the few tumors where angiography still may play an important role. Meningiomas diagnostically appear as lesions with an angiographic stain (tumor blush) and have both dural and pial blood supply (Fig. 3-9). The characteristics of the stain are classically compared with an unwanted guest (or in-law) who comes early and stays late. Depending on the location of the tumor, you may have to perform internal carotid, external carotid, and vertebral injections (Table 3-2). In the typical convexity or sphenoid wing menin-

gioma, the middle meningeal artery is enlarged (seen by primitive radiologists before angiography as enlarged meningeal grooves on the lateral skull film). At present preoperative embolization of meningiomas is sometimes performed to decrease the vascularity of the tumor. Make your referring neurosurgeon's day by decreasing the intraoperative blood loss. Polyvinyl alcohol (PVA) particles are most commonly used as the embolant (100 to 250 micromillimeters in size), but gelfoam, cyanoacrylate, and trisacryl gelatin microspheres (Embospheres) are also employed by some.

Skull base meningiomas in particular often require preoperative embolization. The skull base is the one region where meningiomas can become unresectable because of collateral damage to vital structures (e.g., the cranial nerves and carotid artery in the cavernous sinus meningioma, the vertebrobasilar vessels for foramen

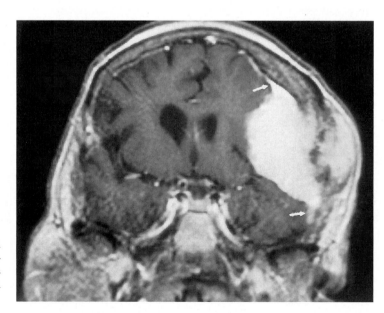

Fig. 3-6 Osseous involvement by meningioma. Enhanced T1WI demonstrates evidence of an osseous meningioma expanding the left calvarium outward as well as inward. Arrows depict the dural tail on either side of this lesion. There is a soft-tissue component extending under the galeal layer.

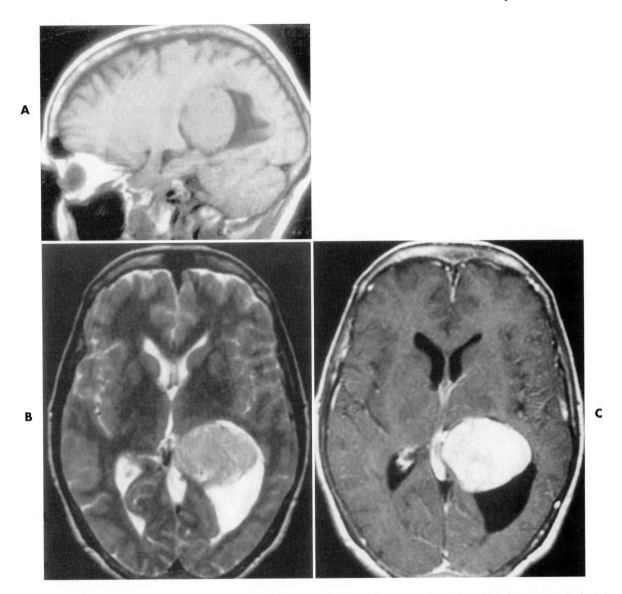

Fig. 3-7   Intraventricular meningioma. **A,** Sagittal T1WI shows a well-defined large mass in a dilated left lateral ventricular trigone. **B,** The mass, typical of a meningioma, is isointense to gray matter. It is centered on the choroid. **C,** Big time enhancement! Classic meningioma!

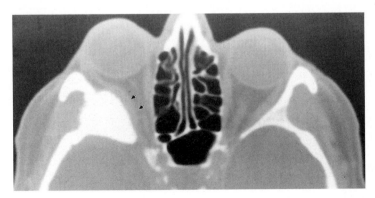

Fig. 3-8   Bony reaction from meningioma. Bone-targeted CT scan shows enlargement and hyperdensity of the right sphenoid wing with buckling of the right lateral rectus *(arrows)* from this sphenoid wing meningioma.

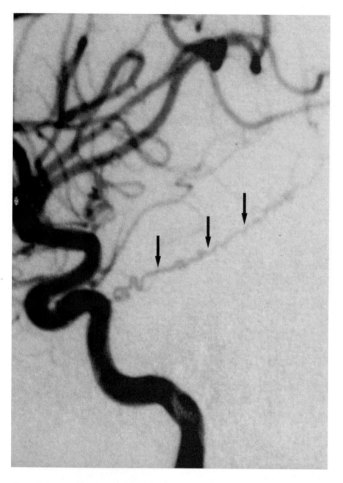

Fig. 3-9 Tentorial meningioma. The artery of Bernasconi Cassanari is enlarged in this case.

agnosed when a meningioma exhibits intraparenchymal invasion or markedly rapid growth. Histopathologically they are defined by malignant cytology, 20 or more mitoses per high powered field, or sarcomatous degeneration. They, as well, have restricted diffusion compared to benign meningiomas. They most likely arise from benign tumors gone awry and when they aggressively invade the brain it gives you the same sinking feeling as opening a blood-tinged egg. The papillary variety of meningioma undergoes malignant differentiation more commonly than the rest. Anaplasia may occur, accounting for the classification of Simpson's grade III meningiomas. The higher grade is associated with a higher rate of recurrence. Survival varies with the site, size, grade, and extent of surgical removal of the tumor.

Radiation-induced meningioma Radiation therapy induces five times more meningiomas than it does gliomas or sarcomas. The diagnosis of radiation-induced meningioma is made if the meningioma arises in the radiation field, appears after a latency period (of years), was not the primary tumor irradiated, and is not seen in a patient with neurofibromatosis. These tumors have been associated with low-dose radiation treatment for tinea capitis and have mean latency periods of about 35 years. Multiple meningiomas (? the double-yolked egg?), occur in up to 30% of previously irradiated patients with meningiomas and in 1% to 2% of nonirradiated patients with meningiomas. Recurrence rates are higher in radi-

magnum lesions, the optic nerves at the optic canal). You take a risk—like eating raw eggs.

On MRS, meningiomas are characterized by high levels of alanine and absent N-acetyl aspartate. No glutamine is seen. One can use the presence of taurine and/or gamma-aminobutyric acid (GABA) in schwannomas to distinguish meningiomas from schwannomas.

Atypical meningioma *Atypical meningiomas* are classified as WHO grade II. Histopathologically they must have increased mitotic rates (four or more mitoses per 10 high power fields) or small cells with high nucleus/cytoplasm ratio, prominent nucleoli, sheet like growth, and foci of necrosis. Accordingly, 2.4% of meningiomas are thereby classified as atypical and these tumors have lower apparent diffusion coefficient (ADC) values on diffusion-weighted images than typical meningiomas. They recur more frequently. They look radiographically like benign meningiomas.

Malignant meningiomas *Malignant meningiomas* (WHO grade III) occur uncommonly and are usually di-

Table 3-2 Blood supply to meningiomas

Location of meningioma	Commonly seen blood supply (origin of vessel)
Convexity	Middle meningeal artery (ECA)
	Artery of the falx (branch of ophthalmic artery)
Sphenoid wing	Middle meningeal artery (ECA)
Tentorium and cerebellopontine angle	Tentorial artery (artery of Bernasconi-Casanari, or "Italian" artery) from meningohypophyseal trunk (ICA)
Olfactory groove	Branches from ophthalmic artery
Foramen magnum and clivus	Anterior meningeal artery (vertebral)
	Dorsal meningeal artery from meningohypophyseal trunk (ICA)
Posterior fossa dura and falx cerebelli	Posterior meningeal artery (vertebral and MMA or ascending pharyngeal branches)

ECA, external carotid artery; *ICA*, internal carotid artery; *MMA*, middle meningeal artery

ation-induced meningiomas than in non–radiation-induced tumors.

The differential diagnosis of primary tumors that mimic meningiomas is broad (see Box 3-1).

Mesenchymal meningeal tumors   As noted in Box 3-1 there are a number of mesenchymal tumors that can affect the meninges. These are all relatively rare lesions, which may have either osseous (osteoma, osteosarcoma, etc), chondroid (chondroma, chondro-sarcoma, etc), muscular (leiomyoma, rhabdomyosarcoma, etc), fatty (lipoma, liposarcoma, etc), or fibrous (fibroma, malignant fibrous histiocytoma) matrices associated with them. If you remember that the fibrous falx can be ossified (with bone and marrow fat), you can recall these tumors more readily.

Hemangiopericytoma   The term "angioblastic meningioma," used in our first edition, has been replaced by the entity "hemangiopericytomas" in the new WHO classification of meningeal mesenchymal tumors (actually this happened in 1993, one year before we published our first edition, but we're slow readers—shhhhh!). These tumors, derived from smooth muscle pericyte cells around the capillaries of the meninges, are more aggressive than most meningiomas, have a higher rate of recurrence, and can metastasize. Hence some consider them malignant and most say they are distinct from meningiomas. They tend to be large (over 4 cm in size), lobular, and extraaxial supratentorial masses. Hydrocephalus, edema, and mass effect are not uncommon with this entrée. Precontrast CT shows heterogeneous, hyperdense tumors that enhance. Hyperostosis and/or calcification is rare. Hemangiopericytomas affect men more than women, unlike most MENingiomas.

Meningioangiomatosis   Meningioangiomatosis is a rare bird indeed straddling the intra- and extraparenchymal domain with a lesion that can appear in the cortex (90%) or meninges. Most often associated with neurofibromatosis type 2, it grows slowly and contains calcification. Intracortical foci of proliferating small vessels and fibroblasts accompany the meningeal process. Cysts may coexist. The entity is seen in the young and is a potential source for seizures owing to its cortical location.

Melanocytic lesions

Within this category one finds diffuse melanocytosis, melanocytoma, neurocutaneous melanosis, and malignant melanoma. The brown pigmentation should remind you of Hershey's syrup, poured over the dura. The melanin containing cells are leftovers from neural crest origin. These diagnoses are difficult to make because metastatic melanoma to the dura does occur and must often be excluded. The melanocytoma is the most common of the lot and is seen in adults, whereas melanocytosis is more of a pediatric disorder. Although the latter

is a diffuse process, the former usually presents as a posterior fossa mass (a Hershey's kiss). Hyperintensity on T1WI is the only hope for sealing this diagnosis, but the presence of this finding varies with melanin content. Spread of melanocytosis through the Virchow Robin spaces is possible.

Malignant melanoma of the meninges may bleed or spread from the dura to the adjacent nerves, brain, or skull. Neurocutaneous melanosis shows melanocytic nevi of the skin (especially about the face), syringomyelia, and CNS lipomas. Prognosis is poor as is malignant melanoma of the meninges with distant metastases (death by chocolate!).

Tumors of Neurogenic Origin

Schwannomas

Think of jelly beans when you consider nerve sheath tumors. This metaphor works because, just as there are so many colors and flavors to jelly beans, there are many varieties of schwannomas and neurofibromas arising from many of the cranial and peripheral nerves. Also, just as one sometimes gets a sticky conglomerate of multiple moist jelly beans, sometimes you get a plexiform neurofibroma that infiltrates aggressively. In the end, jelly beans are sweet and neurogenic tumors are nice and benign and seldom pose much danger to the patient. Of course there is the occasional nasty vestibular schwannoma that wraps itself all over adjacent vessels and nerves—as disgusting as those "Bertie Bott's ear wax flavored jelly beans" of Harry Potter fame.

The three neurogenic tumors (schwannomas, neurofibromas, neuromas), are similar in appearance. Histologically schwannomas arise from the perineural Schwann cells. These cells may differentiate into fibro-blastic or myelin-producing cells. Two types of tissue may be seen with schwannomas, Antoni A and Antoni B tissue. The Antoni A tissue consists of densely packed palisades of fibrous and neural tissue and typically has a darker signal on T2WI because of the compactness of the fibrils. Antoni B tissue is a looser, myxomatous tissue that is typically brighter on the T2WI. Note that, depending on the degree of Antoni A and B tissue within schwannomas, the signal intensity of these lesions may directly simulate that of meningiomas. Other terms used for schwannomas include *neurilemmomas* and *neurinomas*, but the most accurate term is *schwannoma*.

Cellular (Antoni A dominated and favoring the cranial nerves V and VII, pelvis, retroperitoneum, and mediastinum), plexiform (found in the skin and subcutaneous tissue and associated with neurofibromatosis type 2), and melanotic (pigmented, seen in younger patients, favoring spinal nerves over cranial nerves) varieties of schwannomas have been described. Fifty percent of patients with psammomatous melanotic schwannomas have Carney's complex, a syndrome characterized by facial pigmentation, cardiac myxomas, and endocrinologic disorders including Cushing syndrome, acromegaly, pheochromocytoma, or adrenal hyperplasia (NAME syndrome for nevi, atrial myxoma, mucinosis of skin, and endocrine overactivity). Over 10% of melanotic schwannomas may become malignant. Malignant schwannomas may also be seen in patients with neurofibromatosis type I.

The distinction between meningiomas and schwannomas is a common one that radiologists must make (see Table 3-1). In some instances it is impossible to distinguish between the two. Both meningiomas and schwannomas may track along the course of the nerves, and therefore the extent of a tumor is not helpful in distinguishing the two. As described previously, the dural tail is a helpful sign in suggesting a diagnosis of meningioma. In 81% of cases the border of a vestibular schwannoma makes an acute angle with the petrous bone: meningiomas usually make an obtuse angle. A curious finding has been described with vestibular schwannomas; arachnoid cysts coexist in 7% to 10% of cases, usually with the larger tumors (Fig. 3-10). These must be distinguished from cystic degeneration (and preponderance of Antoni B tissue) of the tumor, which is also a frequent phenomenon. Schwannomas may therefore be very bright on a T2WI; unusual for meningiomas.

One of the distinguishing features of vestibular schwannomas from meningiomas is the expansion of the internal auditory canal (IAC) seen in schwannomas. The porus acousticus (the bony opening of the IAC to the cerebellopontine angle cistern) is typically flared and

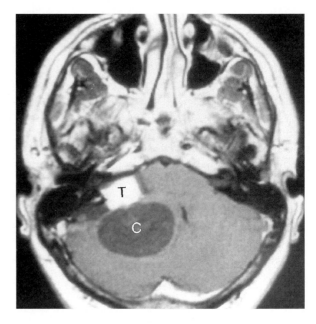

Fig. 3-10   Acoustic schwannoma with arachnoid cyst. A cyst (C) associated with enhancing acoustic schwannoma (T) is seen on this enhanced T1WI.

enlarged with vestibular schwannomas, whereas the amount of tissue seen in the IAC with meningiomas is usually small or absent. Vestibular schwannomas account for more than 90% of purely intracanalicular lesions, but only 5% to 17% of them are solely intracanalicular (Fig. 3-11). Approximately 10% to 20% of vestibular schwannomas present only in the cerebellopontine angle cistern without an IAC stem (Box 3-2). Approximately 75%

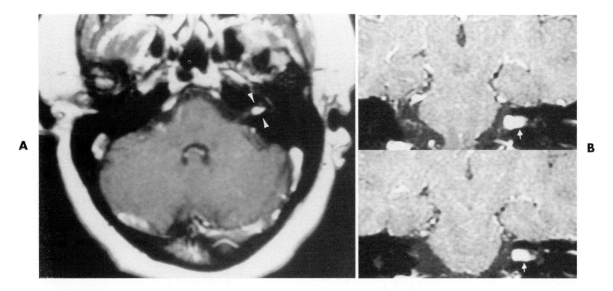

Fig. 3-11   Intracanalicular acoustic schwannoma. **A,** Postcontrast T1WI shows an enhancing left intracanalicular acoustic schwannoma *(arrowheads)*. **B,** Left intracanalicular acoustic schwannoma: Post gadolinium enhanced T1 weighted coronal scans show an intracanalicular mass *(arrows)* on the left side. Perform a fat saturated scan to ensure that this does not represent fat.

Box 3-2 Cerebellopontine Angle Masses

Vestibular schwannoma (75%)
Meningioma (10%)
Epidermoid (5%)
Facial nerve schwannoma (4%)
Aneurysm (vertebral, basilar, posterior inferior
    cerebellar artery)
Brain stem glioma
Arachnoid cyst
Paraganglioma
Hematogenous metastasis
Subarachnoid spread of tumors
Lipoma
Hemangioma
Choroid plexus papilloma
Ependymoma
Desmoplastic medulloblastoma

of vestibular schwannomas have a canalicular and cisternal portion (Fig. 3-12). Think of a little boy who stuck a jelly bean in his ear for a vestibular schwannoma—you would have a waxy intracanalicular piece of the candy inside his ear and a colorful cisternal piece hanging out.

On MR, schwannomas are usually isointense to slightly hypointense compared with pontine tissue on all pulse sequences. Enhancement is nearly always evident and homogeneous in around 70% of cases. Peritumoral

edema may be seen in one third of cases, usually in the larger schwannomas. Less common features of schwannomas include calcification, cystic change (Fig. 3-13), and hemorrhage. Subarachnoid hemorrhage is a rare presentation of vestibular schwannomas.

Schwannomas occur most commonly along cranial nerve VIII. The superior vestibular branch of cranial nerve VIII is the most common origin of the vestibular schwannoma (not "acoustic neuromas"), slightly more common than inferior vestibular nerve. Nonetheless, the patients typically have hearing loss. After lesions of cranial nerve VIII, schwannomas of cranial nerves VII (Fig. 3-14) and V are the most common site of intracranial neurogenic tumors, although ANY cranial nerve may be involved (Fig. 3-15). Jelly beans come in the colors of the rainbow!

Postoperatively, it is not unusual to see linear gadolinium enhancement in the internal auditory canal after vestibular schwannoma resection. This can be followed expectantly. For those cases with progressive, nodular, or masslike enhancement more careful follow-up is required to exclude recurrence.

Trigeminal schwannomas may arise anywhere along the pathway from the pons to Meckel's cave to the cavernous sinus, to and beyond the exit foramina (ovale, rotundum, and superior orbital fissure). Outside the brain,

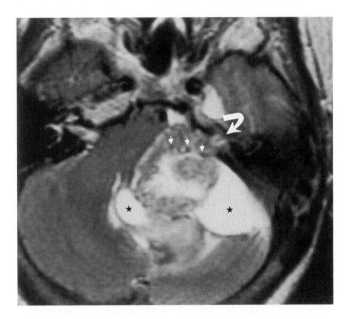

Fig. 3-13   Cysts associated with a vestibular schwannoma. This T2 weighted scan demonstrates a heterogeneous mass extending into the internal auditory canal *(curved arrow)* with associated cysts posterolaterally and posteromedially *(stars)*. Lower signal foci *(arrows)* may represent intratumoral hemorrhage. The brain stem is markedly compressed and shifted to the right side. The mass effect associated with the cyst as well as its elliptical margins ensures that this does not represent a dilated subarachnoid space.

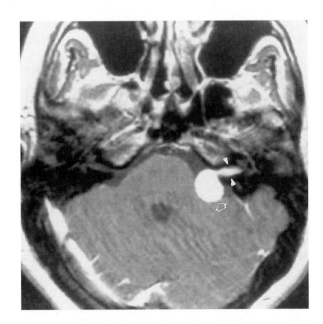

Fig. 3-12   Cerebellopontine angle and intracanalicular acoustic schwannoma. Note the brightly enhancing mass with both a cisternal *(open arrow)* and intracanalicular *(arrowheads)* portion. The ipsilateral prepontine cistern is enlarged.

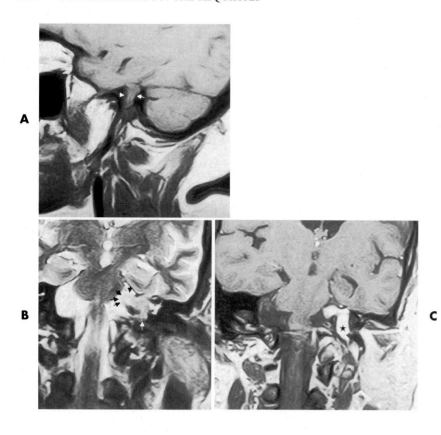

Fig. 3-14   Facial nerve schwannoma. **A,** Sagittal T1WI shows a markedly thickened descending portion of the facial nerve *(arrows).* **B,** The mass is difficult to appreciate on the coronal T2WI were it not for the well-placed arrows delineating its course (This is a new feature on the Geimensillip scanner). **C,** The course of this enhancing mass suggests a facial nerve schwannoma by virtue of its tympanic segment and descending portion *(star).*

the schwannomas of cranial nerve V most commonly occur along the second division. These tumors present with facial pain ("Does your face hurt?" "No." "Well it's killing me.") that is burning in nature.

Jugular schwannomas more commonly grow intracranially than extracranially and typically smoothly erode the jugular foramen. The border of the bone is sclerotic as opposed to the paraganglioma that has a much more irregular and nonsclerotic margin. Schwannomas compress the jugular vein whereas paragangliomas (glomus jugulare tumors) invade the vein. Growth into the posterior fossa is the rule. Jugular foramen schwannomas most commonly present with hearing loss and vertigo rather than cranial nerve IX symptoms. Whether the schwannoma arises from one cranial nerve or the next, the imaging appearance (like the shape and consistency of the jelly bean) is similar.

Neurofibromas

Neurofibromas, strictly speaking, refer to the tumors that are associated with neurofibromatosis. They are classified as WHO grade I and all ages and sexes are represented. They may occur sporadically as well, though less commonly than schwannomas. The skin and subcutaneous tissues are affected more often than peripheral nerves; spinal nerve neurofibromas are rare and cranial nerve involvement is uncommon. These lesions contain Schwann cells, perineural cells, and fibroblastic cells and

may occur in a plexiform aggressive subtype, which appears as a network of diffusely infiltrating masses. Once again, Antoni A or B tissue may predominate in the lesion and will alter the T2WI characteristics. Do not think about neurofibromas for neurofibromatosis type II (NF-2), only type I. NF-2 is a misnomer. Classically, in "neurofibromatosis" type II bilateral acoustic **schwannomas** are seen. Plexiform neurofibromas in the cranial nerves or peripheral nervous system may occur neurofibromatosis type 1 (NF-1). Plexiform neurofibromas, because of their extensiveness, can be distinguished from neuromas and schwannomas. They are generally found in the extremities or in the soft tissues of the head and neck. They have a significant rate of malignant dedifferentiation.

Neuromas

By strict pathologic definition neuromas refer to a posttraumatic proliferation of nerve cells rather than a true neoplasm. The perineural lining and fibroblastic tissue seen in the other lesions just described are not present. These lesions are less common than schwannomas. They are usually seen in the cervical spine when nerves are avulsed, or in an operative bed. Again, one must know where to look for these lesions. Unfortunately, in the common vernacular most people mean "schwannoma" when they say "neuroma" (e.g., "acoustic neuroma," which is a double misnomer as these are truly "vestibular" lesions). On scanning these masses look like small schwannomas.

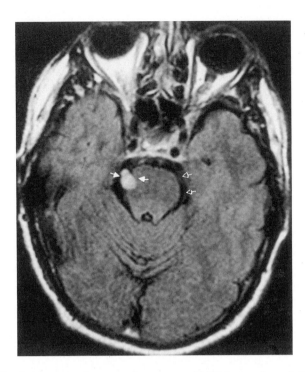

Fig. 3-15   Fourth nerve schwannoma. FLAIR image through the brain stem demonstrates an extraaxial mass along the right side of the upper pons. One can faintly see the normal fourth nerve *(open arrows)* on the left side coursing around the brain stem. The right-sided lesion *(arrow)* represents a fourth nerve schwannoma.

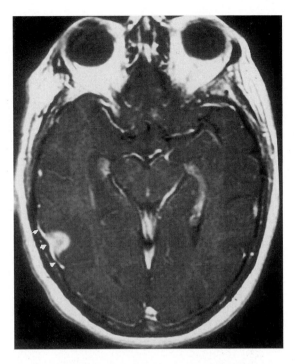

Fig. 3-16   Metastasis with a dural tail: Postgadolinium enhanced T1-weighted scan in a patient with adenocarcinoma of the lung demonstrates a metastasis peripherally in the right temporal lobe. Although a dural tail *(arrows)* is suggestive of a meningioma, it is not pathognomonic for it.

Metastases

Dural metastases

Dural metastases are like chunky peanut butter spreading out along the bread, coating it in an ominous film. Dural metastases usually spread out along the dura as hematogenously disseminated en plaque lesions from extracranial primary tumors (Fig. 3-16). Lung, breast, and prostate cancer, and melanoma are known to produce dural metastases. Some of the dural metastases may arise from spread of adjacent bone metastases. Breast carcinoma is the most common neoplasm to be associated with purely dural metastases. Lymphoma is next most common but is unique in that the dural lymphoma may be the primary focus of the neoplasm (Fig. 3-17). Dural plasmacytomas will look nearly identical to dural lymphoma and should be considered in the same food group (Fig. 3-18). In children dural metastases are most commonly associated with adrenal neuroblastomas and leukemia. These tumors are also famous for lodging in the cranial sutures, widening them in an infant.

The "chunks" in the chunky peanut butter suggest that the dural metastases may not be homogeneously smooth but may have nodularity to them. Subarachnoid seeding (see following section) may also be present and may create more chunks. Again, breast and lung metastases predominate in this realm.

Occasionally, one can identify an adjacent parenchymal metastasis with dural spread (Fig. 3-19), and, alternatively, an osseous-dural metastasis (breast, prostate primaries) occasionally invades the parenchyma (Fig. 3-20). On MR the T1WI and T2WI characteristics are variable; however, typically the lesion is hypointense on T1WI and hyperintense on T2WI (Fig. 3-21 as an exception to the rule). On CT these lesions are identified as isodense thickening of the meninges. Contrast enhancement is prominent. This is a diagnosis where contrast-enhanced T1WI or FLAIR scans can make the diagnosis in a "jiffy," (get it, peanut butter?)

Have you ever eaten peanut butter on a hard boiled egg? Maybe not, but rarely metastases have been known to spread to a dural-based meningioma.

Inflammatory lesions that may simulate dural metastases include granulomatous infections (mycobacterial, syphilitic, and fungal), Erdheim Chester disease, sarcoidosis, and Langerhans cell histiocytosis.

Subarachnoid seeding

Think of sugar and sesame seeds when you think of seeding of the subarachnoid space (SAS). Usually one is dealing with tiny nodules of implanted tumor seedings. When the process is diffuse we use the term "sugar-coating" of the subarachnoid space because the whole pial surface is studded with sugar granules, which are

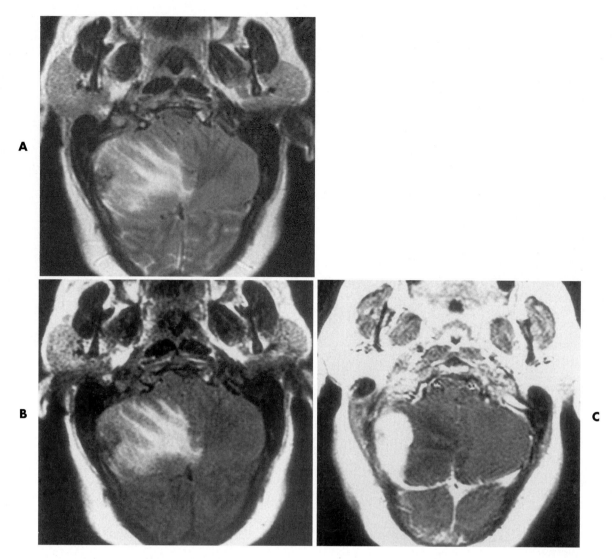

Fig. 3-17   Dural lymphoma. **A,** See the low signal dural mass on the T2WI that is eliciting the intraparenchymal edema? No? **B,** How about now on the FLAIR? No? Are you a neurologist? **C,** Then you cannot miss it (unless cortically blind) on the enhanced scan. Lymphoma will nearly always enhance (unless the neurosurgeons are reluctantly treating it with massive doses of steroids). Include meningioma, sarcoidosis, plasmacytoma, and other dural metastases in the differential diagnosis.

less distinct than sesame seeds. A combination of sugar and sesame seeds (hey, a great idea for a new bagel delight!) may also occur. SAS seeding may occur with primary CNS tumors or primary tumors of other origins (Table 3-3). Lymphoma and leukemia are the most common tumors to seed the CSF. However, because they only rarely invade the meninges and do not incite reactions in the CNS, lymphomatous clusters are infrequently identified by neuroimaging techniques; the diagnosis is usually made by multiple spinal taps for CSF sampling. Myelomatous involvement of the subarachnoid space occurs in less than 1% of patients with multiple myeloma but, because this is a second edition to our book, we thought we would include the zebras this time (Fig. 3-22). CSF seeding is associated with a mean survival of 1 to 2

months without and 6 to 10 months with treatment. The differential diagnosis could include arachnoiditis, Guillain Barré syndrome, sarcoidosis, infectious granulomatous meningitides, Lyme disease, and CMV radiculitis.

When a lesion has spread to the SAS, you may see it only on contrast-enhanced studies, and MR is much more sensitive than CT. However, unenhanced and enhanced FLAIR imaging has been shown to be increasingly effective at identifying subarachnoid disease, including metastatic disease. The malignant cells in the CSF and/or the associated elevated protein in the CSF will cause the usually low signal of CSF to be bright on a FLAIR scan. Although this may be a difficult diagnosis to make in the basal cisterns where "f-ing" (FLAIR and flow) artifacts abound, the presence of such high signal over the con-

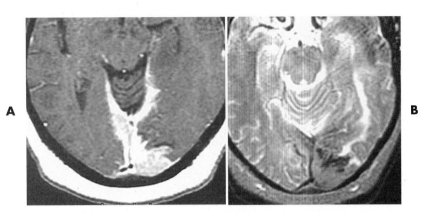

Fig. 3-18   Plasmacytoma of the dura. **A,** The gadolinium-enhanced scan looks just like one would expect for a meningioma with marked enhancement and a dural-based lesion. The irregular margins (saw-toothed appearance) suggesting pial spread would be funky for a meningioma though. **B,** Even the T2WI shows low signal that simulates a meningioma or lymphoma or sarcoidosis. The way to score on this shot is to have a history of a plasma cell dyscrasia.

vexities implies subarachnoid seeding, subarachnoid hemorrhage, or meningeal inflammation. FLAIR may even be positive in lymphoma and leukemia, where enhanced scans fail most dramatically. FLAIR with contrast enhancement increases the yield even higher!

The typical locations where one identifies SAS seeding are at basal cisterns, in the interpeduncular cistern, at the cerebellopontine angle cistern, along the course of cranial nerves, and over the convexities (Fig. 3-23). One may see various manifestations of subarachnoid seeding, including the sugar-coated linear appearance to the enhancement of the surface of the brain (especially cerebellum) and spinal cord, or a nodular sesame seed (tahini for the Desert Storm readers) appearance of tumor deposits on nerve roots, both cranial and spinal. Often one identifies a peripheral intraparenchymal metastasis contiguous with the dural surface of the brain, from which cells are shed into the CSF. With subarachnoid seeding secondary hydrocephalus may be present. Check those temporal horns.

The other terms you will see for the same entity include meningeal carcinomatosis or carcinomatous meningitis. Clinically the patients present with multiple cranial neuropathies, radiculopathies, and/or mental sta-

tus changes secondary to hydrocephalus or meningeal irritation. The cranial neuropathies may be irreversible. Although an initial CSF sample is positive in only 50% to 60% of cases, by performing multiple taps the positive cytology (and headache) rate approaches 95%. Patient survival is usually less than 6 months with this finding except in cases of hematologic malignancies. Breast, lung, and melanoma are the most common non-CNS primaries to seed the CSF.

In 1% of healthy individuals and 25% of individuals with congenital brain malformations there are nests of glial tissue within the subarachnoid space, so called leptomeningeal heterotopias. The occurrence of this tissue accounts for the oh-so-rare primary leptomeningeal gliomas, such as a leptomeningeal oligodendroglioma or primary diffuse leptomeningeal gliomatosis.

Chloroma

Granulocytic sarcoma (chloroma) is a tumor of immature granulocytes found in association with myelogenous leukemias. This soft-tissue mass can occur virtually anywhere and may predate the diagnosis of leukemia. In the CNS, the orbit and epidural space are affected most commonly but dural infiltration or even intraaxial involvement may be seen. The lesion, though eliciting bright vasogenic edema, may be intermediate intensity on T2WI, thought to be due to the high concentration of myeloperoxidase. It enhances. The term chloroma refers to its greenish color akin to chlorophyl. Chloromas portend a blast crisis. They are radiosensitive.

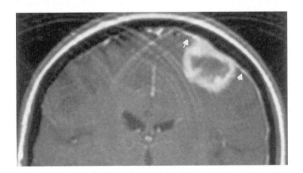

Fig. 3-19   Leiomyosarcoma with dural-based metastasis. Post-gadolinium coronal scan shows a high left frontal intraparenchymal metastasis, which demonstrates dural invasion *(arrows)* along its superomedial margin. (Ignore the phase-ghosting artifact.)

Choroid Plexus Masses

Choroid plexus papilloma

Choroid plexus papillomas (WHO grade I) comprise 3% of intracranial tumors in children and 10% to 20% of those presenting in the first year of life. Eighty-six percent of these tumors are seen in patients less than 5 years old. In children they occur at the trigone and/or atria of the lateral ventricles (80% of pediatric choroid plexus

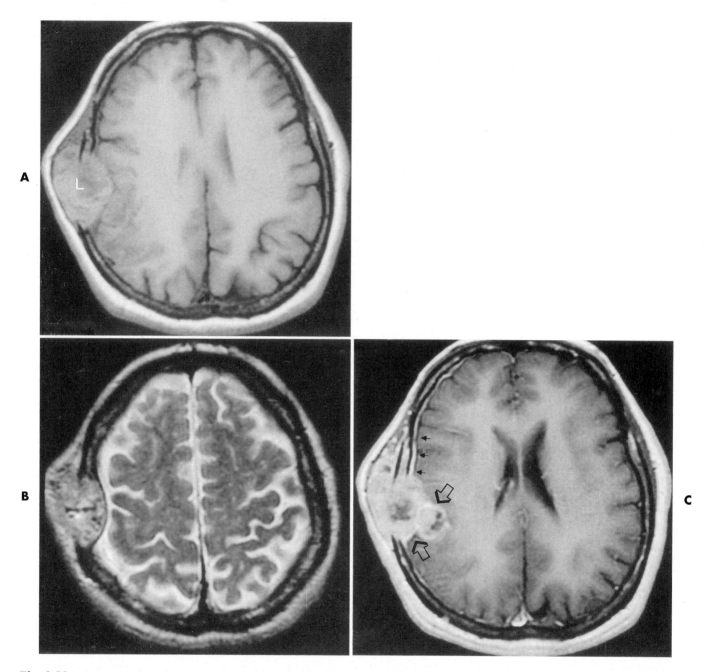

Fig. 3-20 Intraparenchymal growth of renal cell carcinoma metastasis. **A,** T1-weighted scans show a lesion (L) centered on the calvarium with extracalvarial as well as epidural spread. **B,** The T2-weighted scan again demonstrates the center of the lesion to be at the bone. **C,** However, with contrast, at a more inferior location, there is a medial nodule, which extends through the dura into the intraparenchymal compartment *(open arrows)*. Dural enhancement more peripherally is denoted by small black arrows.

papillomas); in adults they are usually seen in the fourth ventricle. Overall, 43% are located in the lateral ventricle, 39% the fourth ventricle, 11% the third ventricle, and 7% in the cerebellopontine angle cistern. Multiple sites are present in 3.7% of cases. If they are seen at the foramen of Luschka, it may be due to extension from the fourth ventricle or the cerebellopontine angle cistern, or from primary involvement in this location from a

choroidal tuft. Simian virus 40 (SV40) has been implicated in the evolution of these tumors. This same virus has been implicated in ependymomas.

The tumors present with hydrocephalus and papilledema caused by overproduction of CSF (four to five times more than normal) or obstructive hydrocephalus caused by tumor, hemorrhage, high-protein CSF, or adhesions obstructing the ventricular outlets. Lately, the obstructionists

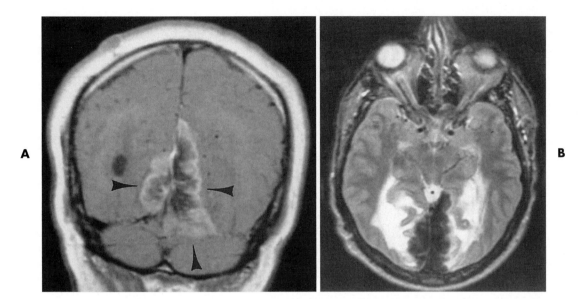

Fig. 3-21   Mucinous adenocarcinoma metastatic to the dura. **A,** Coronal unenhanced T1WI shows a dural-based mass with low signal centrally and peripheral high signal intensity *(arrowheads)*. The lesion was calcified on CT. (Observant readers will note the subcutaneous sebaceous cyst in the right upper part of the scalp.) **B,** On axial T2WI the lesion has low intensity but incites high signal intensity edema.

have gained the majority from the overproductionists as far as the explanation for hydrocephalus. Calcification occurs in 20% to 25% of the cases, and hemorrhage in the tumor is seen even more frequently than calcification. The tumor is typically hyperdense on unenhanced CT, with a mulberry appearance. It is usually of low signal on T1WI and mixed intensity on T2WI unless hemorrhage has occurred. These tumors enhance dramatically. Between the

calcification, flow voids, and/or hemorrhage, the tumor has a heterogeneous appearance, sometimes with a salt-and-pepper appearance from vessel supply. Overall, you should view these lesions like a branch of mulberries centered at the glomus. The red color of the berries brings to mind a highly vascular lesion.

Table 3-3 Sources of subarachnoid seeding	
CNS primary	**Non-CNS primary**
Children	
Choroid plexus papilloma	Neuroblastoma
Ependymoma (blastoma = PNET)	Leukemia
Malignant astrocytomas	Lymphoma
Medulloblastoma (PNET)	
Pineal region tumors	
Retinoblastoma	
Adults	
Glioblastoma multiforme	Breast
Oligodendroglioma	Gastrointestinal
Lymphoma	Genitourinary
	Leukemia
	Lung
	Lymphoma
	Melanoma

PNET, primitive neuroectodermal tumor

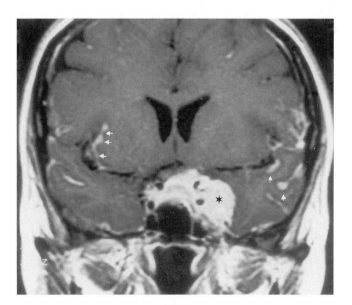

Fig. 3-22   Metastatic multiple myeloma. This patient had disseminated metastatic multiple myeloma with a large mass in the left cavernous sinus *(star)* extending to the suprasellar cistern. Note the subarachnoid seeding as evidenced by the nodular enhancement *(arrows)* in both sylvian fissures.

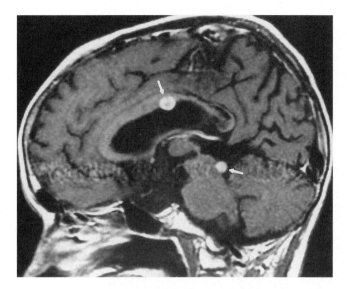

Fig. 3-23 Subarachnoid seeding from a brain stem glioma. Post-contrast T1WI shows contrast-enhancing nodules *(arrows)* in the roof of the lateral ventricle and in the superior vermian cistern. The keen observer will notice the "overly pregnant" belly of the pons.

Choroid plexus carcinomas

Choroid plexus carcinomas (WHO grade III) are much less common than papillomas, with malignant change occurring in fewer than 10% to 20% of cases. They are usually seen in the lateral ventricles. CSF dissemination is the rule with choroid plexus carcinomas, occurring in more than 60% of cases, but even benign papillomas may seed the CSF. It is difficult to distinguish a benign papilloma from a malignant one. Parenchymal invasion may suggest carcinoma (Fig. 3-24). One can have primary melanomas of the choroid plexus as well.

The 5 year survival for completely resected choroid plexus papillomas is 100%; for carcinomas it is more like 40%.

Choroid plexus hemangiomas

Choroid plexus hemangiomas are benign neoplasms of the choroid plexus usually seen in the lateral ventricle. Although the tumor enhances markedly and may calcify, it is usually seen as an incidental finding in an asymptomatic patient. There is an association with Sturge-Weber syndrome. In this syndrome choroidal hemangiomas ipsilateral to the leptomeningeal vascular malformation may be present (see Chapter 9).

Choroid plexus xanthogranuloma

Another benign condition of the choroid plexus is the xanthogranuloma. This incidental lesion may have fat density/intensity within it and is also centered on the glomus of the trigone. Curiously, they are frequently bright on DWI scans (Fig. 3-25). They are of no clinical impact, only rarely causing visual disturbance. Box 3-3 lists common choroid plexus neoplasms. For choroid plexus inflammatory processes, consider Box 6-9.

Non-neoplastic Masses

Epidermoids

There is some confusion involved with putting epidermoids and dermoids into a "tumor" chapter because most people think of these lesions as congenital epidermal inclusion cysts and dermal inclusion cysts. They really are not truly neoplastic and merely reflect two entities of ectodermal origin, one with just desquamated skin (epidermoid) and one with skin appendages like hair follicles and sebaceous cysts (dermoid). Epidermoids and dermoids grow slowly and are histologically benign. Teratomas, usually lumped in the same category, however are true neoplasms of multipotential germ cells. So despite their variable origins, we have fallen into the same old trap of placing these lesions into a heading together, to be consistent with other authors. Remember, to err is human; to blame it on someone else is even more human.

To distinguish these entities, think about different types of salad dressings—you can have vinegar (epidermoids, which appear to be of singular density), oil and vinegar (dermoids, which have fat and fluid), or oil and vinegar and croutons (teratomas, which have fat, fluid, and solid components).

Epidermoids are collections of epithelium with desquamated debris (keratin and cholesterin) resulting from inclusion of ectodermal rests at the time of neural tube closure early in the embryonic development. The walls are lined by simple stratified squamous epithelium, and the lesion has a pearly appearance. Men and women are affected equally, with a peak incidence in the 20- to 40-year age range. Epidermoids often occur in the cerebellopontine angle cistern (where they may present with trigeminal neuralgia and facial paralysis), the suprasellar cistern, the prepontine cistern, or the pineal region (Fig. 3-26). Extradural epidermoids are nine times less common than intradural ones and arise within the diploic space, the petrous bone, and the temporal bone, where they appear as well-defined bony lesions with sclerotic borders (Fig. 3-27).

Epidermoids are typically of low density on CT. This is to be distinguished from dermoids or teratomas that may have fat, bone, calcification, or other dermal appendages associated with them. Epidermoids expand to fill the interstices of the CSF space. An epidermoid is a lesion that is quite aggressive in insinuating itself around normal brain structures and often has scalloped borders. (You'll find vinegar in nearly all salad dressings.) CT demonstrates a nonenhancing lobulated lesion. Sometimes epidermoids are hard to distinguish from arachnoid cysts, particularly in the cerebellopontine angle cis-

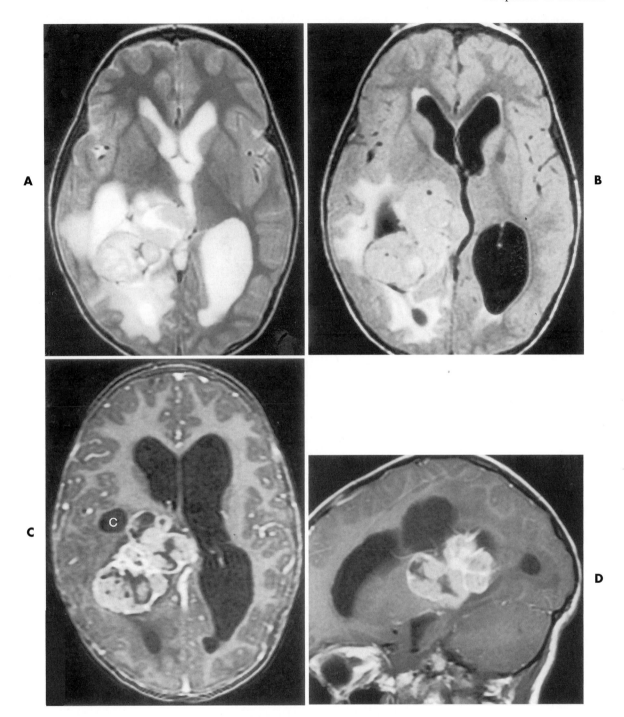

Fig. 3-24   Choroid plexus papilloma. **A,** This choroid plexus mass has a lot of peripheral high signal on T2WI **(A)** and FLAIR **(B),** signifying edema of the parenchyma. **C,** Note the hydrocephalus and central necrosis of the tumor, as well as an extraventricular cyst (C) on the enhanced T1WI. **D,** A mulberry-like shape to the mass, centered on the trigone, is typical of choroid plexus papillomas and carcinomas.

tern (Table 3-4). Classically, epidermoids do not enhance, but rarely the wall may show mild enhancement.

A stereotypical appearance on CT is that of displacement of the brain stem posteriorly by what appears to be just a dilated cistern anteriorly (see Fig. 3-26). In fact, this cistern is really a CSF-density epidermoid with mass effect.

MR has been very helpful in distinguishing between epidermoids and arachnoid cysts, a distinction that is sometimes blurred on CT. On MR these lesions are hypointense on T1WI and hyperintense on T2WI, similar to CSF; however, the intensity on the proton density–weighted images (PDWI) is usually inhomogeneous and often hyperintense to CSF. The advent of FLAIR imaging

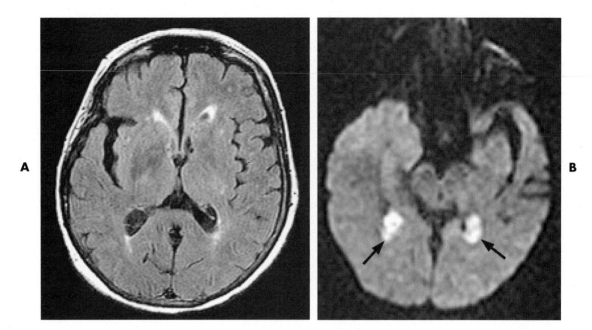

Fig. 3-25 Xanthogranulomas of the choroid plexus. Although the FLAIR scan **(A)** may be relatively unremarkable, the DWI **(B)** shows the bright signal in the xanthogranulomas of the choroid plexus. The presence of protein, cholesterol, or other compounds has been cited for why these are bright on DWI.

has made this an easy diagnosis because epidermoids are bright on FLAIR whereas arachnoid cysts are dark, dark as spinal fluid (Fig. 3-28). On diffusion-weighted images (DWI) these lesions are usually very bright and easily distinguishable from arachnoid cysts, which are dark. Once again, the lesion does not demonstrate enhancement unless it has been previously operated or secondarily infected. A flow-sensitive scan (steady-state free precession scanning) may demonstrate the lack of transmission of CSF pulsations in the epidermoid, signifying that the lesion is not truly cystic, à la an arachnoid cyst, but is a solid insinuating mass. Rarely, epidermoids may be bright on T1WI—this usually is due to high protein and viscosity in the lesion.

Dermoid

The high intensity of fat and signal void of calcification on T1WI suggests a diagnosis of oil and vinegar—a dermoid or teratoma (Fig. 3-29). Dermal appendages such as hair follicles, sebaceous glands, and sweat glands are found histologically in dermoid cysts (but hopefully not in your salad dressing). These lesions more typically occur in the midline as opposed to the epidermoids, which are generally off the midline. Male patients are more commonly affected, and patients are younger than those with epidermoids. The presence of fat may be suggested by an MR chemical shift artifact seen as a hyperintense and hypointense rim at the borders of the lesion in the frequency-encoding direction. Fat suppression scans decrease the intensity on T1WI (see Fig. 3-29C). The possibility of a ruptured dermoid should be considered when multiple fat particles are seen scattered on an MR or when lipid is detected in the CSF. (Rule out pantopaque droplets.) Usually the lesions are very well defined.

Teratoma

Teratomas are congenital neoplasms containing ectodermal (skin, brain), mesodermal (cartilage, bone, fat muscle, and endodermal (cysts with aerodigestive mucosa) elements. Malignant transformation to a sarcomatous neoplasm rarely occurs.

The pineal and suprasellar regions are common sites for teratomas. One will see a lesion of mixed density and intensity. The presence of an enhancing nodule in this neoplasm may help distinguish it from a dermoid. Infected or postoperative dermoids and epidermoids may show some peripheral enhancement however.

Box 3-3   Choroid Plexus Neoplasms

Choroid plexus papilloma
Choroid plexus carcinoma
Ependymoma
Hemangioma
Lymphoma
Meningioma
Metastasis

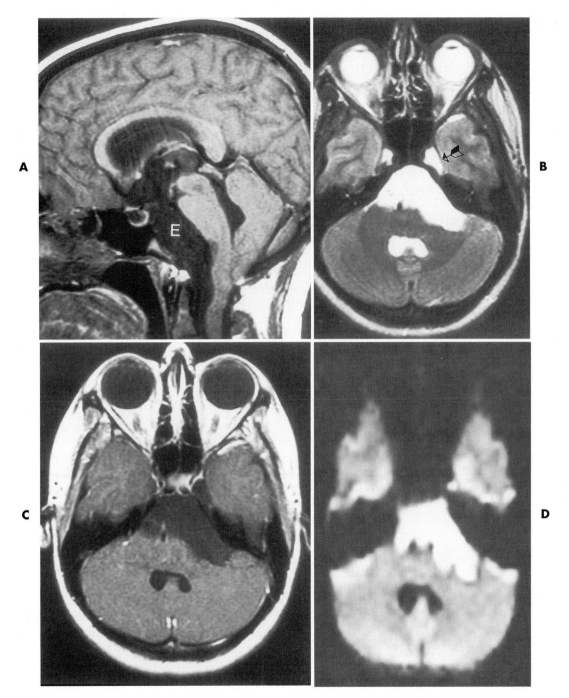

Fig. 3-26   Epidermoid. **A,** Sagittal T1-weighted scan without contrast demonstrates a low intensity mass (E) similar to CSF anterior to the brainstem. Note the scalloped margin to the lesion at the pons-medulla-cervicomedullary region. **B,** On the T2-weighted scan the lesion again has signal intensity similar to cerebrospinal fluid. Note Meckel's cave enlargement *(funky arrow)*—is it involved or merely dilated? **C,** No enhancement *(no arrow)* is seen on the postgadolinium T1-weighted scan. **D,** Aha! The diffusion weighted scan shows that there is restricted diffusion within the mass and it is dissimilar to cerebrospinal fluid based on its very high signal intensity. (Compare with CSF in fourth ventricle). This is classic for an epidermoid.

Lipomas

Just as oil alone does not merit a classification as a food, lipomas alone probably should not be placed in a chapter on neoplasms because they are most frequently developmental or congenital abnormalities associated with abnormal development of the meninx primitiva, a derivative of the neural crest. Although they are only rarely true neoplasms, we mention them here to abide by Grossman's first Postulate; an easily understood workable falsehood is more useful than a complex, incom-

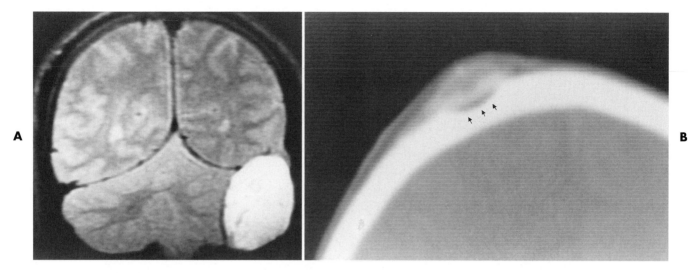

Fig. 3-27   Extradural epidermoids. **A,** T2WI shows a bright lesion displacing the hypointense dura medially in the left posterior fossa. **B,** Axial CT in a different patient shows a bony lesion scalloping the outer table of the skull *(arrows)* with a small superficial soft-tissue mass.

prehensible truth. Lipomas are particularly common in association with agenesis of the corpus callosum, and 60% are associated with some type of congenital anomaly of the associated neural elements. The most common intracranial sites for lipomas are the pericallosal region, the quadrigeminal plate cistern, the suprasellar cistern, and the cerebellopontine angle cistern. Because the tissue is histologically normal but located in an abnormal site, lipomas should best be termed choristomas, not neoplasms. Fat defines the lipoma; look for low density

on CT, high intensity on T1WI, and low intensity on conventional T2WI that suppresses even further when fat suppression techniques are applied.

INTRAAXIAL TUMORS

Although many lesions occur in both compartments of the brain, it is useful to separate primary intracranial tumors into those occurring in the infratentorial and supratentorial space. In addition, it is helpful to separate the lesions into those occurring primarily in children versus those occurring primarily in adults. In children 60% to 70% of intracranial tumors occur infratentorially, whereas the vast majority occur supratentorially in adults. Although the organization of this section of the chapter may make you queasy and produce dyspepsia, remember, *you* bought the book—we only wrote it. We want to make sure you get your money's worth.

One thing that gets our goat is when trainees refer to brain tumors as gliomas. This is not a term befitting readers of our book. You are now a sophisticate, an afficionado of neuroradiology—banish "glioma" from your vocabulary and use a more precise term. The category of gliomas of the brain includes astrocytomas, glioblastoma multiforme (GBMs), oligodendrogliomas, ependymomas, subependymomas, medulloblastomas, neuroblastomas, gangliocytomas, and gangliogliomas. We are sure that you do not mean to lump all these crazy tumors under the umbrella of "glioma." You probably meant to say "astrocytoma." Because surely (and stop calling me Shirley!) an ependymoma does not look like

Table 3-4	Differentiation of epidermoid and arachnoid cyst	
Characteristic	**Arachnoid cyst**	**Epidermoid**
CT density	CSF	Slightly higher than CSF
Margins	Smooth	Scalloped
Calcification	No	25%
Blood vessel involvement	Deviates	Insinuates between vessels
Intrathecal contrast	May take up but can be delayed	No uptake, defines borders
Characteristic on MR sequence sensitive to CSF pulsation (steady-state free precession)	Pulsates	Does not pulsate
Diffusion	Dark	Bright
ADC	Increased	Decreased
FLAIR	Dark	Bright

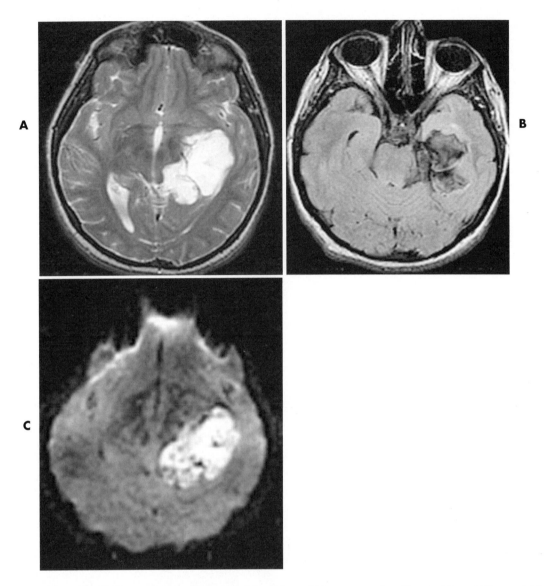

Fig. 3-28   Epidermoid. **A,** The T2W scan cannot distinguish this epidermoid from an arachnoid cyst of the middle cranial fossa. **B,** FLAIR scan shows signal intensity that exceeds that of the vitreous of the eye and therefore is unlike CSF (they usually have the same intensity). **C,** Lest you doubt the authors' veracity, we herein provide the DWI scan where the epidermoid is bright. See, we told you so!

an oligodendroglioma, which certainly does not look like a ganglioglioma. Crank up your level of sophistication— you're a reader of *Neuroradiology: THE REQUISITES.* For the *non-readers* of our book we recommend Grossman's 2nd postulate; "There's no sense in being precise when you don't know what you're talking about." Use gliomas.

It is customary to evaluate each of these lesions individually rather than to lump them together in a glioma group. "Gliomas" account for 35% to 45% of all intracranial tumors, with GBM accounting for 55%, astrocytomas 21%, ependymomas 6%, medulloblastomas 6%, oligodendrogliomas 5%, and gangliogliomas 2%. Metastases account for 40% of intracranial neoplasms.

Pediatric Infratentorial Neoplasms

Astrocytic tumors
Juvenile pilocytic astrocytomas (JPA)   Cerebellar JPAs are the most common infratentorial neoplasm in the pediatric age group and are classified as a WHO grade I astrocytic tumor (Table 3-5). These tumors can be likened to a blow-pop with a bubble gum center surrounded by candy (e.g., cyst and nodule). They are seen in children. They are benign. They have a solid central piece, and a separate peripheral portion. In general, pilocytic astrocytomas are well outlined from normal brain, are usually round, and usually are not ominous in ap-

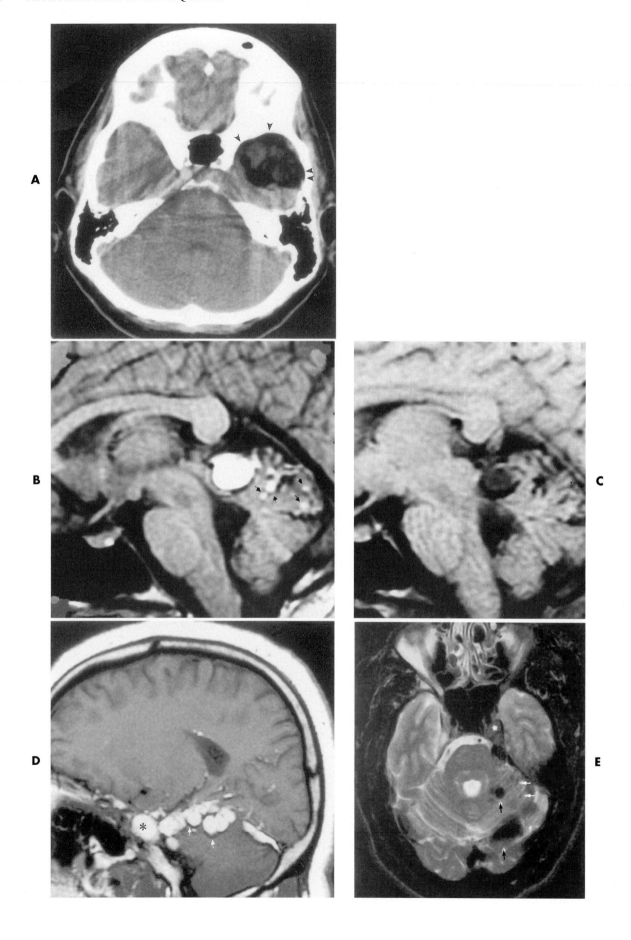

Fig. 3-29 The many faces of dermoids. **A,** This fatty mass seen on CT scan could represent a meningioma with fatty degeneration, a teratoma, or a dermoid. It is extraaxial in location and scallops bone *(arrowheads).* **B,** T1-weighted scan of a different ruptured dermoid shows high signal intensity along the superior surface of the cerebellum. **C,** Fat-suppressed T1WI confirms lesion is fatty. **D,** A larger mass is seen in the Meckel's cave region anteriorly *(asterisk).* Chemical shift artifact *(arrows)* is seen along the inferior margin of the fat droplets extending posteriorly. **E,** This T2-weighted fat suppressed scan demonstrates the dark signal suppressed fat *(star)* in the left Meckel's cave region as well as dark signal intensity large *(arrows)* and small fat deposits along the cerebellar folia representing rupture of this dermoid tumor.

◄ ────────────────────────

pearance (Fig. 3-30). The lesions, when removed completely, are associated with an excellent prognosis (5-year survival rate >90%). Sixty percent of pilocytic astrocytomas occur in the posterior fossa, but they also favor the optic pathways and hypothalamus. Anaplasia is less common when the tumor is cystic than solid, and therefore the prognosis varies according to tumor morphology. The typical cerebellar astrocytoma in the pediatric age group is cystic (60% to 80%), whereas in older patients it is more likely to be solid. A mural nodule may be present with a similar appearance to the hemangioblastomas of adults. Occasionally the astrocytomas in the posterior fossa are solid, without a cystic component, and may simulate other pediatric posterior fossa masses (Table 3-6).

On MR, astrocytomas show hypointensity on T1WI and hyperintensity on T2WI/FLAIR. The cystic portion of the tumor has signal intensity similar to CSF on T1WI and T2WI, but may be hyperintense to CSF on the PDWI or FLAIR because of a larger amount of protein. The lesion is very well defined. The solid portion of the JPA enhances strongly. This is a case where a low grade tumor

Table 3-5 WHO classification of astrocytic tumors

Tumor	Grade	Peak age (years)
Pilocytic Astrocytoma	I	0-20
Subependymal Giant Cell Astrocytoma	I	10-20
Pleomorphic Xanthoastrocytoma	II	10-20
Diffuse Astrocytoma	II	30-40
Fibrillary	II	30-40
Protoplasmic	II	30-40
Gemistocytic	II	30-40
Anaplastic Astrocytoma	III	35-50
Glioblastoma	IV	50-70
Giant cell glioblastoma	IV	40-50
Gliosarcoma	IV	50-70

shows marked enhancement and high metabolic activity on PET scanning.

The fibrillary form of cerebellar astrocytomas is more infiltrative and solid and has a worse prognosis than the pilocytic form. Fortunately, pilocytic astrocytomas constitute 85% of cerebellar astrocytomas and fibrillary the remaining 15%. Fibrillary astrocytomas occur in older children than the pilocytic type and are the predominant histologic finding in brain stem gliomas.

Pilocytic astrocytomas also occur in the hypothalamic-optic chiasm–third ventricular region, where they are often associated with neurofibromatosis. The astrocytomas in this region often infiltrate the third ventricle and present with hydrocephalus. Diencephalic syndrome characterized by weight loss despite normal intake, loss of adipose tissue, motor hyperactivity, euphoria, and hyperalertness may occur in cases of chiasmatic/hypothalamic astrocytomas and kids sucking on blow pops with a sugar buzz. Failure to thrive, nystagmus, elevated growth hormone levels, and other visual symptoms may coexist.

Brain stem "gliomas" Brain stem astrocytomas are usually treated with radiation and do not have as high a survival rate as juvenile pilocytic astrocytomas. Nonetheless they are usually WHO grade II diffuse astrocytic tumors with a 25% 10-year survival rate. The masses may be isolated to one part of the brain stem, may grow exophytically (20% of cases), or shed cells into the CSF. Tectal and exophytic brain stem gliomas have a better prognosis than midbrain or medullary ones, and exophytic ones may benefit from surgical resection. Typically these astrocytomas are of the diffuse fibrillary type and anaplasia develops in 50% to 60%. Pontine brain stem gliomas are most common. These masses may be inapparent on CT because of beam-hardening artifact in the posterior fossa, the decreased soft tissue resolution of CT, and their subtle expansion of the anatomy. By contrast, MR provides high sensitivity for the lesion and is well suited to preradiation therapy planning with its multiplanar capability. The lesions are high in intensity on T2WI/FLAIR amid the normal decreased signal intensity of the white matter tracts of the brain stem (Fig. 3-31). They may (33%) or may not (67%) enhance. Cystic degeneration may occur. Subtle enhancement that cannot be seen with CT may be apparent. Symptoms occur late in the course of the disease because the tumor infiltrates rather than destroys histopathologically. Brain stem astrocytomas also do not produce hydrocephalus until they are far advanced. As they enlarge they often appear to encircle the basilar artery. The food analogy for a brain stem astrocytoma might be a Polish sausage with its plump shape (encircling the rat's tail?).

Brain stem astrocytomas may occur in adults; however, 80% of the time they are childhood lesions. They comprise 20% of posterior fossa masses in children, less

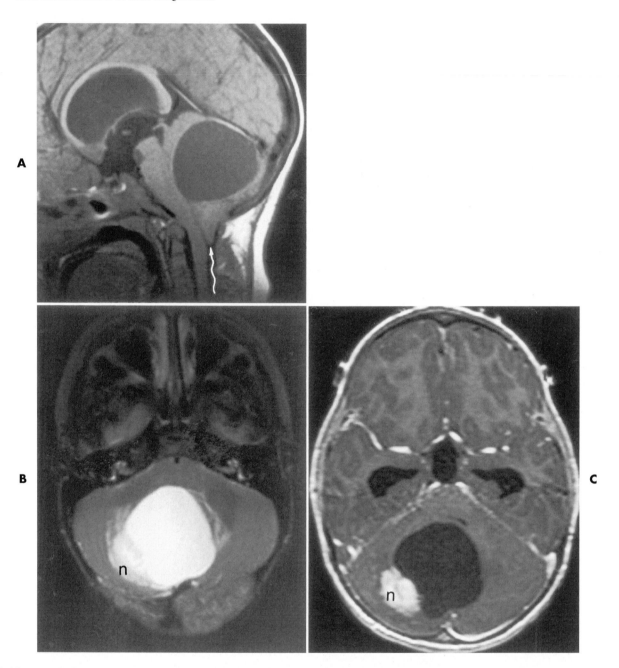

Fig. 3-30 Cyst of pilocytic astrocytoma. **A,** The large cystic mass in the posterior fossa that causes cerebellar tonsillar herniation *(squiggly arrow)* and hydrocephalus in this child with a pilocytic astrocytoma. **B, C,** T2WI shows the dominant feature of the cyst with a small mural nodule (n) which enhances in Fig. 3-30C.

common than cerebellar astrocytomas and medulloblastomas. Other lesions that expand the brain stem in a child include tuberculosis (most common worldwide), lymphoma, rhombic encephalitis (caused by *Listeria*), and demyelinating disorders (acute disseminated encephalomyelitis and multiple sclerosis).

Embryonal tumors

Medulloblastomas/PNET There has been a recent impetus to rename medulloblastomas and other similar cell line tumors "primitive neuroectodermal tumors (PNETs)" (Box 3-4). The rationale is that there really is no such cell line as the "medullo cell" (at least that is what the pathologists tell us). In fact, the latest WHO classification lists these as "embryonal tumors" (Table 3-7). In common vernacular, however, the PNET of the posterior fossa is referred to as medulloblastoma. The analogy to food must be a peanut because of the name but one can think of this class of tumors as typically a solid and dense mass like a peanut. And since they often spread to the subarachnoid space, the peanut butter/sugar and sesame/Tahini analogy works.

Table 3-6   Distinctions among medulloblastoma, ependymoma, and astrocytoma in posterior fossa

Feature	Medulloblastoma	Ependymoma	Astrocytoma
Unenhanced CT	Hyperdense	Isodense	Hypodense
Enhancement	Moderate	Minimal	Nodule enhances, cyst does not
Calcification	Uncommon (10%-21%)	Common (40%-50%)	Uncommon (<10%)
Origin	Vermis	4th ventricle ependyma	Hemispheric
T2WI	Intermediate	Intermediate	Bright
Site	Midline	Midline	Eccentric
Subarachnoid seeding	15%-50%	Uncommon	Rare
Age (yr)	5-12	2-10	10-20
Cyst formation	10-20%	15%	60-80%
Foraminal spread	No	Yes (Luschka, Magendie)	No
Hemorrhage	Rare	10%	Rare
MRS			
Metabolite			
NAA	Low	Intermediate	Intermediate
Lactate	Absent	Often present	Often present
Choline	High	Less elevated	High

Medulloblastomas are one of the most common posterior fossa masses in the pediatric population, accounting for more than one-third of posterior fossa neoplasms and 50% of cerebellar tumors in children. They are quite malignant and have earned the highest class of aggressiveness (grade IV) by Peter Townsend of the WHO. These tumors are usually seen in the midline arising from the vermis and then growing into the inferior or superior velum of the fourth ventricle. Medulloblastomas typically occur in the 5- to 12-year age range, boys twice as commonly as girls, and pa-

tients usually have hydrocephalus. Brain stem dysfunction may also be present.

On nonenhanced CT the lesions are homogeneous hyperdense well-circumscribed masses in the midline associated with the vermis (Fig. 3-32). In older children and adults, medulloblastomas have a greater predilection for the cerebellar hemispheres. The homogeneity of density and hyperdensity on CT are the best findings to suggest medulloblastoma over ependymoma. Occasional calcification and cystic degeneration may occur (see Table 3-6). The fourth ventricle, when seen, is displaced

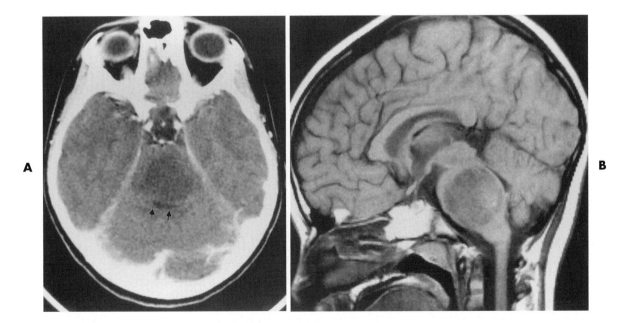

Fig. 3-31   Brain stem glioma. **A,** Pontine brain stem glioma on this enhanced CT compresses the fourth ventricle *(arrows)*. Note lack of enhancement of the tumor. **B,** Sagittal T1WI better defines the extent of the tumor on this midline scan.

Table 3-7 WHO classification of embryonal tumors

Tumor	Grade	Peak age (years)
Medulloepithelioma	IV	0-5
Ependymoblastoma	IV	0-2
Medulloblastoma		
Desmoplastic	IV	0-16, 2nd peak 21-40
Large cell	IV	0-16, peak at 7 years
Medullomyoblastoma	IV	2.5-10.5
Melanotic	IV	0-9
Supratentorial PNET		
Neuroblastoma	IV	0-10
Ganglioneuroblastoma	IV	0-10
Atypical teratoid/ rhabdoid tumor	IV	0-5

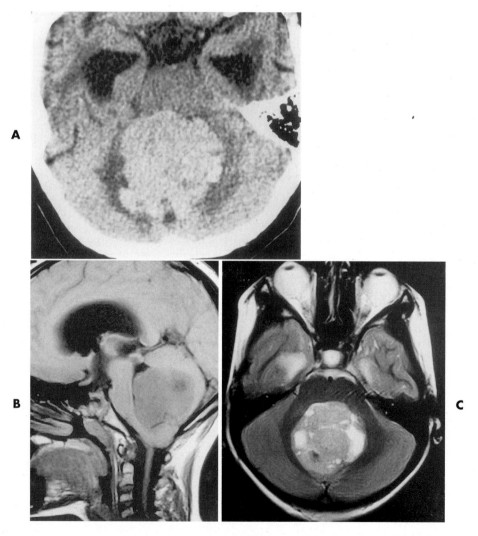

Fig. 3-32   A medulloblastoma that read our book (textbook case, literally). **A,** The unenhanced CT shows a hyperdense mass in the posterior fossa. There is minimal surrounding edema. Note the enlarged temporal horns from hydrocephalus. **B,** Infiltration of the inferior vermis, inferior medullary velum, and fourth ventricle is identified on the sagittal T1WI. **C,** The lesion is intermediate in signal on T2WI.

anteroinferiorly, and there often is obstructive hydrocephalus. The mass shows moderate contrast uptake. Medulloblastomas have a 10% to 21% incidence of calcification. Cystic change, initially thought to be rare, occurs in 10% to 20% of pediatric cases and 59% to 82% of adult cases.

Sagittal images with MR are optimal for visualizing the origin of the tumors from the vermis. The masses are usually hypointense on T1WI and isointense on T2WI. The lesions are typically very well defined and do not demonstrate a large amount of edema (Fig. 3-33). A distinguishing feature between medulloblastomas and ependymomas is that the ependymoma classically en-

larges the fourth ventricle while maintaining its shape whereas medulloblastomas distort the fourth ventricle.

With medulloblastomas, sugar coating or sesame seeding subarachnoid space spread may be present. It has been reported to occur in 15% to 50% of medulloblastomas in children. For this reason MR scanning with contrast of the entire spinal axis is recommended to identify subarachnoid seeds. It has been shown that, for sugar-coating of the cord with tumor, MR is the superior study, but for evaluation of drop lesions on distal spinal nerve roots CT myelography may be competitive. We prefer MR because CT myelography in young children often requires extended sedation and/or general anesthesia. Galen's rule: First do no harm.

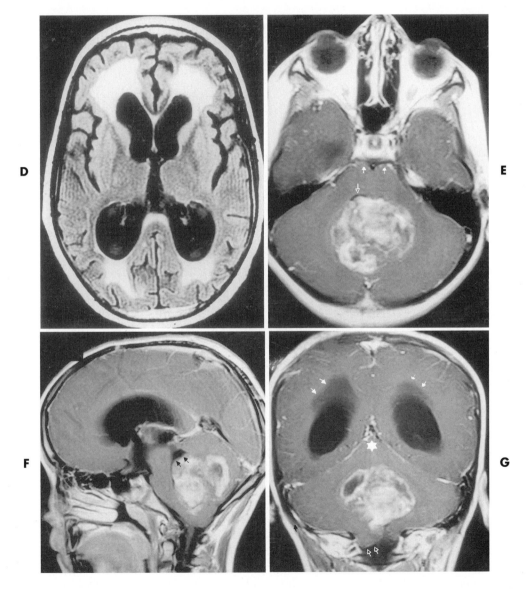

Fig. 3-32 *Continued.* **D,** Hydrocephalus with bright transependymal CSF flow is seen in the supratentorial space on FLAIR. **E,** Axial enhanced T1WI demonstrates compression of the fourth ventricle *(open arrow)*. Note how the brainstem is pushed up against the clivus *(small arrows)*. **F,** A cupping meniscus sign *(arrows)* reflects the obstruction at the top of the fourth ventricle. **G,** Effacement of the superior vermian *(star)* sulci and transependymal CSF flow due to hydrocephalus *(arrows)* are displayed on the coronal postcontrast scan. The right cerebellar tonsil *(open arrows)* is herniating through the foramen magnum. (Figures courtesy of Stuart Bobman, M.D., Naples Florida)

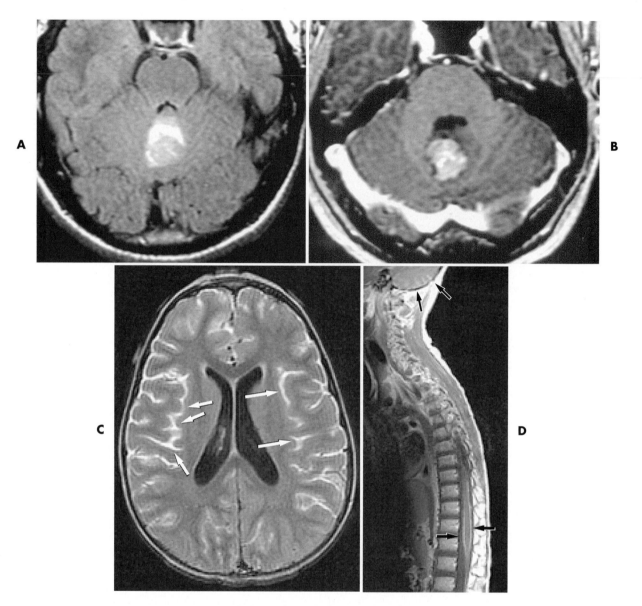

Fig. 3-33   Medulloblastoma. **A,** The vermian mass is hyperintense on FLAIR and in the midline. **B,** It enhances. **C,** Seeding by medulloblastoma may be noted by high signal in the subarachnoid space *(arrows)* on FLAIR scanning, coupled with mild hydrocephalus. Postgadolinium FLAIR scans can be exquisitely sensitive to subarachnoid seeding. **D,** The images of the spine confirm subarachnoid dissemination in the posterior fossa *(arrows)* as well as on the thoracic spinal cord and conus medullaris.

As opposed to some PNETs in adults (cerebral neuroblastoma, adult medulloblastoma), hemorrhage within pediatric medulloblastomas is relatively uncommon.

The spectroscopic signature of a PNET can distinguish it from other posterior fossa masses in children. PNETS show low *N*-acetyl aspartate (NAA):Choline and choline containing compounds (Cho), and creatine-phosphocreatine (CR):Cho ratios compared with low-grade astrocytomas and ependymomas which have higher NAA:Cho ratios. The Cr:Cho ratio is highest for ependymomas compared to astrocytomas and PNETs. Lactate is usually not present in PNETs but is often seen in pilocytic astrocytomas and ependymomas.

Turcot's syndrome (5q21 gene) and nevoid basal cell carcinoma syndrome (9q31 gene) are associated with a high rate of medulloblastomas. The presence of dural calcification in a child less than 10 years of age and a posterior fossa mass should raise the spectre of nevoid basal cell carcinoma (Gorlin's) syndrome.

Medullomyoblastoma   Medullomyoblastomas arise in the vermis and look just like any other type of medulloblastoma. Histologically there is focal myogenic differentiation possibly arising from primitive neuroectodermal tissue. Melanotic medulloblastomas, like medullomyoblastomas occur in the vermis, and have a worse prognosis than the nonmelanotic medulloblastomas.

Rhabdoid tumors/atypical teratoid tumor Rhabdoid tumors are WHO grade IV highly aggressive, heterogeneous looking tumors that may have hemorrhage, necrosis, calcification, or cyst formation (Fig. 3-34). They are dense precontrast on CT. They occur in the same time frame as primitive neuroectodermal tumors, i.e., in the first years of life. Enhancement is patchy. Subarachnoid dissemination is not uncommon (34%), even at presentation and death is predictable within one year of diagnosis. Fifty two percent occur in the posterior fossa,

39% supratentorial, 5% peripineal, and 2% multifocal or intraspinal.

Ependymal tumors

Ependymoma Ependymomas are like sticky buns. They seem to get stuck to every thing they touch and are very hard to clean up. Invariably some sticky goo gets stuck on the counter. In a similar fashion the surgeons find it hard to scrape ependymomas clean, because they stick to the coatings of the brain.

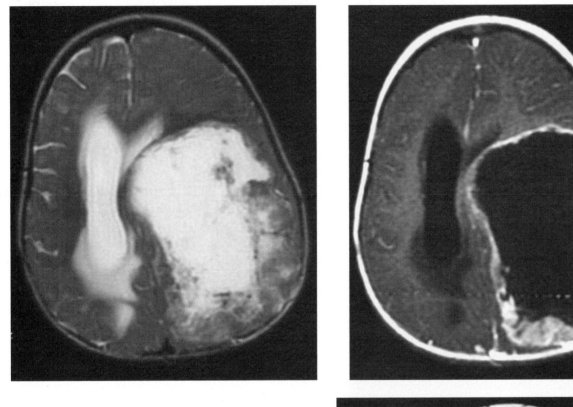

A

B

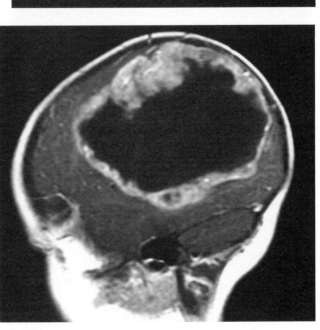

C

Fig. 3-34   Rhabdoid tumor. **A,** This is a huge predominantly cystic mass in the left hemisphere. Note however that there is solid tissue posterolaterally. Check out that mass effect. **B,** The rim of the mass enhances, and the periphery belies the "grade IV" nature of this aggressive mass. Hydrocephalus is present. **C,** These tumors are often over 4-5 cm when discovered.

Table 3-8 WHO classification of ependymal tumors

Tumor	Grade	Peak age (years)
Ependymoma		
Cellular	II	0-9, 2nd peak 30-50 (spinal)
Papillary	II	0-9
Clear cell	II	0-9
Tanycytic	II	30-50
Anaplastic ependymoma	III	0-9
Myxopapillary ependymoma	I	30-40
Subependymoma	I	40-60

Ependymomas are one of a variety of ependymal tumors (Table 3-8) that may occur throughout the brain and spinal cord.

Posterior fossa ependymomas usually are associated with the fourth ventricle, although lesions arising primarily in the foramina of the fourth ventricle do occur and may present as masses outside the fourth ventricle (see Table 3-6). Only 20% of ependymomas arise intraparenchymally, usually in the supratentorial space. The prognosis with ependymomas varies depending on the site; filum terminale (WHO grade I) is best, followed by spinal cord, followed by supratentorial space, followed by posterior fossa (WHO grade II). There is a 50% 5-year progression free survival rate with posterior fossa ependymomas.

Ependymomas have a greater incidence of calcification (40% to 50%) than other posterior fossa pediatric neoplasms (Fig. 3-35). The calcification is typically punctate. When cysts are present (15%), they are small. On unenhanced CT noncalcified infratentorial ependymomas are typically hypodense to isodense without being cystic. The lesions demonstrate mild enhancement, to a lesser degree than the medulloblastomas. Hydrocephalus is usually present due to blockage of the fourth ventricular outflow.

While ependymomas usually present before age 10, a second ependymoma peak in the fourth and fifth decades of life is seen. Once again, they often arise as midline lesions that fill the fourth ventricle without displacing it. A classic appearance of a posterior fossa ependymoma is a calcified fourth ventricular mass that extends through and widens the foramina of Luschka and Magendie. When seen in the cerebral hemispheres, the lesions are large and are cystic 50% of the time.

On MR the lesions are hypointense on T1WI and tend to be intermediate in intensity on T2WI. Particularly when the lesion is in its infantile form (the ependymoblastoma), it may have signal intensity characteristics that are similar to those of normal brain tissue (Fig. 3-36). Hemorrhage is present in about 10% of cases. Hypointensities on T2WI may be due to calcification.

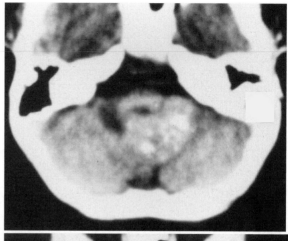

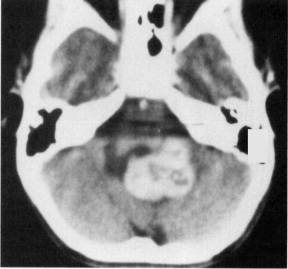

Fig. 3-35 CT of ependymoma. **A,** Noncontrast CT reveals calcification and tumor extending out of the left foramen of Luschka. **B,** After contrast the tumor enhances. Observe that it is virtually impossible to distinguish calcification from enhancement on an enhanced image at these windows.

Ependymomas are another of the brain tumors that have a high incidence of subarachnoid seeding, and the use of contrast material is essential to the detection of subarachnoid spread.

Anaplastic ependymomas Anaplastic ependymomas have an unfavorable prognosis with more rapid growth rate and more frequent contrast enhancement. The prognosis is worse with younger age, incomplete resection, subarachnoid dis-semination, high cell density, and a higher rate of mitoses histopathologically.

Adult Infratentorial Neoplasms

Astrocytic tumors

Astrocytoma, anaplastic astrocytoma, glioblastoma multiforme Astrocytomas are one of the more common pediatric neoplasms of the posterior fossa and the

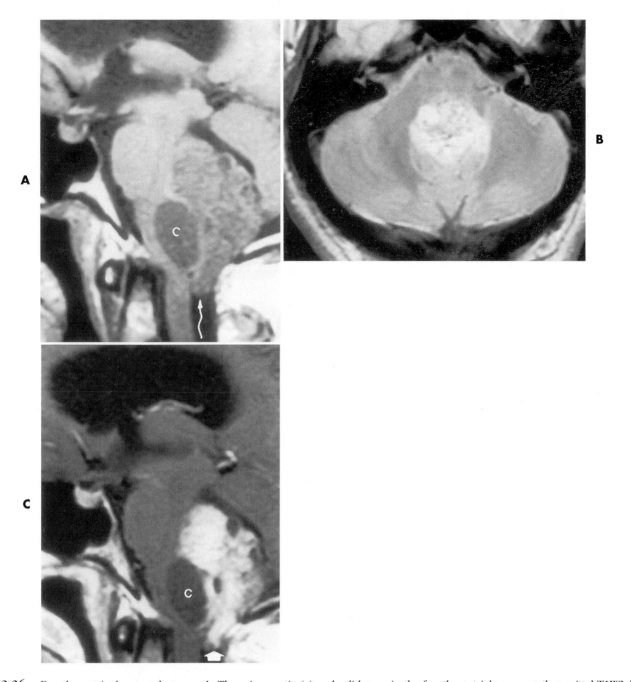

Fig. 3-36   Fourth ventricular ependymoma. **A,** There is a cystic (c) and solid mass in the fourth ventricle seen on the sagittal T1WI. Tumor herniates through the foramen magnum *(squiggly arrow).* **B,** It fills and expands the fourth ventricle and is heterogeneous on T2WI. **C,** Note how it oozes through the foramen of Magendie *(fat arrow)* inferiorly to squirt into the cervicomedullary junction. Cystic components (c) are more evident on this enhanced T1WI.

most common supratentorial adult primary tumor. They will be discussed in depth later but do occur with some regularity in the adult posterior fossa as well. Although the astrocytomas of the posterior fossa in children are often benign in behavior (JPA), those in the posterior fossa of the adult are most commonly GBMs. The GBMs frequently incite a large amount of edema and have tremendous mass effect, often presenting with hydrocephalus caused by obstruction of the fourth ventricle.

On CT, astrocytomas are generally hypodense before contrast and show a varying degree of enhancement. Central necrosis is a hallmark of cerebellar GBM. Irregular ring enhancement is another typical appearance.

MR demonstrates an ill-defined mass that is hypointense on T1WI and hyperintense on T2WI and FLAIR. The degree of edema is sometimes striking because the lesion infiltrates the white matter tracts in the brain stem.

Embryonal tumors

Medulloblastoma/PNET   Although medulloblastomas are typically a pediatric lesion, they may develop in young adults as well (20% of all medulloblastomas reported). As opposed to the pediatric tumors, medulloblastomas in young adults tend to be eccentric in the posterior fossa, residing in the cerebellar hemispheres in more than half the cases. They tend to have a more aggressive course than the pediatric tumors and are less well-defined lesions. A rare variety of medulloblastoma known as the desmoplastic medulloblastoma may arise in an extraaxial location, especially in the cerebellopontine angle. It is an exotic dish, fit for serving to unsuspecting visiting professors, leading to gastric discomfort.

CT of medulloblastomas typically demonstrates a slightly hyperdense, well-circumscribed mass before enhancement. The medulloblastoma enhances to a moderate degree in children and to a lesser degree in adults, possibly because of a more desmoplastic stroma in adults. As noted previously, calcification and cystic portions of the mass are identified more commonly in adults.

Medulloblastomas typically have an intermediate signal on T2WI. On precontrast T1WI they are isointense to gray matter; however, calcification and cystic components may demonstrate either a signal void or CSF intensity, respectively. They enhance.

Medulloblastoma is one of the tumors that have a special propensity for subarachnoid seeding. For this reason the entire craniospinal axis should be imaged with MR after contrast.

Ependymal tumors

Subependymoma   Subependymomas are variants of ependymomas that contain subependymal neuroglia. These tumors are graded WHO grade I and resemble ependymomas in all ways but often do not present until late adulthood. They arise intraventricularly or periventricularly and are frequently multiple at autopsy. They most often arise in the lateral recesses of the fourth ventricle (50% to 60%) but can be seen in the lateral ventricles (30% to 40%) attached to the septum pellucidum (Fig. 3-37). Lateral ventricular subependymomas often arise in patients older than 10 to 15 years. The lesion appears isodense on CT, isointense on T1WI, and hyperintense on T2WI though they may be heterogeneous lesions. Most (>60%) subependymomas do not enhance, but descriptions of lesions with minimal, moderate, and marked enhancement lead to a nonspecific characterization. They are rarely seen in the spinal canal as intra- or extramedullary intradural masses. Usually subependymomas are isodense to gray matter on CT and isointense on all MR pulse sequences. Cyst formation, calcification, and hemorrhage may occur when the tumors are large; larger tumors occur along the lateral ventricles. They have a benign course with slow growth and a lack of invasiveness. Surgical resection is curative.

Neuronal, mixed neuronal/glial tumors

Gangliogliomas   Gangliogliomas of the cerebellum tend to have cystic components but may be solid, mixed, or calcified masses. Over half of them show contrast en-

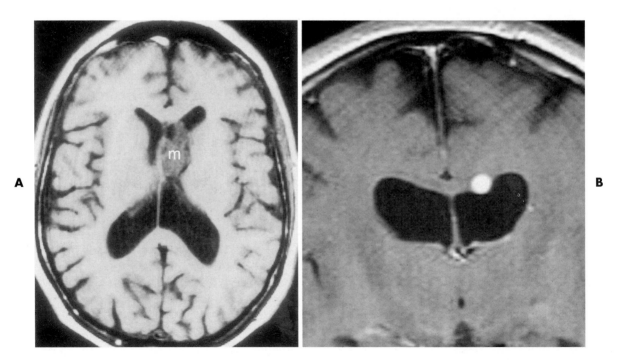

Fig. 3-37   Supratentorial subependymoma. **A,** A mass (m) is attached to the septum pellucidum and enlarges the left frontal horn. It is well defined. Although this was a subependymoma, one should probably include a neurocytoma, low grade astrocytoma, and ependymoma in the differential diagnosis. **B,** Different lesion, outer surface of ventricle, enhancing, but the same diagnosis.

hancement. The grade of the ganglioglioma may be predicted by FDG-PET or 201Tl-SPECT activity (usually low uptake). (More on ganglios in a section below, where they belong).

Cerebellar liponeurocytoma   Cerebellar liponeurocytomas occur in adults with a mean age of 51 years. Fat can be seen in these tumors. They otherwise look like medulloblastomas in adults and can be found in the vermis or the cerebellar hemispheres. Prognosis is great!

Hemangioblastomas

The most common primary intraparenchymal tumor in the infratentorial space in adults is a cerebellar hemangioblastoma (HB). This is a benign tumor, WHO grade I, readily curable with surgery. More than 83% of HBs occur in the cerebellum; the remainder are split among the spinal cord, medulla, and cerebrum in a 4:2:1 ratio. Approximately 10% of posterior fossa masses are HBs. They are far outnumbered by vestibular schwannomas and metastases. Men are more commonly affected than women, and the patients are usually young adults. The common symptoms are headache, ataxia, nausea, vomiting, and vertigo. Polycythemia caused by increased erythropoietin production may be a clinical finding in 40% of cases and is more common with solid HBs. A spinal HB may present with subarachnoid hemorrhage. Twenty-five percent of HBs occur in association with von Hippel-Lindau disease.

The stereotypical findings of an HB are that of a cystic mass with a solid mural nodule (55% to 60% of cases), which is highly vascular and has serpentine signal voids of feeding vessels (Fig. 3-38). (Think of a red strawberry amidst whipped cream.) However, solid HBs (40%) and, less commonly, purely cystic HBs occur as well. You will see a cystic mass in the hemisphere or vermis of the cerebellum with a slightly hyperdense mural nodule on the unenhanced CT scan. The mural nodule demonstrates striking enhancement. The cyst and its walls do not enhance. A purely solid HB also demonstrates strong enhancement (Fig. 3-39).

On angiographic examination a vascular nodule amidst an avascular mass, usually with serpentine vessels, may be identified with or without draining veins. Because sometimes the differential diagnosis includes a meningioma of the tentorium, absence of dural vascular supply strongly mitigates against the diagnosis of a tentorial meningioma. In addition, because the multiple HBs associated with von Hippel–Lindau (VHL) syndrome may be very small, the angiogram may help as a screen for lesions. VHL has been mapped to a gene on the third chromosome (3p25-26).

The MR scan demonstrates findings similar to those of the CT scan, with varying components of cystic and solid tissue. However, the advantage of MR is in showing the large vessels feeding the mural nodule of the HB and the presence of any subtle hemorrhage that may have occurred. The tumors usually reach the pial surface of the brain and therefore may simulate the appearance

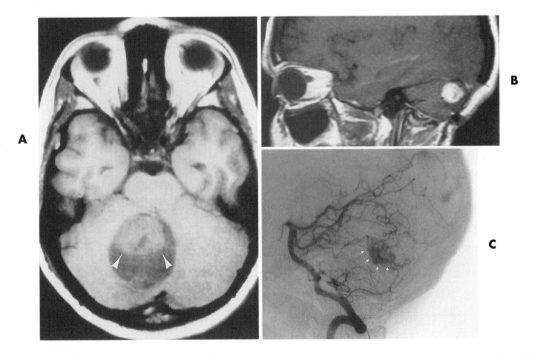

Fig. 3-38   Hemangioblastoma of the cerebellum. **A,** Note the HB with both a cyst and a mural nodule *(arrowheads)* on this unenhanced axial T1WI. **B,** Postcontrast T1WI demonstrates an enhancing solid HB with small flow voids along its circumference in a different patient. **C,** Vertebral artery angiogram shows tumor stain *(arrows)* in another cerebellar HB with vascular supply from the posterior inferior cerebellar artery and branches of the superior cerebellar artery.

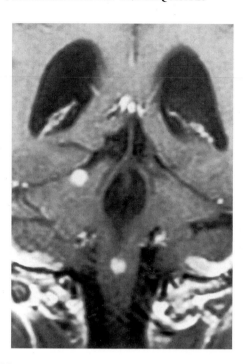

Fig. 3-39 Multiple hemangioblastomas. Peripheral nodules of enhancement are seen on this enhanced coronal T1WI in this patient with multiple hemangioblastomas and von Hippel-Lindau disease.

of a meningioma. The mural nodules of HBs may be multiple in a single lesion rather than multiple HBs. Treatment requires removal of the solid nodule of the lesion only, because the cyst is not really neoplastic. Prognosis is very good with a 5-year survival rate of more than 85%.

Because the description above is nearly the same for JPAs you may ask how to distinguish the two. First and foremost is age—JPAs are seen in the 5 to 15 age range versus 30 to 40 for HBs. Given a 23 year old with a cystic solid mass, go with four findings (1) apial attachment would suggest HB, (2) a tiny nodule with a huge cyst is more likely HB, (3) (if pushed) an arteriogram will show the nodule to be hypervascular with HB and hypovascular with JPA, and (4) multiplicity and association with other findings of VHL syndrome suggests HB.

HBs associated with the VHL syndrome (Box 3-5) generally present at an earlier age. VHL syndrome is inherited as an autosomal dominant trait, with nearly 90% penetrance. HBs associated with VHL syndrome may be multiple in the cerebellum, brain stem, and spinal cord. Current criteria for establishing the diagnosis of VHL syndrome are (1) more than one CNS (including retinal) HB, (2) one CNS HB and one visceral lesion (e.g., renal angiomyolipoma, renal cell carcinoma), or (3) one manifestation of VHL syndrome and a positive family history. One difficulty in analyzing patients with VHL disease occurs when the patient has a known renal cell carcinoma or metastatic pheochromocytoma. Often it is impossible to distinguish hypervascular metastases (which may be

single or multiple) from HBs (which also may be single or multiple).

Metastases

The most common infratentorial neoplasm to occur in the adult population is a metastasis (Fig. 3-40). When

---

Box 3-5 Lesions Associated with VHL Syndrome

CNS

Cerebellar HB (66%–80%)
Spinal HB (28%–40%)
Medullary HB (14%–20%)
Extraaxial HB (<5%)
Retinal HB (50%–67%)

RENAL

Cysts (50–75%)
Hypernephroma (25–50%)
Hemangioblastoma
Adenoma

PANCREATIC

Cysts (30%)
Adenoma
Adenocarcinoma
Islet cell tumor

LIVER

Hemangioma
Cyst
Adenoma

SPLEEN

Angioma

ADRENAL

Pheochromocytoma (10%)
Cyst

LUNG

Cyst

BONE

Hemangioma
Endolymphatic sac tumor (<10%)

CARDIAC

Rhabdomyoma

EPIDIDYMIS

Cyst
Cystadenoma

POLYCYTHEMIA (25–40%)

HB = Hemangioblastoma

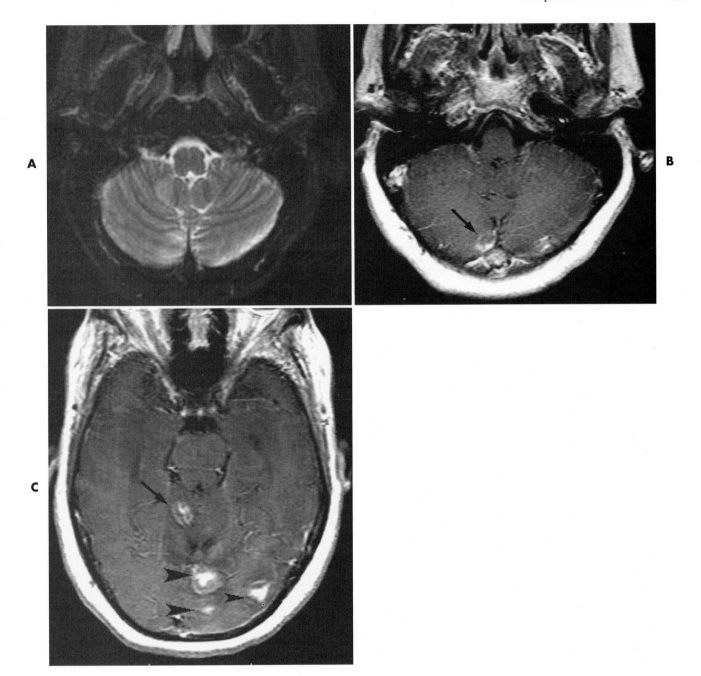

Fig. 3-40   Multiple posterior fossa metastases. **A,** T2 weighted examination shows subtle high-signal intensity in the posterior right cerebellum and in the right nodulus. **B,** With contrast enhancement, the ring enhancing metastasis *(arrow)* is well seen. **C,** Additional metastases are seen in the superior vermis of the cerebellum *(arrow)* and in the occipital lobes *(arrowheads)* at the gray matter-white matter junction.

you think of metastases, think of meatballs or, continuing a Middle East theme, falafel. A plate of spaghetti with multiple meatballs makes sense but the ground beef is detrimental to your HDL/LDL ratio and hence your health. Only one meat or falafel ball provokes a lot of thought, just as a single metastasis becomes thought-provoking because the differential diagnosis becomes much broader with a solitary lesion.

"Meatastatic" lesions are usually seen as well-defined, round masses (like the aforementioned meatballs),

which are identified near the gray-white junction (Fig. 3-41). These lesions show contrast enhancement and are one of the lesions of the brain that often causes nodular or ring enhancement. The most common primary extracranial tumors in adults to metastasize to the infratentorial part of the brain are lung and breast carcinomas. Bronchogenic carcinomas spread to the CNS in 30% of cases, although squamous carcinoma is the least frequent subtype to metastasize to the brain. It is estimated that CNS metastases develop in 18% to 30% of pa-

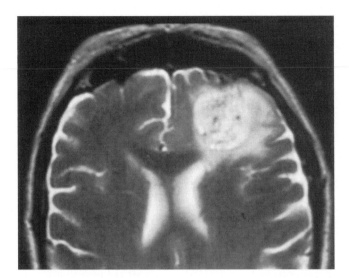

Fig. 3-41   Large metastasis. The gray-white junction is the classic location for where to find a metastasis. A large amount of edema for the size of the mass is another salient feature.

tients with breast cancer. Other neoplasms that have a propensity for metastatic spread to the brain include melanoma (third most common, after lung and breast), renal cell carcinoma, and thyroid carcinoma. Virtually all metastases evoke some vasogenic edema; however, the amount is variable. Sometimes, like a smashed meatball that rolled off the table and onto the floor, the metastasis may be ill defined and infiltrative, and evoke an incredible amount of brain swelling.

Unless the metastatic deposit is hemorrhagic, calcified, hyperproteinaceous, or highly cellular, where it would be hyperdense on noncontrast CT, most metastases are low density on unenhanced CT. Rarely, one may identify calcification in metastatic deposits (Box 3-6). Metastatic deposits may have variable intensity on T2WI. Some lesions are isointense to gray matter on T2WI and can be readily distinguished from the high intensity of the edema they elicit. Other metastatic deposits, however, are hyperintense to gray matter on T2WI. Occasionally one may identify signal intensity characteristics that suggest a primary diagnosis. Hemorrhagic metastases (uncooked meatballs) are usually seen as areas of high signal intensity on T1WI and T2WI with a relative absence of hemosiderin deposition (Box 3-7).

Hemorrhagic metastases must be differentiated from occult cerebrovascular malformations or nonneoplastic hematomas (Table 3-9; Fig. 3-42). Some primary neoplasms such as melanoma, renal cell, choriocarcinoma, and thyroid have a particular propensity to hemorrhage, be it at the primary site or within metastases. However, because lung and breast cancers are so much more common than these primary tumors, a hemorrhagic metastasis is most often from breast or lung. With a single hemorrhagic lesion, primary brain tumors such as GBM and

Box 3-6   Calcified CNS Tumors

METASTASES
Chondrosarcoma
Mucinous adenocarcinoma
    Breast
    Colon
    Ovary
    Stomach
Osteosarcoma

PRIMARY CNS TUMORS
Astrocytoma
Choroid plexus papilloma
Craniopharyngioma
Ependymoma
Ganglioglioma
Meningioma
Neurocytoma
Oligodendroglioma
Pineal region tumors (see Table 3-14)

NEOPLASMS POST RADIOTHERAPY

oligodendroglioma should be considered along with a solitary hemorrhagic metastasis.

In the case of melanoma one may think about all the various varieties of meatballs to account for its various imaging appearances. You have spicy meatballs (melanotic melanomas), uncooked meatballs (hemorrhagic melanomas), soyballs (nonhemorrhagic melanomas) and garden variety meatballs (nonhemorrhagic, nonmelanotic melanomas). One can identify nonhemorrhagic melanotic metastases as lesions that have high intensity on T1WI and isointensity to hypointensity on T2WI caused by intrinsic paramagnetic effects. Although some investigators believe that the paramagnetic effect is due to paramagnetic cations, others believe it to be due to free radicals and still others an inherent characteristic of melanin. However, an *amelanotic* melanoma (without melanin) without hemorrhage may have signal intensity characteristics similar to those of other nonhemorrhagic

Box 3-7   Hemorrhagic Metastases

Breast cancer
Choriocarcinoma
Lung cancer
Melanoma
Renal cell carcinoma
Retinoblastoma
Thyroid cancer

Table 3-9 Features of recently bled occult cerebrovascular malformations versus hemorrhagic metastases

Feature	Hemorrhagic occult cerebrovascular malformations (cavernomas)	Hemorrhagic metastases
Edema	Only with acute episode, resolves by 8 wk	Persistent
Mass	Variable but resolves	Moderate to large, persistent
Hemosiderin ring	Complete	Incomplete or absent
Nonhemorrhagic tissue	Absent	Present
Enhancement	Minimal and central	Nodular, ring, or eccentric
Progression of hemorrhagic stages	Orderly	Delayed
Follow-up	Decreases in size with time	Increases in size with time
Calcification	Approximately 20%	Rare

metastases: low signal on T1WI and high signal on T2WI. Furthermore, hemorrhagic melanoma metastases, be they melanotic or amelanotic, have signal intensity similar to other hemorrhagic nonmelanotic lesions. In fact, the real issue may be the percent content of melanin in the melanoma metastasis; those containing more than 10% melanotic cells demonstrate the typical melanotic MR imaging pattern (bright on T1WI, dark on T2WI). If the content is less than 10% melanin-containing cells, a variety of MR imaging patterns can be present. About half of patients with amelanotic lesions show the characteristic melanotic MR imaging pattern, likely because of hemorrhage.

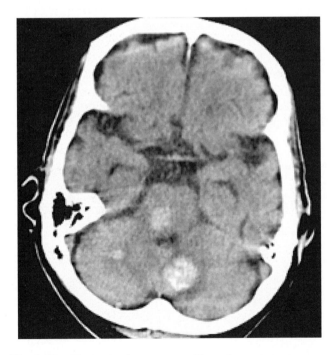

Fig. 3-42 Hemorrhagic metastases. Hyperdense masses are seen in the brain stem and cerebellum. Although one might consider cavernomas in the differential diagnosis, this patient had renal cell carcinoma. The edema around the mass in the cerebellum can be seen.

Supratentorial Pediatric Neoplasms

Astrocytic tumors

Pleomorphic xanthoastrocytoma (PXA) These tumors are seen in children and young adults (first three decades of life). Two thirds occur in patients less than 18 years old. The lesion shows a preference for the periphery of the temporal lobes as they arise from subpial astrocytes. They may show a base at the meninges in more than 70% of cases. Owing to their predilection for the temporal lobes, they cause seizures in most cases. Homogeneous enhancement of the cortical mass is common. Cyst formation occurs in about one-third to one-half of cases, but hemorrhage and calcification are distinctly uncommon. Margins may be well or poorly defined. These tumors may rarely have anaplastic transformation but are considered WHO grade II lesions though circumscribed. Survival is over 80% at 5 years. These tumors are hard to distinguish from DNETs but enhance more frequently. PXAs have a meningeal attachment and no cortical dysplasia—these features also help distinguish them from DNETs. We like to use their abbreviations because, as word salads, pleomorphic xanthoastrocytomas and dysembryoplastic neuroepithelial tumors, can fill you up, and taste the same.

Embryonal tumors

Supratentorial PNET Cerebral neuroblastomas are now called supratentorial PNETs. If there are ganglion cells present they may be termed cerebral ganglioneuroblastomas, but either way they are WHO grade IV, aggressive tumors. The younger the age at diagnosis, the worse the prognosis. These tumors often show cyst formation, calcification (50% to 70%), and hemorrhage and are usually seen in children. They can be seen as hyperdense on unenhanced CT scans. They have a high rate of recurrence and subarachnoid seeding. Usually they are large lesions, 3 to 10 cm in diameter, and inhomogeneous in density and intensity; they enhance in a heterogeneous fashion (Fig. 3-43). Occasionally, they

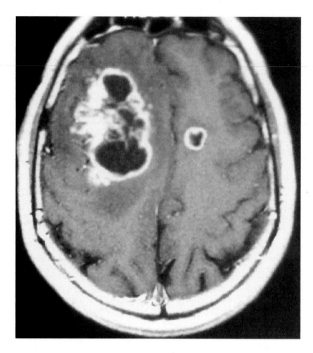

Fig. 3-43 Multifocal cerebral neuroblastoma (a zebra). Note the irregular enhancement and cystic-necrotic portions to the tumors in this patient with an unusual case of multifocal cerebral neuroblastoma. Usually these lesions are solitary and well circumscribed.

arise in a suprasellar or periventricular location, but cerebral neuroblastomas are most commonly found in frontal, parietal, and occipital lobes. The tumors do not incite much edema and are usually well circumscribed. Eighty percent arise in patients less than 10 years old (25% before 2 years old), but they can be seen in young adults. Three-year survival rate is 60%, 5 year is 34%, and recurrence is common (40%).

Medulloepithelioma Medulloepitheliomas are aggressive grade IV embryonal tumors that occur more often supratentorially than infratentorially in infants. The temporal lobes are affected more often than parietal lobes, but this tumor has also been described in the globe. Cysts, calcification, hemorrhage, necrosis, and enhancement occur with tumor progression, which occurs very rapidly. Subarachnoid dissemination occurs in due time.

Ependymoblastoma Another in the WHO grade IV pediatric embryonal tumors (PNET), the ependymoblastoma favors the supratentorial compartment as opposed to ependymomas. The tumors are large at discovery with enhancement, edema, and areas of peripheral necrosis and cyst formation. Nonetheless they are relatively well-circumscribed. They invade the leptomeninges and usually appose the ventricles, having arisen in periventricular neuroepithelial precursor cells. Death due to CSF dissemination usually occurs within 6 to 12 months of presentation and presentation is in young children and neonates.

Neuronal, mixed neuronal/glial tumors

Ganglioglioma Gangliogliomas are most commonly seen in children and young adults (64% to 80% occur in patients < 30 years old). They are the most common mixed glioneural tumors of the CNS (see Table 3-10). They are low-grade tumors with good prognoses. Presentation most commonly is with a seizure. The tumors affect female more than male patients and are characterized by a benign, slow-growing course often associated with bony remodeling that testifies to their indolent growth. The most common sites for these tumors are within the temporal lobes (85%), frontal lobes, anterior third ventricle, and cerebellum. They also frequent the spinal cord and optic nerves. The lesions are cystic in 38% to 50% of cases and are typically hypodense or isodense on CT. One third show calcification and half have faint enhancement (Fig. 3-44). MR features vary depending on cyst formation. If cysts are present, then the ganglioglioma may be hypointense on T1WI and bright on T2WI. A mural nodule may coexist. One could visualize a jello mold (cystic) with small fruit (solid) portions for this delicacy of a neoplasm. The tumor is well defined and avascular at angiography. A cystic ganglioglioma can be distinguished from an arachnoid cyst in that it is clearly intraparenchymal and has higher signal intensity than CSF or arachnoid cysts on PDWI or FLAIR. Epidermoids may have similar intensity properties but are distinguished as being extraaxial.

In children under 10 years old gangliogliomas are larger and more cystic (83% of cases) than those occurring after 10 years of age. More edema may be seen by virtue of the larger size. Solid enhancing components are the rule in both age groups.

The tumor is comprised of neuronal ganglion cells and astrocytic glial cells, hence its name. However, its behavior is defined by the degree of dedifferentiation of the glial portion of the tumor and therefore it may con-

Table 3-10 WHO classification of neuronal and mixed neuronal-glial tumors

Tumor	Grade	Peak age (years)
Gangliocytoma	I	0-30
Ganglioglioma	I or II	0-30
Anaplastic ganglioglioma	III	0-30
Desmoplastic infantile astrocytoma/ganglioglioma	I	0-2
Dysembryoplastic neuroepithelial tumor	I	10-20
Central neurocytoma	II	20-30
Cerebellar liponeurocytoma	I or II	45-55
Paraganglioma of filum terminale	I	30-70

vert into an aggressive lesion, the anaplastic ganglioglioma. The histologic grade of a ganglioglioma may be predicted by FDG-PET and thallium-SPECT studies. The presence of vasogenic edema also is correlated with worse histologic grade, but most gangliogliomas do not produce much edema.

Gangliocytoma   As opposed to ganglio**gliomas**, which may undergo malignant degeneration and a more ag-gressive growth pattern, ganglio**cytomas** have no glial component and no potential for malignant change. Pure Jello. Gangliocytomas are usually located in the cerebral cortex or the cerebellum. In the cerebellum, some people call these tumors Lhermitte-Duclos syndrome, but others believe this entity is a dysplasia not a neoplasia. They may be hyperdense on noncontrast CT and show little to no enhancement. Gangliocytomas are often isoin-

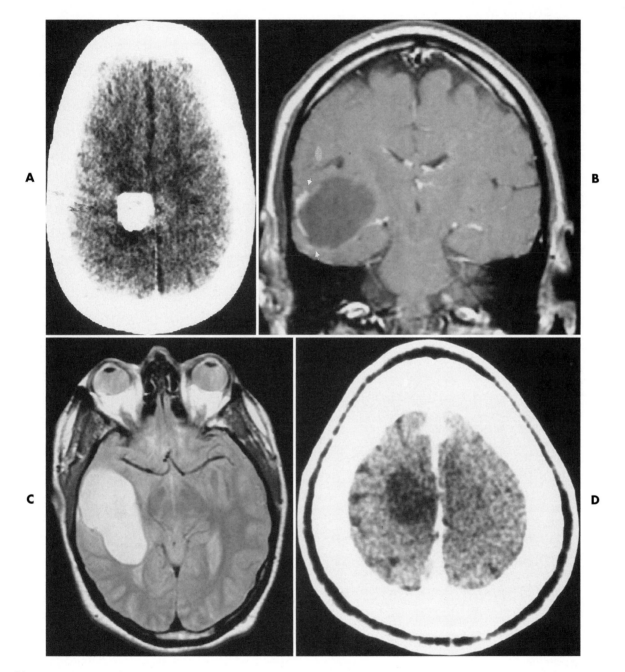

Fig. 3-44   Multiple faces of ganglioglioma. **A,** Axial unenhanced CT shows a well-defined calcified mass in the superficial portion of the right hemisphere without significant edema. **B,** Enhanced coronal T1WI shows a cystic mass in the right temporal lobe with a small peripheral area of rim enhancement *(arrows)*. Ganglio-gliomas may simulate arachnoid cysts in their appearance and need not show enhancement. **C,** Note how well circumscribed the lesion is, without white matter edema, on the PDWI. **D,** Another ganglioglioma demonstrates low density on CT.

Illustration continued on following page

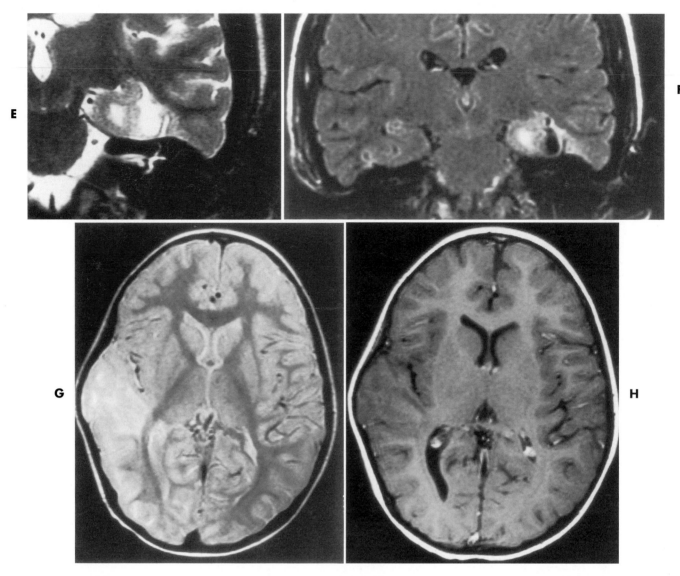

Fig. 3-44 *Continued.* **E,** Yet another in our amazing series of gangliogliomas shows a cystic and solid left temporal lobe mass as seen on T2WI. **F,** FLAIR confirms the infiltration of the hippocampus. The mass did not enhance. **G,** Different case showing bony remodeling of the right temporal bone, squamosal portion, due to the slow growth of the mass on long TR scan. Note the loss of the gray white matter interface. **H,** Absence of enhancement characterized this mass. (You'll never see even half this number of cases in private practice; so stick to academia, our students.)

tense on T1WI and T2WI and are best seen by their hyperintensity on FLAIR.

Desmoplastic infantile ganglioglioma (DIG) This is a variant of the ganglioglioma that is usually seen in the first 2 years of life. The tumors typically occur in the frontal and parietal lobes and have a meningeal base. Cyst formation is the rule and peripheral rim or nodular enhancement usually is present as well. Some may show a calcified rim. Although this lesion may look like a huge necrotic glioblastoma multiforme in an infant, it has a good prognosis with benign histology (WHO grade I). The tumor has both glial and ganglionic derivation (no wonder they call it ganglioglioma). The desmoplasia accounts for the rim of low signal intensity tissue on T2W scans. The differential diagnosis will include DNETs and PNETs, but the incidence of calcification and hemorrhage is higher in cortical PNETS (Fig. 3-45).

Desmoplastic infantile astrocytoma (desmoplastic cerebral astrocytoma of infancy) probably represents a variant of DIG and is a newly described tumor that has features of glial and mesenchymal histology. Absence of neuronal components histologically distinguishes this tumor from a DIG. It is a benign form of astrocytoma found in early life. In general, there is a dural based mass with cystic change. Although the dural-based mass will enhance, the cyst does not, not even on the periphery. Mass effect and vasogenic edema are rare. It also presents in the first 18 months of life and is usually seen supratentorially.

Dysembryoplastic neuroepithelial tumor Dysembryoplastic neuroepithelial (neuroectodermal) tumors (DNET or DNT) are most commonly found in the temporal (50% to 62%) and frontal (31%) lobes and usually cause seizures. The lesion is a neuroepithelial tumor that looks like a ganglioglioma and most present by the second and third decade of life in patients with chronic seizures. They are located peripherally in the brain with the cortex involved in nearly all cases and the subcortical white matter in most cases (Fig. 3-45). Half have poorly defined contours. On MR, this tumor is characterized by the presence of cysts, usually multiple. Look for bright, bright T2W signal. Contrast enhancement is observed in less than a third of the cases (distinguishing it from a DIG) and mass effect is variable. The lesion is often hypodense on CT and grows very slowly. The presence of multiple cysts and the rarity of the lesion in the infratentorial compartment may help to distinguish a DNET from a ganglioglioma (Table 3-11). DNETs usually do not have edema associated with them and they may remodel the calvarium. They are reported to have coincident focal cortical dysplasias with them in over 50% of cases. They rarely recur after resection, even if partial. Good actors! WHO grade I. If you stop to think about these tumors, remember to start again.

Another location for DNET is the septum pellucidum. A recent report has described 10 DNETs as nonenhancing, cystic well-defined masses arising from the septum pellucidum and growing intraventricularly in young patients.

Supratentorial Adult Neoplasms

Astrocytic tumors

Astrocytoma If one took all patients with a single mass in the supratentorial compartment, the odds would be nearly even that the lesion would be an astrocytoma or a metastasis. This is because metastases are more often multiple, and astrocytoma are the most frequent primary solitary intraaxial mass in the adult.

The grading of astrocytomas by pathology groups is variable; the latest WHO classification separates malignant gliomas into circumscribed astrocytomas (grade I) diffuse astrocytomas (grade II), anaplastic astrocytomas (grade III), and GBM (grade IV) on the basis of histologic criteria (Box 3-8) and gross/imaging appearance. The var-

ious varieties of astrocytomas remind us of various forms of steak (porterhouse, sirloin, New York Strip, T-bone, etc.). Circumscribed lesions include the pilocytic astrocytomas (Fig. 3-46), subependymal giant cell astrocytomas, and PXA. Fibrillary, gemistocytic, and protoplasmic astrocytomas are classified as diffuse grade II tumors. Then come the nasties, anaplastic astrocytoma and glioblastoma multiforme, that are of the highest grade, sort of like the way steaks are graded. Syndromes associated with astrocytomas are listed in Box 3-9.

The Grade I pilocytic and fibrillary astrocytomas have been described earlier in sections on cerebellar and brain stem astrocytomas. Diffuse astrocytomas Grade II are more likely to show absence of enhancement. They can occur anywhere (Fig. 3-47) but one third are in the frontal lobes and one third in the temporal lobes. They are the most common variety to attack the brainstem. Cystic change and calcification may occur (Fig. 3-48). Gemistocytic astrocytomas are found exclusively in the cerebral hemispheres and are a rare variety of supratentorial gliomas that in 80% of cases ultimately convert to GBMs. Mean survival time is more than 3.5 years, slightly better than another variety of astrocytoma, the monstrocellular (or magnocellular) type. The borders are relatively well defined for a glioma in both these varieties, but no other features are distinctive.

Anaplastic astrocytoma Anaplastic astrocytomas (AA) occur most commonly in the fourth and fifth decades of life and usually evolve from lower grade astrocytomas. They have ill-defined borders with prolific vasogenic edema. They are much more likely to show contrast enhancement, but if necrosis is seen, bump the lesion up to a GBM. When all astrocytomas are considered, anaplasia occurs in 75% to 80% with ultimate dedifferentiation into GBM occurring in 50% of cases. Typical time for progression from AA to GBM is 2 years—short enough to drive you to drinking and another AA. Histopathologically, when one finds a GBM there is evidence of a diffuse astrocytoma that may have predated the GBM in 35% of cases.

Glioblastoma multiforme The majority of GBMs in the elderly are felt to be primary tumors, that is, they do not evolve from lower grade astrocytomas. The clinical course is short, a few months. Secondary GBMs that arise from dedifferentiation of lower grade astrocytomas occur in a younger age group and with a more protracted clinical prodrome over years in duration. Genetic markers may help distinguish between primary (*EGFR* gene positive, TP53 negative, MDM2 positive) and secondary (*EGFR* gene negative, TP53 positive, MDM2 negative). Of the astrocytomas, GBM (WHO grade IV) is the most common variety, nearly twice as frequent as the anaplastic astrocytomas and the grade I astrocytomas and accounting for 50% to 60% of astrocytic tumors and 15% of intracranial neoplasms. Depicted as a meat, GBM

Text continued on page 142

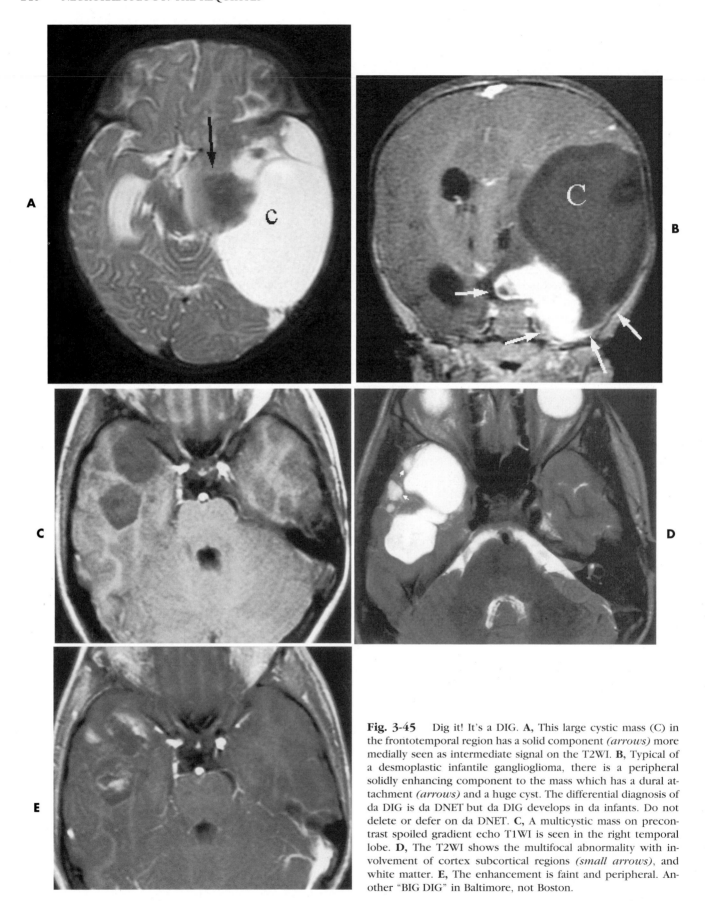

Fig. 3-45 Dig it! It's a DIG. **A,** This large cystic mass (C) in the frontotemporal region has a solid component *(arrows)* more medially seen as intermediate signal on the T2WI. **B,** Typical of a desmoplastic infantile ganglioglioma, there is a peripheral solidly enhancing component to the mass which has a dural attachment *(arrows)* and a huge cyst. The differential diagnosis of da DIG is da DNET but da DIG develops in da infants. Do not delete or defer on da DNET. **C,** A multicystic mass on precontrast spoiled gradient echo T1WI is seen in the right temporal lobe. **D,** The T2WI shows the multifocal abnormality with involvement of cortex subcortical regions *(small arrows),* and white matter. **E,** The enhancement is faint and peripheral. Another "BIG DIG" in Baltimore, not Boston.

Table 3-11 Differentiation of temporal lobe lesions

Tumor	Age	Demarcation	Edema?	Percent of Tumors Causing Temporal Lobe Seizures	Hemorrhage	Cyst Formation	Enhancement	Cortical Involvement	Calcification
Ganglioglioma	0-30	Well	Very little	40%	Rare	Common	Uncommon	Common	Variable
Low grade astrocytoma	0-30	Well	Yes	26%	Rare	Common	Uncommon	Uncommon	Variable to uncommon
DNET	10-20	Well	None	18%	Common	Common, dominant multiple	Uncommon to variable	Always	Common
Oligodendroglioma	30-60	Less well	Yes	6%	Variable	Variable	Common	Variable	Common
PXA	10-35	Well, but malignant change in 20%	Uncommon	4%	Rare	Common	Common in mural nodule	Common, meningeal attachment	Rare
Desmoplastic infantile ganglioglioma	0-1	Well	Occasionally	<3%	No	Common	Common in nodule desmoplasia	Dural attachment	None

DNET = Dysembryoplastic neuroepithelial tumors, PXA = pleomorphic xanthoastrocytomas

141

Box 3-8 Pathologic Criteria for Grading Gliomas

Number of mitoses
Presence of necrosis
Vascular endothelial proliferation
Nuclear pleomorphism
Cellular density

would be my liver and onions. Even the thought of this combination makes me ill and the vision of the solid tumor (liver) with daughter lesions (onions around the meat) brings to mind this lethal neoplasm. GBM is the most lethal of the gliomas, having a 10% to 15% 2-year survival rate. These tumors can appear anywhere in the cerebrum but are seen most commonly in the frontal (23%), parietal (24%), and temporal (31%) lobes. The occipital lobes are frequently spared.

GBM is characterized on imaging by the presence of necrosis within the tumor. Histologic grade seems roughly to parallel patients' age in the adults; the older the patient is, the more likely the lesion is to be a higher grade astrocytoma. Other factors that correlate with higher grade are ring enhancement, enhancement in general, marked mass effect, and intratumoral necrosis. Recent reports have found that relative cerebral blood volume (rCBV) correlates well with astrocytoma histology and vascularity; the higher the rCBV the more likely one is dealing with a GBM. At the same time, hemorrhage, as depicted by gradient echo scans, and the presence of

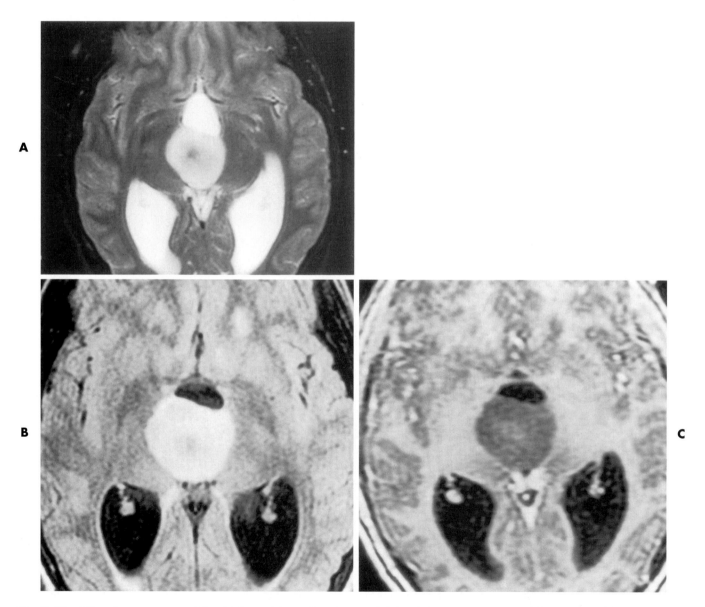

Fig. 3-46   Pilocytic astrocytoma of the third ventricle. **A,** Note how well-defined the mass is on T2WI **(A)** and FLAIR **(B).** The lesion is very bright on these pulse sequences and does not enhance (C). The lesion causes obstructive hydrocephalus.

Box 3-9 Syndromes Associated with Brain Tumors

BASAL CELL NEVUS SYNDROME (CHROMOSOME 9Q31)

Gorlin syndrome—basal cell nevi and carcinomas, odontogenic keratocysts, ribbon ribs, phalangeal deformity and pitting, falcian calcification, craniofacial deformities, scoliosis, and **medulloblastoms**

COWDEN SYNDROME (CHROMOSOME 10Q23)

Multiple hamartomas, mucocutaneous tumors, fibrocystic breast disease, polyps, thyroid adenoma, **Lhermitte-Duclos syndrome**
von Hippel Lindau (see Chapter 9)

LI-FRAUMENI SYNDROME (CHROMOSOME 17P13)

Increased rate of breast cancers, soft tissue sarcomas, osteosarcomas, leukemia
Autosomal dominant with **astrocytomas > PNET > choroid plexus tumors**
CNS tumors in 13.5%

MAFFUCCI SYNDROME

Enchondromas, soft tissue cavernomas

NEUROFIBROMATOSIS 1 AND 2 (SEE CHAPTER 9)

OLLIER SYNDROME

Multiple enchondromas

TUBEROUS SCLEROSIS (SEE CHAPTER 9)

TURCOT SYNDROME (CHROMOSOMES 5Q21, 3P21, 7P22)

Colonic familial polyposis, **glioblastoma, rare medulloblastoma**

---

lactic acid on MRS have been linked to a higher grade. Despite these trends it is not possible for the radiologist to supplant the pathologist in grading the tumors (and the pathologists often ain't so great, either). Leave it to the USDA to grade the steaks.

GBMs infiltrate wildly and are mapped as high signal intensity on long TR images. Enhancement may be solid, ringlike, or occasionally inhomogeneously mild (Fig. 3-49). The tumor frequently crosses the corpus callosum, anterior commissure, or posterior commissure to reach the contralateral hemisphere. Of the adult astrocytomas a GBM is the most common to have intratumoral hemorrhage and subarachnoid seeding (2% to 5% of cases). Occasionally, it coats the ventricles.

MRS has recently shown that there is a strong relationship with choline levels in homogeneous nonenhancing astrocytomas and the Ki-67 labeling index. This in turn corresponds well to grade of tumor. Cho/creatine and Cho/NAA ratios traditionally have been the

best predictors of histologic grade of tumors, along with the presence of lactate in the higher grade masses.

Giant cell glioblastomas are WHO grade IV tumors that were previously called monstrocellular sarcomas and comprise <5% of all GBMs. They are glioblastomas that have multinucleated giant cells in abundance, TP53 mutations, and a fibrous network that causes a more localized appearing tumor. Consider this a well-demarcated GBM.

Gliosarcomas Consider this a nasty GBM-mesenchymal tumor that even Hannibal Lecter might be willing to pass up. They constitute 2% of all GBMs and favor the supratentorial space. Despite their name they may be well-defined, superficial, and strongly enhancing.

Multicentric astrocytomas Multicentric astrocytomas may be due to true metachronous independent lesions, but more often than not represent contiguous spread of gliomatous tissue in which the connection is inapparent on imaging but present on pathologic study. Multiple independent glioblastomas occur in 2.3% of GBMs, so only use your cellular phone on one side of your head, for heaven's sake, and use it on your nondominant hemisphere. NF-1 is associated with multifocal astrocytomas.

DWI has proven very useful in differentiating the cystic or necrotic component of a tumor from the central necrosis of a pyogenic abscess. On DWI, most cystic/necrotic tumors are dark in intensity corresponding to unrestricted diffusion; for some unknown reason pyogenic abscesses are often bright on DWI. The restricted diffusion may have something to do with the viscosity of the pus. Would that we can say that this holds true for all abscesses—the use of this finding with lesions like toxoplasmosis or some fungal abscesses is not as reliable. The MRS people believe that the presence of resonances attributed to lactate, valine, alanine, leucine, acetate, succinate, and unidentified metabolites (at shifts of 2.2, 2.9, 3.2, 3.4, and 3.8 ppm) in abscesses can be differentiated from spectra with necrotic tumor where there are only resonances attributable to lactate—not.

When you see a lesion involving the corpus callosum (Box 3-10), you should put GBM and lymphoma near the top of the list of neoplasms (Fig. 3-50). Because of the compact nature of the white matter fibers in this structure, it is uncommon to have edema spread across the corpus callosum. Infarcts involving the corpus callosum are unusual because the blood supply is said to be bilateral through the anterior cerebral arteries (now in dispute!). Radiation damage generally spares the corpus callosum. The only other lesion of note that affects the corpus callosum is trauma; there is a propensity for shearing injuries in this location because of its relative fixed location spanning the interhemispheric fissure.

The extent of a neoplasm is not defined by its enhancing rim. In fact, radiation oncologists treat the entire area of abnormal T2WI/FLAIR high intensity with radiation followed by a coned-down portal encompassing

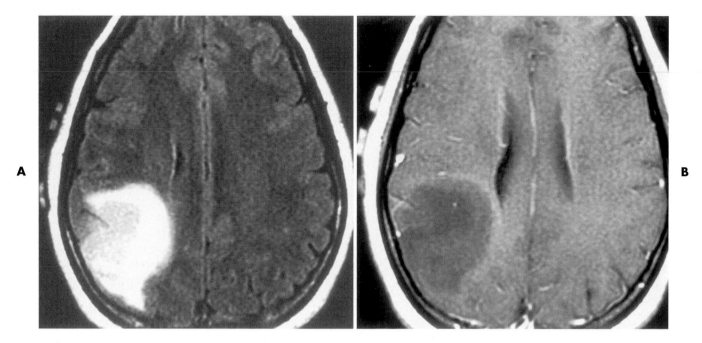

Fig. 3-47 Grade II astrocytoma. **A,** The mass is somewhat well-defined on FLAIR, but still is pretty bulky. **B,** It does not enhance.

the enhancing portion with a 2-cm rim around the enhancing edge. Microscopic infiltration clearly extends beyond the confines of enhancement, and the high signal intensity on T2WI may not represent tumor in all instances. Neoplastic cells can definitely be present histopathologically in brain tissue appearing entirely normal on imaging studies.

Subependymal giant cell astrocytomas Another variant of "glioma" is the subependymal giant cell astrocytoma (SGCA or SEGA). Classically this lesion is seen in

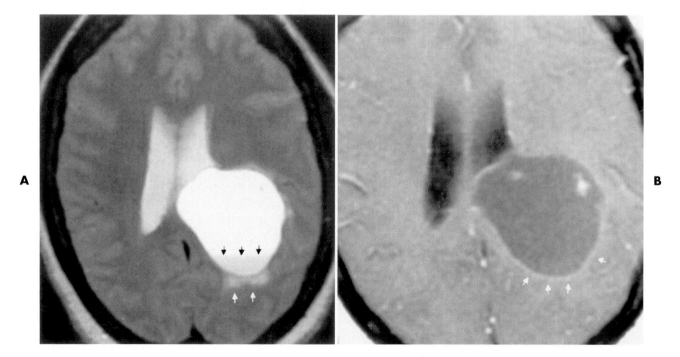

Fig. 3-48 Low-grade astrocytoma. **A,** T2-weighted scan demonstrates a cystic mass compressing the posterior aspect of the left lateral ventricle with a small fluid level within it *(black arrows)*. Note the minimal edema *(white arrows)* present posterior to the lesion. **B,** After contrast administration only a thin rim of enhancement *(arrows)* is seen with focal nodules anteriorly. Final path: low-grade astrocytoma.

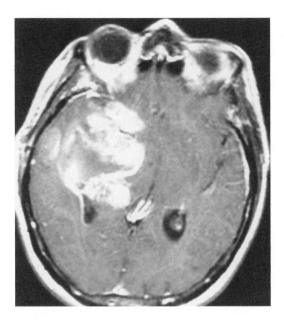

Fig. 3-49 Glioblastoma multiforme. This GBM demonstrates irregular enhancement and mass effect with displacement of midline structures to the left side. Bad actor.

2- to 20-year-old patients with tuberous sclerosis. Patients with tuberous sclerosis may have areas of subependymal nodules or tubers (which may be calcified on CT), subcortical tubers, and other hamartomatous lesions. Subependymal giant cell astrocytomas typically occur near the foramina of Monro and in contradistinction with tubers demonstrate moderate to marked enhancement (Fig. 3-51). This tumor may occur in isolation without tuberous sclerosis, but it is an uncommon variant. The tumor is slow growing (WHO grade I) and projects into the ventricular system, where it appears to be a calcified intraventricular mass (Box 3-11). The outflow of the lat-

---

Box 3-10 Corpus Callosum Mass Lesions

NEOPLASMS

GBM
Lymphoma
Metastases

WHITE MATTER DISORDERS

Multiple sclerosis
Progressive multifocal leukoencephalopathy
Adrenoleukodystrophy
Marchiafava-Bignami disease
PRES

ACUTE SHEARING INJURIES

STROKE

LIPOMA

---

eral ventricle may be obstructed, leading to trapping of one or both lateral ventricles with noncommunicating hydrocephalus. Because many subependymal nodules show enhancement on MR, but not on CT, CT can actually be more specific than MR in distinguishing large subependymal nodules from SGCA by virtue of this feature.

Neuronal, mixed neuronal/glial tumors

Central neurocytoma Many of the neoplasms previously called intraventricular oligodendrogliomas may actually be neurocytomas (WHO grade II tumor of neuronal origin) (Table 3-12). Both calcify frequently, may be cystic, and favor the lateral or third ventricle (often with an attachment to the septum pellucidum) (Fig. 3-52). Edema is rare. Central neurocytomas peak in the third decade of life, mean age 29 years. They are isointense to gray matter on all MR pulse sequences and show mild to moderate enhancement with prominent vascular flow voids. Intraventricular neurocytomas hemorrhage more frequently than oligodendrogliomas, which may suggest that diagnosis. Usually, however, the radiologist cannot differentiate the two. Electron microscopy and immunohistochemical markers for synaptophysin can distinguish intraventricular oligodendrogliomas from neurocytomas. The pathologic distinction is not moot; neurocytomas have a more benign course than oligodendrogliomas and may not require radiation therapy. Oligodendrogliomas show a predilection for the septum pellucidum as well. The analogy here would be those candy dots that are attached to paper; like the mass attached to the septum pellucidum.

Oligodendroglial tumors

Oligodendroglioma Oligodendrogliomas comprise just 4% to 1; 8% of intracranial gliomas but are typified by their high rate of calcification (40% to 80%) (Fig. 3-53). Peak age range is in the fifth and sixth decade, and the tumor favors men by a 2:1 margin. The tumor, when pure, has a benign course (classified as WHO grade II).

Oligodendrogliomas are the ribeye steak of glial tumors. They may have calcification (bones), soft tissue (meat), and cystic areas. Oligodendrogliomas appear differently depending on the contribution of the astrocytic or spongioblastic component. Juxtaposition of patterns may be seen.

Enhancement, when present in oligodendrogliomas, is variable (present in 50% to 67%). Hemorrhage occurs in 20% of cases, as does cyst formation. When the tumor encysts, it has a higher rate of malignant astrocytic behavior. On MR the tumor is hypointense on T1WI and hyperintense on T2WI/FLAIR except in the areas of calcification (Fig. 3-54). Heterogeneity of signal is the watchword. On CT the lesions are hypodense or isodense on unenhanced scans (unless hemorrhage or cal-

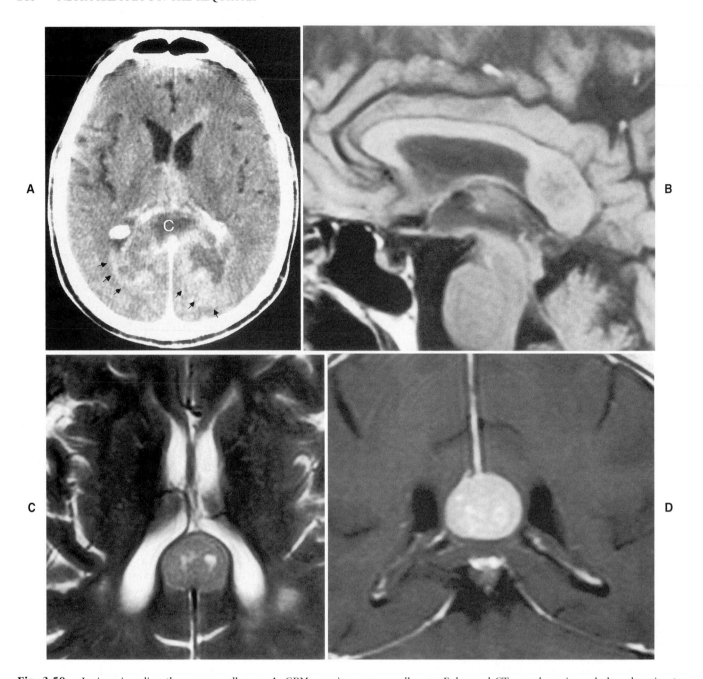

Fig. 3-50   Lesions invading the corpus callosum. **A,** GBM crossing corpus callosum. Enhanced CT reveals an irregularly enhancing tumor in a garland wreath pattern *(arrows)* crossing the splenium of the corpus callosum. Note that the genu of the corpus callosum also shows subtle enhancement denoting tumor infiltration. C marks the splenium of the corpus callosum, which appears to be somewhat necrotic. **B,** Lymphoma of the splenium: Sagittal T1-weighted scan shows expansion of the splenium with abnormal signal intensity. **C,** The T2-weighted scan shows a focal mass in the splenium without significant edema. **D,** The lesion enhances strongly on coronal T1WI. Would this favor lymphoma over an intermediate grade astrocytoma? Try diffusion. (Case courtesy of Stuart Bobman).

cification is present) and the skull may be eroded. Edema associated with the mass is typically absent, a distinguishing point from other more aggressive tumors. Subarachnoid seeding has been reported with oligodendrogliomas.

Mixed tumors Oligodendrogliomas are often histologically mixed (50%) with astrocytic forms; when present, it acts as a medium-grade neoplasm with a high rate

of recurrence. The term used for this tumor is oligoastrocytoma and like the oligodendrogliomas and anaplastic oligos populate the frontal and temporal lobes. Calcification in oligoastrocytomas occur less frequently (14%) but enhance more frequently (50%). Median survival for same grade oligoastrocytomas is 6.3 years as opposed to oligodendrogliomas' 9.8 years. If anaplasia occurs with oligoastrocytomas, the median survival drops to 2.8 years.

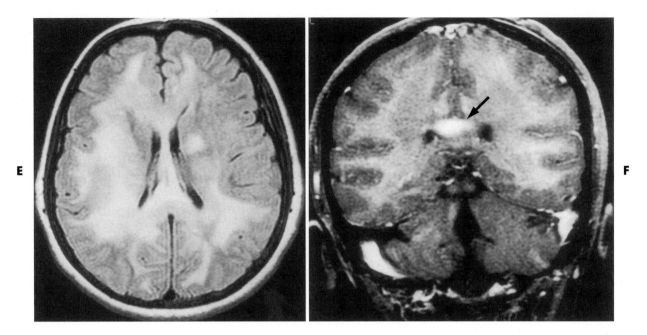

Fig. 3-50 *Continued.* **E,** This poor woman had lupus, was on immunosuppressives, and still developed a diffusely infiltrative process affecting both hemispheres, well seen on axial FLAIR. **F,** Although there is subtle generalized enhancement of the white matter on the coronal study, note the more prominent loss of the blood brain barrier in the splenium of the corpus callosum *(arrow).* This was another case of lymphoma.

Anaplastic oligodendroglioma   Anaplastic oligodendrogliomas have a worse prognosis than WHO grade II oligodendrogliomas. They account for one-fourth to one-half of all oligodendrogliomas with a mean age of 49 years old. Over 90% are found in either the frontal lobe

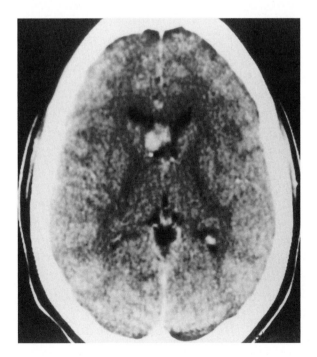

Fig. 3-51   Subependymal giant cell astrocytoma. Note the enhancing mass near the foramen of Monro on the right side with a component of the tumor that extends intraventricularly on this enhanced CT. The septum also seems to be infiltrated.

or temporal lobe. Hemorrhage, necrosis, calcification, cystic degeneration, and avid enhancement alone or in combination may occur in these "surf and turf" delicacies. Five year survival is approximately 30%.

Neuroepithelial tumors of uncertain origin

Gliomatosis cerebri   Gliomatosis cerebri is a pattern of disease in which at least two lobes of the cerebral hemisphere (especially the cortex) may be diffusely infiltrated with tumor with a relative lack of mass effect and distortion (i.e., preservation of neuronal architecture) (Fig. 3-55). Peak age is 40 to 50 years, but they occur in all adult age groups. WHO classification is grade III, analogous to AA. It is not uncommon to have the frontal and temporal lobes involved with the basal ganglia and thalami. Gliomatosis cerebri is bilateral in nearly half the cases. Brainstem involvement is not unusual with the midbrain and pons being affected four times more commonly than the medulla. The WHO classification places the lesion as a subgroup of neuroepithelial tumors of undefined origin along with astroblastomas and chordoid gliomas of the third ventricle. Greenfield's textbook of neuropathology still calls these tumors of "pleomorphic glial cell" origin manifested by "more than one type of glial cell lineage."

A CT may be interpreted as normal in appearance, but you may see loss of the gray-white differentiation and subtle mass effect. The more sensitive T2-weighted MR shows diffuse increased signal intensity throughout. Both gray and white matter may be involved, and the lesion may spread bilaterally. Enhancement, if present at all, is

Box 3-11 Intraventricular Masses by Site

	Lateral	Third	Fourth
NEOPLASMS			
Choroid plexus papilloma/ca	Common, pediatric		Common, adult
Craniopharyngioma		Common from suprasellar growth	
Ependymoma			Common
Medulloblastoma			Common, growth from vermis
Meningioma	Common, glomus, atrium		Along choroid plexus
Metastases	Yes	Yes	Yes
Chordoid glioma	Rare	Typical	Not reported

minimal. The prognosis is equivalent to that of a high-grade glioma and, in fact, gliomatosis cerebri may show an explosive growth rate signifying its transformation to a GBM. Survival is reported to be 48% at 1 year, 27% at 3 years.

Chordoid glioma These are tumors of the hypothalamus and anterior third ventricle described in 1998 that are assigned WHO grade II, a glial tumor of unknown origin. The lesion is slow-growing, solid, well-circumscribed, and avidly enhancing (Fig. 3-56). They look like little olives sitting at the third ventricle . . . ovoid, sharply delineated, no pimento. They are hyperdense to gray matter on CT and reasonably isointense on standard T1WI and T2WI, but may have central necrosis or cystic regions. They occur in adults over age 30 and can cause acute hydrocephalus due to their obstructive nature. They may attach to the hypothalamus and have a propensity to regrow if not totally removed.

Astroblastoma Astroblastomas are rare tumors of variable aggressiveness and of unknown origin. They are tumors of young adulthood affecting the cerebral hemispheres. They are well-circumscribed tumors with peripheral enhancement, central necrosis, and usually large

Table 3-12 WHO classification of oligodendroglial tumors and mixed gliomas

Tumor	Grade	Peak age (years)
Oligodendroglial Tumors		
Oligodendroglioma	II	30-55
Anaplastic oligodendroglioma	III	45-60
Mixed Glioma		
Oligoastrocytoma	II	35-45
Anaplastic oligoastrocytoma	III	40-50

size. Prognosis is good as long as the surgeon does a complete whack . . . of the tumor and is not a whack himself.

Metastases

Parenchymal metastases Metastases are the most common masses in the supratentorial space in the adult, making up 40% of intracranial neoplasms. Meatballs occur on top of the spaghetti (supratentorial) more commonly than buried below (infratentorial). Fifty percent

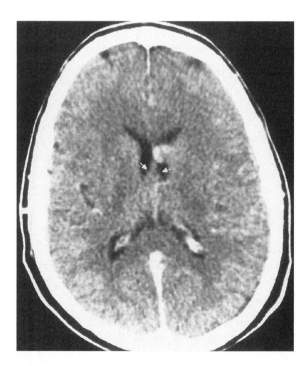

Fig. 3-52 Central neurocytoma. Axial enhanced CT portrays a calcified mass in the frontal horn of the left lateral ventricle. There is septal infiltration *(arrows)*, typical of an intraventricular neurocytoma. On the basis of a preliminary frozen section this mass had been called an oligodendroglioma. Special stains confirmed neurocytoma (see text). But it can look like an SGCA.

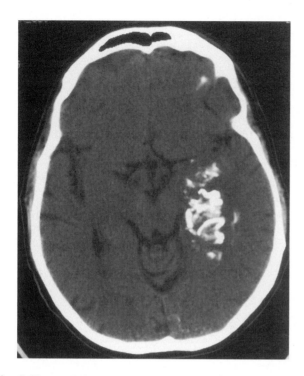

Fig. 3-53   Calcification in an oligodendroglioma. Although unenhanced CT may seem anachronistic at times for the evaluation of a patient with a brain tumor, this lesion shows typical calcification in this low grade tumor. The serpentine nature of the calcification should raise the suspicion of an arteriovenous malformation or even Sturge Weber, so you still have to get the MR anyway.

are solitary and 50% are multiple with just 20% having two lesions. Just as in the infratentorial compartment, the primary tumors that spread to the supratentorial part of the brain are lung (50%) (Fig. 3-57), breast (15%), melanoma (11%), kidney, and gastrointestinal primary tumors. Solitary metastases favor a breast, uterine, gastrointestinal primary whereas hemorrhagic ones favor kidney, melanoma, thyroid, breast, and choriocarcinoma. Cystic or calcified metastases favor lung, breast, and gastrointestinal primary sites (Fig. 3-58). If the primary site is not clinically or radiographically apparent, the differential diagnosis becomes an astrocytoma. A solitary lesion warrants thought.

Remember to peruse the calvarium (bones in the meatballs) for metastatic disease as you look at the scans. In an informal survey of two knuckleheads, it is our perception that bony metastases of the skull occur more frequently than parenchymal metastases in many primary tumors. This is certainly true for prostate metastases where parenchymal metastases without bony disease are virtually reportable. Furthermore, a recent study has indicated that breast primary tumors that are estrogen and progesterone receptor positive have a much higher rate of osseous metastases than brain ones (and the skeletal ones occur earlier in the course of the breast cancer). Those who are receptor negative develop brain and meningeal but not calvarial metastases.

Metastases usually appear as relatively well-defined masses that demonstrate enhancement and moderate

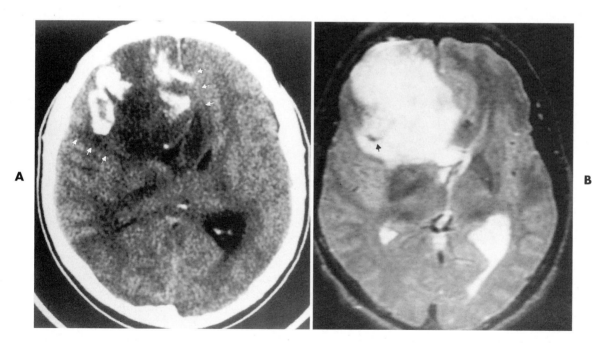

Fig. 3-54   Calcified oligodendroglioma. **A,** Axial unenhanced CT demonstrates a calcified mass *(arrows)* in the right frontal lobe with considerable mass effect on the ventricular system. Calcification in the tumor extends across midline just posterior to the falx. **B,** High signal intensity tumor without evidence of the calcification that was easily seen on the CT scan is present on T2WI. One small hypointense focus *(arrow)* on the posterolateral aspect may result from the calcification.

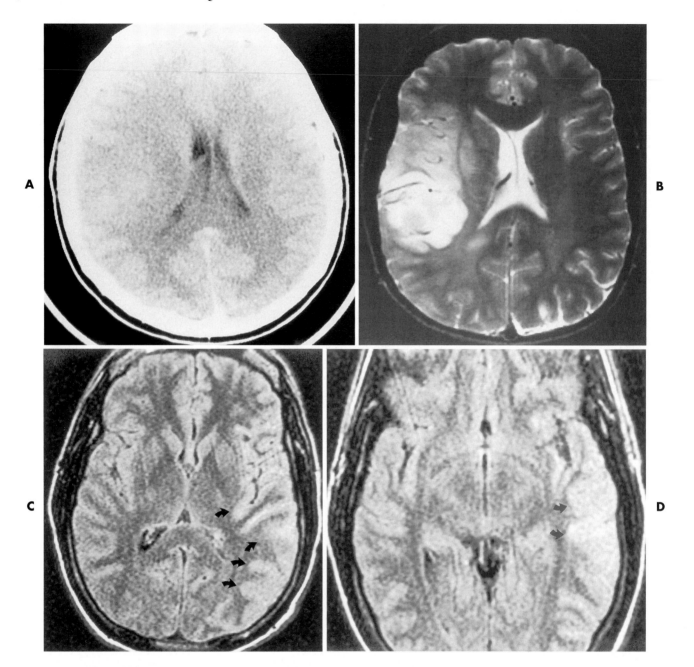

Fig. 3-55   Gliomatosis cerebri. **A,** Axial enhanced CT shows subtle loss of the gray matter-white matter differentiation in the right temporal and frontal lobe. There is mild compression of the right lateral ventricle. **B,** Lesion is clearly seen on the T2WI performed the same day. Note the high signal intensity throughout the right temporal lobe not respecting the gray-white boundaries. **C,** This case of gliomatosis cerebri illustrates how the lesion has become less difficult to define now that MR dominates the realm of CNS imaging. The FLAIR sequence (c) has taken the mystery out of the mass. You can see the diffuse infiltration of the cortex of the left temporal and occipital lobes *(arrows)* on this case. (Close up for myopic readers in **D**).

edema. They characteristically lodge at the gray matter–white matter boundary because of the small caliber of vessels in this region and may extend into the cortex or white matter. The lesions tend to follow vascular flow dynamics, being deposited in the carotid system more commonly than in the vertebrobasilar system (80% to 20%) and favor the middle cerebral artery distribution. Metastases lodge at the gray-white interface in 80% of

cases, basal ganglia in 3%, and cerebellum in 15%. (Remember that 80% of all statistics are made up.)

Metastases are typically hypodense on noncontrast CT and hypointense on T1WI unless hemorrhagic (Fig. 3-59) or hypercellular. Although hypointense (when visible) on unenhanced T1WI, they may be of variable signal intensity on T2WI depending on the presence of hemorrhage, intratumoral necrosis, cyst formation, high

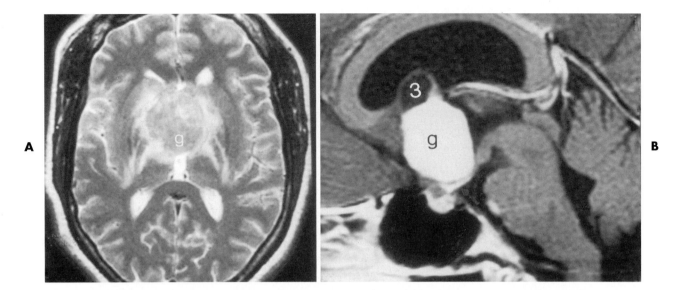

Fig. 3-56   Third ventricular chordoid glioma. This newly described lesion (g) is characterized by its location (hypothalamus or third ventricle), isointensity on T2WI **(A)**, and marked enhancement **(B)**. The third ventricle (3) appears to be partially trapped. (Courtesy of Marty Pomper, M.D., Baltimore MD)

nuclear/cytoplasm ratios, or paramagnetic content. Nearly all metastases enhance to a variable degree, but the pattern may be solid, ringlike, regular, irregular, homogeneous, or heterogeneous. As opposed to gliomas, metastases are better defined and have sharper borders. The vasogenic edema is often out of proportion to the size of the metastasis except in cortical metastases, where edema may be minimal or absent. When edema is absent, T2WI may miss metastases. Contrast becomes

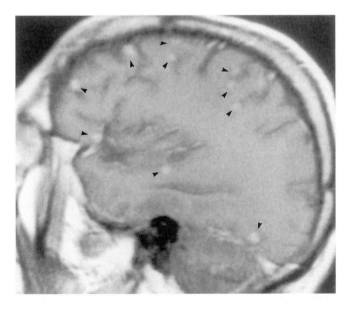

Fig. 3-57   Multiple small cell carcinoma lung metastases. The preponderance of small enhancing lesions *(arrowheads)* at the gray-white junction on this sagittal post contrast scan suggests a diagnosis of metastatic disease.

essential for identification of lesions in this situation (i.e., cortical metastases) (Fig. 3-60).

Because solitary metastases in a noneloquent area of the brain may be treated surgically, it is very important to demonstrate to clinicians whether there are one, two, three, or multiple metastases. Recently, some investigators have shown improved detection and visibility of metastases with the use of triple-dose MR contrast agents. The number of lesions and their conspicuity increased with increasing contrast dosage. The question is: do the numbers increase faster than the cost of the contrast? Where the maximum limit of contrast dosage will stop, no one knows yet. Still others believe that one should delay imaging after contrast administration by up to 30 minutes to increase lesion conspicuity.

One technique used to increase the conspicuity of metastases is to apply magnetization transfer suppression to the postcontrast T1-weighted scans. This suppresses more of the high protein background and can make the enhancing meatballs show up brighter on a darker background. To some, this is a poor man's triple dose gadolinium study at one third the cost. Some advocate using gadolinium and FLAIR scanning. Because the CSF and brain tissue is of low intensity with FLAIR scans, tumors appear more conspicuous than on conventional FLAIR or T2-weighted scans. Anyway you slice your meatballs, it is important to address such issues especially when dealing with presumed solitary, resectable metastases (to exclude additional metastatic deposits).

The neurosurgeons will remind you that they are ready and willing to resect some metastases purely because of unresponsive mass effect, impending herniation, and the proximity of their offspring to a college

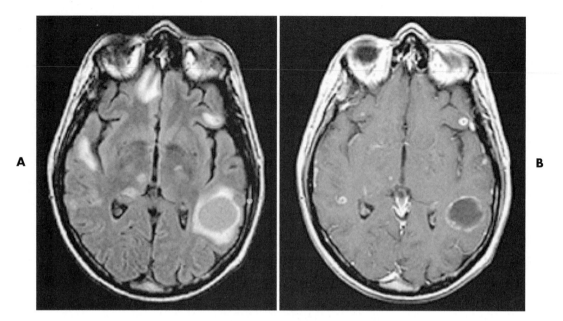

Fig. 3-58 Supratentorial meatballs. **A,** Cystic and solid metastases are present in this patient. The cystic lesion in the left temporal lobe does not have the same intensity as CSF due to high protein. **B,** The masses enhance along the periphery and the posterior right temporal lesion reveals its nature. The differential diagnosis would include a brain abscess and a diffusion-weighted scan could be useful if bright (suggesting an abscess and differentiating the two).

education. Recent studies have suggested benefit in resecting (or gamma-knifing) as many as three separate well-circumscribed metastases—especially if Princeton University is on the "short list" for matriculation.

Paraneoplastic syndromes Paraneoplastic conditions of the brain may occur in association with non-

CNS primary tumors. Among these, limbic encephalitis, an abnormality affecting the temporal lobes and causing memory and mental status changes, has been described extensively. The appearance simulates a herpes simplex encephalitis, usually bilateral (though it may be unilateral in 40%) and extensive disease in the tempo-

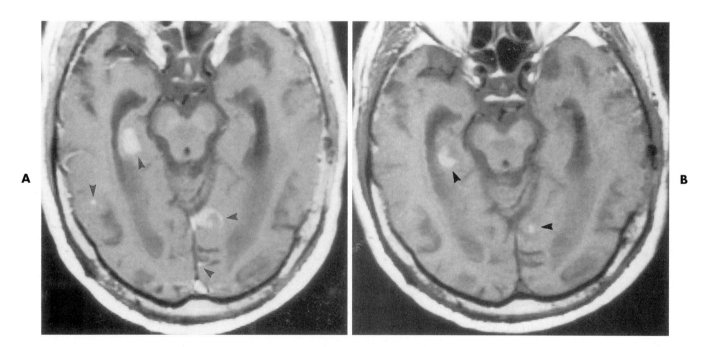

Fig. 3-59 Melanoma metastases. **A,** Enhanced MR shows many small peripheral masses (*arrowheads*) in the brain. **B,** Ooops. Some were bright on precontrast T1WI. This was a case of metastatic melanoma where the high signal was due to melanin or hemorrhage.

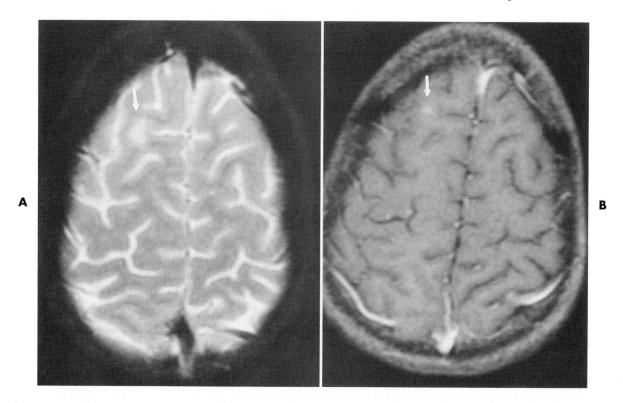

Fig. 3-60   Cortical metastasis. **A,** Axial T2WI was interpreted as normal by the resident nervous about neuroradiology boards. However, one can easily identify the focal high signal intensity *(arrow)* edema, suggesting a metastasis when the postcontrast **(B)** scan is seen side-by-side. (The arrows help! The resident wasn't that bad, but is now confined to Guantanamo Bay.) Patient had cortical metastases from lung cancer.

ral lobes, which is bright on T2WI and may show enhancement (Fig. 3-61). Atrophy of the temporal lobe may coexist but hemorrhage is exceedingly uncommon. (We were told never to say "never," but we have never seen hemorrhage in our vast experience of one case.) Abnormal signal intensity in the brainstem and/or hypothalamus may be seen in about 10% to 20% of cases of limbic encephalitis. Many different primary tumors have been associated with limbic encephalitis: small cell carcinoma of the lung is classic; testicular germ cell, thymic, ovarian, breast, hematologic, and gastrointestinal malignancies have also been reported. The etiology is not well understood. Another paraneoplastic syndrome is that of cerebellar atrophy with clinical manifestations of ataxia. Ovarian carcinoma and lymphoma may cause this finding.

There is a series of antibodies that indicate paraneoplastic syndromes that reads like a Hip Hop lexicon (anti-Yo, anti-Hu, anti-Ma, anti-Ri, anti-CAR, anti-Ta [also called anti-Ma2], anti-What's up?). If you hear these terms, know to look closely at the temporal lobes and cerebellum! The anti-Hu antibodies are most common in the paraneoplastic form of limbic encephalitis, but anti-Ta and anti-Ma antibodies can also be seen. Anti-Hu antibodies are directed against the nuclei of neurons and can cause a syndrome of encephalomyelitis and/or sensory neuropathy. The anti-Hu antibodies are frequently associated with small cell lung carcinoma whereas anti-Ta are seen with testicular germ cell tumors. The anti-Yo antibody produces a syndrome of cerebellar degeneration secondary to the antibodies' assault on the Purkinje cells of the cerebellum. An association with ovarian carcinoma is high. Anti-Ri antibodies cause opsoclonus and ataxia and are seen often with breast and lung cancers. Finally, the anti-CAR antibodies attack retinal neurons and cause a retinopathy. They are seen with small cell carcinomas. Treatment of the primary tumor usually results in improvement of the paraneoplastic syndrome.

Tumors of hematopoietic origin
Lymphomas   The most common type of lymphoma to affect the brain is diffuse histiocytic lymphoma (also known as reticulum cell sarcoma, microglioma, primary cerebral lymphoma). CNS lymphoma is often associated with an immunodeficient state including that resulting from acquired immunodeficiency syndrome (AIDS), organ transplantation, Wiskott-Aldrich syndrome, Sjögren syndrome, and prolonged immunosuppressive therapy. I think of lymphoma as the rotten apple of the smorgasbord. You can have scattered rotten apples seen as multiple masses, rotten apple sauce coating your ventricles (Fig. 3-62), rotten apple juice that looks like clear

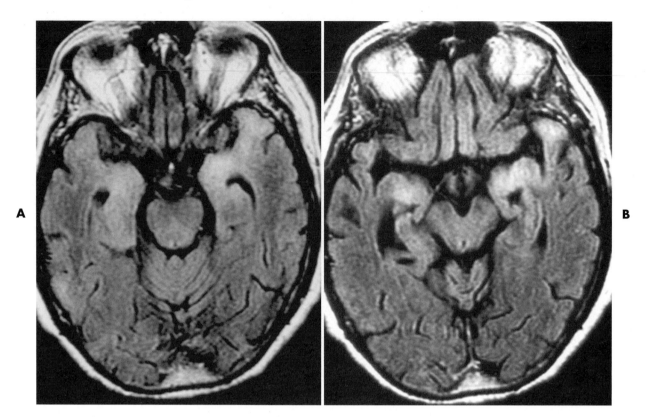

Fig. 3-61   Limbic paraneoplastic encephalitis. **A,** Bilateral mesial temporal lobe hyperintensity is present on the FLAIR scan in this patient with ovarian cancer. **B,** Atrophy argues against acute herpes encephalitis.

CSF but is infiltrated with tumor cells, or one large rotten apple pie occupying much of your brain. Because of the AIDS epidemic in this country, lymphoma is projected in the next decade to become the most common primary malignancy of the brain, as it occurs in 6% of AIDS patients.

It is thought that the dysfunction of suppressor T cells in immunosuppressed patients leads to this B-cell lymphocytic neoplasm. Primary lymphoma of the brain (where no other sites are discovered) is usually supratentorial, although infratentorial primary lymphoma is not rare. Lymphomas tend to be located in deep gray matter nuclei or in the periventricular white matter. Coating of the ventricles (seen in 38% of cases) and spread across the corpus callosum are features of lymphoma that are suggestive of, although not specific for, the diagnosis. The other diagnosis seen in a similar population is toxoplasmosis; however, toxoplasmosis usually does not abut an ependymal surface as lymphoma does (Table 3-13).

Recent studies have shown that thallium scanning is an excellent means for distinguishing toxoplasmosis from CNS lymphoma. The latter is thallium avid; the former does not show activity with thallium scanning. This is an excellent, though underutilized means to distinguish these two entities and effect an early course of

therapy directed at the correct diagnosis. Do it! Another suggested way to differentiate the two, while sticking with your MR scanner, is to perform perfusion scans. Lymphomas have higher regional cerebral blood volume compared with surrounding tissue whereas toxoplasmosis is hypovascular. (See chapter on Infections.)

Secondary lymphoma most commonly involves the leptomeninges and CSF (apple juice); but this is rarely detectable on CT or MR, even with enhancement. Hydrocephalus may be the only telltale sign. Dural invasion is a rarity. When one has parenchymal extension by secondary lymphoma, it is usually supratentorial and is more commonly multifocal. Dense enhancement is the norm; however, ring enhancement may also occur. Non-Hodgkin lymphoma is more common than Hodgkin's, which rarely affects the brain.

The classic teaching used to be that lymphoma was one the lesions that is typically hyperdense on noncontrast CT and enhances to a moderate degree (Fig. 3-63). Such generalizations are no longer valid because AIDS-related lymphoma has come into ascendance. Lymphoma in AIDS patients has a variety of appearances, most commonly hyperdensity on noncontrast CT and variable enhancement. Nonetheless, if you see a hypodense infiltrative mass on a noncontrast CT in an adult positive for human immunodeficiency virus, still con-

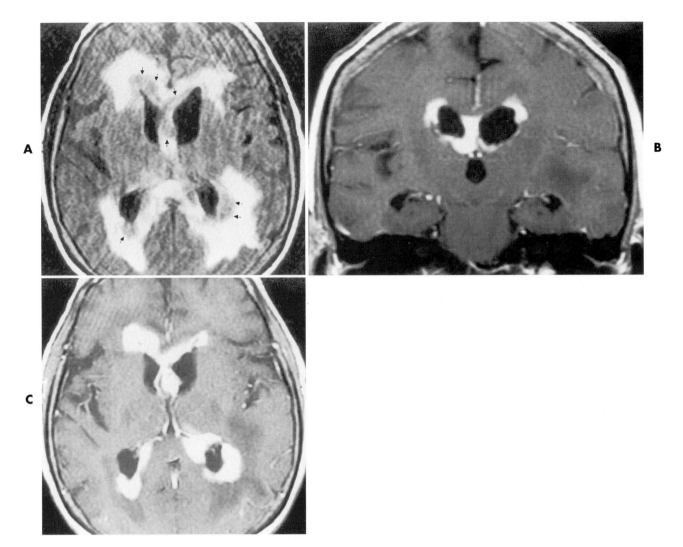

Fig. 3-62   Ependymal spread of lymphoma. The combination of low signal *(arrows)* on FLAIR **(A)** and ependymal enhancement **(B** and **C)** should suggest the diagnosis of lymphoma in this case. Encasement of the ventricles and invasion of the septum pellucidum is evident.

sider lymphoma. Hemorrhage is distinctly uncommon in lymphomas.

MR findings in CNS lymphoma are varied. Periventricular and deep gray matter abnormalities are most common, with masses less than 2 cm in size in patients with AIDS and greater than 2 cm in size in non-AIDS patients. Multiple lesions (20% to 81%) occur more commonly in patients with AIDS, making the distinction with toxoplasmosis even more difficult. The signal intensity is variable on T2W scans with approximately 50% of cases isointense to slightly hypointense. Heterogeneity is the norm. Gadolinium enhancement is marked and homogeneous in over 90% of cases, but beware when steroids are given as treatment as these drugs may suppress the enhancement. Ring enhancement is often seen in immunodeficient patients but is rarely seen in the immunocompetent population.

Lymphomas are said to have low ADC due to their dense cellularity restricting water diffusion (Fig. 3-64). Though somewhat bright on DWI, one should not confuse the mass with a light-bulb bright stroke, which is confined to a vascular distribution.

Intravascular malignant lymphoma (angiotropic malignant lymphoma) is a deadly disease that presents with a different spectrum of imaging findings than classical parenchymal lymphoma. One may see infarct-like lesions, focal parenchymal enhancement, and/or dural/arachnoid enhancement. The lesions in this entity are multifocal.

Sarcoma
The most common forms of sarcomas in the CNS are found along the meninges (meningosarcomas, angiosarcomas, and fibrosarcomas) and have a propensity to invade the brain. Of the primary parenchymal sarcomas, gliosarcoma is most common and has features of a GBM

Table 3-13	Lymphoma versus toxoplasmosis in AIDS	
Feature	**Lymphoma**	**Toxoplasmosis**
Multiple lesions	81%	61%
Size	Diameter 1-3 cm in 75%, >3 cm in 25%	Diameter < 1 cm in 52%, 1-3 cm in 36%, >3 cm in 12%
Mean no. of lesions	3.9	3.3
Homogeneous CT enhancement	76% if <1 cm, 50% if >1 cm	77% if <1 cm, 23% if >1 cm
Hyperdensity on unenhanced CT	33% of lesions	None, unless hemorrhage
T2WI	55% isointense	All hyperintense
Periventricular distribution	50% of patients	3% of patients
Subependymal	38%	None
Radiation therapy effect	Very sensitive	Gornicht helfen
Basal ganglia involvement	Uncommon	Common
Hemorrhage	Rare	More common esp. after treatment
Thallium 201 SPECT scan	Positive	Negative
MR perfusion	Increase	Decrease
MRS	Marked increase in choline and lipid, low NAA	Markedly elevated lactate
Steroids	Melts like butter	Don't bother

From Dina TS: Primary CNS lymphoma versus toxoplasmosis in AIDS, *Radiology* 179:823-828, 1991.

and a sarcoma. The prognosis cannot get much worse than a GBM, but gliosarcomas are said to have a higher rate of distant metastases. They tend to occur in the temporal lobe and often invade dural surfaces. Sarcomas are the horsemeat of the banquet—tough, hard, and indigestible.

Pineal Region Masses

The pineal gland grows steadily until age 2 and then the size stabilizes into early adulthood. No difference in size exists between males and females. The normal pineal gland is calcified in 7% to 10% of patients from 8 to 10 years old, 30% of patients in their mid-teens, and peaks by age 20 to 40 at 33% to 40% of individuals. A calcified pineal gland before the age of 6 should be viewed with suspicion for adjacent tumor and calcified glands over 1.0 cm in size are also worrisome. African Americans have a lower rate of pineal calcification than Caucasian Americans. Fijians and Indians have the highest rates.

Pineal region masses constitute 1% of all CNS tumors. They are generally separated into two categories: those of germ cell origin (60%) and those of pineal cell origin (Table 3-14). The manifestations of pineal region masses are based on their site near many critical structures: the aqueduct, the tectal plate, the midbrain, the vein of Galen. Remember also that the pineal gland may regulate human response to diurnal daylight rhythms. Think of breakfast food items.

Pineal region masses may cause hydrocephalus through obstruction of the aqueduct of Sylvius, precocious puberty, or paresis of upward gaze (Parinaud's syndrome).

Tumors of germ cell origin

Germinoma   The most common pineal tumor of the germ cell line is the germinoma, accounting for 60% of pineal germ cell tumors and 40% of pineal region masses. It has also been termed seminoma and dysgerminoma in the medical literature. This tumor, as in all germ cell tumors, has a distinct male predominance when seen in the pineal region (in some series as high as 33:1) and a slight female predilection when seen suprasellarly. The tumor may be multifocal in suprasellar and pineal locations. It is a tumor of adolescence and young adulthood, rarely seen in patients older than 30 years. Germinomas are far more common in the Asian population. Parinaud's

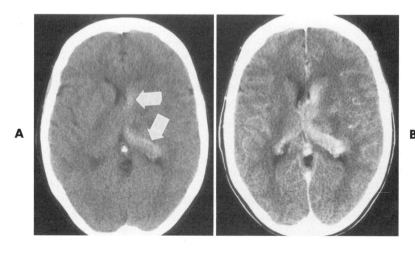

A   **B**

Fig. 3-63   Periventricular lymphoma: Pre (**A**) and post (**B**) contrast CT scans demonstrate the classic findings of lymphoma; a hyperdense mass on an unenhanced scan *(arrows)*, which shows enhancement after iodinated contrast administration (**B**) and infiltrates the ependymal surface of the ventricular system.

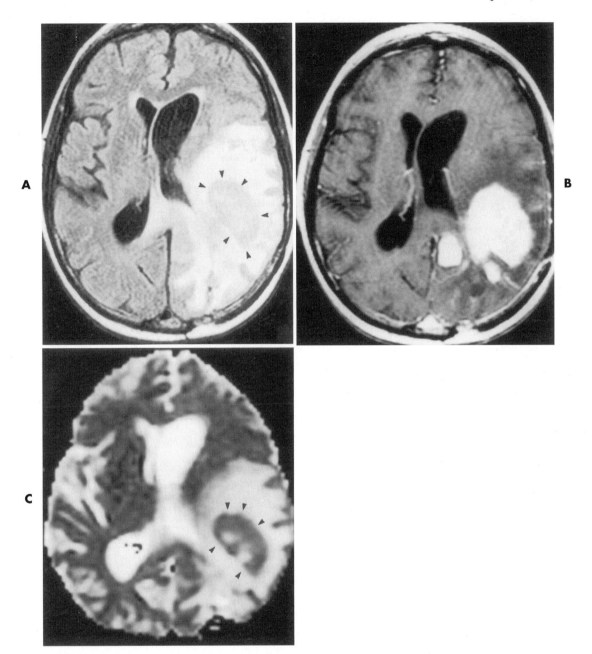

Fig. 3-64   Low ADC value in lymphoma. **A,** Through the bright edema on the FLAIR scan, one can make out a lower intensity mass *(arrowheads)* in the Wernicke area. Abnormal signal crossing the corpus callosum should send off alarm bells. **B,** The mass enhances dramatically and clearly does not look like a stroke. **C,** ADC map shows low signal indicating restricted diffusion in the tumor *(black arrowheads)* and surrounding high intensity vasogenic edema. Hypercellular/small cell tumors can show reduced ADC.

syndrome, paresis of upward gaze, and/or hydrocephalus due to aqueductal obstruction are the most frequent symptomatology in the pineal site with diabetes insipidus and visual field deficits in the suprasellar location. Precocious puberty secondary to expressed hormones may also occur.

The characteristic appearance of the germinoma is that of a hyperdense mass on unenhanced CT, which enhances markedly (Fig. 3-65). The tumor engulfs the pineal gland, and this has led to some confusion re-

garding whether the tumor calcifies. It is currently believed that there is a high incidence of pineal gland calcification in patients with germinomas but that the tumor itself does not calcify. On MR the germinoma has intermediate signal intensity on T1WI and, because of the tumor cells' high nucleus/cytoplasm ratio, a slightly hypointense signal (similar to gray matter) on T2WI. The mass enhances. Germinomas are very radiosensitive and also respond well to chemotherapy. CSF seeding is not uncommon. The best imaging study to evaluate for CSF

Table 3-14 Pineal region masses: differential diagnosis

Characteristic	Pineoblastoma	Pinecytoma	Germinoma	Choriocarcinoma	Teratoma	Yolk Sac Tumor	Astrocytoma
Age/Sex	Child/M = F	Child or adult/M = F	Child/M >> F	Child/M > F	Child/M = F	Child, male > female	Child, adult/ M = F
Density on unenhanced CT	Hyperdense	Hyperdense	Hyperdense	Variable (hemorrhage predilection)	Variable (fat, calcification, teeth)	Hypodense	Isodense
Calcification	Engulfs pineal	Engulfs pineal	Accelerates pineal calcification	Rare	Frequent	Absent	Absent
Enhancement	Moderate	Moderate	Marked	Moderate	Minimal	Rare	Variable
Heterogeneity	Homogeneous	Homogeneous	Homogeneous	Heterogeneous	Heterogeneous	Heterogeneous	Homogeneous
SAS seeding	Frequent	Infrequent	Frequent	Infrequent	Infrequent	Rare	Infrequent
Serum Markers	? Melatonin	? Melatonin	Placental alkaline phosphatase, sometimes HCG	HCG, human placental lactogen	HCG and alpha-fetoprotein	Alpha fetoprotein	None
Hemorrhage	Yes	No	Yes	Yes, yes	Possible	No	No
Other	Large, irregular shape	Small	Boys, Boys, Boys, isointense to gray matter	Hemorrhage is the word	Variable density and intensity, 3rd molar		Tectal plate location, aqueductal obstruction

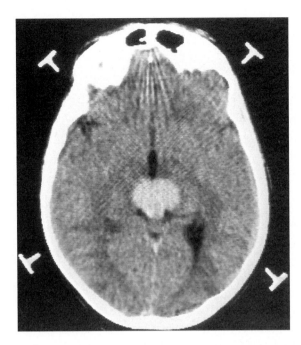

Fig. 3-65 Germinoma in stereotactic biopsy frame. A hyperdense mass in the pineal region is seen on this enhanced CT.

seeding is contrast-enhanced MR of the entire neuroaxis; nonetheless, repeated CSF cytologic studies are still more sensitive than imaging.

Most of the remaining CNS germinomas occur in the suprasellar cistern regions (Fig. 3-66), but some have been reported to occur in the basal ganglia and thalami as well. In these locations they still are hyperdense on

CT but seem to have a higher rate of cystic degeneration and calcification. Ipsilateral cerebral hemiatrophy and brain stem hemiatrophy can occur when the germinomas are located in these sites.

Germinomas with cystic components respond more slowly to radiotherapy than those that are predominantly solid. The location, size, and presence of CSF seeding did not influence long-term response.

Teratoma The other tumors of the germ cell line may have unique appearances. Teratomas may have fat, bone, calcification, cysts, sebaceum, or other dermal appendages associated with them. The lipid and calcification or bone have distinctive CT and MR densities or intensities. A chemical shift artifact may signal the presence of fat rather than blood on the T2WI. Enhancement is irregular because of the nonenhancing fatty or calcified component. Teratomas are the second most common pineal region germ cell neoplasm, but they also abound in the suprasellar cistern. In neonates they may diffusely invade a hemisphere or the sacral spine.

Choriocarcinoma Choriocarcinoma has a distinctive feature: it is commonly hemorrhagic. Teratomas and choriocarcinomas as well as embryonal cell carcinoma and endodermal sinus tumors are more common in male patients and have a worse prognosis. Choriocarcinoma is HCG and human placental lactogen positive on immunohistochemistry. The others are not.

The pineal gland is often referred to as the "third testicle" because of the prevalence of the germ cell line of tumors in males. It is also the "third eye"; retinoblastomas occur here as part of the retinoblastoma oncogene

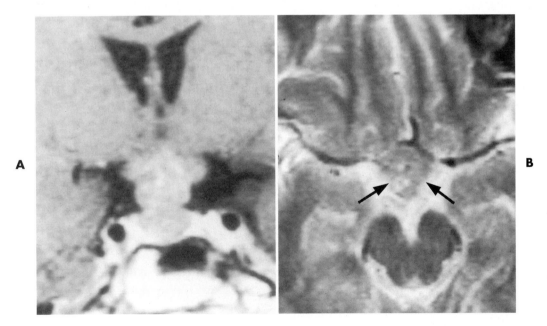

Fig. 3-66 Suprasellar germinoma. **A,** An enhancing suprasellar mass is seen infiltrating the optic chiasm on the coronal scan. The patient, whose name was Euridepes had precipitous diabetes insipidus and a sodium of zipidous and a nonserendipidous germinoma. **B,** Axial T2WI shows the low signal you would expect for this tumor *(arrows)*.

complex. The occurrence of bilateral retinoblastomas in association with pineoblastomas (see following section) has been termed trilateral retinoblastoma (though the third primitive neuroectodermal tumor may also occur in a suprasellar location). This occurs in 3% of patients with bilateral retinoblastomas. There is a high rate of subarachnoid seeding.

Others   Yolk sac tumors often show more cystic change than other germ cell line lesions. Embryonal carcinoma is solid most commonly. Alpha-fetoprotein titers are negative in embryonal cell tumors but positive in yolk sac tumors. Placental alkaline phosphatase characterizes the embryonal tumor.

Tumors of pineal cell origin

Pineoblastoma   The incidence of intrinsic pineal cell tumors, pineocytomas and pineoblastomas, is nearly evenly split between male and female patients and the tumors account for 15% of pineal region neoplasms. The pineoblastoma occurs in a younger age group (peak in first decade of life) than the pineocytoma and is classified as WHO grade IV. Pineoblastomas may occur in association with retinoblastomas and interphotoreceptor retinoid-binding proteins can be seen in pineoblastomas. Their appearance at imaging is nearly identical, but pineoblastomas may be slightly more invasive and larger than pineocytomas and have a higher rate of subarachnoid seeding. Again, because these tumors are of the round cell variety with high nucleus/cytoplasm ratios, they often will be dense on unenhanced CT and intermediate in signal intensity on T2WI (Fig. 3-67). They enhance vividly. Calcification is not common yet may be intrinsic to the tumor rather than within the pineal gland itself. Alternatively, the pineal gland calcification may appear exploded as it is displaced peripherally by the pineal tumor. We say germinomas "engulf" the pineal gland, pineoblastomas "explode" the gland.

The 5-year prognosis for pineoblastomas is 58%.

Pineocytoma   Pineocytomas are slower growing pineal parenchymal neoplasms, WHO grade II, that have a peak incidence at 10 to 19 years of age but can occur in any age group. In fact the mean age is in the 30s. These tumors are smaller than the pineoblastomas, often less than 3 cm in size, and they may demonstrate a higher rate of calcification or cyst formation than their nastier brother the pineoblastoma. The 5-year prognosis is 86%.

Because the signal intensity characteristics of pineal parenchymal tumors, malignant germ cell tumors, germinomas, and gliomas may overlap, some investigators have suggested that serum markers may be more specific than imaging features for histology. It is true that some tumors secrete characteristic markers, and these are summarized in Table 3-14.

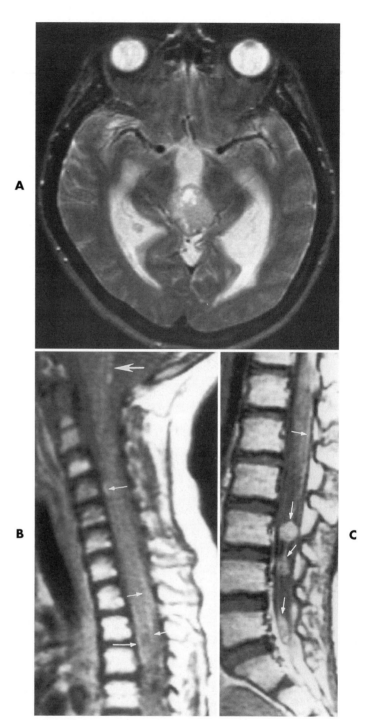

Fig. 3-67   Pineoblastoma. **A,** Axial T2WI shows a pineal mass that is intermediate in signal intensity with some heterogeneity to the lesion. Low signal is characteristic of the highly cellular PNETs. Note the dilatation of the third ventricle and occipital horns of the lateral ventricles caused by the compression of the aqueduct, signifying hydrocephalus. Subarachnoid seeding *(arrows)* in the form of sugarcoating **(B)** or gumdrops on the cauda equina **(C)** is not unusual in pineoblastomas.

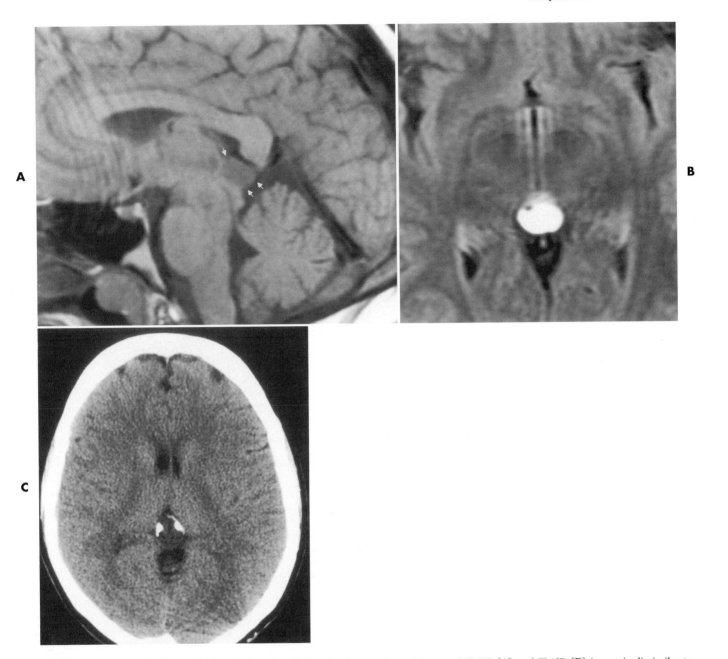

Fig. 3-68   Cyst or cystic tumor? Although the signal intensity *(arrows)* on the sagittal T1WI **(A)** and FLAIR **(B)** image is dissimilar to cerebrospinal fluid, this may still represent a benign pineal cyst. Only her neurosurgeon knows for sure. **C,** What to do? This cystic lesion in the pineal gland displaces the pineal calcification apart. Is it a benign cyst or a neoplasm? In the absence of an enhancing mass or hydrocephalus, one should probably follow this lesion conservatively to assess growth. If necessary, shunting can be performed though this patient did not have hydrocephalus.

Pineal cyst   Pineal and tectal gliomas, cavernous hemangiomas, meningiomas, and benign cysts also populate this area, but they are peripheral to the pineal gland. Pineal cysts are particularly common, and because some pineal masses (pineocytomas) may be cystic, it is important to attempt to identify a solid portion to the lesion to distinguish the two (Fig. 3-68). Cysts in the pineal region are like those mysterious chocolates in the Godiva box; you never know what's inside them, which ones are good, which ones are bad. Contrary to what has previously been written, pineal cysts may compress or occlude the aqueduct, and may be calcified. They may be round or oblong and can be equal to or greater than 2 cm in size. The key to distinguishing a pineal cyst from a cystic astrocytoma is the lack of growth during long-term follow-up. Because pineal cysts are often surrounded by the two limbs of the internal cerebral veins, one must be careful not to misread vascular enhancement as solid mass enhancement.

Benign pineal region cysts can masquerade as any number of pineal region neoplasms and as such are a pain in the habenula. They can be found in up to 40% of individuals on autopsy studies and probably form in late childhood and regress in late adulthood. The cysts may demonstrate peripheral calcification or enhancement, fluid-fluid levels, hemorrhage, mass effect, and growth with time. Another potential pitfall is that, despite their CSF content, pineal cysts do not have the same intensity as CSF on FLAIR, T1W, or PDW series. This may be due to hemorrhage, hemorrhagic debris, or high protein seen histologically in these cysts. They may cause symptoms of headache, diplopia, nausea and vomiting, papilledema, seizures, and Parinaud syndrome (paralysis of upward gaze, lid retraction, abnormal pupillary movements). Hydrocephalus may be produced by the benign cyst and sometimes you can have pineal apoplexy where your pineal cyst acutely hemorrhages. In follow-up a benign pineal cyst usually stays the same size (75%) but some regress and some enlarge by as much as 2 to 3 mm. The point is that they should be treated with respect, watched carefully, and if need be, resected just as one would treat a neoplasm in this location. Obviously there is no risk of subarachnoid space seeding and the follow-up may be less rigorous.

Non-neoplastic Masses

Why discuss nonneoplastic masses in a chapter on neoplasms? The nonneoplastic mass lesions are like meat substitutes, mock meat, garden burgers, veggie burgers, soy. Some can be easily distinguished from true meat, and some are so good that it is hard to tell them from the real thing. Most cysts are readily distinguishable from tumors, but Lhermitte-Duclos could just as easily be a tumor (sweetbreads).

Cysts

Colloid cyst A colloid cyst (neuroendodermal or paraphyseal cyst) arises in the anterior portion of the third ventricle near the foramen of Monro. They occur with an incidence of three cases per one million individuals per year. Positional headaches or hydrocephalus may be the presenting complaints in 30- to 40-year-old patients. Sudden death due to acute hydrocephalus is one scenario. Usually the lesion is hyperdense on CT because of high protein concentration; the same factor may account for its high signal seen 50% of the time on T1WI (Fig. 3-69). The rim of the cyst may faintly enhance. The lesion is lined by simple to pseudostratified epithelium, and is well circumscribed. Theories of evolution (no we

are not talking Big Bang here!) include those who believe colloid cysts arises congenitally as a result of encystment of the ependyma, as persistence of the paraphysis (a piece of the diencephalic roof behind the interventricular foramen), or as one of many neuroepithelial cysts. The endodermal (not neuroectoderm) origin of the lesion has led to the modern theory that the colloid cyst, like the Rathke cyst, is of respiratory epithelial origin perhaps from primitive craniopharyngeal origin. (The debate has led to a Supreme Court ruling not to discuss this in our children's public school classrooms). MR is predictive of the ease at which colloid cysts can be aspirated; if the signal intensity is dark on T2W scans (signifying a high viscosity hyperproteinaceous or cholesterol-laden cyst) it will be a bear to aspirate. Rarely colloid cysts may occur within the body of the lateral ventricles, fourth ventricle, or outside the ventricular system. Treatment may include biventricular shunting, cyst resection, or endoscopic coagulation.

Neuroepithelial cyst Neuroepithelial cysts that may simulate neoplasms often occur within the ventricles. Generally, they are centered on the choroid plexus and may occur anew or in association with previous infections or hemorrhages in the ventricle. The fluid in these cysts simulates CSF on CT and MR but may be bright on T1WI owing to cholesterol debris or high protein concentration. These cysts are lined by epithelium. They can also occur in the spinal canal, parenchyma (Fig. 3-70), or extraaxial intracranial space.

Neuroenteric cyst Neurenteric cysts are lined by cells of endodermal origin and rarely occur in the CNS. When they are seen in the CNS, they usually occur in the intradural extra-medullary spaces of the cervicothoracic region although intracranial cases have been reported. They are typified by bright signal on T1WI secondary to high protein concentration. They will not enhance. Differential diagnosis would include epidermoid cysts, Rathke cleft cysts, and traumatized arachnoid cysts.

When one sees an intraventricular cyst, the differential diagnosis should include a choroid plexus cyst, an ependymal cyst, a colloid cyst, and a cysticercal cyst. Ependymal cysts occur in the frontal horns of the lateral ventricles and are asymptomatic unless they obstruct the foramen of Monro.

Lhermitte-Duclos

Lhermitte-Duclos disease involves a masslike lesion usually seen in the cerebellum as a diffusely infiltrative process. It is unclear whether this lesion is in fact a neoplasm, hamartoma, or dysplasia, but it has the appearance of a tumor. It is correctly classified as WHO grade I and termed a dysplastic gangliocytoma. We put it here since it was placed here before in the first edition and as Emer-

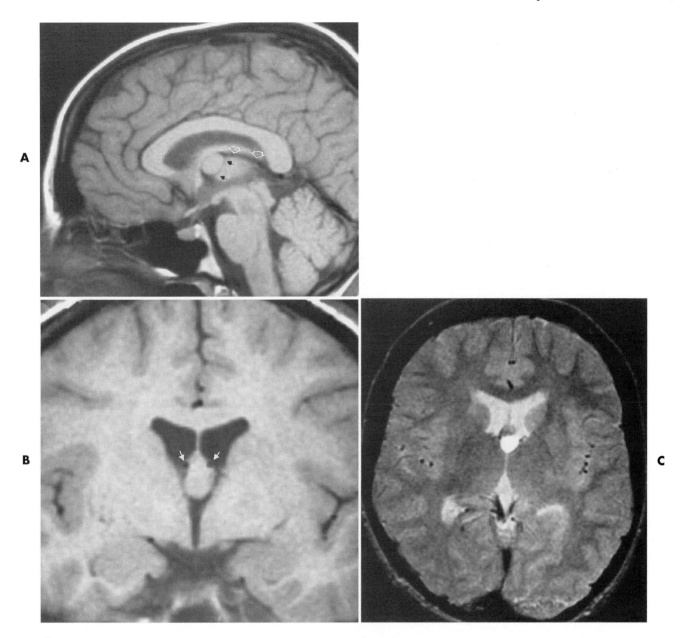

Fig. 3-69   Colloid cyst. **A,** Sagittal midline image demonstrates a well-defined mass *(arrows)* with signal intensity similar to that of white matter. On T1WI the colloid cyst may be variable in its intensity. The internal cerebral vein *(open arrows)* can be seen posterior and superior to the cyst. **B,** In a section just behind the foramen of Monro, note the splaying of the internal cerebral veins *(arrows)* by the colloid cyst. **C,** Axial T2WI shows the high signal intensity mass in the midline at the foramen of Monro.

son said, "A foolish consistency is the hobgloblin of little minds." But we also placed it as a neoplasm under the gangliocytoma category so we're covered for posterity and covering our posterior. The lesion affects cerebellar gray and white matter and is hyperintense on T2WI (Fig. 3-71). Other names for this entity include diffuse ganglioneuroma, Purkinjeoma diffuse hypertrophy, granule cell hypertrophy, and dysplastic gangliocytoma. Lhermitte-Duclos disease usually presents in patients in their early twenties, with symptoms of increased intracranial pres-

sure and/or ataxia. Cowden syndrome, which is associated with multiple hamartomas and neoplasms (especially of the breast) is associated with almost 50% of cases of Lhermitte-Duclos. It is transmitted on chromosome 10q23.

Choristomas

Choristomas are masses of normal tissues in aberrant locations, containing smooth muscle and fibrous tissues. They may be hypervascular. Cases have been described in extraaxial locations including the sella and

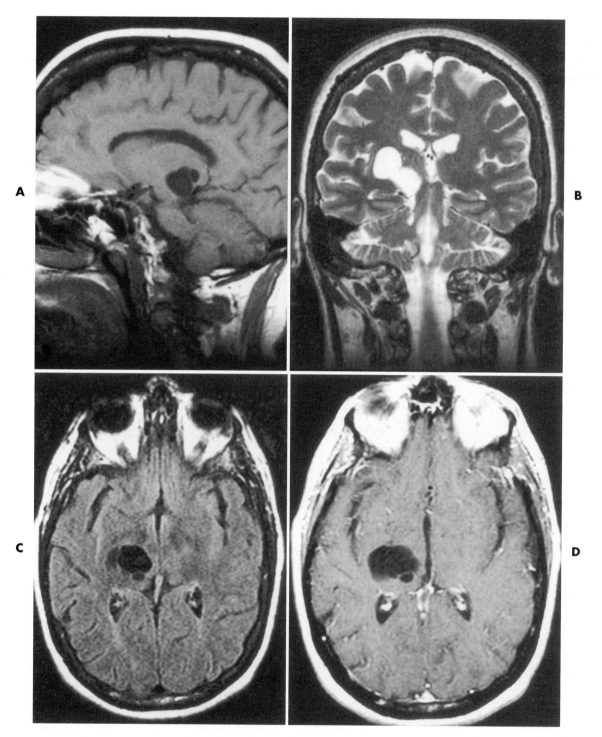

Fig. 3-70 Neuroepithelial cyst. **A,** Unenhanced T1-sagittal scan shows a multi-loculated cystic lesion in the right thalamus. **B,** Coronal T2-weighted scan shows no significant mass effect and high signal similar to CSF. **C,** The FLAIR scan also shows intensity identical to cerebrospinal fluid. **D,** There is no contrast enhancement. This may represent a neuroepithelial cyst, which is a benign lesion that does not require surgical intervention. Differential point: Arachnoid cysts are usually not intraparenchymal, but can exist along perivascular spaces. This could be a huge Virchow Robin space in fact.

parasellar regions as well as the internal auditory canals associated with the facial and vestibulocochlear nerves. Choristomas may enhance and hence may simulate schwannomas.

Amyloid

Amyloid may be deposited in the dura and may simulate meningiomas, dural lymphomas, or plasmacytomas, with reasonably low signal intensity on T2WI. Intra-

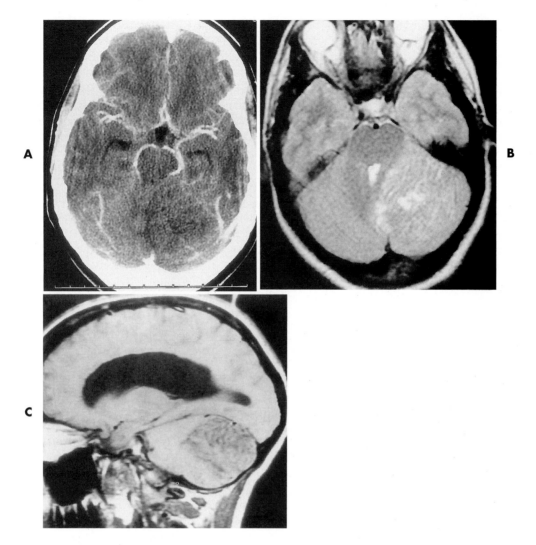

Fig. 3-71 Lhermitte-Duclos disease. **A,** Enhanced CT reveals a nonenhancing mass lesion in the superior left cerebellum. Note the slight low density within the nonenhancing mass. **B,** T2WI of the lesion again demonstrates the obvious mass effect and high intensity striations within the mass. Notice that the intervening tumoral parenchyma has similar intensity to normal cerebellum. **C,** In a different case of Lhermitte-Duclos disease, the sagittal T1WI displays a serpentine low intensity pattern with mass effect. These findings are virtually pathognomonic of Lhermitte-Duclos. (Remember them and win a bottle of '61 Pétrus at Radiology Rounds in "Monte Carlo.")

parenchymal amyloidomas are dense on CT and bright on T1-weighted MR images. Mixed to low intensity on T2-weighted sequences and contrast enhancement have been reported.

Heterotopias and focal areas of abnormal sulcation may also present as masslike lesions. These entities are described more fully in Chapter 9.

Pretreatment Evaluation

The ability of neuroradiologists to predict the grade of a tumor varies by the criteria used. Certainly the presence of necrosis should imply a glioblastoma multiforme and a nonenhancing tumor without edema would imply a low-grade astrocytoma. Although enhancement seems to be a good criterion to suggest higher grade, it is about

as accurate as checking the patient's age. The older the patient the more likely the tumor is of higher grade. It is rare to see an octogenarian with a low-grade astrocytoma and equally unusual to see a child with a glioblastoma multiforme.

Recently, there have been several intriguing reports showing that perfusion scanning can separate high from low-grade tumors. Just as GBMs have neovascularity histologically, so also do they have higher cerebral blood flow on perfusion imaging. This has been used to direct biopsies into the "more malignant" region. By the same token, PET scanning has been used to determine grades of tumor with higher blood flow and/or glucose metabolism corresponding to higher grade. Lower ADC, higher choline, higher cerebral blood volume are other findings that may indicate higher grade. Once again, no neuroradiological interpretation is going to stop a neurosurgical biopsy of a presumed astrocytoma. However, we may be able to eliminate some cases of sampling error by directing that biopsy to the high perfusion, high activity, high grade region. Maybe then the neurosurgeons will throw us a bone every once in a while.

The other recent additions to our armamentarium are the true functional studies. For lesions adjacent to eloquent cortex (by this we mean near the speech, memory, or motor areas) it is helpful to the neurosurgeons for us to show them where these critical areas are so that they can reduce the operative morbidity associated with the resection. Because the surgeons are not going for a complete resection of a GBM, only a gross resection, it would be nice if the patient could spend the remaining months of their life conversant with their family. Functional MRI can be used preoperatively to define the speech areas in relation to the tumor or even intraoperatively to direct the surgical resection to include the maximum amount of tumor and minimal amount of eloquent cortex.

Magnetoencephalography (MEG) is another technique that affords the temporal resolution of the EEG to map the brain superimposed on a co-registered MRI. Right now the war between the better spatial resolution fMRI and the better temporal resolution MEG is being won by fMRI on the basis of greater availability of MR scanners. It used to take the latest new-fangled scanner to do fMRI. Now any practitioner with a decent gradient system MR machine can do tire-kicker motor and auditory mapping. Trust us—even we can do it. A word of caution, the BOLD fMRI contrast effect may be reduced near an astrocytoma secondary to (1) compression of vessels, (2) vasoreactive substances (nitric oxide), (3) neurotransmitter substances expressed by tumors, (4) reduced neuronal function, and (5) invasion of vascular structures by the tumor.

A Look Into the Future

Pretreatment evaluation in the coming decade may also include an assessment of the genetic code for the tumor. Thirty percent of astrocytomas express a deficiency in *TP53*, a tumor suppressor gene on chromosome 17p, which encodes the p53 protein, and many CNS tumors show gains to chromosomes 7 (especially epidermal growth factor receptor) and 20. Platelet-derived growth factors (*PDGF*) and loss of a tumor suppressor gene on chromosome 22q may also contribute to the genetic predisposition to grade II astrocytomas. *P16* and *RB* (chromosome 13q) genes help to control E2F-1 transcription factor, which regulates the G1 cell cycle. These genes are inactivated in 90% of all astrocytomas. These genes and other tumor suppressor genes on 9p and 19q are also associated with conversion of grade II astrocytomas to anaplastic astrocytomas. Epidermal growth factor receptor (*EGFR*) gene amplification in association with in-

activation of tumor suppressor genes on chromosome 10 are found in the progression from anaplastic astrocytoma to glioblastoma multiforme.

TP53 upregulates expression of p21 that blocks the cell cycle in the G1 phase and BAX that promotes cellular apoptosis. This will cause cell cycle arrest and cellular apoptosis—a good thing when one has a cancerous clone running amok in the brain. PDGF overexpression may synergistically turn off the *TP53* gene and vice versa, leading to the oncogenesis.

The *RB* (retinoblastoma) gene is important in cell cycle arrest and is modulated by genes at many other sites. One of these, *CDKN2A*, a gene on chromosome 9p, is deleted in over 50% of high grade tumors. A tumor suppressor gene on chromosome 10, *MMAC1/PTEN* (mutated in multiple advanced cancers 1/phosphatase and tensen homologue), is a target for GBM therapy.

Oligodendrogliomas show allelic losses at the 1p and 19q chromosomes, whereas anaplastic astrocytomas and oligoastrocytomas have losses also at 9p and 10. It has been suggested that some of these genetic combinations may be predictive of the favorable responses of some of the anaplastic oligodendrogliomas to procarbazine, lomustine, and vincristine. We may therefore be able to use the genetic codes of the tumors to determine which drugs to use against them.

What does all this letter and number salad mean to the neuroradiologist? As molecular imaging takes off, we predict that in the future we will be imaging these hot genes, imaging drugs or viruses directed at these dangerous genes. Adeno-viruses, which can replicate in cells deficient with TP53, have already been developed that selectively kill these tumor cells. Other therapies directed at vascular endothelial growth factor (VEGF) will likely employ perfusion imaging as part of the protocol. Already there are therapeutic trials aimed not at the cancer cells themselves, but at the vascular factors that promote their growth. Interferon has an antiangiogenic effect and has been used to suppress vessel growth in some tumors. Endostatin, which is the most effective blocker of angiogenesis currently being studied, may also be able to shut down the blood supply to tumors and/or prevent their metastases (less of an issue with astrocytomas than with breast or lung cancers). Note that these strategies are not directed at the tumor cells and are not cytotoxic. They are meant to starve the tumor instead—working well with our food analogy. Retroviruses encoding mutant VEGF factors have been implanted and have shown suppression of angiogenesis in rats. As go rats, so will go man (the other rodent form).

Posttreatment Evaluation

Postoperative
Determining whether residual neoplasm is present in the postsurgical tumor bed is one of the most daunting

Box 3-12   5-Year Survival Rates by Tumor Type

Neoplasms	Survival (%) at 5 years
GBM	3.4%*
Pilocytic astrocytoma	86.9%
Diffuse astrocytoma	48.6%
Anaplastic astrocytoma	30.0%
Oligodendroglioma	61.7%
Ependymoma	63.5%
Embryonal type	51.2%
Mixed glioma	58.7%

*Whoa! That's bad!

Table 3-15   Scar versus residual tumor

Feature	Scar	Tumor
Enhancement within 1–2 days	No	Yes
Enhancement after 3–4 days	Yes	Yes
Change in size with time	Decreases	Increases
Type of enhancement	Linear, outside preoperative tumor bed	Nodular, solid
Mass effect edema	Decreases	Increases

tasks facing a neuroradiologist. What hangs in the balance are prognostic considerations for the patient (Box 3-12), potential repeated surgeries, nonsurgical therapeutic decision-making, and the wrath of neurosurgeons regarding your analysis of their fine work. Nothing infuriates the surgeon more than a postoperative scan after a "complete resection" that is interpreted by the radiologist as a small biopsy. They want to say they have a clean plate after the meal. Forget the individual rice granules! Here is how you can avoid this pitfall and why it is such a problem.

Surgical margin contrast enhancement almost always present after the second postoperative day, is usually thin and linear. The margin may become thicker or more nodular after a week. It thus becomes difficult to tell whether enhancing tissue in a surgical bed is due to granulation tissue or marginal tumor enhancement (provided that the tumor enhanced preoperatively). The granulation tissue enhancement may persist for months postoperatively, but intraparenchymal enhancement and mass effect after 1 year should be viewed with suspicion. Dural enhancement is nearly always seen even at 1 year and can persist as long as decades after surgery. Enhancement appears sooner and persists longer on MR than on CT.

This has led neurosurgeons to scan patients soon after operation, before this scar tissue has time to develop, to identify residual tumor. A scan within 48 hours showing enhancement in the surgical bed should lead one to suggest residual neoplasm (Table 3-15). Unfortunately, the hemorrhagic blood products from the surgery usually have not resolved by 48 hours, and one is forced to interpret enhancement on CT and MR against a bright background of blood products. Herein lies the difficulty and points up the absolute requirement of precontrast scans in the same plane and location as the postcontrast studies. These scans are viewed side by side to detect the extra thickness of enhancement along a hematoma cavity.

Clearly the best way to distinguish blood from granulation tissue from recurrent or residual tumor is to scan sequentially. Blood resolves, granulation stays the same or decreases in size, and tumor grows. Unfortunately, neurosurgeons and neurooncologists can have the patience of a 6-month-old child who is hungry; and they scream just as loudly at you. Recommending follow-up scans only irritates them, but that is the most reasonable suggestion. Serve them Gerbers.

If a follow-up scan is not an option, consult Table 3-15, and show it to the surgeon as you lay your head on the block.

Postradiation

Patients placed on the radiation rotisserie to have their brains cooked for primary brain tumors, skull lesions, and/or intracranial metastasis frequently exhibit central and cortical parenchymal loss. The radiologist's challenge in the postradiotherapy evaluation is to differentiate residual or recurrent tumor from radionecrosis (where the brain has been fried to a crisp). Several factors influence the development of radiation necrosis. These include total dose, overall time of administration, size of each fraction of irradiation, number of fractions per irradiation, patient age, and survival time of patients. As patients survive longer with more effective treatment, the incidence of radiation necrosis will rise, because it is usually a late effect of treatment (Fig. 3-72). The signs and symptoms of radiation necrosis are nonspecific and do not differentiate it from recurrent tumor.

The effects of irradiation have been separated into those occurring early (within weeks) and late (4 months to many years later) (Table 3-16). The former is transient, may actually occur during radiotherapy, and is usually manifested by high signal intensity in the white matter caused by increased edema (beyond that associated with the tumor). The delayed effects are separated into early delayed injury (within months after therapy) or late injury (months to years after therapy). Early delayed injury

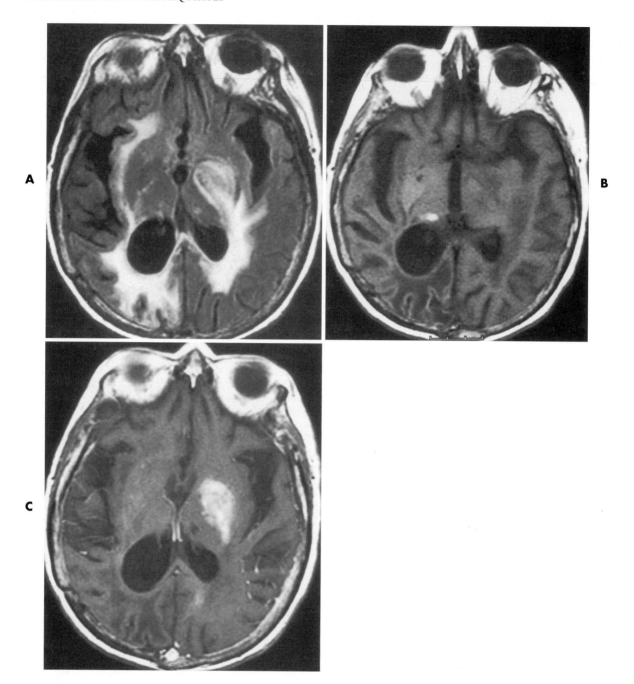

Fig. 3-72   Radiation necrosis. This patient had resection of an anaplastic astrocytoma of the right occipital lobe and was treated with radiation therapy. **A,** FLAIR scan demonstrates high signal intensity without mass effect in the right temporal and occipital lobe with dilatation of the right occipital horn of the lateral ventricle. Note the high signal intensity in the left basal ganglia. **B,** T1-weighted scan shows a high intensity focus in the pulvinar region of the right thalamus secondary to a telangiectasia from radiation therapy. The right basal ganglia are bright but the left are dark. On the post contrast scans **(C)** the left basal ganglia enhance. This was an area of radiation injury.

is also a transient effect and is of little consequence other than recognizing it as such (as opposed to tumor growth) directly after therapy. The late effects are usually irreversible, affect white matter to a much greater extent than gray matter, and histologically involve vascular changes that include coagulative necrosis and hyalinization. The late injury to the brain may be focal or diffuse and occurs in approximately 5% to 15% of irradiated patients. Seventy percent of focal late radiation injuries occur within 2 years after therapy.

Pathologically the mechanism of late injury is vascular with fibrinoid necrosis of small arteries and arterioles. Demyelination is a concomitant feature with myelin dropout.

Table 3-16 Types of radiation injuries

Feature	Early	Early delayed	Late delayed
Time course	During therapy	<3 mo after therapy	>3 mo after therapy
Manifestation	Transient increase in white matter edema	Transient increase in white matter edema	Focal or diffuse longer lasting white matter changes
Contrast enhancement	No	Rare	Not uncommon
Long-term sequelae	None	None	Vasculitis, demyelination
Calcification seen	No	No	Yes, in children
Disseminated necrotizing leukoencephalopathy	No	No	Rarely, with chemotherapy
Symptoms reversible	Yes	Yes	No
Telectangiectasia	No	No	Yes
Hemorrhage present	No	No	Often

Unfortunately, it is exceedingly difficult to make the diagnosis of focal radiation injury. CT or MR may demonstrate a mass lesion associated with edema, low in attenuation on CT and high in signal on T2WI, which usually enhances. Some connoisseurs of radiation necrosis note a soap-bubble and swiss-cheese interior pattern to the lesion, but it is still all dead meat to us. The possibility of focal radiation injury needs to be raised when the lesion is found in the appropriate temporal sequence to treatment. If the lesion is remote from the primary tumor site, then the diagnosis is more easily suggested. Unfortunately radiation necrosis favors the primary tumor site, probably because of predisposing vascular effects (see Fig. 3-72). The diagnosis of radiation necrosis is made by surgical biopsy but may be suggested by PET scan. Distinguishing radiation necrosis from tumor has been the justification of many PET ventures and has caused more radiation than Chernobyl. The bottom line is where there is radiation there is often tumor. A summary of the invaluable work in this field is found in Table 3-17.

With residual or recurrent tumor 18–fluorodeoxyglucose PET has increased activity (greater than normal brain tissue) whereas radiation necrosis shows low activity. Overall accuracy of PET is approximately 85% for distinguishing residual or recurrent tumor from radiation necrosis. Some have recently challenged this number as having been artificially inflated by members of the "mushroom cloud community" (nuclear medicine docs). The accuracy rates are better for high-grade tumors than for low-grade tumors, probably because of inherent differences in tumor growth activity. Removal of the necrotic irradiated nonneoplastic tissue and steroid therapy are the treatments of choice and may be curative. Focal hemorrhage without necrosis also occurs as a result of radiation.

Thallium-201 SPECT has also been advocated for differentiating tumor recurrence from radiation necrosis in patients who have undergone gamma knife radiosurgery and/or in those who receive XRT. Although sensitivity for tumor is high, specificity is moderate with this technique. Some have suggested that ^{11}C-methionine PET can better outline tumors as areas of increased accumulation of ^{11}C-methionine, regardless of grade of tumor.

Some investigators are using MR spectroscopy and perfusion imaging to determine whether necrotic areas after radiotherapy are due to tumor or radiation. Areas of radiation damage without neoplasm show markedly reduced choline levels whereas tumor is usually associated with elevated choline residues. Furthermore, radiation

Table 3-17 Distinction between tumor versus radiation necrosis

	Residual or recurrent tumor	Radiation necrosis
Timing	Immediate or delayed	Months to years
Mass effect/edema	Present	Present
Enhancement	Yes	Yes—soap bubbles or swiss cheese
PET (18-FDG)	Positive	Negative
SPECT (Thallium-201, ^{11}C-Methionine)	Positive	Negative
MRS	Elevated choline	Decreased choline
Perfusion weighted MR	Elevated rCBV	Decreased rCBV

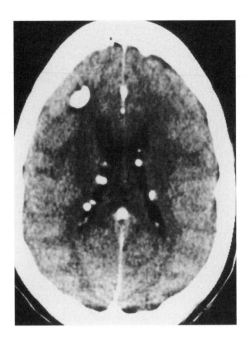

Fig. 3-73 Multiple periventricular and watershed calcifications are noted at the junction of the gray and white matter in a different patient who was irradiated for acute lymphoblastic leukemia.

damage is hypoperfused; most high-grade tumors show increased flow. Relative cerebral blood volume maps appear to be complementary to MRS in detecting nonviable tissue. These techniques haven't quite replaced PET yet, but they are on the rise in academic circles.

Diffuse late injury to the brain (baked Alaska) takes the form of severe demyelination, particularly in periventricular and posterior centrum semiovale regions. CT demonstrates decreased white matter density, but T2WI

is more sensitive and shows high signal intensity in the white matter. Usually the abnormality does not show enhancement. It is estimated that with whole brain irradiation, diffuse white matter changes may occur in 38% to 50% of patients. The incidence increases with increasing patient age. Clinical findings do not correlate well with severity of white matter injuries.

Disseminated necrotizing leukoencephalopathy is a severe form of radiation-related injury usually seen in conjunction with chemotherapy, whether intrathecal or intravenous. Most patients with disseminated necrotizing leukoencephalopathy do extremely poorly. This entity is described more fully in Chapter 7.

Radiation may induce a mineralizing microangiopathy, causing calcification in the basal ganglia or dentate nuclei, with rare cerebral cortical involvement associated with atrophy of intracranial structures (Fig. 3-73). This generally occurs more than 6 months after radiation and is more common in children than in adults. The cause is thought to be an intimal injury to small vessels with associated tissue hypoxia and dystrophic calcification. Frank radiation vasculitis in large vessels may also be seen as focal narrowed segments on angiograms (Fig. 3-74).

Telangiectasias or other occult cerebrovascular malformations may occur as a delayed complication to radiation therapy (see Fig. 3-72). This may manifest by hemosiderin laden deposits in the brain most evident on T2* scans. In children, a vasculopathy leading to intracranial hemorrhage can be seen in radiated brains with or without concomitant chemotherapy.

Graft-versus-host disease
Disorientation, tremors, and myoclonus may be the clinical presentation of graft-versus-host disease (GVHD). MR

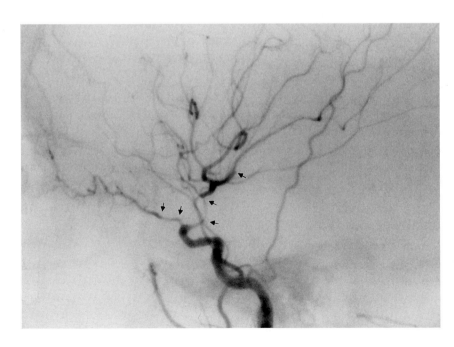

Fig. 3-74 Radiation vasculitis. Common carotid arteriogram shows segmental narrowing of the ophthalmic and supraclinoid vessels *(arrows)* in this patient previously irradiated for a craniopharyngioma.

images may show abnormal signal in the brain stem and deep white matter. The findings may resolve after steroid treatment.

Patients treated for potential allograft transplant rejection may receive the mouse monoclonal antibody (Orthoclone OKT3). Rarely seizures, lethargy, and mental status changes may occur as part of a "cytokine release syndrome" as the T cells are knocked for a loop. This leads to increased capillary permeability, which may be accompanied by symmetrical patchy increase in signal intensity on T2WI white matter bilaterally. This simulates the findings seen in hypertensive encephalopathy or cyclosporine toxicity (posterior reversible encephalopathy syndrome) but may have less of a posterior predilection. Contrast-enhanced MR can display patchy enhancement, even extending to the cortex.

The tone of this chapter reminds us of a joke. A cannibal goes to the cannibal market because he has a yen for some brains for dinner. He looks at the selection in the frozen meat case and sees "Lawyers' brains—$3.49 a pound," "Artists' brains—$3.49 a pound," "Politicians' brains—$3.49 a pound," and "Neuroradiologist's brains—$24.99 a pound." Now the cannibal shopper calls to the cannibal grocer indignantly, "Hey! What's the big idea? Why is the neuroradiologist brain so damn expensive. You can't be telling me that neuroradiologists are so much smarter than the others. I don't believe it!"

"On the contrary," replies the grocer, "do you know how hard it is to find enough neuroradiologists to get even one pound of brain? Sheesh."

And so it goes.

SUGGESTED READINGS

Aoki S, Sasaki Y, Machida T et al: Contrast enhanced MR images in patients with meningioma: importance of enhancement of the dura adjacent to the tumor, *AJNR* 11:935-938, 1990.

Aprile I, Iaiza F, Lavaroni A, et al: Analysis of cystic intracranial lesions performed with fluid-attenuated inversion recovery MR imaging, *AJNR* 20:1259-1267, 1999.

Atlas SW: Adult supratentorial tumors, *Semin Roentgenol* 25:130-154, 1990.

Atlas SW, Grossman RI, Gomori JM et al: Hemorrhagic intracranial malignant neoplasms: spin-echo MR imaging, *Radiology* 164:71-77, 1987.

Bradley WG Jr, Waluch V, Yadley RA et al: Comparison of CT and MR in 400 patients with suspected disease of the brain and cervical spinal cord, *Radiology* 152:695-702, 1984.

Breger RK, Papke RA, Pojunas KA et al: Benign extraaxial tumors: contrast enhancement with Gd-DTPA, *Radiology* 163:427-429, 1987.

Castillo M, Davis PC, Takei Y, Hoffman JCJ: Intracranial ganglioglioma: MR, CT, and clinical findings in 18 patients, *AJNR.* 11:109-114, 1990.

Castillo M, Scatliff JH, Bouldin TW et al: Intracranial astrocytoma, *AJNR* 13:1609-1616, 1992.

Chiechi MV, Smirniotopoulos JG, Mena H: Intracranial hemangiopericytomas: MR and CT features, *AJNR* 17:1365-1371, 1996.

Claussen C, Laniado M, Schorner W et al: Gadolinium-DTPA in MR imaging of glioblastomas and intracranial metastases, *Am J Neuroradiol* 6:669-674, 1985.

Coates TL, Hinshaw DB Jr, Peckman N et al: Pediatric choroid plexus neoplasms: MR, CT, and pathologic correlation, *Radiology* 173:81-88, 1989.

Cohen MD, Klatte BC, Smith JA et al: Magnetic resonance imaging of lymphomas in children, *Pediatr Radiol* 15:179-183, 1985.

Curati WL, Graif M, Kingsley DPE et al: Acoustic neuromas: Gd-DTPA enhancement in MR imaging, *Radiology* 158:447-451, 1986.

Dina TS: Primary CNS lymphoma versus toxoplasmosis in AIDS, *Radiology* 179:823-828, 1991.

Earnest F IV, Kelly PJ, Scheithauer BW et al: Cerebral astrocytomas: histopathologic correlation of MR and CT contrast enhancement with stereotactic biopsy, *Radiology* 166:823-827, 1988.

Elster AD, DiPersio DA: Cranial postoperative site: assessment with contrast-enhanced MR imaging, *Radiology* 174:93-98, 1990.

Filippi CG, Edgar MA, Ulug AM et al: Appearance of meningiomas on diffusion-weighted images: correlating diffusion constants with histopathologic findings, *AJNR* 22:65-72, 2001.

Fleege MA, Miller GM, Fletcher GP, Fain JS, Scheithauer BW: Benign glial cysts of the pineal gland: unusual imaging characteristics with histologic correlation [see comments], *AJNR* 15:161-166, 1994.

Gao P, Osborn AG, Smirniotopoulos JG et al: Epidermoid tumor of the cerebellopontine angle, *AJNR* 13:863-872, 1992.

Goergen SK, Gonzales MF, McLean CA: Intraventricular neurocytoma: radiologic features and review of the literature, *Radiology* 182:787-792, 1992.

Hasso AN, Smith DS: The cerebellopontine angle, *Semin Ultrasound CT MR* 3:280, 1989.

Haughton VM, Rimm AA, Czervionke LF et al: Sensitivity of Gd-DTPA-enhanced MR imaging of benign extraaxial tumors, *Radiology* 166:829-833, 1988.

Healy ME, Hesselink JR, Press GA et al: Increased detection of intracranial metastases with intravenous Gd-DTPA, *Radiology* 169:619-624, 1987.

Helmke K, Winkler P: [Incidence of pineal calcification in the first 18 years of life], *ROFO Fortschr Geb Rontgenstr Nuklearmed* 144(2):221-226, 1986.

Ho VB, Smirniotopoulos JG, Murphy FM et al: Hemangioblastoma, *AJNR* 13:1343-1352, 1992.

Kleihues P, Cavenee WK, ed: *WHO Classification of Tumours: Tumors of the Nervous System*, IARC Press 2000, Lyon, France.

Koeller KK, Dillon WP: Dysembryoplastic neuroepithelial tumors: MR appearance, *AJNR* 13, 1319-1325, 1992.

Krol G, Sze G, Malkin M et al: MR of cranial and spinal meningeal carcinomatosis: comparison with CT and myelography, *AJNR* 9:709-714, 1988.

Kucharczyk W, Brant-Zawadzki M, Sobel D: Central nervous system tumors in children: detection by magnetic resonance imaging, *Radiology* 155:131-136, 1985.

Latack JT, Kartush JM, Kemink JL et al: Epidermoidomas of the cerebellopontine angle and temporal bone: CT and MR aspects, *Radiology* 157:361-366, 1985.

Lee Y-Y, Glass JP, van Eys J et al: Medulloblastomas in infants and children: computed tomographic follow-up after treatment, *Radiology* 154:677-682, 1985.

Lee Y-Y, Tassel PV: Intracranial oligodendrogliomas: imaging findings in 35 untreated cases, *AJNR* 10:119-127, 1989.

Mafee MF: Acoustic neuromas and other acoustic nerve disorders: role of MR and CT—an analysis of 238 cases, *Semin Ultrasound CT MR* 8:256-283, 1987.

Mulkens TH, Parizel PM, Martin J-J et al: Acoustic schwannoma: MR findings in 84 tumors, *AJR* 160:395-398, 1993.

Nelson M, Diebler C, Forbes WSC: Pediatric medulloblastoma: atypical CT features at presentation in the SIOP II trial, *Neuroradiology* 33:140-142, 1991.

Ostertun B, Wolf HK, Campos MG, et al: Dysembryoplastic neuroepithelial tumors: MR and CT evaluation [see comments], *AJNR* 17:419-430, 1996.

Parizel PM, Snoeck HW, van den Hauwe L, et al: Cerebral complications of murine monoclonal CD3 antibody (OKT3): CT and MR findings, *AJNR* 18:1935-1938, 1997.

Park MS, Suh DC, Choi WS, Lee SY, Kang GH: Multifocal meningioangiomatosis: a report of two cases, *AJNR* 20:677-680, 1999.

Peterman SB, Steiner RE, Bydder GM: Magnetic resonance imaging of intracranial tumors in children and adolescents, *AJNR* 5:703-709, 1984.

Pomper MG, Passe TJ, Burger PC et al: Chordoid glioma: a neoplasm unique to the hypothalamus and anterior third ventricle, *AJNR* 22:464-469, 2001.

Poussaint TY, Kowal JR, Barnes PD, et al: Tectal tumors of childhood: clinical and imaging follow-up, *AJNR* 19:977-983, 1998.

Powers TA, Partain CL, Kessler RM et al: Central nervous system lesions in pediatric patients: Gd-DTPA-enhanced MR imaging, *Radiology* 169:723-726, 1988.

Ricci PE, Karis JP, Heiserman JE, Fram BK, Bice AN, Drayer BP: Differentiating recurrent tumor from radiation necrosis: time for re-evaluation of positron emission tomography? [see comments], *AJNR* 19:407-413, 1998.

Russell DS, Rubinstein LJ: *Pathology of tumors of the nervous system*, ed 5, Baltimore, 1989, Williams & Wilkins.

Schwaighofer BW, Hesselink JR, Press GA et al: Primary intracranial CNS lymphoma: MR manifestations, *AJNR* 10:725-729, 1989.

Sheporaitis LA, Osborn AG, Smirniotopoulos JG et al: Intracranial meningioma, *AJNR* 13:29-37, 1992.

Smirniotopoulos JG, Rushing EJ, Mena H: Pineal region masses: differential diagnosis, *Radiographics* 12:577-596, 1992.

Smith MM, Thompson JE, Castillo M, et al: MR of recurrent high-grade astrocytomas after intralesional immunotherapy, *AJNR* 17:1065-1071, 1996.

Smith GB, Petersen RC, Ivnik RJ, Malec JF, Tangalos EG: Subjective memory complaints, psychological distress, and longitudinal change in objective memory performance, *Psychology & Aging* 11:272-279, 1996.

Smith MM, Thompson JB, Castillo M: Radiation-induced cerebral osteogenic sarcoma [letter], *AJR* 167:1067, 1996.

Smith MM, Thompson JE, Thomas D, et al: Choristomas of the seventh and eighth cranial nerves, *AJNR* 18:327-329, 1997.

Spagnoli MV, Goldberg HI, Grossman RI et al: Intracranial meningiomas: high-field MR imaging, *Radiology* 161:369-375, 1986.

Sze G, Krol G, Olsen WL et al: Hemorrhagic neoplasms: MR mimics of occult vascular malformations, *AJNR* 8:795-802, 1987.

Tien RD, Barkovich AJ, Edwards MSB: MR imaging of pineal tumors, *AJNR* 11:557-565, 1990.

Truwit CL, Barkovich AJ: Pathogenesis of intracranial lipoma: an MR study in 42 patients, *AJNR* 11:665-674, 1990.

Tzika AA, Vajapeyam S, Barnes PD: Multivoxel proton MR spectroscopy and hemodynamic MR imaging of childhood brain tumors: preliminary observations, *AJNR* 18:203-218, 1997.

Valk PB, Dillon WP: Radiation injury of the brain, *AJNR* 12:45-62, 1991.

Wang Z, Sutton LN, Cnaan A, et al: Proton MR spectroscopy of pediatric cerebellar tumors, *AJNR* 16:1821-1833, 1995.

Wiegel B, Harris TM, Edwards MK et al: MR of intracranial neuroblastoma with dural sinus invasion and distant metastases, *AJNR* 12:1198-1200, 1991.

Williams RL, Meltzer CC, Smirniotopoulos JG, Fukui MB, Inman M: Cerebral MR imaging in intravascular lymphomatosis, *AJNR* 19:427-431, 1998.

Wilms G, Lammens M, Marchal G et al: Thickening of dura surrounding meningiomas: MR features, *J Comput Assist Tomogr* 13:763-768, 1989.

Yang PJ, Knake JE, Gabrielsen TO et al: Primary and secondary histiocytic lymphomas of the brain: CT features, *Radiology* 154:683-686, 1985.

Zimmerman RA: Imaging of intrasellar, suprasellar, and parasellar tumors, *Semin Roentgenol* 25:174, 1990.

Zimmerman RA, Bilaniuk LT. Age-related incidence of pineal calcification detected by CT. *Radiology* 142:659-662, 1982.

Vascular Diseases of the Brain

The evaluation of stroke using radiologic assessment is now considered routine and essential. This was not always the case. Before the CT era (BCT) the diagnosis was made by astute neurologic examination followed by treatment that consisted of rehabilitation (if you were lucky) and holy water (if you were not so lucky). The clinical examination for the diagnosis of acute stroke can be incorrect in over 10% of cases (one reason radiologists are not out on the street selling apples). Angiography, computed tomography (CT), CT angiography (CTA), and magnetic resonance (MR) imaging including MR angiography (MRA), diffusion and perfusion techniques, and for the lucky few even xenon CT have made accurate diagnosis of this disease mundane, and have aided in therapeutic decision making. The approval by the FDA in 1996 of thrombolytic therapy with tissue plasminogen activator (tPA) for intravenous use as well as the positive results reported from the use of intraarterial Pro-urokinase (urokinase) have dramatically changed our approach toward acute ischemic stroke. It has also put the impetus on radiologists to rapidly and accurately evaluate the patients. This chapter first discusses primary ischemic abnormalities and then turns to the hemorrhagic causes of stroke. Our goals are to provide a foundation to understand the diseases and problems that exist under the gamut of stroke. Can this chapter bring order to chaos (or will it bring chaos to order)? Will the reader find satisfaction at its end? Will Bill and Hillary live happily ever after (BTW we asked the same question in our first edition)? Does Pinocchio have a wooden backside? Enough with these existential problems—we know you are radiologists and we know we are not John Paul Sartre.

Stroke is actually a lay term denoting a sudden loss of neurologic function. This term has little clinical relevance because the source of the event is not defined. Yet, it does connote a notion to which the public and press can relate, and in an information age where diseases compete for bucks, it is obviously a trademark for a most important category of diseases. Is "brain attack" any better? The authors want to make love not war. We suggest the better approach is to elucidate precisely the cause of the neurologic deficit, hence the pivotal role of radiology.

ISCHEMIC CEREBROVASCULAR DISEASE (STROKE)

Ischemic stroke has been recognized (as with almost everything else in medicine) since the work of Hippocrates. Its etiology has been aggressively debated and is as controversial as its recognition is old. Thromboembolic disease consequent to atherosclerosis is the principal cause of ischemic cerebrovascular disease. Ischemic stroke has been classified by subtypes. These are listed in Box 4-1 and are based upon a classification of stroke from a multicenter clinical *T*rial of a drug *O*rg 10172 in *A*cute *S*troke *T*reatment. Hence the name TOAST classification system. Large-artery atherosclerosis, cardioembolism, and lacunes account for the most common causes of ischemic stroke. There are several issues with respect to classification. Outcomes may differ regarding subtype. For example, large artery lesions have a higher mortality than lacunes. Recurrent strokes are

most common in patients with cardioembolic stroke, which also have the highest 1 month mortality. Treatment and its evaluation can be based upon specific subtype so that carotid endarterectomy or stenting is the treatment for large vessel disease whereas anticoagulation therapies are useful in patients with small-vessel disease. This uniformity in evaluation is useful both in clinical practice and in treatment trials. Significant stenosis is defined as that greater than 50%. High-risk and medium-risk categories for cardioembolism are given in Box 4-2. Stroke of determined etiology includes nonatherosclerotic vasculopathies, hypercoagulable states, or hematologic disorders.

Neurologists studied stroke in order to learn
If ischemic classifications could be discerned
After thinking of most
Someone smelled TOAST
It improved diagnosis but not atherosclerosis so they
got burned

Other definitions A transient ischemic attack (TIA) is a sudden functional neurologic disturbance limited to a vascular territory that usually persists for less than 15 minutes, with complete resolution by 24 hours. Although TIAs have a variety of different causes, the common pathway is temporarily inadequate blood supply to

---

Box 4-1 TOAST Classification of Subtypes of Acute Ischemic Stroke

Large-artery atherosclerosis (embolus/thrombosis)
Cardioembolism (high-risk/medium-risk)
Small-vessel occlusion (lacune)
Stroke of other determined etiology
Stroke of undetermined etiology
   a. Two or more causes identified
   b. Negative evaluation
   c. Incomplete evaluation

Box 4-2 Risk of Cardioembolism

HIGH-RISK SOURCES

Mechanical prosthetic valve
Mitral stenosis with atrial fibrillation
Atrial fibrillation
Left atrial/atrial appendage thrombus
Sick sinus syndrome
Recent myocardial infarction (<4 weeks)
Left ventricular thrombus
Dilated cardiomyopathy
Akinetic left ventricular segment
Atrial myxoma
Infective endocarditis

MEDIUM-RISK SOURCES

Mitral valve prolapse
Mitral annulus calcification
Mitral stenosis without atrial fibrillation
Left atrial turbulence
Atrial septal aneurysm
Patent foramen ovale
Atrial flutter
Lone atrial fibrillation
Bioprosthetic cardiac valve
Nonbacterial thrombotic endocarditis
Congestive heart failure
Hypokinetic left ventricular segment
Myocardial infarction (>4 weeks, <6 months)

a focal brain region. Almost one third of patients with a TIA eventually have cerebral infarction, with 20% of these infarctions occurring within 1 month of the initial TIA. In addition, patients with a clinical TIA may have actual evidence of infarction based on MR. Thus proceeding with the workup after the TIA is urgent.

A lacunar infarction is a small cerebral infarct that becomes cystic and is produced by occlusion of a small end artery (Fig. 4-1). These lesions have a predilection for the basal ganglia, internal capsule, pons, or corona radiata. They can result in specific clinical neurologic syndromes. Although originally thought to arise from small-vessel atherosclerosis and lipohyalinosis associated with hypertension, many other causes have been proposed including emboli, hypercoagulable states (e.g., polycythemia, use of oral contraceptives), vasospasm, and small intracerebral hemorrhages. The important point is that the term *lacunar infarction* should be reserved for small strokes, about 5 mm in diameter (with a limit of up to 15 mm), regardless of their cause. Small, while not perfect, may be better in this case.

Although running the risk of losing all but the most punctilious readers, we will persist in briefly describing the pathology of atherosclerosis. You should at least feel that you are getting your money's worth. The process begins in the first decade of life in the aorta with subendothelial fatty deposition (fatty streak) consisting of smooth muscle cells, foam cells, T lymphocytes, and an extracellular matrix of among other things lipid and collagen. Fat is discharged from the smooth muscle and foam cells into the extracellular space. This may precipitate intimal thickening, associated with the proliferation of smooth muscle cells in the vessel wall, and inflammatory changes including fibrosis and scarring. An

aspirin a day keeps the fatty streaks at bay. A fibrous plaque consisting of collagen, lipid, smooth muscle cells, and fibroblasts develops and is the characteristic lesion of advanced atherosclerosis. The endothelial surface of the fibrous plaque degenerates with subsequent ulceration and discharge of lipid and/or calcified debris into the vessel lumen. Platelets may accumulate on the ulcerated intimal surface and become exposed to collagen, which causes thrombus formation and possible platelet emboli. Fibrous plaques have variable size, with some becoming large and fibrotic, producing luminal narrowing, whereas others accumulate lipid and cholesterol. Arterial bifurcations are subject to the greatest mechanical stress and are especially prone to atherosclerosis.

The principal causes of ischemic stroke are emboli, however, the sources of emboli are variable. They can arise from arterial stenosis and occlusion, atherosclerotic debris and ulceration, or cardiac sources (an embolus from a cardiac source occurs in about 15% to 20% of ischemic strokes). The extent to which narrowing of the arterial lumen contributes to stroke is more problematic. However, reduction in flow may decrease the ability to "wash out" emboli before they produce ischemia.

Hemodynamically significant narrowing occurs when the diameter of the vessel is decreased by 50% to 60%. Other definitions of "hemodynamically significant" used in the literature include stenosis greater than 70% or residual carotid artery lumen of less than 1.5 mm (corrected for magnification). The hemodynamically significant lesion is manifested by a pressure gradient across it. However, flow reduction does not occur until the diameter is decreased approximately 90%. The disparity between flow reduction that occurs with high grade stenosis and a hemodynamically significant lesion is the

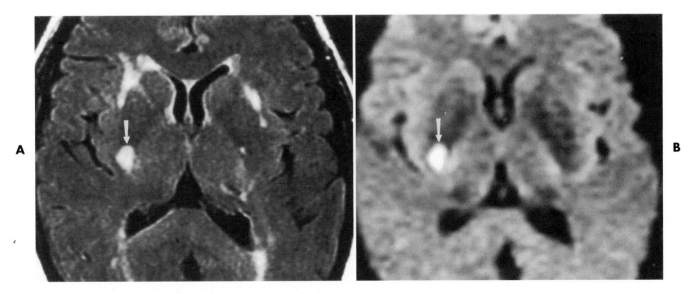

Fig. 4-1   Lacunar infarction. **A,** Periventricular high signal intensity foci and a focal lacunar infarction (*arrow*) in the internal capsule are demarcated on the FLAIR scan. **B,** The acuity of the lesion is exemplified by the bright signal (*arrow*) on the diffusion-weighted image. Note that the white matter foci are not of the same age.

result of the autoregulation in the brain, which decreases cerebrovascular resistance so that only with very high grade stenosis is blood flow to the brain decreased. Even with complete occlusion of the vessel lumen, infarction may not occur because of the redundancy of collateral circulation. On the other hand, patients with complete internal carotid occlusions in the neck may still have cerebral infarctions from emboli. Emboli may be multiple and simultaneous or a single embolus may break up and produce multiple infarctions.

The bad news is that there usually are multiple regions of atherosclerotic involvement in cerebrovascular disease. The silver lining is that even though 35% of those patients more than 50 years old may have widespread atherosclerosis, only one third of these persons have symptoms. This is one case where it is better to finish in the lower two thirds.

When does primary occlusion result in stroke? The most obvious situation is in the case of a watershed infarction. Vascular watersheds are generally the most distal arterial territories, where communication between the principal routes of supply connect (see Chapter 2). Major watershed zones are found between the anterior and middle cerebral arteries and the middle and posterior cerebral arteries. All other things being equal, reduction in flow affects these zones to the greatest extent. The areas of particular interest are in the posterior parietal region (middle and posterior cerebral watershed), the basal ganglia region, and the frontal lobes between the anterior and middle cerebral arteries. In other sites the brain is selectively jeopardized by hypotensive changes due to increased susceptibility to ischemia (perhaps because of increased metabolic rate) as well as lack of redundancy of blood supply. These include the occipital lobes, cerebellum, hippocampus (Ammon's horn), globus pallidus, and amygdala (anterior choroidal–posterior cerebral watershed). The third, fourth, and fifth cortical layers are particularly vulnerable to ischemia.

Interest in the detection and treatment of extracranial occlusive carotid artery disease has been accelerated because of the reported results in two large trials for the treatment of symptomatic and asymptomatic patients. The North American Symptomatic Carotid Endarterectomy Trial (NASCET) and Asymptomatic Carotid Atherosclerosis Study (ACAS) confirmed the benefit of carotid endarterectomy in patients with high-grade carotid stenosis (≈60% or more). In combination with these studies the implementation of vascular stenting for extracranial occlusive vascular disease and MRA has set off a modern day "gold rush" to identify and treat patients who walk (or even crawl) with asymptomatic disease. This subject is controversial especially with patients at 50% to 69% stenosis.

One other issue with respect to carotid stenosis is the method of measurement. In the NASCET study the percent stenosis was measured as:

The diameter of lumen at the point of the maximal stenosis divided by the diameter of the lumen of the normal artery distal to the stenosis times 100% whereas in the European Carotid Surgery Trial (ECST) the percent stenosis was measured as:

The diameter of lumen at the point of the maximal stenosis divided by the estimated "true" lumen diameter at the point of stenosis.

Both methods have their strengths and weakness. The former method may underestimate stenosis when the distal lumen narrows as a result of the severe proximal stenosis that limits flow. The latter method has problems because the observer must extrapolate what is thought to be the true lumen (Fig. 4-2).

Depending upon the belief$ of surgeons and physicians caring for the particular patient, extracranial occlusive vascular disease may be worked up solely with noninvasive imaging techniques including ultrasound, MRA, CTA, or noninvasive imaging, which may be followed by catheter angiography. In ambiguous, discordant, or problematic cases catheter angiography is usually performed.

Radiologic Workup

Let us set the stage. Since our last edition, we have observed that many radiologists and scientists have made a career out of developing and implementing new meth-

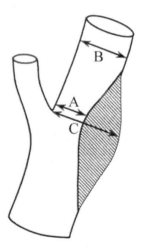

NASCET % STENOSIS = 100 [B-A] / B

ECST % STENOSIS = 100 [C-A] / C

Fig. 4-2 Drawing of North American Symptomatic Carotid Endarterectomy Trial (NASCET) and European Carotid Surgery Trial (ECST) criteria for evaluation of carotid stenosis. *A* is the diameter of the residual lumen at the point of maximal stenosis; *B* is the diameter of the normal artery distal to the stenosis; *C* is the estimated "true" lumen at the point of stenosis. (Courtesy of P. Kim Nelson, M.D. and Danko Vidovitch, M.D.)

ods to identify and evaluate stroke. We start with a review of the techniques available for the assessment of stroke beginning with conventional approaches followed by the newer more specific methods

Noncontrast CT is the most efficient method for the workup of acute stroke (within 24 hours of the ictus) and TIAs. The problem is that for the most critical time period the hyperacute stage (0 to 6 hours) (and the stage where therapy has its greatest impact) it is usually not very conclusive. Although conventional MR is more sensitive than CT in the detection of early infarction (82% versus 58%), it is equally weak within the hyperacute phase. However, with the addition of diffusion and perfusion weighted MR (see Diffusion/Perfusion Section) the sensitivity for detection of ischemic stroke has radically improved. The goals of imaging in stroke are: (1) to make a definitive diagnosis of stroke and determine if there is salvageable brain; (2) to determine whether there is a nonischemic cause for the patient's neurologic presentation such as a brain tumor, primary intraparenchymal hemorrhage, or subarachnoid hemorrhage; and (3) to identify any hemorrhagic component to the infarction.

Carotid ultrasound/transcranial Doppler Ultrasound uses sound waves to image structures or measure the velocity and direction of blood flow. Color-coded Doppler ultrasound can depict the residual lumen of the extracranial carotid artery more accurately than conventional duplex Doppler. However, the results from color coded Doppler ultrasound examination are operator dependent and controversial. Problems include distinguishing high grade stenosis from occlusion, calcified plaques interfering with visualization of the vascular lumen, inability to show lesions of the carotid near the skull base, difficulty with tandem lesions, and inability to image the origins of the carotid or the vertebral arteries. In the NASCET study, Doppler measurements were 59.3% sensitive and 80.4% specific for the detection of stenosis greater than 70%. A battery of ultrasonic noninvasive carotid studies including indirect tests monitoring the superficial and deep orbital circulations and direct studies using imaging and function has been advocated to increase the accuracy particularly in significant vascular disease.

Transcranial Doppler ultrasound is a noninvasive means used to evaluate the basal cerebral arteries through the infratemporal fossa. It evaluates the flow velocity spectrum of the cerebral vessels and can provide information regarding the direction of flow, the patency of vessels, focal narrowing from atherosclerotic disease or spasm, and cerebrovascular reactivity. It can determine adequacy of middle cerebral artery flow in patients with carotid stenosis and evidence of embolus within the proximal middle cerebral artery. It is very useful in the detection of cerebrovascular spasm following subarachnoid hemorrhage or after surgery, and can rapidly assess the results of intracranial angioplasty or papaverine infusions to treat vasospasm.

MRA is another important noninvasive test to study both the extracranial and intracranial circulation. (MRA has already been discussed in Chapter 1 but for the malignantly lazy we will repeat the most salient features.)

Magnetic resonance angiography (MRA) (Fig. 4-3) The inherent appeal of MRA is obvious. Conventional neuroangiography is an invasive procedure with a very low but significant morbidity and mortality. There are three different techniques used to generate MRA—time-of-flight (TOF), phase contrast (PC), and contrast enhanced angiography. Once the imaging data is gathered it may be processed by several display techniques. The one most commonly used is termed maximal intensity projection (MIP), which finds the brightest pixels along a ray and projects them along any viewing angle. MIP is fast and insensitive to low-level variations in background intensity.

TOF The principle is that protons not immediately exposed to a radio frequency (RF) pulse (unsaturated spins) flow into the imaging volume and have higher signal than the partially saturated stationary tissue (which has lost signal secondary to the RF pulse). This is a T1 effect and has been termed "flow related enhancement." The images can be acquired as individual slices (2D) acquisition or as a volume (3D) acquisition. In either case flowing blood will appear bright. The 2D TOF techniques are very sensitive to slow or moderate flow (as flow related enhancement is maximized) whereas 3D techniques are better than 2D MRA for rapid flow and have higher resolution. 3D techniques are used almost exclusively for intracranial arterial evaluation. 2D TOF has also been implemented in the coronal plane for evaluation of venous thrombosis. Pitfalls still occur with high intensity thrombus.

PC The principal of PC involves using bipolar flow-sensitizing gradients of opposite polarity to tag moving spins, which are then identified owing to their position change at the time of each gradient application. The operator chooses the flow velocities that the angiogram will be sensitive to, termed the VENC, which varies in neuroradiology from 30 cm/sec for arterial flow to 15 cm/sec for venous flow. Complex subtraction of data from the two acquisitions (one of which inverts the polarity of the bipolar gradient) will cancel all phase shifts and phase errors except those due to flow. This technique provides excellent background suppression to differentiate flow from other causes of T1 shortening such as methemoglobin or fat. This technique is less often implemented but is useful in cases of suspected venous thrombosis to differentiate between flow and thrombus. In TOF images both thrombus containing methemoglobin and flow can be bright whereas only flow will have signal on PC images.

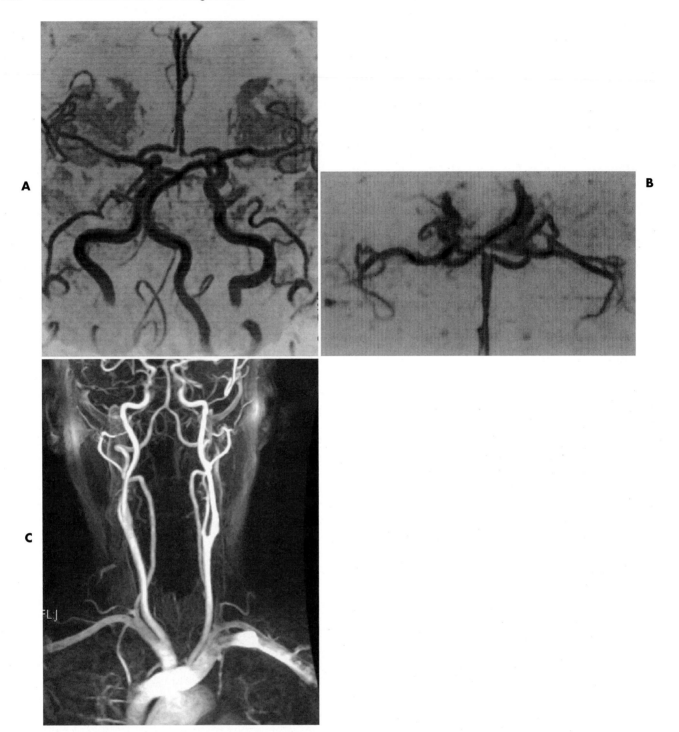

Fig. 4-3 Montage of MRA. **A,** TOF MRA of circle of Willis. One can appreciate the major intracranial vessels and bifucations. **B,** Phase contrast study of same patient. Background is suppressed in by phase contrast. Vessels are not quite as sharp. **C,** Contrast enhanced MRA of the great vessels of the neck and head. Although requiring contrast the examination produces unambiguous images of the carotid bifurcations.

Contrast enhanced MRA (CEMRA) (see Fig. 4-3) A new and potentially important improvement in MRA has been the use of paramagnetic contrast enhancement in association with 3D TOF imaging. The procedure generally requires very fast pulse sequences com-

bined with software that can time the intravenously administered bolus of contrast. This method has many advantages over the noncontrast approach. The use of paramagnetic vascular enhancement abolishes the signal loss secondary to spin saturation from slow flow or in-plane flow. The result is a high resolution image of the extra or intracranial vessels including the aortic arch. Timing is critical as enhancement of veins confounds the ability to demonstrate arterial anatomy. This methodology may be useful to exclude aneurysm or other vascular malformations and study the carotid bifurcation as well as the aortic arch. CEMRA may also be able to delineate the exact location of extracranial ulceration, large vessel intracranial vascular occlusions from embolic disease, intracranial stenosis, and narrowing of vessels from vasculitis. It also can decrease ambiguity in cases with flow reversal such as subclavian steal (Fig. 4-4).

Indications and limitations of MRA MRA is the best (but some might argue that CT angiography is competitive) noninvasive technique for evaluating the extracranial vasculature for the presence of a hemodynamically significant lesion of the carotid arteries, dissection of the vertebral and carotid arteries, extracranial traumatic fistula, extracranial vasculitis such as giant cell arteritis, or congenital abnormalities of the vessels such as fibromuscular disease. Intracranial MRA is used to detect aneurysms particularly in those cases where there is a relatively low probability of occurrence. This includes asymptomatic relatives of patients with aneurysms and patients with headache where concern is raised about aneurysm. The accuracy of MRA for aneurysms greater than 3 mm has been reported to be about 90% plus, however, the accuracy falls to less than 40% for small aneurysms less than 2 to 3 mm in diameter.

Other situations where MRA could provide information is in the follow-up of unruptured aneurysms, and in cases where a diagnosis is important but treatment or conventional angiography is contraindicated, or in the follow-up of treated aneurysm. Additional indications for MRA include the workup of intracranial stenosis (controversial), intracranial vasculitis (very controversial), stroke, venoocclusive disease, congenital AVMs, vascular compression syndromes, and definition of the blood supply to vascular neoplasms. However, conventional angiography remains the definitive diagnostic modality both for the diagnosis of intracranial aneurysm including those patients presenting with acute third nerve palsy and for therapeutic planning.

The limitations of extracranial MRA include a tendency to overestimate stenosis particularly if 2D TOF methods are used. It is also difficult to detect tandem lesions with MRA. Ulcers are poorly seen and the methodology is less sensitive to very slow flow, perhaps suggesting occlusion in vessels that possess trickle flow. This problem is circumvented by using cMRA. This is the important difference between a surgical stenosis and nonsurgical vascular occlusion. The patients must be cooperative as motion degrades the images. In the case of carotid stenosis, only performing the extracranial MRA

can preclude diagnosis of additional vascular lesions such as an aneurysm or AVM in the brain. In addition, patients with a history of transient ischemic attacks or recent neurologic deficits may have unrecognized embolic occlusions, which are difficult to detect with MRA. Surgery in such cases can be associated with hemorrhagic complications.

MRA images, particularly the intracranial portion of the examination, are challenging to interpret. The distal vessels are suboptimally visualized so that conditions affecting these vessels, such as involvement in vasculitis, may be difficult to detect. Careful examination of all images, preferably after the image is segmented so that each vessel can be viewed independently without overlap of other vessels, is important to the successful delineation of intracranial lesions. In comparison with CT angiography (see following section), intracranial MRA generally involves no or low doses of contrast agents, no radiation, can be repeated multiple times (if no contrast is used) during the same examination, and may have a larger acquisition volume (although multidetector CT alleviates this problem) commonly including the origin of the posterior inferior cerebellar artery.

Computed tomographic angiography (CTA) (Fig. 4-5) CTA is emerging as an alternative to MRA for imaging both the extracranial and intracranial blood vessels. It requires the placement of a small catheter usually in the antecubital vein with injection of approximately 50 to 125 mL of iodinated contrast material. After a short delay following contrast injection, imaging commences and a 3D data set is acquired. Computer postprocessing is necessary for MIP images and excluding the bony base of the skull structures. CTA is fast and noninvasive but does require the injection of intravenous iodinated contrast. It is probably as good as MRA at detecting aneurysms 3 mm or larger (i.e., those having the greatest likelihood of rupture). CTA: (1) is fast (less than 30 seconds); (2) is less motion sensitive than MR; (3) is without the flow related effects seen in MRA; (4) can easily visualize slow flow or turbulent flow in aneurysms (particularly large aneurysms); (5) involves no MR compatibility problems with intubated patients or aneurysm clips; (6) is helpful in diagnosis of dissection and pseudoaneurysms in the neck, and (7) can present a multiplanar view of the vascular anatomy from any perspective including the relationship of the aneurysm to the bony skull. It can also detect calcification in the neck of an aneurysm, provide bony surgical landmarks, and detect intraluminal thrombus, all of which may be useful for the surgeon to know. It has been advocated for evaluation of intracranial stenoocclusive lesions in patients with acute stroke.

The limitations of CTA include: (1) risks of intravenous iodinated contrast injection; (2) significant time for postprocessing of data; (3) exposure to radiation;

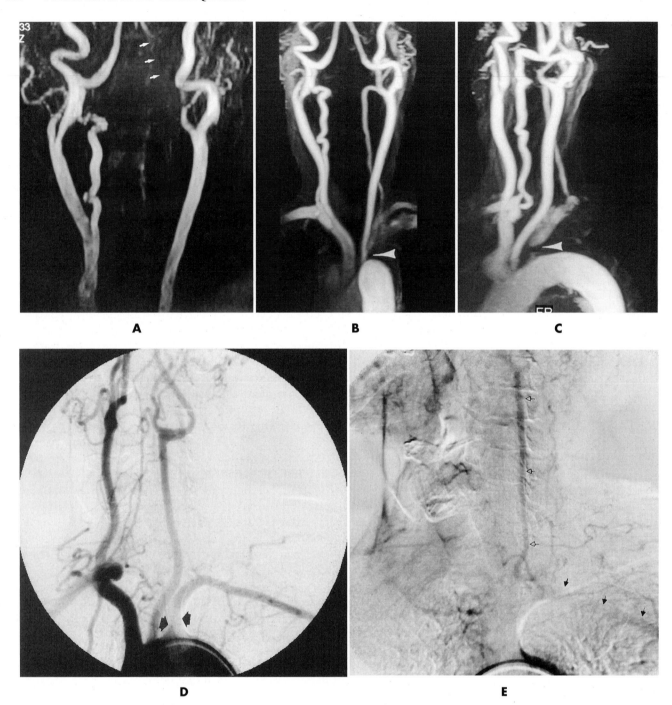

Fig. 4-4   Subclavian Steal. **A,** Time of flight MRA fails to adequately demonstrate the proximal left vertebral artery. You can just make out a portion of the vessel *(arrows)*. **B,** Gadolinium enhanced MRA now shows the left vertebral artery, the victim of slow flow. The cause is a stenosis of the proximal left subclavian artery *(arrowhead)* which is hard to believe on this projection, but much more plausible *(arrowhead)* on the oblique view (**C**). **D,** Arch injection depicts the significant stenosis of the proximal left subclavian artery *(arrows)*. Contrast does go beyond the stenosis; however, there is no antegrade filling of the left vertebral artery. **E,** On the late phase of the arch injection, retrograde flow is noted down the left vertebral artery *(open arrows)* and into the left subclavian artery *(closed arrows)*.

(4) vessels at the base of the skull may be obscured by enhancement in the cavernous sinus or bone at the base of the skull; (5) in subarachnoid hemorrhage the high density of blood can obscure the bleeding aneurysm; (6) the acquisition volume (not a problem if multidector

CT is available) can potentially miss the take-off of the posterior inferior cerebellar arteries unless specifically directed to this area (MRA may have similar problems); (7) aneurysm clips in the postoperative patient produce artifacts that may obscure anatomic detail (MRA has sim-

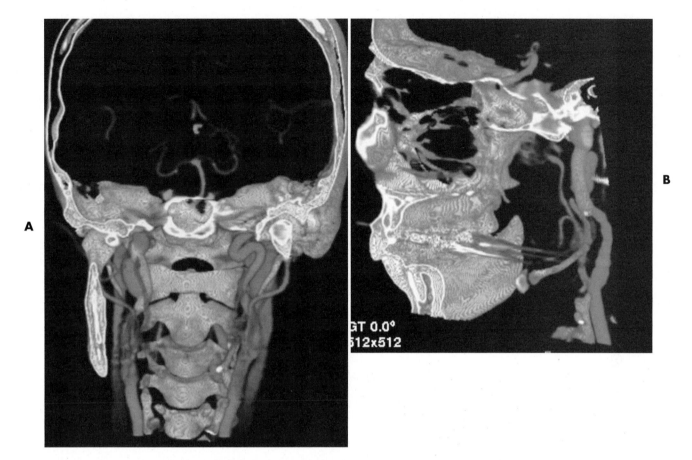

Fig. 4-5   CTA of carotid bifurcation. **A,** AP. **B,** Lateral. When you're dealing with a normal bifurcation all techniques look outstanding. This CTA is as good as any MRA or conventional arteriogram for saying that this woman is not a candidate for endarterectomy.

ilar problems); (8) calcifications in the walls of the vessels, in the anterior clinoid processes, and other areas can produce artifacts; (9) there is only one opportunity to perform the study as opposed to MRA, which can be repeated, and (10) the 3D reconstruction process is operator dependent. Presently, CTA is used as a screening tool, primarily to rapidly show aneurysms in symptomatic patients and to screen asymptomatic patients at risk for cerebral aneurysms. It also has champions in cases of angionegative evaluation of subarachmoid hemorrhage (SAH), to mediate between discordant ultrasound and MRA, for angiography patients at high risk for bifurcation disease, and in neck trauma.

Role of Angiography

Arterial catheter angiography is the definitive imaging modality for vascular lesions of the brain and great vessels of the neck but has been relegated to a secondary role in the diagnosis of stroke. Patients are referred for angiography for the following reasons (a) if the MRA, CTA, or/and carotid ultrasound is poor; (b) if MRA is contraindicated that is, the patient has a pacemaker; (c) if test results are equivocal; (d) to better discern tandem lesions; (e) to evaluate aneurysm or vascular malformations responsible for an intracranial hemorrhage; and (f) for the evaluation of vasculitis. One example of the importance of aggressively pursuing angiography is in the case of vasculitis. Drug therapy, usually in the form of immunosuppressives, is not without risk! Angiographic evidence suggestive of vasculitis can guide surgical planning for definitive diagnosis or can itself serve as a justification for treatment. With modern methods of imaging, angiography continues to be an important diagnostic tool, but its use must be well defined. The converse of this is also true: failure to perform an arteriogram can result in misleading and incorrect diagnoses. Angiography is a safe (but not harmless) study and in many situations provides crucial information. The incidence of all complications for femoral artery catheterizations is approximately 8.5% with the range of permanent complications (the most significant of which is stroke) from 0.1% to 0.33%, a 2.6% incidence of transient complications, and a 4.9% incidence of local complications.

Angiography is an excellent albeit invasive method for determining whether a lesion is hemodynamically significant in the carotid circulation. At present, the concept of hemodynamically significant lesions is not entirely consistent with current thoughts that the vast majority of strokes result from embolic occlusions. However, the hemodynamically significant lesion, with its decreased flow, may be insufficient to clear small emboli. Collateral circulation is also important in providing blood flow. Autoregulation dilates small arterioles to maintain blood flow. The brain can also increase the extraction fraction of oxygen to maintain function and metabolism. There is, however, evidence of an association between high-grade carotid stenosis (70% or greater) (Fig. 4-6) in patients with ipsilateral TIAs or nondisabling stroke, and the incidence of subsequent stroke within 2 years of the TIA. In addition to the obvious hemodynamic problem, it is likely that high-grade stenosis predisposes to embolic events. The embolus lodges in an already hemodynamically compromised region of the brain. This issue is far from resolved, so we have listed in Box 4-3 the angiographic findings associated with hemodynamically significant carotid disease.

Lesion location, as usual, is important, with most disease occurring at the carotid bifurcation. Patients with asymptomatic internal carotid disease may have a better prognosis than those with asymptomatic occlusion of the middle cerebral artery. This may be related to the copious colateral for the internal carotid (anterior communicating, posterior communicating, and leptomeningeal arteries) whereas the middle cerebral artery only possesses leptomeningeal colaterals.

The incidence of hemodynamically significant lesions of the aortic arch is extremely low (0.6%). Such lesions are usually apparent during attempts at selective catheterization or result in slow antegrade flow in the great vessels of the neck and can be detected on angiographic review. Arch injections are useful when attempts at selective catheterization fail and the dyspeptic angiographer must ascertain whether this problem is the result of the technique (poor hands versus reduced synaptic transmission in the angiographer), an anatomic variant, or proximal occlusion of the vessel. With digital subtraction methods, the amount of contrast can be reduced substantially, and with the use of nonionic con-

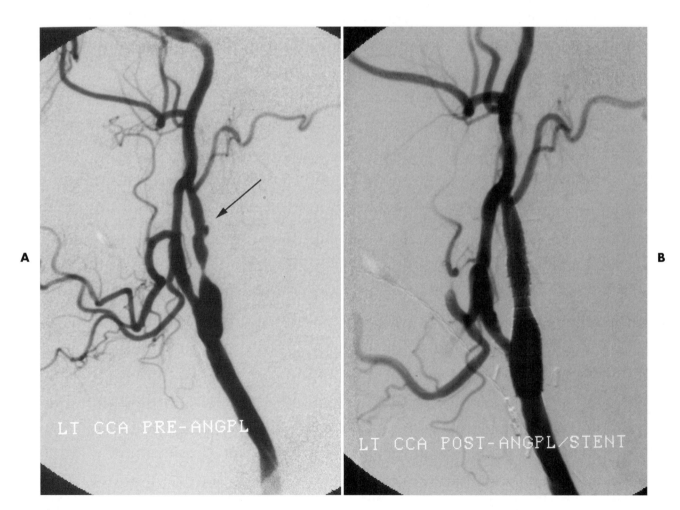

Fig. 4-6   A, Common carotid angiogram showing high-grade stenosis of the left internal carotid artery. Notice the ulceration in a distal plaque (*arrow*). **B,** The patient underwent an angioplasty and stenting procedure. Observe the improved flow and the obliteration of the ulcer by the stenting. (Courtesy of P. Kim Nelson, M.D.)

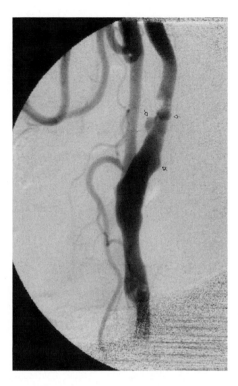

Fig. 4-7   Ulceration. Multiple ulcers *(arrows)* are seen in the internal carotid artery, which is narrowed by atheromatous disease.

Box 4-3   Angiographic Findings in Hemodynamically Significant Lesions of the Extracranial Carotid Arteries

Lesions with 50%–70% reduction of vessel lumen diameter
Less than 2 mm residual lumen corrected for angiographic magnification
External carotid artery opacification leads internal carotid artery opacification
Delayed ocular choroidal blush (>5.6 sec for patients >30 yr old)
With injection of contralateral carotid or vertebral arteries, angiographic filling of ipsilateral carotid circulation

trast, complications are minimized. The risk of complications from the arch injection is still higher and is related in part to catheter whipping and plaque dislodgement during injection. The low diagnostic yield together with higher potential complications bestows extremely limited use on the arch injection.

Arch disease has been implicated as a cause of brain ischemia in the syndrome of subclavian steal (see Fig. 4-4). This occurs when a subclavian stenosis proximal to the origin of the vertebral artery leads to retrograde flow down the ipsilateral vertebral artery, "stealing" blood from the circle of Willis, with subsequent distal subclavian artery filling from the retrograding vertebral artery. Similar brain ischemia can be seen with occluded vertebral arteries. The symptoms of cerebral ischemia, when present in this syndrome, are thus not related to the steal phenomenon but simply to decreased antegrade flow. This again points out the limited use of the arch injection.

The accuracy of diagnosing ulceration is on the order of 50% to 85%. It is particularly difficult on the basis of angiography to distinguish ulceration from irregularity, but MRA reeks when it comes to this diagnosis. The most reliable angiographic sign is the penetrating niche, but depression between adjacent plaques and intraplaque hemorrhage may produce a similar appearance (Fig. 4-7). Luminal bulging secondary to destruction of the media with an intact intima can also appear as an ulcer. One should appreciate that the association of ulcer and stroke is also controversial. Many asymptomatic plaques are ulcerated, and many symptomatic plaques are not. Generally, however, ulceration is frequently found on the symptomatic side in association with significant stenosis. The best approach presently is for the radiologist to describe the plaque as smooth or irregular, and if an undermined niche is present, the term *ulceration* can be used. It is in the province of the physician caring for the patient to base therapy on the severity of findings and

on the patient's symptoms. No studies have documented any greater risk of angiography during an acute stroke. The vascular supply to the symptomatic region should be the first order of business. What is the current role of angiography in hyperacute stroke? It is primarily used in an interventional mode for thrombolysis and stenting. Remember therapeutic thrombolysis helps pay the mortgage or a portion of the month's rent in New York.

CT and MR Findings

CT has improved and become more sensitive than initially thought to the subtle findings in acute stroke (Fig. 4-8). Within 6 hours of some infarcts, faint loss of definition of gray-white borders may be observed. This includes obscuration of the lentiform nucleus (hypodensity) (in middle cerebral artery infarction) or loss of definition of regions of the cortex (cortical or insular ribbon sign). The latter has been described in the region of the insular cortex associated with middle cerebral infarction. It can also be seen in other regions of the brain. The implementation of PACS workstations enables use of variable nonstandard window width and center level settings (approximately 8 and 32 Hounsfield units respectively) facilitating detection of early hypointensity in acute infarction (Fig. 4-9). High density in the proximal middle cerebral artery has been noted as an early sign of infarction representing either an acute thrombus or calcified em-

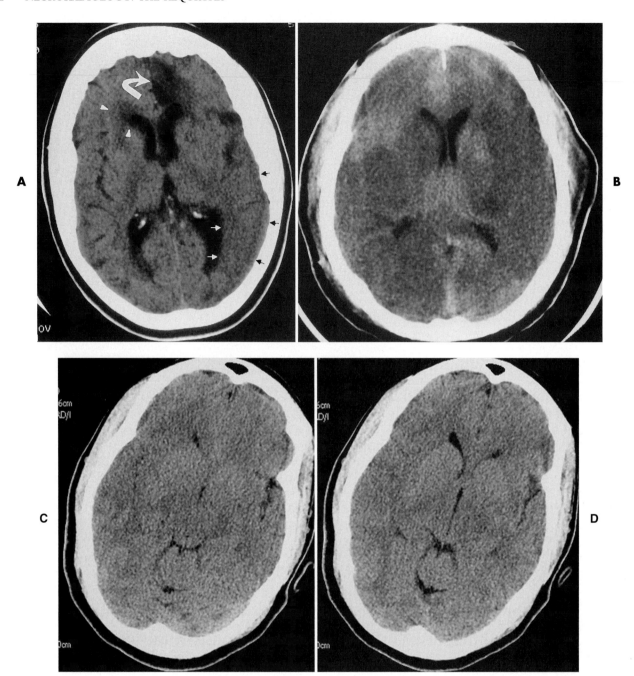

Fig. 4-8   CT of stroke. **A,** Early (24 hours old) subtle left middle cerebral artery infarction *(black arrows)* with loss of normal sulci (compare to other side), slight mass effect on lateral ventricle *(white arrows),* and loss of gray/white interface. This patient also demonstrates previous old left frontal anterior cerebral artery infarction with low density (malacic changes) in the frontal region *(curved arrows)* and dilatation of the left frontal horn. There are also periventricular white matter changes *(arrowheads).* **B,** Massive cerebral infarction following a cardiac arrest (48 hours before CT). Note the marked low density throughout both hemispheres involving anterior, middle, and posterior cerebral artery vascular distributions. There is compression of the ventricles. The high density areas represent spared cerebral tissue. **C** and **D,** Insular ribbon sign. Observe the loss of the insular gray and white matter of the right in this acute right-middle cerebral artery infarction.

bolus lodged in the middle cerebral artery (Fig. 4-10). High density may also be observed in the basilar artery and in the venous sinuses secondary to thrombus.

Within 12 to 24 hours, an indistinct area of low density is apparent in the appropriate vascular distribution.

Mass effect may be feeble initially. The region starts to become circumscribed after 24 hours with more apparent mass effect. Look for sulcal asymmetry or minimal compression of one ventricle. Mass effect usually peaks between 3 and 5 days after the ictus. Enhancement is

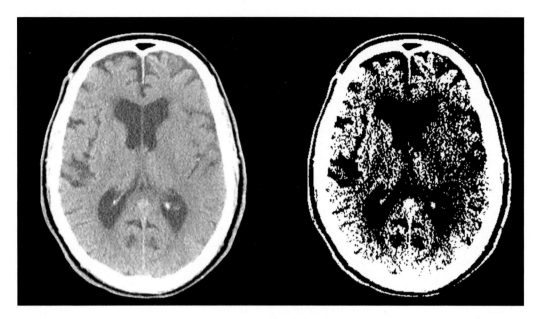

Fig. 4-9   Left middle cerebral stroke seen best with non "standard windows." The image on the left is filmed with the standard window level 30 HU and width 90 HU (range −15 to 75). Note that the left middle cerebral stroke is very difficult to appreciate although the *cognoscenti* appreciate the subtle loss of gray-white differentiation. The image on the right is filmed with a center level of 30 HU and a narrower width 20–30 HU (range 10 to 40). Observe the obvious hypodensity in the left middle cerebral artery distribution. (Courtesy M. Lev, M.D.)

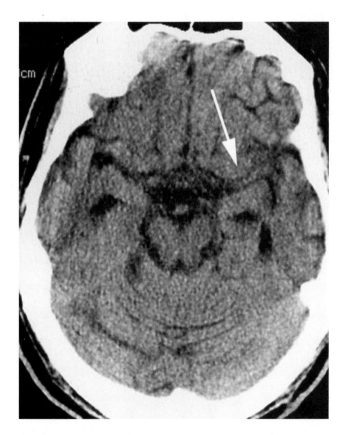

Fig. 4-10   Acute thrombosed vessel on CT. Note high density in the vessel *(arrow)*.

unusual before the third day, but when present can mask low density of the infarcted region. For enhancement to occur, two criteria must be met: (1) the blood-brain barrier must be abnormal and (2) the contrast must be able to reach this locale. Thus, if parenchymal enhancement is seen within 24 hours of the ictus, one must presume that the embolus has moved distally or lysed, or that there is excellent collateral circulation to reach the locale. Perfusion into this region of defective blood-brain barrier increases the probability of hemorrhage into the infarcted tissue. The usual duration of CT enhancement of infarction is a few weeks.

Mass effect starts to decrease after about 5 days and is usually gone in 2 to 4 weeks. Persistence of mass effect beyond 6 weeks strongly implies that another lesion, most likely tumor, should be considered. In about 50% of cases, between the second and the third week, the infarct changes from low density to isodensity. This has been termed the CT "fogging" effect and appears to result from hyperemia from reperfusion, petechial hemorrhage, and extensive macrophage activity in the necrotic brain. At this time enhancement can be identified in 70% of lesions. Enhancement may be gyriform if the infarct is cortical or can have a ring configuration if the lesion involves the basal ganglia, cortex, or brain stem. We have also identified "fogging" in the Pinocchio syndrome, associated with extreme rationalization and hypertrophy of the bulbocavernous, a case report of an ex-President.

The lesion reverts to a well-circumscribed region of low density, which is noted after 4 weeks. At this time, there is usually absence of enhancement and no mass effect, and parenchymal loss is seen in the affected vascular territory. If laminar necrosis (breakdown of cortical cell layers) occurs there may be deposition of paramagnetic compounds and/or calcium, which can produce hyperdensity (hyperintensity on T1WI) in chronic infarcts. Although in rare cases infarcts may enhance longer than this, persistent enhancement reduces the probability of simple infarction and favors the diagnosis of tumor or inflammatory lesions.

The term *luxury perfusion* is used to describe increased circulation through an area of infarcted brain. This is demonstrated angiographically by early venous drainage and a transient angiographic blush (Fig. 4-11). This is seen between the first and third week following the ictus. The wise reader may ask, "Who is doing angiography for strokes at this time?" The simple authors reply that strokes are not always that easy to detect and that luxury perfusion may be misdiagnosed (as a vascular malformation or other hypervascular lesion including tumor) in patients with conditions other than stroke presenting with transient neurologic problems.

Findings may be seen on MR in the first few hours after infarction. Swelling of the cortex is observed on T1WI and FLAIR without changes in signal intensity. On FLAIR images, arteries with slow flow/no flow may be hyperintense and outlined by the hypointensity of CSF. By 8 hours, high intensity develops on T2WI, and at 16 hours, low intensity is noted on T1WI. Arterial enhancement is an early marker of infarction. Arterial enhancement is rarely seen in deep white matter or deep gray matter infarction. Gradient-moment nulling technique should not be used when one is looking for arterial enhancement, because it can cause high intensity in normal arteries.

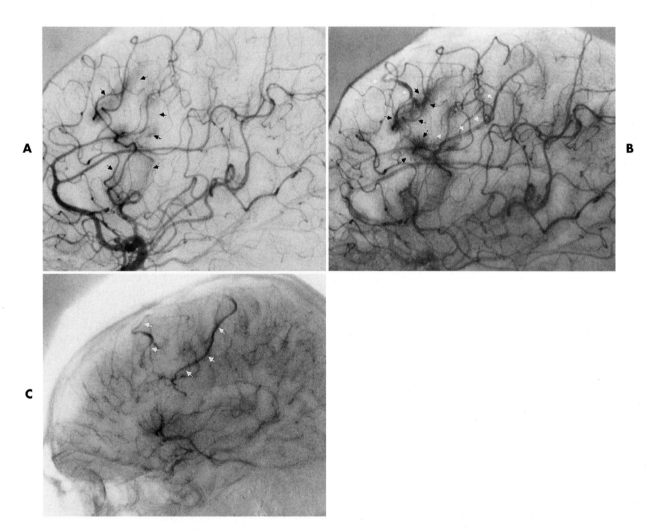

Fig. 4-11 Luxury perfusion in a patient with sickle cell disease. (Courtesy Mark Mishkin, M.D.) **A,** Lateral angiogram in the midarterial phase demonstrates the vascular stain *(arrows)* seen in luxury perfusion. **B,** Late arterial phase again demonstrates the stain *(black arrows)* as well as early veins *(white arrows),* which are characteristic of luxury perfusion. **C,** Early venous phase shows those veins *(arrows)* again.

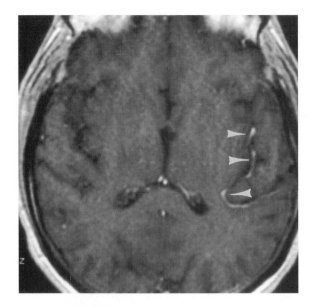

Fig. 4-12 Arterial enhancement (? An anachronism). This enhanced T1WI in a patient with an early left MCA stroke shows arterial enhancement likely secondary to slow flow in the artery.

Enhancement in arteries appears to be more sensitive than T2WI in the first hours of acute infarction but is rarely used these days because of the implementation of diffusion weighted imaging (see following section). Because normal rapid arterial flow produces a flow void, arterial enhancement represents slow flow, and this can be detected in approximately 50% of ischemic lesions (Fig. 4-12). It is not a very specific finding as it may be observed with the presence or absence of arterial occlusion. Slow flow from an incomplete occlusion or a complete occlusion with relatively slow retrograde collateral flow (leptomeningeal) produces this arterial enhancement. Reappearance of the flow void suggests reestablishment of faster flow. Arterial enhancement ceases in 7 to 11 days. This suggests the establishment of either significant collateral flow or lysis of a proximal embolus. The loss of arterial enhancement is coupled to a certain extent with the onset of parenchymal enhancement but parenchymal enhancement is generally observed earlier than the loss of arterial enhancement.

Both cerebral blood volume and mean transit time are reported to be increased in cortical areas showing vascular enhancement. It has been hypothesized that vascular enhancement in association with acute stroke indicates a state of impaired cerebral hemodynamics.

In cases where there is middle cerebral artery occlusion impaired diffusion (see following discussion) in the complete middle cerebral artery distribution has been seen. This is associated with a poor prognosis. In patients with middle cerebral artery occlusion, the presence of arterial enhancement has been shown to indicate the presence of good collateral circulation. It

can be viewed perhaps as a simple statement regarding perfusion.

It is interesting that parenchymal enhancement in the acute phase is inversely proportional to the extent of high signal on T2WI. Infarcts with little collateral supply are the most severe and have the greatest area of high signal abnormality, whereas early and intense enhancement in acute infarction implies good collateral circulation. Noncortical infarctions enhance between 4 and 7 days, whereas cortical infarctions enhance after 6 days. The early enhancement in noncortical infarction is probably due to their watershed vascular pattern, enabling contrast to reach the infarcted tissue early. In addition, cortical watershed infarcts and reversible ischemic neurologic deficits may demonstrate even earlier and/or more intense enhancement, indicating good tissue perfusion of contrast.

Paramagnetic enhancement in infarction may last 6 to 8 weeks. Just as with iodine enhancement, persistence beyond this period requires further investigation and skepticism regarding infarction as the diagnosis.

Lacunar infarction   (see Fig. 4-1) Initially this infarct appears as a small, low-density region on CT or high intensity on T2WI. A few days after the event there is transient enhancement for approximately 1 week. At approximately 4 weeks, the lesion appears as a sharply demarcated low-density region or as a focal area of high intensity on T2WI.

Cerebellar infarction   Cerebellar infarction is a special case. The frequency of cerebellar infarction is less than 5% and has a male predominance and a mean age of 65 years (+/−13 years). The clinical findings suggesting cerebellar infarction include the abrupt onset of posteriorly located headaches, severe vertigo, dysarthria, nausea and vomiting, nystagmus, ipsilateral dysmetria, and unsteadiness of gait. Cerebellar infarction can be treacherous, with delayed alteration of consciousness seen in 90% of patients, with mass effect. This can occur rapidly (within a few hours) or up to 10 days after the ictus. The cerebellum swells with (1) an infarction involving more than one third of its volume, (2) a basilar artery occlusion with poor collateral supply, (3) an embolus with reperfusion, and (4) a massive superior cerebellar artery infarction. CT or MR findings reveal low density, high intensity on T2WI with mass effect in the appropriate vascular distribution. The imaging pitfall lies particularly with CT because beam-hardening artifact or partial volume averaging masks subtle regions of low density. The opposite also can occur where the cerebellar fissures get confused with stroke. It is important to visualize the fourth ventricle with particular attention to subtle asymmetry (Fig. 4-13). Check for the presence of hydrocephalus manifested by enlargement of the temporal horns (an early sign of obstructive hydrocephalus). Subtle imaging characteristics (minimal mass effect and

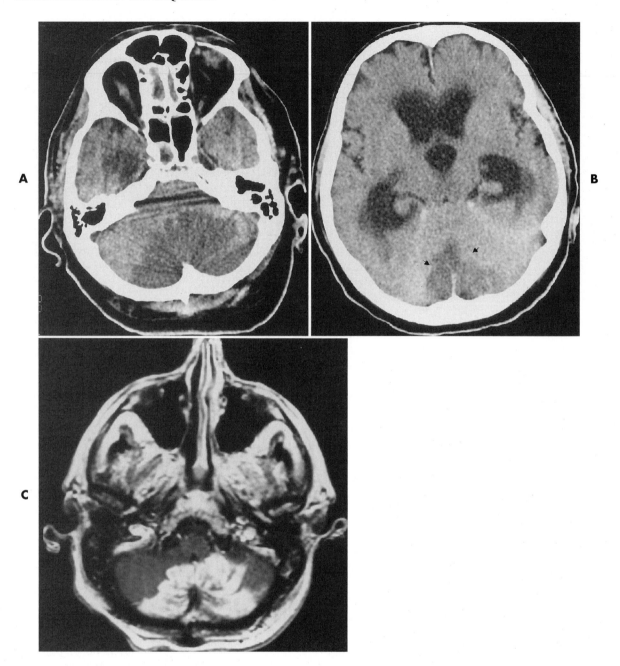

Fig. 4-13 Acute cerebellar infarction. **A,** There is an acute cerebellar infarct on this CT having a variegated anterior border and producing significant mass effect with compression of the pons and fourth ventricle. **B,** Higher section revealing acute hydrocephalus from compression of the fourth ventricle by the cerebellar mass effect. The superior vermis is also involved *(arrows)* and the swollen cerebellum compresses the superior vermian cistern (not visualized). **C,** Enhancement on T1WI in the infarcted cerebellum is seen.

slight enlargement of the ventricles) can rapidly evolve to large mass lesions with compression of the brain stem and cerebellar herniation. The superior vermis can herniate upward through the tentorium, whereas the tonsils and inferior vermis may herniate downward into the foramen magnum. Treatment of acute cerebellar infarction producing such mass effect involves ventricular drainage and cerebellar decompression.

Small cerebellar infarctions (particularly in the poste-

rior inferior cerebellar artery distribution) have a more benign course and are the result of small arterial branch occlusions. These are detected on CT or MR and are unassociated with mass effect. The principal cause is thromboembolic disease from a cardiac source or from atherosclerotic disease in the vertebrobasilar system. In younger patients with cerebellar infarction, perform MR supplemented with MRA and pay special attention to the vertebral arteries, to rule out vertebral dissection (dis-

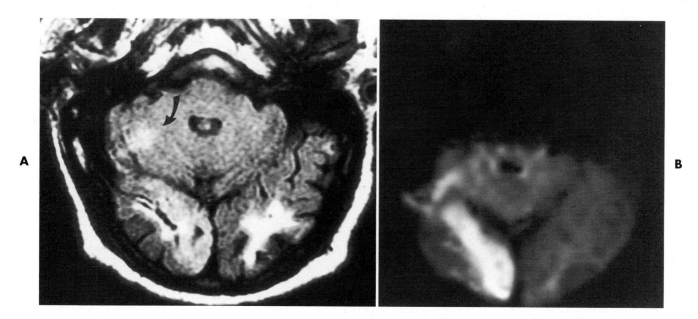

Fig. 4-14   Posterior circulation infarcts. **A,** The presence of vascular lesions in the cerebellum *(curved arrow)* and the occipital lobes go hand and hand. **B,** The DWI shows its enormous value in identifying that the acute lesion is in the right occipital lobe. Note the artifact that limits DWI around the sphenoid sinus region and anterior brainstem. Observe the absence of high signal from the left cerebellum.

cussed later in the chapter). When an infarction is identified either in the posterior fossa or in the occipital lobes, carefully inspect the other area. Remember that the vertebrobasilar system supplies both territories and that emboli can affect both regions at the same time (Fig. 4-14).

His neurologic exam was weak and full of hokey
So the neurologist ordered MR to rule-out the strokey
When asked why diffusion
He said please perfusion
The HMO fired his ass for being too pokey

Diffusion/perfusion   Diffusion imaging is a technique that is sensitive to the movement of water molecules (Brownian motion). Water protons in a swimming pool can have a ball changing position and direction in any way they want (isotropic diffusion). The distance traveled by the particular water molecule we are watching (self diffusion) depends upon how long we watch it. If the observation time is short, the paths of most molecules will not be affected by cellular barriers (membranes, proteins, etc.), however, when the observation time is long enough to produce an encounter with a barrier there is restricted diffusion. The effect of this diffusion can be measured as a change in signal intensity on MR. This measurement can be made by applying two gradient pulses to dephase and rephase the water molecules. Those molecules that diffuse the greatest distance (i.e., subject to the greatest gradient strength difference) will be unable to rephase completely and will lose signal. The signal loss is dependent upon the diffusion co-

efficient of the molecule and the strength and duration of the gradient pulses. This can be defined mathematically by the following *equation:*

$$S(b) = S_o \cdot e^{-bD}$$

where D is the diffusion coefficient, S_o is the signal intensity of the unweighted image, $S(b)$ is the signal intensity of the images for various b values, and the b value is specific for the particular pulse sequence used to measure diffusion. b is a function of the diffusion gradient strength, the duration of the diffusion gradient pulse and the time of the diffusion measurement. The b value can be defined as:

$$\gamma^2 G^2 \delta^2 (\Delta - \delta/3)$$

Where γ is the gyromagnetic ratio of hydrogen (a physical constant), Δ is the spacing between gradient pulses, G is the diffusion gradient strength, and δ is the diffusion gradient pulse duration.

In biologic systems, water molecules are restricted from walking very far because membrane barriers and proteins get in their way, and thus the term "apparent" is applied to modify the word "diffusion" connoting the uncertainty of the water motion. The apparent diffusion coefficient (ADC) can be calculated by using images with varied gradient strengths (different b values). The ADC can be calculated if there are at least two b values one of which may be set to 0 close to 0, that is, no diffusion weighting. ADC is the negative slope of a linear regression line that correlates a b value with the natural log of the signal intensity acquired at that particular b value.

Two *b* values are generally used in the clinical setting, however, four or more *b* values should be measured for accuracy. Commonly used values include a maximum *b* value of 800 to 1200 sec/mm^2, TE 90 to 120 msec, and a low *b* value of about 2 to 10 sec/mm^2 with an identical TE.

Diffusion images can either be created to be directionally sensitive (with a T2 component), directionally insensitive (the cube root of the product of three directions—with a T2 component), or directly correlated to ADC values (no T2 component). Most diffusion weighted imaging in clinical practice is currently the diffusional average image (D_{avg}) (D_{avg} = trace of the diffusion tensor/3).

Substances with high ADC will lose signal more rapidly than those with low ADC. Thus CSF appears dark on diffusion weighted images as the water molecules can diffuse relatively large distances freely (isotropic diffusion). Contrast this to the region of the splenium of the corpus callosum where diffusion is limited in the anterior-posterior direction by the orientation of the myelin fiber tracts thus producing high intensity on appropriately diffusion oriented images. This strong bias for diffusion parallel to white matter fiber orientation is referred to as diffusion anisotropy. If a diffusion measurement is made using a diffusion sensitizing gradient in the direction perpendicular to white matter fiber tracts the measurement (reflecting the restricted diffusion in the perpendicular plane) could be confused with acute white matter ischemia. These perpendicular tracts will appear bright. Conceptually, diffusion is a three-dimensional event and thus it can be described by a mathematical entity, the tensor, which can account for three-dimensional movement, thus the effects of diffusion anisotropy are minimized by using the trace (an image of the average from three or more diffusion directions) of the diffusion tensor.

Here is the beef (and we will hold the prions)—in acute and hyperacute ischemic stroke we see blood flow reduction with cellular dysfunction and then structural breakdown. The cellular swelling is associated with reduction in the extracellular space, and cytotoxic edema with the redistribution of extracellular water to the intracellular space, and/or increased tortuosity of the extracellular space, and/or changes in viscosity, and/or changes in temperature, and so on, contributing to the observed decrease in the ADC (bright on DWI). Cytotoxic and vasogenic edema are both bright on T2WI but only the former is associated with decreased water diffusion. Whatever the cause, the net effect is an increase in the signal on diffusion-weighted images and a very bright region seen on the image. Conversely, if ADC maps are displayed (images where intensity is related to ADC values), reduced diffusivity will show up as a zone of lower intensity.

Based upon diffusion characteristics one can differentiate acute versus chronic infarction (see Fig. 4-14). This is sometimes difficult on standard T2 weighted or FLAIR images as both acute and chronic infarction will be high intensity on both studies. It can be useful in the detection of acute lacunar or subcortical infarction and their separation from unidentified bright objects (UBOs) of other etiologies. ADC maps are particularly helpful in situations where there are abnormalities in which the tissue has increased water content (e.g., an old infarct). This will produce an area of brightness (Fig. 4-15) (but not very bright—how bright?—about 500 on the SATs) on the diffusion weighted image that is termed "T2 shine-through." This is because DWI have T2 weighting, which shines through. The ADC map, however, will correctly separate the acute lesion (lower intensity) from the old infarct (higher intensity) (see Fig. 4-15). Other potential sources of confusion with DWI may be areas of hemorrhage and susceptibility. The ADC may also be decreased by nonischemic etiologies (Box 4-4) many of which are reversible.

Diffusion weighted imaging (DWI) is a rapid pulse sequence with a total imaging time of usually less than 1 minute. It can be performed using a variety of imaging techniques including echoplanar, line scan diffusion imaging (sequential acquisition of multiple one dimensional lines of data) and navigated spin-echo diffusion imaging—both useful in systems without strong gradient systems, diffusion-weighted-half-Fourier acquisition single-shot turbo-spin echo imaging, or diffusion-weighted-fast spin-echo imaging just to name some of the technical options available for DWI.

DWI can detect cerebral ischemia within about 2–3 minutes of its onset (if you are a cat or rodent) and about 30 minutes for humans. Contrast this to conventional MR, which is positive, if you are lucky within a few hours after an cerebral infarction (Fig. 4-16). DWI is a very sensitive and specific technique and as stated at the beginning of the chapter there is now an effective treatment for cerebral ischemia that works most successfully (with the lowest probability of producing hemorrhage) in the first 3 (to possibly 6 hours) after the onset of ischemia. It has been able to detect multiple acute stroke lesions in 17% of cases probably the result of multiple emboli or embolic breakup. In contrast, only about 2% were reported in the literature before implementation of DWI, thus, the concept of marrying a technique that potentially can provide information about the extent of irreversible ischemia to a method of therapy (thrombolysis).

The duration of restricted diffusion (low ADC, bright on DWI) is about 10 to 14 days. The ADC then normalizes (pseudonormalization) following that it becomes elevated (encephalomalacia) (see Table 4-1).

The dogma is that all cases of diminished diffusion in the hyperacute ischemic state represents complete infarction. Of course, nothing is perfect except perhaps the authors' wives. Ditto for diffusion. No absolute threshold in lower ADC values is available to predict tissue infarction. There are now documented cases of reversible hyperacute diffusion abnormalities. These exceptions probably represent spontaneous cases of successful reperfusion. There have been reports of a rare case of infarction without DWI abnormality but this finding has also been associated with what was a clinical TIA. DWI can be negative and then develop into infarcted tissue or negative DWI can occur with extensive abnormalities on perfusion weighted images (see following section). Indeed, the exact worth of DWI in determining tissue viability and ischemic reversibility as well as arbitrating therapeutic intervention remains to be proven. This is particularly true in assessing tissue viability in patients ongoing early treatment. DWI lesion volume measured within 48 hours has been suggested to be a reasonable predictor of outcome in stroke.

Perfusion imaging (Fig. 4-17) Perfusion imaging differs from diffusion imaging in that its aim is to characterize microscopic flow at the capillary level. The brain parenchymal blood flow is the ratio of the cerebral blood volume (CBV) to the transit time of the blood through the parenchyma. Conventional radiologic techniques including catheter angiography, positron emission tomography (PET), xenon CT, CT perfusion, and single photon emission computed tomography (SPECT) have been used for estimation of tissue perfusion, but MRI perfusion imaging may offer significant advantages including higher spatial resolution and minimal or no invasiveness. Techniques include the use of either exogenous contrast agents (gadolinium) termed dynamic susceptibility contrast (or contrast agent bolus tracking) or endogenous contrast from deoxyhemoglobin (blood oxygen level dependent—BOLD), or magnetic labeling (spin tagging) of arterial water. The technique most of-

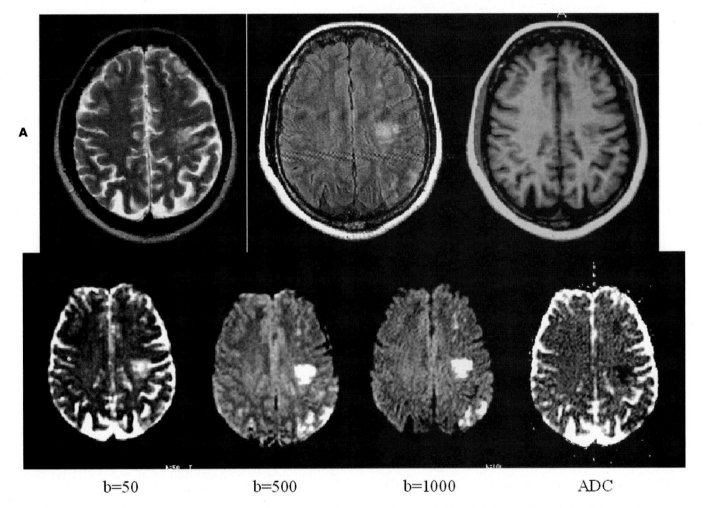

b=50   b=500   b=1000   ADC

Fig. 4-15   Diagnosis of new and old strokes with a little help from your friends (DWI and ADC images). **A,** Subtle left posterior frontal acute infarction without swelling. Top images show T2, FLAIR, and T1WI. There is no mass effect and the question is "new or old." Only the diffusion and ADC images can tell for sure. In the bottom row, the first three images are diffusion weighted at various b values. Observe how bright the infarct becomes with increased diffusion weighting. The ADC image is low intensity indicating restricted diffusion as opposed to "T2 shine-thru" and thus the lesion is a new infarction.

Illustration continued on following page

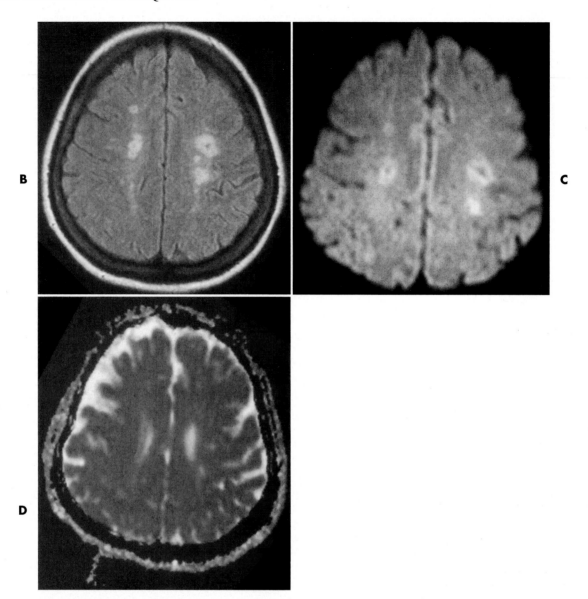

Fig. 4-15 *Continued.* **B,** Flair image of old ischemic changes in the white matter. Observe the high intensity in all of the lesions. **C,** Diffusion-weighted image show corresponding high intensity secondary to "T2 shine-thru." **D,** ADC map at a slightly lower level shows no evidence of low ADC confirming shine-thru.

Box 4-4 Nonischemic Causes for Decreased ADC

Abscess
Cortical spreading depression
Lymphoma and other Tumors (Epidermoid, PNET)
Multiple sclerosis
Metabolic diseases (e.g. Canavans)
Seizures
Severe hypoglycemia
Trauma

---

ten used is dynamic susceptibility, which provides quantitative relative or absolute measures of perfusion. Dynamic susceptibility is the perfusion method commonly used and is discussed later. BOLD, although commonly used for functional imaging, has not been clinically implemented. Arterial spin labeling inverts arterial spins before their entering an imaging slice. It can generate absolute blood flow quantification and is entirely noninvasive requiring neither a power injector nor exogenous paramagnetic contrast. It can be repeated indefinitely and quantifies cerebral blood flow as opposed to cerebral blood volume. There are several methods that enable spin tagging but the problem is that it is limited

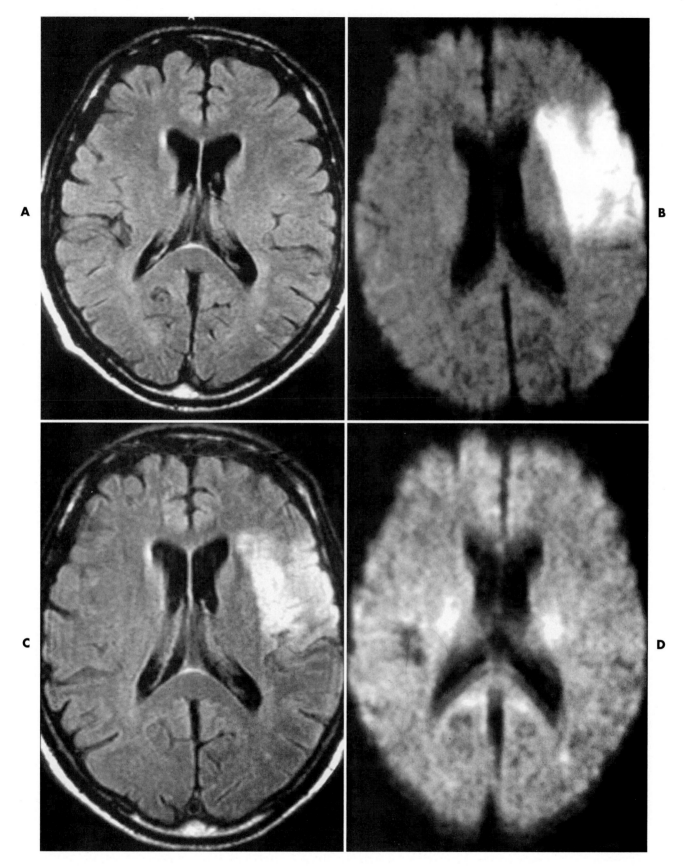

Fig. 4-16   **A,** FLAIR image in a patient 4 hours after speech arrest and right arm hemiparesis. Observe that there is no significant abnormality. **B,** Diffusion weighted images shows a large bright area representing a middle cerebral artery infarct. **C,** Two weeks later the infarct is obvious on FLAIR but way too late for the patient. **D,** Diffusion is now negative.

Table 4-1   Ischemic stroke—MR intensity, DWI, ADC

Stage	T1WI	T2WI	DWI	ADC
Hyperacute (0–6 hrs)	Isointense—maybe some loss of sulci	Isointense	Bright	Low
Acute (6 hrs–4 days)	Low intensity—mass effect	High intensity	Bright	Low
Subacute (4–14 days)	Low intensity	High intensity	High intensity 2° to T2 shine through	Pseudonormalization
Chronic	Smaller area of low intensity—encephalomalacia	High intensity	High intensity 2° to T2 shine through	High

to a small number of slices. We shall thus focus on dynamic susceptibility perfusion.

Presently the most commonly used methodology involves the use of contrast agent bolus tracking with gadolinium either injected with a power injector or by hand over a brief period of time (less than 5 seconds). When observed using susceptibility weighted imaging the intravascular gadolinium bolus produces decreased signal intensity from the susceptibility effects in the capillary bed's blood vessels that can be followed every second or

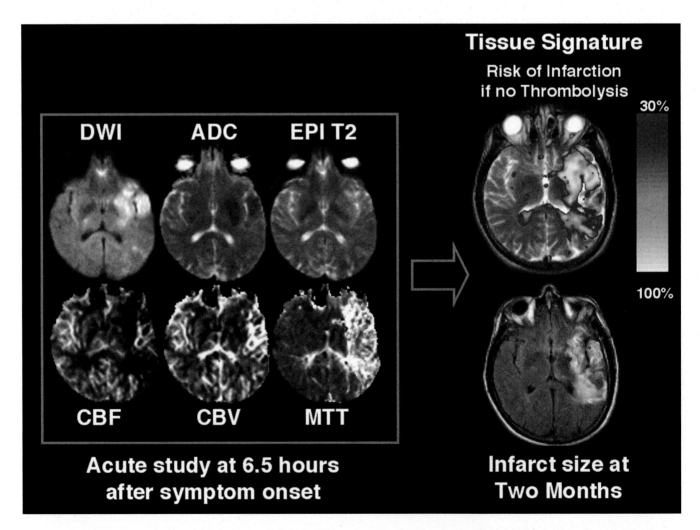

Fig. 4-17   Acute left MCA stroke (6.5 hours after symptom onset). Top row reveals diffusion (high) and ADC (low) abnormality consistent with stroke. Note the T2 weighted image is normal. Perfusion metrics including cerebral blood flow (CBF), cerebral blood volume (CBV), and mean transit time (MTT) are all varyingly abnormal. The infarct size appears to correlate with CBV. Using these measurements, one can create tissue signatures so that it is possible to estimate the risk of infarction if there is no thrombolysis. (Courtesy of G. Sorensen, M.D.)

so with fast gradient echo techniques. Fig. 4-17 demonstrates this effect. The signal loss is related to the concentration of the contrast agent and proportional to the cerebral blood volume. If the blood-brain barrier (BBB) is not intact, the effect of leakage of gadolinium can affect the measurement. However, as you will learn in ischemic stroke the BBB is intact in the hyperacute stage and even in the first 24 hours. The common parameters used to assess perfusion include the relative cerebral blood volume (rCBV), relative cerebral blood flow (rCBF), time to peak (TTP), and relative mean transit time (rMTT). These are related in the following equation:

$$rCBF = rCBV/rMTT$$

Regions with prolonged rMTT and a marked decrease in rCBV have a high probability of irreversible ischemic injury. These measures can be mapped to the brain. The limitations of the technique include its invasiveness (need a venous line—ouch!), susceptibility artifacts from air-filled sinuses affecting the lower imaging slices, and the intensive data processing required. rMTT is dependent on the proximity and severity of the stenosis. A proximal stenosis will produce a larger rMTT than a distal one. Increased rMTT is the result of any hemodynamic problem be it acute (i.e., an embolus) or chronic oligemia (primary middle cerebral artery stenosis). In addition, rMTT may be altered in regions where collateral circulation is the primary route of blood supply. It is generally a visual measurement of asymmetry and thus bilateral lesions can confound the interpretation.

The CBF of the normal brain ranges between 45 and 110 mL/min/100 g of tissue. Cerebral oligemia (about 20 to 40 mL/min/100g) is defined as underperfused asymptomatic region of brain that will recover spontaneously whereas an ischemic hypoperfused brain is symptomatic and at risk to develop irreversible infarct without revascularization. The ischemic threshold identified in animal experiments when there is cessation of action potential generation occurs around 20mL/min/100g and the infarction threshold, associated with irreversible neuronal damage, is at approximately 10 mL/min/100 g.

The theory goes that the perfusion weighted image is the sum of the ischemic core and the ischemic penumbra. The core is the most damaged tissue where there is presumably energy failure, inability to maintain ionic gradients, and irreversible damage. The ischemic penumbra is tissue that is injured and at risk for death but is potentially salvageable. There is some evidence that subtraction of perfusion from diffusion images can demonstrate the area of ischemic penumbra. Another way to think about these concepts is that the penumbra contains tissue with normal diffusional properties (but with impaired perfusion measured by rCBF or MTT) surrounding the core of tissue with diffusional abnormality. Diffusional abnormalities can grow between day 1 and day 2. This confirms the notion that there is salvageable tissue after 3 to 6 hours following the acute event.

Perfusion imaging in combination with diffusion has been advocated in a treatment algorithm for acute stroke. In such a scenario the larger the difference between the perfusion and diffusional abnormalities the greater the need for acute intervention with thrombolytic agents. If there is no perfusional abnormality, or it is equal to the diffusional lesion, then the probability that thrombolysis will be effective is low. This is very controversial. Presently perfusion imaging has still not been fully implemented in the clinical setting for a variety of reasons including equipment (hardware/software), reimbursement, efficacy, and inertia.

What measure best correlates with the size of the final infarct? It depends upon many factors including what literature you read. It seems that MTT maps tend to overestimate the final infarct size whereas the rCBV maps appear to have the best correlation with the size of the infarct. However, this is controversial, with some reports indicating that rCBV underestimated final infarct volume whereas rCBF overestimates it. Such differences may, in part, be related to when the measurement is made (12 hours versus 24 hours).

A few words regarding treatment Therapy has become the mantra of the contemporary stroke neurologist and interventional neuroradiologist. The first issue is to exclude hemorrhage (see section on Hemorrhage in this chapter), determine the extent of infarcted tissue as well as demonstrate that there is salvageable brain tissue (using perfusion/diffusion methodology). There is an increased risk of fatal hemorrhage when there is decreased density in greater than one-third the middle cerebral artery territory (thrombolytics in large MCA infarcts even with an ischemic penumbra are contraindicated). Intravenous tPA has been reported to induce hemorrhage in 6% to 20% of cases. Urokinase treatment has also been associated with hemorrhage. This complication is the result of reperfusion to microvascular bed of nonviable brain parenchyma and has been reported to occur early (3 to 5 hours) in therapeutic intervention in patients with low CBF (<35% of normal). The time of ischemia is critical, that is, "time is brain." What is generally reported is a 3 to 6 hour window for successful treatment of middle cerebral artery infarction. However, this is a range and with good collateral circulation there is evidence that the ischemic process is reversible beyond those limits. The effective therapeutic window for revascularization of the posterior circulation is longer than the 3 to 6 hour window (maybe up to 36 hours).

There is a great deal of controversy regarding what methodology should be used to determine if patients should be treated. The issue is the clock is ticking. The patient does not get through the emergency room to radiology at warp time. Some argue that if the plain CT shows no hemorrhage the patient needs to be treated. Others would argue to get the dog off the MR and put the patient on for diffusion/perfusion measures and then treat if indicated. The next edition will provide the definitive approach.

Since the approval of tPA in 1996, the impact on stroke has been negligible ($\leq 1.1\%$). It is legitimate to ask why this is the case especially if we are spending megabucks on brain attack campaigns and wish to implement the latest and greatest techniques (perfusion/diffusion imaging). For one thing it is a pain to get to the hospital within the 3 to 6 hour time frame (only 3.6% to 16% of patients are eligible for treatment) combined with having no true algorithm for patient selection and consequently a low rate of therapeutic efficacy (12% to 30%).

Proton spectroscopy   In finishing we thought a few words were useful on this technique relative to stroke—lactate, *N*-acetyl-aspartate (NAA). How is that for a few words—You guessed it—NAA is decreased and lactate is elevated within the first 24 hours. Elevated lactate is observed in ischemic areas of the brain whereas NAA is associated with neuronal death. Much more work is necessary to determine its exact role but biochemical markers are the real deal, however, their implementation needs work.

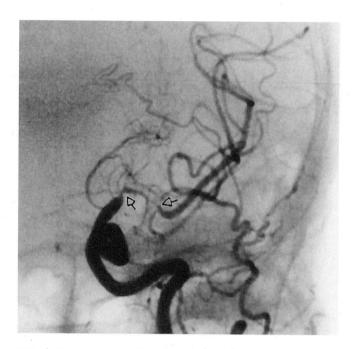

Fig. 4-18   Vasculitis. AP arteriogram reveals abrupt narrowing of the M1 segment of the middle cerebral artery *(open arrows)* in a patient with herpes zoster vasculitis. The anterior cerebral artery was occluded.

VASCULITIDES

The vasculitides are a most interesting assorted group of diseases. Most have an immunologic basis resulting in vascular injury. You should appreciate that only about 10% of patients undergoing cerebral angiography for vasculitis actually have it angiographically documented. Part of the problem is the resolution of angiography (500 μm) can only detect involvement of medium and large vessels. X-ray vision does not help when superradiologist is technique limited.

Inflammatory changes within and surrounding the vessel wall result in narrowing and obliteration of the vascular lumen with subsequent thrombotic occlusion or necrosis and rupture of the vessel. The pathologic features in this lesion include spasm, edema, cellular infiltration, and proliferation. The vessel can be compressed by thickened meninges or fibrosis. These inflammatory changes result in the classic angiographic picture of segmental narrowing and dilatation. Long segments of vessels are involved circumferentially (Fig. 4-18). When seen in the cerebral arteries these features strongly favor vasculitis, although other disease processes can produce this picture. Atherosclerosis tends to occur eccentrically, with shorter segments of involvement than inflammatory vasculitis. Tuberculosis and *Haemophilus influenzae* infections often cause a basilar meningitis involving the internal carotid and basilar artery together with their proximal branches, although convexity vessels may also be affected. Tertiary meningovascular syphilis affects both arteries and veins, particularly in the middle cerebral distribution. Vasospasm, neoplasms, and embolic occlusions (particularly after lysis) can at times have an angiographic appearance similar to vasculitis.

MR is quite sensitive detecting abnormalities in patients with vasculitis but falls short in specificity. MRA is very limited in this diagnosis both because of technique and its limited ability to visualize distal vessels. Usually there are multiple abnormal regions (which vary in size and location) that can include infarction (cortical and subcortical), hemorrhage (intraparenchymal, subarachnoid, even subdural), and/or nonspecific white matter lesions. Enhancement occurs in some but not all of these lesions. Perfusion imaging has been suggested to improve both sensitivity and specificity in detecting vasculitis. It has the ability to detect microcirculatory abnormalities, but more importantly can provide evidence that there is no perfusional abnormality thus effectively eliminate the diagnosis of vasculitis. Other techniques that may increase our sensitivity include diffusion imaging, PET, and SPECT imaging.

The correlation between MR and angiography is modest, at best, and the modalities should be viewed as complimentary. Thus biopsy is indicated on two counts: (1) to make the diagnosis in clinically suspicious but angiographically negative cases and (2) to confirm the diagnosis or to offer another diagnosis. However, physicians are reluctant to recommend brain biopsy and patients are not so thrilled about the prospects either. Thus, without tissue many patients are diagnosed and treated based

Box 4-5   CNS Vasculitis

NONINFECTIOUS

Necrotizing Vasculitides
  PACNS (Primary angiitis of the central nervous system)
  Polyarteritis nodosa
  Giant cell arteritis
  Takayasu's arteritis
  Wegener's granulomatosis
  Lymphomatoid granulomatosis
Neurosarcoidosis
Vasculitis Associated with Collagen Vascular Diseases
  Systemic lupus erythematosus
  Scleroderma
  Rheumatoid arthritis
  Sjogren's syndrome
Drug-Related Vasculitis
Others
  Susac's syndrome (retinocochleocerebral vasculopathy)
  Behcet's syndrome
  Sneddon syndrome
  Eales disease
  Degos disease (malignant atrophic papillosis)

INFECTIOUS

Haemophilus influenzae
Syphilis
Tuberculosis
Herpes Zoster
HIV
Other

---

with a predilection for small arteries and arterioles (200 to 500 mm in diameter). It strikes middle-aged persons with complaints of headache and signs of focal or global neurologic dysfunction. This can be a rapidly progressive disease and is frequently fatal. The sedimentation rate is elevated in more than two thirds of patients, and cerebrospinal fluid (CSF) demonstrates elevated protein and pleocytosis in more than 80% of cases.

The vasculitic process results in multiple regions of deep white matter infarction, hemorrhage, or tumorlike masses that may be easily imaged on MR. Lesions are usually multiple and supratentorial, involving both hemispheres. Lesions detected on MR have a positive angiographic correlation; however, not all lesions seen angiographically have positive MR findings. Angiography is more sensitive than MR at detecting vessel involvement. The arteriogram may be abnormal in about 85% of cases; however, in 15% of cases angiography may be negative because disease is at the precapillary arteriole level.

Herpes zoster has been implicated as a cause of PACNS. Herpes zoster ophthalmicus can cause a granulomatous vasculitis identical to PACNS, affecting the proximal segments of the anterior and middle cerebral arteries on the ipsilateral side of the zoster ophthalmicus and producing a delayed contralateral hemiparesis. There is also an association between PACNS, herpes zoster infection, and lymphoma.

Polyarteritis Nodosa (Periarteritis Nodosa) (Fig. 4-19)

Polyarteritis nodosa is a multisystem disease characterized by necrotizing inflammation of the small and medium size arteries with CNS involvement occurring late in the disease in more than 45% of cases. The CNS manifestations include encephalopathy, seizures, and focal deficits. It is an immune-mediated disease with about 30% of patients having hepatitis B surface antigen. The diagnosis is confirmed by nerve, muscle, or kidney biopsy, which demonstrates multiple small aneurysms or arteritis. Polyarteritis is closely related to allergic angiitis and granulomatosis (Churg-Strauss) disease and a polyangiitis overlap syndrome (combination of Churg-Strauss and polyarteritis nodosa).

Imaging findings include cortical or subcortical infarction as well as nonspecific high intensity T2WI lesions in the white matter. Intracranial hemorrhage (SAH, intraparenchymal) and vascular dissection have been reported. Aneurysms, which are common in the renal and splanchnic vessels, are unusual in the CNS.

Giant Cell Arteritis

Giant cell arteritis (temporal arteritis) tends to involve systemic vessels larger than those affected by PACNS.

---

upon clinical presentation and radiologic findings. This is not perfect either. Subjecting patients to long term steroid therapy poses other risks as well. It also lets everyone, including legal scholars with large overhead and tuition bills, to second guess the physician. One last word regarding angiography is that it appears to be more sensitive than MR in documenting response to treatment.

The vasculitides can be divided into noninfectious and infectious causes (Box 4-5). The infectious issues are also discussed in Chapter 6.

NECROTIZING (GRANULOMATOUS) VASCULITIDES

Primary Angiitis of the Central Nervous System

Primary angiitis of the central nervous system (PACNS), also known as noninfectious granulomatous angiitis of the central nervous system or granulomatous angiitis of the nervous system, affects parenchymal and leptomeningeal vessels of the central nervous system

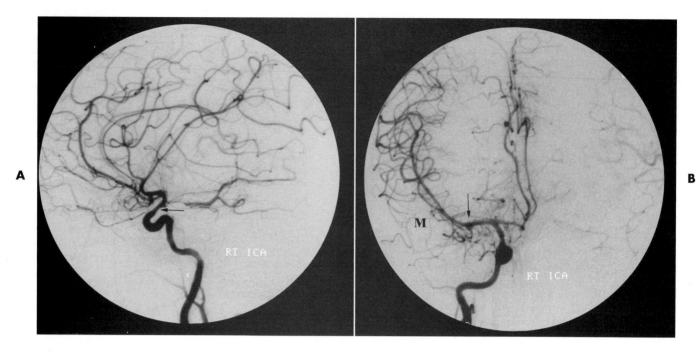

Fig. 4-19   Polyarteritis nodosa vasculitis. (Courtesy of D. Vitovitch, M.D.) **A,** Lateral oblique angiogram shows supraclinoid carotid artery narrowing (*arrow*). **B,** AP arteriogram reveals an inflammatory aneurysm of the right MCA (*arrow*) and mass effect on the branches of the MCA by a mass (hematoma) in the sylvian region (M).

The media is predominantly stricken as opposed to PACNS, where there is relative sparing of the media. The temporal artery is usually affected, whereas PACNS is confined to the intracranial vessels. The population is generally older than that with PACNS, and the disease is chiefly self-limited. Polymyalgia rheumatica occurs in about 40% of patients with giant cell arteritis. Patients are seen most commonly with visual loss and headache, usually with tenderness, swelling, and nodularity over their temporal arteries. Visual loss has been attributed to involvement of the ophthalmic and/or posterior ciliary arteries. The lesions tend to be scattered along the artery so that angiography may be useful in demonstrating vasculitic changes in the temporal artery and in guiding the biopsy. Intracranial arterial involvement is rare but has been reported.

Wegener Granulomatosis (also see Chapter 10)

This granulomatous necrotizing systemic vasculitis affects the kidneys, upper and lower respiratory tracts, but can affect the brain producing stroke, visual loss, and other cranial nerve problems. The peak incidence is in the fourth to fifth decade with a slight male predominance. The vasculitis affects small and medium-size arteries and veins while sparing larger vessels. High intensity abnormalities on T2WI occur in about 28% of cases. History plus positive c-ANCA tests help make the diagnosis.

Neurosarcoidosis

Vasculitis can be demonstrated in patients with neurosarcoidosis. Such a meningovascular form of sarcoid is uncommon. It is characterized by frank granulomatous invasion of the walls of the arteries with or without ischemic changes in the supplied brain parenchyma. The angiographic picture is similar to PACNS. These patients usually have a history of systemic sarcoid, although sarcoid can rarely affect only the CNS. Leptomeningeal involvement with enhancement is usually present in such situations. Sarcoid is more extensively covered in Chapter 6.

VASCULITIS ASSOCIATED WITH COLLAGEN VASCULAR DISEASES

Systemic Lupus Erythematosus

Cerebral vasculitis is rarely associated with collagen vascular disease. The primary CNS lesion seen at autopsy in patients with CNS systemic lupus erythematosus is perivascular inflammation or endothelial cell proliferation. However, true vasculitis is rarely if ever present. The causes of stroke in these patients include cardiac valvular disease (Libman-Sacks endocarditis), an increased tendency toward thrombosis (or reduced thrombolysis) related to antiphospholipid antibodies such as lupus anticoagulant and/or anticardiolipin antibodies, atherosclerosis accelerated by hypertension or long-term steroid use, and vasculitis from infection or as a primary process. Although it is a controversial subject, vasculitis has been reported in 7% of patients with lupus. Pathologically this involves the small arterioles and capillaries with hyalinization, endothelial proliferation, and perivascular inflammation.

On T2WI, high signal is recognized in the white matter, sometimes in a vascular distribution but also involving cortical and subcortical areas, particularly in the occipital region. Such high-intensity regions have been reported in a symmetric distribution in young female patients with diffuse CNS lupus. Periventricular white matter appears to be relatively spared even in patients with diffuse CNS lupus, which may differentiate it from multiple sclerosis, where there is a predilection for periventricular lesions. Atrophy is commonly found in these patients, related either to the encephalopathy itself or to the effect of steroid treatment. Data suggest that some lesions may evolve within a 7- to 10-day course in patients with rapidly changing neurologic symptoms and that certain lesions may be responsive to steroid therapy. Subarachnoid hemorrhage and intraparenchymal hemorrhage have also been reported in CNS lupus. The presence of saccular and fusiform aneurysms has also been observed.

Sjögren Syndrome

This autoimmune disease is characterized by focal or confluent lymphocytic infiltrates in the exocrine glands producing clinical features of dry eyes and dry mouth, however, 25% of these patients have central nervous system complications. Stroke is a well reported complication of Sjögren. The etiology of the stroke may be a small vessel vasculitis, however, these patients also have antiphospholipid antibodies (another risk factor). Cerebral angiography has been reported as positive in about 20% of cases.

OTHER ARTERIAL DISORDERS AND CAUSES OF STROKE

Drug-Related Vasculitis

Certain drugs have been implicated in producing vasculitis and stroke in those under 35. Amphetamines are documented sources of inflammatory vasculitis with vessel wall necrosis and subsequent hemorrhage. This necrotizing arteritis ("speed arteritis") is similar to periarteritis nodosa.

Cocaine has been implicated in vasculitis affecting the CNS. Such reports are rare considering its relatively common use and tend to be confounded by multiple other drugs used by such abusers. Proposed mechanisms for cocaine-induced strokes include increased platelet aggregation with thrombosis, hypertension, direct or indirect arterial constriction, or migraine phenomena induced by the drug. Cocaine induced hypertensive episodes have been thought to be responsible for pre-existing aneurysmal rupture and bleeding from arteriovenous malformations. Chronic use of cocaine may lead to major vascular occlusion and a moyamoya picture. The use of cocaine has been implicated specifically in infarction of the spinal cord and retina, and in intraparenchymal, intraventricular, and subarachnoid hemorrhage.

Cocaine in the brain
Causes considerable pain
With little to gain
Except a hemosiderin stain

Heroin-induced vasculitis is also rare and may be related to contaminants used to prepare it. Sympathomimetic amines such as ephedrine, phenylpropanolamine, and pseudoephedrine can produce angiographic features of vasculitis and hemorrhage. These compounds are commonly found in over-the-counter drugs and have led to strokes in children and young adults. 3,4-methylenedioxymetamphetamine (MDMA or "ecstasy") alters serotonin concentrations and predisposes to cerebro-vascular accidents.

INFECTIOUS VASCULITIS

Neurosyphilis (Fig. 4-20) (also see Chapter 6)

Neurosyphilis can cause arteritis of intracranial and extracranial vessels. This occurs in meningovascular syphilis resulting from chronic meningitis, which damages the large and medium sized arteries blood vessels (Heubner's arteritis) producing focal neurologic deficit whereas small artery vasculitis (Nissl's endarteritis) produces an encephalopathic presentation. It occurs 6 to 8 years after initial infection; however, in patients with HIV infection meningovascular neurosyphilis occurs earlier in the course of syphilis (often within one year of primary infection). Occlusion of branches of the vertebral and/or basilar arteries or other cerebral vessels by this vasculitis produces appropriate neurologic findings. Such a vasculitic pattern can occur in the brain or spinal cord and can be confused with atherosclerotic vascular changes.

HIV Vasculitis (see Chapter 6) (Fig. 4-21)

This has been seen in children with HIV infection without strokes. In children these vessels may be calcified and dilated. It has also been seen later in the course of adult HIV although these cases can be confounded by infection and drugs. Various sized vessels have been reported to be involved and hemorrhage has been reported.

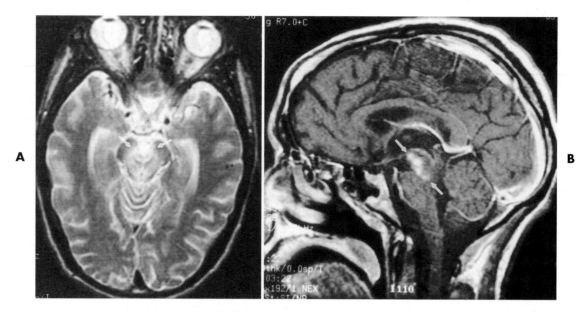

Fig. 4-20   Syphilis. **A,** Abnormal signal intensity (*white arrows*) is seen in the interpeduncular cistern affecting the rostral midbrain on the T2WI. **B,** Intraparenchymal (*white arrows*) and leptomeningeal enhancement is present. DDx: TB, sarcoid, fungus, lymphoma—the usual suspects. But Ol' Syph was the bad boy this time.

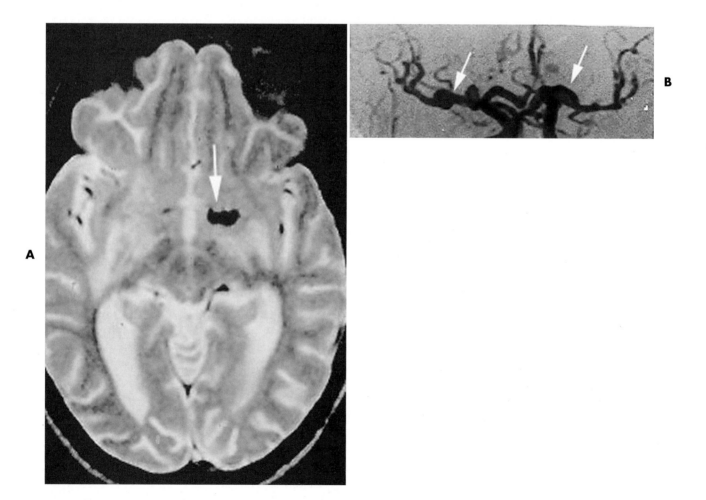

Fig. 4-21   HIV vasculitis. **A,** Observe the high intensity on T2WI in the subinsular region. Arrow is on what appears to be a dilated/fusiform aneurysm of the middle cerebral artery. **B,** MRA revealing dilatation of both middle cerebral arteries (*arrows*). (Courtesy of R. Quencer, M.D.)

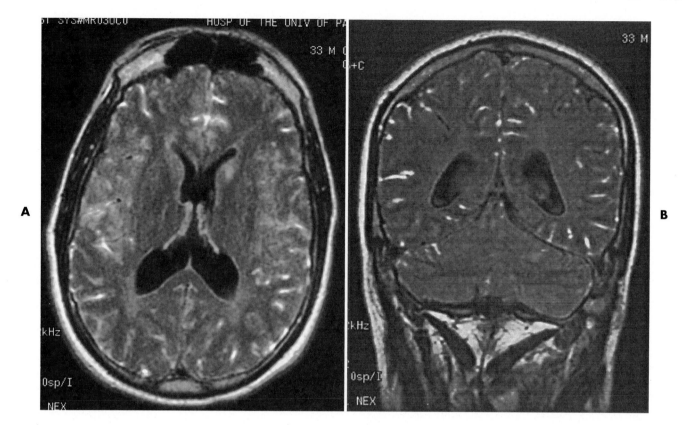

Fig. 4-22 Susac's syndrome (retinocochleocerebral vasculopathy). This was a most confusing case. The patient presented with a subacute onset of visual difficulties, hearing loss and confusion. The T2WI showed nonspecific white matter abnormalities but the FLAIR postcontrast images revealed extensive leptomeningeal enhancement suggesting diffuse vasculitis. **A,** Postgadolinium FLAIR shows leptomeningeal enhancement and a high intensity abnormality in the left caudate. **B,** Coronal postgadolinium FLAIR nicely illustrates the widespread leptomeningeal enhancement.

Other Retinocochleocerebral Vasculopathy (Susac's Syndrome) (Fig. 4-22)

First reported in 1979, this syndrome consists of acute or subacute multifocal encephalopathic symptoms, visual loss, and hearing loss secondary to microangiopathy affecting the arterioles of the brain, retina, and cochlea. The disease usually follows a fluctuating monophasic course that lasts from months to years and has a presumed immune-mediated etiology. Attention should be focused on the presence of retinal arteriolar occlusions, mid- to low-frequency unilateral or bilateral sensorineural hearing loss, and high intensity MR abnormalities on T2WI. The T2 lesions may be smaller than the typical MS lesion and in contrast to MS have a propensity for the basal ganglia and thalamus. Post contrast FLAIR has been particularly sensitive in revealing leptomeningeal disease. Treatment consists of steroids, immunosuppressive agents, and calcium channel blockers.

Behçet's Disease

You should not feel sorry for poor little Hulusi Behçet (a Turkish dermatologist)—his disease is discussed in the infection chapter. The disease is a multisystem vasculitis with a venous predominance. It has a preference for the brain stem and diencephalon (midbrain-diencephalon junction) (see Fig. 6-35). Vasculitis is a characteristic feature with narrowing, occlusion, and aneurysm formation reported in about a third of cases (12% arterial versus 88% venous). The small intraaxial veins of the brain stem are particularly vulnerable because of the poor venous collateral. Cortical involvement in Behçet's disease is rare in contrast to other vasculitides.

Sneddon Syndrome

This is a heterogeneous group of diseases consisting of patients with cerebrovascular disease and fixed deep bluish-red reticular skin lesions on the legs and body (livedo racemosa). Patients may have antiphospholipid antibodies, verrucous endocarditis, and some have an occlusive intracranial vascular disease with Moyamoya-type collaterals.

Eales Disease

This disease is seen in young men and characterized by retinal hemorrhages secondary to retinal vasculitis and CNS involvement including stroke.

Malignant Atrophic Papulosis (Degos Disease)

This occlusive vasculitis affects the skin, brain, bowel, and eye. Skin lesions consist of umbilicated papules with a white necrotic center. High intensity lesions in the brain on T2WI that can enhance have been noted.

Fibromuscular Dysplasia

Fibromuscular dysplasia (FMD) consists of nonatheromatous fibrous and muscular thickening alternating with dilatation of the arterial wall, which produces an appearance characterized as a "string of beads" (Type 1 FMD) (Fig. 4-23). Less common appearances include unifocal or multifocal tubular stenosis (Type 2) or lesions confined to only a portion of the arterial wall (Type 3). Although all layers of the artery may be involved, the media is most commonly affected with hyperplasia producing arterial narrowing. Thinning of the media is associated with disruption of the internal elastic lamina, producing saccular dilatations (pseudoaneurysm picture). It involves the cervicocephalic arteries in about 30% of cases with the most common CNS vessel affected being the internal carotid artery, approximately 2 cm or more from the bifurcation (in 90% of cases). Involvement of the external carotid and vertebral arteries also occurs. The vertebral artery is involved in approximately 12% of FMD. Multiple vessel involvement is common (bilateral carotid involvement occurs in 60% of cases), whereas intracranial FMD is rare. Dilated regions are always wider than the normal lumen, and narrowing is usually less than 40% diameter stenosis. LMDs have difficulty diagnosing FMD, so that it is left to the university M.D., Ph.D., but it's not a BFD except in VIPs.

The etiology of FMD is unknown. The condition predominantly affects women (approximately 80% of cases) with a mean age of 50 years. It is controversial whether these lesions are related to symptoms and findings such as headache, TIAs, stroke, vascular dissection, or subarachnoid hemorrhage. However, there appears to be an association between intracranial aneurysms and FMD. The differential diagnosis of FMD includes atherosclerotic disease, vascular spasm secondary to the catheter, and standing waves. Atherosclerotic disease is usually asymmetric and has a propensity for the bifurcation. Catheter spasm can be identified at the tip of the catheter, and standing waves do not usually have the constrictive picture characteristic of FMD. Dilatation of the vessel is not seen with catheter spasm.

Moyamoya

Slow occlusion and high-grade stenoses of the distal internal carotid arteries and their proximal first-order branches (the circle of Willis) in some cases result in the development of an extensive network of collateral blood supply. The principal sources of collateral blood consist of leptomeningeal collateral vessels from the three main cerebral arteries, the perforating basal ganglionic vessels, and transdural anastomoses from the external carotid artery via a rete mirabile (plexus of vessels). These collateral vessels produce an appearance on angiography termed moyamoya, which in Japanese translates to "hazy like a puff of cigarette smoke." Moyamoya is commonly seen in Japanese patients but also occurs in neighborhood bars, at some airports, and in Veterans Administration hospitals. The cause of the occlusions is unknown, although extensive collateral vessels can be demonstrated in sickle cell disease, atheromatous disease, radiation arteriopathy, neurofibromatosis, and other lesions that cause progressive obliteration of the proximal intracranial carotid arteries. The disease may be divided into pediatric and adult subgroups on the basis of clinical course and disease features. In children, moyamoya has a more progressive course, presenting with symptoms of cerebral ischemia including TIAs and stroke, whereas in adults intraparenchymal and subarachnoid hemorrhages are the most common presentations.

Cerebral angiography demonstrates the previously mentioned distal internal carotid artery and proximal

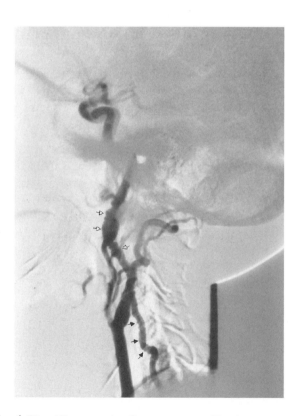

Fig. 4-23   Fibromuscular disease. "String of beads" appearance of both the carotid *(open arrows)* and vertebral arteries *(closed arrows)* on this lateral right common carotid arteriogram with reflux up the right vertebral artery.

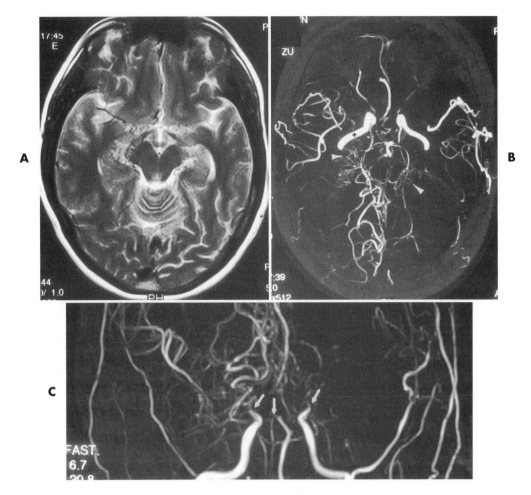

Fig. 4-24   Moyamoya. **A,** Do you notice the tiny flow voids in the subarachnoid space and in the hippocampi? **B,** Collapsed view of the MRA shows absence of supraclinoid distal internal carotid arteries (*plus sign on petrous carotid*) with moyamoya development along the proximal posterior cerebral arteries *(arrowheads).* **C,** The occluded carotids and basilar arteries are outlined by the *arrows* on this AP projection image from the MRA.

first-order branch occlusions with the extensive collaterals from the vertebral and external carotid arteries (Fig. 4-24). The lenticulostriate arteries and other perforating arteries are dilated, producing the characteristic moyamoya appearance. MR demonstrates loss of the distal internal carotid artery flow void and what appear to be hypointense holes in the basal ganglia noted on T1WI, (either hypointense or hyperintense on T2WI, depending on the flow velocity). These holes are the extensive basal ganglionic vascular collateral network, and this appearance is classic. MRA confirms a tangle of vessels in the basal ganglia and the proximal occlusions. Mid and distal anterior choroidal artery aneurysms have been seen through the smoke in moyamoya.

Sickle Cell Disease

Patients with sickle cell disease have an incidence of cerebrovascular occlusive disease ranging from 5% to 17%. Children are at higher risk than adults. Only those

patients with the most severe hematologic disease have cerebrovascular complications. A common misconception is that occlusion of the capillaries, small venules, and arterioles by sickled red blood cells is responsible for the infarction in these patients. Although this may happen, it is clearly not the important pathophysiologic element in the vast majority of cases. Instead, infarction is most likely related to stasis and ischemia in the vasa vasorum, leading to intimal and medial hyperplasia with eventual significant narrowing or occlusion of the internal carotid or the proximal anterior and middle cerebral arteries. The posterior circulation is usually spared. The vessels appear stenotic or are occluded with prominent collateral circulation, producing at its extreme a moyamoya picture. Treatment with blood transfusions to suppress the level of hemoglobin S to less than 30% can decrease the recurrence of stroke within 3 years from 67% to 10% or less.

Cerebral angiography reveals large-vessel disease in up to 87% of cases with CNS presentations. At the time of initial infarction, the angiographic manifestations in some cases may be minor with only mild luminal irregularity and slight arterial narrowing. Careful inspection of the angiogram is necessary to detect these changes. In other cases, florid vascular changes can be identified with significant narrowing and embolic vascular occlusions if the study is performed just after the cerebrovascular event. Subarachnoid hemorrhage has been reported in 1% to 2% of patients with sickle cell although this is related in most cases to aneurysms and not to sickle cell disease. There may be a tendency for multiple aneurysms with a propensity for the posterior circulation in sickle cell disease. Angiographic contrast media may precipitate a sickle cell crisis. Because cerebral angiography is associated with additional complications in this patient group, protective measures such as exchange transfusions (decreasing the percentage of hemoglobin S to <20%), volume expansion before angiography, supplemental oxygen, and a warming blanket are useful in minimizing angiographic risks.

MR and CT demonstrate areas of infarction, and MRA can detect areas of major vascular compromise or occlusion (Fig. 4-25). High-intensity abnormalities on T2WI have been found in the subcortical region in patients both with and without stroke. Their appearance is indistinguishable from multiple sclerosis, but their clinical presentation is as different from multiple sclerosis as night and day. The cause of these lesions is unknown, but in the case of small-vessel ischemia sickling is a possible explanation (as opposed to large-vessel disease mentioned previously). Furthermore, in some patients white matter lesions may be present without significant large-vessel changes.

Drug Abuse

You need not have vasculitis to experience the effects of drug abuse. It has been frequently implicated as a cause of both ischemic and hemorrhagic stroke. The drugs implicated include cocaine (and its alkaloidal form, "crack"), amphetamines, heroin, anabolic steroids, alcohol, lysergic acid diethylamide (LSD), and heavy use of marijuana (enough to prevent election to a major political office even if you do not inhale). A common pathway in many drug-related strokes is hypertension, but drug users also have a reasonably high rate of stroke secondary to bacterial endocarditis.

Lymphomatoid Granulomatosis (Neoplastic Angioendotheliosis) (Fig. 4-26)

This malignant lymphoma is restricted to the intracranial vessels. It presents with recurrent strokes or stroke-like symptoms, encephalopathy, and seizures. There are multiple high intensity lesions on T2WI and angiography shows evidence of medium sized vascular occlusions. Brain biopsy is needed to establish the diagnosis.

Pregnancy

The risk of stroke is increased 13 times in pregnancy or puerperium. Conditions responsible for this increase

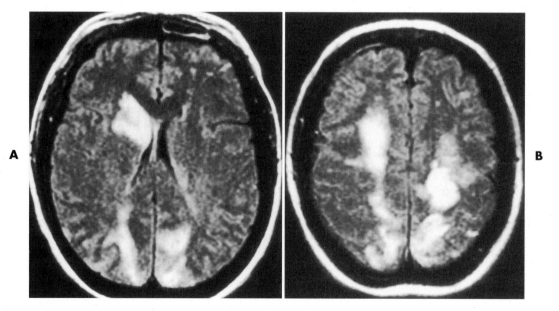

Fig. 4-25 Sickle cell disease. **A,** The caudate head on the right has been wiped out. Subcortical infarctions are also revealed on the FLAIR image. **B,** Watershed distribution infarctions are present bilaterally.

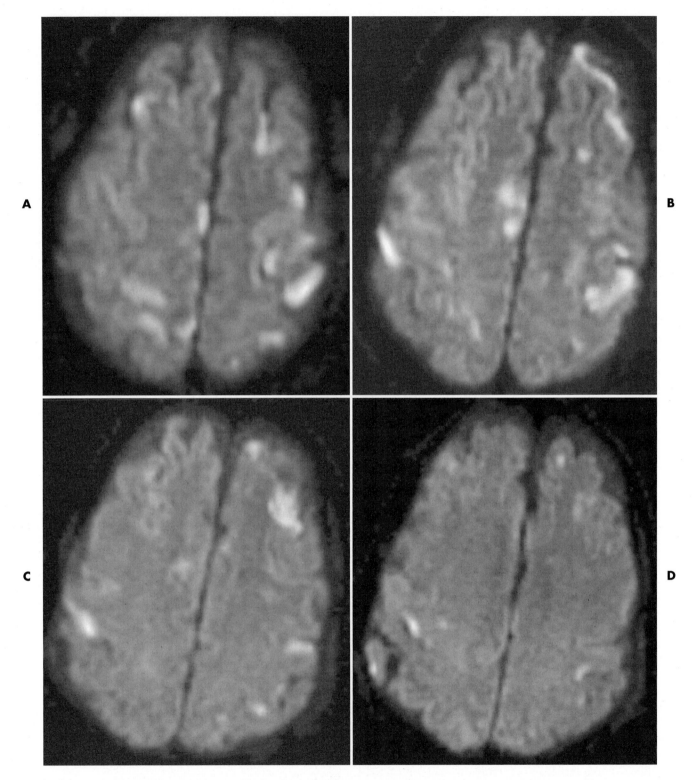

Fig. 4-26   Neoplastic angioendotheliosis. **A–D,** Montage of diffusion-weighted images revealing what appear to be multiple diffusional abnormalities. This could be the result of an embolic shower, but in this patient with encephalopathy, the biopsy proved to be malignant lymphoma of the intracranial vessels. This should be in your differential diagnosis of multiple intracranial occlusions.

include hypercoagulability, embolism, migraine, vasculitis, and vasospasm, which result in arterial occlusion or venous thrombosis. In patients with preeclampsia and toxemia, vasospasm has been observed. A condition termed postpartum cerebral vasculopathy is quite similar (probably the same) to eclampsia and posterior reversible encephalopathy syndrome (PRES) has also been described with headaches, seizures, encephalopathy and focal neurologic findings. There is a proclivity for the posterior cerebral artery distribution. High intensity on T2WI can be seen in the white matter of the parietooccipital region and brain stem. These changes may be related to hypertension with increased vascular permeability or vasospasm, and they may be reversible.

Radiation Vasculopathy

Radiation can induce structural damage to arteries including endothelial degeneration, intimal fibrosis, and fibroblastic proliferation of the media. Radiation vascular injury should be considered as a cause of stroke months to years after therapy. Vascular occlusion of the extracranial portion of the internal carotid artery rarely occurs after neck irradiation. Cerebrovascular lesions involving the internal carotid artery and its principal branches can be identified in patients where the radiation portal is centered at the base of the skull. Telangiectasias and cavernous malformations have been associated with radiation therapy. These have been discussed in Chapter 3. Other factors influence this condition and are discussed in Chapters 3, 6, and 7.

Carbon Monoxide Toxicity

The diagnosis of acute carbon monoxide intoxication can be suggested by the circumstances in which the patient is found down and is confirmed by identifying carboxyhemoglobin in the blood. Characteristically, carbon monoxide poisoning exhibits low or high signal on T1WI and high intensity on T2WI in the globus pallidus bilaterally (see Chapter 8). On CT, low density is identified in the globus pallidus bilaterally. White matter, cortical, and hippocampal lesions as well as enhancement in the globus pallidus have also been reported (Fig. 4-27). A delayed encephalopathy begins 2 to 3 weeks after recovery and occurs in 3% of patients, resulting in additional findings of high intensity on T2WI in the corpus callosum, subcortical U fibers, and internal and external capsules associated with low intensity on T2WI in the thalamus and putamen (see Chapter 7 regarding postanoxic encephalopathy). The high intensity white matter findings are thought to represent in some cases a reversible white matter process with subsequent improvement in the patient's neurologic status. In other instances, patients may enter a persistent vegetative state with extensive demyelination of the cen-

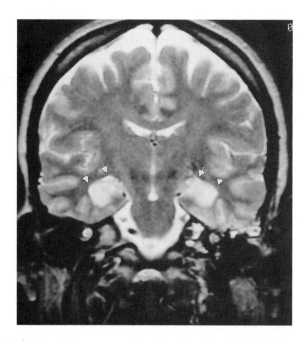

Fig. 4-27   Carbon monoxide poisoning. Coronal T2WI demonstrates bilateral hippocampal high intensity lesions *(arrows)* in this patient after a suicide attempt. (Courtesy S. Bobman, M.D., Fort Myers, Florida.)

trum semiovale. The low intensity observed in the thalamus and putamen is the result of iron deposition.

Migraine

Stroke rarely can be seen in patients with migraine. It is usually in the distribution of the anterior or middle cerebral arteries but has been reported in the posterior circulation. Angiography is generally contraindicated in patients undergoing a migraine attack but not in migraineurs. High intensity abnormalities in the subcortical white matter on T2WI have been reported in migraineurs; however, this may be controversial. Several of such reported sightings were noted by nonradiologists who might have confused *état criblé* and *je ne sais quoi*. They also reported the appearance of little green men jumping over the semilunar ganglion.

Intracranial hemorrhage is the primary event in 15% to 20% of strokes. We now consider CT and MR characteristics of hemorrhage and attempt to explain why we see what we do with these modalities.

HEMORRHAGE: IMAGING TECHNIQUES AND CONCEPTS CT

CT

The x-ray attenuation values of a substance or a structure determine its visibility on CT. There is a linear relationship between CT attenuation (density) and hematocrit values. The attenuation of whole blood with a hematocrit of 45% is approximately 56 Hounsfield units (HU). Normal gray matter ranges from 37 to 41 HU, and normal white matter is from 30 to 34 HU. Thus, freshly extravasated blood in a patient with a normal hematocrit can immediately be demonstrated on CT. The increased attenuation of whole blood is based primarily on the protein concentration of the blood (mostly hemoglobin). If one is imaging hemorrhage in an anemic patient, whatever the cause, there is a possibility that the acute hemorrhage will be isodense to brain. Likewise, in infants with high hematocrit or patients with polycythemia the sinuses and vessel may appear abnormally dense. Hemorrhage associated with hemoglobin values less than 10 g/dL may be undetectable based on density alone. The effect of protein concentration on x-ray attenuation is easily noted by the appearance of the lens (which has the highest protein concentration in the body) and is bright on CT.

After the extravasation of blood, a clot forms with a progressive increase in the density of the hemorrhage for approximately 72 hours (Fig. 4-28). Clot formation and retraction with the extrusion of low-density serum increase hemoglobin concentration. After approximately the third day, the attenuation values of the clot begin to decrease and during the next few weeks, the hemorrhage fades to isodensity. The clot loses density from the periphery to the central region. This is the result of the biochemical changes that are occurring in the clot. The red blood cells containing desaturated hemoglobin are undergoing lysis, dilution, and subsequent digestion of the blood products by peripheral macrophages. After 1 month (rarely 2 months), no high density should be demonstrated from a single intraparenchymal hemorrhage. It is obvious from our understanding of MR (see following subsection) that the blood products do not disappear in the brain just because the clot has become isodense on CT.

In a simple intraparenchymal hemorrhage the initial low attenuation surrounding the high-density hemorrhage is caused by the serum from the retracted clot. This hypodense rim is not large. The circumferential hypodensity increases and reaches a maximum at approximately 5 days because of vasogenic edema. With an uncomplicated hemorrhage, less atrophy is seen than with infarction. The CT picture of gradual fading of the high-density hemorrhage is very different from the MR, in which certain hallmarks persist indefinitely. After approximately 2 months there is commonly just a little hypodense slit representing the residua of the hemorrhagic event. Interestingly, unenhanced CT has rarely observed high density rims around the old hemorrhage in the time frame of approximately 1 to 2 months post ictus. This actually represents hemosiderin deposition detected by CT.

CT allows one to see acute and subacute hemorrhage in the nonanemic patient. It is fast, relatively easy to perform, not cumbersome, and accurate in most regions of the brain. Less favorable situations occur when the hemorrhage is small, thin, or in the lower brain stem and posterior fossa. Lesions in the brain stem may be obscured by beam-hardening artifact. Thin, flat collections of blood (particularly subarachnoid and extracerebral hemorrhages) may not be visualized because of partial volume averaging. Thin sectioning perpendicular to the clot provides the best method for detection. The collection must be twice the width of the slice thickness to be unaffected by partial volume averaging. This is usually a minor problem because axial imaging is perpendicular to the falx and major cisterns.

The use of intravenous iodinated contrast in hemorrhage is unnecessary in most situations. However, it is useful when one is dealing with a small hemorrhage associated with mass effect out of proportion to that hemorrhage. Here the differential diagnosis involves hemorrhage into a tumor, either primary or metastatic, venous infarction, or arterial hemorrhagic infarction. Venous or arterial hemorrhagic infarction characteristically follows a vascular distribution, although venous infarction may have a variable territorial distribution. Thrombosis of a vein or sinus is positive proof of this cause of hemorrhage. In these cases, one need not give contrast. The diagnosis of tumor with hemorrhage often requires contrast both to verify the presence of tumor and perhaps to identify additional lesions. The differential diagnosis of hemorrhagic infarction versus hemorrhagic tumor at times can be difficult. Both may have mass effect and edema. Hemorrhagic infarctions have cortical hemorrhage and follow a vascular distribution, whereas intratumoral hemorrhage occurs in the tumor. We believe that in most situations unenhanced CT should be followed when necessary by enhanced MR.

An enhancing ring in an uncomplicated intraparenchymal hemorrhage may appear from approximately 6 days to 6 weeks after the initial event (see Fig. 4-28D). This is not associated with mass effect and disappears from 2 to 6 months after the first scan. Diagnostically, a problem arises if the patient, for whatever reason, was not scanned within the first week or so after the ictal event. One is then presented with a ring-enhancing lesion, the differential diagnosis of which might include (to the simple son) tumor (primary or metastatic), abscess and other inflammatory conditions, infarction, and multiple sclerosis. Most of these conditions would be associated with edema and mass effect (the wise son). This situation may be clarified by appropriate history and clinical findings as well as by a repeated CT (Rabbi Hillel). Serial imaging is useful in differentiating benign hemorrhage from tumors and abscesses because benign hemorrhages decrease in mass effect and enhancement over

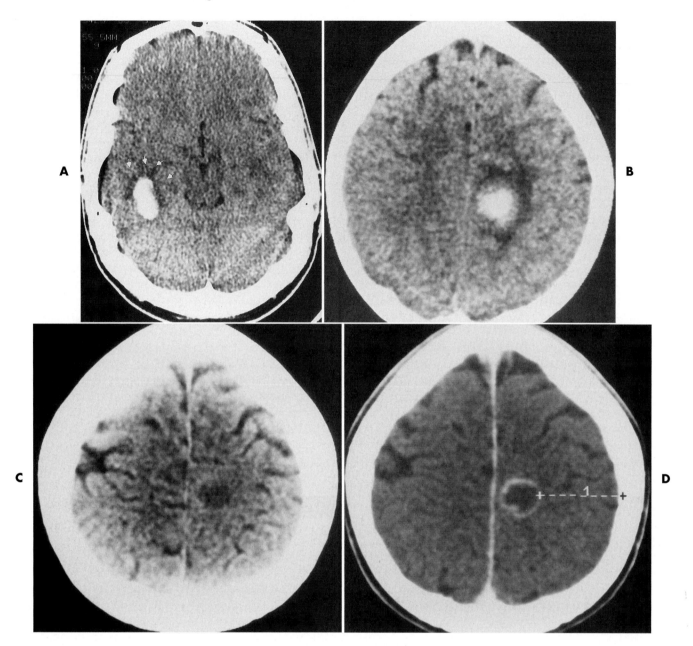

Fig. 4-28 **A,** CT of acute hemorrhage. Observe the high-absorption hemorrhage in the right temporal region. Subtle amount of low absorption *(arrows)* represents serum extruded into the surrounding brain after clot retraction. This image was performed within 24 hours of the ictus. **B,** Acute hemorrhage 3 days after the ictus. CT shows high density in the left parietal region with surrounding low density (edema and serum). **C,** Two weeks later. The hematoma is now low density secondary to the breakdown, absorption, and dilution of the previously concentrated protein. **D,** Ring enhancement is observed at this time as well.

time without treatment. MR, however, definitively separates hemorrhage from a nonhemorrhagic ring-enhancing lesion. MR is the present-day alchemist; it has turned iron into "gold" ($) and thus relegated CT to the Bronze Age.

MR of Blood

MR has dramatically altered our diagnostic prowess in the assessment of hemorrhagic conditions. It has provided the radiologist with the ability to render rather sophisticated diagnostic opinions. Understanding the MR characteristics of the various stages of hemorrhage is essential in this pursuit. The progression of imaging hallmarks is well understood, although the specific time intervals for these changes are variable. MR of hemorrhage is more than "dark, bright; bright, dark." Let us now briefly consider some of the biophysical mechanisms necessary to understand the MR appearance of blood. Although substantially simplified, the following explanation is still rather complex. We strongly recommend that you persist in reading the separate mechanisms, which will eventually all be connected in the Imaging Scenarios subsection at the end. Go for it! But if you prefer not to slog through the details, Table 4-2 summarizes the salient features of MR of hemorrhage. You can rejoin the group at the section entitled Hemorrhagic Conditions.

Structure of hemoglobin Hemoglobin, the primary oxygen carrier in the bloodstream, is composed of four protein subunits. Each subunit contains one heme molecule consisting of a porphyrin ring and an iron atom, which provides the binding site for oxygen (Fig. 4-29). Binding of oxygen to the heme molecule of an individual subunit produces a conformational change in that and adjacent subunits. The iron atom (Fe^{21}) sits near the center of the porphyrin ring and is bound to one of the nitrogens of the amino acid histidine. Oxygen (O_2) binds to the Fe^{21} on the opposite side of the porphyrin ring. Oxyhemoglobin functionally has no unpaired electrons and is diamagnetic.

When a hemoglobin subunit loses its O_2 to form deoxyhemoglobin, the protein undergoes a small but significant change in its tertiary structure. The histidine ligand of the heme pulls the Fe^{21} atom of deoxyhemoglobin out of the plane of the porphyrin ring and causes the porphyrin itself to dome. Because of the doming, water molecules are effectively prevented from approaching close enough (3 Å) to the paramagnetic iron to undergo proton-electron dipole-dipole interactions. The water molecules around deoxyhemoglobin are unable to bind to the heme iron as they do in methemoglobin (see following subsection).

Deoxyhemoglobin (which has four unpaired electrons) can be oxidized to methemoglobin via several different mechanisms. Normally an enzyme system within the red blood cell (RBC) rapidly reduces methemoglobin back to deoxyhemoglobin, but this process requires glucose and the reduced form of nicotinamide-adenine dinucleotide phosphate (NADPH). However, in hemor-

				Table 4-2 Stages of hemorrhage on MR and CT[*]			
Stage	**CT**	**T1WI**	**T2WI**	**Mass effect**	**Time course**	**Explanation**	
Hyperacute	High density	Low intensity	High intensity with peripheral low intensity	+++	<6 hours	CT: High protein T1WI, T2WI: Central oxyhemoglobin in with peripheral deoxyhemoglobin	
Acute	High density	Isointense to low intensity	Low intensity	+++	≈8 to 72 hours	T1WI: High protein, susceptibility (deoxyhemoglobin) T2WI: Susceptibility (deoxy-Hb) CT: High protein	
Early subacute	High density	High intensity	Low intensity	+++/++	≈3 days to 1 wk	T1WI: PEDDI (intracellular met Hb), High protein T2WI: Susceptibility (intracellular met-Hb), High protein CT: High protein	
Late subacute	Isodense	High intensity	High intensity with rim of low intensity	±	≈1 wk to months	T1WI: PEDDI (free met-Hb), absence of susceptibility effects (from intracellular met-Hb), dilution of high protein T2WI: PEDDI (free met-Hb), absence of susceptibility effects, dilution of high protein, susceptibility effects from hemosiderin and ferritin in peripheral rim CT: Absorption of high protein	
Chronic	Low density	Low intensity	Low intensity	−	Months to years	T1WI: Susceptibility effects from hemosiderin and ferritin (T2 effect on T1WI) T2WI: Susceptibility effects from hemosiderin and ferritin CT: Atrophy	

[*]This appearance is classic at 1.5 T; however, with decreasing field strength the susceptibility effects are diminished.

Note that time course is variable but progression usually follows the stages.

Hb, Hemoglobin; PEDDI, proton-electron dipole-dipole interaction; range of mass effect: − (mass effect absent) to +++ (greatest amount of mass effect).

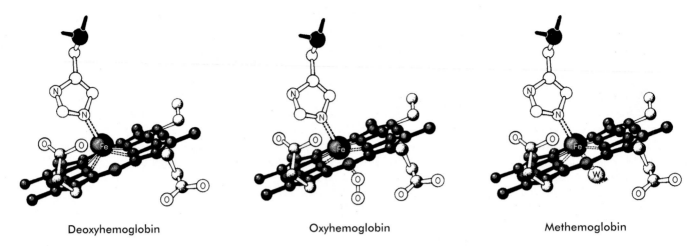

Deoxyhemoglobin   Oxyhemoglobin   Methemoglobin

Fig. 4-29   Subunit of hemoglobin. Note the change in Fe position in deoxyhemoglobin, oxyhemoglobin, and methemoglobin. The Fe in deoxyhemoglobin is domed and water cannot approach within 3 Å. In methemoglobin water (w) can closely approach Fe (which is close to the plane of the porphyrin ring) to produce PEDDI.

rhage, this mechanism deteriorates and oxidation to methemoglobin takes place. The Fe^{3+} atom (in methemoglobin) is closer to the plane of the porphyrin ring than the Fe^{2+} atom of deoxyhemoglobin, allowing a water molecule to bind to the heme iron. The Fe^{3+} atom of methemoglobin has five unpaired electrons.

Before we can appreciate how these small electronic changes dramatically influence what is seen on MR, other parts of the puzzle need to be understood.

Susceptibility effects   When placed in a magnetic field, certain substances generate an additional smaller magnetic field, which either adds to or subtracts from the externally applied field. The proportionality constant between the strength of the external field and the induced field is a measure of the "susceptibility" of the substance. Diamagnetic substances, those with no unpaired electrons, generate very weak fields that subtract from the externally applied fields. Paramagnetic materials such as deoxyhemoglobin and methemoglobin generate much larger local fields surrounding the paramagnetic molecule that add to the externally applied field. As described previously, the Fe^{21} atoms in deoxyhemoglobin possess four unpaired electrons whereas the Fe^{31} atoms in methemoglobin possess five unpaired electrons.

When deoxyhemoglobin or methemoglobin is encapsulated within RBCs, the effective local field is greater within the RBC than outside the cell because of the greater susceptibility of the paramagnetic hemoglobin solution compared with saline solution or plasma. Remember that protons precess at a rate proportional to the strength of local magnetic field. Therefore, the protons within the RBC precess faster than those outside because of the increased effective field. There may additionally be intracellular magnetic field gradients. Thus after a 90-degree pulse the phase of the transverse magnetization accumulates faster for spins inside the RBC than

outside. As the water protons diffuse (and they do) through these locally varying gradients during the time to echo (TE), they accumulate varying amounts of phase change depending on the time spent at different effective field strengths. These phase dispersions produce signal loss. Susceptibility effects for imaging magnets are roughly proportional to the square of the main magnetic field.

Assume, for example, that two protons, one inside the cell and the other outside the cell, exchange positions just before the 180-degree pulse. Proton 1 inside the cell has accumulated more phase change than proton 2 before the 180-degree pulse. After exchanging positions (diffusion), proton 1 will have a lower effective field and will precess slower. Therefore, at TE the transverse magnetization of proton 1 will not have precessed back to its starting position. Proton 2, now within the cell and in an area of higher effective field, will precess faster and at TE will have precessed beyond its starting position. Thus, the two spins will be out of phase with each other, resulting in a diminished signal (Fig. 4-30). Clearly with longer TE there will be more time for diffusion, greater phase incoherence, and hence a greater loss of signal.

It should be noted, however, that if significant signal loss results from a very large susceptibility effect, hypointensity may occur at short TEs and further incremental signal loss may not be detectable on increasing TE. T1WI and PDWI still have a finite TE (i.e., 20 milliseconds) and thus susceptibility effects may be observed, albeit smaller than with longer TE images. Gradient-refocused echo images (check Chapter 1 to recall that there is no 180-degree refocusing pulse) are more sensitive to susceptibility changes, because the resultant local field gradients are superimposed on the applied phasing and rephasing gradients.

Proton-electron dipole-dipole interaction   The paramagnetic iron atom in methemoglobin generates a

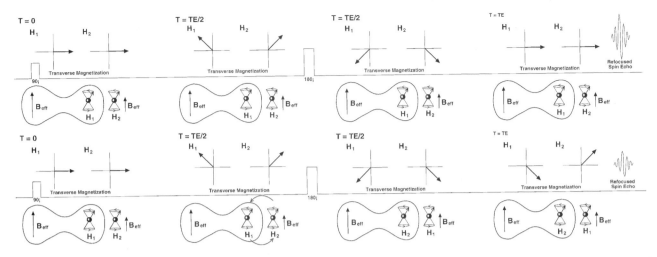

Fig. 4-30   Effect of diffusion on protons. Two sets of circumstances are diagrammed. *Upper set* demonstrates what occurs when protons do not diffuse through varying magnetic fields. You can appreciate proton H_1 inside an RBC (coronal view of RBC) and proton H_2 outside the RBC. RBC contains deoxyhemoglobin and therefore has a slightly increased magnetic field inside it (B_{eff}) compared with the B_{eff} outside the RBC. A spin echo experiment is then carried out with a 90-degree and a 180-degree pulse. Note that in the upper diagrams (without diffusion of protons) the net magnetization vector of the proton inside the RBC is in phase at the TE with the proton outside the RBC. This results in a nicely formed spin echo. Lower experiment is carried out with an exchange of protons *(lower row second RBC from left)*. Here, before the 180-degree pulse, there is diffusion of the H_2 proton into the RBC and at the same time diffusion of the H_1 proton outside the RBC. What is observed is that at TE the spins are still out of phase and the spin echo produced is diminished in magnitude, resulting in less signal (hypointensity) on T2WI. You can appreciate that if there are small, locally varying fields, such as with intracellular deoxyhemoglobin, intracellular methemoglobin, and hemosiderin, and protons diffuse into these varying fields, then the spin echo experiment cannot completely rephase all these protons and signal loss will occur. The longer the interecho interval (the interval between radiofrequency pulses), the more time the protons have to sample local inhomogeneous areas. A consequence of this is that protons will have greater loss of phase with respect to each other and therefore have more signal loss (increased hypointensity on T2WI).

local field approximately 1000 times greater than the local field generated by the proton nucleus. If a proton moves close enough to this field (within 3 Å), a spin transition can be induced. Water binding to the heme is required, to have a significant proton-electron dipole-dipole interaction (Fig. 4-31). Because the number of heme molecules is relatively small compared with the number of water molecules, this effect would be small except that the exchange rate of the water molecules is rapid relative to repetition time, allowing many water molecules to bind to the heme during the course of imaging. Both T1 and T2 are shortened by proton-electron dipole-dipole interaction. Remember that in biologic systems T1 is much longer than T2. Although relaxation times are not additive, their reciprocals (relaxation rates) are. When added to the smaller relaxation rate (1/T1), the proton-electron dipole-dipole interaction effect contributes proportionally more to the observed relaxation rate than it would if added to the larger 1/T2. The bottom line is that proton dipole interactions are best observed on T1WI, where T1 shortening produces high signal intensity.

Although the iron atom of deoxyhemoglobin also generates a local magnetic field, no significant proton-electron dipole-dipole effect is observed. As mentioned previously, in deoxyhemoglobin the heme iron moves out of the plane of the porphyrin ring, making binding of the water molecules to the heme difficult. A large susceptibility effect is seen with intracellular methemoglobin, as with deoxyhemoglobin on T2WI, and with gradient-refocused images, which are most striking at intermediate hematocrit levels but which are clearly present in clots with hematocrits of 90%.

Effect of protein   The molecular basis of T1 relaxation has been ascribed primarily to rotational interactions of the water molecules. The hydrogen nucleus of the water molecule consists of a single proton. Because this positively charged particle rotates on its axis, a magnetic field or magnetic moment is generated, which either adds to or subtracts from the externally applied field. As other protons rotate through this magnetic field, the change in the local field strength induces transitions in the orientation of the proton spin, thereby producing T1 relaxation. These same rotational interactions also produce T2 relaxation.

For such a rotational interaction to produce efficient relaxation (short T1), the frequency of rotation of the water proton needs to approximate the Larmor frequency. In pure water, the water molecules rotate rapidly and a relatively small number of molecules rotate at the resonance frequency so that T1 is long. The addition of protein slows the rotation of the water molecules, in-

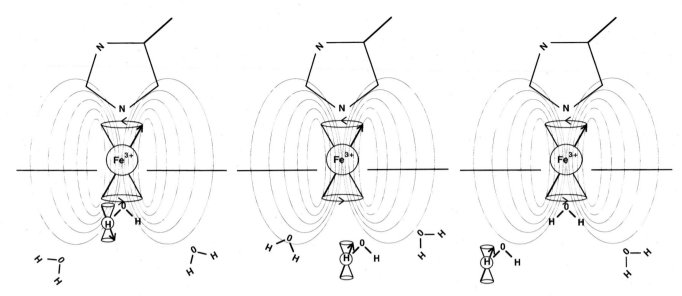

Fig. 4-31 Proton-electron dipole-dipole interaction. This diagram, proceeding from left to right, demonstrates water protons approaching within 3 Å of the unpaired electrons of the iron atom of the methemoglobin molecule *(far left)*. Proton-electron dipole-dipole interaction results from this close contact, with shortening of both T1 and T2. Note that the proton on the left had a spin (↑) down position, while the water proton in the center has come off the Fe and is relaxed (spin up). The diagram on the right shows a new water proton approaching the Fe.

creasing the percentage of protons precessing at the Larmor frequency. The much larger protein molecule has an intrinsically slower rate of rotation arising from Brownian motion because of its much larger mass. A strongly bound hydration shell of water molecules surrounds the protein molecule with a zone of "structured" water possessing slower rotational rates than the "bulk" (unbound) water molecules. Thus with the addition of protein, more molecules are rotating closer to the resonance frequency, resulting in greater T1 shortening. As mentioned previously, a slowing of the rotational rate of the water molecules by the addition of protein also produces a decrease in T2.

In summary, essentially two effects are created by the hemoglobin molecule: (1) the paramagnetic effect secondary to the iron within the heme molecule, which can produce susceptibility effects in the case of deoxyhemoglobin and proton-electron dipole-dipole interactions with methemoglobin, and (2) the diamagnetic effects of the protein portion (apoprotein) of the hemoglobin molecule.

Imaging Scenarios

Hyperacute hemorrhage (Fig. 4-32) Rarely, (as when the patient hemorrhages on the CT or MR table) do we have an opportunity to visualize hemorrhage within its first hours (hyperacute stage). In these first 3 to 6 hours the intact red cells still contain mostly oxyhemoglobin. The T2WI image (if the patient is lucky enough to get to the MR this early) is hyperintense with peripheral hypointensity. The periphery of the hematoma contains red blood cells containing hemoglobin that has started to desaturate and thus the hypointense periphery.

Acute hemorrhage (Fig. 4-33) After the initial accumulation of oxyhemoglobin, there is clot formation with retraction and reabsorption of serum. The inability of the isolated hematoma to easily rid itself of metabolic wastes, together with the possibility of increased lactic acid and carbon dioxide, tends to shift the oxyhemoglobin dissociation curve to the right (Bohr effect), which at any oxygen pressure will result in less hemoglobin saturation and more deoxyhemoglobin. The oxyhemoglobin molecules thus rapidly deoxygenate to yield deoxyhemoglobin. This can be appreciated very early after an ictus (within hours). The high protein content of the clot, as evidenced by the hyperdensity noted on CT, shortens T1 relative to CSF, causing the hematoma to be hyperintense relative to CSF and isointense to the brain parenchyma on the T1WI. Not infrequently the hematoma is observed to be hypointense to brain parenchyma on T1WI. This is caused by the very short T2 (susceptibility effects), which is so pronounced that it affects the T1WI. Because solvent water molecules are unable to approach close enough to the Fe^{2+} heme of deoxyhemoglobin; no additional T1 shortening is caused by proton-electron dipole-dipole interactions.

On T2WI there is marked hypointensity secondary to susceptibility effects. These arise from the local field inhomogeneity produced by encapsulation of the paramagnetic deoxyhemoglobin within the RBC. This effect

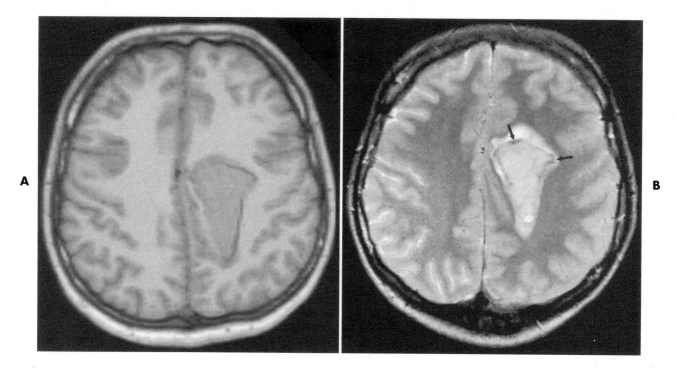

Fig. 4-32   MR of hyperacute hemorrhage (within 4 hours). **A,** T1WI reveals isointense mass with slight rim of hypointensity. **B,** T2WI show the hemorrhage is mostly hyperintense with peripheral hypointensity (*arrows*) representing deoxyhemoglobin in intact red blood cells, and the beginning of vasogenic edema (surrounding hyperintensity). (Courtesy of G. Hotson M.D.)

is magnified on gradient-refocused images, which are more sensitive to susceptibility effects. The protein also shortens T2, rendering the clot hypointense relative to CSF. The result is the profound hypointensity of the acute hematoma on T2WI and gradient-refocused images. Here

it may have a variable intensity on T1WI, but hypointensity, sometimes in a rim, is observed on T2WI because of the susceptibility effects of deoxyhemoglobin.

Care must be exercised in interpreting acute hematomas on diffusion weighted images. The hypointense appear-

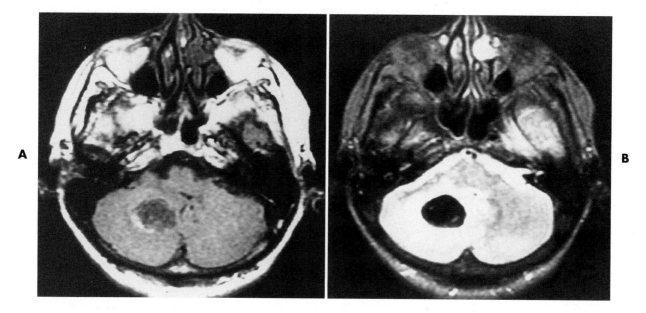

Fig. 4-33   MR of acute hemorrhage. **A,** T1WI of this posterior fossa hemorrhage performed within 48 hours of the ictus. Hemorrhage appears slightly hypointense to cerebellum (T2 effect of deoxyhemoglobin on T1WI). There is a small amount of peripheral high intensity. **B,** T2WI demonstrates marked hypointensity of this acute hemorrhage. This appearance is caused by deoxyhemoglobin in intact RBCs.

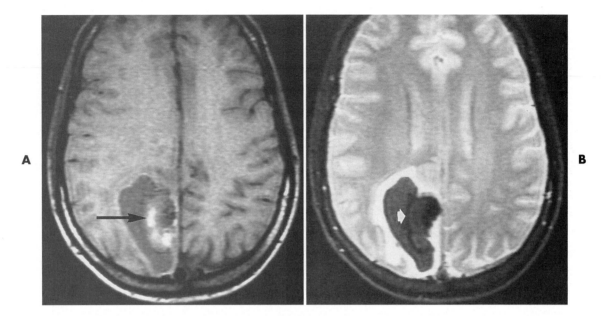

Fig. 4-34   Early subacute hemorrhage. **A,** Peripheral high signal *(arrow)* is seen on the T1WI. **B,** On the T2WI note the marked hypointensity *(arrow)* in the region that was of high signal intensity. This represents the intracellular methemoglobin stage. You can also appreciate that the hemorrhage peripheral to the arrow is in the acute stage, being isointense on the T1WI (**A**), and on this T2WI appears hypointense. Furthermore, surrounding this hemorrhage is a high intensity region composed of edema and serum from the retracted clot. In **A** you will also note a thin rim of high intensity representing early methemoglobin formation in the periphery of the outer clot.

ance of these lesions is most likely related to the absence of signal from the effect of the susceptibility induced signal loss (effectively T2 shine-through) rather than the presence of restricted diffusion.

Early subacute hemorrhage   (Fig. 4-34) Within 3 to 7 days there is oxidation of the deoxyhemoglobin to

methemoglobin inside the RBC (at the periphery of the clot). Unlike deoxyhemoglobin, water molecules are able to approach within 3 Å of the paramagnetic heme of methemoglobin, permitting proton-electron di-pole-dipole interactions that shorten T1. This effect, in concert with the T1 shortening from the high pro-

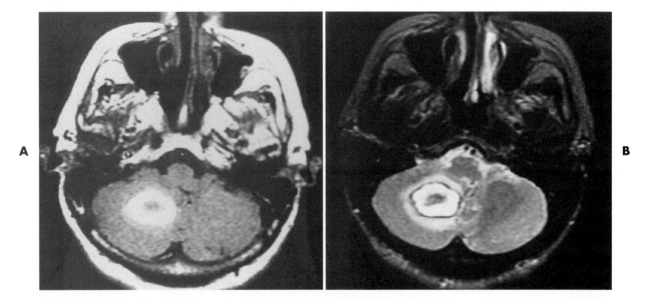

Fig. 4-35   Late subacute hemorrhage. **A,** T1WI of the same patient as in Fig. 4-19 taken approximately 1 week later. Note the high signal intensity peripherally around the hematoma. **B,** T2WI with high signal intensity peripherally, representing vasogenic edema. This surrounds a hypointense rim (hemosiderin and ferritin). Inside this rim is high signal intensity from free methemoglobin, and centrally a hypointense area appears, probably representing some residual deoxyhemoglobin. Appearance of the hypointense rim on T2WI and the high intensity on T1 and T2 inside the rim stages the hemorrhage to the late subacute phase.

tein concentration, gives methemoglobin its characteristic hyperintensity on T1WI. Because the paramagnetic methemoglobin remains encapsulated within the RBC, marked hypointensity is also seen on the T2WI and gradient-refocused images because of the same susceptibility mechanism described previously for deoxyhemoglobin. The proton-electron dipole-dipole interaction also shortens T2, but this effect is insignificant compared with the much larger susceptibility effects. Oxidation of deoxyhemoglobin to methemoglobin proceeds peripherally to centrally in the first week after the ictus.

Late subacute hemorrhage (Fig. 4-35) Methemoglobin is less stable than deoxyhemoglobin, and the heme group can spontaneously be lost from the protein molecule. This free heme and/or other exogenous compounds (including peroxide and superoxide) can produce RBC lysis. Concomitantly there is protein breakdown and dilution of the remaining extracellular methemoglobin. Hyperintensity persists on the T1WI despite the decrease in the protein concentration because of the T1-shortening effects of the heme of methemoglobin even at relatively low concentrations. The hematoma signal intensity increases on T2WI, approaching that of CSF, because of a loss of local field inhomogeneity on RBC lysis and a decrease in the protein concentration. In addition, the T2-shortening effects of the paramagnetic heme caused by proton-electron dipole-dipole interactions are rather small and

unimportant except at the highest concentrations. Paralleling the breakdown of the methemoglobin is an accumulation of the iron molecules hemosiderin and ferritin within macrophages at the periphery of the lesion. The iron cores of hemosiderin and ferritin contain approximately 2000 iron molecules ferromagnetically coupled to produce a "superparamagnetic" substance that exhibits a very large susceptibility effect. The result is a black ring surrounding the lesion, visible on T1WI but increasingly prominent on T2WI and gradient-refocused images. The appearance in this stage is clearly seen by the end of the second week.

Chronic hemorrhage (Fig. 4-36) After months there is nearly complete breakdown and resorption of the fluid and protein within the clot. The iron atoms from the metabolized hemoglobin molecules are deposited in hemosiderin and ferritin molecules, which are unable to exit the brain parenchyma because of restoration of the blood-brain barrier. The susceptibility effects of the superparamagnetic iron cores of hemosiderin produce hypointensity on all spin sequences but are most prominent on the T2WI and gradient-refocused images, where "blooming" of the hypointensity is observed.

HEMORRHAGIC CONDITIONS

We want to welcome back those who shunted the so-called physics of hemorrhage.

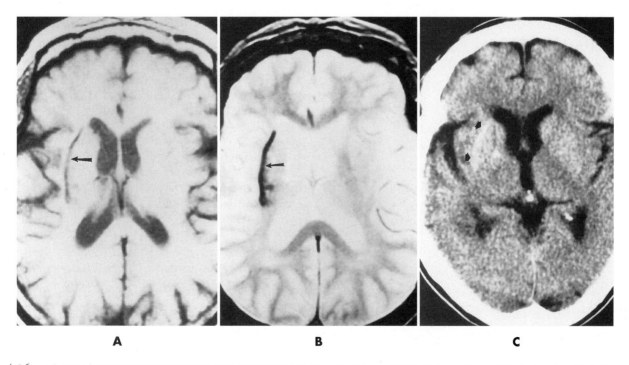

A **B** **C**

Fig. 4-36 Chronic hemorrhage (subcortical slit hemorrhage) (>5 years old). **A,** T1WI demonstrates a thin hypointensity in the external capsule *(arrow).* **B,** T2WI with marked hypointensity from hemosiderin and ferritin in the chronic (slit) hemorrhage *(arrow).* **C,** On the CT note the high density of that hemorrhagic cavity *(arrows).* This high density is from iron in the walls of the slit.

Intraparenchymal Hemorrhage

Intraparenchymal hemorrhage accounts for only about 10% of strokes, with a median age of about 56 years as opposed to ischemic stroke, which has a median age of about 65 years. Hypertension is the presumed cause of nontraumatic intraparenchymal hemorrhage in 70% to 90% of cases. Box 4-6 lists the principal causes of primary intraparenchymal hemorrhage. The location of this hemorrhage is variable, although approximately half to two thirds of intraparenchymal hemorrhage occurs in the basal ganglionic-thalamic (especially in the putamen) region (Fig. 4-37). Approximately 10% to 50%

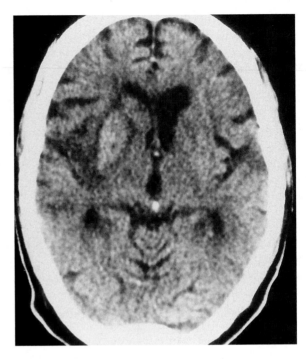

Fig. 4-37 Hypertensive ganglionic hemorrhage. CT of an acute basal ganglionic hemorrhage with high density in the right basal ganglia surrounded by low density with compression of the ipsilateral ventricle.

Box 4-6 Hemorrhagic Causes of Stroke

PRIMARY INTRACEREBRAL HEMORRHAGE

Aneurysm (Mycotic, Congenital)
Hemorrhagic Infarction (Arterial, Venous)
Hypertensive, Arteriosclerotic Hemorrhage
Neoplasms (Primary or Metastases)
Trauma
Vasculitis
Vascular Malformations
Amyloid Angiopathy
Drugs
    Cocaine
    Amphetamine
    Phenylpropranolamine
    L-asparaginase
Hematologic Causes
    Antithrombin III deficiency
    Protein C + S deficiency
    Antiphospholipid antibodies
    Factor VII deficiency
    Factor IX deficiency
    Factor VIII deficiency
    von Willebrand factor deficiency
Acquired coagulopathies
    Thrombocytopenia and platelet dysfunction
    Disseminated intravascular coagulopathy
    Uremia
    Multiple myeloma
    Myeloproliferative disorders
    Lymphoproliferative disorders
    Leukemia

SUBARACHNOID HEMORRHAGE

Aneurysm
AVM, Non-aneurysmal perimesencephalic hemorrhage
Dural Malformation
Hemorrhagic Tumor
Trauma
Vascular dissection

AVM, Arteriovenous malformations.

---

of intraparenchymal hemorrhage may be lobar, 10% to 15% of hemorrhages occur in the brain stem, and approximately 5% to 10% of hemorrhages happen in the cerebellum. The numbers do not add up because they represent estimates from different series and are reasonable approximations of the brain regions affected.

Intraparenchymal hemorrhages may also result from vascular lesions including amyloid angiopathy, microaneurysms, and fibrinoid arteritis, which may be superimposed on hypertensive changes. It is not only hypertension but actually the rapidity in the change of blood pressure that also predisposes to hemorrhage. It is one reason why cocaine and other drugs are associated with an increased incidence of intracranial bleeding. Charcot-Bouchard aneurysms are miliary aneurysms that occur on small arteries (100 to 300 mm in diameter) commonly located in the basal ganglia and are seen in hypertensive patients. These aneurysms were thought to be responsible for intracranial hemorrhage. This lesion has been reevaluated with modern histopathologic techniques with the conclusion that Charcot-Bouchard aneurysms are distinctly uncommon and are most likely not a common cause of intraparenchymal hemorrhages.

Lobar hemorrhages occur in the subcortical region of any lobe. The most common causes include hypertension, vascular malformations, tumor, trauma, and blood dyscrasias, although in a large group of these hemorrhages there is no apparent cause. Amyloid angiopathy may account for some of these cases (see following discussion in this section). Lobar hemorrhages may carry a better prognosis than the ganglionic-thalamic group. The presence of acute hemorrhage in a lobar distribution warrants a compulsive workup. Particular attention should be directed to ruling out other causes of hemorrhage including vascular malformations and tumors. In addition to conventional CT and MR, phase-contrast MRA can be useful. Remember, in the face of hemorrhage, time-of-flight techniques are of limited value because of the short T1 of hemorrhage containing methemoglobin, which would be the same high intensity as flowing blood. Phase-contrast angiographic techniques suppress the high signal intensity of stationary methemoglobin so that normal and abnormal vascularity can be seen. For whatever reasons phase contrast angiography, like Salman Rushdie, is often cited but rarely seen. Finally, angiography is the definitive diagnostic study when you come up empty on CT, MR, and MRA for the cause of a lobar hemorrhage. In this situation, a small arteriovenous malformation or vasculitis may be the culprit.

Enhancement can be useful in lobar hemorrhage to identify tumor as the cause. It may be possible to differentiate an enhancing tumor nidus from the high intensity of the hemorrhage. Pitfalls include ring enhancement around a hematoma and the inability to discern a small area of tumor enhancement in the large area of hemorrhage.

Hemorrhagic Infarction

Hemorrhagic infarction is a secondary event with blood extravasating into infarcted tissue. Initially the cerebral artery is occluded, in most cases by an embolus. After occlusion with infarction, the embolus undergoes lysis, and if there is perfusion breakthrough, hemorrhage occurs in the infarcted region. Hemorrhagic transformation is delayed for at least 6 to 12 hours but is present in most cases by 48 hours. Hemorrhagic transformation may develop 1 week or more after ictus (late hemorrhagic transformation), when collateral circulation has been reestablished. In fact, most infarctions have some petechial hemorrhage and the distinction between pale infarction and mild hemorrhagic infarction is arbitrary. Autopsy studies suggest that up to 42% of infarcts are hemorrhagic. The hemorrhagic component results from diapedesis of RBCs through the ischemic endothelium. Not only does there need to be a change in vascular permeability, but also blood must be able to get to the damaged vessels from either collateral circulation or partial lysis of the proximal embolus.

High-field MR is much more sensitive than CT at identifying acute hemorrhagic cortical infarction (Fig. 4-38). Hemorrhagic infarction can have a serpentine morphology after cortical gyrations. When the serpent is seen,

bite the apple, spit the worm out, notice its convoluted configuration, and call it a hemorrhagic infarct (not a hemorrhagic tumor). The hypointensity of deoxyhemoglobin on T2WI in the acute stage is highlighted by the hyperintensity of the infarcted tissue with its increased water content. Gradient-echo imaging has increased sensitivity for hemorrhagic infarction. In the subacute phase, one notes gyriform high intensity on T1WI. Petechial infarction has been emphasized here, but large hematomas can also occur in hemorrhagic infarction. It has recently been reported that in acute hemorrhagic stroke decreased ADC tends to persist longer than in nonhemorrhagic stroke lesions. This has been hypothesized to be related to high viscosity of the hemorrhage or to cytotoxic edema. The etiology of the persistent reduction of ADC in chronic hemorrhagic stroke is related to the increased cellularity of infiltrative inflammatory cells as well as the increased clot viscosity.

The evolution of hemorrhagic cortical infarction is similar to intraparenchymal hemorrhage. Laminar necrosis can occur in hemorrhagic cortical infarction and appear bright on T1WI.

Venous Thrombosis

Venous infarction secondary to thrombosis is, together with vascular dissection, an underdiagnosed lesion. In both cases, hemosiderin deposition is not usually observed. Rather the vessels generally recanalize and one may demonstrate return of the normal flow void.

Venous thrombosis progresses to infarction in about 50% of cases. The etiology of the infarction appears to be, at least partially, based on decreased cerebral blood flow produced by the venous thrombosis. ADC has been documented to be decreased in some cases supporting decreased cerebral blood flow as the mechanism. The other hypothesis regarding infarction is the production of vasogenic edema and hemorrhage into the extracellular space from the elevated venous pressure and subsequent breakdown of the blood-brain barrier. It is possible that both mechanisms may contribute to the infarction and MR appearance.

Venous infarction can be very epileptogenic and is associated with headache, papilledema, and focal neurologic deficits. Venous thrombosis is linked with many systemic conditions, listed in Box 4-7. It has been implicated as the cause of dural arteriovenous malformations and of pseudotumor cerebri. Tumors such as meningiomas can grow and slowly obliterate a dural sinus. Venous thrombosis was a particularly tricky call before MR. Numerous findings were described in the CT literature, including (1) the cord sign, representing a high density cord or dot delineating a clot in the vein; a triangle of high density (clot) can also be seen in the sagittal sinus (noncontrast CT); (2) the delta sign (one

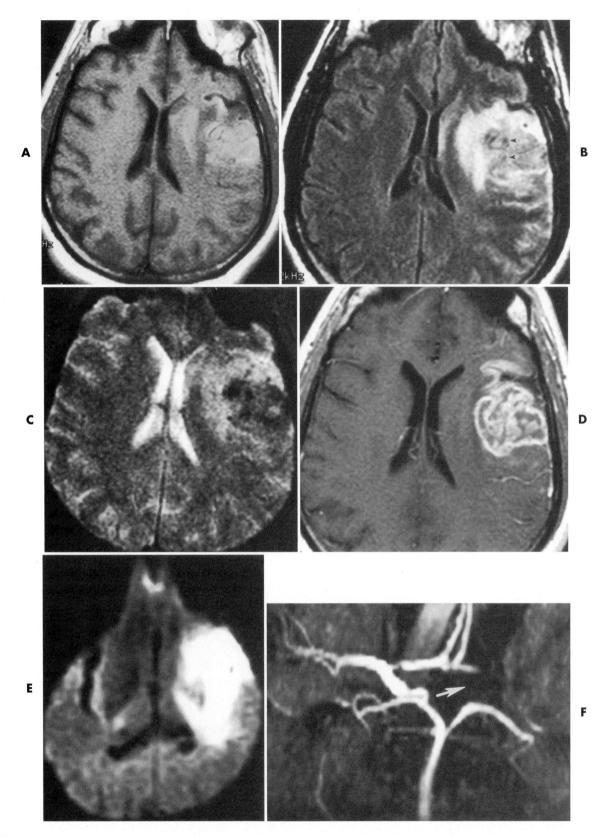

Fig. 4-38   Hemorrhagic infarction. **A,** Unenhanced T1WI shows an area of hemorrhage in the left temporal lobe. **B,** The lesion is bright on FLAIR but the hemorrhage has lower intensity in the hemorrhagic portion (*arrowheads*). **C,** Blooming of the hemorrhage is typical of a gradient echo sequence. **D,** Gyriform enhancement implies that the lesion is subacute in age. **E,** The DWI dates the lesion to the first 10 days. Between the enhanced scan and the DWI we'd call it about a week old. **F,** Etiology? Occluded left MCA (*arrow*) on MRA.

of the most overrated signs in radiology- (see Chapter 18), in which enhancement is noted around a clot in the sinus; and (3) the appearance of medullary veins, indicating collateral venous drainage.

Intracerebral hemorrhage and hemorrhagic infarction are complications of sinus and cortical vein thrombosis. Some hallmarks of hemorrhage are associated with venous thrombosis. Think about it in cases where subcortical hemorrhage is seen or in situations with bilateral hemorrhage, gyriform hemorrhage, or hemorrhagic infarctions not in an arterial distribution. Hemorrhage from venous thrombosis may be small or large. Locations of hemorrhages are variable, depending on the site of thrombosis. Hemorrhages are generally proximal to the draining sinus.

Acutely thrombosed cerebral veins lack a flow void and are isointense on T1WI. The absence of the flow void in a cerebral vein should make one suspect venous thrombosis. On the T2WI, hypointensity is seen as a result of deoxyhemoglobin. This situation may be confusing if only the T2WI is assessed, because hypointensity is observed in acute thrombosis and in normally flowing blood. Gradient-echo images sensitive to flow are useful to separate acute thrombosis (black because of lack of flow) from normally flowing blood (high intensity on the gradient-echo images).

When imaging slowly flowing venous blood, we must also take into account flow-related enhancement and even-echo rephasing. The former produces high intensity in the vessel on the T1WI in the first few slices of the sequence perpendicular to the imaging plane, whereas the latter gives high intensity on even echoes in a double- or quadruple-echo sequence. Flow-related enhancement is seen in vessels perpendicular to the imaging plane, whereas thrombus containing methemo-

globin should be high intensity in any plane. Switching from the sagittal to axial plane obviates the high intensity from flow-related enhancement, whereas thrombus continues to have increased intensity. Even-echo rephasing is identified on T2WI and is not responsible for high intensity on T1WI. Another problem may be gradient-moment nulling, which eliminates the appearance of a flow void in some slow-flowing veins.

These high intensity effects become a problem in diagnosing subacute thrombosis. In this situation methemoglobin in the thrombosed vessel generally produces high intensity on both T1WI and T2WI (Fig. 4-39). Time-of-flight gradient-echo images sensitive to flow may not be useful here because thrombus composed of methemoglobin and blood flow both appear as high intensity. If time-of-flight techniques are used, modification of the technique to produce black blood by presaturation of moving spins (bolus tracking) can be helpful. This would show displacement of the saturated spin (absence of signal), whereas stationary methemoglobin would be high signal. Phase-contrast angiography is particularly useful in this instance and in situations where assessment of vessels, in the face of high intensity from hemorrhage, is required. Phase-contrast angiography provides virtually complete suppression of high signal from the hemorrhage so that only flow (high or low signal depending on how the gradients are applied) is imaged and provides a fast accurate assessment of venous thrombosis. With phase-contrast angiography, anything that has flow is either white or black depending on the direction of flow and the gradient polarity. The converse is that if there is no flow, you will see neither black nor white; rather, stationary tissue will be gray. It is important to

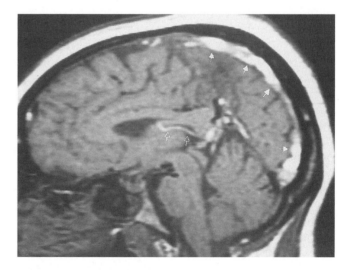

Fig. 4-39   Venous thrombosis. This patient has thrombosis of the sagittal sinus *(closed arrows)*. *Open arrows* demonstrate a thrombosed internal cerebral vein. Thrombosis is also present in the vein of Galen and straight sinus.

set the velocity encoding low (5 to 15 cm/sec) so that slow flow can be detected.

Venous infarction can most often be diagnosed without MRA because in most instances the spin-echo images provide the appropriate information. Sagittal (parasagittal) images are particularly useful for transverse sinus thrombosis.

Cerebral Amyloid Angiopathy

Cerebral amyloid angiopathy (CAA) results from deposition of amyloid (an eosinophilic, insoluble extracellular protein) in the media and adventitia of small and medium-sized vessels of the superficial layers of the cerebral cortex and leptomeninges, with sparing of the deep gray nuclei. Amyloid deposition increases with age but does not correlate with hypertension. The principal risk factor is aging, a very difficult condition to treat but significantly more palatable than the alternative. Amyloid accumulates Congo red dye and exhibits yellow-green birefringence when examined with polarizing light. Pathologic examination reveals microaneurysms and fibrinoid degeneration. There is loss of elasticity with increased fragility of the vessels secondary to replacement of the elastic lamina by amyloid deposits. Hemorrhages are usually lobar, involving the frontal and parietal lobes including the subjacent white matter. Subarachnoid and subdural hemorrhages have also been reported as a result of the superficial vessels involved in CAA. CAA is rarely found in the cerebellum, white matter, basal ganglia, and brain stem. There is a propensity for recurrent hemorrhage or multiple simultaneous hemorrhages. Gradient-echo imaging with emphasis on T2* effects (see Chapter 1) is useful in demonstrating the multiplicity of hemorrhages in this condition. At times, you can observe diffuse punctate regions of hypointensity on these gradient echo images. The differential diagnosis includes hypertension, multiple cavernous malformations including those secondary to radiation therapy, or previous traumatic brain injury. It is presently a diagnosis of exclusion. CAA may be responsible for up to 10% of nontraumatic intraparenchymal hemorrhages (Fig. 4-40). Patchy white matter changes have been seen that are indistinguishable from the garden-variety high signal abnormality on T2WI (unidentified bright object), probably the result of hypoperfusion of deep white matter from CAA. Associations with CAA include dementia (30% to 40% of patients), Alzheimer disease (85%), Down syndrome, dementia pugilistica, late postirradiation necrosis, Jacob-Creutzfeldt disease, spongiform encephalopathy of Kuru, and leukoencephalopathy associated with severe white matter changes and sparing of subcortical U fibers. It is not associated with systemic amyloidosis. There are a few case reports of nonhemorrhagic mass or lesions in CAA.

CADASIL (Cerebral Autosomal Dominant Arteriopathy with Subcortical Infarction and Leukoencephalopathy)

The authors made an editorial decision to include this disease with other white matter problems (Chapter 7). However, let us add a few additional words. The most frequent clinical manifestations in this inherited arterial disease are subcortical transient ischemic attacks or strokes usually occurring at the young age of 40 to 50. The disease progresses to death within 20 years. These patients deteriorate clinically a subcortical dementia, urinary incontinence, and pseudobulbar palsy. The MR reveals diffuse symmetric white matter high intensity in the periventricular region with involvement of the external capsule and small strokes in the basal ganglia, pons, and other subcortical regions. The cortex and cerebellum are usually spared. The white matter high intensity becomes severe as these patients age (over 55) and is greater in symptomatic patients.

Intratumoral Hemorrhage

Underlying tumors have been reported in up to 10% of cases of intracranial hemorrhage, whereas hemorrhage has been noted in about 1% of brain tumors. Brain tumors associated with hemorrhage are usually malignant as with primary astrocytoma (anaplastic astrocytoma, glioblastoma multiforme), or metastatic (most commonly bronchogenic carcinoma, melanoma, choriocarcinoma, or thyroid or renal cell carcinoma) (see Chapter 18). Other tumors associated with hemorrhage include oligodendroglioma, meningioma, pituitary adenoma, hemangioblastoma, and acoustic schwannoma.

The MR picture of hemorrhage into a tumor does not progress in the same temporal and morphologic fashion as a simple intraparenchymal hemorrhage (Fig. 4-41). The patient cares about this differential: tumor versus nonneoplastic hemorrhage. We hope the following discussion raises your consciousness. With tumoral hemorrhage, the deoxyhemoglobin state may be prolonged with central hypointensity existing for more than a week, and one does not usually encounter a complete rim of hemosiderin. The hemosiderin deposition may appear in a dot-dash fashion or may be completely absent. There is generally more edema and mass effect than are consistent with a simple hematoma; persistent vasogenic edema is also present. Another clue is that there may be multiple foci of hemorrhage in a mass or that the hemorrhage is irregular. In some cases, the hemorrhage can involve structures such as the corpus callosum, which would be most unusual for hypertensive hemorrhage. High intensity surrounding nonneoplastic hemorrhage should normally disappear within 4 to 8 weeks. Furthermore, with simple hemorrhage, mass effect clearly should be gone at this time, and

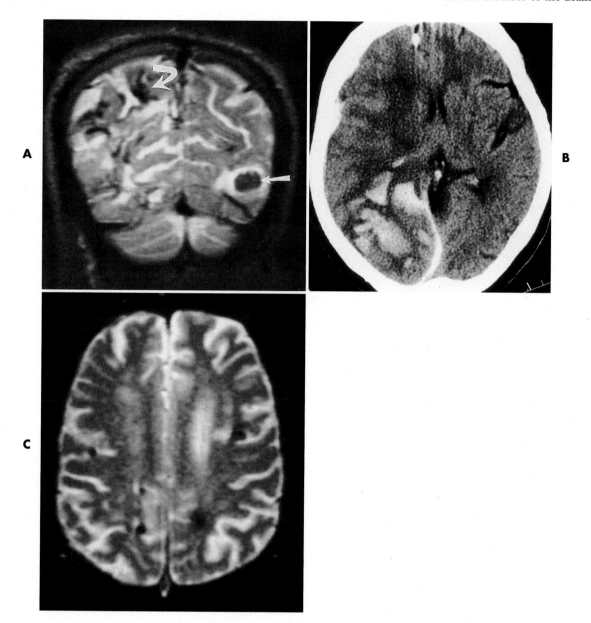

Fig. 4-40 Amyloid angiopathy. **A,** Cerebral amyloid angiopathy. Coronal T2WI in occipital region depicts an acute hemorrhage *(arrow)* on the left associated with some edema. In the right occipital region note the appearance of hemosiderin *(curved arrow)* in an old hemorrhage. In elderly patients with multiple recurrent hemorrhages think about the diagnosis of CAA. **B,** CT of a different patient with amyloid angiopathy had a lobar hemorrhage with an associated subdural hematoma (not that unusual in the entity). **C,** Amyloid angiopathy. Gradient echo image revealing multiple hypointense lesions consistent with hemorrhage. This case is amyloid angiopathy, but the differential diagnosis includes multiple cavernomas.

in most cases, parenchymal loss should be noted. The signal characteristics of small tumors can be overwhelmed by a hemorrhage, and the only atypical feature may be the remaining vasogenic edema. The differential diagnosis includes hemorrhagic cavernous malformation, metastatic melanoma, thrombosed aneurysm, fungal infection, septic embolic infarction, and venous infarction.

Enhancement can be useful in the case of primary tumors by demonstrating enhancement peripheral to the hemorrhagic component of the lesion, and in metastatic disease by revealing additional distant lesions. Suspect intratumoral hemorrhage under appropriate clinical circumstances such as in patients who have known malignancy, in elderly nonhypertensive persons, and in patients who had progressive symptoms before the hemorrhagic ictus.

Vascular Dissection

Vascular dissection occurs when an intimal tear in a blood vessel permits blood to go into the arterial wall

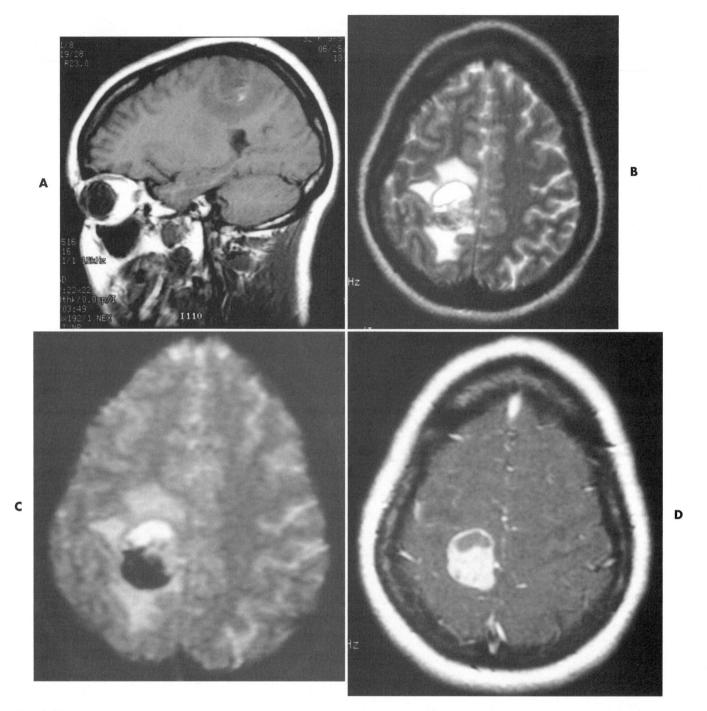

Fig. 4-41   Recent intratumoral hemorrhage in an astrocytoma. The clues are a large amount of edema (**A** and **B**), incomplete hemo-siderin rim (**B** and **C**), and enhancement in a portion of the mass that is not hemorrhage (**C** and **D**). **A,** T1WI sagittal of a posterior frontal-parietal mass lesion. Observe the punctuate hemorrhage (high intensity) and the generous edema around the lesion. **B,** Axial T2WI. Observe the deoxyhemoglobin (hypointensity) and absence of a complete hemosiderin rim medially. There is a large amount of edema surrounding the hemorrhage. **C,** Gradient echo image shows the marked hypointensity (deoxyhemoglobin) of the hemorrhage. Note that part of the mass is not hypointense (thus not hemorrhagic). **D,** Postcontrast T1WI shows that that medial portion of the mass that was not hemorrhagic in **C** enhances. This strongly suggests that there is an underlying neoplasm.

and divide its layers producing either stenosis or pseudoaneurysm formation. These can occur either spontaneously or following injury (albeit very minor). Vascular dissection of the carotid or vertebral artery is an often overlooked cause of stroke, particularly in young patients. Dissection usually affects the extracranial great vessels but can occasionally occur in intracranial vessels. One or more vessels may be involved. Symptoms differ in that extracranial dissection can present with neck and face pain, headache, Horner's syndrome, cranial nerve involvement, and ischemic symptoms that occur days to weeks after the dissection. The association of ptosis and miosis with headache and preservation of ipsilateral facial sweating (Raeder's syndrome) can occur with cervical internal carotid dissections, because the sympathetic fibers for sweat follow the external carotid artery whereas those controlling the dilator pupillae and superior palpebral muscle follow the internal carotid artery. Dissection may occur after blunt trauma to the neck but has also been reported with maneuvers that produce abrupt head-turning or hyperextension of the neck including scoping out the opposite sex, chiropractic manipulation, and sports injury. Other reported circumstances include coughing, sneezing, vomiting, ventilation associated with resuscitation or anesthesia, respiratory tract infection, automobile accidents, or after direct puncture of the vessel from stab or gunshot wounds.

Intracranial dissections are generally associated with earlier symptoms (hours to days) including ischemia and subarachnoid hemorrhage after transmural or subadventitial dissection. Dissecting aneurysms may also act as mass lesions compressing the brain. Predisposing factors include fibromuscular disease, elastic tissue disease (Ehlers-Danlos IV syndrome—cerebrovascular malformations, joint hypermobility, cutaneous hyperextensibility; Pseudoxanthoma elasticum—cerebrovascular arterial occlusive disease and fistulas, angioid streaks of the ocular fundus, and skin lesions), arterial hypertension, Marfan syndrome, homocystinuria, autosomal dominant polycystic kidney disease, osteogenesis imperfecta type

I, and migraine. Five percent of patients with a spontaneous dissection of the carotid or vertebral arteries have at least one family member who has had a history of spontaneous dissection. Vascular dissection should be considered when stroke occurs in patients without significant risk factors! In addition, the risk of a recurrent dissection in an initially unaffected artery is about 2% during the first month and decreases to 1% per year, which continues for a decade or more. This is another case in which you must think (and continue to think) of the diagnosis and perform the appropriate study.

In most cases of extracranial dissection, there is a residual lumen. Thrombus rapidly fills the false lumen. MR can detect the intramural hemorrhage, which is usually high signal on T1WI, and can demonstrate the residual patent lumen of the vessel with low signal flow void (Fig. 4-42). The intensity characteristics of the intramural hemorrhage follow those of parenchymal hemorrhage, but hemosiderin deposition is rare. Fat-suppression imaging may be useful to distinguish periarterial fat from intramural subacute hemorrhage. The key is to note narrowing in the flow void in the vessel. MR is also useful for following the dissection to visualize when the hemorrhage is reabsorbed, when the normal lumen dimensions are reestablished, and if there is progression to pseudoaneurysm.

The principal complications of extracranial vascular dissection, stroke, and TIAs, result from luminal compromise and embolic phenomena. Treatment (anticoagulation) is directed toward preventing recurrent emboli. Most dissections of the great vessels of the neck heal

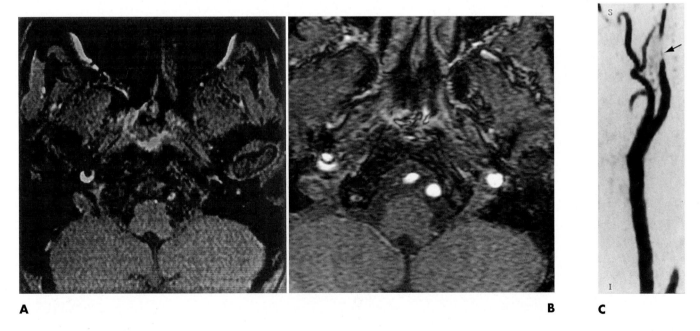

A   **B**   **C**

Fig. 4-42   Carotid dissection. **A,** Axial T1 with fat saturation demonstrates high intensity surrounding the right carotid flow void and representing methemoglobin in a carotid dissection. **B,** Source image from **C** shows the carotid dissection and flow in the residual lumen. **C,** MRA. Observe the tapering of the distal right carotid (*arrow*) where the vessel is dissected.

spontaneously. The treatment for dissecting aneurysms in the cervical region is stenting whereas, intracranial dissecting aneurysms are associated with subarachnoid hemorrhage are usually treated by occluding the vessel to prevent initial or recurrent hemorrhage. Rarely, aneurysms of the cervical vertebral artery develop as a result of dissection; usually it is the intracranial segment of the vertebral that is involved.

The angiographic appearance shows a variety of presentations including segmental tapering by the intramural hematoma, which markedly reduces the lumen of the involved vessel. This angiographic finding has been termed the "string sign" (see Fig. 4-42C). Aneurysmal dilatation of the vessel may also be observed. Although rare, a double lumen (true lumen and intramural dissection) represents a dissecting aneurysm and is the only sign that is specific for dissection. Other angiographic findings include total vascular occlusion, an intimal flap, a ripple appearance (wavy ribbonlike sign), proximal or distal dilatation, and retention of contrast material in the vessel wall.

Siderosis of the CNS

Siderosis of the CNS is a result of chronic recurrent hemorrhages (e.g., bleeding from cranial or spinal dural AVMs, tumors, postoperative manipulation) and presents with hearing loss, cerebellar dysfunction, pyramidal tract signs, and progressive mental deterioration. Cranial nerves II, V, VII, and VIII are involved, with nerve VIII being the most vulnerable. Pathologically, hemosiderin deposits in reactive macrophages are demonstrated in the leptomeninges, subpial tissue, spinal cord, and on the cranial nerves. Before the advent of MR, this diagnosis was almost exclusively made at autopsy. MR beautifully reveals the marked hypointensity on T2WI, particularly with gradient echo images, around the leptomeninges and on the cranial nerves (Fig. 4-43). Hemosiderin deposition has also been noted on the ventricular ependyma after neonatal intraventricular hemorrhage.

Aneurysms and Subarachnoid Hemorrhage

Aneurysms   An aneurysm is a focal dilatation of an artery. Many different types of aneurysms involve the CNS and are listed in Box 4-8. The most frequent aneurysm encountered in the CNS is the berry aneurysm, which we will discuss in detail in a moment. Fusiform aneurysms are atherosclerotic dilatations, usually of the vertebral and/or basilar artery (Fig. 4-44). Dissecting aneurysms may occur after trauma (traumatic aneurysms) or may occur spontaneously. Organized hematoma from a vessel that has bled is termed pseudoaneurysm. There are no true vessel walls, and the hematoma is confined by the adventitia. These are pathologically distinguished by concentric rings of fibrin and organized blood. Neoplastic aneurysms result from tumor emboli and subsequent growth of the neoplasm through the vessel wall. This can be seen with atrial myxoma and choriocarcinoma. Mycotic aneurysms are the result of endocarditis with septic emboli to the vasa vasorum with secondary destruction of the vessel wall so that all that is left is the intima. Such aneurysms may be saccular or fusiform and tend to be peripheral in the middle cerebral artery distribution. Multiple peripheral aneurysms should suggest this diagnosis.

A berry or saccular aneurysm forms because of a con-

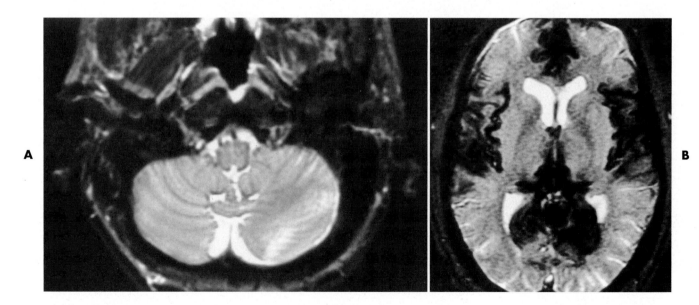

Fig. 4-43   Hemosiderosis/ Siderosis. **A,** Subtle: The FSE on this scan still depicts a dark periphery to the brain stem. **B,** Flagrant (or subtle for frequent flyers to Louisville): A different case with a gradient echo scan shows fulminant hemosiderin deposition in the meninges.

Box 4-8   Aneurysms

Dissecting
Fusiform or atherosclerotic
Mycotic
Neoplastic
Pseudoaneurysm
Saccular or berry
Traumatic

genitally thin or absent tunica media and either absent or extremely fragmented internal elastica of the arterial wall. This occurs at branching points where the parent vessel is curving. Aneurysms are typically found at locations where the blood would be flowing straight if not for the vascular curve. The wall of an aneurysm is composed of only an intima and adventia with a variable amount of fibrohyalin tissue between these layers and may have calcification in it. Larger aneurysms can contain organized clot with a lamellated architecture. Clot can form in any aneurysm, although it is more prominent in larger ones, and such aneurysms may be a source of distal emboli. Arterial stress plays an important role in the formation and growth of aneurysms. Increased flow in AVMs can induce aneurysm formation both on the arterial and venous side (varicosities). In these situations (where an aneurysm and AVM coexist) it is usually the aneurysm that ruptures. Aneurysms may enlarge in time, with the larger aneurysms generally tending to bleed more frequently. The average age of patients with an aneurysmal bleed is approximately 50 years.

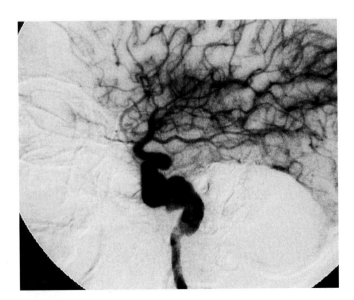

Fig. 4-44   Carotid arteriogram demonstrates large fusiform aneurysm of the internal carotid artery in a patient with arteriomegaly.

The prevalence of intracranial aneurysm has been estimated to be between 1% and 6 % in adult autopsy series but between 0.5% and 1% for incidental aneurysms in patients undergoing cerebral angiography. The frequency of aneurysms depends on which series one quotes and whether such series include only ruptured or both ruptured and unruptured aneurysms. From the International Cooperative Study published in 1990, the frequency of ruptured aneurysms was anterior communicating/anterior cerebral artery (39%), internal carotid artery (including posterior communicating, ophthalmic segment) (30%), middle cerebral artery (22%), and vertebrobasilar circulation (8%). The remaining aneurysms were unclassified. Multiple berry aneurysms, usually two or three in number (but as many as 13 have been reported), occur in about 20% to 30% of cases, most frequently on the middle cerebral artery. Aneurysms vary widely in size and shape. Some are as small as 1 to 2 mm, whereas those 25 mm or more are termed giant aneurysms. In general, aneurysms smaller than 9 mm are statistically less likely to bleed especially those 3 mm or less. The question is often raised regarding treatment or followup in these very small aneurysms. Philosophically, this depends on how you like having a time bomb between your ears versus the possibility that third grade goes into the suction tube. Aneurysms tend to rupture from their dome and those that rupture tend to be irregular with daughter sacs with variable wall thickness.

Although most aneurysms occur sporadically, there is also a familial incidence (7% to 20% of patients with aneurysmal subarachnoid hemorrhage have a first- or second-degree relative with a confirmed intracranial aneurysm), with siblings having the highest association. Remember to tell your children how important genes really are. Certain conditions, particularly connective tissue disorders or abnormalities of blood flow, have an increased propensity for aneurysms. Box 4-9 lists disorders that have been associated with aneurysm in which MRA could play a screening role.

This an improved the quality of life for entrepreneurs who perform executive screening by MRA or CTA for occult aneurysm with COB (cash on the barrel). Before the age of 50 men have a higher incidence of SAH but postmenopausal women have a higher incidence than men. Cigarette smoking, which decreases the effectiveness of alpha1-antitrypsin (an inhibitor of elastase), is associated with 3 to 10 times the risk of aneurysmal SAH. Binge drinking increases the risk of SAH. Controversy exists over what role hypertension plays in the genesis and rupture of aneurysms.

Presently, the diagnosis of aneurysm presenting as subarachnoid hemorrhage (SAH) is definitively made on conventional angiography. This is because the patient is betting his or her life on the results of the study. It is that simple! SAH the sequela of a ruptured aneurysm car-

Box 4-9 Disorders Associated with Intracranial Aneurysms

3M syndrome
Alkaptonuria
Anderson-Fabry disease
Autosomal dominant polycystic kidney disease (10% of asymptomatic patients)
Behcet's disease
Coarctation of the aorta
Collagen vascular disease
Ehlers-Danlos syndrome type IV
Familial idiopathic nonarteriosclerotic cerebral calcification syndrome
Fibromuscular dysplasia
Hereditary hemorrhagic telangiectasia
Homocystinuria
Marfan's syndrome
Moyamoya disease
Neurofibromatosis type 1
Noonan's syndrome
Pseudoxanthoma elasticum
Sickle Cell Disease
Systemic Lupus Erythematosus
Takayasu's disease
Tuberous sclerosis
Wermer's syndrome
α-Glucosidase deficiency
α1-Antitrypsin deficiency

ries a significant morbidity and mortality rate. Approximately 12% of patients with SAH die before reaching the hospital. Forty percent of hospitalized patients die within one month after the ictus and one third of the survivors have major neurologic deficits. The annual rupture rate of aneurysm has been estimated to be 0.5% to 2% with a tendency toward rupture increasing with size particularly those greater than 10 mm. Rebleeding occurs in approximately 20% of untreated patients within 2 weeks of initial hemorrhage, in 30% by 1 month, and in 40% by 6 months. Rebleeding is associated with a mortality rate in excess of 40%. New aneurysms have been reported to develop in at least 2% of patients with previously ruptured aneurysm. The incidence of SAH in the United States is about 1 in 10,000, but is 6 to 10 times higher in patients with previous SAH who have a new aneurysm.

To make the diagnosis, meticulous technique is required. Each vessel must be scrutinized separately. In patients in whom an aneurysm is to be ruled out, all four vessels must be injected. Injection of one vertebral artery with excellent reflux down the other may be adequate but care must be taken to identify the contralateral posterior inferior cerebellar artery origin and to ascertain whether visualization of that entire vessel is sat-

isfactory. Depending on the age of the patient and the extent of atherosclerosis, the catheter can be placed in the common or internal carotid artery and vertebral arteries. The positive side of a common carotid injection is in the ability to visualize the external circulation and to identify a dural malformation, which rarely can be the cause of SAH.

The radiologist should answer the following questions for the interventional neuroradiologist/surgeon when possible: (1) Is there an aneurysm? (2) What is the exact location of the aneurysm? (3) Is there one or more than one? (4) If there is more than one aneurysm, which one bled? (5) What is the size of the aneurysm? (6) From what vessel is the aneurysm arising? (7) Does the aneurysm have a neck, and what is the orientation of the neck and the dome? (8) What is the ratio of the neck to the dome (for treatment with coils). (9) What is the relationship of branch vessels to the aneurysm (and its dome). (10) Is the aneurysm the source of the patient's SAH? (11) What is the status of the circle of Willis? (12) Is any other lesion associated with the aneurysm (e.g., extracranial occlusive vascular disease, vasculitis, AVM)? (13) Is there vasospasm?

There are certain standard views in addition to the anteroposterior and lateral projections for the evaluation of common aneurysms. These are provided in Table 4-3 and should serve as a beginning guide to best display the most frequent types of aneurysms. After the anteroposterior and lateral views, additional projections can be performed with magnified, coned-down, rapid (three to six images per second), arterial sequences only. Rotational angiography (where the image intensifier moves around the patient during a prolonged contrast injection) is also performed to eliminate vascular overlap and provide stereoscopic images. When in doubt, do not shout, turn the head about, and work it out (shoot another run with a different projection).

Vascular loops Certain characteristics may help distinguish an aneurysm from a vascular loop. A vascular loop has the same wash-in and wash-out as the parent vessel. With modern arterial digital subtraction, such sequences can be ascertained on the display monitor when the arterial and venous images are viewed. Aneurysms have different flow dynamics, particularly with delayed wash-out compared with the parent vessel. Vascular loops are usually completely regular in shape, whereas aneurysms generally have asymmetry or slight irregularity. A vessel seen end-on has more density than parent vessels, whereas aneurysms have a density equal to or less than the parent vessel.

Infundibular dilatation Another problem encountered is that of differentiating an infundibular dilatation from a true aneurysm. This is most commonly seen at the origin of the posterior communicating artery. There are several criteria for classifying a dilated vascular ori-

Table 4-3 Additional angigraphic projections for common aneurysms*	
Aneurysm location	**Angiographic projection**
Anterior cerebral/anterior communicating artery	1. Head turned 25-35 degrees away from side being injected
	2. Cross-compression of contralateral carotid filmed in either AP or oblique projection
	3. Submental or base view
Internal carotid/posterior communicating artery	1. Contralateral AP oblique: Head turned between 25-55 degrees away from side of injection
	2. AP oblique: Head turned 25-30 degrees toward side of injection
Middle cerebral artery	1. Head cocked laterally with ipsilateral middle cerebral projected superiorly
	2. Supramagnified AP with genu of middle cerebral artery projected through orbit
	3. Submental or base view
Posterior inferior cerebellar artery, Basilar	1. Contralateral AP oblique: Head turned 45 degrees away from side of injection, Townes projection

*In addition to the standard anteroposterior and lateral projections. AP, Anteroposterior.

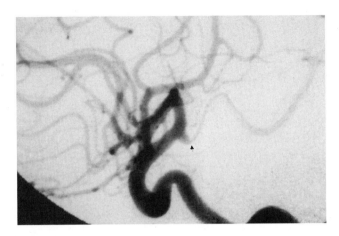

Fig. 4-45   Posterior communicating artery infundibulum. Arteriogram shows a smooth tapering posterior communicating artery infundibulum with the posterior communicating artery taking off at its apex *(arrow)*.

gin as an infundibulum (Fig. 4-45). The artery should originate directly from the apex of the infundibulum. The dilatation should not be larger than 3 mm, and the infundibulum should be tentlike or cone-shaped rather than saccular. No irregularity or aneurysmal neck should be present. There is evidence that some infundibula may grow and become true aneurysms.

Aneurysmal rupture   In the case of multiple aneurysms certain findings can indicate which aneurysm has bled. The best indication of the aneurysm that has bled is finding a hematoma associated with it. CT confirms the diagnosis of SAH and can suggest the probable location of the bleeding aneurysm by showing where the greatest amount of hemorrhage lies. Blood in the interhemispheric fissure and lateral ventricle is most consistent with an anterior communicating artery aneurysm. Hemorrhage in the sylvian fissure is most compatible with a middle cerebral artery aneurysm, whereas blood in the fourth ventricle suggests a posterior inferior cerebellar artery aneurysm rupture. This is not foolproof, however. On CT, the subarachnoid blood fades away (see following section). MR is particularly useful because

it is able to show hemorrhage on T1WI in the wall of the aneurysm that has bled (unfortunately uncommon). Angiographic findings associated with aneurysmal rupture include (1) the proximity to the most significant spasm; (2) the irregularity of the aneurysm; (3) the tendency that, in general, the larger the aneurysm (especially if it is >9 mm), the greater the tendency to bleed; (4) mass effect around the aneurysm (although with CT or MR this is obvious); and (5) tapering of the apex of the aneurysm (Murphy's tit) (Fig. 4-46 [don't get your hopes up, this is an allegedly scientific book]).

Subarachnoid hemorrhage   Fifty percent to 70% of SAH is the result of rupture of intracranial aneurysms. Other causes of SAH include secondary leakage of blood from a primary intraparenchymal hemorrhage, trauma, intracranial AVM, hemorrhagic tumor, dural AVM, spinal cord AVM, blood dyscrasias, or bleeding diatheses, amyloid angiopathy, moyamoya disease, or complications of pregnancy. Fifteen percent of patients with SAH have no aneurysm found and no other cause noted after four-vessel angiography.

After reading this description of hemorrhage, you probably have the worst headache of your life. What is the appropriate workup for this presentation? You confront the publisher, who ascertains that you have appropriate insurance (a forgone conclusion because you paid big bucks for this so-called neuroradiology text). You are taken to the emergency room and a CT is performed. If the CT is positive, you have bought the angiogram (and at its current price, you think that you also bought the equipment). If the CT is negative, a lumbar puncture awaits you. Are you sure you still have the headache? If the tap is bloody (provided it is nontraumatic) and/or there is xanthochromia (yellow discoloration caused by blood product breakdown in the cerebrospinal fluid that takes several hours to occur) of the

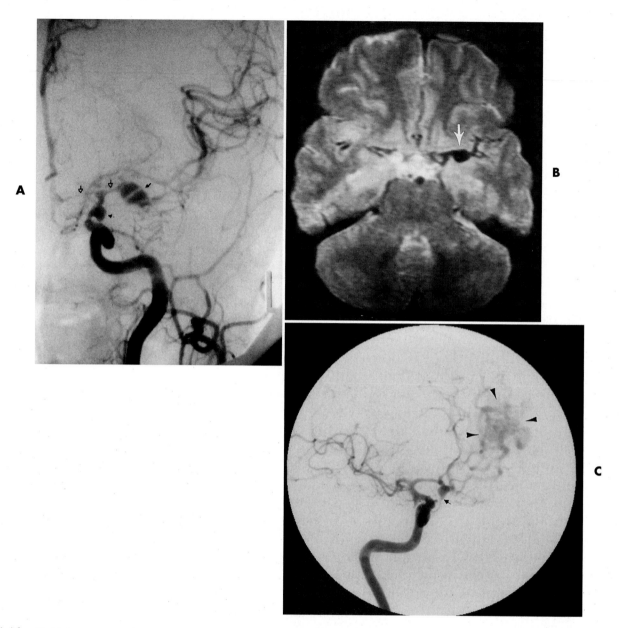

Fig. 4-46 Multiple aneurysms in a patient with SAH. **A,** Aneurysms of the posterior communicating and middle cerebral arteries *(black arrows)* are demonstrated. *Open arrows* show spasm of M1 and A1. **B,** On T2WI you can appreciate the aneurysm of the middle cerebral artery *(arrow)*; however, you cannot appreciate evidence of acute hemorrhage. **C,** Murphy's tit. Anteroposterior arteriogram shows an anterior communicating artery aneurysm with a small protrusion *(arrow)* from the body of the aneurysm representing Murphy's tit and suggesting that this is the origin of the patient's subarachnoid hemorrhage. Note an associated arteriovenous malformation *(arrowheads)* from the left anterior cerebral artery.

CSF supernatant, guess what? You will also get an angiogram. If the tap is negative and there is a strong clinical suspicion, you may still get an angiogram or perhaps a CTA in the emergency room or an MRA (at the freestanding imaging center).

CT findings in SAH demonstrate blood (high density) within cisterns and subarachnoid spaces in 90 to 95% of patients within the first 24 hours following SAH. This can at times be subtle. Carefully assess the insular and other cisterns for slightly increased density in patients

with this presentation (Fig. 4-47). The sensitivity of CT for SAH decreases to 80% within 3 days, 70% within 5 days, 50% within one week, and 30% within 2 weeks. CT is also useful in directing the arteriogram. Use the Willie Sutton approach: go where the payoff (blood) is first. Generally, the greatest concentration of blood is where the aneurysm is. Finally, CT will direct your attention to other possible sources for the patient's presentation, including intraparenchymal hemorrhage and traumatic subdural hematoma in a patient without a his-

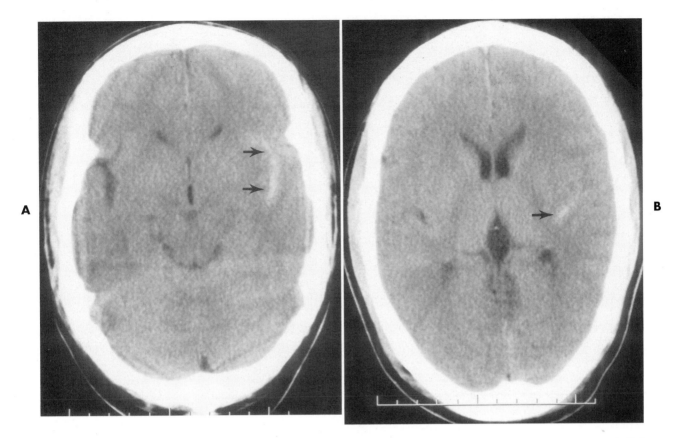

Fig. 4-47   CT of insular subarachnoid hemorrhage. **A,** Observe the increased density of blood in the insular cistern (*arrows*). **B,** Be careful sometimes the only inkling of subarachnoid blood is increased density in one sulcus (*arrow*).

tory (or unable to give a history) of trauma. CT is necessary before lumbar puncture to determine whether there is significant mass effect (from unsuspected tumor, infarction, extraaxial collection, acute hydrocephalus), which can produce herniation or require timely therapy. Why not begin with an MR? CT is easier, faster, and more specific.

Most imaging centers now perform routine FLAIR images (Fig. 4-48). It is essential in those patients with appropriate histories to carefully survey the sulci for increased intensity. This can also be subtle. On FLAIR images SAH can be seen as high intensity in the sulci secondary to blood protein shortening the T2 of the CSF. Even with FLAIR, MR still has problems with reduced specificity for SAH. Remember patients present with a constellation of symptoms including headache and meningismus and not the diagnosis of SAH.

On conventional T1 and T2WI acute SAH is not visible. CSF has an oxygen pressure of approximately 43 mm Hg. At this level, because of the sigmoid shape of the oxyhemoglobin dissociation curve, hemoglobin is approximately 72% saturated. Therefore, only 28% of the hemoglobin is in the deoxygenated form. The hematocrit of a SAH is usually low (5%), and thus the low hematocrit together with the small amount of deoxyhemoglo-

bin makes acute hemorrhage difficult to detect on MR. Oxyhemoglobin has no unpaired electrons and therefore behaves like other nonparamagnetic substances, being isointense to the brain on T1WI and T2WI*If the diagnosis of subarachnoid hemorrhage is entertained, MR is not the imaging modality of choice and CT should be the first study performed although by the next edition things could be different. We shall take the conservative approach, unlike the political the pundits who called Florida for Al Gore, we would rather be right than have a patient sleep with the fishes.*

Most of the time the RBCs are cleared from the CSF so that normally one does not detect subarachnoid methemoglobin if the patient is imaged a few days after an ictus. MR can be useful in determining which aneurysm has bled after SAH if one demonstrates multiple aneurysms on MR or angiography. The aneurysm that has bled may have high intensity of methemoglobin in its wall or nearby.

MRA/CTA has utility in the following situations: (1) headache and low probability of aneurysm, (2) a familial history of aneurysm (such as polycystic kidney disease), (3) follow-up of unruptured aneurysms, (4) situations in which a diagnosis is important but treatment is contraindicated, or (5) situations in which angiography

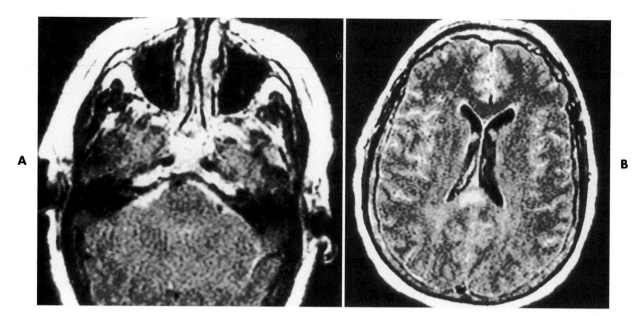

Fig. 4-48 SAH on MR **A,** FLAIR scanning has improved MR's ability to detect subarachnoid hemorrhage. The CSF should be dark in the basal cisterns (**A**) and the sylvian fissures (**B**). CSF pulsation artifacts can make the CSF in the posterior fossa region problematic.

is contraindicated. We have not mentioned acute third nerve palsy because of the medical-legal consequences. If the MRA iş negative, we still feel that a conventional angiogram is called for. If MRA/CTA is positive, you need a four-vessel study anyway. So, why perseverate?

The rate of rehemorrhage is at least 4% (but may be as high as 20%) within the first 24 hours. It is between 1% and 2 % per day for the first 2 weeks. Vasospasm, occurs at 3 to 15 days after SAH, and is one of the chief causes of morbidity and mortality. It has been reported in up to 75% of cases by angiography. Noninvasive methodology used to detect vasospasm includes transcranial Doppler and CTA. Recently severe vasospasm has been treated with hypervolemia, hypertension, hemodilution, nimodepine, intraarterial papaverine infusion, and/or balloon angioplasty.

Treatment of unruptured cerebral aneurysms may be surgical or by endovascular coil embolization. The morbidity (5% to 15%) and mortality (2%) of treatment between the two methods is similar. The methodology is beyond the scope of this book (and the expertise of the authors). In a recent preliminary study, it appeared that coil embolization of unruptured aneurysms was associated with significantly fewer complications than surgical aneurysm clipping. However, certain aneurysm locations are better treated with particular techniques (Table 4-4).

Nonaneurysmal perimesencephalic SAH The syndrome of nonaneurysmal perimesencephalic SAH is a condition that carries an extremely low probability of finding an aneurysm (obviously). The clinical presentation is of the sudden onset of headache in patients, with a mean age of 53 years. These cases have an un-

complicated clinical course without rehemorrhage. The radiologic criteria consist of (1) hemorrhage centered immediately anterior to the midbrain with or without extension of blood into the anterior part of the ambient cistern or to the basal part of the sylvian fissure, (2) no blood filling the anterior interhemispheric fissure and no extension to the lateral sylvian fissure (except for minute amounts of blood), and (3) absence of frank intraventricular hemorrhage (Fig. 4-49). Repeated CT scanning 1 week after the ictus reveals disappearance of the hemorrhage in almost all cases. The cause of perimesencephalic hemorrhage is unknown; however, it may result from capillary or venous rupture. When angiography is performed and is negative in the face of perimesencephalic hemorrhage, repeated angiography may be un-

Table 4-4 Aneurysm location vs treatment	
Artery	**Treatment**
Distal Internal Carotid Artery	Endovascular or Surgery
Periophthalmic	Endovascular or Surgery
Middle Cerebral	Surgery
Anterior Communicating	Endovascular or Surgery
Posterior Communicating	Endovascular or Surgery
Basilar	Endovascular
Posterior Inferior Cerebellar	Endovascular
Pseudoaneurysm in the neck	Stenting
Pseudoaneurysm or dissection in the brain	Endovascular occlusion
Dissection in the neck	Medical or Stenting

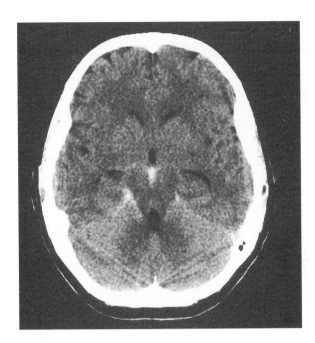

Fig. 4-49   CT of nonaneurysmal perimesencephalic hemorrhage. Hemorrhage is centered in the perimesencephalic cistern with slight extension into ambient cistern. No aneurysm was found at angiography.

necessary (indeed CTA may be useful) and the patient may have a better prognosis.

Angiographically negative SAH   What is the approach to the case of angiographically negative SAH? Start with the obvious. Was the hemorrhage identified on CT or just lumbar puncture? If it was only lumbar puncture, then one should question the validity of the spinal tap results, particularly if no xanthochromia is reported. Does the patient have sinusitis, and does the physician who performed the puncture have Parkinson disease? If it is a true SAH, were all four vessels injected? If not, go back and inject them. Make sure you subtract each run and assess all the vessels slowly and carefully! Dural malformations will be identified only if a common carotid or selective external injection is done. Think of the nonaneurysmal causes of SAH. In the vast majority of cases the aneurysm is on the original film series and for reasons such as poor choice of angiographic projection, or inadequate gray matter or defects in visual association areas of the radiologist, the aneurysm may be cryptic. When looking at the angiogram for subtle aneurysms or vasculitis, radiologists gather like flies to fecal material. Repeated angiography approximately a week or two later is sometimes useful, particularly when there is spasm on the initial angiogram, which may preclude filling of the aneurysm. Many times the aneurysm is seen on the repeated study. You should go back and look at the original study; it was probably there. Humiliating, but it is always a learning experience. The bot-

tom line here is to be compulsive about your projections and your reading. Using modern angiographic methodology about 5% to 10% (educated guess) of cases will be negative on the first angiogram and positive on the repeat. Compromising any component of the angiogram can result in your patient's purchasing ranch tickets.

ARTERIOVENOUS AND OTHER VASCULAR MALFORMATIONS

Vascular malformations have been traditionally divided into four categories: (1) capillary telangiectasias, (2) cavernous hemangiomas, (3) venous angiomas, and (4) true AVMs.

Capillary Telangiectasias (Fig 4-50)

These lesions have a propensity for the pons, although they may be seen in other regions of the brain. Such lesions are angiographically occult but can be identified on enhanced MR or CT. They vary in size but average about 3 cm in diameter. Between the telangiectasias is normal brain. Cerebral capillary telangiectasias are rarely seen in hereditary hemorrhagic telangiectasia disease (HHT or Osler-Weber-Rendu disease see AVM below).

These lesions are difficult to diagnose because the vast majority do not hemorrhage and therefore have no characteristic blood products associated with them. They are usually observed as nodular enhancement after contrast on the T1WI and may be isointense on T2WI. Gradient echo images reveal hypointensity but are not often done with standard imaging protocols. They can occasionally present with other vascular lesions. The differential diagnosis of such an enhancing nodule in the pons includes demyelination, neoplasia, inflammation, and numerous other conditions. In most cases they are pure curiosities put there by the Greatest Neuroradiologist to stimulate academic discussions and to create appropriate uncertainty.

Cavernous Angioma (Cavernous Hemangioma, Cavernous Malformation)

Cavernous angiomas appear as high density regions on noncontrast CT. They may have associated calcification and enhance. Pathologically they are considered congenital vascular hamartomas consisting of a sinusoidal collection of blood vessels without interspersed normal brain as opposed to other vascular malformations. Besides blood products of various ages, calcification and gliosis are also present. Before the advent of MR, CT findings were compatible with low-grade tumor, hematoma, granuloma, and inflammatory conditions such as tuberculomas and sarcoidomas. Angiographically, no feeding arteries are seen, although occasionally

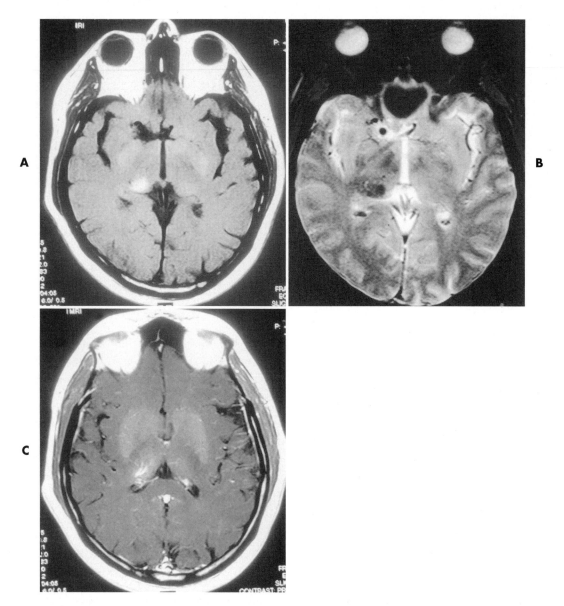

Fig. 4-50 Telangiectasia and venous angioma. **A,** High signal is seen in the right pulvinar could represent hemorrhage or calcification. **B,** The gradient echo scan shows low intensity—which doesn't help much in the battle between hemosiderin and calcification. **C,** But the post contrast scan shows enhancement of the capillary telangiectasia as well as an associated venous angioma (commonly seen together).

an early vein or subtle blush may be visualized, particularly after prolonged injection of contrast (10 mL for the vertebral and 13 to 15 mL for the carotid injection for a 3-second injection duration). By and large these lesions are angiographically occult. Some of these lesions have been histologically examined and in the past treated with radiation therapy for what were thought to be low-grade gliomas. MR has provided increased sensitivity to the diagnosis of these malformations (Fig. 4-51). Such lesions may be asymptomatic or may present with neurologic symptoms after hemorrhage. They may also produce seizures and a constellation of neurologic findings similar to tumor. In the workup of a seizure disorder if the spin-echo pulse sequence reveals no abnormality, gradi-

ent-echo imaging (with its increased sensitivity to susceptibility effects) is a useful additional pulse sequence to try to visualize small cavernous malformations.

On MR, you will see copious amounts of hemosiderin (low intensity on T2WI or gradient-echo images emphasizing T2*) surrounding various circumscribed regions of hemorrhage (methemoglobin). As opposed to simple intraparenchymal hemorrhages, which tend to collapse ultimately into slitlike cavities, cavernous malformations are round, have a matrix, and do not collapse. As opposed to tumors, in cavernous malformations there is a complete rim of hemosiderin. These lesions may bleed, perhaps because of associated venous thrombosis. In such cases, they behave like other hemorrhagic lesions.

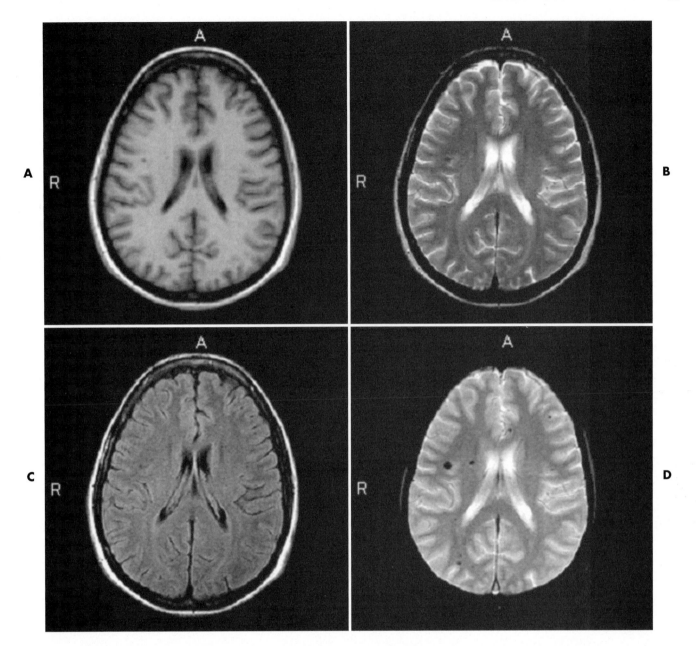

Fig. 4-51   Multiple pulse sequences showing cavernomas. **A,** Fast spin echo T2W is modestly successful in demonstrating cavernomas. **B,** The FLAIR scan is usually somewhat less sensitive because the CSF is dark making the hemosiderin containing lesions less conspicuous. **C,** By virtue of the presence of the proton electron dipole dipole interaction, the methemoglobin of the cavernoma appears bright on the T1WI (not seen here). However hemosiderin is still dark. **D,** Gradient echo scans will be more sensitive to the susceptibility effects of the hemosiderin. Look at this image and then back titrate to see how many of the lesions are visible on the other sequences.

Edema from an acute hemorrhage should disappear within 4 to 6 weeks, and then the characteristic features of the cavernous malformation manifest. Cavernous angiomas may be multiple (16% to 33% of cases), and the condition tends to be familial.

The term *occult cerebrovascular malformation,* which is sometimes used synonymously with cavernous hemangioma, is perhaps more appropriate for radiologists (than pathologists) to use because it is based on the MR characteristics of this lesion rather than on histopathology. *Occult* refers to the lack of findings on an angiogram, although in today's world the angiogram should be occult in the diagnosis of these lesions. These lesions can occur in any location, including the spine, and have even been reported extracranially; however, they have a propensity for the cerebral hemispheres and brain stem. Regardless of whether all these lesions are histopathologically true cavernous hemangiomas, their MR characteristics are similar and they appear to have a common clinical course. These lesions usually do not produce life-threatening hemorrhages; rather, their effects result from the location of the lesion and at times their slow expansion (most hemorrhages with this lesion are small and of low pressure).

Venous Malformation (Venous Angioma or Developmental Venous Anomaly)

Venous malformation consists of a network of dilated medullary veins converging in a radial fashion to a large vein that drains into either deep or superficial veins. The surrounding brain parenchyma is normal. The incidence of venous angioma has been reported to be 2.6%. Angiographically, there should be neither an abnormal number of arteries nor enlargement of feeding arteries. Early venous filling and even a blush have been reported, although most commonly one sees persistence of normally filling aberrant veins. These malformations are hypothesized to represent an anatomic variant of the venous drainage of the periependymal zones. They usually occur in the paraventricular region; however, they can also be observed subcortically and juxtacortically. Venous angiomas are diagnosed on MR by observing linear structures with flow voids, usually around the ventricle, with a transcerebral course, and uniform enhancement. This enhancement is in a rather characteristic fashion (caput medusae, umbrella shape), unlike flow voids in normal arteries or arteries of AVMs (Fig. 4-52). The vast majority of these lesions are asymptomatic and do not bleed, although rarely hemorrhage has been reported to occur from venous angiomas especially in the posterior fossa under stresses of increased pressure. Occasionally a venous angioma is associated with a cavernous hemangioma.

One important aspect of this lesion is that the venous angioma is a compensatory drainage route for normal brain. Sacrifice of this pathway can produce venous infarction of brain tissue being drained. These are not surgical lesions unless misdiagnosed. Careful and critical assessment of neurologic symptoms such as seizures, headache, and vertigo, or parenchymal hemorrhage, should be made before they are attributed to venous angioma.

Arteriovenous Malformations

True AVMs contain one or more enlarged feeding arteries and have enlarged early draining veins. They are considered congenital anomalies of blood vessels that arise in fetal life but usually become symptomatic in the third or fourth decade of life. They have a tendency to hemorrhage at a rate that has been estimated in a study from Finland to be 4% annually with an annual mortality rate of 1% and a mean interval between hemorrhagic events of 7.7 years. A recognized complication of AVMs is the steal phenomenon. In this situation, blood supply preferentially seeks the AVM and normal brain parenchyma is thus relatively undersupplied. Steal can produce focal neurologic symptoms, seizures, and ultimately parenchymal loss in the affected part of the brain. Aneurysms of vessels supplying AVMs can occasionally be detected and, if there has been a recent hemorrhage, are usually the source of bleeding. It is interesting that if the AVM is treated, the aneurysm will regress, suggesting that the increased flow was responsible for its creation and growth.

The AVM consists of a feeding artery or arteries, which are usually dilated, and a cluster of entangled vascular loops (the core or nidus) connected to abundant vascular channels where the arterial blood is shunted, finally terminating in an enlarged draining vein or veins. AVMs

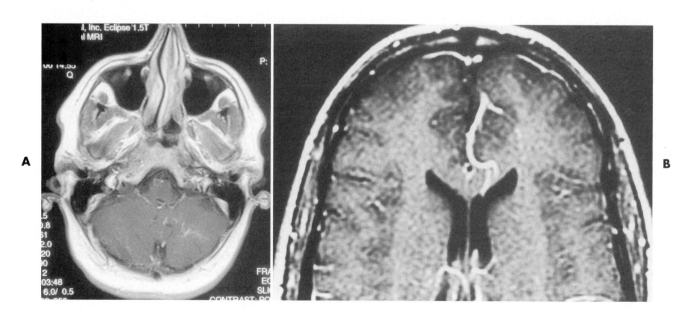

Fig. 4-52   Venous angioma (Developmental venous anomaly-DVAs). Left cerebellum (**A**) and left frontal (**B**) DVAs are well-depicted after gadolinium administration. These are generally hard to see on unenhanced sequences.

Table 4-5 AVM classification*	
Size	**Score**
<3 cm	1
3-6 cm	2
>6 cm	3
Eloquent	
No	0
Yes	1
Cortical drainage	
No	0
Yes	1

*Spetzler

can be supplied by many different vascular distributions such as from both anterior and middle cerebral arteries; from anterior, middle, and posterior cerebral arteries; and from both hemispheres. External carotid branches can also supply superficial AVMs with dural components. It is important to map completely the anatomy of these lesions. AVMs have been classified according to their size, location, and venous drainage (see Table 4-5). The higher the score the worse the prognosis.

The diagnosis of AVM can be made on CT or MR. On CT, the tangled vessels in the brain parenchyma are high density without contrast (blood pool effect) and have a serpentine, punctate, or an irregular mélange configuration (Fig. 4-53). Curvilinear or speckled calcification may

be present. These lesions enhance. On MR curvilinear flow voids secondary to fast flow are observed on most pulse sequences, and dilated feeding arteries can also be noted. The exact appearance is dependent on the blood flow and the particular pulse sequence. MRA is useful for mapping the AVM. Both three-dimensional time-of-flight and three-dimensional phase-contrast techniques are useful. Enhancement increases the conspicuity of the AVM, particularly the venous portion. In lesions that have high signal associated with hemorrhage, phase-contrast MRA techniques are necessary to provide the best demonstration of the AVM.

The definitive study is cerebral angiography. The diagnosis is made by demonstrating an enlarged feeding artery, the core or nidus, and the enlarged draining veins. Early venous filling should be searched for in cases of small AVMs. One approach is to start with the venous films and trace backward to see whether any of the veins are present in the arterial phase (early draining vein). AVMs can be associated with dilated medullary veins. In occasional cases, angiography fails to document surgically proven AVMs (cryptic AVM). This may be due to (1) the mass effect from the hemorrhage on the vascular malformation (particularly in the rare situation of a bleed from a venous angioma), (2) thrombosis of the vascular lesion after hemorrhage, or (3) a very small (cryptic) AVM. If the initial angiogram is negative, repeated angiography, performed after the mass effect has decreased, can reveal evidence of the lesion such as an early draining vein.

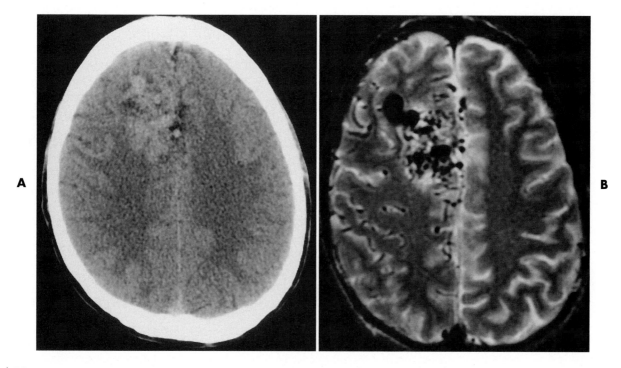

Fig. 4-53 Arteriovenous malformations. **A,** Unenhanced CT with high density in the right frontal region caused by the blood pool of the enlarged veins and perhaps some calcification. **B,** T2WI with flow voids from the obvious AVM.

AVMs can markedly enlarge draining veins, an extreme example of which is the vein of Galen malformation (Fig. 4-54; also see in utero ultrasound Chapter 9). In fact, vein of Galen malformation has multiple causes. It can be the result of a pial AVM with deep venous drainage, a direct arteriovenous fistula, or a combination of both. In these cases, obstruction may be present in the distal vein of Galen or venous sinuses. Arterial supply is variable but commonly is from dilated thalamoperforating arteries, anterior cerebral branches, and branches from the posterior cerebral artery including the posterior choroidal arteries. The symptoms depend on whether there is a fistula or pial malformation and on the age of the patient. Pediatric, adolescent, and adult presentations of vein of Galen aneurysms include headaches, seizures, and other focal neurologic syndromes. With increasing age, there is usually more malformation and less fistula. In neonates, congestive heart failure and seizures are produced from large arteriovenous fistulas. Steal phenomenon and parenchymal loss may be demonstrated in children with untreated vein of Galen malformations. Hydrocephalus is a common problem, in most cases caused by venous hypertension and perhaps increased CSF production secondary to increased choroidal blood flow. Mass effect from the enlarged vein of Galen on the posterior third ventricle and aqueduct has also been proposed as a cause of the hydrocephalus. The prognosis is grim for the pediatric group.

A few syndromes are associated with vascular malformations. You will read about Sturge-Weber in Chapter 9. Wyburn-Mason syndrome is a disorder of retinal, cutaneous, mandibular, and brain stem vascular malformations. Klippel-Trenaunay-Weber syndrome is a hemihypertrophy syndrome with angiomatosis of the extremity and the brain. It may be part of the Sturge-Weber spectrum. HHT (Osler Weber Rendu disease) is an autosomal dominant (endoglin gene on chromosome 9 and activin receptor-like kinase gene on chromosome 12) vascular disorder has mucocutaneous telangiectases and visceral arteriovenous malformations. Two percent of cerebral AVM have been reported to be associated with HHT and 5% to 10% of patients with HHT have AVMs. These AVMs are multiple in over 50% of cases. These lesions tend to be cortical in location and small (micro AVM). As stated above capillary angiomas may also be seen. Foix-Alajouanine, a dural malformation of the spine associated with spinal venous hypertension, is discussed in Chapter 17. An affinity for eponyms, Grossman-Yousem syndrome, is also associated with sophomoric humor, microacademia, and hyporoyaltyism.

Treatment of any AVM depends on its size, location, and angioarchitecture. It consists of endovascular therapy, surgery, and radiation therapy, or combinations thereof. In cases of AVM, less that 3 cm in diameter stereotactic radiotherapy is the treatment of choice (depending of location) with cure rates of 80% to 90% within 2 to 3 years. An immediate complication associated with treatment, either surgical or embolic, of AVMs with extensive steal (resulting in hypoperfusion of the normal brain) is brain swelling and/or hemorrhage. This

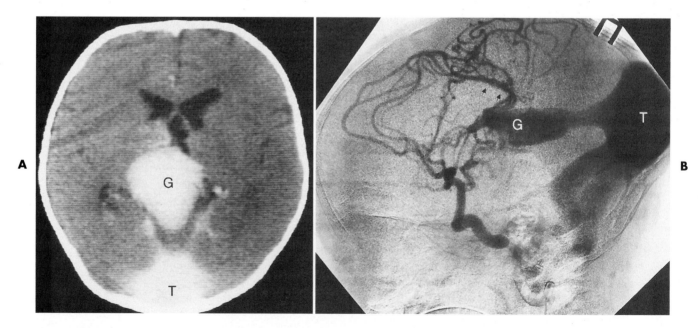

Fig. 4-54 Vein of Galen malformation. **A,** Enhanced CT shows an obviously enlarged, homogeneously enhancing vein of Galen *(G)* and an enlarged torcular *(T)*. **B,** Lateral angiogram demonstrates the vein of Galen "aneurysm" *(G)* and torcular *(T)*. Direct fistulous communications are present between anterior cerebral arteries *(arrows)* and aneurysm. Other vessels also supply the lesion. Note the absent filling of the middle cerebral artery produced by the fistula's stealing blood supply from the middle cerebral artery.

is secondary to normal perfusion pressure breakthrough related to marked hemodynamic changes after obliteration of the AVM. In this situation the chronically hypoperfused brain may be unable to autoregulate because of long-standing ischemia and the abrupt change in hemodynamics after obliteration of the AVM. Staged embolization is advocated to prevent perfusion break-

through from occurring. The rate of cure for endovascular obliteration is about 10% to 20%. Other complications associated with AVM treatment include retrograde thrombosis of the feeding vessels and hemorrhage from an incompletely treated residual nidus.

Another type of vascular malformation is the dural AVM or fistula (Fig. 4-55). These lesions have been pos-

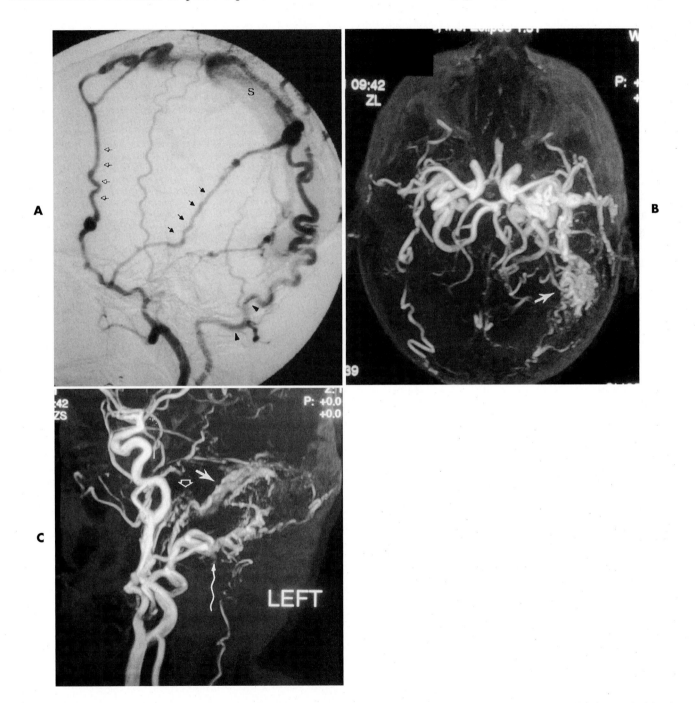

Fig. 4-55   Dural AV fistula (**A**) and dural AVM (**B** and **C**). **A,** External carotid arteriogram reveals a large dural AV fistula supplied by the anterior *(open arrow)* and posterior *(closed arrows)* divisions of the middle meningeal artery and the occipital artery *(arrowheads)*. Note the filling of the sagittal sinus (S). **B,** Collapsed view from an MRA shows a dural AVM *(arrows)* with a nidus centered on the sigmoid sinus. **C,** Projection image of the left carotid circulation shows upward retrograde filling of the sigmoid sinus *(arrow)* with feeders from ascending pharyngeal *(open arrow)* and occipital *(squiggly arrow)* branches.

tulated to be the consequence of sinus (or venous) thrombosis with subsequent recanalization and development of a collateralized network of prominent vessels feeding into a venous sinus. At times, increased flow and decreased venous drainage of the sinus can result in blood being routed via cortical veins. This can result in intraparenchymal hemorrhage, SAH, venous infarction, and elevated intracranial pressure.

Symptoms from dural malformations depend on the location, size of the malformation, and venous drainage pattern. Parasellar malformations draining into the cavernous sinus with retrograde flow in the superior ophthalmic vein (supplied from the meningohypophyseal trunk, accessory meningeal artery, middle meningeal artery, branches of the ascending pharyngeal artery, and other vessels) can create a clinical picture similar to carotid-cavernous fistulas. In this case there is no history of trauma (although cavernous carotid aneurysm rupture can also produce a carotid-cavernous fistula), but dural malformations can have enlargement of the cavernous sinus and superior ophthalmic vein, associated with proptosis and ophthalmoplegia. Visual loss results from glaucoma. Dural malformations in this location can spontaneously improve or can improve after incomplete embolization or even after diagnostic angiography (with current Medicare billing you may be tempted to put in a separate charge for the spontaneous thrombosis, although with the new reimbursement rate it may not be worth the paperwork). At times patients appear to become more symptomatic as the malformation is thrombosing.

Other common symptoms in dural malformations are headache, bruit, or tinnitus (posterior fossa drainage). Pulse-synchronous tinnitus occurs if the malformation has a component near the petrous pyramid. Headaches and hydrocephalus are related to venous hypertension. A rare complication of dural malformation is a dementia-like syndrome (venous hypertensive encephalopathy) secondary to the elevated venous intracranial pressure with associated diminished cerebral perfusion. This is a potentially reversible dementia and should be in your differential diagnosis of dementing illness.

Dural malformations and fistulas are difficult to diagnose on CT or MR. Findings include sinus thrombosis and dilated cortical veins. In the absence of such findings, the images may be entirely normal. Occasionally, one may see a prominent middle meningeal artery or vein over the convexity or an enlarged foramen spinosum. Angiography is the key to the diagnosis of this lesion. This must include selective catheterization of vessels that have meningeal supply including the middle meningeal artery, accessory meningeal artery, ascending pharyngeal artery, internal carotid artery, and vertebral artery. Dural malformations can be treated with success by embolization (arterial and/or venous), although permanent closure may demand use of tissue adhesives,

which are riskier than particulate embolic agents. These increased risks include skin necrosis, cranial nerve palsy, and visual loss. Another approach to reduce venous hypertension is to reopen by stenting the previously thrombosed sinus with restoration of normal flow patterns.

We thought that after finishing this chapter you would be so-o-o-o happy you could sing. Try the following tune to be sung to the melody of "A Few of My Favorite Things" from *The Sound of Music*. (If you pretend to be Julie Andrews, we will pretend to be Rodgers and Hammerstein.)

> Vascular lesions and leaky adhesions,
> Trauma and tumors and vitreous humors,
> Dural-based lesions on sphenoid bone wings:
> These are a few of the hem'rhagic things!
> Hemoglobin turns deoxy, then it turns to met;
> Ferritin forms on the edge of the mass and then it's
>   dark rings you get
> Acoustic neuromas and clivus chordomas,
> Hypo then iso then hyper, that's right—oh,
> Soon you will note hemosiderin rings;
> These are a few of the hem'rhagic things!
> When the catheter moves, when the patient strokes,
> We simply remember our hem'rhagic things,
> And then we don't feel so bad!

We know—Keepa the day job!

SUGGESTED READINGS

Adams HJ, Bendixen B, Kappelle LJ, et al: Classification of subtype of acute ischemic stroke. Definitions for use in a multicenter clinical trial. TOAST. Trial of Org 10172 in Acute Stroke Treatment, *Stroke* 24(1):35-41, 1993.

Alhalabi M, Moore P: Serial angiography in isolated angiitis of the central nervous system, *Neurology* 44(7):1221-1226, 1994.

Anderson SC, Shah CP, Murtagh FR: Congested deep subcortical veins as a sign of dural venous thrombosis: MR and CT correlations, *J Comput Assist Tomogr* 11:1059-1061, 1987.

Anderson G, Ashforth R, Steinke DE, et al: CT angiography for the detection of cerebral vasospasm in patients with acute subarachnoid hemorrhage, *AJNR* 21(6):1011-1015, 2000.

Atlas SW, Mark AS, Grossman RI, et al: Intracranial hemorrhage: gradient-echo MR imaging at 1.5T: comparison with spin-echo imaging and clinical applications, *Radiology* 168:803-807, 1988.

Atlas S, Thulborn K: MR detection of hyperacute parenchymal hemorrhage of the brain, *AJNR* 19(8):1471-1477, 1998.

Atlas S, DuBois P, Singer MB, et al: Diffusion measurements in intracranial hematomas: implications for MR imaging of acute stroke, *AJNR* 21(7):1190-1194, 2000.

Baird A, Warach S: Magnetic resonance imaging of acute stroke, *J Cereb Blood Flow Metab.* 18(6):583-609, 1998.

Baird A., Loveblad K, Schlaug R, et al: Multiple acute stroke syndrome: marker of embolic disease, *Neurology* 54(3):674-678, 2000.

Bizzi A, Brooks RA, Brunetti A, et al: Role of iron and ferritin in MR imaging of the brain: a study in primates at different field strengths, *Radiology* 177:59-65, 1990.

Bradley WG, Schmidt PG: Effect of methemoglobin formation on the MR appearance of subarachnoid hemorrhage, *Radiology* 156:99-103, 1985.

Bragoni M, Di Piero V, Priori R, et al: Sjögren's syndrome presenting as ischemic stroke, *Stroke* 25(11):2276-2279, 1994.

Broderick JP, Brott TG, Tomsick T, et al: Ultra-early evaluation of intracerebral hemorrhage, *J Neurosurg* 72:195-199, 1990.

Brooks RA, Di Chiro G, Patronas N: MR imaging of cerebral hematomas at different field strengths: theory and applications, *J Comput Assist Tomogr* 13:194-206, 1989.

Bruggen NV, Syha J, Busza AL, et al: Identification of tumor hemorrhage in an animal model using spin echoes and gradient echoes, *Magn Res Med* 15:121-127, 1990.

Chalela J, Alsop D, Gonzalez-Atavales JB, et al: Magnetic resonance perfusion imaging in acute ischemic stroke using continuous arterial spin labeling, *Stroke* 31(3):680-687, 2000.

Chimowitz MI, Awad IA, Furlan AJ: Periventricular lesions on MR: facts and theories, *Stroke* 20:963-967, 1989.

Clark RA, Watanabe AT, Bradley WG, et al: Acute hematomas: effects of deoxygenation, hematocrit, and fibrin-clot formation and retraction on T2 shortening, *Radiology* 175:201-206, 1990.

Crain MR, Yuh WTC, Greene GM, et al: Cerebral ischemia: evaluation with contrast-enhanced MR imaging, *AJNR* 12:631-639, 1991.

Di Chiro G, Brooks RA, Girton ME, et al: Sequential MR studies of intracerebral hematomas in monkeys, *AJNR* 7:193-199, 1986.

Ebisu T, Tanaka C, Umeda M, et al: Hemorrhagic and nonhemorrhagic stroke: diagnosis with diffusion-weighted and T2-weighted echo-planar MR imaging, *Radiology* 203(3):823-828, 1997.

Edelman RR, Johnson K, Buxton R, et al: MR of hemorrhage: a new approach, *AJNR* 7:751-756, 1986.

Essig M, von Kummer R, Egelhof T, et al: Vascular MR contrast enhancement in cerebrovascular disease, *AJNR* 17(5):887-894, 1996.

Forbes K, Pipe J, et al: Evidence for cytotoxic edema in the pathogenesis of cerebral venous infarction, *AJNR* 22(3):450-455, 2001.

Futrell N, Millikan C: Frequency, etiology, and prevention of stroke in patients with systemic lupus erythematosus, *Stroke* 20:583-591, 1989.

Gammal TE, Adams RJ, Nichols FT, et al: MR and CT investigation of cerebrovascular disease in sickle cell patients, *AJNR* 7: 1043-1049, 1986.

Giang D: Central nervous system vasculitis secondary to infections, toxins, and neoplasms, *Semin Neurol* 14(4): 313-319, 1994.

Gillard J, Barker P, van Zijl PC, et al: Proton MR spectroscopy in acute middle cerebral artery stroke, *AJNR* 17(5):873-886, 1996.

Goldberg HI, Grossman RI, Gomori JM, et al: MR diagnosis of cervical internal carotid artery dissecting hemorrhage, *Radiology* 158:157-161, 1986.

Gomori JM, Grossman RI, Bilaniuk LT, et al: High-field MR imaging of superficial siderosis of the central nervous system, *J Comput Assist Tomogr* 9(5):972-975, 1985.

Gomori JM, Grossman RI, Goldberg HI, et al: Occult cerebrovascular malformations: high-field MR imaging, *Radiology* 158:707-713, 1986.

Gomori JM, Grossman RI, Hackney DB, et al: Variable appearances of subacute intracranial hematomas on high-field spin-echo MR, *AJNR* 8:1019-1026, 1987.

Gomori JM, Grossman RI, Yu-Ip C, et al: NMR relaxation times of blood: dependence on field strength, oxidation state, and cell integrity, *J Comput Assist Tomogr* 11:684-690, 1987.

Gomori JM, Grossman RI: Mechanisms responsible for the MR appearance and evolution of intracranial hemorrhage, *Radiographics* 8:427-439, 1988.

Gonzalez R, Schaefer P, Buonanno FS, et al: Diffusion-weighted MR imaging: diagnostic accuracy in patients imaged within 6 hours of stroke symptom, *Radiology* 210(1):155-162, 1999.

Grossman RI, Gomori JM, Goldberg HI, et al: MR imaging of hemorrhagic conditions of the head and neck, *Radiographics* 8:441-453, 1988.

Grossman RI, Kemp SS, Ip CY, et al: Importance of oxygenation in the appearance of acute subarachnoid hemorrhage on high field magnetic resonance imaging, *Acta Radiol* 139:56-58, 1988.

Hackney DB, Atlas SW, Grossman RI, et al: Subacute intracranial hemorrhage: contribution of spin density to appearance on spin-echo MR images, *Radiology* 165:199-202, 1987.

Haley EC Jr, Kassell NF, Torner JC: The International Cooperative Study on the Timing of Aneurysm Surgery: the North American experience, *Stroke* 23:205-214, 1992.

Hart RG, Easton DJ: Dissections, *Stroke* 16:925-927, 1985.

Hecht-Leavitt C, Gomori JM, Grossman RI, et al: High field MRI of hemorrhagic cortical infarction, *AJNR* 7:581-586, 1986.

Jacobs K, Moulin T, Bogousslavsky J, et al: The stroke syndrome of cortical vein thrombosis, *Neurology* 47(2):376-382, 1996.

Johnston S, Wilson C, Halbach VV, et al: Endovascular and surgical treatment of unruptured cerebral aneurysms: comparison of risks, *Ann Neurol* 48(1):11-19, 2000.

Johnston S, Selvin S, Gress DR, et al: The burden, trends, and demographics of mortality from subarachnoid hemorrhage, *Neurology* 50(5):1413-1418, 1998.

Joshi V, Pawel B, Connor E, et al: Arteriopathy in children with acquired immune deficiency syndrome, *Pediatr Pathol* 7(3):261-275, 1987.

Kassell NF, Torner JC, Haley EC Jr, et al: The International Cooperative Study on the Timing of Aneurysm Surgery: part 1—overall management results, *J Neurosurg* 73:18-36, 1990.

Kassell NF, Torner JC, Jane JA, et al: The International Cooperative Study on the Timing of Aneurysm Surgery: part 2—surgical results, *J Neurosurg* 73:37-47, 1990.

Koc Y, Gullu I, et al: Vascular involvement in Behçet's disease, *J Rheumatol* 19(3):402-410, 1992.

Koeppen AH, Dentiger MP: Brain hemosiderin and superficial siderosis of the central nervous system, *J Neuropathol Exp Neurol* 47:249-270, 1988.

Kushner JM, Bressnman SB: The clinical manifestations of pontine hemorrhage, *Neurology* 35:637-643, 1985.

Lev M, Farkas J, Gemmete JJ, et al: Acute stroke: improved nonenhanced CT detection—benefits of soft-copy interpretation by using variable window sidth and center level settings, *Radiology* 213(1):150-155, 1999.

Liem M, Gzesh D, Flanders AE, et al: MRI and angiographic diagnosis of lupus cerebral vasculitis, *Neuroradiology* 38(2):134-136, 1996.

Macchi PJ, Grossman RI, Gomori JM, et al: High field MR imaging of cerebral venous thromboisis, *J Comput Assist Tomogr* 10:10-15, 1986.

Maldjian J, Listerud J, Moonis G, et al: Computing diffusion rates in T2-dark hematomas and areas of low T2 signal, *AJNR* 22(1):112-118, 2001.

Marks MP, Lane B, Steinberg GK, et al: Hemorrhage in intracerebral arteriovenous malformations: angiographic determinants, *Radiology* 176:807-813, 1990.

Mason WG, Latchaw RE, Yock DH: Spontaneous hemorrhage during cranial computed tomography, *AJNR* 1:266-268, 1980.

Matias-Guiu X, Alejo M, Sole T, et al: Cavernous angiomas of the cranial nerves, *J Neurosurg* 73:620-622, 1990.

Matsubara S, Manzia J, ter Brugge K, et al: Angiographic and clinical characteristics of patients with cerebral arteriovenous malformations associated with hereditary hemorrhagic telangiectasia, *AJNR* 21(6):1016-1020, 2000.

Miyazawa N, Hashizume K., Uchida M, et al: Long-term followup of asymptomatic patients with major artery occlusion: rate of symptomatic change and evaluation of cerebral hemodynamics, *AJNR* 22(2):243-247, 2001.

Morgenstern L, Hankins L, Grotta JC, et al: Anterior choroidal artery aneurysm and stroke, *Neurology* 47(4):1090-1092, 1996.

Norman D, Price D, Boyd D, et al: Quantitative aspects of computed tomography of the blood and cerebrospinal fluid, *Radiology* 123:335-338, 1977.

North American Symptomatic Carotid Endarterectomy Trial Collaborators: Beneficial effect of carotid endarterectomy in symptomatic patients with high-grade carotid stenosis, *N Engl J Med* 325:445-453, 1991.

Ostergaard L, Sorensen A, Chesler DA, et al: Combined diffusion-weighted and perfusion-weited flow heterogeneity magnetic resonance imaging in acute stroke, *Stroke* 31(5):1097-1103, 2000.

Osumi A, Tien R, Felsberg GJ, et al: Cerebral amyloid angiopathy presenting as a brain mass, *AJNR* 16(4 suppl):911-915, 1995.

Pantano P, Toni D, Caramia F, et al: Relationship between vascular enhancement, cerebral hemodynamics, and MR angiography in cases of acute stroke, *AJNR* 22(2):255-260, 2001.

Perl JN, Tkach J, Porras-Jimenez M, et al: Hemorrhage detected using MR imaging in the setting of acute stroke: an invivo model, *AJNR* 20(10):1863-1870, 1999.

Petty G, Engel A, Younge BR, et al: Retinocochleocerebral vasculopathy, *Medicine* 77(1):12-40, 1998.

Pomper M, Miller T, Stone JH, et al: CNS vasculitis in autoimmune disease: MR imaging findings and correlation with angiography, *AJNR* 20(1):75-85, 1999.

Provenzale J, Sorensen A: Diffusion-weighted MR imaging in acute stroke: theoretic considerations and clinical applications, *AJR* 173(6):1459-1467, 1999.

Provenzale J, Allen N: Neuroradiologic findings in polyareritis nodosa, *AJNR* 17(6):1119-1126, 1996.

Reneman L, Habraken J, Majoie CBL, et al: MDMA (Ecstasy) and its association with cerebrovascular accidents: preliminary findings, *AJNR* 21(6): 1001-1007, 2000.

Requena I, Arias M, Lopez-Ibor L, et al: Cavernomas of the central nervous system: clinical and neuroimaging manifestations in 47 patients, *J Neurol Neurosurg Psychiatry* 54:590-594, 1991.

Rigamonti D, Spetzler RF, Medina J, et al: Cerebral venous malformations, *J Neurosurg* 73:560-564, 1990.

Rinne J, Hernesniemi J, Puranen M, et al: Multiple intracranial aneurysms in a defined population: prospective angiographic and clinical study *Neurosurgery* 35(5):803-808, 1994.

Rippe DJ, Boyko OB, Spritzer CE, et al: Demonstration of dural sinus occlusion by the use of NM angiography, *AJNR* 11:199-201, 1990.

Roda JM, Alvarez F, Isla A, et al: Thalamic cavernous malformation, *J Neurosurg* 72:647-649, 1990.

Salgado AV, Furlan AJ, Keys TF: Mycotic aneurysm, subarachnoid hemorrhage, and indications for cerebral angiography in infective endocarditis, *Stroke* 18:1057-1060, 1987.

Schievink W: Spontaneous dissection of the carotid and verebral arteries, *N Engl J Med* 22:898-906, 2001.

Schievink W, Wijdicks E, Parisi JE, et al: Sudden death from aneurysmal subarachnoid hemorrhage, *Neurology* 45(5):871-874, 1995.

Scott WR, New PFJ, Davis KR, et al: Computerized axial tomography of intracerebral and intraventricular hemorrhage, *Radiology* 112:73-80, 1974.

Seeger JF, Gabrielsen TO, Giannotta SL, et al: Carotid-cavernous sinus fistulas and venous thrombosis, *AJNR* 1:141-148, 1980.

Shrier D, Tanaka H, Numaguchi Y, et al: CT angiography in the evaluation of acute stroke, *AJNR* 18(6):1011-1020, 1997.

Sigal R, Krief O, Houtteville JP, et al: Occult cerebrovascular malformations: follow-up with MR imaging, *Radiology* 176:815-819, 1990.

Singer M, Chong J, et al: Diffusion-weighted MRI in acute subcortical infarction, *Stroke* 29(1):133-136, 1998.

Som PM, Patel S, Nakagawa H, et al: The iron rim sign, *J Comput Assist Tomogr* 3:109-112, 1979.

Sorensen A, Copen W, Østergaard L, et al: Hyperacute stroke: simultaneous measurement of relative cerebral blood volume, relative cerebral blood flow, and mean tissue transit time, *Radiology* 210(2):519-527, 1999.

Storen E, Wijdicks E, Crum BA, et al: Moyamoya-like vasculopathy from cocaine dependency, *AJNR* 21(6):1008-1010, 2000.

Suzuki S, Inoue T, Haga S, et al: Stroke due to a fusiform aneurysm of the cervical vertebral artery: case report, *Neuroradiology* 40(1):19-22, 1998.

Thijs V, Lansberg M, Beaulieu C, et al: Is early ischemic lesion volume on diffusion-weighted imaging an independent predictor of stroke outcome? A multivariable analysis, *Stroke* 31(11):2597-2602, 2000.

Thulborn KR, Brady TJ: Iron in magnetic resonance imaging of cerebral hemorrhage, *Magn Res Q* 5:23-38, 1989.

Thulborn KR, Sorensen AG, Kowall NW, et al: The role of ferritin and hemosiderin in the MR appearance of cerebral hemorrhage: a histopathologic biochemical study in rats, *AJNR* 11:291-297, 1990.

Thulborn KR, Waterton JC, Matthews PM, et al: Oxygenation

dependence of the transverse relaxation time of water protons in whole blood at high field, *Biochem Biophys Acta* 714:265-270, 1982.

Tsuruda JS, Shimakawa A, Pelc NJ, et al: Dural sinus occlusion: evaluation with phase-sensitive gradient-echo MR imaging, *AJNR* 12:481-488, 1991.

Ulmer JL, Elster AD: Physiologic mechanisms underlying the delayed delta sign, *AJNR* 12:647-650, 1991.

Wang P, Barker P, Wityk RJ, et al: Diffusion-negative stroke: a report of two cases, *AJNR* 20(10):1876-1880, 1999.

Weingarted K, Zimmerman RD, Deo-Narine V, et al: MR imaging of acute intracranial hemorrhage: findings on sequential spin-echo and gradient-echo images in a dog model, *AJNR* 12:457-467, 1991.

White P, Wardlaw J, Easton V, et al: Can noninvasive imaging accurately depict intracranial aneurysms? A systematic review, *Radiology* 217(2):361-370, 2000.

Yousem DM, Balakrishnan J, Debrun GM, et al: Hyperintense thrombus on GRASS MR images: potential pitfall in flow evaluation, *AJNR* 11:51-58, 1990.

Yuh WTC, Crain MR, Loes DJ, et al: Cerebral ischemia: evaluation with contrast-enhanced MR imaging, *AJNR* 12:631-639, 1991.

Yuh W, Ueda T, Maley JE, et al: Diagnosis of microvasculopathy in CNS vasculitis: value of perfusion and diffusion imaging, *J Magn Reson Imaging* 10(3):310-313, 1999.

Zimmerman RD, Leeds NE, Naidich TP: Ring blush associated with intracerebral hematoma, *Radiology* 122:707-711, 1977.

Zimmerman RS, Spetzler RF, Lee SK, et al: Cavernous malformations of the brain stem, *J Neurosurg* 75:32-39, 1991.

Head Trauma

Traumatic brain injury (TBI) has an incidence of over 500,000 cases per year, and is the leading cause of disability and death in children and young adults in the United States. The annual cost of TBI including direct costs and lost income is estimated to be above $25 billion. It has a peak incidence in 15 to 24 year olds with males being injured two to three times more frequently than females. More indication that the smarter sex will continue to prevail.

Imaging of head trauma has a primary role both in diagnosing the extent of the traumatic injury and in expediently determining the appropriate therapy. The most efficient method of triage for acute trauma remains computed tomography (CT). It is fast and usually very accurate at detecting acute hemorrhage (high density on un-

enhanced scan) (Fig. 5-1). CT is excellent for assessing facial and skull fractures. Neurosurgeons are interested in knowing the precise source of the patient's clinical problems with respect to the trauma. Their most overriding concern is whether there is a treatable lesion. Such lesions could be an epidural hematoma, a large subdural hematoma, or a significantly depressed skull fracture. CT does have some pitfalls of which the radiologist should be aware, particularly during the 12-hour board examination. Not all hemorrhage is high density. Isodense to low density hemorrhages are seen in patients who are severely anemic or in those patients with disseminated intravascular coagulopathy (Fig. 5-2). CT does not easily detect extracerebral hemorrhages of the infratemporal region, subfrontal region, or posterior fossa. It also is less sensitive than magnetic resonance imaging (MR) in detecting diffuse axonal injury and vascular injury.

When trauma is evaluated with CT, imaging should include brain, subdural, and bone windows routinely. The wide window setting aids in separating high-density blood from the high density of bone, and is particularly useful in acute subdural and epidural hematomas, which can be thin and difficult to differentiate from the calvarium. Bone windowing is essential in the search for fractures, as is the combination of coronal and axial images with very thin sections (1.5 mm) particularly of the skull base, temporal bone, orbit, or face (Fig. 5-3).

CLINICAL EVALUATION OF TRAUMATIC BRAIN INJURY

Patients with TBI have been classified into mild, moderate, severe, or very severe brain injury. Mild brain injury is defined as transient loss of or alteration of consciousness, a brief amnestic period of less than 60 minutes, followed by a rapid return to their previous level of consciousness. In moderate brain injury, the al-

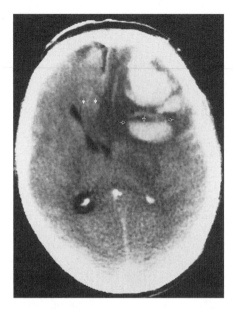

Fig. 5-1 CT of acute traumatic intraparenchymal hematoma. Multiple large intraparenchymal hematomas are identified as high-density mass lesions associated with edema in the frontal region. Subfalcine herniation is present *(arrows)*. Also, note hemorrhagic cavity with blood level that can be observed in traumatic intraparenchymal hemorrhage *(open arrows)*.

teration of consciousness is for more than one hour. Moderate brain injury is also defined in circumstances when the level of consciousness is less than an hour but when the patient has focal neurologic deficits. Posttraumatic amnesia can be up to 24 hours. In severe brain injury the patient is immediately incapacitated with an inability to follow simple commands, associated with coma, motor deficits and pathologic reflexes. Posttraumatic amnesia persists for 1 to 7 days or longer. Very se-

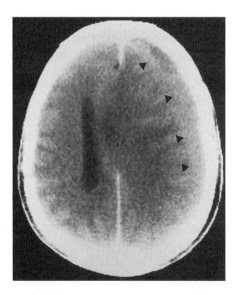

Fig. 5-2 CT of isodense subdural hematoma. Note that the density of the subdural hematoma *(arrowheads)* is similar to that of cortex.

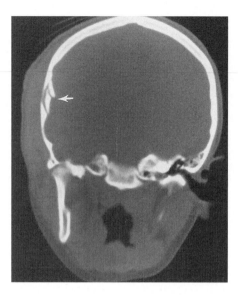

Fig. 5-3 Comminuted fracture of right temporal bone *(white arrow)*.

vere brain injury is associated with immediate unconsciousness or unresponsiveness. The patient is unable to follow simple commands. Many patients die within minutes after the injury. Of those surviving all sustain permanent damage, the degree varying by the magnitude of the injury.

The Glasgow Coma Scale (GCS) was devised to provide a uniform approach to the clinical assessment of patients with acute head trauma. It attempts to assign numeric values (1 to 5) to eye opening, the best motor response, and the best verbal response as a predictor of outcome. Scores of 13 to 15 are considered to correspond to mild injury, 9 to 12 moderate injury, and 8 or lower severe injury. This scale measures levels of arousal and awareness and does correlate with survival and outcome from coma in severe head injury. It may not correlate with long-term prognosis from mild or moderate head injury (a total score of 3 to 4 is associated with a 97% chance of death or persistent vegetative state, whereas a total of 15, the highest score, has normal findings). One issue is the marked heterogeneity of brain lesions in the severe TBI patients, thus individuals with the same GCS could have markedly different outcomes depending upon the nature of the causative lesion.

A frequent issue involves the evaluation of patients with minor head injury (little or no loss of consciousness, GCS 13 to 15). Approximately two thirds of patients with head trauma in the United States are classified as having minor head injury, but less than 10% of these cases have positive CT, and less than 1% require neurosurgery. The following findings in patients with head trauma were associated with positive CT—headache, vomiting, over 60 years of age, drug or alcohol intoxication, deficits in short-term memory, physical evidence of trauma above the clavicles, coagulopathy, and seizure.

Of course, the patient would not be seen in the ER following minor head injury if they were normal (except if they had been to see their neighborhood serpent lawyer).

MR is more sensitive than CT in detecting all the different stages of hemorrhage (i.e., acute, subacute, and chronic but within the first 4 hours, for hyperacute hemorrhage, CT may be more sensitive than low field MR). However, detecting acute subarachnoid hemorrhage is difficult if fluid attenuated inversion imaging (FLAIR) imaging is not performed with the MR exam (Fig 5-4). MR's multiplanar capability enables excellent visualization of the inferior frontal and temporal lobes and the posterior fossa (Fig. 5-5). It is more sensitive than CT in demonstrating diffuse axonal injury (see discussion under Primary Injury) and following this lesion temporally. MR and magnetic resonance angiography (MRA) are the methods of choice for imaging vascular dissection; however, in penetrating wounds of the neck, angiography may be more efficient. MR does not miss the CT-isodense subdural hematoma. It potentially may be difficult to differentiate small amounts of intracranial air from acute hemorrhage (both are hypointense on T2WI). Major drawbacks of MR are the increased imaging time necessary to perform the procedure, the cumbersome nature of imaging and monitoring the trauma patient (particularly one on a ventilator), and the location of most MR centers outside the main hospital or emergency area. It is less sensitive than CT in detecting fractures and other bony lesions. In short, the complete MR evaluation (CMR or the big ca$ino) including FLAIR, diffusion, and gradient echo images enable detection of most of the critical traumatic lesions including ischemia, subarachnoid and intraparenchymal hemorrhage, and nonhemorrhagic shearing injuries. Although MR is more sensitive in most traumatic situations, the ease and speed of CT, and its high sensitivity in detecting treatable lesions, make it, in most circumstances, the imaging modality of choice in the acutely injured patient.

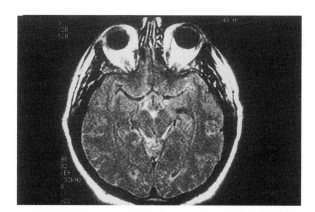

Fig. 5-4 FLAIR of subarachnoid hemorrhage. Note that the cerebrospinal fluid around the midbrain on this FLAIR scan is bright instead of dark. The patient had subarachnoid hemorrhage. Often the ventricular CSF remains dark.

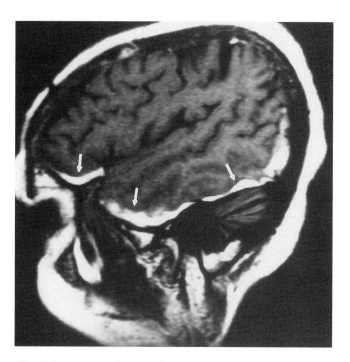

Fig. 5-5 Sagittal T1WI demonstrating inferior frontal and inferior temporal lobe subdural hematoma extending along the tentorium posteriorly (*white arrows*).

Skull films have little role in the triage or care of the patient with significant head trauma. They are useful only to ascertain whether linear skull fractures are present. CT is excellent at demonstrating depressed or comminuted skull fractures; however, fractures parallel to the plane of the scan slice such as those involving the vertex of the skull may be missed. Always assess the scout view from the CT for evidence of fracture or high cervical injury.

At present angiography is indicated to define the anatomy of traumatic fistulas, particularly before therapeutic endovascular obliteration and, in some cases, for diagnosis of vascular dissection and pseudoaneurysm. Another indication for angiography is the question of an expanding hematoma in the neck.

An organized approach to the categorization of head trauma is essential in examining patients undergoing diagnostic imaging. Accurate classification enables prediction of prognosis and institution of appropriate therapeutic management. Open head injury involves the intracranial contents communicating through the skull and scalp. In closed head injury, there is no communication between the intracranial contents and the extracranial environment.

CLASSIFICATION OF INJURY

Traumatic brain damage may be separated into two major categories: (1) primary injury, and its associated primary complications, are directly related to immediate impact damage and (2) secondary complications (not present at the time of injury) resulting from the primary injury over time. Why all the fuss? Well you obviously cannot prevent the primary injury. We know that may not exactly be true. Indeed, one of the author's wives suggested that her 16-year-old wear a helmet when he was learning to drive. Importantly, secondary lesions are preventable or treatable.

Primary Injury

Primary injury is the consequence of brain damage occurring at impact. It may result in contusions of the brain and diffuse axonal injury (DAI). Contusions may be defined as bruises that are associated with petechial hemorrhages, and are the most common primary intraaxial lesion. DAI is produced by stress-induced movements of the head that severely disrupt axons either completely or incompletely. Primary complications involve lesions that are produced at impact and progress over time. These include mass lesions, such as extraparenchymal or intraparenchymal hemorrhage, and brain swelling.

Primary injury can be divided further into focal or diffuse injury. Focal injuries represent contusions and other mass lesions such as epidural or subdural hematomas, which may generate shift of the midline brain structures and herniation with compression of and damage to the brain stem. The simplest form of DAI is concussion, which may be defined as a transient paralysis of neurologic function associated with loss of consciousness occurring at the time of injury. In its fulminant form, there is diffuse disruption of axons throughout the brain, resulting in permanent coma (persistent vegetative state) or death.

Two different mechanisms are principally responsible for primary injury: (1) direct contact between the skull and an object (contact phenomena) and (2) inertial injury resulting from the differential accelerations between white and gray matter. The former is responsible for scalp laceration, skull fractures, intracerebral and extracerebral hematoma, and contusion. Contact phenomena generate stress waves, which create skull base fractures, contusions, and hemorrhages remote from the site of contact. Severe contact injury is associated with subdural hematoma and massive intraparenchymal hemorrhage ("burst" lobe). Inertial injury results in DAI and pure subdural hematoma after shearing of bridging veins.

Secondary Complications

Secondary complications are temporally removed from the original trauma and result in brain injury including raised intracranial pressure (ICP), hypoxia, infection, and infarction secondary to brain herniation.

CORRELATION OF IMAGING AND OUTCOME

Knowledge of the pathophysiologic cascades, which occur after TBI, has been primarily obtained from the study of severe human TBI. Victims of severe TBI are usually monitored invasively, have abnormalities readily visualized on routine CT and MR imaging, and have a high enough mortality rate that the brains can be inspected pathologically. In this population, secondary neuronal damage is known to commonly occur from hemorrhagic complications, raised ICP, diffuse brain edema, hypoxia, and hypotension. Treatment of these mechanisms has resulted in decreased mortality after severe TBI. These mechanisms of secondary injury trigger excitatory amino acid release, generation of free radicals, increase in calcium concentration, cytokine release, caspase (proteases that cleave proteins that induce apoptosis) activation, mitochondrial dysfunction, breakdown of the cytoskeleton, and additional neuronal death. Many of these specific cascades have been targeted with pharmacologic treatments.

Apoptosis is the transcription-dependent method of cell death, which has been shown to occur in numerous physiologic and pathologic conditions. Recent evaluation of human victims of severe TBI who have died has demonstrated the presence of cells undergoing apoptosis.

The development of brain swelling leading to raised intracranial pressure was thought to be related to the inability of the blood vessels to autoregulate generating vascular engorgement and increased vascular volume. Recent information suggests that in the acute period (hours to days) cytotoxic swelling detected by diffusion weighted imaging (DWI) is the most important factor responsible for increased intracranial volume. Vasogenic edema plays little or no role.

Following traumatic head injury there is a transient decrease in high-energy phosphates, which may be related to cerebral ischemia. N-acetyl-aspartate (a neuronal and axonal marker) is reported to be decreased in head injury (in part related to DAI), and this may correlate with outcome.

There are certain predictors of raised ICP and impending death. The state of the mesencephalic cistern is an important predictor of outcome, especially in patients with intermediate GCS. The risk of death in the severely injured patient is increased twofold if the mesencephalic cistern is compressed or obliterated. The risk of elevated ICP is increased threefold if the cistern is obliterated. Subarachnoid hemorrhage also increases the possibility of death twofold. Two thirds of deaths in head injury are associated with acute subdural hematoma and DAI. Ten percent to 42% of patients with severe head injury have normal-appearing CT scans, and elevated ICP develops in 10% to 15% of these patients.

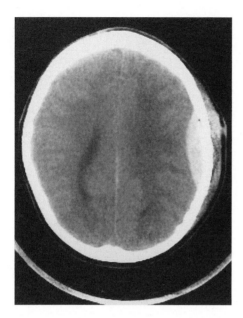

Fig. 5-6   CT of acute epidural hematoma. Note the convex shape of the epidural hemorrhage.

Local reductions in blood flow that do not approach an ischemic threshold have been noted with moderate brain injury whereas ischemia is part of the severe TBI. DWI has been advocated as a method to separate moderate injury (diffusion negative) from more severe injury (diffusion positive).

EPIDURAL HEMATOMA

The potential space between the inner table of the skull and the dura is the epidural space. The most common cause of epidural hematoma is head trauma with skull fracture of the temporal bone (90% of cases) crossing the vascular territory of the middle meningeal artery or vein. In children, the greater elasticity of the skull permits meningeal vascular injury without fracture. Tears of the middle meningeal artery (60% to 90%) or venous structures (middle meningeal vein, venous sinus, or diploic veins) (10% to 40%) result in the extravasation of blood and acute epidural hematoma. The blood appears to have the consistency of dark red jelly. After injury there may be a lucid interval (50% of patients) before deterioration (as opposed to DAI, where coma occurs immediately after the injury). Slower bleeding from the meningeal vein or dural sinus temporally delays symptoms. Chronic epidural hematoma has also been observed. Epidural hematomas are usually biconvex and are the result of the firm adherence of the dura to the inner table and its attachment to the sutures. (Fig. 5-6). Most frequently, these hematomas are observed in the temporal parietal region. When fractures run through

the middle meningeal artery and vein, occasionally a fistula may develop between the two. Pseudoaneurysm of the meningeal artery may also occur. Epidural hematomas of the posterior fossa result from tearing of the venous sinus and may be continuous with the supratentorial and infratentorial space. Epidural hematoma may be associated with child abuse or occur after ventricular decompression of hydrocephalus by shunting (more commonly this produces subdural hematomas). Venous epidural hematoma is most often noted in the pediatric population and carries a lower incidence of skull fracture.

CT reveals a high density extraaxial mass acutely. There may be some low density in the acute hemorrhagic mass, probably representing serum extruded from the clot. In these cases, perform bone window settings to look for fractures and examine the scout image for fractures and upper cervical spine subluxations not visible on axial sections. Chronic epidural hematomas reveal low density and enhancement, and they may be concave. Chronic epidural hematomas must be distinguished from other epidural masses such as infection, inflammation, and tumor, and from subdural lesions such as empyemas.

On MR, the extraaxial hemorrhage has different appearances depending on the interval between the traumatic event and imaging. If imaged shortly after trauma, acute hemorrhage demonstrates low intensity on T2-weighted images (T2WI) and isointensity on T1-weighted images (T1WI), whereas if the hemorrhage is imaged a few days after the incident (subacute hematoma), it is high intensity on T1WI (Fig. 5-7). Intensity is not usually an is-

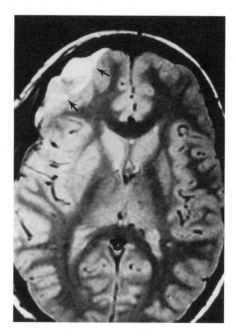

Fig. 5-7   Subacute epidural hematoma. MR (PDWI) of right elliptical collection *(arrows)* in the frontal region. This was high signal on T1WI as well.

sue because the morphology of the extraaxial mass in the setting of acute trauma makes the diagnosis obvious. One may visualize the medial dural margin as a hypointense rim on all pulse sequences. Linear fractures are poorly visualized on MR, but cortical veins and arteries are displaced inward as in any extraaxial lesion.

SUBDURAL HEMATOMA

Hemorrhage into the potential space between the pia-arachnoid and the dura is termed a subdural hematoma. Acute subdural hematomas result from significant head injury and are caused by the shearing of bridging veins (Fig. 5-8). This occurs because of rotational movement of the brain with respect to fixation of these veins at the adjacent venous sinus. The subdural portion of the vein is not ensheathed with arachnoid trabeculae as is the subarachnoid portion and therefore is the weakest segment of the vein. Acute subdural hematomas also occur in the setting of the burst lobe (Fig. 5-9). Intracerebral clot is in direct continuity with the subdural hematoma. Penetrating injury can also result in acute subdural hematoma.

Subdural hematomas are seen in approximately 30% of patients with severe closed head trauma. They may be classified as simple (without associated brain parenchymal injury and complicated (with parenchymal injury). In the latter the subdural component of the lesion is relatively insignificant compared with the parenchy-

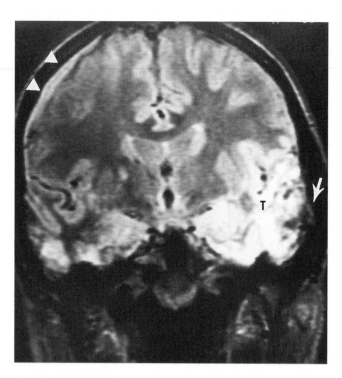

Fig. 5-9 Burst temporal lobe with associated acute subdural hematoma. Coronal PDWI image demonstrates evidence of acute subdural hematoma *(white arrow)* associated with the burst left temporal lobe *(T)*. A subacute subdural hematoma *(arrowheads)* is identified over the right convexity. There is also evidence of contusion of the right temporal lobe.

mal injury. Because of this, acute subdural hematoma is associated with a 35% to 50% mortality rate, and of those who survive most have functional limitations. Simple acute subdurals have a better prognosis than complicated ones. The worst prognosis in acute subdural hematoma occurs in head trauma secondary to motorcycle injury (Harley-Davidson syndrome), in postoperative patients with ICP greater than 45 mm Hg, in cases with the presence of severe mass effect, in rapid accumulation of the subdural, in delay (greater than 4 hours) in evacuation of significant lesions, and in patients older than 65 years (impaired regenerative capacity). Control of ICP is very important.

The patient population can be divided into two groups on the bases of age and mechanism of injury. In young patients (<40 years) the usual cause of injury is an automobile accident associated with a small acute subdural hematoma. In elderly patients, the most common injury is the fall. After a lucid interval, there is neurologic deterioration. The subdural hematomas in this group of patients are larger because of the generalized loss of brain parenchyma. In addition, discovery may be delayed (2nd term in office). Subdurals and epidurals are contrasted in Table 5-1 (compare Fig. 5-6 with Fig. 5-8).

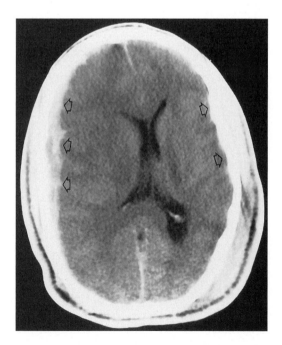

Fig. 5-8 CT demonstrates bilateral acute subdural hematomas *(open arrows).* Lesions are concave medially.

Table 5-1   Subdural vs. Epidural

Type	"Bleeder"	Acute Shape	Chronic Shape	Nontraumatic Etiologies
Subdural Hematoma	Bridging veins	Crescentic	Elliptical	Aneurysm Amyloid Menkes Disease Postshunt Coagulopathy
Epidural Hematoma	Middle meningeal artery, middle meningeal vein, venous sinus	Biconvex	Crescentic	Postoperative

The temporal nomenclature of the subdural hematoma is arbitrary. Lesions occurring at the time of the initial injury are considered acute, although symptoms may take up to a few days to become manifest. Those lesions becoming symptomatic between approximately 3 days to 3 weeks are subacute whereas those lesions that are diagnosed after 3 weeks are considered chronic (Fig. 5-10). The subacute and chronic subdural hematomas have a predilection for elderly persons with tethered veins from atrophy as the brain shrinks inward. These lesions may grow large and produce herniation. Subdural hematomas generally arise over the convexities but can also occur in the posterior fossa, middle cranial fossa, and/or along the tentorium (Fig. 5-11).

Imaging Characteristics of Subdural

Acute subdural hematomas on CT are high-density concave extracerebral masses. The thickness of the hematoma can range from pencil-thin to large and can at times be convex inwardly. Rarely, acute subdural hematomas have been reported to be isodense or low density on CT. This may be correlated with significant anemia (hemoglobin level 8 to 10 g/dL), disseminated intravascular coagulopathy, or tears in the arachnoid membrane, leading to dilution of the red blood cells with cerebrospinal fluid (CSF).

Subacute and chronic subdural hematomas may display layering with dependent cells and cellular debris and an acellular supernatant (Fig. 5-12). The dependent portion is of higher density than the supernatant. The lesion usually is concave but occasionally may be convex when chronic, with inward displacement of the convexity veins, which course along the inner surface of the arachnoid. As opposed to epidural hematomas, subdural hematomas are not confined by the cranial sutures. Intermediate window settings on CT are useful in separating thin subdural hematomas from the bony calvarium. This is obviously not an issue with MR.

Subacute subdural hematomas may be isodense to low density; however, mass effect is common in significant hematomas. Subacute and chronic subdural lesions enhance (but who gives contrast in this setting). This is caused by the vascularization of the subdural membranes (usually being thick outside and thin inside), formed between 1 to 3 weeks following injury, which enhance. These vessels are not associated with tight junctions. They leak contrast and may easily be torn resulting in various blood products and growth of the subdural. Repeated episodic bleeding results in fibrous septations and compartments within the hematoma. Delayed enhanced

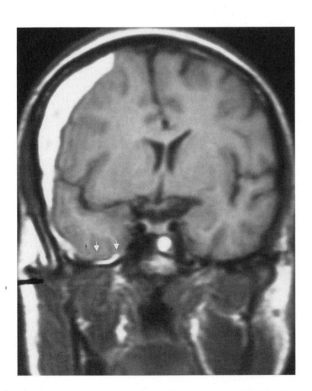

Fig. 5-10   Right subacute subdural hematoma on T1WI. Observe the extension to the floor of the right middle cranial fossa *(arrows).*

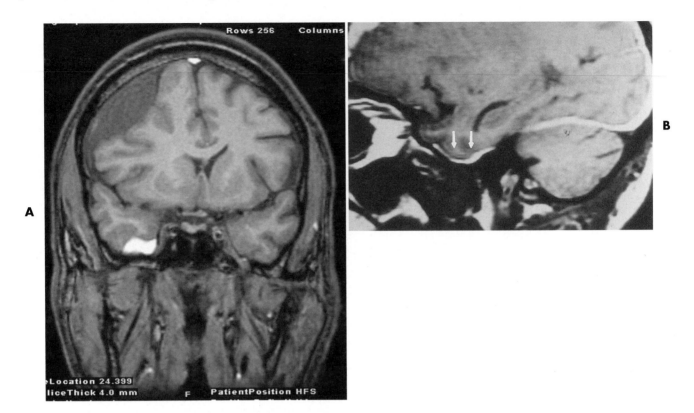

Fig. 5-11 Infratemporal subdural hematoma. **A,** This small subacute hematoma along the base of the temporal lobe would be invisible on CT because of beam hardening artifact, partial volume averaging, and reduced contrast sensitivity. Large right-frontal epidural is also present. **B,** Different patient with a similar finding: The sagittal T1WI allows detection of the small subdural hematoma along the floor of the middle cranial fossa and the extension over the tentorium and along the occipital lobe. The subdural turns the corner and extends up to the parietal region.

scans may reveal contrast layering in extracerebral collections. Hematomas may also occur between the leaves of the tentorium. Tentorial subdurals fade out laterally and stop abruptly at the medial margin of the tentorium (Fig. 5-13).

Chronic subdural hematomas are usually low density (Fig. 5-14). Levels observed in these lesions may be caused by rebleeding into the chronic subdural collection. There may be no history or an insignificant history of head trauma. Other contributing conditions include coagulopathy, alcoholism, increased age, epilepsy, and surgery for ventricular shunts. Over 75% of chronic subdurals occur in patients over 50 years of age. Chronic subdurals occur in infants as a result of birth injury, vitamin K deficiency, child abuse, or coagulopathy. Rarely, chronic subdural hematomas may ossify or contain fat.

It is easy to be fooled on CT in patients with isodense subdural hematomas, particularly if the lesions are bilateral. In such a situation both lateral ventricles are compressed and may appear symmetric. There are two keys to this difficult diagnosis. First, look carefully at the brain parenchyma and note whether it is appropriate for the

patient's age. Large subdurals usually occur in older patients who have prominent sulci. Anytime that sulci are poorly visualized (especially in your mother-in-law) think subdural. Second, look at the gray matter-white matter interface. If this is visualized and buckled inward from its normal position, then consider an extraaxial mass (Fig. 5-15). Infiltrating intraaxial masses obliterate the interface. Contrast is helpful in isodense subdural by visualizing the inwardly displaced cortical veins.

On MR, subdural hematomas follow the intensity of blood. Acute subdural hematomas are isointense on T1WI and hypointense on T2WI (Fig. 5-16 and see also Figs. 5-11 and 5-12). Subacute subdural hematomas generally have high intensity on T1WI and T2WI. However, over time, the high intensity on the T1WI gradually diminishes and the extracerebral collection becomes isointense to brain. Such a collection can be confused with an extracerebral process such as a subdural empyema. Both would enhance, and clinical correlation would be important. Chronic subdural hematomas rarely have significant amounts of hemosiderin deposition except after recurrent hemorrhages (Fig. 5-17).

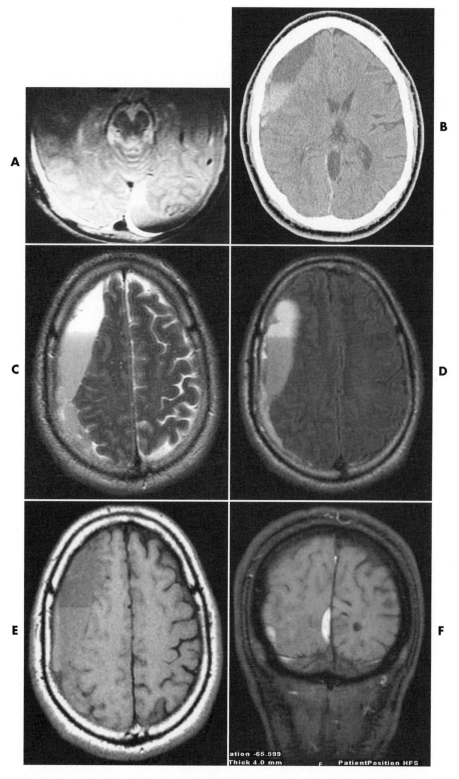

Fig. 5-12 **A,** T2WI of layered left subdural hematoma. High intensity and lower intensity gradients inferiorly can be identified in this layered subdural hematoma. (You are correct; there is also a subdural hematoma on the right.) **B,** This poor chap shows a blood fluid layer over the right frontal convexities on the ED CT. **C,** The clinicians rushed him to the MR where axial T2WI **(C), D,** FLAIR, and **E,** T1WI show the layering of the serum anteriorly (dark on T1WI, bright on T2WI) and the deoxyhemoglobin posteriorly (isointense on T1WI, dark on T2WI). **F,** The coronal fat suppressed T1WI scan also showed an interhemispheric subacute hematoma (bright on T1WI).

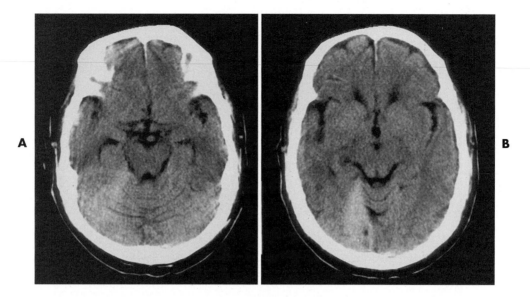

Fig. 5-13   CT of tentorial subdural hematoma. Observe the high density on the left (inferior) image **(A)** is lateral to the medial high density on the right (superior) image **(B).** That is why it is called a TENTorium. The hemorrhage is contained within the leaves of the tentorium.

SUBDURAL HYGROMA

Collections of fluid within the subdural space that have similar imaging characteristics to CSF, although they may have higher protein, are termed hygromas. They result from trauma and either can occur acutely as a tear in the arachnoid membrane with CSF collecting in the subdural space, or can result from the degradation of a subdural hematoma. Problems may arise in distinguishing subdural hygromas from atrophy (Fig. 5-18; also see Fig. 6-1). An anatomic approach is useful in this situation. The superficial cortical veins lie within the cortical sulci in close approximation to the underlying pia and overlying the arachnoid and dura. The veins first

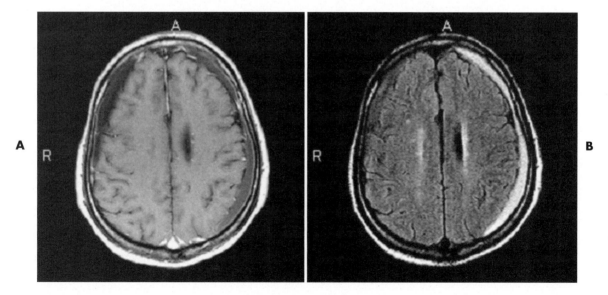

Fig. 5-14   MR of chronic subdural hematomas. **A,** T1WI of bilateral chronic subdural hematomas of different intensities secondary to protein content. **B,** FLAIR image shows the left-sided subdural to be high intensity and the right to be iso- to high intensity. The intensity differences reflect the protein content of the fluid.

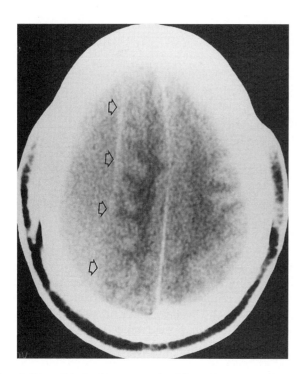

Fig. 5-15 CT of white matter buckling. *Open arrowheads* at right identify the edge of an isodense subdural hematoma. Note the significant amount of white matter buckling with preservation of the gray-white interface.

penetrate the arachnoid and then the inner layer of dura to reach the sagittal sinus. In atrophy, the arachnoid remains closely applied to the dura whereas the cortex shrinks away from the dura. The cortical veins are tethered in their course to the sagittal sinus, first by the arachnoid and then by the dura. In subdural hygroma, the collection is between the dura and the arachnoid, forcing the arachnoid inward along with the cortical veins. Atrophy is present if you can see cortical veins (flow voids on MR) on the surface of the brain and extending across the fluid collection at some distance from the sagittal sinus. Veins on the calvarial surface can be identified in atrophy. These veins lie just beneath the arachnoid membrane. If the cortical veins are not detected crossing the fluid collection, then most likely it is a subdural hygroma. MR makes the diagnosis of hygroma a slam-dunk being able to discern high protein (FLAIR) and small amounts of residual hemorrhage (gradient echo).

Inward displacement of cortical veins and associated mass effect by the hygroma differentiates it from atrophy but not from an arachnoid cyst, which has been postulated also to have (in some cases) a traumatic cause. Arachnoid cysts but not hygromas remodel bone. Subdural hygromas may be unilateral or bilateral. It is impossible on imaging at times to distinguish chronic subdural hematoma from chronic subdural hygroma, especially because the former may evolve into the latter.

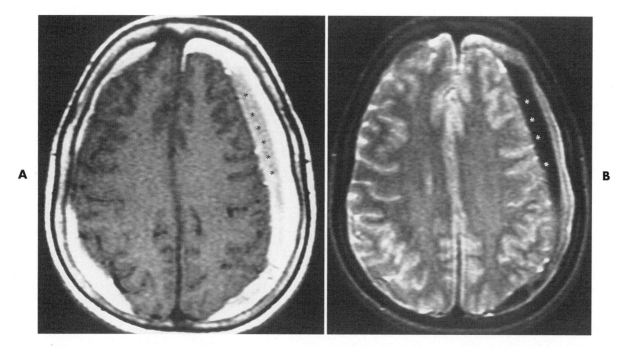

Fig. 5-16 Subdural hematomas. **A,** T1WI demonstrates acute and subacute hematoma. Acute hematoma is isointense to gray matter (*asterisks*) whereas the subacute hematoma is high intensity on T1WI and is bilateral. **B,** T2WI shows marked hypointensity of the acute subdural hematoma and the higher intensity of the subacute subdural hematoma. Acute subdural hematoma in both cases is marked by *asterisks*. Subacute subdural hematoma is peripheral.

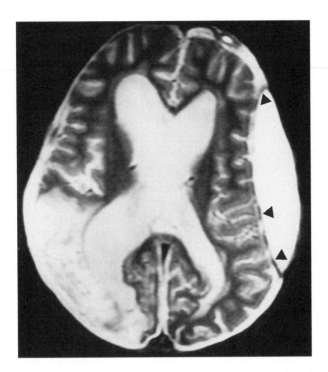

Fig. 5-17 T2WI reveals hemosiderin, seen as marked hypointensity *(arrowheads)* in a chronic subdural hematoma that has become convex. There is evidence of contralateral subdural hematoma and infarction secondary to old trauma.

HEMORRHAGIC CONTUSION

Contusions are brain parenchymal bruises where petechial hemorrhage (because of the gray matter vascularity) is visualized in the cortex. The hemorrhage may extend bidirectionally into the white matter, subdural, and subarachnoid space. Focal edema is associated with the hemorrhage. Contusions may be wedge shaped and involve the crowns of the gyri. Two mechanisms of injury include direct trauma (where the head is not in motion) resulting from depressed skull fracture, and acceleration (e.g., boxing injury) or deceleration (e.g., car accident where the head strikes the dashboard) of the skull. In the case of head motion there is an increased propensity for cortical injury adjacent to roughened edges of the inner table of the skull, along the floor of the anterior cranial fossa, the sphenoid wings, and petrous ridges. The inferior, anterior, and lateral surfaces of the frontal and temporal lobes are particularly vulnerable (Fig. 5-19). Contusions occurring at the site of impact are referred to as coup contusions whereas diametrically opposed contusions are termed contrecoup contusions. These terms are controversial, but we like them because they are simple and connote location (our usage) as opposed to mechanism (purist rationale [we ain't no purists for sure] for discouraging use of the terms). Contusion of brain may also occur along the falx and tentorium. Intermediate-coup contusions are those of the deeper structures of the brain. Gliding contusions are those occurring along the superior parasagittal mar-

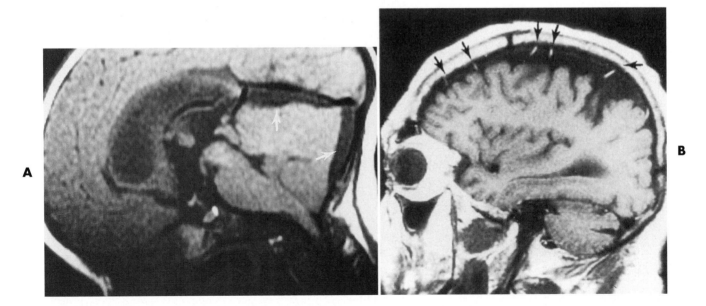

Fig. 5-18 **A,** Sagittal T1WI of acute subdural hygroma *(white arrows)* with mass effect and compression of the fourth ventricle. **B,** Cortical veins in cerebral atrophy. Note the high intensity of the bridging cortical veins on this sagittal T1WI *(arrows)*. The high intensity is secondary to flow-related enhancement. Observe that they cross the extracerebral space of the parietal region. Because these veins are identified coursing through this space, there is no subdural hygroma, and the patient (a politician) has cortical atrophy.

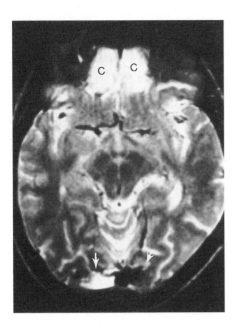

Fig. 5-19 T2WI of inferior frontal contusions *(C)*. Also, note contrecoup injury in occipital regions *(white arrows)*.

gin of the cerebral hemispheres particularly in the frontal lobes (Fig. 5-20). Initially contusions may be difficult to detect on CT with relatively small hypodense cortical/subcortical abnormality. Hemorrhage may be subtle. These lesions become more prominent and obvious over days. On CT, high density is noted at the site of injury. Focal regions of low density representing edema surround the acute hemorrhage. On T2WI acute hemorrhagic contusions are hypointense and surrounded by

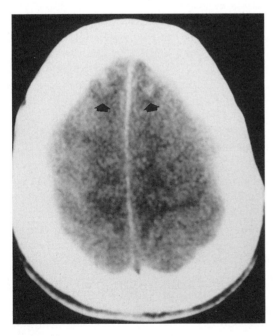

Fig. 5-20 Gliding contusion along the superior margin of the brain bilaterally *(arrows)*.

high intensity. Gradient echo images are more sensitive for detecting these focal hemorrhagic areas as regions of low signal abnormality. Thus, these lesions are similar in appearance to the hematomas described previously.

FLAIR may prove particularly useful with detection of the edema following acute contusion.

In the patient with significant head injury occasional blood-fluid levels may be identified in the brain parenchyma (See Fig. 5-1). Patients with this injury tend to have a poorer outcome. Hemorrhage into contused necrotic brain is responsible for the blood-fluid levels. These lesions are associated with extensive edema, most likely caused by the large parenchymal necrosis. Blood-fluid levels can be seen early after trauma and have also been associated with coagulation defects.

PENETRATING INJURIES

Penetrating injuries produce lacerations of the brain, and they are associated with bullet wounds, stab wounds, or bone fragments (Fig. 5-21). Long-term follow-up of these lesions demonstrates resolution of the hemorrhage, residual hemosiderin, and loss of brain substance (Fig. 5-22). The dura and the surface of the brain may be ad-

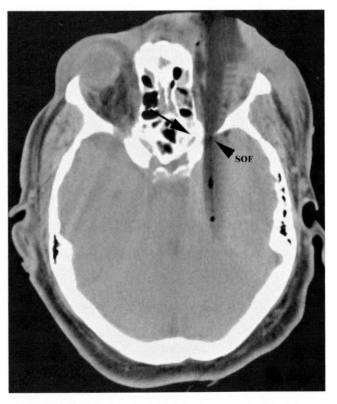

Fig. 5-21 CT of penetrating knife injury through the roof of the orbit. Note the tract through the superior orbital fissure (SOF with *arrowhead*) crossing the path of the optic nerve *(arrow)* and into the medial temporal lobe. These patients should be followed to rule out the development of infection and pseudoaneurysm.

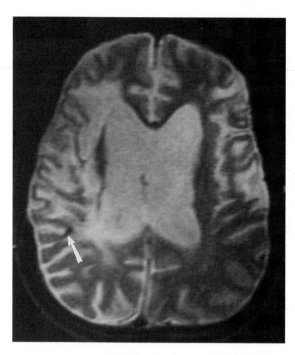

Fig. 5-22 T2WI demonstrating malacic changes in the brain bilaterally with dilatation of the ventricles and hemosiderin from the residual traumatic hemorrhage *(arrow).*

hered to each other by fibroglial scar, a source of seizures in posttraumatic patients.

With any penetrating wound of the head or neck there is the risk of injury to vital structures traversed by the penetrating object. In the brain, the risks are indisputable. Damage to brain parenchyma is deleterious to normal function (except perhaps in the case of malpractice attorneys). Injury to blood vessels in the brain and neck can lead to dissection, acute hemorrhage, and pseudoaneurysms with delayed hemorrhage. With respect to penetrating wounds of the brain, CT is the most efficient method for triage of these emergency patients. It can determine whether a surgical lesion exists (e.g., acute hematoma) and the amount and location of foreign bodies lodged in the brain. In all cases, infection is an ever-present danger. Intracranial air (pneumocephalus) implies a communication between the intracranial compartment and an extracranial air-filled space such as a sinus. Rarely, air can be trapped in the brain with a "ball-valve mechanism" so that the air cavity gradually expands and compresses normal brain. This is termed a pneumatocele.

Vascular dissection of the great vessels of the neck has been previously discussed (Chapter 4) but should be considered in all patients with blunt trauma or penetrating wounds of the neck. Focal neurologic signs after a latent period following head and neck trauma should suggest vascular injury and require MR evaluation. Other sequelae of traumatic vascular injury include laceration,

occlusion, pseudoaneurysm, and arteriovenous fistula (Fig 5-23). Puncture wounds of the neck may be associated with the development of vertebrovenous fistulas, which can be delayed in appearance (weeks to months) (see Fig. 5-23 D). Patients may have neck bruits. The diagnosis is made on vertebral angiography, which reveals diffuse filling of the paravertebral venous plexus in the arterial phase. These fistulas can be treated by balloon occlusion, usually with preservation of the vertebral artery. In cases of acute penetrating neck wounds, perform a simple aortic arch injection and attempt to visualize all the great vessels of the neck. If a question arises concerning a particular vessel, selective catheterization can be done. This procedure is rapid and can determine whether there has been significant arterial injury or whether there is an active bleeding site. MR is generally more cumbersome because the patient usually needs close monitoring and may not be particularly cooperative.

DIFFUSE AXONAL INJURY (DAI)

The cause of this important lesion has been recently elucidated. The less classically oriented reader can skip to the next paragraph, but those with perspicacity will enjoy the brief historical interlude. The first pathologic description of a particular histologic aspect of diffuse axonal injury (DAI), axonal retraction balls, was made by Santiago Ramón y Cajal in 1907. Holbourn in 1943 and 1945 hypothesized that degeneration in white matter resulted from shearing of nerve fibers at the time of original injury. In 1956, Strich made the association of white matter degeneration with a chronic vegetative state after severe head injury. In 1982, Generelli experimentally produced traumatic coma and histologic lesions similar to those seen in fatal injuries by angular acceleration.

DAI is the injury responsible for coma and poor outcome in most patients with significant closed head injury resulting from automobile accidents (although it can result from other kinds of trauma as well). At the time of injury the stress induced by rotational acceleration/deceleration movement of the head causes some regions of the brain to accelerate or decelerate faster than other regions resulting in axonal injury. Axons may be completely disrupted together with adjacent capillaries, or some axons may be incompletely disrupted, the so-called injury-in-continuity. Patients with severe DAI are unconscious from the moment of injury and may remain in a persistent vegetative state or be severely impaired. In the most severe cases of DAI specific anatomic structures are characteristically involved and are sites of maximum shear strain (Box 5-1). These regions include the body (usually lateralized to one side and on the inferior surface) and the splenium (most common location) of the corpus callosum. The unbending falx, which is

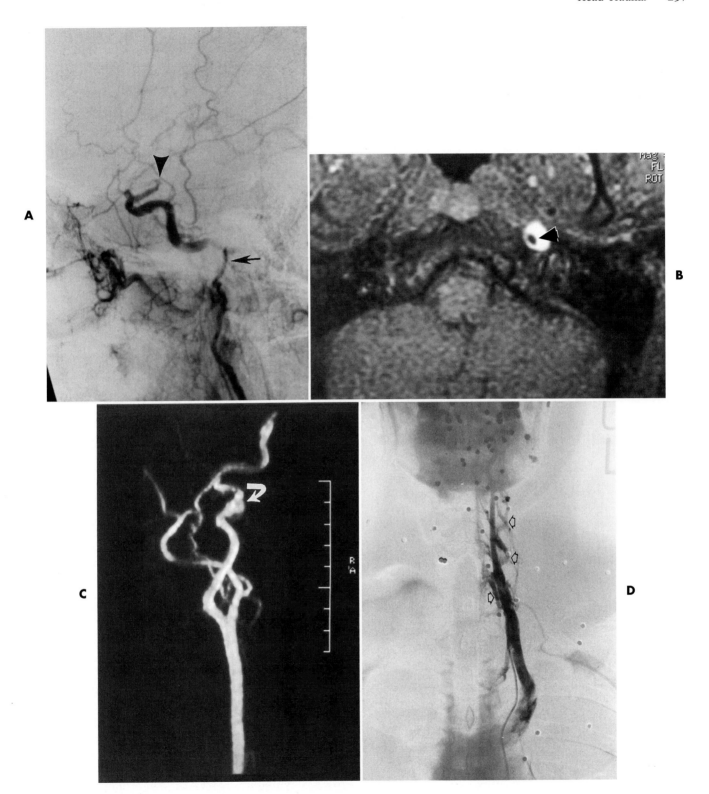

Fig. 5-23   **A,** Lateral common carotid arteriogram with irregularity and narrowing of the distal portion of the extracranial carotid artery *(arrow).* The intracranial portion of the internal carotid *(arrowhead)* fails to fill above the ophthalmic artery because of a large embolus, which is a complication of the extracranial vascular dissection. **B,** Fat suppressed T1WI shows a wall hematoma in the dissected left internal carotid artery *(arrowhead on residual lumen).* **C,** A pseudoaneurysm of the high cervical internal carotid artery on the MIPPED MRA is denoted by the *white curved arrow.* **D,** Vertebrovenous fistula. Left vertebral arteriogram with filling of the vertebral artery and epidural venous plexus *(open arrows).* Notice the pellets from the shotgun injury.

broader posteriorly, prevents the cerebral hemispheres from moving across the midline whereas anteriorly the falx is shorter so that the brain can transiently move across the midline. The fibers of the splenium and posterior corpus callosum are thus under greater risk of shearing than the anterior fibers. If the lesion is midline, you may note disruption of the septum pellucidum and ventricular blood secondary to disruption of subependymal veins and capillaries. Lesions are also seen in the dorsolateral quadrant of the rostral part of the brain stem, adjacent to the superior cerebellar peduncle. Brain stem DAI tends to be associated with more profound injury. It may be inconspicuous on initial CT. Diffuse damage to other axons, including those in the internal capsule and subcortical white matter, may also be present. The most severe DAI results in lesions in all of these locations. The mildest form tends to have lesions at the white/gray junctions of the frontal and temporal lobes. In 11% of patients with DAI, associated intracranial hematoma can be identified. Pathologic findings depend on length of survival. Within days axonal swelling (retraction ball) develops, within weeks microglial clusters are observed, and within months wallerian degeneration takes place. Rotationally induced shear-strain may also produce cortical contusion and lesions in the deep gray matter.

CT is not nearly as sensitive as MR in detecting DAI in the brain. On CT, one may visualize focal punctate regions of high density that may be surrounded by a collar of low-density edema (Fig. 5-24). These are hemorrhagic shearing injuries most likely associated with complete axonal disruption. On CT, it may be difficult to detect nonhemorrhagic shearing injury. MR reveals high intensity on T2WI/FLAIR, which may or may not be associated with hemorrhage (Fig. 5-25). Eighty percent of DAI lesions are nonhemorrhagic. Both hemorrhagic and nonhemorrhagic shearing injuries are easily visualized by MR. Lesions may be ovoid or elliptic, with the long axis parallel to fiber bundle directions. Gradient echo images further enhance our sensitivity in detecting hemorrhagic shearing injury. DWI may be positive (Fig. 5-25 J and K) This can be detected in cases of mild head injury and normal CT. It can be an explanation for the postconcussion syndrome (see following sec-

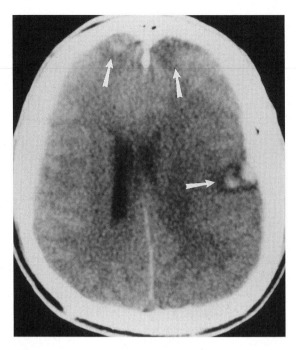

Fig. 5-24   CT reveals multiple high-density regions surrounded by areas of low density *(arrows)*. This is what hemorrhagic DAI looks like on CT.

tion). SPECT scanning seems particularly sensitive in detecting abnormalities in mild head injured patients with postconcussion syndrome.

A variant of the axonal injury is a rent at the pontomedullary junction or in the cerebral peduncles produced by severe hyperextension. Associated injuries include fractures of the petrous bone, fracture dislocations of the cervical vertebrae, and ring fractures of the foramen magnum.

OUTCOME

Cognitive deficits resulting from TBI include decreased speed in information processing, poor attention, concentration, and memory, and impaired logical reasoning skill, as well as more focal deficits including impairment of language or constructional abilities. (Residual function still enables one to qualify to be a radiology department chairperson.) Reports indicate that following head injury, patients may display extended and persistent postconcussive symptoms (subjective complaints including difficulty concentrating, memory problems, headache, or dysequilibrium, and is associated with deficits in information processing or neuropsychologic testing). The correlation of head injury symptoms and their sequelae is controversial yet there is growing evidence that head injury even mild in nature may have greater consequences than previously assumed. Indeed, TBI is now considered

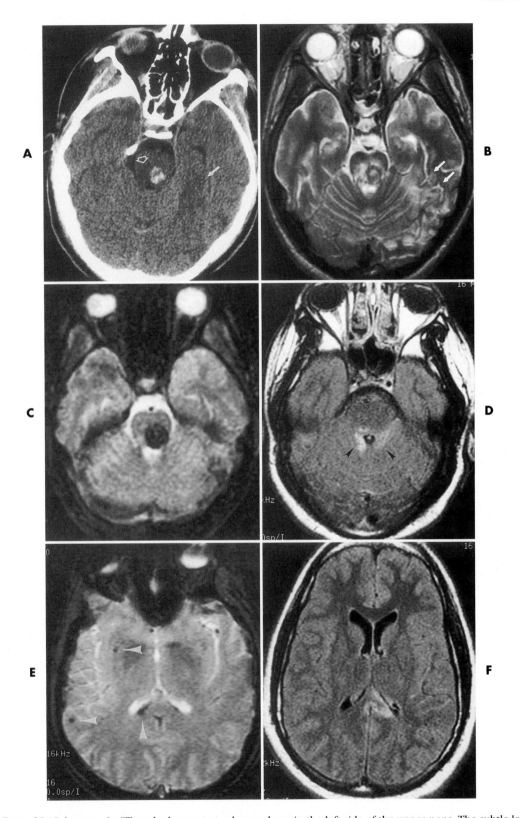

Fig. 5-25   Gallery of DAI damage: **A,** CT study demonstrates hemorrhage in the left side of the upper pons. The subtle low density more posteriorly *(open arrows)* is edema extending to the midbrain tectum. A left temporo-occipital contusion is also present *(arrow)*. **B,** The same section on T2WI shows evidence of diffuse edema of the brainstem and the involvement of the cortex of the posterior temporal lobe seen as higher intensity *(arrows)*. **C,** Blooming of the hemorrhagic byproducts is typical of a gradient echo performed at the same level. **D,** High intensity *(arrowheads)* on the FLAIR scan corresponds to tears in the superior cerebellar peduncles leading to the brainstem. **E,** Typical DAI lesions along the corpus callosum and gray-white junctions are pointed out by Dr. Arrowhead. **F,** Hemorrhage in the cisterns around the splenium and injury to the splenium itself are seen on this FLAIR scan.

Illustration continued on following page

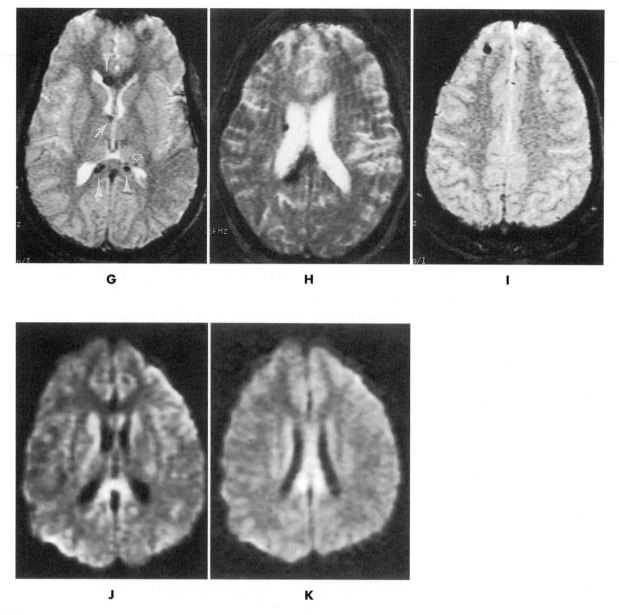

Fig. 5-25 *Continued.* **G,** Gradient echo image demonstrates multiple shearing injuries in the genu and splenium of the corpus callosum *(arrowheads)*. A spot in the pulvinar *(open arrow)* and the foramen of Monro *(arrow)* completes the DAI picture (at least Fig. 5-25 G). **H,** The top of the splenium is a frequent site for DAI and often accounts for concomitant intraventricular hemorrhage. **I,** Subcortical foci high up are typically seen as well. **J** and **K,** DWI high intensity (seen here in the splenium) may be present due to T2 shine through or because of cellular death and myelin disruption.

a risk factor in the development of Alzheimer disease. Apolipoprotein E genotype increases the susceptibility in patients subjected to head trauma to progress to Alzheimer disease.

There are many reports describing loss of brain parenchymal volume as the sequelae of TBI in particular structures including the caudate nucleus, corpus callosum, hippocampus, fornix, and thalamus. These injuries result in enlargement of the ventricles (width of the third ventricle, bicaudate span of the lateral ventri-

cles, area of lateral ventricles, total ventricular volume, temporal horn or ventricular/brain ratio). Posttraumatic thalamic atrophy has been correlated with the presence of cortical and subcortical (but nonthalamic) lesions. This suggests that such traumatic lesions may be responsible for transneuronal degeneration.

Injury to the hippocampus and dilatation of the temporal horn have been correlated with verbal memory (hippocampus) and intellectual outcome (temporal horn). The bottom line is that head injury results in brain volume loss and that in cases where you observe premature diffuse parenchymal loss think previous TBI (also HIV, radiation therapy, and so on).

The prevalence of cavum septum pellucidum has been observed to be increased in professional boxers and soccer players. This has been related to repetitive head trauma with tearing of the septal walls and secondary CSF dissection of the septi forming a cavum.

SECONDARY COMPLICATIONS HERNIATION SYNDROMES

As you know, the brain lives in a rigid container (the skull) and is compartmentalized by inelastic dural reflections (tentorium, falx cerebri, falx cerebelli). Swelling or mass lesions, when large enough, force the brain from one compartment into another location. Herniations of brain from one region to another can produce both brain and vascular damage. Five basic patterns can be encountered (Fig. 5-26): inferior tonsillar and cerebellar herniation, superior vermian herniation (upward herniation), temporal lobe herniation, central transtentorial herniation, and subfalcine herniation.

When mass effect occurs in the posterior fossa, the fourth ventricle is compressed, producing obstructive hydrocephalus (dilated temporal horns are particularly sensitive indicators of such hydrocephalus). The cerebellar tonsils and cerebellum are usually pushed inferiorly through the foramen magnum. On CT or MR, the obvious finding is absence of the normal CSF around the foramen magnum and the presence of tonsillar and cerebellar tissue in that site (Fig. 5-27). In circumstances where there is superior cerebellar mass effect (or when supratentorial mass effect is rapidly reduced such as in immediate decompression of a larger subdural hematoma), forces are exerted, producing upward herniation of the vermis (Fig. 5-28). Cerebellar tissue can be identified obliterating the superior vermian and quadrigeminal cisterns.

To understand transtentorial herniation, one must appreciate the anatomy around the tentorium. The medial surface of the temporal lobe (uncus, hippocampus) slightly overhangs the tentorium. The brain stem passes through the tentorial hiatus. The posterior cerebral artery circles the midbrain in the crural and ambient cistern just above the tentorium and medial to the temporal lobe. The anterior choroidal artery courses between the dentate gyrus of the temporal lobe and medial edge of the tentorium. Cranial nerve III originates from the midbrain, crosses the interpeduncular cistern below the posterior cerebral artery and above the superior cerebellar artery, and is medial to the uncus.

Transtentorial herniation is produced by mass lesions whose vector force is directed inferiorly and medially.

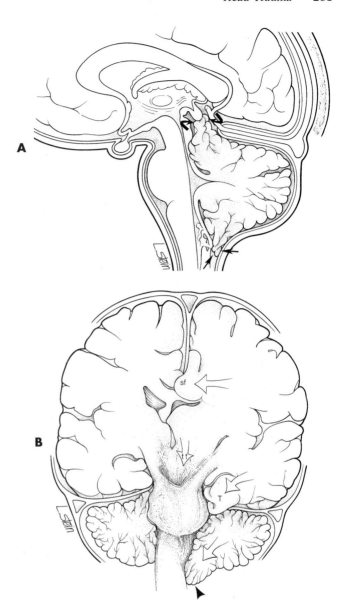

Fig. 5-26 Herniations of the brain. **A,** Sagittal diagram of cerebellar herniation with *curved arrows* demonstrating upward herniation of the superior cerebellum and superior vermis, with the *straight arrows* demonstrating tonsillar and inferior vermian herniation. **B,** Coronal diagram with temporal lobe herniation *(T),* central transtentorial herniation *(tt),* tonsillar herniation *(arrowhead),* and subfalcine herniation *(sf).* Lines of force are demonstrated by large *open arrow.* Note the pressure on the brain stem from these herniation patterns.

The temporal lobe shifts over the tentorium, compressing to a variable extent the oculomotor nerve (with ipsilateral pupillary dilatation), the posterior cerebral and anterior choroidal arteries, and the midbrain. Compression of the contralateral cerebral peduncle against the edge of the tentorium by a supratentorial mass produces ipsilateral motor weakness and is termed Kernohan-Woltman notch phenomenon (false localizing sign). It is

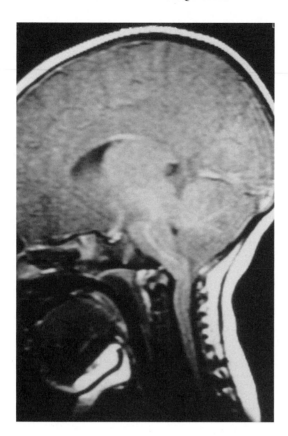

Fig. 5-27 Sagittal T1WI in a child with massive cerebral swelling. Notice the herniation of the cerebellum into the foramen magnum.

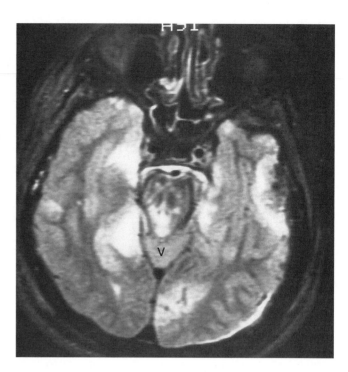

Fig. 5-28 Axial T2WI with obliteration of the superior vermian cistern by the superior vermis *(V)* that is being elevated because of a posterior fossa hemorrhage. Also, note bilateral evidence of contusion and left posterior subdural hematoma. Notice that the brain stem with abnormal signal from DAI is compressed bilaterally by swollen temporal lobes. There is also high intensity in the left medial occipital region, perhaps from compromise of the posterior cerebral artery secondary to herniation.

associated with high intensity on T2WI in the midbrain from compression and occlusion of perforating arteries at the tentorial notch. Vascular compression of the posterior cerebral and anterior choroidal arteries by the medial temporal lobe against the tentorium or by the petroclinoid ligament results in infarction in these vascular distributions. Attention should be directed to the posterior cerebral artery distribution and diencephalon, respectively, for evidence of ischemia or infarction in situations where supratentorial mass effect is significant (Fig. 5-29). Direct central caudal transtentorial herniation forces the diencephalon and midbrain down through the incisura. Herniation can result in small hemorrhages in the brain stem. Hemorrhages in the tegmentum of the pons and the midbrain caused by uncal herniation have been termed Duret's hemorrhages.

Another herniation pattern is the subfalcine variety. Here, supratentorial mass effect can be directed medially, causing the cingulate gyrus to shift beneath the falx cerebri with possible compression of the anterior cerebral artery or internal cerebral veins (Fig. 5-30).

Herniations are not difficult to recognize on CT or MR. It is important to look at the foramen magnum and to make sure that space is adequate. Move progressively su-

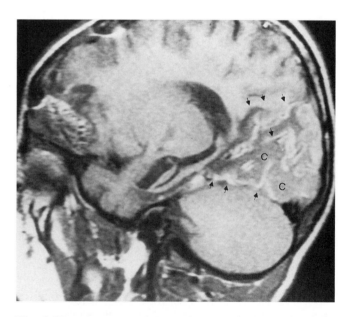

Fig. 5-29 Transtentorial herniation secondary to trauma produced this hemorrhagic cortical infarction *(arrows)* in the distribution of the posterior cerebral artery on this sagittal T1WI. Low intensity is noted in the edematous swollen cortex *(c)*.

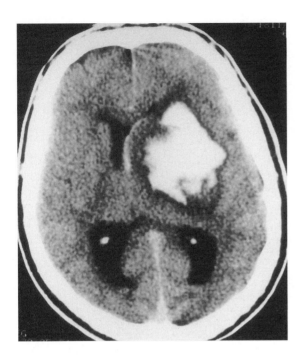

Fig. 5-30   CT of acute hemorrhage with mass effect and subfalcine herniation. The left lateral ventricle is shifted across the midline. There is compression of the foramen of Monro with dilatation of the occipital horns bilaterally.

periorly (or inferiorly from the vertex if you are someone who likes starting on top) while assessing the regions just mentioned. It is important to alert the physicians caring for the patient with incipient herniation even if the patient does not appear to be in acute distress.

VASCULAR DISSECTION

Extracranial dissection may result from direct or indirect trauma or manipulation of the neck. Dissection may also occur intracranially. Extracranial dissection usually occurs within the media or adventitia. Patients with dissection may have an underlying vascular abnormality including fibroelastic thickening, fibromuscular hyperplasia, cystic medial degeneration, Marfan syndrome, Ehlers-Danlos syndrome, homocystinuria, or syphilis. In extracranial dissection neurologic deficits most often occur days, weeks, or months after the injury and are the result of embolic events. Rarely is there immediate complete obliteration of the vascular lumen. In such a case neurologic deterioration is related to the absence of circle of Willis collateral circulation. Treatment is controversial but may include anticoagulation, particularly in nonpenetrating injuries. Vascular dissection is an overlooked cause of stroke in the young patient.

Intracranial dissection may be the result of trivial trauma, blunt trauma, or penetrating injury to the in-

tracranial vessel. The most common intracranial dissection is of the supraclinoid carotid midway between the cavernous carotid and bifurcation and may extend into the anterior or middle cerebral artery. It is a subintimal lesion that results in significant luminal reduction and immediate neurologic deficit. Intracranial vascular dissection can produce subarachnoid hemorrhage. It is associated with a very high mortality rate (75%). Other vascular lesions associated with trauma are pseudoaneurysms, which may occur in any dissected vessel, both intracranially and extracranially, and are prone to bleed.

On angiography the diagnosis of extracranial dissection is obvious, with an irregular, narrowed carotid exhibiting a tapered configuration (string sign) (see Fig. 5-23). As opposed to aortic dissection, the double lumen sign is rarely present. Clots may be visualized in the distal portion of the vessel. The tapered appearance is also noted intracranially. In many instances, complete occlusion of the intracranial vessel is observed. These dissections occur in the internal carotid and not in the common carotid. The catheter should be kept in the common carotid so that confounding factors such as catheter-induced spasm and iatrogenic dissection are eliminated from consideration.

On MR the residual lumen of the vessel and the hemorrhage into the wall of the vessel are seen (see Fig. 5-23). In most cases the hemorrhage appears as high intensity (subacute hematoma). This high signal intensity most likely relates to the temporally delayed relationship of the dissection to the symptoms and subsequent imaging.

Trauma to the cavernous carotid artery can produce direct communication between the carotid artery and cavernous sinus. The fistula may drain from the cavernous sinus into the orbit through the superior and inferior ophthalmic veins, posteriorly through the petrosal veins, inferiorly through veins around the foramen ovale, or superiorly through middle cerebral veins. If there is cortical venous drainage, patients are particularly prone to intraparenchymal hemorrhage. "Stealing" of blood by the fistula can occur in the carotid artery on the ipsilateral side. Venous hypertension with edema can occur, particularly if venous drainage is compromised. This situation has been noted in the brain stem in patients with such fistulas. Other complications of carotid cavernous fistula include subarachnoid hemorrhage, intraorbital hemorrhage, epistaxis, otorrhagia, glaucoma, dilated conjunctival vessels, progressive proptosis, ophthalmoplegia, and increased ICP. The diagnostic findings and angiographic workup of this condition are discussed in Chapter 10.

Fat embolism is associated with long-bone fracture or its surgical repair. Patients present with confusion a few days after the initial injury. Diffuse white matter ischemia results either directly from massive fat embolism or in combination with hypoxia from pulmonary complica-

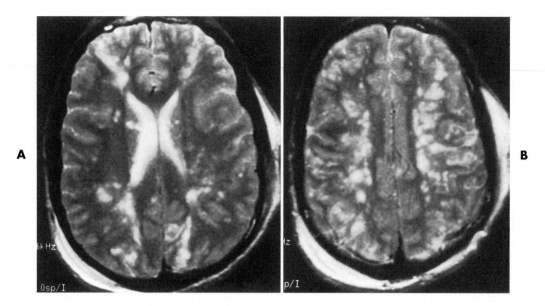

Fig. 5-31 Sequelae of fat emboli. **A,** This young soul (literally now) had fat emboli after manipulation for treatment of an acute hip fracture. Note the stunning array of punctate areas of high intensity on the T2WI in watershed (**A**) and subcortical (**B**) zones. The course was complicated by cardiopulmonary collapse from the event.

tions (Fig. 5-31). DWI is positive because of the extensive small vessel ischemia and hypoxia.

BRAIN DEATH

Brain death is defined as the irreversible cessation of all cerebral and brain stem functions. The absence of cerebral blood flow (from increased ICP) is generally accepted as a definite sign of brain death (although we have had some fellows with blood flow who we swore were brain dead possessing absent cephalic reflexes, suck reflex intact, Throckmorton, and hyperflatulence). In the clinical setting of absence of spontaneous respirations, no brain stem reflexes, and a flat EEG, serial EEG, or radionuclide perfusion studies (SPECT, ^{99m}Tc HMPAO) confirm the diagnosis of brain death. MR criteria include (1) transtentorial and foramen magnum herniation, (2) absence of the intracranial vascular flow void, (3) poor gray/white matter differentiation, (4) no intracranial enhancement, (5) intravascular enhancement (carotid artery), and prominent nasal and scalp enhancement (hot nose sign). Absence of the cerebral flow on time-of-flight (TOF) MR angiography (MRA) has also been reported to be specific to brain death.

CHILD ABUSE

Radiologists must display increased sensitivity to the diagnosis of child abuse. Caffey first recognized this in

1946 in children with long-bone fractures and chronic subdural hematomas. Attention should be directed to the presence of skull fractures, particularly depressed fractures with a history of "mild trauma," fractures that cross the midline, and those involving the occiput without a known significant event. The detection of any of these fractures should raise the possibility of child abuse. Bone window settings are important with CT to detect such fractures. Shaken baby syndrome is caused by sudden acceleration-deceleration forces in the process of violent shaking. There may be little evidence of external injury but retinal hemorrhages (intraretinal and preretinal) are present in many instances associated with subdural (particularly interhemispheric) hematomas and/or subarachnoid hemorrhage. Contusions and diffuse cerebral swelling are also noted (Fig. 5-32). Hematomas in the upper cervical spinal cord have been described. The abused child can have epidural, subdural, subarachnoid, intraparenchymal, and intraventricular hemorrhages as well as DAI. MR is useful in determining the ages of these lesions by noting the various stages of blood products (acute, subacute, and/or chronic). Other common clinical features include seizures, ecchymoses, vitreous hemorrhage, and hemiparesis. Box 5-2 lists the central nervous system abnormalities associated with the shaken baby syndrome.

Global ischemia from strangulation, smothering, aspiration, or other conditions generating hypoxia produces distinctive CT findings. There is loss of the gray-white junction and generalized low density of the cerebral cortex (Fig. 5-33). The basal ganglia may show high or low density. The cerebellum is more resistant to

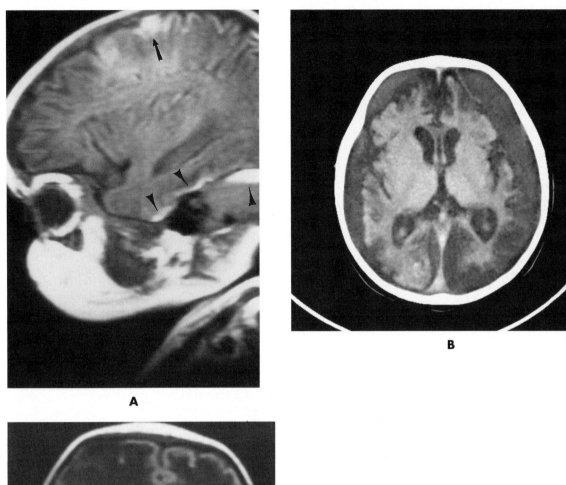

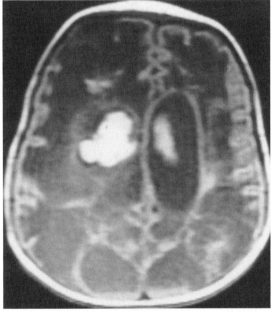

Fig. 5-32   Child abuse. **A,** Sagittal T1WI demonstrating gyral contusion *(arrow)* and floor of middle cranial fossa and tentorial subdural hematomas *(arrowheads).* **B,** Chronic subdural hema-tomas bilaterally and encephalomalacia are the sequelae of long-standing child abuse. The emotional damage is as devastating as the physical damage. **C,** T1WI of repeated traumatic events in a child. Note multiple cystic areas throughout the brain with some central high intensity *(hemorrhage).*

hypoxia and therefore demonstrates normal density in this situation. This starkly contrasts with the cerebrum, which reveals diffusely low density. In rare instances, the white matter may appear high density. MR can reveal diffuse cerebral swelling with loss of the normal

sulci. Hypoxic injury from global oligemia has been classified into three patterns. In pattern I the lesions are confined to the watershed zones, in pattern III lesions involve the cortex and basal ganglia diffusely, and pattern II has some combinations of I and III. Contrast en-

Box 5-2 Shaken Baby Syndrome

SKELETAL

Skull fracture (diastatic, communinuted, linear)
Vertebral compression fracture, fracture dislocation, disc space narrowing, spinous process fracture
Cervical spinal cord hematoma

BRAIN INJURY

Contusion
Diffuse cerebral swelling
Subdural (interhemispheric)
DAI
Subarachnoid hemorrhage
Epidural
Intraventricular hemorrhage

ORBIT

Retinal hemorrhage
Vitreous hemorrhage

hancement has been observed in the globes in pattern III because of disruption of the blood-ocular barrier.

The result of significant cerebral insults from repeated traumatic events is the malacic atrophic brain with or without collections of hemorrhages in different compartments and of varying ages (see Fig. 5-32).

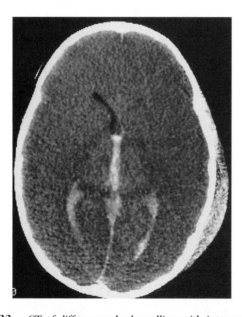

Fig. 5-33 CT of diffuse cerebral swelling with intraventricular hemorrhage. Loss of differentiation on CT between gray and white matter and the inability to visualize basal ganglionic structures are features of hypoxic insult to the brain. Intraventricular hemorrhage is noted in the third and lateral ventricles.

SKULL FRACTURE

There are several types of common skull fractures: (1) linear, (2) diastatic, (3) comminuted, and (4) depressed. Linear skull fractures alone have little clinical significance. Associated lesions, including contusion, shearing injury, or extracerebral collection, which are demonstrated on MR/CT, are far more consequential. Depressed fractures are usually comminuted and can produce underlying brain damage. Comminuted fractures commonly have a depressed fragment. It is important for the radiologist to comment on the extent of the depression (usually defined in relation to the thickness of the skull table), and associated brain injury. Attention should be focused on open fractures, and fractures through air filled sinuses which increase the risk of intracranial infection. Longitudinal fractures of the temporal bone have a high correlation with temporal lobe injury.

In children, most linear fractures heal in time whereas in adults evidence of these fractures is present for years after injury, although the margins are less distinct. When the dura is torn with the skull fracture, the arachnoid can insinuate itself into the cleft of the fracture. Rarely, the pulsations of the CSF enlarge the cleft between the fracture fragments, producing either linear widening of the fracture margins or multiloculated cysts with smooth, scalloped margins. This appearance has been termed a "growing fracture" or "leptomeningeal cyst" and is seen most commonly in children.

FACIAL AND ORBITAL TRAUMA

CT is the most efficient imaging modality for visualizing facial fractures. Axial and coronal images are essential for detecting the full extent of the injury and should be performed with thin sections (3 mm or less). The approach that we take is to describe all the fractures seen on CT and the associated soft tissue injury. Certain classic fracture eponyms have attained historical notoriety and at times are useful in describing what tends to be a complex of fractures. The limitation of such description is the imprecision at indicating associated soft tissue and hemorrhagic components. We will cover just a few of the more common fractures.

Signs of facial and orbital trauma include soft tissue swelling about the face or orbit, and fluid and blood in the maxillary or paranasal sinuses. In orbital fractures, note the location of the fracture, its extent, whether muscle or fat is entrapped in the fracture site, and associated orbital hemorrhage including subperiosteal hematomas. In the orbit, the most common fracture is the so-called blowout fracture resulting from a direct (blunt) injury resulting in fracture of the orbital wall and decompres-

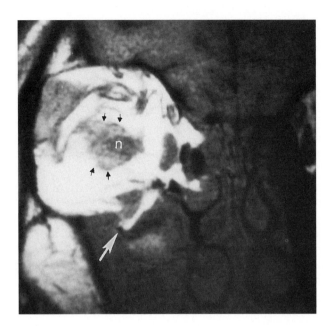

Fig. 5-34   Optic nerve sheath hematoma. Coronal T1WI with nerve sheath hematoma *(arrows)* around optic nerve *(n).* Notice the orbital floor fracture *(large arrow)* and the opacified maxillary sinus.

sion of the orbital contents. This can involve the orbital floor, with the fracture usually through the orbital plate of the maxilla medial to the infraorbital groove (Fig. 5-34). The fracture is commonly hinged on the medial side, appearing on coronal CT as a "trapdoor," or, if the fracture splits the floor, as a "bomb-bay door." Medial orbital blowout fractures involve the lamina papyracea of the ethmoid bone. Rarely the blowout can occur upward into the frontal sinus. Besides entrapped tissue, air may be noted in the orbit (orbital emphysema), and air fluid levels in the involved sinuses. This can be an excellent indicator of a subtle ethmoidal fracture. Blowout floor fractures are associated with enophthalmos, diplopia, (on upgaze), and ocular injuries but generally do not involve the orbital rim. Focus on the rectus muscles and orbital fat, which may be displaced through the fracture site. At times (particularly in children), this can result in entrapment syndromes with limitation of movement of the globe. Entrapment can cause a Volkmann-type of ischemic contracture secondary to ischemia and fibrosis. Hematomas involving the orbital muscles can also produce limitations in range of motion. Involvement of the orbital rim indicates a more severe injury. This is particularly true when it is the superior rim that would be associated with intracranial injury (particularly in children). The weakest portion of the roof is near the superior orbital fissure and optic foramen. As children pneumatize their paranasal sinuses, the incidence of orbital floor fractures increases.

A direct blow to the maxillary sinus can cause a "blow-in" fracture, with elevation of the orbital floor into the orbit. These fractures cause proptosis and restrict ocular motility. These injuries require surgical intervention. Blow-in fractures with superior orbital rim fractures are associated with frontal lobe contusion and epidural hematoma. The Lewinsky fracture (a delicatessen of a near-fatal injury—in the "blow-in blow-out" category) endemic in Washington, D.C. associated with Peyronies disease, confabulation, apraxia of language, and lip biting results in a severe disability, loss of stature (both national and international—except perhaps in France or Brazil).

Ocular trauma can result in perforation of the globe and ocular hypotony (flat tire sign) (Orbit Chapter picture) (Fig. 10-18). Double perforation (anterior and posterior) is associated with a poor prognosis. Ocular hypotony should not be confused with a second posterior perforation. Hemorrhage can occur within the anterior chamber (hyphema) and vitreous. Increased density can be observed in these locations on CT acutely. Ophthalmologic evaluation in the face of hyphema is limited and imaging is helpful to discern the extent of orbital injury. Other injuries involving the globe include foreign bodies, cataract, lens dislocation, or retinal or choroidal detachment. Retinal detachment points to the optic nerve whereas choroidal detachment is biconvex and does not extend to the optic nerve. Choroidal hemorrhage may appear as a globular high-density mass. Always identify the lens on CT in cases of trauma. Orbital/facial trauma can cause rapid equatorial expansion of the globe, which tears the zonular fibers anchoring the lens. The lens may sublux (partial tear) or dislocate (complete circumferential tear). Decubitus films showing lens mobility are useful to reveal a complete dislocation.

Orbital hemorrhage can occur in the intraconal space, within the nerve sheath (subdural), in the extraconal space, subperiosteal, and sub-Tenons' (between the sclera and Tenons' capsule, which is a fibrous membrane adjacent to the orbital fat). Retrobulbar hemorrhage occurring within the intraconal space appears as a four-leaf clover on coronal images. Extraconal hemorrhage tends to be linear. Sub-Tenons' hemorrhage conforms to the shape of the globe and extends from the ciliary body to the optic nerve. Subperiosteal orbital hemorrhage is rare and can produce displacement of the globe and proptosis. The orbital roof is the most common location and they are seen predominantly in children and young adults. Occasionally these lesions may not resolve but evolve into hematic cysts (cholesterol granuloma). Fracture of the orbital roof can predispose to pseudomeningocele (Fig. 5-35). CT can be problematic with a variety of density patterns whereas MR can reveal methemoglobin (high intensity), which is helpful to differentiate this result from previous trauma.

MR can have a special role in detecting optic nerve sheath hematomas (see Fig. 5-34). These tend to be more obvious on MR than on CT. Diagnosis is important be-

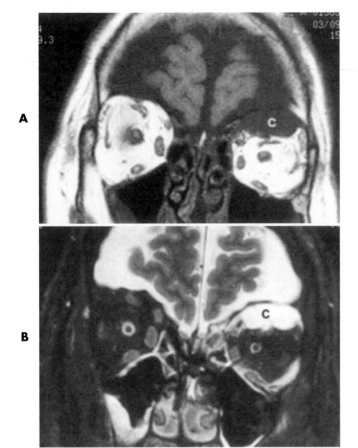

Fig. 5-35 Complication of an old orbital roof fracture. **A,** Meningocele *(c)* is present in the right superior orbit compressing the superior rectus muscle. While a resolving hematoma/seroma could look similarly, the corresponding **(B)** CT showed the communication with the subarachnoid space.

cause vision can be rapidly lost and operative nerve sheath decompression can be restorative. On MR, hemorrhage can be observed along the nerve sheath, which may be swollen and irregular. On CT, the nerve sheath complex may be enlarged. Orbital hemorrhage on CT reveals a haziness in the low-density orbital fat.

The zygomatic arch can be fractured alone or as part of the zygomaticomaxillary complex (tripod) fracture, which includes (1) fracture of the lateral wall of the orbit, usually as diastasis of the zygomaticofrontal suture; (2) fracture of the inferior orbital rim and floor, at times injuring the infraorbital nerve; and (3) fracture of the zygomatic arch. The zygoma can be displaced posteriorly and medially, causing difficulty with the normal motion of the jaw. When this occurs, the lateral wall (at times the anterior and posterior walls as well) of the maxillary sinus is involved (the fourth foot in the tripod) in addition to the floor of the orbit. "Simple" fractures are those without displaced fragments whereas "complex" ones are associated with displaced and rotated fracture frag-

ments that may produce secondary airway or vascular injury.

Naso-Orbital-Ethmoid Complex Fracture (Facial Smash)

This is an injury involving direct trauma to the midface and nasal bones. Concerns include telecanthus (widening of the interorbital distance due to rupture of the medial canthal ligament), transection of the nasolacrimal system associated with epiphora or lacrimal mucocele, and CSF rhinorrhea.

LeFort has classified maxillary fractures into three basic forms based on laboratory experiments on skulls (Fig. 5-36). Classically, all LeFort fractures are symmetric and bilateral, and involve the nasal region and the pterygoid plates. A LeFort I (transmaxillary fracture) refers to a fracture that extends around both maxillary antra, through the nasal septum and the pterygoid plates. The maxilla is free from the rest of the facial bones (floating palate) and is usually displaced posteriorly. LeFort II, or pyramidal fracture, starts at the bridge of the nose and extends obliquely lateral to the nasal cavity, traversing the medial wall of the orbit, the floor of the orbit, the inferior orbital rims, the maxillary antra, and the pterygoid plates. It results in disarticulation (usually posteriorly) of the nose and maxilla from the remainder of the face (the "sat-on" facial appearance). In the LeFort III fracture (cranial-facial separation) the nose, zygoma, and maxilla are disarticulated from the skull. The fracture lines run from the nasofrontal area across the medial, posterior, and lateral orbital walls, the zygomatic arch, and through the pterygoid plates. Such a fracture is very uncommon but can be seen in cases of severe head injury. Finally, combinations of the tripod and LeFort I, II, or III fractures can occur.

TRAUMATIC CRANIAL NERVE INJURY

This can occur following head trauma and knowledge of the anatomy is useful in the search for the lesion. Cranial nerves 1 through 7 are the ones most often involved. The first cranial nerve can be injured in frontal brain trauma or from surgery. This can result in anosmia, which is no picnic (but does have value in public toilets). Fractures of the optic canal/orbital apex or direct injuries to the optic nerve result in visual loss (injury to the optic nerve). Chiasmal injury has been reported secondary to mechanical, contusive, compressive, or ischemic mechanism. Fractures of the sella, clinoid processes, or facial bones should initiate a careful evaluation of the chiasm. Also, be mindful of associated pituitary stalk or hypothalamic injuries. Third nerve injury can occur in the absence of skull fracture from rootlet

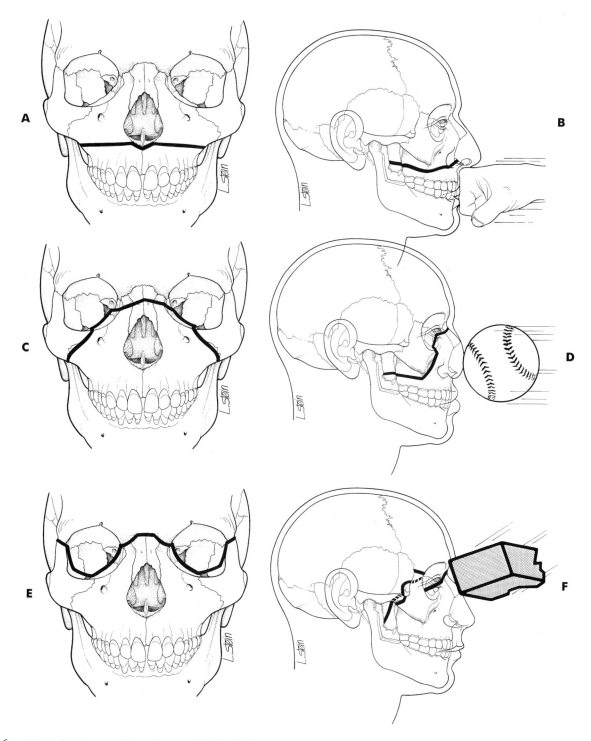

Fig. 5-36   LeFort fractures. **A,** Frontal view of LeFort I fracture. **B,** Lateral view of LeFort I fracture. **C,** Frontal view of LeFort II fracture. **D,** Lateral view of LeFort II fracture. **E,** Frontal view of LeFort III fracture. **F,** Lateral view of LeFort III fracture.

avulsion and distal fascicular damage secondary to a shearing type mechanism. Hemorrhage at the exit site of the nerve and high intensity in the midbrain can be identified by MR. Horner syndrome from traumatic carotid dissection should also be considered with third nerve symptoms. Isolated fourth nerve palsy is common

(43% of trochlear lesions) following traumatic injury. The trigeminal nerve can be injured in orbital floor, roof, or apex fractures. The sixth cranial nerve can be affected from basilar skull fractures (Dorrello's canal), and injuries to the cavernous sinus/orbital apex or secondary to increased intracranial pressure. It has been acknowledged to be particularly sensitive to injury because of its long intracranial course. The seventh nerve can also be injured from longitudinal or transverse fractures through the petrous bone involving the facial canal (also see Chapter 12). Associated injuries will include disruption of the ossicular chain, hematotympanum, otorrhea, and injury to the temporomandibular joint. Mechanisms of posttraumatic peripheral facial nerve palsy include transection, extrinsic compression by bony fragment or hematoma, or intrinsic compression within the facial canal secondary to intraneural hematoma/edema. Enhancement has been identified in the distal intrameatal segment, labyrinthine and proximal tympanic segments and in the geniculate ganglion.

SUGGESTED READINGS

Adams JH, Brierley JB, et al: The effects of systemic hypotension upon the human brain. Clinical and neuropathological observations in 11 cases, *Brain* 89(2):235-268, 1966.

Anderson CV, Wood DM, et al: Lesion volume, injury severity, and thalamic integrity following head injury, *J Neurotrauma* 13(1):35-40, 1996.

Antonyshyn O, Gruss JS, et al: Blow-in fractures of the orbit, *Plastic & Reconstructive Surg* 84(1):10-20, 1989.

Aoki N: Chronic subdural hematoma in infancy, *J Neurosurg* 73:201-205, 1990.

Ashikaga R, Araki Y, et al: MRI of head injury using FLAIR, *Neuroradiology* 39(4):239-242, 1997.

Awwad EE, DiIorio G, Martin DS, et al: Fat deposition adjacent to chronic subdural hematoma: CT demonstration, *J Comput Assist Tomogr* 14:665-667, 1990.

Ball WS Jr: Nonaccidental craniocerebral trauma (child abuse): MR imaging, *Radiology* 173:609-610, 1989.

Bartynski WS, Wang AM: Cavernous sinus air in a patient with basilar skull fracture: CT identification, *J Comput Assist Tomogr* 12:141-142, 1988.

Bhimani S, Virapongse C, Sabshin JK, et al: Intracerebral pneumatocele: CT findings, *Radiology* 154:111-114, 1985.

Bigler ED, Blatter DD, et al: Hippocampal volume in normal aging and traumatic brain injury, *AJNR* 18(1): 11-23, 1997.

Bixler RP, Ahrens CR, Rossi RP, et al: Bullet identification with radiography, *Radiology* 178:563-567, 1991.

Boyko OB, Cooper DF, Grossman CB: Contrast-enhanced CT of acute isodense subdural hematoma, *AJNR* 12:341-343, 1991.

Cajal SR: *Degeneration and regeneration of the nervous system,* vol 2, New York, 1959, Hafner (translated and edited by RM May).

Cecil KM, Hills EC, et al: Proton magnetic resonance spectroscopy for detection of axonal injury in the splenium of the corpus callosum of brain-injured patients, *J Neurosurg* 88(5):795-801, 1998.

Chambers EF, Rosenbaum AE, Norman D, et al: Traumatic aneurysms of cavernous internal carotid artery with secondary epistaxis, *AJNR* 2:405-409, 1981.

Chan KH, Mann KS, Yue CP, et al: The significance of skull fracture in acute traumatic intracranial hematomas in adolescents: a prospective study, *J Neurosurg* 72:189-194, 1990.

Chen CJ: Intraocular contrast enhancement in Adams pattern III hypoxic brain damage: MRI, *Neuroradiology* 42(1):54-55, 2000.

Chirico PA, Mirvis SE, et al: Orbital "blow-in" fractures: clinical and CT features, *J Comput Assist Tomogr* 13(6):1017-1022, 1989.

Choi SC, Muizelaar JP, Barnes TY, et al: Prediction tree for severely head-injured patients, *J Neurosurg* 75:251-255, 1991.

Costeff H, Groswasser Z, Goldstein R: Long-term follow-up review of 31 children with severe closed head trauma, *J Neurosurg* 73:684-687, 1990.

Fueredi GA, Czarnecki DJ, Kindwall EP: MR findings in the brains of compressed-air tunnel workers: relationship to psychometric results, *AJNR* 12:67-70, 1991.

Gennarelli TA, Spielman GM, Langfitt TW, et al: Influence of a type of intracranial lesion on outcome from severe head injury, *J Neurosurg* 56:26-36, 1982.

Gennarelli TA, Thibault LE, Adams JH, et al: Diffuse axonal injury and traumatic coma in the primate, *Ann Neurol* 12:564-574, 1982.

Gentry LR, Godersky JC, Thompson B, et al: Prospective comparative study of intermediate-field MR and CT in the evaluation of closed head trauma, *AJNR* 9:91-100, 1988.

Gentry LR, Thompson B, Godersky JC: Trauma to the corpus callosum: MR features, *AJNR* 9:1129-1138, 1988.

Grabowski EF, Zimmerman RD. Disseminated intravascular coagulation and the neuroradiologist, *AJNR* 12:344, 1991.

Gudeman SK, Kishore Pulla RS, Becker DP, et al: Computed tomography in the evaluation of incidence and significance of post-traumatic hydrocephalus, *Radiology* 141:397-402, 1981.

Han JS, Kaufman B, Alfidi RJ, et al: Head trauma evaluated by magnetic resonance and computed tomography: a comparison, *Radiology* 150:71-77, 1984.

Hanstock CC, Faden AI, et al: Diffusion-weighted imaging differentiates ischemic tissue from traumatized tissue, *Stroke* 25(4):843-848, 1994.

Hartling RP, McGahan JP, Lindfors KK, et al: Stab wounds to the neck: role of angiography, *Radiology* 172:79-82, 1989.

Haydel M, Preston C, et al: Indications for computed tomography in patients with minor head injury, *N Engl J Med* 13(343):100–105, 2000.

Heros RC: Cerebellar infarction resulting from traumatic occlusion of a vertebral artery, *J Neurosurg* 41:111-113, 1979.

Holbourn AHS: Mechanics of head injuries, *Lancet* 2:438-441, 1943.

Holbourn AHS: The mechanics of brain injuries, *Br Med Bull* 3:147-149, 1945.

Howard MA, Gross AS, Dacey RG, et al: Acute subdural hematomas: an age-dependent clinical entity, *J Neurosurg* 71:858-863, 1989.

Ishige N, Pitts LH, et al: The effects of hypovolemic hypotension on high-energy phosphate metabolism of traumatized brain in rats, *J Neurosurg* 68(1):129-136, 1988.

Ishii K, Onuma T, et al: Brain death: MR and MR angiography, *AJNR* 17(4):731-735, 1996.

Ito J, Marmarou A, et al: Characterization of edema by diffusion-weighted imaging in experimental traumatic brain injury, *J Neurosurg* 84(1):97-103, 1996.

Jend HH, Jend-Rossmann I: Sphenotemporal buttress fracture, *Neuroradiology* 26:411-413, 1984.

Jeret JS, Mandell M, et al: Clinical predictors of abnormality disclosed by computed tomography after mild head trauma [see comments], *Neurosurgery* 32(1):9-15; discussion 15-16, 1993.

Jones RM, Rothman MI, et al: Temporal lobe injury in temporal bone fractures, *Arch Otolaryngol—Head & Neck Surg* 126(2):131-135, 2000.

Jordan B, Jahre C, et al: CT of 338 active professional boxers, *Radiology* 185(2):509-512, 1992.

Kawamoto H, Arita K, et al: Fluid-attenuated inversion recovery (FLAIR) in a patient with parasagittal white matter shearing injury, *Acta Neurochirurgica* 139(6):566-568, 1997.

Koltai PJ, Amjad I, et al: Orbital fractures in children, *Arch Otolaryngol—Head & Neck Surg* 121(12):1375-1379, 1995.

Kraus GE, Bucholz RD, Smith KR, et al: Open depressed skull fracture missed on computed tomography: a case report, *Am J Emerg Med* 9:34-36, 1991.

Lesoin F, Viaud C, Pruvo J, et al: Traumatic and alternating delayed intracranial hematomas, *Neuroradiology* 26:515-516, 1984.

Levin HS, William D, Crofford MJ, et al: Relationship of depth of brain lesions to consciousness and outcome after closed head injury, *J Neurosurg* 69:861-866, 1988.

Lipper MH, Kishore PRS, Enas GG, et al: Computed tomography in the prediction of outcome in head injury, *AJNR* 6:7-10, 1985.

Lobato RD, Rivas JJ, Cordobes F, et al: Acute epidural hematoma: an analysis of factors influencing the outcome of patients undergoing surgery in coma, *J Neurosurg* 68:48-57, 1988.

Lustrin ES, Brown JH, et al: Radiologic assessment of trauma and foreign bodies of the eye and orbit, *Neuroimaging Clin North Am* 6(1):219-237, 1996.

Masuzawa T, Kumagai M, Sato F: Computed tomographic evolution of posttraumatic subdural hygroma in young adults, *Neuroradiology* 26:245-248, 1984.

Mauriello JA Jr, Lee HJ, et al: CT of soft tissue injury and orbital fractures, *Radiol Clin North Am* 37(1):241-252, 1999.

McCabe C, Donahue S: Prognostic indicators for vision and mortality in shaken baby syndrome, *Arch Ophthalmol* 118(3):373-377, 2000.

Meyer CA, Mirvis SE, Wolf AL, et al: Acute traumatic midbrain hemorrhage: experimental and clinical observations with CT, *Radiology* 179:813-818, 1991.

Miller EC, Holmes JF, et al: Utilizing clinical factors to reduce head CT scan ordering for minor head trauma patients, *J Emergency Med* 15(4):453-457, 1997.

Mittl RL, Grossman RI, et al: Prevalence of MR evidence of diffuse axonal injury in patients with mild head injury and normal head CT findings, *AJNR* 15(8):1583-1589, 1994.

North CM, Ahmadi J, Segall HD, et al: Penetrating vascular injuries of the face and neck: clinical and angiographic correlation, *AJNR* 7:855-859, 1986.

Numerow LM, Krcek JP, Wallace CJ, et al: Growing skull fracture simulating a rounded lytic calvarial lesion, *AJNR* 12:783-784, 1991.

O'Sullivan RM, Robertson WD, Nugent RA, et al: Supraclinoid carotid artery dissection following unusual trauma, *AJNR* 11:1150-1152, 1990.

Orrison WW, Gentry LR, et al: Blinded comparison of cranial CT and MR in closed head injury evaluation, *AJNR* 15(2):351-356, 1994.

Pozzati E, Grossi C, Padovani R: Traumatic intracerebellar hematomas, *J Neurosurg* 56:691-694, 1982.

Reed D, Robertson WD, Graeb DA, et al: Acute subdural hematomas: atypical CT findings, *AJNR* 7:417-421, 1986.

Ross BD, Ernst T, et al: 1H MRS in acute traumatic brain injury, *J Magnetic Resonance Imaging* 8(4):829-840, 1998.

Sahuquillo-Barris J, Ciuro JL, Vilalta-Castan J, et al: Acute subdural hematoma and diffuse axonal injury after severe head trauma, *J Neurosurg* 68:894-900, 1988.

Sartoretti-Schefer S, Scherler M, et al: Contrast-enhanced MR of the facial nerve in patients with posttraumatic peripheral facial nerve palsy, *AJNR* 18(6):1115-1125, 1997.

Sartoretti-Schefer S, Wichmann W, et al: MR differentiation of adamantinous and squamous-papillary craniopharyngiomas, *AJNR* 18(1):77-87, 1997.

Sato Y, Yuh WTC, Smith WL, et al: Head injury in child abuse: evaluation with MR imaging, *Radiology* 173:653-657, 1989.

Sortland O, Tysvaer A: Brain damage in former association football players. An evaluation by cerebral computed tomography, *Neuroradiology* 31(1):44-48, 1989.

Sosin DM, Sacks JJ, et al: Head injury-associated deaths in the United States from 1979 to 1986 [see comments], *JAMA* 262(16):2251-2255, 1989.

Sosin DM, Sacks JJ, et al: Head injury-associated deaths from motorcycle crashes. Relationship to helmet-use laws, *JAMA* 264(18):2395-2399, 1990.

Strich SJ: Diffuse degeneration of the cerebral white matter in severe dementia following head injury, *J Neurol Neurosurg Psychiatry* 19:163-185, 1956.

Stringer WL, Kelly DL: Traumatic dissection of the extracranial internal carotid artery: clinical and scientific communications, *Neurosurgery* 6:123-130, 1980.

Tang R, Kramer L, et al: Chiasmal trauma: clinical and imaging considerations, *Surv Ophthalmol* 38(4):381-383, 1994.

Thornbury JR, Campbell JA, Masters SJ, et al: Skull fracture and the low risk of intracranial sequelae in minor head trauma, *AJNR* 5:459-462, 1984.

Unger JM, Gentry LR, Grossman JE: Sphenoid fractures: prevalence, sites, and significance, *Radiology* 175:175-180, 1990.

Wilberger JE, Harris M, Diamond DL: Acute subdural hematoma: morbidity, mortality, and operative timing, *J Neurosurg* 74:212-218, 1991.

Young AB, Ott LG, Beard D, et al: The acute-phase response of the brain-injured patient, *J Neurosurg* 69:375-380, 1988.

Zilkha A: Computed tomography in facial trauma, *Radiology* 144:545-548, 1982.

Zimmerman RD, Russel EJ, Yurberg E, et al: Falx and interhemispheric fissure on axial CT. II. Recognition and differentiation of interhemispheric subarachnoid and subdural hemorrhage, *AJNR* 3:635-642, 1982.

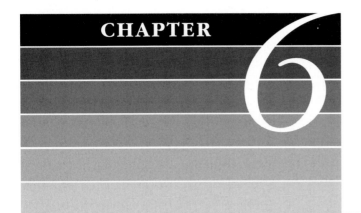

Infectious and Noninfectious Inflammatory Diseases of the Brain

A plethora of infectious and noninfectious inflammatory diseases affects the central nervous system (CNS). The normal brain responds to these insults in a rather limited, unimaginative, and stereotypical manner (as a politician confronted by a sex scandal). This is generally true for all injuries to the CNS. Initially it gets irate (although it may try to claim it never had "injury" there is a characteristic "stain" on MR), ruborous, swollen, and flushed with water (edema). In most cases, there is a concomitant abnormality of the blood-brain barrier with associated enhancement. Later, if the insult results in neuronal death, the tissue shrinks and becomes atrophic (similar to what occurs when politicians are caught). Thus, it is easier for radiologists to understand how magnetic resonance (MR) and computed tomography (CT) can be nonspecific with respect to a particular pathogen than it is for politicians (with requisite cerebral hypoperfusion) to understand the difference between public and private behavior.

However, imaging techniques are relatively sensitive for detecting an abnormality, localizing it, and in many cases categorizing the lesion into infectious or inflammatory disease versus tumor versus vascular disease. Contrast enhancement is usually helpful in evaluating these conditions (lucky for the drug companies!). With the aid of clinical history, physical examination, and the patient's age, the radiologist can more accurately interpret the particular images and, if fortunate, make an educated guess at a probable differential diagnosis.

Localization of lesion(s) is the critical first step in the differential diagnosis. Cherchez la lésion! Is it epidural, subdural, subarachnoid, intraventricular, or intraparenchymal, in the white matter, gray matter, gray-white junction, or deep gray matter? Is it confined to a particular region of the brain such as the temporal lobe? State of the art imaging methodologies including magnetic resonance spectroscopy (MRS), diffusion weighted imaging (DWI), and single-photon emission computed tomography (SPECT) scanning have had little impact in the diagnosis of specific infectious/inflammatory conditions. Nevertheless, we have included them when appropriate—you know for the obsessive-neurotic constipated individuals who believe "scientia pors scientia" and we all know what happened to Rome.

ANATOMY OF THE SPACES AROUND THE BRAIN AND ITS COVERINGS

This chapter begins by briefly defining the anatomy of the spaces of the brain. In most cases, these spaces restrict the infectious and noninfectious inflammatory processes. We then discuss infections restrained by these particular spaces of the brain, from the epidural space to the brain parenchyma and finally centrally to the ventricles. Individual pathogens (virus, bacterium, spirochete, fungus, and parasite) are then described with attention to those features that might increase our ability to make a specific diagnosis. With this approach, however, problems are created in addressing acquired immunodeficiency syndrome (AIDS), its complications, and infections associated with non-AIDS immunosuppression. We have spent a great deal of time perseverating about this issue. Our solution is imperfectly consistent. Toxoplasmosis and cryptococcal infections have been placed in their appropriate infectious groups, parasite and fungus, respectively. All other problems associated with AIDS, including lymphoma, pediatric AIDS, and spinal AIDS, are in the AIDS section, which is situated under viral infections. Non-AIDS immunosuppression infections are located in their appropriate category. The final section of the chapter deals with noninfectious inflammatory diseases.

ANATOMICALLY BOUNDED INFECTIOUS PROCESSES

Three membranes cover the brain; these layers of connective tissue are collectively called the meninges. They are named, from the outermost layer inward, the dura mater, arachnoid mater, and pia mater. The dura mater (pachymeninx) (literally, "tough mother") is composed of two layers of very tough connective tissue. The outermost layer is also the periosteum of the inner table of the skull and is tightly adherent to the skull, especially at the suture lines. The inner layer is covered with mesothelium and lines the subdural space. The two layers separate to form the venous sinuses. The inner layer reflects away from the skull to give rise to the tentorium cerebelli, the falx cerebri, the diaphragma sellae, and the falx cerebelli. The space between the inner table of the skull and the dura mater is the epidural space. The space between the dural covering and the arachnoid is the subdural space. This is a potential space containing bridging veins, which drains blood from the cortex into the venous sinuses, and outpouchings of the arachnoid (arachnoid villi), which project into the venous sinuses.

Beneath the subdural space are two other layers of connective tissue, the arachnoid mater and pia mater, which together constitute the leptomeninges. The arachnoid is a delicate outer layer that parallels the dura and is separated from the pia by the subarachnoid space, which contains the cerebrospinal fluid (CSF). The pia is closely applied to the brain and spinal cord and carries a vast network of blood vessels. Fig. 6-1 illustrates this anatomy.

Epidural Abscess

Epidural abscess is most often the result of infection extending from the mastoids, paranasal sinuses, or cranium into the epidural space. Syphilis is one of the few causes of a primary epidural abscess (pachymeningitis externa). The imaging findings of epidural abscess are those of a focal epidural mass of low density on CT, low intensity or isointensity on T1-weighted images (T1WI), and high signal on proton density-weighted and T2-weighted images (T2WI/fluid attenuated inversion imaging [FLAIR]). Enhancement, particularly on a thickened dural surface or in a ring configuration, may be observed. An epidural abscess can extend into the subgaleal space through emissary veins or intervening osteomyelitis, a finding more frequent when the abscess occurs as a postoperative complication.

Epidural abscesses can cross the midline, distinguishing them from a subdural empyema, which is usually confined by the midline falx. Epidural abscess, like other epidural lesions such as hematoma, can be confined by sutures. A specific site of origin for the infection and its contiguous spread into the extracerebral space also helps establish the diagnosis of epidural abscess (Fig. 6-2).

Subdural Empyema

Disruption of the arachnoid meningeal barrier by infection leads to the formation of CSF collections within the potential compartment of the subdural space. These may present acutely or chronically, and can be sterile or infected at time of presentation. Empyema rather than abscess is the appropriate term for a purulent infection in this potential space. Box 6-1 lists the causes of subdural empyema. Among the several possible mechanisms by which a subdural empyema is thought to form are (1) a distended arachnoid villus could rupture into the subdural space and infect it, (2) phlebitic bridging veins (secondary to meningitis) may infect the subdural space, (3) the subdural space may be infected by direct hematogenous dissemination, and (4) direct extension may occur through a necrotic arachnoid membrane from the subarachnoid space or from extracranial infections.

Clinical signs and symptoms in this group of patients include fever, vomiting, meningismus, seizures, and hemiparesis. The duration of symptoms before presentation ranges from 1 to 8 weeks. Venous thrombosis or brain abscess develops in more than 10% of patients with subdural empyema. The mortality rate from subdural empyema

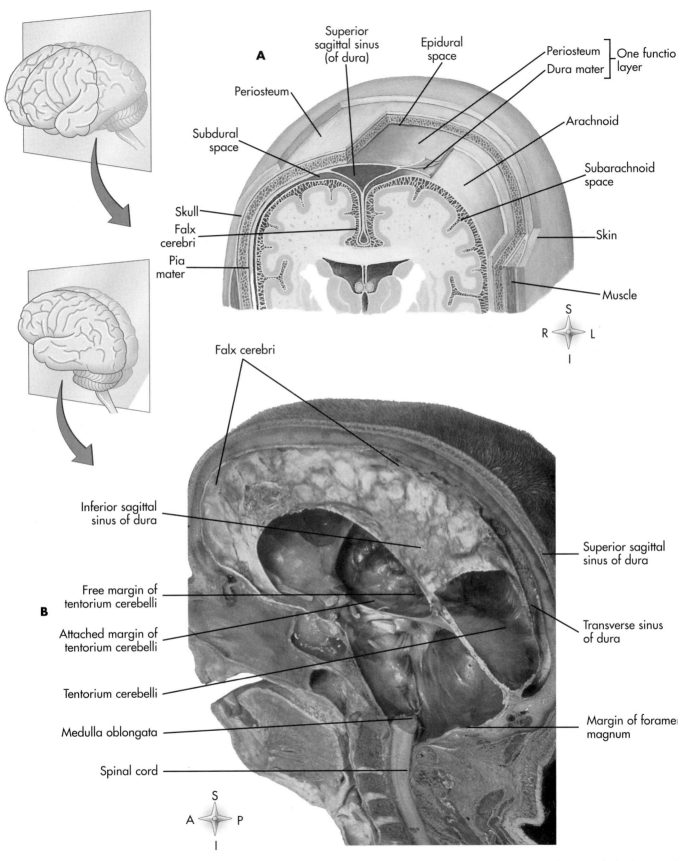

Fig. 6-1 Coverings of the brain. **A,** Frontal section of the superior portion of the head, as viewed from the front. Both the bony and the membranous coverings of the brain can be seen. **B,** The dura mater has been retained in this specimen to show how it lines the inner roof of the cranium and the falx cerebri extending inward.

Illustration continued on following page

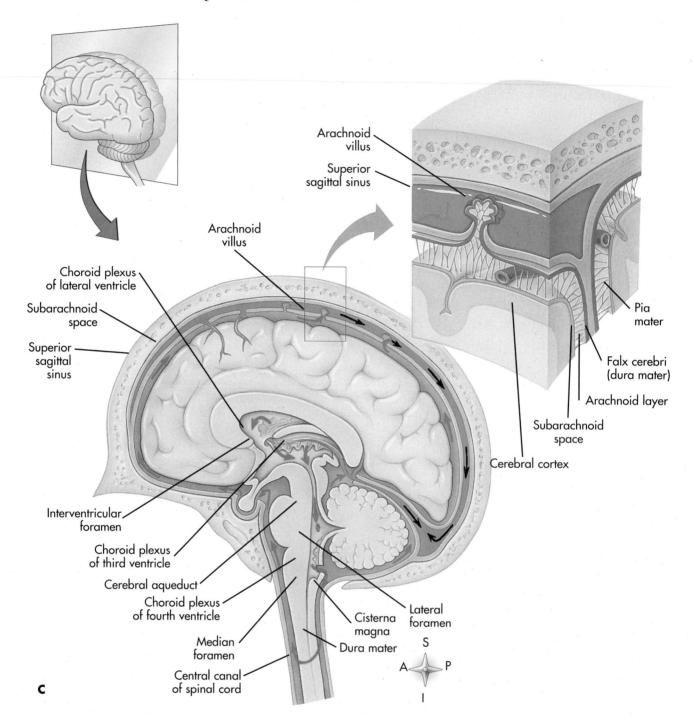

Fig. 6-1 *Continued.* **C,** Flow of cerebrospinal fluid. The fluid produced by filtration of blood by the choroid plexus of each ventricle flows inferiorly through the lateral ventricles, interventricular foramen, third ventricle, cerebral aqueduct, fourth ventricle, and subarachnoid space and to the blood. (From Thibodeau GA, Patton KT: *Anatomy and Physiology,* ed 4, St Louis, Mosby, 1999, pp 376, 379.)

has been reported to range approximately from 12% to 40%. Prompt treatment with appropriate antibiotics and drainage through an extensive craniotomy can result in a favorable outcome. Outcomes research has become avant-garde in medicopolitics recently, so we thought that this would be a propitious chapter, which includes parasites and other pathogens, to introduce the concept.

We assume that you understand the definition of a favorable outcome; however, an alternative to a favorable outcome is the unfavorable income, a result of missed diagnosis, bad disease, or poor health care policies.

Features of subdural empyema are those of extracerebral collections over the convexities and within the interhemispheric fissure, which on MR display isointensity

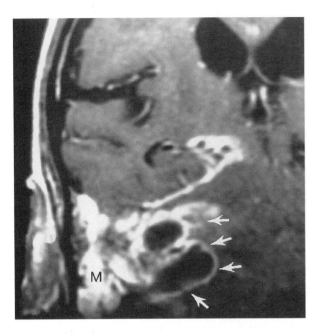

Fig. 6-2   Epidural abscess resulting from mastoiditis (M) on enhanced T1WI. *Arrows* demonstrate medial extent of epidural collection. Enhancement is identified along the tentorium.

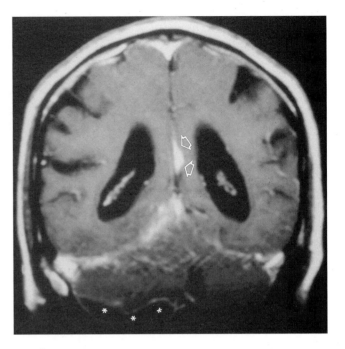

Fig. 6-3   Subdural empyema on enhanced T1WI. *Open arrows* point to thickened subdural collection. Enhancement is also noted along the tentorium. Note the second subdural empyema *(asterisks)* at the edge of the film.

on T1WI and high signal on T2WI/FLAIR, and on CT show an isodense to low density extraaxial mass (Fig. 6-3). Empyema may be distinguished from subdural effusion on diffusion weighted images (DWI) and by their apparent diffusion coefficient (ADC). Empyemas are hyperintense on DWI and have low ADCs whereas sterile effusions are low intensity on DWI and have ADCs similar to CSF. There may be effacement of the cortical sulci and compression of the ventricular system. A rim of enhancement may be observed. This enhancement occurs from granulation tissue that has formed over time in reaction to the adjacent infection. Depending on the changes produced in the contiguous cerebral vessels, gyriform enhancement may also be demonstrated. Coronal MR is a useful aid in confirming the exact location of the collection.

Unfortunately, a chronic subdural hematoma can at times mimic the MR characteristics of a subdural empyema. On CT, chronic subdural hematomas might be low density or isodense and show thick membrane enhancement.

On MR, chronic subdural hematomas can be isointense on T1WI and high intensity on T2WI/FLAIR. This occurs because methemoglobin from the old hematoma is absorbed and degraded. The hematoma consists of fluid and protein, including methemoglobin, so that the sum of these components is isointensity to brain on T1WI, whereas the increased water content produces high intensity on T2WI/FLAIR. MR enhancement is similar to that of CT. Subdural empyema can produce inflammatory changes in the subjacent part of the brain, whereas this does not occur in chronic hematoma. History and symptoms are also useful in distinguishing these different processes. Pick up the telephone before you pick up the Dictaphone.

Leptomeningitis

The pathologic process of meningitis (leptomeningitis) involves inflammatory infiltration of the pia mater and arachnoid mater (Fig. 6-4). Leptomeningeal inflammation most often occurs after direct hematogenous dissemination from a distant infectious focus. Pathogens also gain access by passing through regions that may not have a normal blood-brain barrier, such as the choroid plexus or circumventricular organs. Direct extension from sinusitis, orbital cellulitis, mastoiditis, or otitis media is much less common. After septicemia, bacteria may lodge in venous sinuses and precipitate inflammatory changes, which in turn can interfere with CSF drainage leading to

---

Box 6-1   Causes of Subdural Empyema

Hematogenous dissemination
Osteomyelitis of calvarium
Otitis media, mastoiditis
Paranasal sinusitis
Postcraniotomy infection
Posttraumatic
Purulent bacterial meningitis

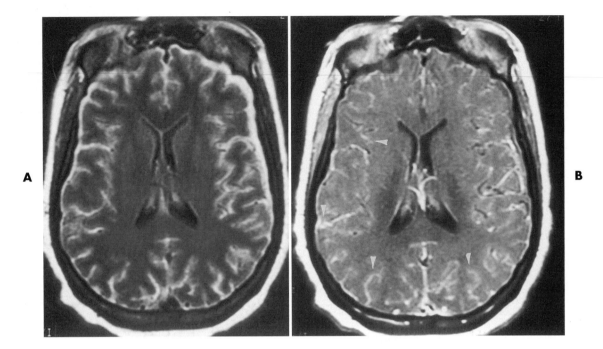

Fig. 6-4   Leptomeningitis: **A,** FLAIR scan with normal CSF intensity (seen in ventricles) has bright CSF in subarachnoid space over convexities. **B,** Note the enhancement on this T1WI deep within the sulci (*arrowheads*). Although some of the enhancement may be attributable to veins especially with edematous meninges, the thickness and smeared margins argues for pial inflammation.

hydrocephalus. With stagnation of CSF flow, bacteria are offered the opportunity to invade the meninges and indulge themselves. Early in the course of infection, there are congestion and hyperemia of the pia and arachnoid mater. Later an exudate covers the brain, especially in the dependent sulci and basal cisterns. The leptomeninges become thickened. Clinical features are related to patient age (Box 6-2). Infants and particularly neonates may have a perplexing clinical picture, lacking physical signs that directly demonstrate meningeal irritation.

Imaging findings in early and in successfully treated cases of meningitis are reported to be normal. Excep-

tions to this in acute meningitis are (1) visualization of distended subarachnoid space, particularly noted in the basal cisterns and along the interhemispheric fissure (most easily recognized in children as abnormal, especially on sequential studies leading to recovery); (2) high intensity of the subarachnoid fluid on FLAIR; (3) acute cerebral swelling (often leading to herniation and death); and (4) communicating hydrocephalus, with enlargement of the temporal horns and effacement of the basal cisterns.

Shortly after the onset of meningitis, it is not uncommon to visualize marked enhancement of the leptomeninges, better visualized on MR than on CT (much more common with bacterial lesions). Postgadolinium FLAIR images appear to be very sensitive for subarachnoid disease. This finding in itself does not appear to be of prognostic significance. Parenchymal abnormalities (uncommon) are primarily those of high signal on T2WI/FLAIR, or of low density on CT. DWI may be abnormal in the sulci and may show abnormality in the cortex. These regions may enhance and pathologically represent areas of infarction and subsequent necrosis secondary to focal vasculitis. Rarely, this represents cerebritis. The vasculitis may involve either arteries or veins; hence, the pattern of infarction differs depending on the location, number, and type of vessels involved. It is more demarcated than cerebritis. Box 6-3 summarizes the spectrum of imaging abnormalities in purulent meningitis.

Box 6-2   Clinical Features of Leptomeningitis

INFANTS	ADULT
Altered state of consciousness	Fever
Anorexia	Kernig's sign
Bulging fontanelle	Headache
Constipation	Meningismus
Failure to thrive	Photophobia
Fever	
Irritability	
Kernig's sign	
Seizures	
Vomiting	

Box 6-3 Imaging Findings in Leptomeningitis

Normal scan
Enlargement of CSF spaces
Poor visualization of basal cisterns
General cerebral swelling
Diffuse meningeal enhancement, +/− Virchow Robin
 spaces
Communicating hydrocephalus
Subdural effusion
Parenchymal high intensity 2° to infarction (+DWI)—
 uncommon

Many additional complications occur as a result of inflammation involving the meninges. These sequelae are better imaged and characterized than are the manifestations of the meningitis itself. Communicating hydrocephalus can occur as both an early and a late manifestation of leptomeningitis, often becoming symptomatic to the point of requiring ventricular shunting. The subacute imaging findings of complicated leptomeningeal infection are those of atrophy, encephalomalacia (infarction), focal abscess, subdural empyema formation, and basilar loculations of CSF (Box 6-4).

Sinusitis can serve as a nidus for leptomeningeal infection and can produce septic thrombosis of adjacent venous sinuses and pseudoaneurysm formation (Fig. 6-5). Labyrinthitis ossificans may occur secondary to infiltration of the cochlear aqueduct by infected CSF.

Neonates represent a special case with respect to the cerebral sequelae of bacterial leptomeningitis. The most commonly encountered organism is gram-negative bacilli, followed by group B *Streptococcus*, *Listeria monocytogenes,* and others. The neonatal meningitides are believed to be acquired as a result of the delivery

---

Box 6-4 Complications of Leptomeningeal Infection

Arterial infarction
Atrophy
Basilar adhesions
Encephalomalacia
Epidural empyema
Focal abscess formation
Hydrocephalus
 Communicating
 Obstructive
Subdural empyema
Subdural hygroma
Venous thrombosis
Ventriculitis

---

process, chorioamneitis, immaturity, or environmental problems (e.g., catheters, inhalation therapy equipment). The lack of a developed immune system at birth makes neonates susceptible to organisms that are normally not very virulent. These children frequently have severe parenchymal brain damage that ultimately produces a multicystic-appearing brain. The imaging findings are those of multifocal encephalomalacia leading to multiple distended intraventricular and paraventricular cysts (Fig. 6-6). In children (1 month to 15 years old), *Haemophilus influenzae* is a common pathogen associated with upper respiratory infections and can produce a virulent meningitis with vascular infarction. Other bacteria in this group are *Neisseria meningitidis* and *Streptococcus pneumoniae.* In adults, *S. pneumoniae* and *N. meningitidis* are the most common bacterial organisms producing meningitis.

The radiologist should appreciate that the diagnosis of bacterial meningitis is a clinical one based on history and physical examination, and confirmed by CSF studies. The radiologist does not identify the organism with imaging (without cheating and looking at the microbiology report or just playing the odds). Imaging is important, however, to rule out a mass lesion or other diagnostic possibilities before spinal tap and to delineate the complications of meningitis. The most common presentation is headache and stiff neck and the differential is migraine versus subarachnoid hemorrhage versus leptomeningitis versus kvetchosis. Subarachnoid hemorrhage is first excluded by CT before LP.

Leptomeningitis versus pachymeningitis (Fig. 6-7) These entities may be legitimately separated by their enhancement pattern on MR. Leptomeningeal enhancement follows the gyri/sulci and/or involves the meninges around the basal cisterns (because the dura-arachnoid is widely separated from the pia-arachnoid here) (see Fig. 6-4, and 6-5A). Pachymeningeal enhancement is thick and linear/nodular following the inner surface of the calvarium, falx, and tentorium and without extension into the sulci or involvement of the basal cisterns (see Fig. 6-7). Infectious meningitis is associated with a leptomeningeal pattern whereas carcinomatous meningitis tends to have a pachymeningeal pattern. The theory behind these observations is that the dura mater does not possess a blood-brain barrier whereas the leptomeninges do. The endothelial cells and cells of the choroid plexus (which do not have a blood-brain barrier) may have specific receptors for the bacterial cell wall. An inflammatory process involving the endothelial cells would open the tight junctions allowing the pathogens to reach the leptomeninges producing leptomeningitis. In carcinomatous meningitis, the tumor cells lack the properties that bacterial cell walls possess. They do not produce the same inflammatory process and blood-brain barrier remains intact. The tumor cells can pass through the capillaries (no

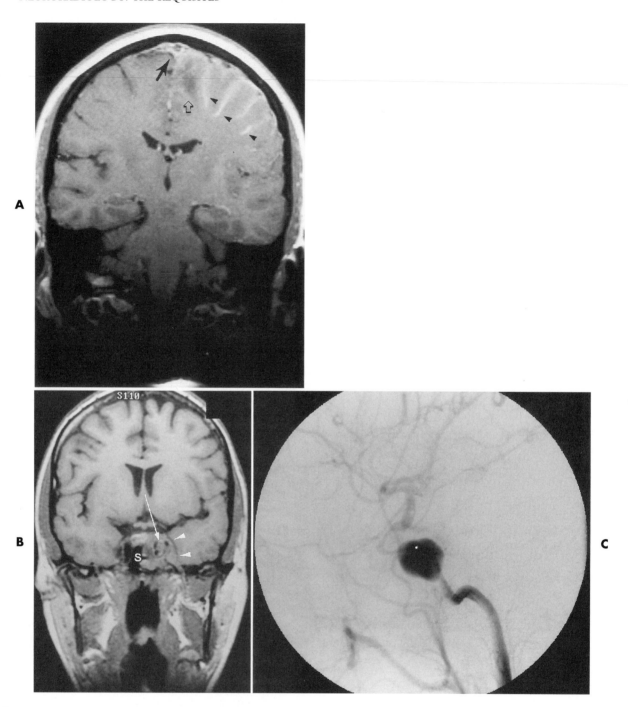

Fig. 6-5   **A,** Septic thrombosis of the sagittal sinus (*arrow*) from meningitis (note enhancing leptomeninges—*arrowheads*) caused an infarct in the left high frontal lobe (low intensity area—*open arrow*). **B,** Meningitis as a complication of sphenoid sinusitis *(s)* produced this cavernous sinus thrombosis with swelling of the sinus *(arrowheads)*. Observe the soft tissue in the cavernous sinus and the unusual pattern of flow voids. *Long arrow* is on the mycotic aneurysm that has developed. **C,** Common carotid angiogram reveals this mycotic aneurysm.

tight junctions) of the dura resulting in dural inflammation. CSF cytology in these cases may be negative. As everyone is aware, the leptomeninges can be involved by tumor. In such cases, the CSF is positive and the tumor cells probably get there via the choroid plexus (no blood-brain barrier) or from extension of superficial parenchymal lesions. The authors express appropriate caution to betting the department on these patterns. Nevertheless, the odds are in your favor. Let us stress that with parenchymal lesions a leptomeningeal pattern is not unexpected. Box 6-5 provides a list of conditions that can produce pachymeningeal versus leptomeningeal enhancement.

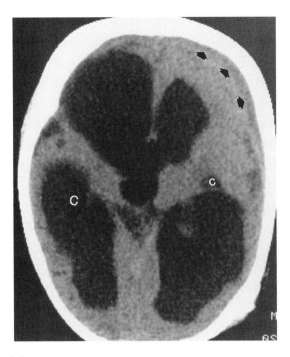

Fig. 6-6 CT of child demonstrates paraventricular cysts *(c)*, porencephaly, central atrophy, and a left subdural empyema *(arrows)*.

Idiopathic hypertrophic cranial pachymeningitis

This is a rare disorder characterized by severe headache, cranial nerve palsies, and ataxia. The peak age is in the sixth decade. The clinical course is chronic with

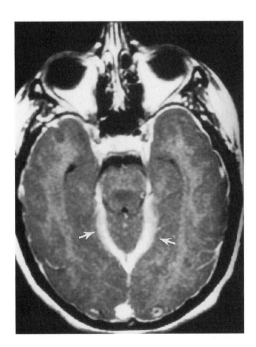

Fig. 6-7 Pachymeningitis. Note that the very thick enhancement of the dura mater of the tentorium *(arrows)* and middle cranial fossa *(arrowheads)* does not extend to the depths of the sulci. This is characteristic of pachymeningitis and distinguishes it from leptomeningitis.

Box 6-5 Conditions That Produce Pachymeningeal and Leptomeningeal Enhancement	
PACHYMENINGEAL	**LEPTOMENINGEAL**
CSF Leak	Acute stroke
Idiopathic Hypertrophic Cranial	Infection
Infection	Inflammatory diseases eg, sarcoid
Inflammatory diseases eg, sarcoid	Metastases
Metastases including those involving the skull	
Pachymeningitis	
Shunting	
Spontaneous intracranial hypotension	
Subarachnoid hemorrhage	

some initial improvement with steroids. The prognosis for loss of vision in patients with optic nerve sheath involvement is poor. On T1WI the dura is obviously thickened sometimes in a pseudotumor fashion and avidly enhances, while on T2WI the dura is hypointense but there is no involvement of the brain (see Fig. 6-7). Thallium-201 SPECT scanning has been advocated as being more sensitive than MR for identifying the inflammatory component and assessing the response to therapy. Biopsy demonstrates an inflammatory infiltrate composed of polymorphonuclear cells. The differential diagnosis includes meningioma, sarcoid, tuberculosis, and syphilis. The syndrome is in the category of orbital pseudotumor, Tolosa-Hunt, and other fibrotic syndromes (clueless diseases).

Box 6-6 Causes of Cerebral Abscess
DIRECT EXTENSION
Otitic
Paranasal sinus
HEMATOGENOUS DISSEMINATION
AV shunts (Osler Weber Rendu)
Cardiac
Drug abuse
Pulmonary infection
Sepsis
TRAUMA
Penetrating injury
Postsurgical
No predisposing posing factors in 25% of cases

Pyogenic Brain Abscess

Cerebral abscess is most often the result of hematogenous dissemination from a primary infectious site. The various causes of cerebral abscess are listed in Box 6-6. The most frequent locations are the frontal and parietal lobes in the distribution of the middle cerebral artery. Intracranial abscess affects predominantly preadolescent (the authors) and middle-age groups (the editors). In part, this is related to the incidence of congenital heart disease, drug abuse, and tympanomastoid and paranasal sinus infections. In all series there is a preponderance of male patients over female (men are again weaker than their counterparts). Abscesses may be unilocular or multilocular, solitary or multiple. A variety of bacterial organisms are commonly cultured from brain abscesses (Box 6-7). In addition, numerous other pathogens can infect the brain when the immune system is compromised.

Abscess formation appears to depend on stasis of bacteria and a focus of ischemic or necrotic brain. Abscess formation has been divided into four stages based on animal work performed with CT: (1) early cerebritis (1 to 3 days), (2) late cerebritis (4 to 9 days), (3) early capsule formation (10 to 13 days), and (4) late capsule formation (14 days and later). The cerebritis phase of abscess formation consists of an inflammatory infiltrate of polymorphonuclear cells, lymphocytes, and plasma cells. By the third day a necrotic center is formed. This deliquescent (we liked the word so check your medical dictionary) region is surrounded by inflammatory cells, new blood vessels, and hyperplastic fibroblasts. In the late cerebritis phase, extracellular edema and hyperplastic astrocytes are seen. Thus the cerebritis phase of abscess formation starts as a suppurative focus that breaks down and begins to become encapsulated by collagen at 10 to 13 days. This process continues with increasing capsule thickness.

The deposition of collagen is particularly important because it directly limits the spread of the infection. Factors that affect collagen deposition include host resistance, duration of infection, characteristics of the organism, and drug therapy. Steroids may decrease the formation of a fibrous capsule and the effectiveness of antibiotic therapy in the cerebritis phase and may reduce antibiotic penetration into the brain abscess. Brain abscesses that are spread hematogenously usually occur at the junction of the gray and white matter. Collagen deposition is asymmetric, with the side towards the white matter and ventricle having a thinner wall, resulting in a propensity for intraventricular rupture or daughter abscess formation, which is sometimes useful to neophytes in distinguishing abscess from tumor. Death from cerebral abscess is due to its mass effect with herniation and/or the development of a ventricular empyema. In the late capsule phase, there is continued encapsulation and decreasing diameter of the necrotic center. Conservative therapy with antibiotics alone has been advocated in conjunction with close monitoring of the clinical and imaging findings in patients with multiple abscesses, in eloquent locations, and in poor surgical candidates.

The characteristics of cerebral abscess depend on the pathologic phase during which the abscess is being examined. In the cerebritis phase, CT demonstrates low-density abnormalities with mass effect. Patchy or gyriform enhancement is present. On MR, one may see low intensity on T1WI and high signal intensity on T2WI/FLAIR (Fig. 6-8), with a typical epicenter at the corticomedullary junction and patchy enhancement. In the late cerebritis phase, ring enhancement may be present. The presence of ring enhancement should not unequivocally imply capsular formation. It is important for the surgeon contemplating drainage to appreciate that a firm, discrete abscess may not be present despite ring enhancement.

Occasionally, a thin rim of high signal on T1WI and low intensity on T2WI/FLAIR may be observed. This may be related to free radical formation (secondary to oxidative effect of the respiratory burst of the bacteria), hemorrhage, or other factors. Duration of symptoms is important in assessing capsular formation. It was suggested, based on CT animal experiments, that the ring lesion of cerebritis may be distinguished from encapsulated abscess by delayed scanning. In the cerebritis phase, contrast was observed to have diffused into the necrotic center, whereas in the well-formed brain abscess this did not occur.

After 2 to 3 weeks a mature abscess appears on T1WI as a round, well-demarcated low-intensity region with mass effect and peripheral low intensity (edema) beyond the margin of the lesion. On T2WI/FLAIR, high intensity is noted in the cavity and in the parenchyma surrounding the lesion (Fig. 6-9). Concentric bands of varying thickness on T2WI/FLAIR have been seen in abscesses. DWI is useful because the high signal intensity of the necrotic center may show reduced diffusion (low ADC)

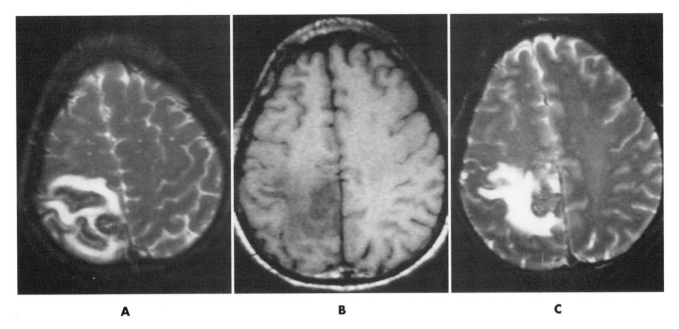

A   **B**   **C**

Fig. 6-8   Early cerebritis. **A,** T2WI/FLAIR with high intensity in right parietal region of a drug addict, 3 days after becoming symptomatic. Note absence of defined margins. **B** and **C,** Late cerebritis (10 days after onset of symptoms). T1WI **(B)** and T2WI/FLAIR **(C)** demonstrate more definition in the forming abscess.

thus differentiating it from necrotic neoplasms (Fig. 6-10). Unfortunately, many abscesses have not read the literature. The low ADC is probably related to high protein, high viscosity, and cellularity (pus) within the abscess cavity.

The vast majority of pyogenic abscesses evoke considerable edema. Remember that the vasogenic edema surrounding the pyogenic abscess will be bright on ADC maps. A ring-enhancing lesion that does not evoke much edema should steer you away from a diagnosis of abscess. A differential diagnosis, including granuloma, primary or metastatic tumor, and demyelinating disease, is more appropriately proffered in such ambiguous cases. Most pyogenic lesions enhance with a thin rim surrounding the necrotic center. Tiny abscesses may appear to have nodular enhancement. Ventricular or subarachnoid spread has been described on FLAIR as having higher intensity than CSF.

On CT, the encapsulated intracerebral abscess shows a low-density center and low density surrounding the lesion (edema). Uniform ring enhancement is virtually always present in pyogenic brain abscess. Occasionally, the abscess may spread into the ventricles because of lower collagen content in the medial wall, producing periventricular enhancement and/or high density within the ventricles. Very rarely does an abscess present as a hemorrhage.

An interesting observation on noncontrast CT is the presence of a complete ring (Fig. 6-11). The noncontrast ring is most often identified in metastases and less often in abscess or glioma. This noncontrast ring surrounding

a low-density center must have a structural component. This is contrasted to ring enhancement, which occurs because of a blood-brain barrier abnormality related to structural alterations in the parenchyma adjacent to a lesion (i.e., a resolving hematoma). A noncontrast ring on CT has been reported to exclude a self-limited nonprogressive process such as a ring-enhancing hematoma or infarct. This finding could help in unknown cases of ring enhancement by narrowing the differential diagnosis. In the era of cost-effective, outcome-generated health care, the noncontrast CT may be all that we are left with. Although at the rate we are going, the skull film may be pronounced the only "cost-effective" imaging study.

Thickness, irregularity, and nodularity of the enhancing ring should raise the suspicion that one is dealing with a tumor (most of them) or an unusual infection (e.g., fungus). However, many exceptions to this rule occur and nodular, irregular pyogenic abscesses are not that infrequent. Some of these represent subacute and chronic abscesses, whereas others are the result of adjacent daughter abscess formation. The ring-enhancing lesion should not be evaluated in a clinical vacuum. The appropriate history is essential for a specific diagnosis. Multiple ring-enhancing lesions are more consistent with hematogenous dissemination of an infectious focus. Multiple rings in a single location can be seen with daughter abscesses but have also been noted with glioma (and other lesions). Box 6-8 is a partial differential diagnosis of the ring-enhancing lesion.

The treated brain abscess may enhance and show high signal on T2WI/FLAIR or low density on CT for long pe-

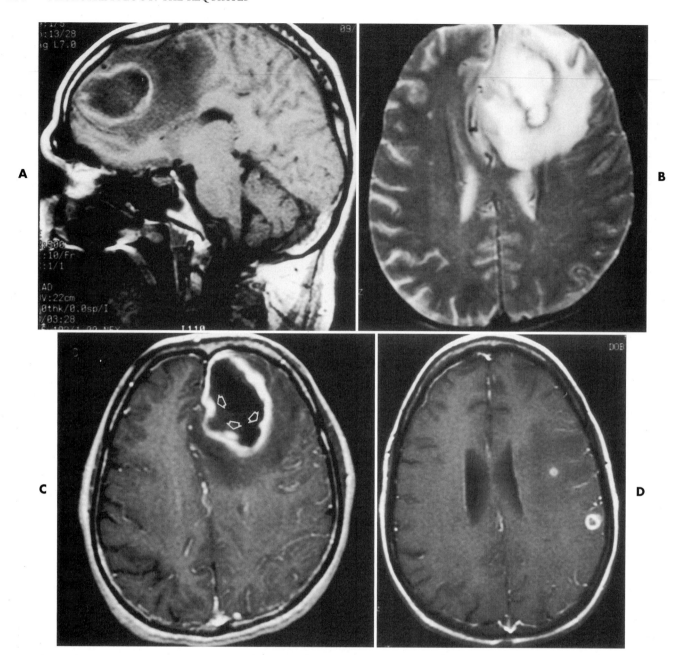

Fig. 6-9   Abscess. **A,** Unenhanced T1WI sagittal image demonstrating frontal high intensity ring with low intensity surrounding the abscess. **B,** Abscess is well defined on this T2WI/FLAIR together with the surrounding high-intensity vasogenic edema. **C,** Ring enhancement on T1WI. Ring is smoother on outside than inside, which is considered a sign of abscess *(arrows)*. This was a streptococcal abscess. **D,** Note the ring enhancement with leptomeningeal/venous engorgement in this patient with multiple abscesses.

riods of time (>8 months) in an otherwise asymptomatic patient.

There are several reports in the literature about proton (1H) magnetic resonance spectroscopy (MRS) in pyogenic abscess. These include resonances from cytosolic amino acids (0.9 ppm), acetate (1.92 ppm), lactate (1.3 ppm), and alanine (1.5 ppm). It is believed (by the same people who are fans of Santa Claus) that the presence of amino acid resonances may distinguish pyo-

genic abscess from necrotic brain tumors. The authors caution our readers not to bet their weekly salary solely on the MRS diagnosis (of anything).

Ventriculitis (Ependymitis)

Ventriculitis can be seen as part of the spectrum of infection including meningitis as a postoperative complication (particularly related to ventricular shunting), or as

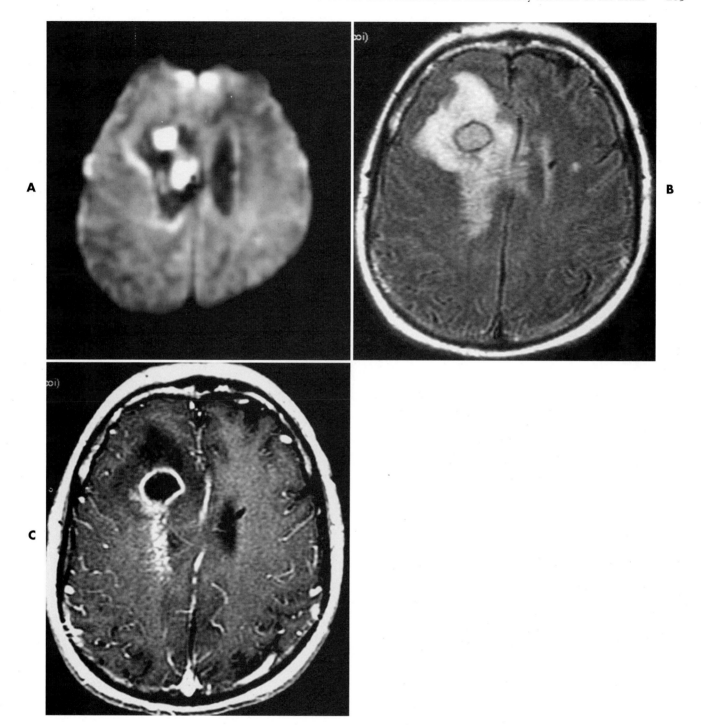

Fig. 6-10   Diffusion positive (low ADC) brain abscess. **A,** DWI typifies the very bright abnormality in brain abscess caused by high protein, high viscosity, and cellularity (pus) resulting in restricted diffusion (low ADC; very bright DWI). **B,** FLAIR image at a slightly different level with a complete ring surrounded by vasogenic edema (increased intensity). **C,** Postcontrast T1WI with complete ring enhancement.

an isolated finding. Organisms are introduced into the ventricle as a result of bacteremia, from abscess, trauma, or instrumentation of the ventricle. The ventricles can be enlarged, and on T2WI/FLAIR high intensity can be observed surrounding the ventricles. The key to the diagnosis is

subependymal enhancement (Fig. 6-12). Choroid plexus enhancement has been reported. Periventricular calcification can be seen on CT after neonatal ventriculitis.

Enhancement of the ependyma is also observed in lymphoma (the most likely diagnosis in patients in-

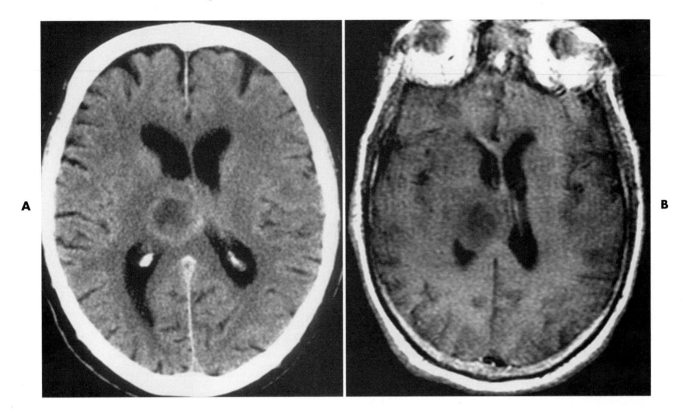

Fig. 6-11 Ring-a-ding-ding. Brain abscess with rings on CT and MR. **A,** Noncontrast CT illustrates the complete ring in the right thalamus indicating a structural abnormality—in this case an abscess. Note the ring is surrounded by low density representing vasogenic edema. **B,** T1WI also shows a complete ring which may be slightly hyperintense (from hemorrhage versus free radicals).

Illustration continued on following page

fected with human immunodeficiency virus [HIV] with subependy-mal enhancement) and other malignant lesions with subependymal spread. This finding would be unusual in toxoplasmosis.

Choroid Plexitis

Capillaries of the choroid plexus, because of their fenestrated epithelium, serve as a conduit through which infections may gain access to the brain. A second barrier between blood and CSF, the choroidal epithelium, possesses tight junctions and prevents passive exchange of proteins and other solutes. Usually, choroid plexitis is seen in association with encephalitis, meningitis, or ventriculitis. It is rarely seen as an isolated infection. Pathogens with a propensity for producing choroid plexitis include *Nocardia* and *Cryptococcus.*

The normal choroid plexus is isodense on CT or isointense to brain on MR and enhances. Calcifications of the choroid plexus produce hypointensity on MR and high density on CT. Asymmetry of the lateral ventricle choroid plexus or bilateral symmetric enlargement of the choroid plexus should alert one to possible choroid plexitis. The differential diagnosis of choroid plexus disease is provided in Box 6-9.

Septic Embolus

The most frequent manifestation of infective endocarditis is stroke, with *Staphylococcus aureus* by far the most common organism. However, sepsis from any cause including pulmonary arteriovenous malformations, pulmonary infection, intravenous drug abuse, infected catheters with cardiac septal defects, and occult infection may produce septic emboli to the brain. Septic emboli are associated with persistent mass effect, edema, and enhancement beyond a 6-week period. This should alert the radiologist to consider septic infarction with development of abscess formation in association with cerebral infarction. Rarely, bland infarction may serve as a nidus for subsequent bacterial colonization from bacteremia and abscess formation. Another diagnostic possibility would be tumor emboli mimicking a stroke. This usually results in hemorrhage or tumoral edema. Cardiac myxoma can embolize and produce acute stroke, and later the tumor grows into the vessel wall to produce aneurysmal dilatation. The vast majority of septic emboli are self-induced by drug users. Septic emboli result in brain abscess, mycotic aneurysm (these occur in distal vessels usually the middle cerebral artery and are less likely to hemorrhage), or obliterative vasculitis (Fig.

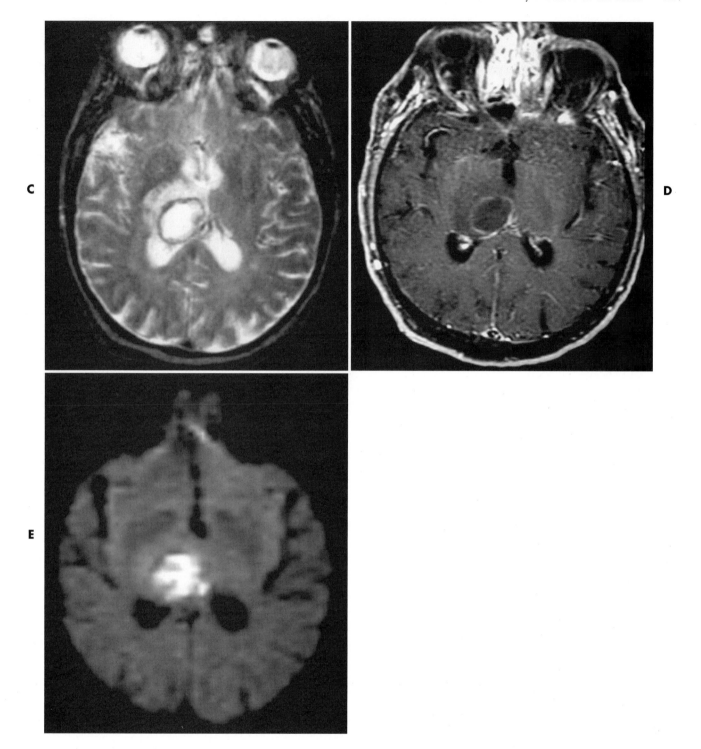

Fig. 6-11   *Continued.* **C,** T2WI with hypointensity in the ring. Surrounding vasogenic edema is high intensity. **D,** Postcontrast T1WI demonstrates the thin ring enhancement consistent with pyogenic brain abscess. **E,** DWI with very bright central region.

6-13). Mycotic aneurysm presents with intracranial or subarachnoid hemorrhage. There is little justification to screen routinely for occult mycotic aneurysms. Rather, angiography should be restricted to cases with subarachnoid hemorrhage or severe headache after control of infection.

SPECIFIC INFECTIOUS PATHOGENS

Thus far, we have covered generic CNS infections with respect to their location and particular imaging appearances. We now consider specific pathogens in normal pa-

Box 6-8   Differential Diagnosis of Ring Enhancement

Fungal, parasitic infection
Granuloma
Infarction
Lymphoma
Metastatic brain tumor
Multiple sclerosis
Primary brain tumor
Pyogenic brain abscess
Radiation necrosis
Subacute hematoma
Thrombosed aneurysm
Tuberculosis

Box 6-9   Differential Diagnosis of Choroid Plexus Lesions

ANGIOMATOUS

Klippel-Trenaunay-Weber syndrome
Primary angiomas and AVMs of choroid plexus
Sturge-Weber syndrome

CONGENITAL

Megachoroid plexus in meningomyelocele

INFECTION

Cryptococcus
Nocardia
Other

INFLAMMATION

Rheumatoid nodule
Sarcoid granuloma
Xanthogranuloma

NEOPLASTIC

Astrocytoma
Choroid plexus papilloma
Ependymoma
Lymphoma
Meningioma
Metastases
Neurocytoma
Oligodendroglioma
Primitive neuroectodermal tumor
Subependymal giant cell astrocytoma
Subependymoma
Teratoma

tients, in patients with AIDS, and in immunosuppressed patients without AIDS. Making the winning diagnosis in immunosuppressed patients is challenging because of their clinical state and the propensity for multiple pathologic processes to occur in tandem. The bottom line is that many infections today occur in a complex environment. The radiologist must attempt to unravel the vagaries of the imaging findings in the context of the clinical findings.

This section is not intended to be a comprehensive catalog of every infectious agent; rather, a tasting menu approach has been chosen so that you may have a sample of a variety of these diseases dim sum. (See the fortune cookie at the end of the chapter.)

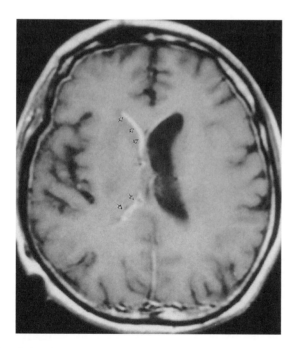

Fig. 6-12   Ependymitis. Enhancement of the ependyma *(arrows)* on T1WI.

Viral

Herpes simplex   Herpes simplex virus is the most common cause of fatal endemic encephalitis. The survivors of infections with this virus have severe memory and personality problems. Early diagnosis and therapy with antiviral agents can favorably affect the outcome. Both the oral strain (type 1) and the genital strain (type 2) may produce encephalitis in human beings. Type 2 is responsible for infection in the neonatal period, presumably acquired either transplacentally or during birth from mothers with genital herpes. This strain may cause a variety of teratogenic problems including intracranial calcifications, microcephaly, microphthalmia, and retinal dysplasia. It carries a high morbidity and mortality rate, with CNS infection either primary or part of a disseminated infection. Sequelae from neonatal herpes also include multicystic encephalomalacia, seizures, motor deficits, mental and motor retardation, and poren-

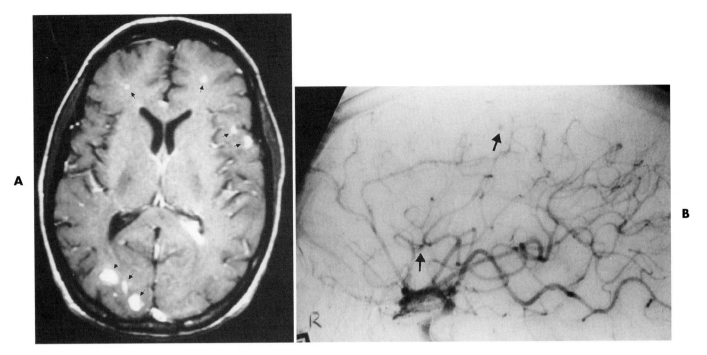

Fig. 6-13   Subacute bacterial endocarditis. **A,** Enhanced T1WI in a patient with subacute bacterial endocarditis. Note the multiple enhancing abscesses at the corticomedullary junction *(arrows).* **B,** Lateral angiogram in a patient with subacute bacterial endocarditis. Two mycotic aneurysms *(arrows)* on branches of middle cerebral artery are identified.

cephaly. The features of intracranial neonatal herpes are different from those in adults and are summarized in Box 6-10. The early findings in neonatal herpes are subtle regions of low density on CT in various regions in the brain parenchyma including gray matter and cerebellum. These regions enlarge rapidly, with meningeal and gyriform enhancement. Later gyri may demonstrate strikingly high density on noncontrast CT. Calcification can appear between 17 and 21 days after disease onset and can be variable in location. Thalamic hemorrhage has been observed. Atrophy is also seen early in this disease. The normal low intensity on T1WI of neonatal white matter and high intensity on T2WI/FLAIR limit the sensitivity of MR in this disease. Loss of gray-white contrast is

an early abnormality that can be incorrectly interpreted as poor quality images. The MR correlate of the high density in the cortex on CT is hypointensity on T2WI/FLAIR. The cause of these characteristic cortical changes is not understood, but increased cortical blood volume (with deoxyhemoglobin), calcification, and other associated paramagnetic ions may be possible causes.

The type 1 virus is responsible for the fulminant necrotizing encephalitis seen in children and adults. It has an incidence of one to three cases per million. The clinical picture (just like board examination toxicity) is one of acute confusion and disorientation followed rapidly by stupor and coma. Seizures, viral prodrome, fever (in more than 95% of cases), and headache are common presentations. Focal neurologic deficits such as cranial nerve palsies are found in less than 30% of cases. Those patients with left temporal disease become symptomatic earlier because of their language impairment and thus may have more subtle imaging findings at the time of presentation.

The pathologic findings are stereotypic. The virus asymmetrically attacks the temporal lobes, insula, orbitofrontal region, and cingulate gyrus. Approximately one third of CNS herpes infections are due to primary infection (usually in persons younger than 18 years of age) whereas two thirds are the result of reactivation confirmed by the presence of preexisting antibodies. One proposed route of entry has been through the nasal airway to the olfactory tracts. A possible explanation

---

Box 6-10   Features of Neonatal Herpes Simplex Infection

Atrophy
Hydrocephalus
Increased density in cortical gray matter
Intracranial calcification from punctate to gyriform
Microcephalt
Microophthalmia
Multiple cysts
Rapidly increasing low density high intensity
    parenchymal abnormalities

for the focality and latency of herpes simplex type 1 may depend on its known residence in the trigeminal ganglia. This latent virus under certain circumstances becomes reactivated and spreads along the trigeminal nerve fibers, which innervate the meninges of the anterior and middle cranial fossae. A diffuse meningoencephalitis with a predominant lymphocytic infiltration is seen. There is marked necrosis and hemorrhage, with loss of all neural and glial elements. The result in untreated cases, if the patient survives, is an atrophic cystic parenchyma. Laboratory diagnosis is dependent on polymerase chain reaction (PCR) on CSF for herpes.

In type 1 herpes encephalitis, MR findings within the first 5 days of the disease show high intensity on T2WI/FLAIR and either positive or negative DWI (depending upon whether there is superimposed infarction) in the temporal and inferior frontal lobes and progressive mass effect including the cingulated region, whereas CT findings at this time may be subtle (Fig. 6-14). Negative diffusion images may indicate some possibility for reversibility. The earliest CT abnormalities are low-density areas in the temporal lobe and insular cortex. Hemorrhage may be identified. The areas of abnormality in the temporal lobe and insula abruptly end at the lateral putamen, which is characteristically spared. It is most unusual to have isolated frontal or parietal involvement. MR is frequently able to detect asymmetric bilateral temporal lobe involvement. This picture is virtually pathognomonic of herpes simplex infection. Unlike other viral encephalitides (see later discussion), simplex rarely involves the basal ganglia (occurring late and lateral). The full extent of parenchymal damage is difficult to assess during the first 10 days of the disease.

Gyriform enhancement may be visualized; however, enhancement varies with severity and stage of disease. Leptomeningeal enhancement has also been observed. Mass effect may persist for a considerable time (39 days in one case). Residual abnormalities include areas of low density and parenchymal loss at the site of involvement. Diffuse cortical calcification in an infant has also been described.

Herpes simplex encephalitis is a potentially treatable encephalitis where outcome depends on early diagnosis. Untreated herpes has a 70% mortality rate, with only 2.5% of survivors returning to a normal functional life. MR is clearly the imaging modality of choice, and it behooves the radiologist to be alert to this condition at all times. This is one diagnosis you do not want to blow.

Herpes zoster   Herpes varicella zoster virus (VZV) is a DNA virus that affects elderly immunocompetent individuals but has a propensity for infecting immunosuppressed patients, particularly those with lymphoma and AIDS. It is caused by reactivation of latent varicella zoster virus that has remained dormant in cranial nerve and dorsal root ganglia since primary varicella infection (chickenpox). The virus travels along the sensory nerve from the dorsal root ganglion to the skin producing a rash (shingles) with associated severe radicular pain and allodynia (sensitivity to touch). It may be detected in the blood or CSF by methods based upon PCR.

VZV is most common in the thorax followed by the face (Ramsay Hunt syndrome—Herpes zoster oticus). One clinical presentation occurs in patients who initially have involvement of the ophthalmic division of the trigeminal nerve, and then develop contralateral hemiplegia several weeks later. Rarely, VZV can produce infarction of the optic nerve. Pathology reveals an occlusive granulomatous vasculitis involving the intracranial arteries and meningoencephalitis.

Imaging features reported in CNS zoster include high intensity on T2WI/FLAIR or low-density areas on CT, mass effect, gyriform enhancement in the segmental distribution of the vasculitis, or pachymeningeal enhancement in cases of meningoencephalitis. Spherical white matter lesions have been reported to increase the specificity for VZV (Fig. 6-15).

Cerebral angiography can demonstrate the severe vasculitis caused by herpes revealing multiple areas of segmental constriction, usually involving proximal segments of the anterior and middle cerebral arteries without involvement of the extracranial vessels (see Fig. 6-15).

Small vessel vasculitis occurs only in immunocompromised patients, and has become the most common complication involving the CNS. These cases have a previous history of zoster weeks to months before developing chronic progressive encephalitis. Multiple areas of high intensity on T2WI involving the cortex, at the gray-white junction, and in the deep white matter (see Fig. 6-15). These lesions may be hemorrhagic and are multiple. The differential diagnosis is PML, however, zoster lesions do not enlarge and tend to appear more vascular in nature. Other reported presentations include ventriculitis and meningitis. Zoster may also produce myelitis secondary to neurotrophic spread of the virus. This occurs 1 to 2 weeks after the appearance of the rash. Patients present with paraparesis and a sensory level. On MR there is high intensity on T2WI in the dorsal root entry zone and within a significant section of the spinal cord emanating from the root (see Fig 17-5). Patients may improve (especially those that are immunocompetent) but are usually left with a residual neurologic deficit. Aggressive early treatment with acyclovir has been strongly advocated. Ipsilateral, posterior column atrophy has been described in shingles.

VZV is linked to cerebral granulomatous angiitis. Granulomatous angiitis, more recently termed primary angiitis of the CNS (see Chapter 4), has also been reported in immunosuppressed patients, particularly those with lymphoproliferative disorders. There is diffuse infiltration with lymphocytes, giant cells, and mononuclear

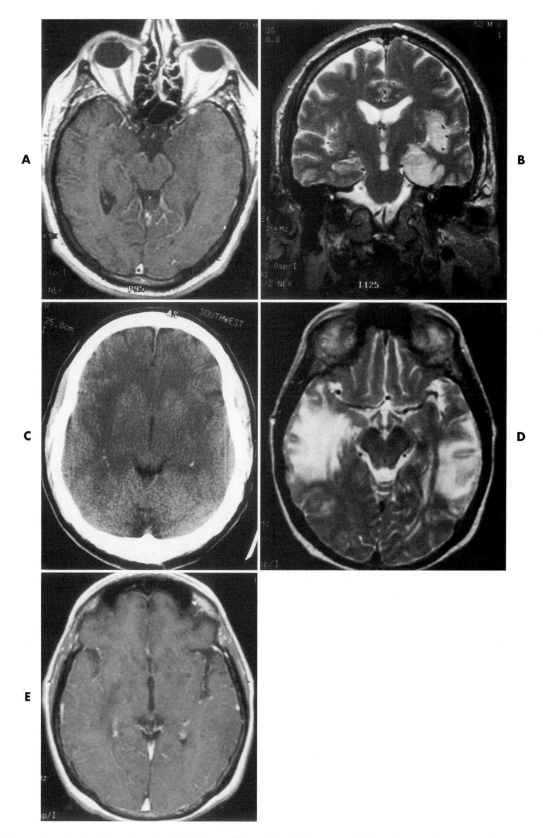

Fig. 6-14   Herpes simplex I gallery. Case 1: **A,** Subtle swelling of the left temporal lobe without enhancement is seen on the postcontrast T1WI. **B,** Coronal T2WI shows sparing of the basal ganglia but involvement of the hippocampus and perinsular region. Case 2: **C,** CT demonstrates bilateral swelling of the medial frontal and insular cortex. **D,** Bilateral disease is clearly evident on the T2WI. **E,** Again no significant enhancement is seen.

Illustration continued on following page

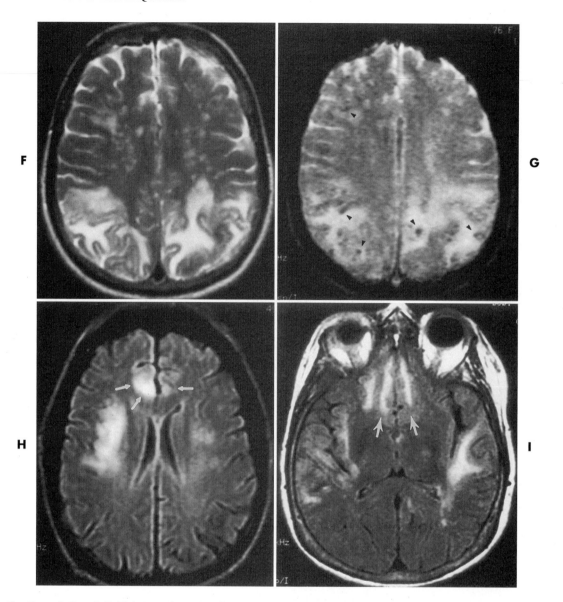

Fig. 6-14 *Continued.* Case 3: **F,** This case shows involvement superiorly of biparietal regions. **G,** The gradient echo scan shows punctate hemorrhages *(arrowheads)* in the cortex. Case 4: **H,** Note the bilateral involvement of the cingulum *(arrows)* as well as the frontal opercular zones. **I,** Gyrus rectus spread *(arrows)* can also be seen with herpes.

cells, of small cerebral arteries and veins (less than 200 μ in diameter). Clinical manifestations include disorientation and impaired intellectual function, with up to 25% of cases progressing to death. MR shows multiple bilateral supratentorial lesions producing infarction, particularly in the deep white matter. Other presentations can be intracranial hemorrhage and a tumorlike appearance. Enhancement is commonly observed in these lesions. These areas correspond to segmental abnormalities in the blood-brain barrier secondary to vasculitis.

VZV can also occur without a rash in immunocompetent individuals. The clinical constellation includes headache, altered mental status, neurologic deficit, CSF pleocytosis (predominantly monocytes), and the pres-

ence of multiple superficial and deep infarcts (some of which may be associated with hemorrhage), and disproportionate involvement of the white matter.

Postvaricella encephalitis   In children postvaricella encephalitis can demonstrate bilateral symmetric regions of symmetric high intensity on T2WI, without enhancement, involving the caudate nuclei, basal ganglia, internal and external capsules, and claustra. Associated clinical symptoms include headache, nausea, vomiting, fever, nuchal rigidity, cerebellar ataxia, and parkinsonism. This may occur 1 to 3 weeks after chickenpox with a differential diagnosis of ADEM. Another MR pattern demonstrated multiple high intensity lesions on T2WI in the gray and white matter, some of which enhance.

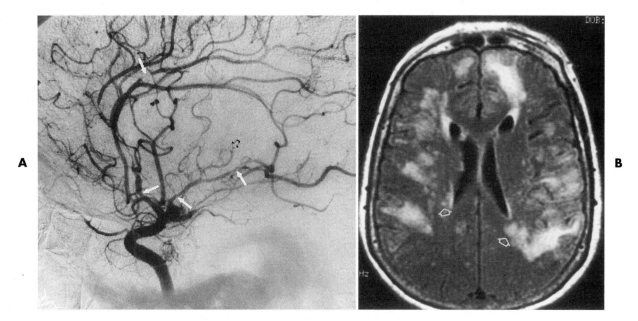

Fig. 6-15   **A,** VZV arteritis. Internal carotid angiogram with multiple areas of vasculitic narrowing *(arrows)* and vascular occlusion *(arrowhead)*. (Is this better than MR angiography or what?) **B,** Multiple segmental areas of abnormal signal intensity at the gray-white junction, some within a vascular distribution, can be seen with herpes zoster arteritis and infection. Spherical white matter lesions *(arrows)* have also been reported.

Subacute sclerosing panencephalitis Subacute sclerosing panencephalitis (SSPE) is a slow viral infection that occurs primarily in children and young adolescents after measles infection 3 to 9 years earlier. Boys (again the weaker sex) are affected twice as often as girls. Risk of SSPE is significantly increased when measles occurs before 18 months of age. SSPE progresses through stages. It starts with language difficulty and behavioral changes. This is followed by intellectual deterioration, ataxia, chorea, dystonic rigidity, seizures, myoclonus, and ocular problems (optic atrophy, cortical blindness, and chorioretinitis). In the final stages the child is unresponsive, displaying severe autonomic dysfunction and the condition progresses to coma and death within months to years. The course occasionally is prolonged and may be associated with one or more remissions.

Supportive laboratory evidence of SSPE includes marked elevation of the CSF γ-globulin content. The electroencephalogram is characterized by periodic high-voltage slow and sharp waves (suppression-burst pattern). Elevated concentrations of neutralizing antibody to measles (rubeola) virus are found in the CSF and serum. The diagnosis is strongly supported by a finding of antibody in unconcentrated CSF. It is rare to isolate rubeola from the brain tissue. Pathologic changes include inflammation, necrosis, and repair with eosinophilic intranuclear inclusions, demyelination, and perivascular lymphocytic infiltration.

MR, unlike what was reported in the ancient CT literature, is frequently abnormal. The findings include high intensity abnormalities on T2WI/FLAIR in the periventricular regions, subcortical white matter, basal ganglia (particularly the putamen, which may account for the movement problems—chorea, dystonia, rigidity), cerebellum, and pons. High signal has also been reported in the frontal and occipital white matter. Lesions progress from the cortex/subcortical white matter to periventricular involvement and diffuse cerebral atrophy. Enhancement and mass effect occur early in the disease. Involvement of the splenium of the corpus callosum on T2WI/FLAIR has been reported. Imaging of SSPE reflects the effects of slow virus infection on brain, resulting ultimately in profound parenchymal loss.

Epstein-Barr virus (EBV) and infectious mononucleosis (IM) EBV can cause a spectrum of neurologic disorders including seizures, neuropathies both cranial and peripheral, myelitis, aseptic meningitis, and encephalitis (incidence between 0.37% and 7.3%). The brain stem and cerebellum are preferred sites of involvement in children and are characterized by high intensity on T2WI/FLAIR. The differential diagnoses in such cases involves brain stem tumor, multiple sclerosis, and acute disseminated encephalomyelitis.

IM, one consequence of EBV infection, is characterized by pharyngotonsillitis, fever, and generalized lymphadenopathy (also see Chapter 14). Usually symptom duration is 1 to 3 weeks followed by uneventful recovery. Severe complications include airway obstruction, meningoencephalitis, and Guillain-Barre syndrome. Multiple cranial nerve palsies including bilateral palsies have been reported secondary to inflammatory tissue compressing the nerves at the foramen. This tissue is high intensity on T2WI/FLAIR and enhances. Arcuate fiber enhancement associated with acute behavioral, perceptual disturbances, and seizure was reported following EBV. Oculomotor nerve enlargement and enhancement associated with dysfunction has also been seen.

Eastern equine encephalitis This mosquito-borne arboviral infection presents with a short typical viral prodrome followed by altered mental status, seizures, and focal findings. High intensity T2W lesions in the basal ganglia, thalamus, and brain stem have been observed early in the course of the disease (Fig. 6-16). Other less common areas of involvement are the periventricular and cortical regions. Meningeal enhancement can occasionally be identified.

These findings are not specific for eastern equine encephalitis and have been described in Japanese encephalitis, measles, mumps, echovirus 25 encephalitides, and Creutzfeldt-Jakob disease. Influenza A may cause thalamic, pontine, cortical, and subcortical abnormalities.

Japanese encephalitis This disease occurs throughout Asia usually in the summer and early fall. It is a fulminant disease with rapid progression to coma. It is caused by a virus with the vector being a mosquito. Clinical signs include high fever, headache, and impaired consciousness. Neurologic signs include extrapyramidal signs (tremor, dystonia, and rigidity). At present there is no specific antiviral therapy, with associated high fatality rate, but it is important to distinguish this viral disease from *Herpes simplex,* which is treatable. It can affect the brain stem, hippocampus, thalamus, basal ganglia, and white matter. On T2WI/FLAIR high intensity, bilateral lesions in the thalami and putamina are reported. Some lesions especially in the thalamus may be hemorrhagic. Enhancement is not usually observed. SPECT scanning shows increased uptake in the thalami and putamina bilaterally matching the MR changes. This is quite different from Herpes, which does not usually involve the basal ganglia.

Nipah viral encephalitis This was previously confused with Japanese encephalitis. It recently caused an epidemic amongst pig farmers in Southeast Asia (another reason to stay away from the pig). These patients all had multiple bilateral high intensity white matter lesions on T2WI/FLAIR, some had additional cortical and brain stem lesions with occasional enhancement and positive diffusion images.

Cat scratch disease This occurs after an inoculation from animal contact particularly with kittens and is caused by the bacteria *Bartonella henselae.* The clinical manifestations are usually self-limited and include lymphadenopathy, fatigue, headache, and anorexia. Encephalopathy has been reported with lesions in the thalami and other brain regions. Vasculitis has also been demonstrated by angiography.

AIDS and HIV Approximately 40% of patients with AIDS have neurologic symptoms during life, whereas the CNS is involved in more than 75% of autopsies. The radiologic approach to this condition is frustrating because of our inability to make specific diagnoses. You should appreciate the common CNS MR manifestations of this illness and its complications. In general, MR in patients with AIDS yields little information in the asymptomatic cases. Indeed, in some cases, despite neurologic disease the imaging may be rather unremarkable. With increasing symptoms atrophic and white matter changes are more obvious. Divide them into encephalitis, meningitis, pure white matter changes, mass lesions (both infectious and neoplastic), and atrophy. Also, appreciate that AIDS may affect the spinal cord as well.

AIDS ENCEPHALOPATHY (PROGRESSIVE DEMENTIA COMPLEX OR AIDS DEMENTIA COMPLEX [ADC]) AND ATROPHY. Brain infection, clinically manifested by a subcortical dementia with cognitive, motor, and behavioral deficits, results from HIV, which is the putative agent responsible for the progressive dementia complex, also known as AIDS encephalopathy (ADC), seen in patients during the course of their disease. Pathologically the white matter and deep gray matter are involved. Diffuse pallor can be identified in the centrum semiovale. The white matter and subcor-

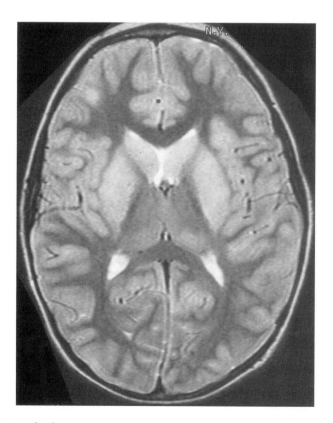

Fig. 6-16 Eastern Equine Encephalitis. T2WI demonstrating increased intensity in the basal ganglia and caudate nuclei bilaterally. (Courtesy of R. Zimmerman, M.D.)

tical gray matter are most severely affected. Inflammatory changes may be minor with only perivascular macrophage infiltrates and microglial nodules. In severe infections, there are multinucleated giant cells with HIV antigen. The major imaging findings on MR are high signal abnormalities on T2WI/FLAIR in white matter, caudate nuclei, basal ganglia, and atrophy (Fig. 6-17). No enhancement is seen in these involved regions. It is thought that the high intensity abnormalities are the result of HIV directly or HIV induced vasculopathy. Cocaine use is a frequent variable found in cases of hyperintensity in the basal ganglia. It has been hypothesized that the changes in the basal ganglia result from a combination of vascular changes from drug use and a direct HIV effect. Investigators using 1H MRS have reported decreased N-acetyl aspartate (NAA) and increased choline (Cho) in cases of AIDS with low CD4 lymphocyte ($<200/\mu$l) counts, neurologic evidence for ADC, and atrophy.

In patients who are cognitively normal and clinically asymptomatic, 1H MRS in the subcortical region demonstrated elevated Cho concentrations early in the disease before symptoms whereas NAA was abnormally low only with severe neuropsychologic impairments.

No significant correlation exists between the imaging findings and state of immunosuppression, the severity of histopathologic white matter changes, atrophy, and the severity of dementia. Protease inhibitor therapy as part of a combination highly active antiretroviral (HAART) drug therapy can result in regression or stabilization of periventricular and subcortical white matter signal intensity abnormalities seen in HIV encephalopathy. Decreased NAA/creatine and a lactate peak have been demonstrated by spectroscopy in basal ganglia, which may be reversible following retroviral therapy.

White matter changes may be symmetric or asymmetric, focal or diffuse, and not associated with mass effect or enhancement. The cortical gray matter is usually not affected. The microglial nodules are not detected by MR, and the imaging findings represent secondary demyelination and gliosis. HIV encephalitis can coexist with cytomegalic inclusion virus (CMV), toxoplasmosis, cryptococcus infection, progressive multifocal leukoencephalopathy, and primary CNS lymphoma. Detection of mass lesions militates against the diagnosis of HIV alone.

CMV in HIV-seropositive patients may produce a progressive encephalopathy characterized by dementia, which yields no specific findings on CT or MR. Histopathologic evidence for CMV is found in one third of AIDS patients and correlates with the clinical syndromes of radiculomyelitis and encephalitis. Atrophy, periventricular or subependymal enhancement, and periventricular low density on CT or high intensity on T2WI/FLAIR may be associated with CMV infection but can be seen in the plethora of other diseases affecting the brain in AIDS (see Fig. 6-17).

MENINGITIS   Meningitis is sometimes manifested by enhancement of the meninges, which may be associated with vasculitic changes and ischemia. Common pathogens include cryptococcus, toxoplasmosis, tuberculosis, and CMV. Meningovascular syphilis occurs rarely in patients with AIDS and should be in the differential diagnosis of vasculitis and stroke syndromes in this patient population (Fig. 6-18). There is widespread thickening of the meninges and perivascular spaces with a lymphocytic infiltration. Angiographic findings of syphilis are those of segmental constriction and occlusion of the supraclinoid carotid artery, the proximal anterior and middle cerebral segments, and involvement of the basilar artery (this large and middle-sized vascular involvement is termed Heubner arteritis). Smaller vessels can also be involved (Nissl arteritis). A spectrum of parenchymal abnormalities has been described, including enhancing nodules (cerebral gumma) with variable intensity patterns and an appearance of mesiotemporal high intensity on T2WI that could be confused with herpes encephalitis (Fig. 6-18E).

WHITE MATTER LESIONS   Progressive multifocal leukoencephalopathy (PML) is described in Chapter 7. It is very difficult to distinguish this condition from primary HIV changes, from lymphoma, and from other infections in patients with AIDS. The key finding in PML is high signal intensity on T2WI/FLAIR in the white matter (although PML can involve the cortex), usually, but not always without enhancement and mass effect; obviously a nonspecific picture. PML characteristically involves the subcortical U-fiber as opposed to HIV or CMV, which tend to involve the white matter more centrally. Furthermore, although PML has a viral etiology, presently there are no known treatments so that diagnosis in this context is no great feat! PML has been described in patients with primary immunologic deficiencies (hyperimmunoglobulinemia M, hypogammaglobulinemia) or secondary immunologic deficiencies (HIV infection or immunosuppressive therapies).

CEREBRAL INFARCTION   The frequency of clinical cerebral infarction in AIDS is between 0.5% and 18% whereas the autopsy frequency is between 19% and 34%. The most common location for infarction is the basal ganglia. The causes for infarction include altered vasoreactivity from HIV in combination with drug use (particularly cocaine), HIV vasculitis, infection (varicella-zoster, cytomegalovirus, tuberculosis, cryptococcosis, syphilis, and toxoplasmosis), marantic endocarditis, disseminated intravascular coagulopathy, or hypoxia. The vascular disease associated with HIV can produce bright signal on T1WI in the basal ganglia.

LYMPHOMA   Primary CNS lymphoma of the brain has an incidence in AIDS patients of about 6%. It is also seen in other types of immunosuppressed patients, particularly allograft recipients (heart, kidney). CT characteristics of this lesion include single or multiple areas of in-

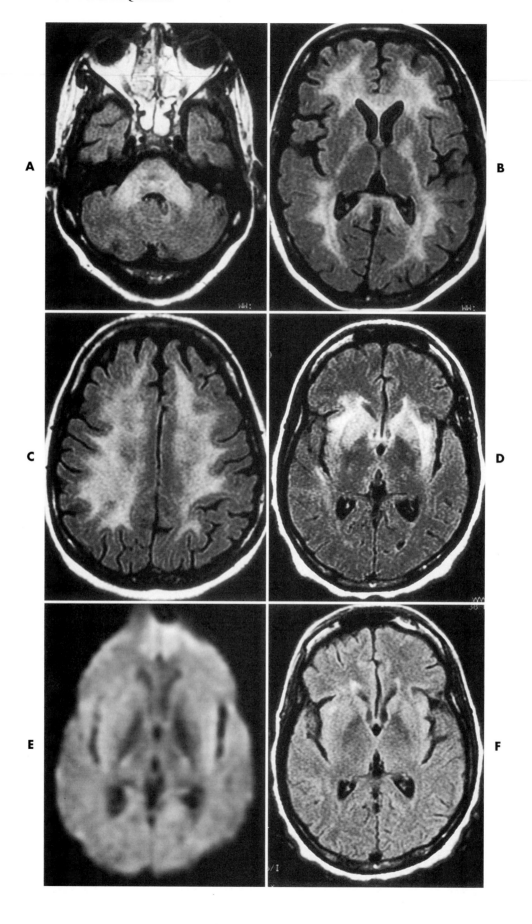

volvement with mass effect without a great deal of edema relative to the tumor size. There is a marked predilection for the basal ganglia, cerebellar hemispheres, thalamus, brain stem, corpus callosum, and subependymal region. The tumor may be isodense, hyperdense, or hypodense (in AIDS) on unenhanced CT. It is unusual for this lesion to demonstrate central necrosis except in AIDS. It usually exhibits homogeneous enhancement on CT. On MR these lesions may be isointense or of low intensity on T1WI and variable intensity on T2WI/FLAIR (Fig. 6-19). Most lesions enhance in a solid or ring fashion, although nonenhancing lymphoma has been reported. CNS lymphoma is exquisitely sensitive to steroids and radiation therapy, but it is prone to recurrence. (As Arnold Schwarzenegger would say, "I'll be back.") Previous therapy with steroids may render the CT scan completely normal. Occasionally lymphoma may be particularly fulminant with lesions doubling in size in approximately 2 weeks. This pattern could clearly be confused with toxoplasmosis or other infectious processes.

Toxoplasmosis vs. lymphoma   It is important to differentiate lymphoma from toxoplasmosis as the former benefits from radiation therapy with more than a fourfold increase in survival rates over the untreated. In addition, it is believed that delaying therapy to embark on a course of antitoxoplasmosis therapy diminishes the benefit of radiation therapy. Certain features might enable one to distinguish CNS lymphoma and toxoplasmosis, and although it is wise not to bet the ranch, trends do emerge. CT is more specific than MR with respect to the diagnosis of lymphoma. High density masses on noncontrast CT (not as frequent in AIDS lymphoma) and periventricular lesions with subependymal spread are findings suggestive of lymphoma. Encasement of the ventricle does not occur with toxoplasmosis but can be seen in patients with lymphoma. On MR lymphoma has a tendency to be isointense to hypointense relative to white matter on T2WI/FLAIR whereas toxoplasmosis is more likely to be hyperintense on T2WI/FLAIR (see Chapter 3; Table 3-7). Toxoplasmosis can have a low-intensity ring surrounded by high intensity on T2WI/FLAIR with ring enhancement. Both lesions may present with solid or multiple lesions, have lesions of various sizes (although toxoplasmosis abscesses tend to be more numerous and smaller than lymphoma), and either ring-enhance or display solid enhancement. Location of the lesions does not separate entities, although toxoplasmosis has a propensity for the basal ganglia and does not

spread in a periventricular pattern or usually involve the ependyma whereas lymphoma has a penchant for the periventricular region and subependymal spread. Toxoplasmosis has a predilection for hemorrhage, which is not the case with CNS lymphoma (except after steroids or radiation therapy) (Fig. 6-20). These diseases can coexist. Thallium-201 SPECT has been reported to show abnormal uptake in lymphoma but not in toxoplamosis. Improved specificity may be gained by performing a quantitative analysis of the scans to exclude lesions with activity not greater than that of scalp. MR perfusion measurement is another technique that has been suggested to differentiate lymphoma (increased perfusion) from toxoplasmosis (decreased perfusion). Another solution to this problem is 1H MRS where toxoplasmosis lesions show markedly elevated lactate and lipid concentrations whereas lymphoma shows moderate increased lactate and lipid and marked increased Cho (secondary to increased cellularity and membrane turnover). Despite what we have just said clinicians usually treat for toxoplasmosis first and image both before and after (very cost effective).

Other reported zebras include leiomyosarcoma (in the brain and spinal cord in patients with latent EBV), central pontine myelinolysis, facial nerve palsy, and optic neuritis.

SPINAL CORD LESIONS   Box 17-2 provides a list of intramedullary lesions occurring in AIDS patients. AIDS-associated myelopathy (vacuolar myelopathy) consists of spinal cord white matter vacuolation and lipid-laden macrophages (its autopsy incidence varies from 3% to 55%). Clinical findings include the insidious onset of urinary incontinence, progressive spastic-ataxic paraparesis, and sensory loss. Viral myelitis (herpes simplex type 2, CMV, and varicella-zoster) has also been implicated in patients with AIDS. Toxoplasmosis can rarely produce a myelitis. The thoracic spinal cord is most frequently involved in AIDS-associated myelopathy generally manifesting late in the disease. Findings on MR of atrophy (most frequent) with or without high signal on T2WI/FLAIR, which usually does not enhance in AIDS cases, should evoke this differential.

MARROW CHANGES IN AIDS   Normally yellow marrow, manifest by high intensity on T1WI, becomes dominant in the clivus by the age of 20. In AIDS patients, there is hemosiderin deposition with a change in marrow intensity to hypointense on T1WI. Clival marrow changes have been correlated with CD4 cell counts.

PEDIATRIC AIDS   At this time only 1% to 2% of AIDS occurs in the pediatric population, yet in 80% of these

---

Fig. 6-17   Pastiche of AIDS. Case 1: **A,** brain stem abnormal signal intensity is well seen on the FLAIR scan. **B,** Diffuse bilateral symmetric white matter involvement is present at the level of the ventricles. Atrophy coexists. **C,** Centrum semiovale disease generally spares subcortical U fibers, a distinguishing feature from progressive multifocal leukoencephalopathy. Case 2: **D,** Basal ganglia involvement was present in this woman with AIDS related dementia. **E,** Note that the disease is not bright on DWI. **F,** After HAART the abnormality on FLAIR resolved and the patient was able to return to her job as a professional blood donor at the Red Cross.

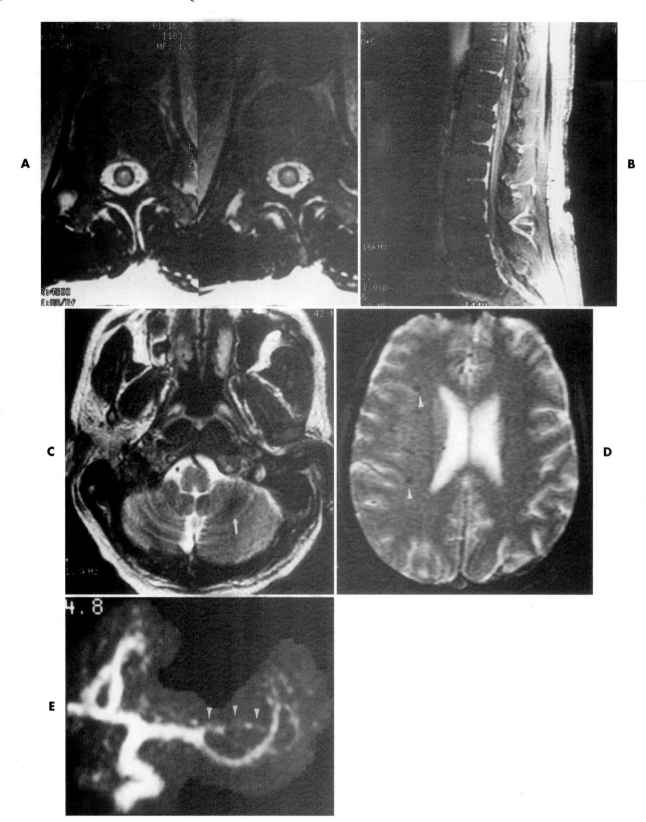

Fig. 6-18 Syphilis. **A,** Abnormal signal in the thoracic cord on axial T2W is indicative of tabes dorsalis. **B,** Enhancement both in the cord *(arrow)* and along the surface of the cord and subarachnoid space is seen. **C,** This prompted a brain study that showed curious hypointensity in the cerebellum *(arrow)* on FSE T2WI. **D,** This prompted gradient echo images that showed punctate areas of hemorrhage *(arrowheads)* in subcortical white matter. **E,** These findings led to an MRA showing vasculitic changes *(arrowheads)* compatible with syphilis. This in turn led to an MRI bill of $5000 to Medicaid. The profee returned from Medicaid was $37.18.

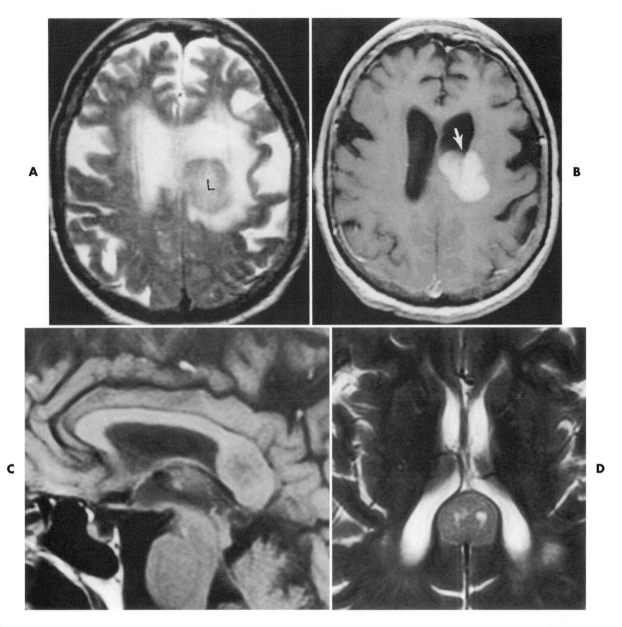

Fig. 6-19 AIDS and lymphoma. Case 1: Lymphoma in AIDS. **A,** T2WI/FLAIR of lymphoma with solid mass lesion and surrounding high intensity. **B,** Enhanced T1WI of the same lesion with encasement of the ventricle *(arrow).* Case 2: **C,** Sagittal T1WI reveals a large mass in the splenium. **D,** It is low in intensity on T2WI, similar to that seen in figure **A.**

Illustration continued on following page

cases CNS involvement including acquired microcephaly, diffuse cerebral atrophy, calcifications, and HIV encephalitis develops. Atrophy has been correlated with diminished brain weight for age and infiltration of microglial nodules and multinucleated giant cells. Scattered areas of gliosis correspond in part to focal white matter abnormalities on T2WI/FLAIR. Calcifications are uncommon before the age of 1 year or when the neurologic examination yields negative results and are a prominent feature of HIV infection in children but not in adults. The calcifications are located in the basal ganglia,

periventricular, frontal white matter, and cerebellum (Fig. 6-21). Vascular ectasia of intracranial vessels and aneurysmal dilatation of the circle of Willis occurs with neonatal AIDS (Fig 6-22). The probable etiology of the aneurysmal dilatation is VZV vasculitis although HIV may also primarily affect the vessels. The incidence of symptomatic vascular disease in pediatric AIDS is a little over 1%, however, at autopsy 25% of cases were observed to have vascular lesions caused by hypoperfusion, thromboembolic disease, and infectious vasculitis. Infections and lymphoma are very uncommon in the pediatric pa-

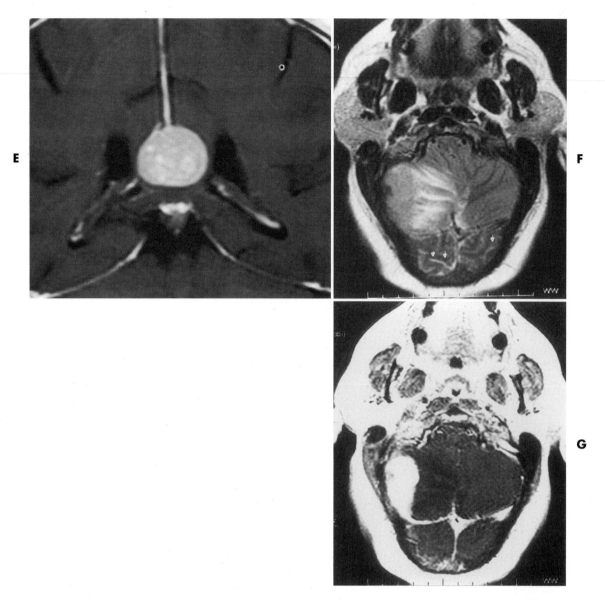

Fig. 6-19 *Continued.* **E,** Coronal enhanced T1WI shows homogeneous gadolinium uptake. Case 3: **F,** Dural based lymphoma with low intensity extraaxial mass is seen with subarachnoid space hyperintensity over inferior occipital region (*arrows* at edge of film, boys!). This implies CSF spread. **G,** Naturally, the lesion enhances.

tients whereas cerebral atrophy, calcification, white matter high intensity on T2WI/FLAIR, and hemorrhage are the predominant findings in this population.

Cytomegalic inclusion virus CMV, a member of the herpesvirus family, causes diseases in both the normal and immunosuppressed patient. It is the most frequent cause of fetal and neonatal viral infection. Transplacental transmission occurs as a result of either recurrent or primary maternal infection. It commonly exists in a latent form in the adult population. Reactivation of latent maternal infection is associated with a 3.4% risk of congenital fetal infection, whereas primary CMV infection poses a 30% to 50% risk of intrauterine infection. The mechanism of injury is ischemia because of insufficient

fetal circulation probably secondary to placentitis and secondary chronic perfusion insufficiency. Injury before 18 weeks results in agyria and between 18 and 24 weeks polymicrogyria (see Fig 9-25).

It has a propensity for the ependymal and subependymal regions. CNS abnormalities associated with CMV include microcephaly, ocular defects, and deafness. Other findings in infants with CMV infection include atrophy, cerebellar hypoplasia, focal white matter lesions, hippocampal abnormalities, ventriculomegaly, hydranencephaly, porencephaly, paraventricular cysts, and gyral anomalies including complete lissencephaly, pachygyria, microgyria, and localized cortical dysplasia (Fig. 6-23). The pathologic hallmark of the infection is the finding

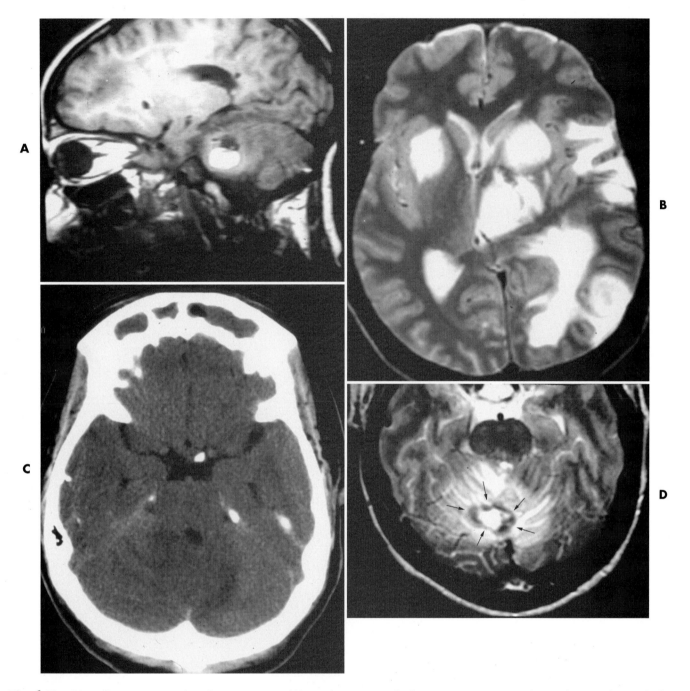

Fig. 6-20   Toxoplasmosis versus lymphoma. **A,** Sagittal T1WI demonstrates high intensity representing hemorrhage in the cerebellum in a toxoplasma brain abscess. **B,** Axial T2WI in same patient reveals basal ganglia and subcortical toxoplasma abscesses. **C,** Noncontrast CT of another case showing low density and mass effect in the cerebellum. **D,** T2WI axial of B. Note the hypointensity in the toxoplasma abscess wall *(arrows).*

Illustration continued on following page

in ependymal, subependymal cells, and white matter of intranuclear inclusions, which demonstrates an "owl eye" picture with distention of the nucleus by the viral inclusions and a surrounding halo.

Bilateral periventricular calcifications have been described in CMV and in infants with toxoplasmosis and with bacterial meningitis complicated by ventriculitis.

Nevertheless, CMV calcifications are usually limited to the subependymal region, whereas neonatal toxoplasmosis has calcifications not only in the periventricular region but also throughout the brain, including a characteristic curvilinear pattern in the basal ganglia. Herpes simplex has rarely been associated with calcifications and rubella has not, although microscopic calcification in relationship

Text continued on page 304

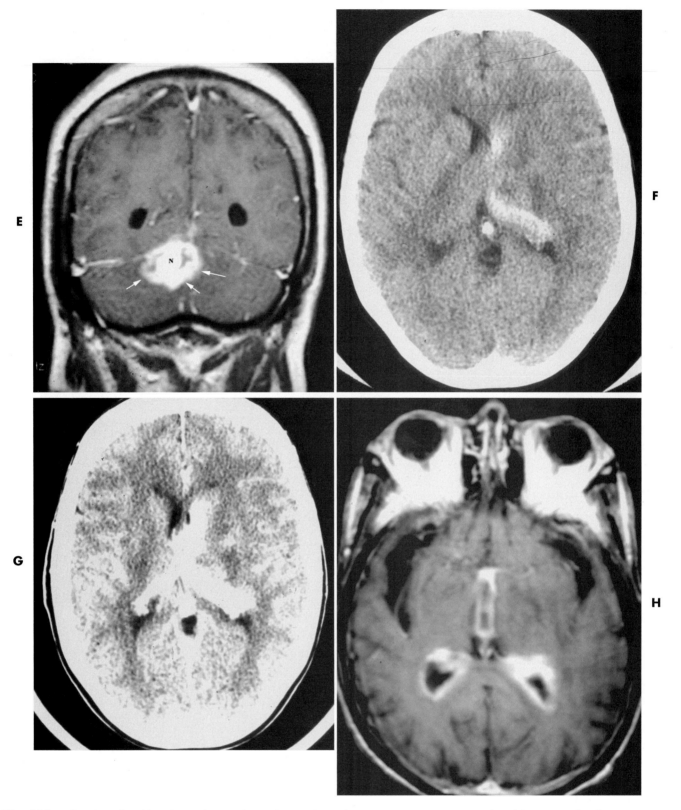

Fig. 6-20 *Continued.* **E,** T1 enhanced coronal reveals complex enhancement (ring *[arrows]* and nodule [N]) in the abscess. **F,** Non-contrast CT shows high-density lymphoma encasing the ventricles. **G,** Enhanced CT exhibits enhancement in the lymphoma. **H,** Lymphoma encasing the ventricles on this enhanced T1WI.

Illustration continued on following page

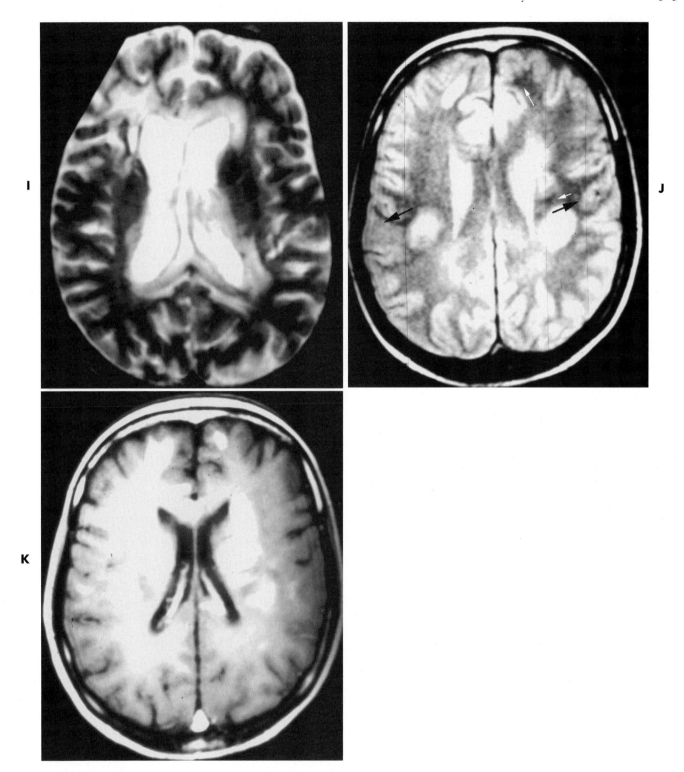

Fig. 6-20 *Continued.* **I,** T2WI of H showing hyperintensity of the lymphoma around the ventricles. **J,** PDWI displays low *(small white arrows),* iso *(large black arrows)* and high (obvious) intensity lymphoma lesions. **K,** T1 enhanced image of J exhibiting enhancement in all varieties of lesions.

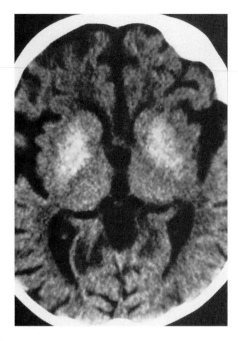

Fig. 6-21 Pediatric AIDS. Calcification in the basal ganglia and atrophy on CT in a child with AIDS.

to blood vessels can be found pathologically. In the differential diagnosis of periventricular calcifications, tuberous sclerosis should also be considered, although calcifications of the subependymal nodules occur in childhood.

The subependymal calcifications of CMV are more obvious on CT. Periventricular low density on CT or high intensity on T2WI/FLAIR, although nonspecific, has also been reported in CMV (Fig. 6-24).

Bacterial

Tuberculosis The incidence of tuberculosis has markedly increased in recent years, particularly in conjunction with AIDS and the emergence of drug-resistant strains of the bacillus. Approximately 5% to 10% of cases of tuberculosis have CNS involvement; however, between 4% and 19% of patients with AIDS have coexisting CNS tuberculosis. Intracranial tuberculosis has two related pathologic processes—tuberculous meningitis and the intracranial tuberculoma. The two conditions are separate clinical entities, with only 10% of patients with tuberculoma having tuberculous meningitis. Tuberculous meningitis is more commonly seen in children associated with primary infection. The pathophysiology of

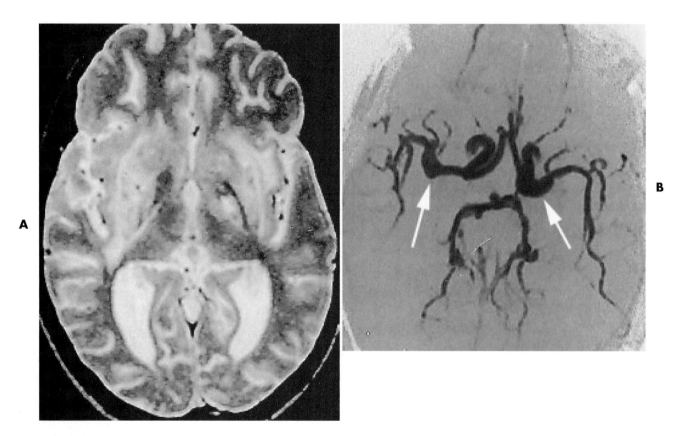

Fig. 6-22 HIV vasculitis. **A,** Axial MR of the brain demonstrating diffuse high signal secondary to HIV infection. **B,** Base view MRA shows dilatation of both middle cerebral arteries *(arrows)* from HIV vasculitis. (Courtesy of Robert Quencer, M.D.)

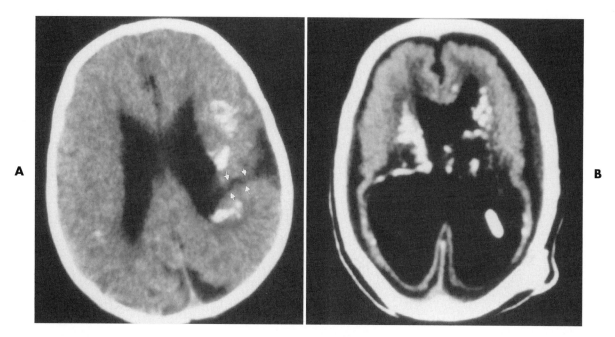

Fig. 6-23   CMV infection. **A,** CT with periventricular calcification and schizencephalic porencephaly *(arrows)*. **B,** CT of another patient with CMV infection, periventricular calcifications, pachygyric-like brain, and hydrocephalus.

tuberculous meningitis begins with an initial focus, which is usually pulmonary but may occur in the abdomen or genitourinary tract. Hematogenous dissemination of the bacilli seeds the leptomeninges and brain parenchyma. When cell-mediated immunity develops, small tubercles are formed. These grow and are walled off by a dense fibrous capsule that centrally has a characteristic caseous necrotic core surrounded by Langhans giant cells, epithelioid cells, and lymphocytes—the tuberculoma. The tuberculoma is a small (1 to 3 mm in diameter) nodule, and can coalesce to form a large lesion. The intracranial tuberculoma produces symptoms from mass effect and associated edema. These are related to the location of the lesion. Signs and symptoms include seizures, raised intracranial pressure, and papilledema; however, patients are usually noted to have a disparity between minimal symptoms and rather significant lesion burden. Worldwide, tuberculoma may be the most common brain stem lesion, and in underdeveloped countries, tuberculoma may account for a significant incidence of intracranial mass lesions (15% to 50%). Tuberculomas may be solitary or multiple. They can occur in the supratentorial and infratentorial regions.

Tuberculomas may be dormant for years. The infection may completely resolve, or the tuberculoma may rupture into the subarachnoid space, discharging its necrotic debris and causing tuberculous meningitis and more properly a meningoencephalitis affecting the brain parenchyma and blood vessels. The basal cisterns are most affected by the exudative meningitis, with an epicenter in the in-

terpeduncular cistern and spread into the prepontine, sylvian, and superior cerebellar cisterns. Obstruction to the normal CSF flow results in hydrocephalus. Inflammatory changes in the blood vessels caused by this process lead to an arteritis and infarction particularly seen in the basal ganglia and internal capsule. Cranial nerve palsy occurs as a result of the basilar meningoneuritis.

Clinical features of tuberculous meningitis in adults include confusion, fevers, headache, lethargy, and meningismus. Lumbar puncture reveals hypoglycorrhachia, increased protein, pleocytosis (predominantly lymphocytes), and negative smears for organisms. This progresses in a subacute fashion with stupor, coma, decerebrate rigidity, cranial nerve palsy, and possible stroke. It is interesting to note that 19% of patients with tuberculous meningitis have no evidence of extrameningeal active disease at the time of diagnosis. The tuberculin skin test is often negative early in the disease. In children, the most common symptoms include nausea, vomiting, and behavioral changes with a medical history that is usually unremarkable.

Imaging features depend on the stage of the infection. In tuberculous meningitis, the basal and sylvian cisterns are poorly visualized without contrast because of the dense exudate. On FLAIR, the basal cisterns can have increased intensity compared with normal, because of the thick proteinaceous exudate. The cisterns enhance uniformly and intensely, and this enhancement can extend into the hemispheric fissures and over the cortical surfaces (Fig. 6-25). Rarely calcification can be appreciated

Text continued on page 308

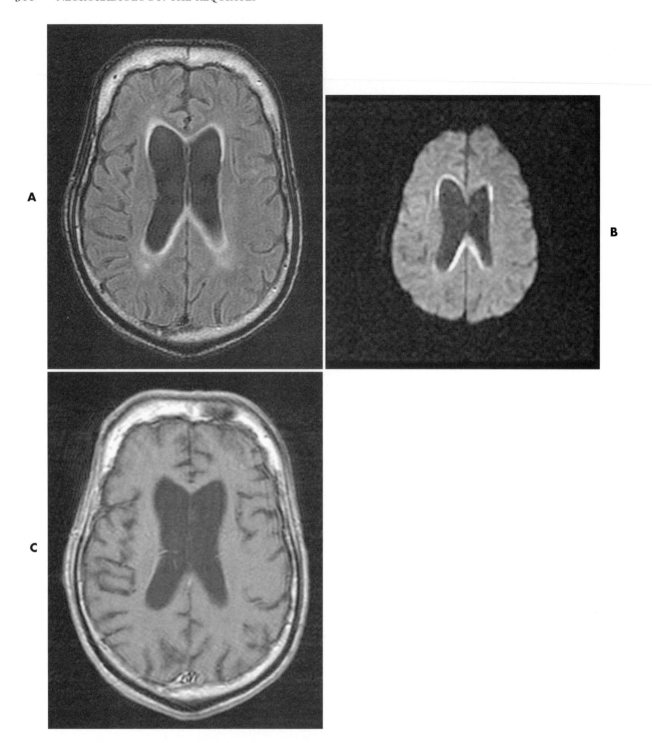

Fig. 6-24 CMV infection in a patient with AIDS. **A,** Axial FLAIR scan shows dilated ventricles and a peripheral rim of hyperintensity. **B,** This periependymal hyperintensity is also bright on DWI (?T2 shine through). **C,** The ependyma enhances in a subtle fashion. This is one of the patterns of involvement with CMV. Sometimes all you see is patchy white matter disease.

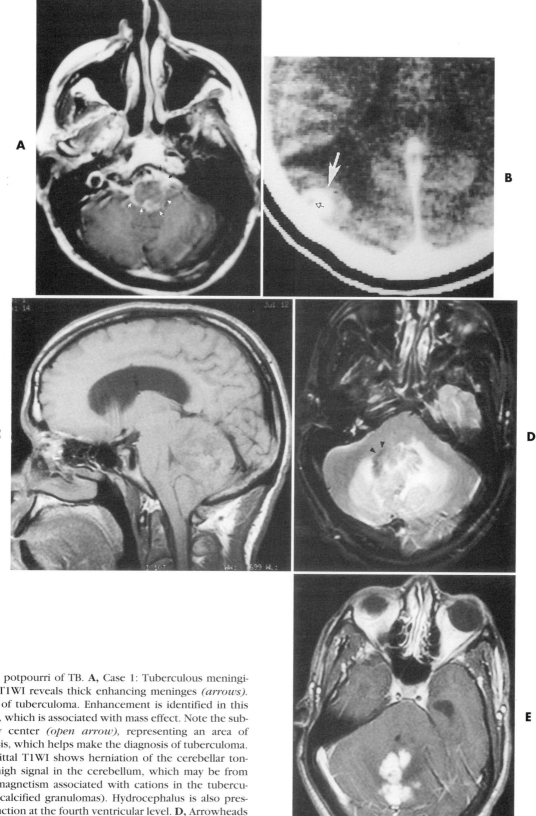

Fig. 6-25   A potpourri of TB. **A,** Case 1: Tuberculous meningitis. Enhanced T1WI reveals thick enhancing meninges *(arrows).* **B,** Case 2: CT of tuberculoma. Enhancement is identified in this lesion *(arrow),* which is associated with mass effect. Note the subtle low-density center *(open arrow),* representing an area of caseous necrosis, which helps make the diagnosis of tuberculoma. **C,** Case 3: Sagittal T1WI shows herniation of the cerebellar tonsils. There is high signal in the cerebellum, which may be from blood or paramagnetism associated with cations in the tuberculous reaction (calcified granulomas). Hydrocephalus is also present with obstruction at the fourth ventricular level. **D,** Arrowheads mark low intensity in the cerebellar inflammatory mass on axial T2WI, not unusual with TB. **E,** Cloverleaf type of enhancement with compression of fourth ventricle is seen on enhanced T1WI.

(particularly on CT) in the basal meninges. Periventricular low density has been observed on CT. Sequelae of tuberculous meningitis include hydrocephalus and infarction secondary to panarteritis of the vessels in the basal cisterns.

The intracranial tuberculoma appears as a nodule that ranges from low to high density on CT. These nodules may be solitary but are commonly multiple and are associated with mass effect and edema. Calcification is uncommon (less than 20%). As it enlarges, the tuberculoma may adhere to dura, causing hyperostosis and thus masquerading as a meningioma. Tuberculoma and tuberculous meningoencephalovasculitis can simulate an infiltrating brain stem glioma. Often concomitant hydrocephalus results from basilar inflammation. The typical tuberculoma would appear as a nodule with a small central area (caseous necrosis) of high signal on T2WI/FLAIR or low density on CT. It is interesting to note that on MR, high intensity may be observed in the wall of tuberculomas on T1WI and low intensity on T2WI/FLAIR. This low intensity rim has also been seen in toxoplasmosis and aspergillosis (Fig. 6-25D). Surrounding the nodule is high intensity on T2WI/FLAIR or low density on CT. This represents edema with mass effect. Enhancement is in rings (with irregular walls with variable thickness) or nodules (which may have punctate nonenhancing centers) (Fig. 6-25B). Noncaseating tuberculomas are often high intensity on T2WI with nodular enhancement whereas caseating lesions are isointense to hypointense on T2WI and ring enhance.

Imaging does not necessarily show tuberculoma in cases of tuberculous meningitis, and obviously not all patients with tuberculoma have meningeal enhancement. However, if you are lucky you will have both and cinch the diagnosis. (TB or not TB, phthisis the question.)

Intracranial tuberculoma has 1H MRS features that primarily result from lipids, a constituent of the cell wall, seen at 0.9 ppm, 1.3 ppm, 2.0 ppm, and 2.8 ppm. Resonances of serine and phenolic lipids (from the granuloma wall) were identified at 7.1 and 7.4 ppm.

Follow-up imaging after appropriate antibiotic therapy shows that the tuberculous nodules decrease in size and may show small areas of punctate calcification on CT at the tuberculoma site. At times, the tuberculoma may be transformed into a calcified nodule that does not enhance. This calcified nodule may completely resorb. In tuberculous meningitis, the degree of hydrocephalus shows no demonstrable improvement. This is the result of the dense adhesions formed from the copious exudate. Other sequelae besides hydrocephalus and infarction are the development of syringomyelia/syringobulbia (rare).

Atypical mycobacterial infections occur in HIV-positive patients; however, there are no specific imaging findings that distinguish these pathogens.

Listeria monocytogenes   This short gram-positive rod pathologically elicits meningitis, meningoencephalitis, and rarely brain abscess. *Listeria* does not present with a distinctive radiologic picture, although it may have a particular predilection for the brain stem, producing abscess, or encephalitis (rhombencephalitis). Rhombencephalitis (inflammation of the brain stem and cerebellum) has a broad differential diagnosis (Box 6-11). The principal problem lies in the difficulties encountered in laboratory diagnosis. CSF specimens often contain only a few *Listeria* organisms, which are easily mistaken for diphtheroids (gram-positive rods) and dismissed as a contaminant or confused with pneumococcus in the CSF.

The diagnosis of *Listeria* infection should be considered in patients with impaired cellular immunity, (or chemotherapy, other related predisposing conditions such as diabetes, alcoholism, renal transplantation, and AIDS) suspected bacterial meningitis, and the imaging findings of meningeal enhancement (or brain abscess) when the findings of bacteriologic studies are negative (Fig. 6-26).

Food-borne transmission of Listeria may account for at least 20% of sporadic cases. The foods associated with this include coleslaw, Mexican-style cheese, raw vegetables, seafood, pasteurized milk, Swiss cheese, raw hot dogs, and undercooked chicken. It is also a cause of neonatal meningitis.

The lesion created hysteria
It involved the brain stem area
The radiologist expressed with precision
In spite of colleagues derision
It enhances and thus it's Listeria

Box 6-11   Differential Diagnosis of Rhombencephalitis

Acute disseminated encephalomyelitis
Behçet disease
Brain stem tumor
Coccidioidomycosis
Legionnaire's disease
Listeria monocytogenes
Lyme disease
Multiple sclerosis
Mycoplasma infection
Rickettsia
Tuberculosis
Viral diseases
   Adenovirus
   Arbovirus
   Herpes simplex
   Herpes zoster
   Influenza A
Whipple disease

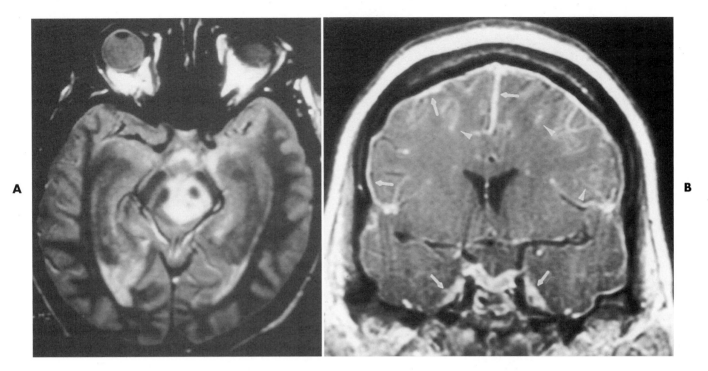

Fig. 6-26 **A,** *Listeria monocytogenes* rhombencephalitis. T2WI/FLAIR with high intensity in brain stem in this patient with altered cellular immunity. **B,** Listeria may cause a meningitis without parenchymal involvement. This is seen on an enhanced scan in a different patient showing patterns of both leptomeningeal *(arrowheads)* and pachymeningeal *(arrows)* involvement.

Rickettsia

Rocky mountain spotted fever This is a seasonal disease seen between late spring and summer in the South Atlantic region of the United States with clinical manifestations of headache, fever, seizures, hearing impairment, neuropathy, altered mental status, lethargy, and coma. A rash is only noted in 50% of cases. Patients greater than 15 years of age tend not to have the cutaneous manifestations. Mortality of 20% is reported in untreated cases. The CNS manifestations include meningoencephalitis and vasculitis. Imaging abnormalities are uncommon, and include basal ganglia infarction, diffuse cerebral edema, diffuse meningeal enhancement, and dilatation of the perivascular spaces in the basal ganglia. Enhancement has been seen in the distal spinal cord, conus medullaris, and cauda equina. Normal imaging studies are associated with improved prognosis.

Spirochetal

Syphilis has already been discussed in the section on AIDS (like the disease, once is more than enough), but we thought we should add a few more words.

At the time he was becoming dummer
The aorta required a plummer
The more he cavorted

So many aborted
What a bummer, dead with the gumma

Lyme disease Lyme disease is an inflammatory disease that can involve multiple systems in the body. It is caused by a spirochete (*Borrelia burgdorferi;* in New York *Borrelia burgdorferi goodman;* noted to have expensive tastes) and transmitted most commonly by the deer tick (*Ixodes dammini;* in New York *Ixodes damn-it*). Three clinical stages have been described: stage 1, constitutional symptoms and an expanding skin lesion (erythema chronicum migrans); stage 2, cardiac and neurologic problems (meningitis, radiculoneuropathy) occurring weeks to months after initial infection; and stage 3, arthritis and chronic neurologic problems that are noted from months to years after infection. These stages may overlap or occur alone. Approximately 10% to 15% of patients with Lyme disease have CNS involvement. Facial nerve palsy can result either from meningitis or as a mononeuritis multiplex. In endemic areas (northeastern United States), it may account for two thirds of childhood facial nerve palsy. It may be associated with optic neuritis (this should ring a bell when you get to the white matter chapter). The pathophysiology includes direct invasion of the parenchyma and/or a vasculitic or immunologic process. Diagnosis is based on clinical findings and serology, although the yield of culture is very low and presently no test indicates active infection.

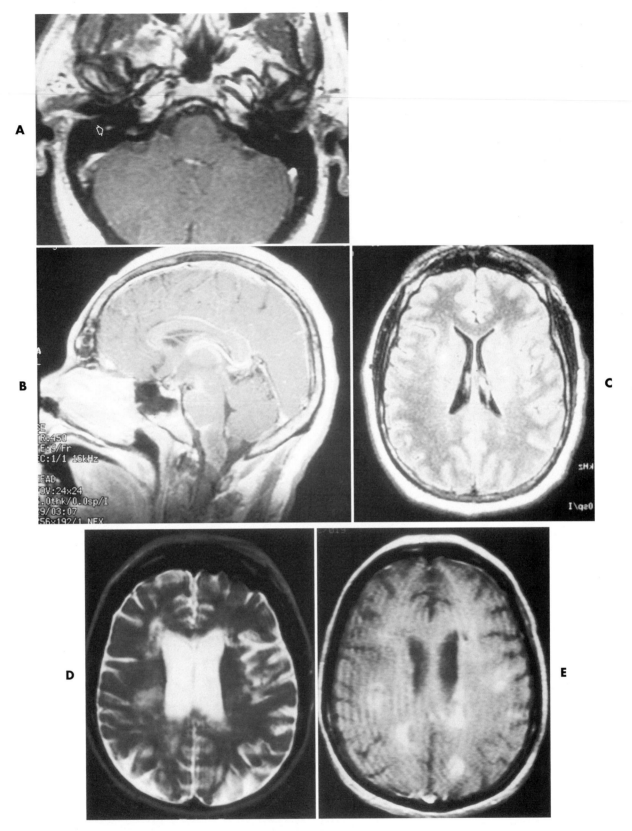

Fig. 6-27 Medley of Lyme disease. **A,** Case 1: Lyme disease. Enhancement and enlargement are identified in the right descending portion of nerve VII on T1WI. Another presentation (parenchymal involvement) is seen in Fig. 7-11. **B,** Case 2: Sagittal enhanced scans demonstrate leptomeningeal enhancement particularly seen in the interpeduncular cistern but also seen coating the pons. **C,** FLAIR scan shows multiple high signal intensity abnormalities in the white matter. **D,** Case 3: Another case showing diffuse white matter change on T2WI. **E,** Many of these lesions enhance. DDx = MS.

On MR, findings include (1) most commonly a normal scan; (2) high signal abnormalities on T2WI/FLAIR, which can vary in size from punctate to large mass lesions; and (3) contrast-enhancing parenchymal lesions, meninges, labyrinth, and cranial nerves (Fig. 6-27). Other abnormalities reported include hydrocephalus, high intensity in the pons, the thalamus and basal ganglia. There may be a predilection for subcortical high intensity abnormalities on MR in the frontal and parietal lobes. Lyme disease should be considered in the differential diagnosis of multiple sclerosis, acute disseminated encephalomyelitis, and vasculitis.

Lyme encephalopathy has been characterized as a cognitive disturbance of mild to moderate memory and learning problems sometimes accompanied by somnolence months to years after the onset of infection. MR with gadolinium in these cases is usually entirely normal. So when all else fails what should a radiologist suggest— you got it—a SPECT scan. Moreover, what is the finding? Yes again, hypoperfusion particularly in the frontal/temporal cortex and subcortical structures including the basal ganglia and white matter. These findings have also been reported in chronic fatigue syndrome, cocaine abuse, HIV encephalopathy, Rasmussen encephalitis, and so on. Following treatment SPECT scans demonstrate increased cerebral perfusion.

Fungal

Fungal infections can produce meningitis, granuloma formation, and rarely encephalitis. We shall discuss the specific entities below.

Cryptococcosis *Cryptococcus* is a yeast with a polysaccharide capsule that distinctively stains with India ink. Sensitive immunologic diagnosis can also be made by detecting cryptococcal antigen or anticryptococcal antibody in the CSF or blood. Pathologic findings include meningitis, meningoencephalitis, or granuloma formation. Hematogenous dissemination from an occult pulmonary focus is the usual vector into the CNS. *Cryptococcus* ranks third behind HIV and toxoplasmosis as a cause of CNS infection in AIDS. CNS cryptococcosis develops in up to 11% of patients with AIDS. MR may be normal (why do you think it is called "crypto-"?), or can demonstrate a spectrum of abnormalities. Recognition of dilated Virchow-Robin spaces in young immunosuppressed patients should raise a red flag concerning the possibility of intracranial cryptococcus (Fig. 6-28). These

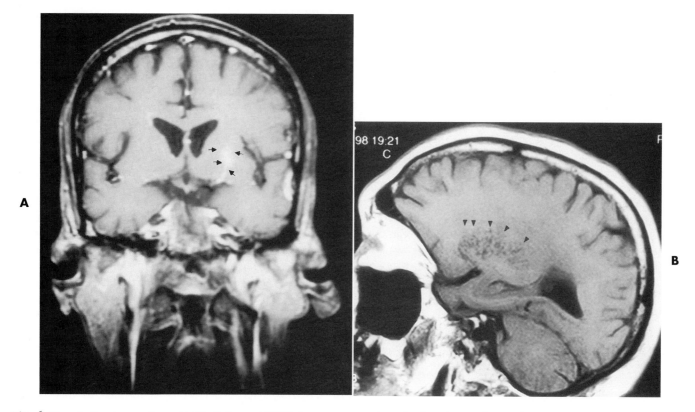

Fig. 6-28   **A,** Cryptococcal meningitis. Enhanced T1WI demonstrates enlarged enhancing Virchow-Robin space in a patient with documented cryptococcal meningitis *(arrows)*. This is unusual because most enlarged Virchow-Robin spaces in cryptococcal meningitis do not enhance. (Is it a venous angioma?) **B,** Dilated Virchow-Robin spaces *(arrowheads)* are depicted on this parasagittal T1WI.

dilated spaces filled with gelatinous cysts, in and adjacent to the basal ganglia and the corticomedullary junction, may or may not enhance. Another important pattern is that of multiple miliary enhancing parenchymal and leptomeningeal nodules with involvement of the choroid plexus in the trigone as well as the spinal cord and spinal nerve roots. Less common findings include widening of the basal cisterns, hydrocephalus, and diffuse atrophy. Diffuse confluent basal cisternal-leptomeningeal enhancement is not usually present in cryptococcal meningitis, differentiating it from tuberculosis or bacterial meningitis. Cryptococcomas occur in 4% to 11% of patients with cryptococcal meningitis presenting as a solid mass or as disseminated lesions predominately in the midbrain and basal ganglia. Contrast is needed to detect leptomeningeal nodules. Numerous bilateral small foci of high signal intensity on T2WI/FLAIR that do not enhance are not pathognomonic of cryptococcosis and can be seen in coccidioidomycosis and candidiasis. The differential diagnosis of basal ganglia lesions in these patients should also include toxoplasmosis and lymphoma.

Other less common fungal infections affecting HIV-positive patients include those caused by *Candida, Aspergillus, Histoplasma,* and *Mucor.*

In HIV negative patients, cryptococcus can produce enlargement and enhancement of the choroid plexus.

Coccidioidomycosis Coccidioidomycosis (Valley Fever) is an endemic fungus infection in the southwestern United States and northern Mexico. The spore is inhaled, and a primary pulmonary focus develops. Hematogenous dissemination to the CNS occurs within a few weeks or months, but dissemination years later has been reported. It can involve the calvarium or skeleton. The intracranial infection may be manifested pathologically by a thick basilar meningitis with meningeal and parenchymal granulomas. The intraaxial granulomas have been reported to have a propensity for the cerebellum. Vasculitis producing occlusion has also been noted. The disseminated cerebral form of coccidioidomycosis occurs predominantly in white men, and diagnosis is confirmed by CSF serology or culture. It is one of the most common causes of eosinophilic meningitis.

On MR, dilated Virchow-Robin spaces similar to *Cryptococcus* (see previous discussion) can be identified (see Fig. 6-28). On PDWI/FLAIR, there is increased signal in the cisterns. Enhancement is noted in the basal meninges, cisterns, and sulci. When ependymitis is present, enhancement is noted around the ventricle. The CT picture is of basal arachnoiditis with obliteration and distortion of the cisterns. These may show increased density before contrast. Associated with this active arachnoiditis is communicating hydrocephalus. Focal areas representing infarction secondary to vasculitis and enhancing nodules can occasionally be observed.

Mucormycosis Prognosis in mucormycosis is directly

related to early recognition of this disease. It affects patients with abnormalities in host defenses, including altered cellular immunity. Particularly prone to this pathogen are diabetic patients with ketoacidosis or debilitated patients with burns, uremia, or malnutrition. It is also seen in HIV patients with a history of drug abuse presenting with basal ganglionic lesions. It has been reported that persons taking the iron chelating agent deferoxamine, such as patients undergoing dialysis, are at increased risk for mucormycosis. Deferoxamine apparently abolishes the normal fungistatic effect of serum on *Mucor.* This fungus is usually inhaled and rapidly destroys the nasal mucosa, forming black crusts (classic eschar). It may then spread into the paranasal sinuses (with or without bone destruction), orbit, and the base of the skull, or may extend through the cribriform plate, resulting in involvement of the anterior cranial fossa. It has a high frequency (50% in some series) of intracranial extension. Clinical symptoms include facial pain, bloody nasal discharge, dark swollen turbinates, chemosis, exophthalmos, cranial nerve palsy progressing rapidly to stroke, encephalitis, and death.

Mucor infection characteristically presents as a rim of soft-tissue thickness along the walls of the paranasal sinus. CT features of sinonasal *Mucor* infection include sinus opacification, air fluid concentrations, increased density or calcification and obliteration of the nasopharyngeal tissue planes (Fig. 6-29). On MR, low intensity may be present in the sinuses on T1WI and T2WI/FLAIR. In some cases, bony destruction is present. Orbital extension from the ethmoid sinuses can produce proptosis and chemosis, and thrombosis of the superior ophthalmic vein, with extension through the orbital apex and subsequent thrombosis of the cavernous sinus. *Mucor* can extend into the infratemporal fossa and pterygopalatine fossa from the maxillary sinus.

Mucor has a striking tendency to proliferate along and through vascular structures producing arteritis with aneurysm, pseudoaneurysm, abscess formation, vascular occlusion, and infarction. This is most frequent in the cavernous portion of the internal carotid but has been seen in the basilar artery. When this virulent fungus extends intracranially (after extension into the orbit or the deep facial structures), low-density abnormalities are noted particularly in the anterior cranial fossa but may be present in any part of the brain. These regions show mass effect and enhancement. *Mucor* may also cause large-vessel cerebral infarction with the associated CT and MR findings. Intracranial abscess, consisting of a low density mass without significant vasogenic edema, evidence of leptomeningitis, or well-defined ring enhancement on CT, has been reported.

Nocardiosis Nocardia, an aerobic fungus resembling Actinomyces, does not produce the sulfur granules seen with actinomycosis. Nocardia is associated with a state of compromised immunity, especially in the setting of steroid therapy. However, it may infect patients with

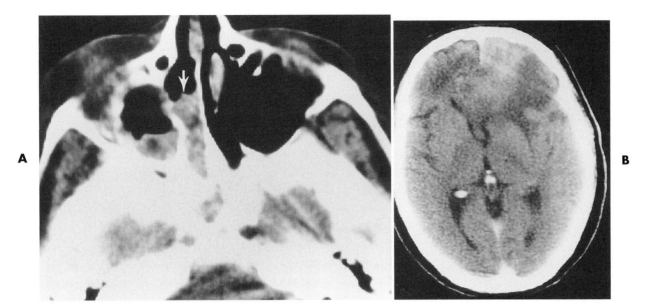

Fig. 6-29   Mucormycosis. **A,** CT showing soft tissue in nasal cavity in a diabetic patient with *Mucor* infection. **B,** *Mucor* grew through the cribriform plate to involve the frontal region, producing a massive frontal cerebritis.

normal immunity as well. Nocardia complicates a spectrum of diseases that includes pulmonary alveolar proteinosis, sarcoidosis, ulcerative colitis, and intestinal lipodystrophy. Hematogenous dissemination occurs from a pulmonary focus into the CNS. This usually results in brain abscess formation; meningitis is rare. The onset of symptoms is often insidious. Nocardial lesions show an enhancing capsule commonly containing multiple loculations (Fig. 6-30). The diagnosis should be considered in the appropriate clinical setting because Nocardia is relatively sensitive to the sulfonamides.

Aspergillosis   In contradistinction to *Nocardia,* where a well-formed capsule is usually apparent, intracranial aspergillosis may or may not demonstrate ring enhancement. This ubiquitous fungus primarily infects the immunocompromised host. It may gain entry into the CNS by inoculation, hematogenous dissemination (most often from a pulmonary focus), or direct extension from the paranasal sinuses.

Pathologically, aspergillosis involves the brain in an aggressive form, producing meningitis and meningoencephalitis with subsequent hemorrhagic infarction. Less malignant presentations include solitary cerebral abscess or isolated granulomas. In aggressive aspergillosis, one histologically visualizes invasion of blood vessels with secondary thrombosis and infarction.

MR shows high intensity lesions on T2WI/FLAIR and at times on T1WI (Fig. 6-31). If the site of origin is the paranasal sinus, one may see decreased intensity on T2WI/FLAIR secondary to calcification or manganese accumulation. There may be evidence of infarction with or without enhancement. The MR findings are nonspe-

cific. CT abnormalities are subtle and include areas of low density with minimal mass effect, poor contrast enhancement, and usually no ring formation. In fact, the presence of true ring enhancement militates against the most aggressive meningoencephalitic variety of aspergillosis. The relatively benign CT picture contrasts sharply with the consumptive nature of this infection. The lack of correlation between the radiographic and pathologic findings is related to the rapidity of the destructive process (inability to form an effective capsule) and to suppression of enhancement by steroid therapy. The clinical setting of immunosuppression, steroid therapy, fever, pulmonary infection, and neurologic findings including a decreasing level of consciousness suggests the aggressive form of intracranial aspergillosis, which implies an extremely poor prognosis.

Candidiasis   *Candida* is the most common cause of autopsy-proved non-AIDS cerebral mycosis. It has a propensity for neutropenic patients who are receiving steroids. *Candida* reaches the CNS by hematogenous dissemination through the respiratory or gastrointestinal tracts. Microscopic pathologic findings include vascular inflammation, thrombosis, infarction, or intraparenchymal microabscess formation, typically in the middle cerebral artery distribution. Noncaseating granulomas have also been observed. The gross pathologic findings induced by this yeast-like fungus include meningitis, pachymeningitis, septic infarction, abscess, or granuloma. These various pathologic presentations consequently generate different images that include hydrocephalus (leptomeningeal disease), enhancing nodules with edema (granuloma), calcified granuloma, infarction, and abscess formation.

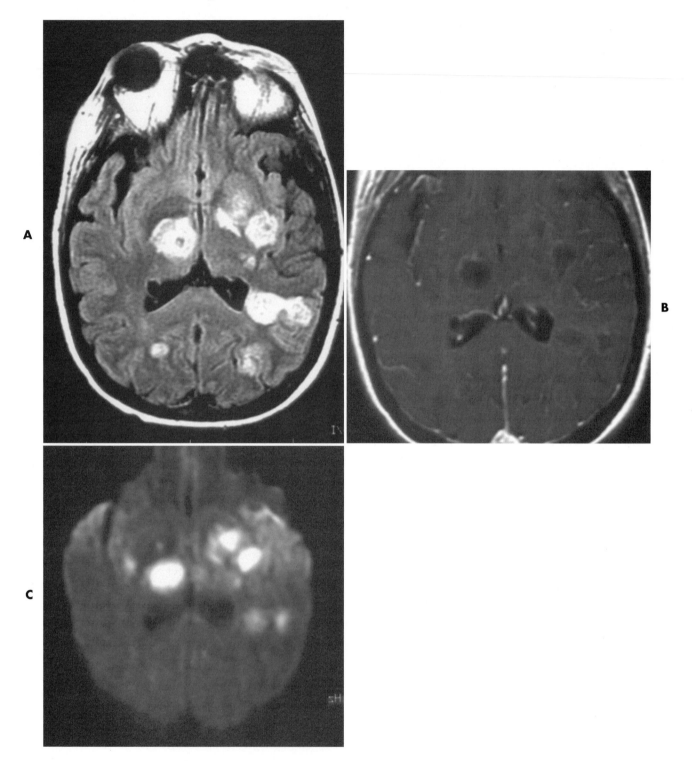

Fig. 6-30   Nocardia. **A,** Flair image reveals multiple lesions in this immunosuppressed patient. **B,** Following contrast observe the rim enhancement. **C,** Diffusion weighted image is positive suggesting very proteinaceous material in the abscesses.

The infectious presentation depends on the state of the host's natural defenses. The inability to mount an effective localizing cell-mediated immune response when challenged favors an aggressive infection rather than granuloma formation. Endophthalmitis is a complication of *Candida* septicemia. This finding in the face of intracranial lesions in the suppressed host strongly supports the diagnosis of CNS candidiasis.

And you thought *Candida* was just another "yeast infection."

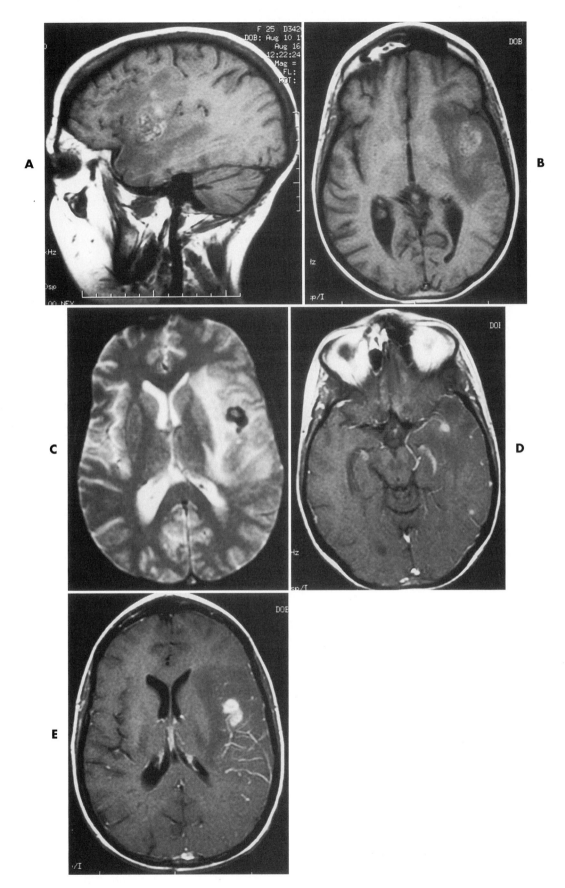

Fig. 6-31 Aspergillus. Hemorrhage seen as high intensity on sagittal (**A**) and axial (**B**) T1WI and low intensity on gradient echo scans (**C**). **D,** and **E,** show enhancing nodules at gray-white junctions and a lot of surrounding edema in the left temporal lobe.

Parasitic

Toxoplasmosis *Toxoplasma gondii* is a ubiquitous protozoan parasite (20% to 70% of the American population is seropositive) infecting the CNS in approximately 10% of patients with AIDS and also affecting adults with compromised cellular immunity (particularly defects in the lymphocyte-monocyte system). Acute toxoplasmosis in immunocompromised patients often occurs from reactivation of remotely acquired latent infection. It can evoke an acute vascular thrombosis with infarction (uncommon) or be well localized in the form of an abscess. Lesions have a propensity for the basal ganglia, corticomedullary junction, white matter, or periventricular region. As opposed to congenital toxoplasmosis, calcification is not common, although it has been reported after therapy. Occasionally, these lesions may be hemorrhagic. On MR, multiple lesions of high intensity on T2WI/FLAIR associated with vasogenic edema and ring or nodular enhancement are seen on T1WI, see Figure 6-20. Reported CT abnormalities have included areas of low density with little or no enhancement, gyriform enhancement, or isodense nodules that enhance. Prompt response to appropriate antibiotic therapy can distinguish toxoplasmosis from lymphoma. (Do not bet the Mouton '45 on differentiating these two entities, because they may coexist—and it is not worth losing this liquid gold; rather, bet the Thunderbird!)

Congenital toxoplasmosis occurs during maternal infection. Its manifestations include bilateral chorioretinitis associated with hydrocephalus (secondary to ependymitis producing aqueductal stenosis) and intracranial calcifications particularly in the basal ganglia and cortex.

Cysticercosis This parasite is endemic in parts of Mexico, Central and South America, Asia, Africa, and Eastern Europe. Human beings are the only known definitive hosts (in which the parasite undergoes sexual reproduction) for the adult tapeworm (*Taenia solium*) and the only known intermediate hosts (in which the larval or asexual stage is present) for the larval form (*Cysticercus cellulosae*), which prospers in the CNS. The parasite is acquired by ingestion of insufficiently cooked pork containing the encysted larvae (one of the benefits of keeping kosher or being Muslim). The larvae develop into the adult tapeworm in the human intestinal tract. The oncospheres (active embryo) released from ova of the adult tapeworm by gastric digestion burrow through the intestinal tract to reach the bloodstream, which carries them to the CNS and to other regions, where they form cysticerci. Humans may also directly ingest the eggs (as an intermediate host) in contaminated food, through self-contamination by the anus-hand-mouth route (yuk!), or by regurgitation of ova. Infestation of the CNS produces many neurologic problems, the most common be-

Box 6-12   Neurologic Problems Associated With Cerebral Cysticercosis

Communicating hydrocephalus
Confusion
Dementia
Headache
Obstructive hydrocephalus
Paresthesias, paresis, paralysis
Psychological disturbances
Seizures
Vertigo
Visual disturbances

ing seizure seen in 30% to 92% of patients (Box 6-12). After several weeks, a cystic covering and a scolex develop in the embryo, which has lodged in the CNS. The interval between the probable date of infection and the first distinctive symptom varies from less than 1 year to 30 years, with the average being approximately 4.8 years. The cysticerci vary in size from pinpoint to 6 cm in diameter. They are located in the brain parenchyma, subarachnoid space, ventricles, or rarely intraspinal locations. Symptoms are related to the site of the parasites. It is not until the larvae die that an acute inflammatory reaction is incited and patients become symptomatic. The parenchymal cysts have a propensity for the cortical and deep gray matter, whereas the subarachnoid cysts can produce basal meningitis, hydrocephalus and mass lesions, particularly in the suprasellar cistern, cerebellopontine angle cistern, sylvian cistern, and cerebral arteritis (in over 50% of cases with subarachnoid lesions) with subsequent infarction usually in the middle cerebral or posterior cerebral distribution. Intraventricular cysts may be free or attached to the wall and become symptomatic when ventricular drainage is obstructed. Spinal cysts are seen in 3% of patients, mostly in the thoracic region, and can cause arachnoiditis and spinal cord compression. Inflammation of the meninges is often more severe in spinal cysticercosis.

CT shows calcification in the brain parenchyma. These are characteristic, with a slightly off-center spherical calcification of 1 to 2 mm in diameter, representing the scolex, surrounded by a partially or totally calcified sphere (7 to 12 mm in diameter). The calcification only occurs in the dead larvae. However, a spectrum of MR and CT findings is associated with cysticercosis (Fig. 6-32). Four stages of cyst formation have been described with imaging that roughly parallel these changes. In the vesicular stage, the larvae are alive and the cyst contains clear fluid. Edema is minimal, and the cyst is surrounded by a thin capsule. On MR, the fluid appears isointense to CSF on all pulse se-

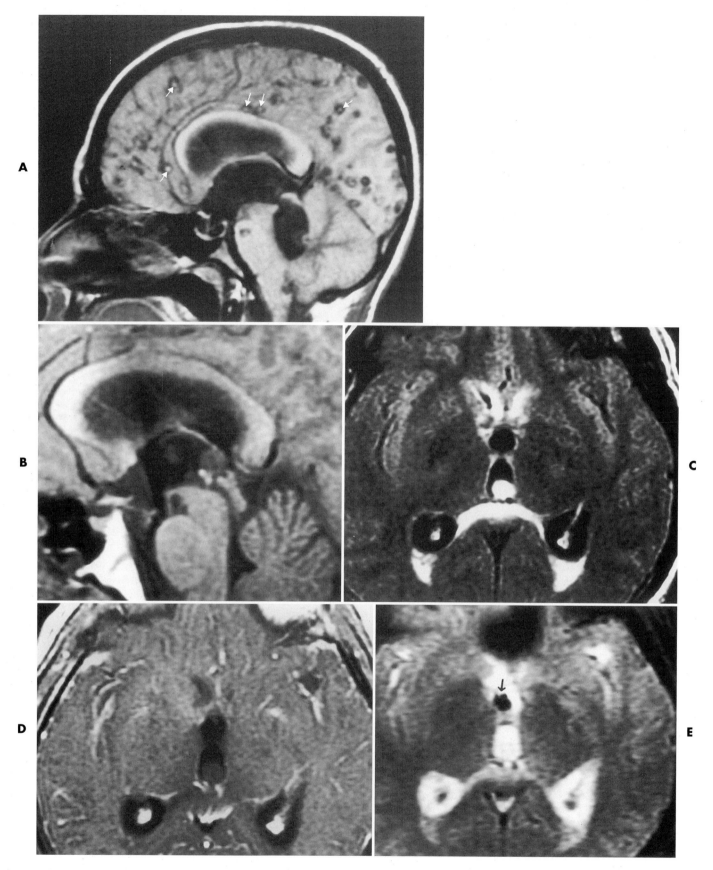

Fig. 6-32 Cysticercosis. **A,** Case 1: Innumerable lesions on T1WI. Scolices *(arrows)* appear of high intensity on this noncontrast image. **B,** Case 2: Intraventricular involvement A cystic lesion is seen on sagittal T1WI **(B),** axial FLAIR **(C),** and enhanced axial **(D)** scans. Note the lack of enhancement. Cysticercosis cysts are usually bright on FLAIR scans. **E,** The piece de resistance—the gradient echo scan shows a calcified cysticercus *(arrow)* in the third ventricle.

quences, and the eccentric scolex (which appears as a mural nodule) can be identified. Little surrounding high intensity on T2WI/FLAIR (edema) or enhancement is appreciated. CT in this stage shows a circumscribed cyst with a density similar to CSF and a denser scolex.

The acute encephalitic phase of the infection is more common in children and is characterized by either multiple diffuse nodular lesions (85%) or localized lesions. In most cases of encephalitis, cysts are located throughout the parenchyma, although they can be localized to one region. The encephalitis phase of the disease lasts from 2 to 6 months, with edema persisting after the enhancement disappears. Diffuse brain edema and ring or nodular enhancement patterns are present. This phase can be fatal. If the patient survives, CT can detect small calcifications as early as 8 months after the acute phase. These lesions occur in the white matter, cerebral cortex, and basal ganglia. Noncalcified nodules of increased density that enhance have also been reported.

In the second (colloidal vesicular) and third (granular nodular) stages the fluid in the cysts becomes turbid and the larvae die, with associated thickening of the capsule. In some cases, there is a strong inflammatory reaction and encephalitis can occur as the cysts move into the colloidal vesicular stage. In the third stage the cyst shrinks between one-third to one-fourth its original size and begins to calcify. In patients without significant reaction to the parasite no enhancement may occur and edema can be minimal. The cyst in these stages can be isointense to hyperintense on T1WI. On T2WI/FLAIR the fluid is isointense to high intensity and the cyst wall is difficult to identify or may be hypointense.

In patients with significant reaction to the cyst, in the second or third stage, foci of high signal and low density associated with surrounding edema are seen. The lesions uniformly enhance as dense nodules or small ring areas. Enhancement is thought to be the result of larval death, reaction to antigen, and release of metabolic products with associated blood-brain barrier abnormality.

In the fourth stage, (nodular calcified stage) focal calcification is seen. CT is more specific than MR, with the brain parenchyma containing calcified dead larvae and low-density cysts. These low-density cysts may or may not enhance. On MR, the lesion is seen as hypointense nodule on T2WI so it can be confused with cavernous malformations. The time it takes for the parasite to evolve through all of the different stages is from 2 to 10 years with an average of approximately 5 years (slightly longer than the normal political parasite).

Ventricular cysticercosis is best noted on MR, where lesions are of higher intensity than CSF to isointense on T1WI and the cyst wall may be identified. The eccentric scolex can be seen as a nodule isointense to brain. The fourth ventricle is the most common location for these lesions. They have the same density as CSF on CT. Intraventricular cysticercosis (7% to 20% of intracranial cysticercosis) produces obstructive hydrocephalus and also causes a granular ependymitis by provoking an inflammatory reaction secondary to toxic substances released from the permeable cyst wall of the dead larvae. The fourth ventricle is the most common ventricle affected. The cyst may be adherent to the wall of the ventricle producing a subependymal rim of high intensity on T2WI/FLAIR. The scolex may be visualized as a small dot within what looks like a dilated ventricle. FLAIR, PDWI, and T1WI are better than conventional T2WI because of the lack of conspicuity on the latter. The differential diagnosis is a dilated ventricle.

Hydrocephalus may also be caused by meningeal involvement, with basilar arachnoiditis and meningeal enhancement. Cysticercosis has been reported rarely to cause obstructive hydrocephalus by presenting as a mass (cysticercotic cyst) of the septum pellucidum. Larvae can have a racemose (grapelike cluster) form that occurs in the subarachnoid spaces (particularly the basal cisterns, sylvian fissures) and ventricles. It may on CT simulate a low-density tumor in the sellar or cerebellopontine angle regions. Widening of a cistern should raise suspicion. The racemose cysticercus does not calcify and lacks a scolex. On MR it appears as a multilobulated mass isointense to CSF. The cyst wall can be visualized as septum-like curved lines on T1WI. There is usually no enhancement of this lesion itself, however, it may evoke extensive leptomeningeal inflammation with fibrosis and chronic granulomatous meningitis. The diagnosis of racemose cysticercosis should be considered in situations where there is a subarachnoid cyst associated with leptomeningeal enhancement in a patient from an endemic region.

Spinal cysticercosis is very rare. So rare that we hesitate to put it in the book, but as we have an international audience, and some of you may be taking boards in the third world (i.e., Louisville) we are obligated to bring this to your attention. It can involve the subarachnoid space, the epidural space, or be intramedullary with similar findings to the spectrum of lesions within the brain. The cysts can compress and compromise the spinal cord. Differential diagnosis here involves arachnoid cyst and epidermoid.

Unusual neuroradiologic features of intracranial cysticercosis include positional cyst alteration, evidence of cortical enhancement with vasculitis and mycotic aneurysm formation, and stroke.

The diagnosis of neurocysticercosis is usually made with the aid of serologic testing for specific antibody in serum, CSF, or both by ELISA. Enhancement has been advocated for meningitis, granulomatous lesions, or cysts with surrounding edema.

Cysticercosis
Produces neurosis,
Convulsions,
Revulsions,
And missed diagnosis!

The jury ruled that she missed the cysti
The radiologist then became quite misty
The plantiff was mean
Saying it could be seen
"The racemose lesion was obvious even to a gypsy"

Cerebral malaria This occurs in about 2% of patients infected with *Plasmodium falciparum*. It is thought that the brain is affected when capillaries are occluded by infected red blood cells containing the parasite. Neurologic manifestations are nonspecific but occur with classic high fever and chills. MR has demonstrated cortical infarction and high intensity on T2WI/FLAIR in the white matter including the splenium of the corpus callosum. The latter changes have been interpreted as occurring as a result of immune mediated cytokine release leading to vasodilatation, swelling, and myelin loss.

Paragonimiasis This is caused by the lung fluke and is endemic in Latin America, East and Southeast Asia, and West Africa. Readers beware of undercooked freshwater crayfish or crabs or eating raw boar meat at your local McDonald's. Brain involvement with Paragonimus has been reported in 2% to 27% of infected patients. The life cycle of this worm is interesting. The adult worm resides in or around bronchioles of cats, dogs, wild carnivores, and humans. The worms arrive in fresh water where miracidia develop. Miracidia invade freshwater snails. After asexual reproduction, cercariae are produced, which invade freshwater crabs or crayfish. The metacercariae infect the final hosts after being ingested and excyst in the small intestine to eventually invade the pleural cavity and lung parenchyma. Brain infection occurs via the perivascular soft tissue in the foramina of the skull base where the worms penetrate meninges and invade brain parenchyma directly. Clinical findings including epilepsy, headache, visual disturbances, and meningeal symptoms. The diagnosis can be made by specific antibody tests by ELISA especially early in the disease.

The initial intracranial lesions of cerebral paragonimiasis include exudative aseptic inflammation, cerebral hemorrhage, or infarction tending to involve one side of the brain. After intracranial invasion, granulomatous lesions are formed around the adult worm. The most characteristic and frequent lesions are multiple, conglomerated and interconnected granulomas, which are located around a focus. These have features of conglomerated rings. Hemorrhage can be detected in some of these patients on MR. In the chronic stage, nearly all the granulomas calcify. The radiologic findings in the chronic stage are "soap-bubble calcifications" on plain radiographs or CT.

The differential diagnosis of these lesions in the early stages include other abscess and tumors (the "tubetti" pasta sign). Clearly the history, region of the world, and circumstance such as visiting professor rounds favor this unusual organism.

Sparganosis This is really a nauseating disease, most common in East Asia, caused by a migrating tapeworm. It usually involves the subcutaneous tissue or muscle of the chest, abdominal wall, or extremities. Humans are infected by drinking water infected with copepods (first intermediate host), eating raw or inadequately cooked infected snakes or frogs (second intermediate host), or by applying the flesh of the infected host to a wound. To pay the price of eating a snake or frog for a disease with no known therapy just is not worth it, even if the meal is part of a survival course at your neighborhood community college. The worm has been reported to be between 1 cm to 1 m long (pretty big worm even by our standards) and can survive in humans up to 20 years.

Cerebral sparganosis causes headache, seizures, and hemiparesis. Chronic granulomatous lesions produce cerebral atrophy with associated myelin loss that result from organizing edema to fibrillary gliosis. Calcification can be seen (multiple punctate or small nodular). Enhancing lesions of different shapes have been described. Enhancement was also visualized near granulation tissue outside the dense collagenous wall around the worm. The worm is not always present inside these dense collagenous walls and the cavities may often be elongated or sinusoidal as opposed to cysticercosis, which are round. Hyperintensity on T1WI in combination with hypointensity on T2WI in subcortical areas may be subacute or chronic petechial hemorrhages. Punctate calcifications are from the calcospherules or from calcification in the degenerated worm's smooth muscle. The lesion is associated with ipsilateral ventricular atrophy.

There is no effective therapy; surgical removal of the live worm is the treatment of choice. Granulomas around the dead worm regress. It is believed that a large enhancing lesion associated with edema or change in location of the enhancing nodule or worsening of imaging findings suggest a live worm.

Eating snakes with sparganosis
Makes a very difficult radiological diagnosis
However the prognosis
Is clearly worse than in halitosis or echinococcocis—
see belowsis

Echinococcosis (Hydatid disease) This is another great disease brought to you by the dog tapeworm. Clinical signs and symptoms include seizures, raised intracranial pressure, and focal neurologic deficits. It is endemic in the Middle East, South America, and Australia caused by ingestion of dog feces that include ova of dog tapeworm (*Echinococcus granulosus*). The ova hatch in the gastrointestinal tract and embryos are spread throughout the body. The embryo matures into a cystic larva (hydatid cyst), which are commonly large and unilocular although other cystic configurations may be seen. Cerebral involvement is seen in 2% to 5% of cases. The most common location is the parietal lobe. The cystic component has an intensity similar to CSF. Severe inflammatory reaction in the brain occurs if the cyst ruptures (surgeons need to be careful here). Scolices and aggregates of scolices (hydatid sand) can be seen on MR within the cyst. Calvarial echinococcal cyst can extend into the intracranial cavity.

Raccoon roundworm encephalitis Raccoons are commonly infected with an intestinal roundworm *Baylisascaris procyonis.* This has been identified in children and adults after ingesting raccoon feces or from areas or articles contaminated by them (logs, wood piles, associated soil, barn lofts that are used as communal toilets, and so on). Its manifestations include encephalitis and ocular findings including neuroretinitis. Periventricular white matter lesions, which may be diffuse, and brain stem lesions have been identified on T2WI/FLAIR. The infection results in atrophy. Eosinophilia in combination with neuroretinitis and MR abnormalities suggests this infection and the definitive diagnosis is made by identification of the larvae from tissue.

Inflammatory Diseases

Sarcoidosis

Sarcoidosis, a systemic granulomatous disease of unknown etiology, primarily occurs in the third and fourth decades of life, affecting the nervous system clinically in approximately 5% of cases of systemic sarcoid and up to 16% in autopsy series. This figure includes involvement of peripheral nerves and myopathy. A very small percentage of patients have only the CNS disease without systemic manifestations. CNS sarcoidosis is an exclusionary diagnosis because even a positive biopsy represents only a nonspecific reaction to a variety of diseases. We have been told that this is controversial and that some pathologists believe that one can make a diagnosis with a positive biopsy finding (particularly if the pathologist is off his lithium). Granulomatous intracranial disease has two principal patterns. The more common presentation is a chronic basilar leptomeningitis with involvement of the hypothalamus, pituitary stalk, optic nerve, and chiasm. The convexities may also be involved. Patients may have unilateral or bilateral cranial nerve (particularly nerve VII) palsy, or endocrine or electrolyte disturbances. In these patients, communicating hydrocephalus develops and signs of meningeal irritation may be present. The granulomatous process frequently spreads from the leptomeninges to the Virchow-Robin spaces, invading and thrombosing affected blood vessels (arteries and/or veins) and producing a granulomatous angiitis similar to primary angiitis of the CNS. The CSF abnormalities are elevated lymphocytes and protein with hypoglycorrhachia. These findings are nonspecific and not diagnostic for this disease.

The second pattern is parenchymal sarcoid nodules.

These granulomatous masses are usually associated with extensive arachnoiditis and microscopic granulomas throughout the brain parenchyma. They have been reported to cause obstructive hydrocephalus when located in the periaqueductal region. These masses may be calcified and avascular. The sarcoid nodules produce signs and symptoms of an intracranial mass. High intensity white matter can be observed in sarcoid, and this can be indistinguishable from multiple sclerosis.

The imaging picture depends on whether there is leptomeningitis, granulomas in the brain, or a mass lesion. On MR, high signal on T2WI/FLAIR in the parenchyma and at the gray-white junction has been recognized. Intraparenchymal sarcoid masses may or may not enhance. Diffuse, focal, and gyriform enhancement of the leptomeninges and basilar enhancement in the hypothalamic region can be observed. An interesting observation is that the enhancement can follow the Virchow-Robin spaces and appear linear (Fig. 6-33). Hydrocephalus, either obstructive or communicating, is common.

Nodules may be calcified, have slightly increased density, or be isodense, and can occur throughout the brain parenchyma with a marked predilection for the skull base, pituitary, pons, hypothalamus, and periventricular region. The nodules are not usually associated with edema. Sarcoid nodules do not cavitate as frequently as tuberculous nodules.

Sarcoid can masquerade as a brain tumor, pituitary lesion, meningioma (with similar imaging features), vasculitis, multiple sclerosis, and even angiographically as a subdural mass. Extraaxial sarcoid is particularly a common mimic of meningioma, with a dural-based mass, occasional hyperostosis, and meningeal enhancement (see Fig. 6-33). Up to 25% of patients can have ophthalmic manifestations including anterior uveitis (most common manifestation), posterior uveitis, lacrimal gland infiltration, optic nerve/sheath involvement, retrobulbar masses, exophthalmos, extraocular muscle thickening, and infiltration of the visual pathways. It can mimic Tolosa-Hunt syndrome. It may affect the spinal cord with lepto-meningeal coating of the cord or appear as an intra-medullary mass. Rarely sarcoid can inflame the cauda equina, causing a polyradiculopathy and demonstrating nodularity and thickening of the nerve roots. Leptomeningeal sarcoid must be distinguished clinically from carcinomatous, lymphomatous, and infectious meningitis. Dramatic response has been noted in some cases with steroid therapy, which can produce a complete disappearance of the enhancing lesions. Sarcoid has replaced syphilis as the great mimic. When you have no idea, think sarcoid.

Wegener Granulomatosis

Wegener granulomatosis is a disease characterized by necrotizing granulomas that can involve multiple organs of the body (upper and lower respiratory tracts, kidneys, orbits, heart, skin, and joints). In 2% to 8% of cases the meninges and brain can be affected. Manifestations include meningeal thickening and enhancement either diffuse or focal in morphology in the brain and spinal cord, infarction, nonspecific white matter abnormalities on T2WI/FLAIR, intraparenchymal granuloma, and atrophy. It produces a vasculitis that results in peripheral neuropathy (frequent), myopathy, intracerebral hemorrhage, subarachnoid hemorrhage, arterial and venous thrombosis. It can involve the pituitary gland and stalk either from direct extension of extracranial disease or as a remote granuloma.

Behçet's Disease

Behçet's disease is a multisystem immune-related vasculitis, with CNS involvement in 5% to 10% of cases, characterized by exacerbations and remissions. The diagnosis requires recurrent oral ulcerations and two of the following to establish a definite diagnosis: recurrent gen-

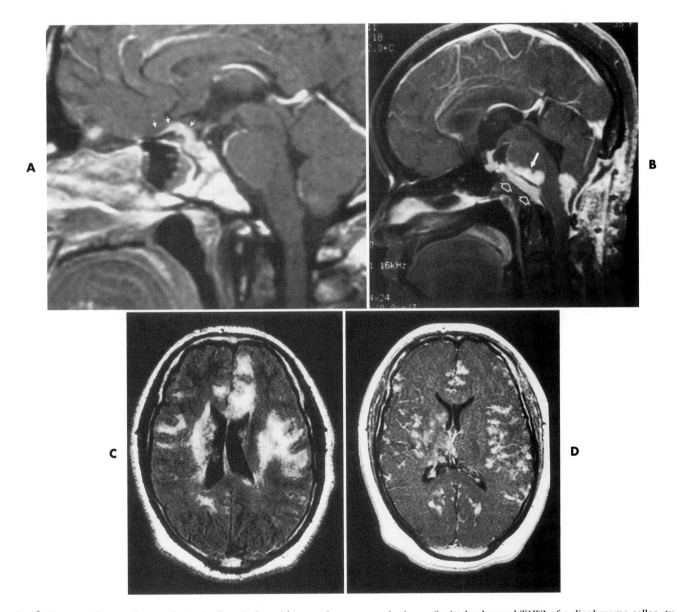

Fig. 6-33   A mélange of sarcoidosis. **A,** Case 1: Sarcoid appearing as a meningioma. Sagittal-enhanced T1WI of a diaphragma sellae, tuberculum sellae-enhancing mass that looks and smells just like a meningioma including a dural tail *(arrows)* and maybe even blistering of the bone. (A blinded taste test was performed by the pathologist, who stated unequivocally that this was sarcoid, probably 1982 vintage.) **B,** Case 2: Leptomeningeal *(arrows)* and dural *(open arrows)* involvement is portrayed nicely on this sagittal enhanced T1WI. **C,** Case 3: Abnormal intensity to the white matter is illustrated on the FLAIR scan. There may be subtle high intensity in the subarachnoid space but all doubt is removed on the enhanced T1WI **(D).** Note the diffuse bilateral nature of the disease, predominantly pial in presentation.

Illustration continued on following page

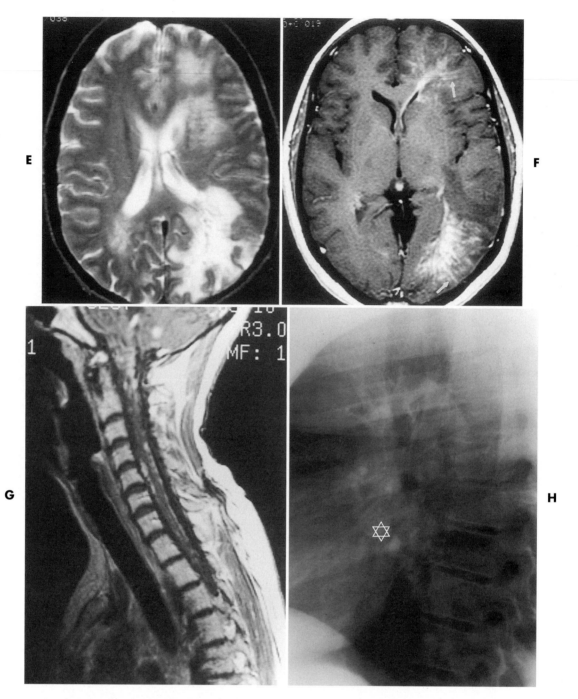

Fig. 6-33 *Continued.* **E,** Case 4: Asymmetric white matter changes are present on T2WI. **F,** Note the linear *(arrows)* perivascular pattern of enhancing sarcoid involvement in this case. Case 5: Spinal **(G)** leptomeningeal and pulmonary **(H)** involvement are seen in this case. Note the hilar adenopathy *(star)*. (Not bad for neuroradiologists, eh?)

ital ulcerations, skin or eye lesions, or a positive pathergy test. The pathology has a clear venous vasculitic component in the CNS particularly the brain stem.

Three patterns of neurologic manifestations are observed: a brain stem syndrome, a meningoencephalitic syndrome, and an organic confusion syndrome. It occurs along the Silk Road from Japan to the Mediterranean, and the Middle East but can be seen in North America, particularly in persons from these ethnic backgrounds. Patients may man-

ifest other signs at the same time as or months to years after the onset of the syndrome complex, including erythema nodosum, polyarthritis, thrombophlebitis, arterial occlusions, pulmonary infarction, ulcerative colitis, portal hypertension, or neurologic, cardiac, or renal complications.

On MR, multiple high intensity lesions can be seen with variable enhancement. The most common finding is a mesodiencephalic junction lesion with edema extending along tracts in the brain stem and diencephalon

(Fig. 6-34). Another pattern is involvement of the pontobulbar region. These lesions can simulate brain stem tumors. Other regions affected include basal ganglia, spinal cord, cerebral hemispheres, and rarely the optic nerve. Enhancement may occur as a ring or nodule, and multiple lesions may be present. Hemorrhage can occasionally be detected in these lesions. The radiologist should appreciate that Behçet disease is associated with venous thrombosis in more than one third of cases, although it rarely occurs in the dural sinuses. Brain stem atrophy has been reported in chronic cases. The vast majority of patients are less than 50 years of age. It is thus difficult to separate these lesions from those of multiple sclerosis, other vasculitides such as primary arteritis of the CNS, and inflammatory diseases such as sarcoid.

Whipple Disease

Whipple disease, a chronic granulomatous disorder with a propensity for the gastrointestinal tract, can primarily involve the CNS (20% of cases). Clinical findings include cognitive changes leading to progressive dementia, ophthalmoplegia, seizures, myoclonus, gait disturbance, and hypothalamic dysfunction. It can be fulminant,

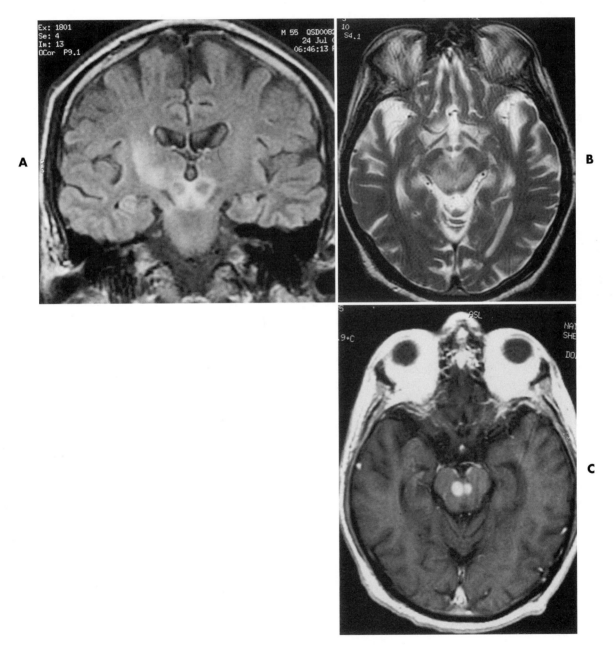

Fig. 6-34   Behçet's disease **A,** Coronal FLAIR portrays the brainstem involvement with at the meso-diencephalic junction. **B,** Diffuse spread in the midbrain-pons region was seen on axial T2WI. **C,** Enhancement was present in red nucleus zone.

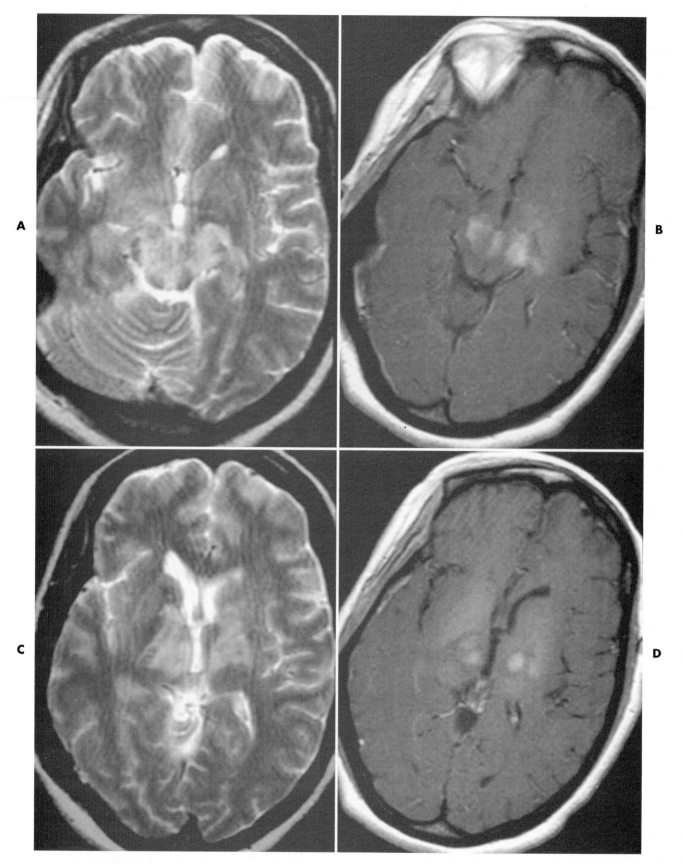

Fig. 6-35 CNS Whipples. **A,** Midbrain hyperintensity is present on T2WI, which shows modest enhancement in **B. C,** The thalamus was also involved and showed enhancement **(D).** This case amazed us because the lesions waxed and waned over 2 years before a definitive diagnosis of Whipple's disease was made, based on the isolation of PAS positive bacteria and a response to antibiotics.

progressing to coma and death. Diagnostic histopathologic features of Whipple disease include periodic acid-Schiff and methenamine-silver staining of macrophages, negative stains for acid-fast bacilli, and ultrastructural demonstration of unique membrane-bound inclusions at different stages of degradation. Delayed hypersensitivity to the Whipple disease gram-positive bacillus (*Tropheryma whippelii*) is thought to be the mechanism of granuloma formation. Electron microscopy shows macrophages containing *Tropheryma whippelii*. The brain lesions are located in the gray matter including the basal part of the telencephalon, the hypothalamus, and the thalamus. However, it has also been reported to involve other regions of the brain including the chiasm, posterior fossa, and the spinal cord.

There is no specific CT or MR finding; however, nodules that are hypointense on T1 and high-intensity on T2 that enhance, together with myoclonus, ophthalmoplegia, progressive dementia, steatorrhea, malabsorption, and arthritis, in a man 40 to 50 years of age should bring this disease to mind (Fig. 6-35). Polymerase chain reaction of peripheral blood mononuclear cells has recently been suggested as a method for making the diagnosis.

Guillain-Barre Syndrome

This is a demyelinating polyneuropathy produced by an immune-mediated mechanism. Patients present with progressive motor weakness and hyporeflexia or areflexia. It may also involve the seventh cranial nerve. There is increased protein in the CSF without pleocytosis and EMG demonstrates nerve-conduction slowing, conduction block, prolonged distal latencies, and prolonged or absent F waves. MR demonstrates enhancement and thickening of the cauda equina and anterior spinal nerve roots (more common and specific for this

---

Box 6-13   **Differential Diagnosis of Radicular Enhancement**
Arachnoiditis
Charcot Marie Tooth
CMV
CSF Metastases
Dejerine Sottas
Disc Herniation with Root Inflammation
Guillain-Barre
Herpes Zoster
Lyme
Neurofibroma
Sarcoid and other Granulomatous diseases
Schwannoma

---

disease, if seen alone) (see Fig 17-7A). Clinical support (plus plasmapheresis and infusion of immunoglobulin) until recovery (which may be incomplete) is the main form of treatment. Polyradiculopathy in AIDs has been associated with cytomegalovirus. Box 6-13 provides the differential diagnosis of radicular enhancement.

Miller-Fisher syndrome is a variant of Guillain-Barre characterized by the acute onset of external ophthalmoplegia, cerebellar ataxia, and areflexia. Contrast enhancement has been observed in the abducens and oculomotor nerves as well as the spinal nerve roots.

WEIRD AND NOT-SO-WONDERFUL DISEASES

We did not know where exactly to put these devastating diseases that most likely have an infectious or postinfectious etiology so we stuck them here. The first three affect children.

Rasmussen Encephalitis

This is seen in children with a mean of 6 to 8 years of age. Focal motor seizures are followed over time by progressive loss of ipsilateral motor function associated with cognitive decline. Histopathology shows perivascular lymphocytic cuffing of round cells, gliosis, and microglial nodules in the cortical layers of the brain. Late in the disease, neuronal loss is noted without inflammatory change. The etiology has been attributed to a viral-induced autoimmune mechanism. Early in the disease imaging can be normal although cerebral swelling has been reported. High intensity lesions on T2WI in the basal ganglia and periventricular white matter have also been observed. Because the therapy of this disease is hemispherectomy, make certain you comment on basal ganglia involvement. Removal of the basal ganglia gives a worse motor prognosis although not removing affected tissue can result in persistent seizures (bad news either way). Late in the disease, diffuse atrophy either progressive or nonprogressive has been noted. The frontal or frontotemporal regions are most commonly involved with a predominant unilateral distribution (Fig. 6-36).

This is another disease in which SPECT scanning may be more sensitive than MR revealing large regions of diminished cerebral perfusion. Crossed cerebellar diaschisis (secondary to disruption of the corticopontocerebellar system) has been reported. This appears as an area of diminished perfusion of the cerebellar hemisphere contralateral to the affected cerebral hemisphere. 1H MRS reveals decreased NAA (yet another "specific finding"—NOT), increased myoinositol, elevated Cho, glutamine, and glutamate.

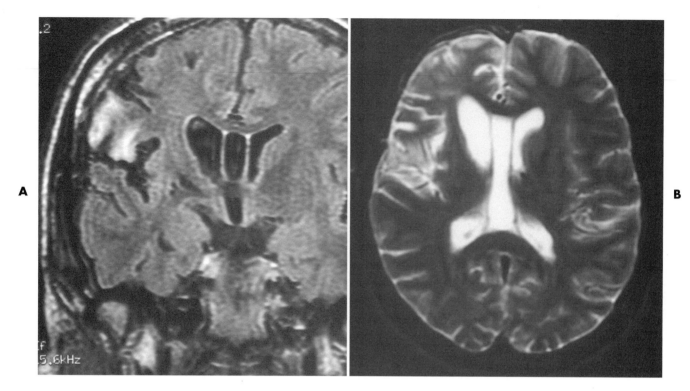

Fig. 6-36   Rasmussen encephalitis. **A,** High intensity on coronal FLAIR in the right frontal region in this 6-year-old with focal seizures. **B,** T2 weighted image with associated right-sided atrophy.

Acute Necrotizing Encephalopathy (ANE) of Childhood

This condition is predominantly reported in children (5 months to 11 years) from Asia and occurs after an infectious encephalitis episode presenting with vomiting, fever, diarrhea progressing to seizures and coma. The patients have evidence of recent infection with various viruses. Clinical findings include elevated liver enzymes, lactate dehydrogenase, and ammonia, elevated CSF pressure, increased CSF protein and myelin basic protein. CT/MR shows multifocal and symmetrical lesions with the thalami affected in all cases and the internal capsules in most. Other reported locations of involvement include the pons, midbrain, cerebellum, and white matter. Those children who survive (70%) have motor and cognitive sequelae and well as residual lesions including atrophy, thalamic hypodensity/hyperintensity and cystic changes in their white matter. The differential diagnosis is provided in Box 6-14.

Hemorrhagic Shock and Encephalopathy Syndrome (HSES)

Mechanisms involved in this syndrome include hypoxic/anoxic damage resulting from an infectious or toxin-mediated mechanism involving microbial toxins acting as superantigens. Hyperpyrexia has been reported to be a factor in the pathogenesis of HSES and children with it have defects in elaboration of heat shock proteins (which are protective against a variety of stresses). The patients range from 2 to 33 months of age and the clinical criteria include shock, coma, seizures, diarrhea (which can be bloody), disseminated intravascular coagulation, anemia, low platelets, elevated liver enzymes, renal dysfunction, acidosis, and negative blood/CSF cultures. CT may display regions of diffuse low density in various regions of the brain (including the basal ganglia, cortical and subcortical regions) and intraparenchymal hemorrhage. MR shows hemorrhagic cortical lesions (hypointensity on T2 and gradient echo images).

Chronic Fatigue Syndrome

This is characterized by varying degrees of chronic fatigue and persistent or recurrent episodes of fever, pharyngitis, myalgia, headache, arthralgia, paresthesias, depression, difficulties with memory, and concentration. The subjective and nonspecific nature of the clinical symptoms combined with the absence of definitive serologic or immunologic finding also make this a ponderous medical judgment. The etiology and the entity itself are very controversial but may be secondary to chronic

Box 6-14   Differential Diagnosis of Acute Necrotizing Encephalopathy (ANE) of Childhood

Acute Encephalopathy with hemorrhagic Shock
Acute poisoning with hydrogen sulfide or cyanide
Carbon monoxide
Glutaric Aciduria Type I
Hemolytic uremia syndrome
Hypoxia
Inflammatory Viral Disease
Leigh Syndrome
Methanol
Methylmalonic Aciduria
Other Mitochondrial myopathies
Reye Syndrome
Sandhoff
Stroke
Symmetrical Thalamic Degeneration with
   Calcifications in infancy
Systemic Lupus Erythematous
Tay Sach
Trauma
Viral and Postinfectious Encephalitis

viral encephalitis. High intensity abnormalities have been seen on T2WI in the white matter (so what), but to date there is no MR pattern of white matter abnormalities specific for chronic fatigue syndrome. SPECT imaging shows multiple perfusion defects throughout the brain.

FORTUNE COOKIE
Man who eat contaminated meat
Better examine his sheet

SUGGESTED READINGS

Abe T, Kojima K, Shoji H, et al: Japanese encephalitis, *J Mag Res Imaging* 8(4):755-761, 1998.

Angelini L, Bugiani M, Zibordi F, et al: Brainstem encephalitis resulting from Epstein-Barr virus mimicking an infiltrating tumor in a child, *Ped Neurol* 22(2):130-132, 2000.

Anlar B, Saatci I, Kose G, et al: MRI findings in subacute sclerosing panencephalitis, *Neurology* 47(5):1278-1283, 1996.

Barinagarrementeria F, Cantu C: Frequency of cerebral arteritis in subarachnoid cysticercosis: an angiographic study, *Stroke* 29(1):123-125, 1998.

Barkovich AJ, Lindan CE: Congenital cytomegalovirus infection of the brain: imaging analysis and embryologic considerations, *AJNR* 15(4):703-715,1994.

Barloon TJ, Yuh WTC, Knepper LE, et al: Cerebral ventriculitis: MR finding, *J Comput Assist Tomogr* 14:272-275,1990.

Bash S, Hathout G, Cohen S, et al: Mesiotemporal T2-weighted hyperintensity: neurosyphilis mimicking herpes encephalitis, *AJNR* 22(2):314-316, 2001.

Benator RM, Magill HL, Gerald B, et al: Herpes simplex encephalitis: CT findings in the neonate and young infant, *AJNR* 6:539-543, 1985.

Berthier M, Sierra J, Leiguarda R: Intraventricular tuberculoma: report of four cases in children, *Neuroradiology* 29:163-167, 1987.

Bonawitz C, Castillo M, Mukherji SK, et al: Comparison of CT and MR features with clinical outcome in patients with Rocky Mountain spotted fever, *AJNR* 18(3):459-464, 1997.

Braun IF, Chambers E, Leeds NE, et al: The value of unenhanced scans in differentiating lesions producing ring enhancement, *AJNR* 3:643-647, 1982.

Burke DG, Leonard DG, Imperiale TF, et al: The utility of clinical and radiographic features in the diagnosis of cytomegalovirus central nervous system disease in AIDS patients, *Mol Diagn* 4(1):37-43, 1999.

Bursztyn EM, Lee BCP, Bauman J: CT of acquired immunodeficiency syndrome, *AJNR* 5:711-714, 1984.

Byun WM, Park WK, Park BH, et al: Guillain-Barre syndrome: MR imaging findings of the spine in eight patients [see comments], *Radiology* 208(1):137-141, 1998.

Callebaut J, Dormont D, Dubois D, et al: Contrast-enhanced MR imaging of tuberculous pachymeningitis cranialis hypertrophica: case report, *AJNR* 11:821-822, 1990.

Campistol J, Gassio R, Pineda M, et al: Acute necrotizing encephalopathy of childhood (infantile bilateral thalamic necrosis): two non-Japanese cases, *Dev Med & Child Neurol* 40(11):771-774, 1998.

Chang KH, Han MH: MRI of CNS parasitic diseases, *J Mag Res Imaging* 8(2):297-307, 1998.

Chang L, Miller BL, McBride D, et al: Brain lesions in patients with AIDS: H-1 MR spectroscopy [published erratum appears in *Radiology* 1996 Feb;198(2):586], *Radiology* 197(2):525-531, 1995.

Chiang FL, Miller BL, Chang L, et al: Fulminant cerebral lymphoma in AIDS, *AJNR* 17(1):157-160, 1996.

Cholankeril JV, Lieberman H: Chronic granulomatous abscess simulating cerebellopontine angle tumor, *AJNR* 5:637-638, 1984.

Chong J, Di Rocco A, Tagliati M, et al: MR findings in AIDS-associated myelopathy [see comments], *AJNR* 20(8):1412-1416, 1999.

Cordoliani YS, Sarrazin JL, Felten D, et al: MR of cerebral malaria, *AJNR* 19(5):871-874, 1998.

Corssmit EP, Leverstein-van Hall MA, Portegies P, et al: Severe neurological complications in association with Epstein-Barr virus infection, *J Neurovirol* 3(6):460-464, 1997.

Danziger A, Price H, Schechter MM. An analysis of 113 intracranial infections, *Neuroradiology* 19:31-34, 1980.

Darling CF, Larsen MB, Byrd SE, et al: MR and CT imaging patterns in post-varicella encephalitis, *Ped Radiol* 25(4):241-244, 1995.

Deresiewicz RL, Thaler SJ, Hsu L, et al: Clinical and neuroradiographic manifestations of eastern equine encephalitis [see comments], *N Engl J Med* 336(26):1867-1874, 1997.

Diebler C, Dusser A, Dulac O: Congenital toxoplasmosis: clinical and neuroradiological evaluation of the cerebral lesions, *Neuroradiology* 27:125-130, 1985.

Drouat S, Abdenabi B, Ghanem M, et al: Computed tomography of cerebral tuberculoma, *J Comput Assist Tomogr* 11:594-597, 1987.

Dubrovsky T, Curless R, Scott G, et al: Cerebral aneurysmal arteriopathy in childhood AIDS, *Neurology* 51(2):560-565, 1998.

Enzmann D, Chang Y, Augustyn G: MR findings in neonatal herpes simplex encephalitis type II, *J Comput Assist Tomogr* 14:453-457, 1990.

Enzmann DR, Britt RR, Obana WG, et al: Experimental *Staphylococcus aureus* brain abscess, *AJNR* 7:395-402, 1986.

Enzmann DR, Placone RC, Britt RH: Dynamic computed tomographic scans in experimental brain abscess, *Neuroradiology* 26:309-313, 1984.

Ernst TM, Chang L, Witt MD, et al: Cerebral toxoplasmosis and lymphoma in AIDS: perfusion MR imaging experience in 13 patients, *Radiology* 208(3):663-669, 1998.

Eustace S, McGrath D, Albrecht M, et al: Clival marrow changes in AIDS: findings at MR imaging, *Radiology* 193(3):623-627, 1994.

Fernandez RE, Rothbert M, Ferencz G, et al: Lyme disease of the CNS: MR imaging findings in 14 cases, *AJNR* 11:479-481, 1990.

Filippi CG, Sze G, Farber SJ, et al: Regression of HIV encephalopathy and basal ganglia signal intensity abnormality at MR imaging in patients with AIDS after the initiation of protease inhibitor therapy, *Radiology* 206(2):491-498, 1998.

Fink IJ, Danziger A, Dillon WP, et al: Atypical CT Findings in bacterial meningoencephalitis, *Neuroradiology* 26:51-54, 1984.

Gamba JL, Woodruff WW, Djang WT, et al: Craniofacial mucormycosis: assessment with CT, *Radiology* 160:207-212, 1986.

Gaston A, Gherardi R, Guyen JPN, et al: Cerebral toxoplasmosis in acquired immunodeficiency syndrome, *Neuroradiology* 27:83-86, 1985.

Geller E, Faerber EN, Legido A, et al: Rasmussen encephalitis: complementary role of multitechnique neuroimaging, *AJNR* 19(3):445-449, 1998.

Gilden DH, Kleinschmidt-DeMasters BK, LaGuardia JJ, et al: Neurologic complications of the reactivation of varicella-zoster virus [published erratum appears in *N Engl J Med* 2000 Apr 6;342(14):1063], *N Engl J Med* 342(9):635-645, 2000.

Gillams AR, Allen E, Hrieb K, et al: Cerebral infarction in patients with AIDS, *AJNR* 18(8):1581-1585, 1997.

Greco A, Tannock C, Brostoff J, et al: Brain MR in chronic fatigue syndrome, *AJNR* 18(7):1265-1269, 1997.

Greenan TJ, Grossman RI, Goldberg HI: Cerebral vasculitis: MR imaging and angiographic correlation, *Radiology* 182:65-72, 1992.

Haanpaa M, Dastidar P, Weinberg A, et al: CSF and MRI findings in patients with acute herpes zoster, *Neurology* 51(5):1405-1411, 1998.

Haimes AB, Zimmerman RD, Morgello S, et al: MR imaging of brain abscesses, *AJNR* 10:279-291, 1989.

Hayes WS, Sherman JL, Stern BJ, et al: MR and CT evaluation of intracranial sarcoidosis, *AJNR* 8:841-847, 1987.

Herman TE, Cleveland RH, Kushner DC, et al: CT of neonatal herpes encephalitis, *AJNR* 6:773-775, 1985.

Ishibashi T, Sato A, Hama H, et al: Liver scarring associated with congenital absence of the right hepatic lobe: CT and MR findings, *J Comput Assist Tomogr* 19(6):997-1000, 1995.

Jensen MC, Brant-Zawadzki M: MR imaging of the brain inpatients with AIDS: value of routine use of IV gadopentetate dimeglumine, *AJR* 160:153-157, 1993.

Jinkins JR, Al-Kawi MZ, Bashir R: Dynamic computed tomography of cerebral parenchymal tuberculomata, *Neuroradiology* 29:523-529, 1987.

Jinkins JR, Siqueira E, Al-Kawi MZ: Cranial manifestations of aspergillosis, *Neuroradiology* 29:181-185, 1987.

Jinkins JR: Dynamic CT of tuberculous meningeal reactions, *Neuroradiology* 29:343-347, 1987.

Jinkins JR: Focal tuberculous cerebritis, *AJNR* 9:121-124, 1988.

Joki-Erkkila VP, Hietaharju A, Numminen J, et al: Multiple cranial nerve palsies as a complication of infectious mononucleosis due to inflammatory lesion in jugular foramen, *Ann Otol Rhinol Laryngol* 109(3):340-342, 2000.

Just M, Kramer G, Higer HP, et al: MR of *Listeria* rhombencephalitis, *Neuroradiology* 29:401-402, 1987.

Kanter MC, Hart RG: Neurologic complications of infective endocarditis, *Neurology* 41:1015-1020, 1991.

Kelley WM, Brant-Zawadzki M: Acquired immunodeficiency syndrome: neuroradiologic findings, *Radiology* 149:485-491, 1983.

Kessler LS, Ruiz A, Donovan Post MJ, et al: Thallium-201 brain SPECT of lymphoma in AIDS patients: pitfalls and technique optimization, *AJNR* 19(6):1105-1109, 1998.

Ketonen L, Koskiniemi ML: Gyriform calcification after herpes simplex virus encephalitis, *J Comput Assist Tomogr* 7:1070-1072, 1983.

Ketonen L, Oksanen V, Kuuliala I: Preliminary experience of magnetic resonance imaging in neurosarcoidosis, *Neuroradiology* 29:127-129, 1987.

Kilpatrick C, Tress B, King J: Computed tomography of rhinocerebral mucormycosis, *Neuroradiology* 26:71-73, 1984.

Kimura K, Dosaka A, Hashimoto Y, et al: Single-photon emission CT findings in acute Japanese encephalitis, *AJNR* 18(3):465-469, 1997.

Kioumehr F, Dadsetan MR, Feldman N, et al: Postcontrast MRI of cranial meninges: leptomeningitis versus pachymeningitis, *J Comput Assist Tomogr* 19(5):713-720, 1995.

Kioumehr F, Rooholamini SA, Yaghmai I, et al: Idiopathic hypertrophic cranial pachymeningitis: a case report, *Neuroradiology* 36(4): 292-294, 1994.

Kocer N, Islak C, Siva A, et al: CNS involvement in neuro-Behcet syndrome: an MR study, *AJNR* 20(6):1015-1024, 1999.

Kramer LD, Locke GE, Byrd SE, et al: Cerebral cysticercosis: documentation of natural history with CT, *Radiology* 171:459-462, 1989.

Kremer S, Besson G, Bonaz B, et al: Diffuse lesions in the CNS revealed by mr imaging in a case of Whipple disease, *AJNR* 22(3):493-495, 2001.

Lester JW, Carter MP, Reynolds TL: Herpes encephalitis: MR monitoring of response to acyclovir therapy, *J Comput Assist Tomogr* 12:941-943, 1988.

Lever N, Haas L: Serial MRI in listeria mesenrhombencephalitis: a case report, *J Neurol Neurosurg Psychiatr* 59(5): 524-527, 1995.

Lim CC, Sitoh YY, Hui F, et al: Nipah viral encephalitis or Japanese encephalitis? MR findings in a new zoonotic disease, *AJNR* 21(3): 455-461, 2000.

Lott T, Gammal TE, Dasilva R, et al: Evaluation of brain and epidural abscesses by computed tomography, *Radiology* 122:371-376, 1977.

Martin N, Masson C, Henin D, et al: Hypertrophic cranial pachymeningitis: assessment with CT and MR imaging, *AJNR* 10:477-484, 1989.

Masson C, Henin D, Hauw JJ, et al: Cranial pachymeningitis of unknown origin: a study of seven cases, *Neurology* 43(7):1329-1334, 1993.

Mathews VP, Smith RR: Choroid plexus infections: neuroimaging appearances of four cases, *AJNR* 13:374-378, 1992.

McIntyre PB, Lavercombe PS, Kemp RJ, et al: Subdural and epidural empyema: diagnostic and therapeutic problems, *Med J Aust* 154:653-657, 1991.

Meltzer CC, Wells SW, Becher MW, et al: AIDS-related MR hyperintensity of the basal ganglia, *AJNR* 19(1):83-89, 1998.

Meyerhoff DJ, Bloomer C, et al: Elevated subcortical choline metabolites in cognitively and clinically asymptomatic HIV+ patients, *Neurology* 52(5):995-1003, 1999.

Miller RF, Harrison MJ, Hall-Craggs MA, et al: Central pontine myelinolysis in AIDS, *Acta Neuropatholog* 96(5):537-540, 1998.

Modi G, Campbell H, Bill P: Subacute sclerosing panencephalitis, *Neuroradiology* 31:433-434, 1989.

Moller HE, Chen XJ, Chawla MS, et al: Sensitivity and resolution in 3D NMR microscopy of the lung with hyperpolarized noble gases, *Magnetic Res Med* 41(4):800-808, 1999.

Moseley IF, Kendall BE: Radiology of intracranial empyemas, with special reference to computed tomography, *Neuroradiology* 26:333-345, 1984.

Murphy JM, Gomez-Anson B, Gillard JH, et al: Wegener granulomatosis: MR imaging findings in brain and meninges, *Radiology* 213(3):794-799, 1999.

Nagaoka U, Kato T, Kurita K, et al: Cranial nerve enhancement on three-dimensional MRI in Miller Fisher syndrome, *Neurology* 47(6):1601-1602, 1996.

Nakazawa G, Lulu RE, Koo AH: Intracerebellar coccidioidal granuloma, *AJNR* 4:1243-1244, 1983.

New FJ, Davis KR, Ballantine HT: Computed tomography in cerebral abscess, *Radiology* 121:641-646, 1976.

Nishioka H, Ito H, Haraoka J, et al: Idiopathic hypertrophic cranial pachymeningitis with accumulation of thallium-201 on single-photon emission CT, *AJNR* 19(3):450-453, 1998.

Noorbehesht B, Enzmann DR, Sullender W, et al: Neonatal herpes simplex encephalitis: correlation of clinical and CT findings, *Radiology* 162:813-819, 1987.

Paskavitz JF, Anderson CA, Filley CM, et al: Acute arcuate fiber demyelinating encephalopathy following Epstein-Barr virus infection, *Ann Neurol* 38(1):127-131, 1995.

Patel DV, Neuman MJ, Hier DB: Reversibility of CT and MR findings in neuro-Behçet disease, *J Comput Assist Tomogr* 13:669-673, 1989.

Pavlakis SG, Lu D, Frank Y, et al: Brain lactate and N-acetylaspartate in pediatric AIDS encephalopathy, *AJNR* 19(2):383-385, 1998.

Penar PL, Kim J, Chyatte D, et al: Intraventricular cryptococcal granuloma, *J Neurosurg* 68:145-148, 1988.

Post MJD, Hensley GT, Moskowitz LB, et al: Cytomegalic inclusion virus encephalitis in patients with AIDS: CT, clinical, and pathologic correlation, *AJNR* 7:275-280,1986.

Post MJD, Tate LG, Quencer RM, et al: CT, MR, and pathology in HIV encephalitis and meningitis, *AJNR* 9:469-476, 1988.

Press GA, Weindling SM, Hesselink JR, et al: Rhinocerebral mucormycosis: MR manifestations, *J Comput Assist Tomogr* 12:744-749, 1988.

Rafto SE, Milton WJ, Galetta SL, et al: Biopsy-confirmed CNS Lyme disease: MR appearance at 1.5T, *AJNR* 11:482-484, 1990.

Renier D, Flandin C, Hirsch E, et al: Brain abscesses in neonates, *J Neurosurg* 69:877-882, 1988.

Rodesch G, Parizel PM, Farber CM, et al: Nervous system manifestations and neuroradiologic findings in acquired immunodeficiency syndrome (AIDS), *Neuroradiology* 31:33-39, 1989.

Rosenblum ML, Hoff JT, Norman D, et al: Nonoperative treatment of brain abscesses in selected high-risk patients, *J Neurosurg* 52:217-225, 1980.

Rowley HA, Uht RM, Kazacos KR, et al: Radiologic-pathologic findings in raccoon roundworm (Baylisascaris procyonis) encephalitis, *AJNR* 21(2):415-420, 2000.

Schmidt S, Reiter-Owona I, Hotz M, et al: An unusual case of central nervous system cryptococcosis, *Clin Neurol Neurosurg* 97(1):23-27, 1995.

Schoeman J, Hewlett R, Donald P: MR of childhood tuberculous meningitis, *Neuroradiology* 30:473-477, 1988.

Schroth G, Kretzschmar K, Gawehn J, et al: Advantage of magnetic resonance imaging in the diagnosis of cerebral infections, *Neuroradiology* 29:120-126, 1987.

Schwartz RB, Komaroff AL, Garada BM, et al: SPECT imaging of the brain: comparison of findings in patients with chronic fatigue syndrome, AIDS dementia complex, and major unipolar depression *AJR* 162(4):943-951, 1994.

Schwartz RB, Garada BM, Komaroff AL, et al: Detection of intracranial abnormalities in patients with chronic fatigue syndrome: comparison of MR imaging and SPECT *AJR* 162(4):935-941, 1994.

Smith AS, Meisler DM, Weinstein MA, et al: High-signal periventricular lesions in patients with sarcoidosis: neurosarcoidosis or multiple sclerosis, *AJNR* 10:485-490, 1989.

Stevens EA, Norman D, Kramer RA, et al: Computed tomographic brain scanning in intraparenchymal pyogenic abscesses, *AJR* 130:111-114, 1978.

Suh DC, Chang KH, Han MH, et al: Unusual MR manifestations of neurocysticercosis, *Neuroradiology* 31:396-402, 1989.

Thebaud B, Husson B, Navelet Y, et al: Haemorrhagic shock and encephalopathy syndrome: neurological course and predictors of outcome, *Intensive Care Med* 25(3):293-299, 1999.

Titelbaum DS, Hayward JC, Zimmerman RA: Pachygyriclike changes: topographic appearance at MR imaging and CT and correlation with neurologic status, *Radiology* 173:663-667, 1989.

Tuite M, Ketonen L, Kieburtz K, et al: Efficacy of gadolinium in MR brain imaging of HIV-infected patients, *AJNR* 14:257-263, 1993.

van der Knaap MS, Valk J, Jansen GH, et al: Mycotic encephalitis: predilection for grey matter, *Neuroradiology* 35(8):567-572, 1993.

van Dyk A: CT of intracranial tuberculomas with specific reference to the "target sign," *Neuroradiology* 30:329-336, 1988.

Weaver S, Rosenblum MK, De Angelis LM, et al: Herpes varicella zoster encephalitis in immunocompromised patients, *Neurology* 52(1):193-195, 1999.

Wehn SM, Heinz ER, Burger PC, et al: Dilated Virchow-Robin spaces in cryptococcal meningitis associated with AIDS: CT and MR findings, *J Comput Assist Tomogr* 13:756-762, 1989.

Weingarten K, Zimmerman RD, Becker RD, et al: Subdural and epidural empyemas: MR imaging, *AJNR* 10:81-87, 1989.

Yang PJ, Reger KM, Seeger JF, et al: Brain abscess: an atypical CT appearance of CNS tuberculosis, *AJNR* 8:919-920, 1987.

Yousem DM, Galetta SL, Gusnard DA, et al: MR findings in rhinocerebral mucormycosis, *J Comput Assist Tomogr* 13:878-882, 1989.

Zee C, Segall HD, Apuzzo MLJ, et al: Intraventricular cysticercal cysts: further neuroradiologic observations and neurosurgical implications, *AJNR* 5:727-730, 1984.

Zee C, Segall HD, Boswell W, et al: MR imaging of neurocysticercosis, *J Comput Assist Tomogr* 12:927-934, 1988.

Zimmerman RD, Leeds NE, Danziger A: Subdural empyema: CT findings, *Radiology* 150:417-422, 1984.

Although NAAs specific function is unknown, it is believed to be present almost exclusively in neurons and their processes (10, 10a, 35). It should be noted, however, that oligodendrocyte-type 2 astrocyte progenitor cells (36) and mature oligodendrocytes (37) also express NAA, and may reduce its specificity to reflect neuronal damage measure, such as the Multiple Sclerosis Functional Composite measure developed by the National MS Societys Clinical Outcome Assessment Task Force.

10. Simmons MS, Frondoza CG, Coyle JT. Immunocytochemical localization of N-acetyl aspartate with monoclonal antibodies. *Neuroscience* 1991;45:37-45.

10a. Tsai G, Coyle JT. N-acetylaspartate in neuropsychiatric disorders. *Prog in Neurobiol.* 1995;46:531-540.

35. Moffett JR, Namboodiri MA, Cangro CB, Neale JH. Immunohistochemical localization of N-acetylaspartate in rat brain. *Neuroreport* 1991;2:131-134.

36. Urenjak J, Williams SR, Gadian DG, Noble M. Proton nuclear magnetic resonance spectroscopy unambiguously identifies different neural cell types. *J Neuroscience* 1993;13:981-989.

37. Bhakoo KK, Pearce D. In vitro expression of N-acetyl aspartate by oligodendrocytes: implications for proton magnetic resonance spectroscopy signal in vivo. *J Neurochem* 2000;74:254-262.

White Matter Diseases

White matter diseases are heterogeneous conditions linked together because they involve the same real estate. Think of white matter as a rental apartment building owned by a cheapskate landlord with a tremendous variety of angry tenants, some of whom temporarily disrupt function (edematous lesions), whereas others are nasty enough to destroy the structural component of the building (lesions producing axonal transections).

Magnetic resonance (MR) imaging is quite sensitive and, when combined with age and other pertinent clinical information, provides a reasonable amount of specificity. The authors assume that readers possess a minimum level of competence to discern whether abnormalities are in the gray or white matter. Remember this is the "Requisites" not "Sesame Street." We are going to start by dividing white matter diseases into demyelinating and dysmyelinating diseases (Box 7-1).

Demyelinating disorders are a common inflammatory component that injures, and in some cases, destroys, white matter. Keep in mind, the white matter starts out normal and is then injured by the particular pathologic process. The oligodendrocyte is the cell responsible for wrapping the axon concentrically to form the myelin sheath and although we speak of white matter diseases as those that affect myelin, in actual fact, there is now a great deal of evidence that myelin is not the only brain tissue damaged in "demyelinating diseases" and axons and neurons are also commonly affected Our appreciation of the nature of these disorders has improved dramatically with more precise histopathology and new magnetic resonance methodology.

We can further divide these diseases based on their presumed etiology (Table 7-1). We shall consider each of them shortly but first we need to give all of our perspicacious readers a dysesthetic diversion—dysmyelinating conditions.

Dysmyelinating disorders involve intrinsic abnormalities of myelin formation or myelin maintenance because of a genetic defect, an enzymatic disturbance, or both. These diseases are rare, usually seen in the pediatric or adolescent population, and often associated with a bizarre appearance on MR. Some diseases such as adrenoleukodystrophy have characteristics of both demyelinating and dysmyelinating processes (although in

Box 7-1 Classification of White Matter Diseases

Primary demyelinating disease
    Multiple sclerosis
        Balo
        Devics
        Schilder's
        Marburg
Secondary demyelinating disease
    Allergic (immunologic)
        Acute disseminated encephalomyelitis
    Viral
        HIV-associated encephalitis
        Progressive multifocal leukoencephalopathy
        Subacute sclerosing panencephalitis
    Vascular (hypoxic/ischemic)
        Binswanger disease
        CADASIL
        Postanoxic encephalopathy
        Reversible posterior, leukoencephalopathy
    Metabolic
        Osmotic demyelination or central pontine
            myelinolysis
    Toxic
        Alcohol
        Radiation
        Marchiafava-Bignami disease
        Disseminated necrotizing leukoencephalopathy
        Drugs including chemotherapeutic agents and
            intravenously abused drugs (metamphetamine,
            cocaine, heroin)
        Toxins (triethyl tin, lead, mercury)
    Traumatic
        Diffuse axonal injury
Dysmyelinating disease
        Alexander's disease
        Krabbe's disease
        Sudanophilic leukodystrophy
        Pelizaeus-Merzbacher disease
        Canavan's disease
        Metachromatic leukodystrophy
        Adrenoleukodystrophy

Table 7-1 Demyelinating diseases categorized by presumed etiology

Autoimmune (Idiopathic)
    Multiple Sclerosis
    Monophasic Demyelination
        Acute Disseminated Encephalomyelitis
            Acute Hemorrhagic Leukoencephalitis
            Optic Neuritis (may be the first presentation of MS)
            Acute Transverse Myelitis (may be the first
                presentation of MS)
Viral
    Progressive Multifocal Leukoencephalopathy
    Subacute Sclerosing Panencephalitis
    HIV-associated encephalitis
Vascular (hypoxic/ischemic)
    CADASIL (Cerebral Autosomal Dominant Arteriopathy with
        Subcortical Infarction and Leukoencephalopathy)
    Postanoxic Encephalopathy
    Reversible Posterior Leukoencephalopathy
    Binswanger Disease
Metabolic/Nutritional
    Osmotic Demyelination
    Marchiafava-Bignami
    Combined Systems Disease (B_{12} deficiency)
Toxic
    Radiation
    Toxins
    Drugs
    Disseminated Necrotizing Leukoencephalopathy
Trauma
    Diffuse Axonal injury

Box 7-1 it is operationally listed in the dysmyelinating category). The term *leukodystrophy* is used interchangeably with *dysmyelinating diseases* and represents primary involvement of myelin. For concerned clinicians-in-training, 99.9% of what you will see in an adult private practice of radiology will be demyelinating disease, but we cannot provide any written guarantees for those of you who are taking the boards as there are still some dyschezic examiners.

PRIMARY DEMYELINATING DISEASE

Multiple Sclerosis

Multiple sclerosis (MS), first described by Charcot in 1868, is the most common demyelinating disease encountered in clinical practice (as well as in imaging) and so excuse our assiduousness. Affecting nearly 350,000 Americans, 100,000 Britons and over 2 million worldwide, it is the leading cause of nontraumatic neurologic disability in young and middle-aged adults.

MS has a peak age range of 30 years with a female predominance, however, it can occur in children and adolescents (3% to 5%) and in those over 50 (9%). The authors feel that age is a state of mind and their maturity level as evidenced by the attempts at so-called humor suggests a long at-risk stage.

Clinical presentation Symptoms range from isolated cranial nerve palsy, optic neuritis, and vague sensory complaints, to paresis and paraplegia of limbs, and myelopathy. Subtle and obvious changes in intellectual capacity are also identified in patients with MS.

Clinical criteria The diagnosis of MS is presently still based upon clinical and paraclinical criteria alone. These parameters were initially proposed to select patients for treatment trials. The clinical diagnosis of MS (according to Schumacher's criteria) is made by history or neurologic examination resulting from two or more white matter lesions with either (1) two or more episodes of worsening, each lasting at least 24 hours and each at least a month apart, or (2) slow stepwise progression of signs or symptoms for at least 6 months.

The criteria designed by Poser and coworkers in 1983 establish two principal groups—definite and probable MS—each with two subgroups, clinical and laboratory supported. Clinically, definite MS is defined by two attacks and clinical evidence of two separate lesions, or two attacks with clinical evidence of one lesion and paraclinical evidence of another separate lesion. Clinically probable MS includes: (a) two attacks and clinical evidence of one lesion; (b) one attack and clinical evidence of two separate lesions; or (c) one attack and clinical evidence of one lesion and paraclinical evidence of another, separate lesion. Paraclinical evidence included CSF, CT, or MR data. MR is by far the best paraclinical test demonstrating abnormalities in 95% of patients with clinically definite MS. This number probably understates the sensitivity of MR as it does not include state-of-the-art spinal cord imaging. Combined brain and spinal cord imaging can increase the sensitivity to almost 100%. Although the diagnosis is first made on clinical grounds, MR has a pivotal role in confirming the clinical diagnosis. A positive study, together with appropriate clinical data, strongly supports the diagnosis of MS. However, you should be aware that there are cases of MR-negative (including brain and spinal examinations) MS, (particularly when residents or neurosurgeons interpret the MR). The demonstration of lesions distributed over time differentiates MS from acute disseminated encephalomyelitis and other monophasic diseases that have a different course and prognosis.

New criteria for the diagnosis of MS have been recently advocated (McDonald Criteria). The recommendations suggest that the terms "clinically definite" and "probable MS" be replaced by MS, "possible MS" (for those at risk for MS, but with equivocal diagnostic evaluation, or "not MS." Table 7-2 clarifies the proposed diagnostic criteria. Table 7-3 defines MR criteria for dissemination of lesions in time. Table 7-4 provides the diagnostic criteria for MS. If the criteria are fulfilled the diagnosis is MS. If they are incompletely met the diagnosis is "possible MS," and if they are not met the diagnosis is "not MS."

Laboratory tests Laboratory tests including visual, auditory, and somatosensory evoked responses, can confirm the presence of lesions, but they are nonspecific and provide no clue to the cause of the abnormal finding. Approximately 70% of patients with MS have elevated cerebrospinal fluid (CSF) levels of IgG and approximately 90% have elevated oligoclonal bands.

Clinical course MS is a disease characterized by a variety of clinical courses. Terminology about clinical classification can be confusing and even contradictory. Relapsing remitting (RR) MS is the most common course of the disease initially occurring in up to 85% of cases. At the beginning, exacerbations are followed by remissions. However, over years additional exacerbations result in incomplete recovery. Within 10 years 50% (and

---

Table 7-3 Multiple Sclerosis: Criteria for dissemination of lesion in time

MRI dissemination in time
  GAD enhancing lesion demonstrated in a scan done at least 3 months after clinical attack at another site
  In absence of gad-enhancing lesion at 3 months, follow-up scan after additional 3 months showing gad-enhancing lesion or new T2WI lesions

McDonald et al. *Annals of Neurology*, 2001, 50:121–127.

Table 7-2 Multiple Sclerosis—definitions

Attack: subjective or objective, >24 hours duration, neurologic disturbance
Time: 30 days between onset of events
CSF: IgG bands in CSF or IgG index
MRI must have three out of four
  One gad enhancing or 9 T2 hyperintense lesions if no gad enhancing lesions
  One or more infratentorial lesions
  One or more juxtacortical lesions
  Three or more periventricular lesions

McDonald et al. *Annals of Neurology*, 2001, 50:121–127.

Table 7-4 Diagnostic criteria for Multiple Sclerosis

Two or more attacks, two or more objective clinical lesions
Two or more attacks, one objective lesion, dissemination in space demonstrated by MRI, CSF, or further clinical attack
One attack, two or more objective lesions, dissemination in time by MRI or second attack
One attack, one objective lesion, dissemination in time and space by MRI or CSF
Insidious neurologic progression suggestive of MS, positive CSF, and dissemination in space and time by MRI

McDonald et al. *Annals of Neurology*, 2001, 50:121–127.

within 25 years 90%) of these cases enter a progressive phase, termed secondary progressive (also termed relapsing progressive) MS. During this phase deficits are progressive without much remission in the disease. Less commonly, the disease is progressive from the start. This entity was first distinguished in 1952 and has been termed primary progressive (also termed "chronic progressive") MS. These patients (5% to 10% of the MS population) may present at a later age with progressive neurologic findings including paraparesis, hemiparesis, brain stem syndromes, or visual loss, and typically have a more severe disability. They may have occasional plateaus and temporary improvements, but do not have distinct relapses. Primary progressive patients tend to have less lesion load, fewer new lesions on monthly T2 weighted images (T2WI), and fewer enhancing lesions when compared to patients with secondary progressive disease, despite progressive declining neurologic status. Progressive-relapsing MS, a rare clinical course, is defined as progressive disease with clear acute relapses, with or without full recovery, and with the periods between relapses characterized by continuing progression. All of these groups also have been lumped together and identified as chronic progressive MS, however, some experts believe the term should be abandoned because of its vague nature and the variable clinical courses and corresponding MR patterns. Benign MS describes those cases, where after initial clinical symptomatology, there is no clinical progression over, approximately, a 10 to 15 year course. Conversely, a rapid progressive disease leading to significant disability or death in a short time after the onset has been termed malignant MS.

Monosymptomatic patient In addition to these well-described clinical patterns of the disease, there exists the dilemma of the monosymptomatic patient. This presentation consists of a single episode of neurologic deficit such as optic neuritis, transverse myelitis, or brain stem syndrome. Seventy-seven percent of patients presenting with an isolated brain stem syndrome have been reported to have asymptomatic supratentorial white matter abnormalities. Progression to MS occurs in about 57% of patients with isolated brain stem syndrome and in 42% of patients with spinal cord syndrome. Fifty percent of patients with optic neuritis had lesions in their brain 3 weeks to 7 years following their attack. The risk of developing MS following optic neuritis has been estimated to be up 75% or more. The presence, as well as the number, of asymptomatic lesions on MR markedly increases the risk of progression to MS not only in cases presenting with optic neuritis but also in isolated brain stem or spinal cord. Those patients presenting with isolated acute syndromes without brain lesions are at lower risk of progressing to MS. MR, thus, possesses good predictive power in patients presenting with clinically isolated syndromes suggestive of MS.

Pathologic findings MS is believed to be an autoimmune disease, however, other mechanisms have been proposed. At this time, its etiology is still unknown. The pathology of MS is manifest by a chronic inflammatory process resulting in myelin loss. Active lesions demonstrate axonal transactions, infiltration with lipid-laden macrophages (Gitter cells), perivascular inflammatory cuffing with T and B lymphocytes, and plasma cells associated with perivascular demyelination. Attempts by the oligodendroglia at remyelination have been observed in both acute and chronic plaques. The extent of this process can vary from a narrow rim around silent lesions to macroscopic satellite zones contiguous with demyelinated lesions, the latter having been termed a "shadow plaque." Remyelination and its relationship, if any, to clinical recovery is still problematic. Inactive plaques are hypocellular without perivascular inflammation.

The classical description of the histopathologic hallmarks of the disease include multifocal lesions demonstrating inflammation with lymphocytes and macrophages, demyelination, gliosis, attempts at remyelination, and "relative sparing of axons." The sparing of axons has recently been questioned and it has been hypothesized that axonal loss (with subsequent neuronal loss) could be responsible for neurologic impairment. Axonal loss appears to be common in acute lesions as well as in more chronic ones. Perhaps, MS should be considered a neuronal disease as well as a demyelinating disease. We will classify MS as a demyelinating disease plus.

Indeed, Charcot suggested the loss of axons almost 150 years ago; however, there was something lost in the translation because most investigators did not consider axonal loss to be a significant cause of disability until very recently. Leave it to the French to get it right—wine, women, and neuronal loss?

MR findings On T1 weighted imaging (T1WI), plaques are iso- or low intensity regions whereas on T2 weighted images (T2WI) the lesions are high intensity (Fig. 7-1). The hypointense lesions on T1WI have been termed "black holes" and have been reported to be associated with areas of greatest myelin loss although this is controversial. On T2WI, tiny nodules or large confluent high intensity lesions are seen. MS lesions have a predilection for certain regions of the brain including the periventricular region, corpus callosum (best visualized on sagittal FLAIR or proton density weighted images [PDWI]), subcortical region (best seen on FLAIR), optic nerves and visual pathways, posterior fossa (including the brain stem and cerebellar peduncles best seen on T2WI), and cervical region of the spinal cord. However, MS lesions can and do occur in any location in the brain. This includes the cortex (6%), where white matter fibers track up to the superficial cortical cells, and the deep gray matter (5%). CAUTION—FLAIR imaging does not

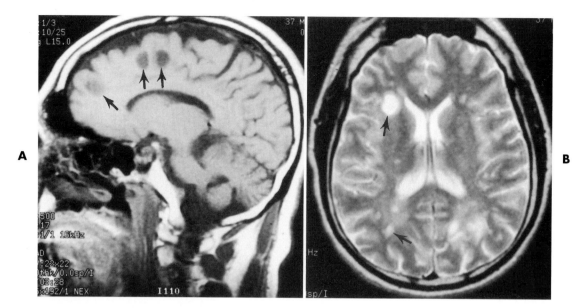

Fig. 7-1   MS. **A,** Sagittal T1WI with hypointense lesions or so-called "black holes" *(arrows).* **B,** Axial T2WI showing multiple hyperintense lesions *(arrows).*

detect lesions in the posterior fossa, brain stem, and spinal cord as well as conventional T2WI. In addition, very hypointense lesions on T1WI may look similar to CSF on FLAIR, that is, not bright—like some of your professors. High intensity lesions at the callosal-septal interface (sagittal MR either PD or FLAIR) have been suggested to have 93% sensitivity and 98% specificity in differentiating MS lesions from vascular disease (Fig. 7-2). The shape of these MS plaques may be variable. However, ovoid lesions are believed to be more specific

for MS. Their morphology has been attributed to inflammatory changes around the long axis of a medullary vein (Dawson's fingers) (Fig. 7-3).

Lesions may display mass effect that can mimic a tumor (tumefactive MS) and have been associated with seizures (Fig. 7-4). There are several hints that aid in suggesting this diagnosis including the history, which is usually acute or subacute in onset in a young adult, and other white matter abnormalities unassociated with the mass lesion (check the spinal cord), and the callosal-

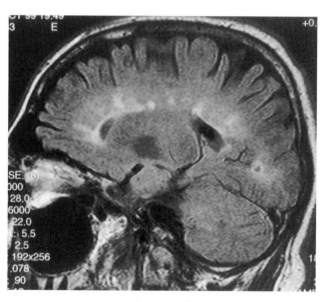

Fig. 7-2   Sagittal FLAIR image with high intensity lesions emanating from the septal-callosal interface.

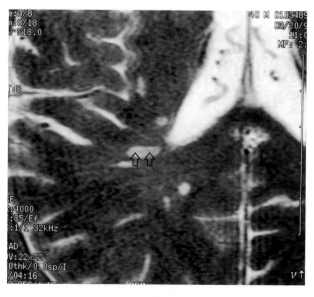

Fig. 7-3   Dawson's finger on 4 Tesla MR. Note both the ovoid appearance of the lesions and the vein *(open black arrows)* actually course through the middle of the ovoid lesion.

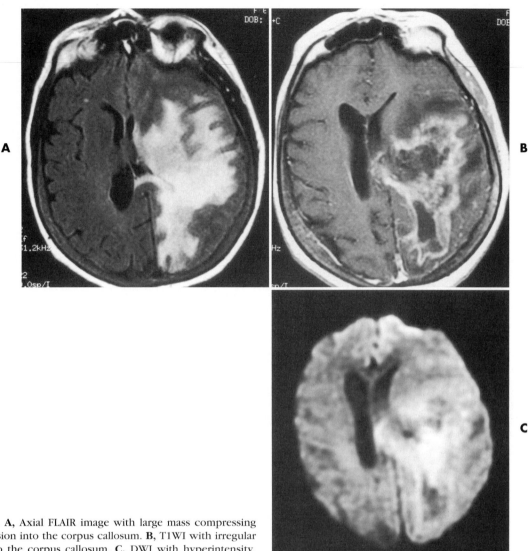

Fig. 7-4   Tumefactive MS. **A,** Axial FLAIR image with large mass compressing the left ventricle with extension into the corpus callosum. **B,** T1WI with irregular enhancement extending into the corpus callosum. **C,** DWI with hyperintensity. This may be due to T2-shine-through or associate cytotoxic edema.

septal interface. Tumefactive MS lesions have a leading edge of enhancement and an incomplete "horseshoe-shaped" ring. Perfusion in tumors is usually increased and in MS it is normally not. Veins are displaced by neoplasms but course through MS lesions. There also have been rare reports of hemorrhage into demyelinating lesions. Some of the many faces of MS are displayed in Fig. 7-5.

Other findings include atrophy of the brain and spinal cord. In general, the longer the course of the disease, the greater the accumulation of MS lesions. This can average between 8% and 10% of the disease burden a year in relapsing remitting MS. The greater the loss of myelin and axons, the more likely the lesion is to be hypointense on T1WI. High intensity on unenhanced T1WI can be observed infrequently, most often in the periphery of the plaque. The cause of this phenomenon is undetermined, but hypotheses include a small amount of paramagnetic accumulation from hemorrhage, myelin cata-

bolites including fat, free radical production from the inflammatory response, or focally increased regions of protein.

Increased iron deposition (in the thalamus and basal ganglia) producing low intensity on T1 and T2WI has been reported in patients with long-standing MS. This latter finding is nonspecific, having been described in a variety of different conditions including Parkinson disease, multisystem atrophy, and other degenerative conditions.

MR criteria for MS   MR criteria for the diagnosis of MS have been reported predominantly in the neurologic literature and are typically based solely on conventional proton density, T2 weighted images, and gadolinium enhanced images. Paty and co-workers proposed that four or more lesions (Paty A criteria) or at least three lesions with one lesion bordering the lateral ventricles (Paty B criteria) are strongly suggestive of MS. Fazekas and colleagues suggested criteria including three or more le-

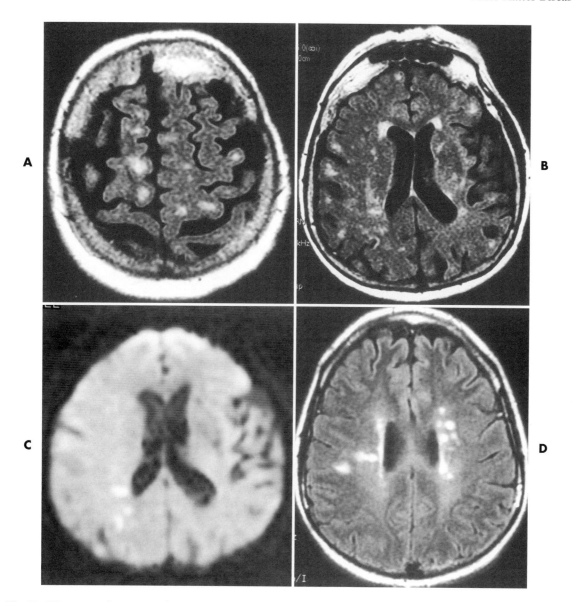

Fig. 7-5 The Ms MS pageant from top to bottom. **A,** Subcortical lesions on FLAIR. **B,** Same as **A** only inferior slice with corresponding DWI (C). **C,** Diffusion image with high intensity from possible cytoxic edema (?acute demyelination). **D,** Periventricular lesions on FLAIR.

Illustration continued on following page

sions with the presence of at least two of the following characteristics: (1) size greater than 5 mm, (2) periventricular, and (3) infratentorial. Although lesions in the centrum semiovale tend to occur with aging and other processes, periventricular lesions do appear to be more specific for MS. Lesions around the temporal horn and fourth ventricle, as well as in the cerebellar peduncle and midbrain, also appear more specific for MS but have a low frequency of occurrence. Yetkin and others reported that 2% to 4% of healthy patients had high intensity periventricular abnormalities, which could not be distinguished from MS. Barkhof and colleagues proposed that the presence of juxtacortical lesions in patients with monosymptomatic neurologic disease was a highly specific prognosticator of progression to MS. McDonald et

al criteria (see Tables 7-2 and 7-3) combine lesion number and location for added specificity.

There is a significant incidence of high intensity abnormalities in the brains of healthy individuals. This number varies depending upon the exact report and the cohort's age. In one study of healthy volunteers, white matter abnormalities were noted in 11% of subjects aged 0 to 39, in 31% aged 40 to 49, 47% aged 50 to 59, 60% aged 60 to 69, and in 83% of those 70 and older. Rudimentary MR criteria may have a role in prioritizing differential diagnoses, however, with all of the caveats related to high intensity abnormalities, the use of MR criteria alone is open to criticism and fraught with error.

Enhancement in MS The enhancement pattern of the initial lesion is usually in the shape of a nodule, which

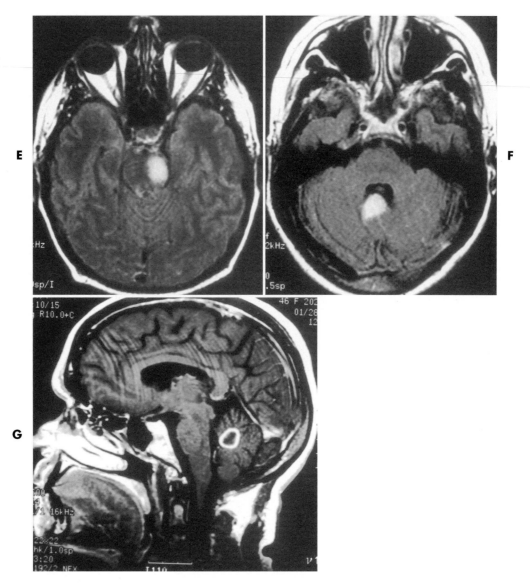

Fig. 7-5   *Continued.* **E,** Brain stem lesion on FLAIR. **F,** Vermian MS with mass and ring enhancement **(G).**

may be ovoid in appearance. Nodular enhancement can evolve to a ring or arc shape (Fig. 7-6.). If lesions recrudesce, they usually have an arc or ring appearance. Many times the center of this type of lesion is lower intensity on T1WI. On T2WI, lesions generally wax and wane in size. Most often, one is left with a residual high intensity lesion on the T2WI. If a lesion is enhancing as a nodule for over 3 months, be a little suspicious—it can happen but you don't want to be an idiot either. Cranial nerves (besides the optic nerve) can also enhance but make sure the patient has MS (Fig. 7-7). Enhancement is more sensitive than either clinical examination or T2WI in detecting disease activity, and potentially can separate clinical groups. Increased sensitivity enables the detection of a treatment effect in smaller patient cohorts over shorter periods, and has been used as a parameter in monitoring the efficacy of treatment. The normal window of enhancement is from 2 to 8 weeks; however, plaques can enhance for 6 months or more. Enhancement cannot be viewed as "an all or none" phenomenon, rather it is dependent on the time from injection to imaging, the dosage of contrast agent, the magnitude of the blood-brain barrier (BBB) abnormality, and the size of the space where it accumulates. Delayed imaging (usually 15 to 60 minutes following injection) increases the detection of enhancing MS lesions (and decrease patient throughput and revenue). Triple doses of gadolinium (0.3 mmol/kg) or a single dose (0.1 mmol/kg) with magnetization transfer (MT) (also see in the New Methods section) to suppress normal brain can increase the number of detectable MS lesions (and fill the coffers of drug companies, while bankrupting radiology departments).

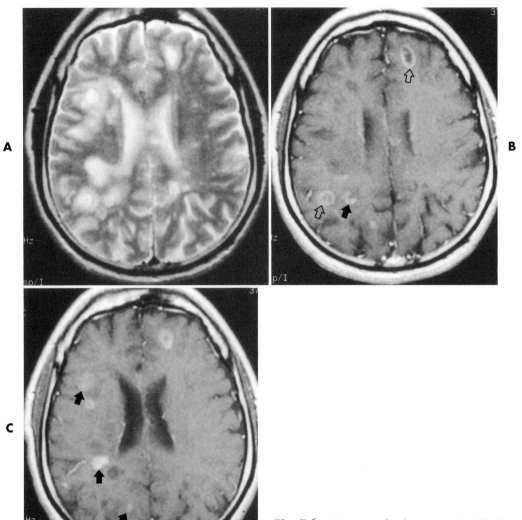

Fig. 7-6   Patterns of enhancement in MS. **A,** Axial T2WI of a patient with MS showing a variety of shaped lesions. **B,** Axial enhanced T1WI with arc *(arrow)* and ring enhancement *(open arrows)*. **C,** Axial enhanced T1WI with nodular enhancement *(arrows)*.

Triple dose gadolinium has been reported to increase lesion detection by 75% when compared to single dose. On the other hand, MT combined with a 20 to 40 minute scan delay increased the number of enhancing lesions detected with single-dose by 47% and with triple-dose by 27%. MT, with a 40 to 60 minute delay following triple-dose Gd-DTPA, resulted in the detection of 126% more enhancing lesions than in standard single-dose imaging. The down side of the MT imaging here is that you need a pre-MT image T1WI (more time, more $$$$) so that high intensity on the postgadolinium T1WI is not confused with preexisting noncontrast hyperintensity.

Enhancement may precede the development of both T2 high intensity and clinical symptoms. We also recognize that there is disease in the normal appearing white matter (NAWM) (see later discussion), which is beyond our resolution to detect by standard imaging and contrast techniques. It is also unlikely that all of the inflammatory change occurs in the 2 to 8 week window of enhancement. A negative correlation between enhancing lesion volume and duration of disease was reported suggesting that the BBB abnormalities are less important over time. Furthermore, when the disease evolves to the secondary progressive stage, decreasing enhancement is observed in spite of growing neurologic problems, again suggesting a diminished role of the BBB abnormality. Last, primary progressive MS displays little enhancement despite progressive neurologic decline suggesting an alternative pathologic process most likely dissociated from BBB abnormality such as primary neuronal loss.

Normal appearing white matter (NAWM)   We have just covered combinations and permutations of visible lesion but the NAWM is also abnormal. What an oxy-

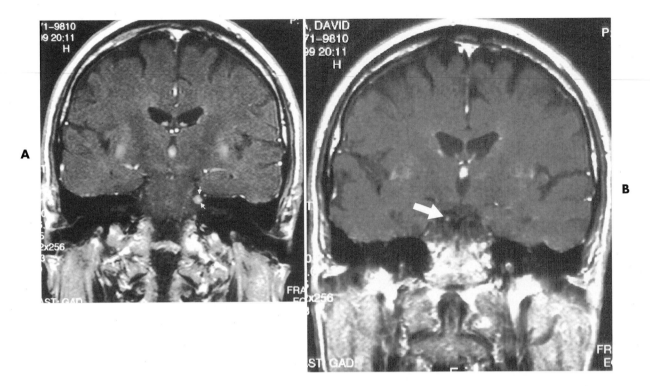

Fig. 7-7   Neural enhancement in MS (courtesy of Robert Quencer, M.D. Miami, Florida). **A,** Coronal postcontrast T1WI revealing enhancement of cranial nerve V *(white arrows).* **B,** Coronal enhanced image with enhancement of right cranial nerve III.

moron the smart child says. Yes, the term is quite relative. There are many new MR methods (see New Methods) that clearly demonstrate that the NAWM in MS is not normal, that is, there are lesions that we cannot detect by conventional MR. This is important, as the extent of disease in MS patients is generally greater than the visible T2 lesion load. In addition, MS lesions tend to have fuzzy borders, that is, even the visible lesions have abnormalities that extend beyond the visible boundaries on T2WI.

Spinal cord disease   MS can affect the spinal cord alone (5% to 24%) or, more commonly, both the brain and the spinal cord. Approximately 60% of spinal cord lesions occur in the cervical region. In one study, most patients had only one spinal lesion; whereas in another large study, 56% of cases had more than one spinal lesion. Spinal cord MS tends not to involve the entire cord, is peripherally located, generally does not respect boundaries between white and gray matter, and can range in length from 2 to 60 mm. Ninety percent of MS lesions are less than two vertebral body segments in length. Spinal cord swelling associated with lesions occurs in 6% to 14% of cases, whereas atrophy ranges from 2% to 40%. Most lesions in patients referred for imaging of spinal cord MS symptoms demonstrate enhancement. In terms of clinical categories spinal cord lesion load is highest in relapsing-remitting and secondary progressive

MS. Primary progressive patients (which have overall low lesion load) have a higher proportion of their lesion load within the spinal cord than secondary progressive patients. Nonetheless, no correlation is found between spinal cord lesion load and Kurtzke's Expanded Disability Status Scale (EDSS). Clinical disability has been correlated with spinal cord atrophy.

Spinal cord imaging   Spinal cord imaging is important in the context of patients presenting with signs and symptoms of MS. Here, it can increase the diagnostic sensitivity by demonstrating MS lesions in the cord in patients who have normal brain MR, as well as find other non-MS lesions and account for neurologic findings that were mistakenly attributed to MS. The latter can include lesions such as an intrinsic tumor or extrinsic compression from an extraaxial tumor or disk/bone disease. It can increase the specificity of the diagnosis in patients with white matter abnormalities in the brain. In this case, brain lesions plus spinal cord lesions may increase the likelihood of MS. Moreover, false positive lesions in the spinal cord rarely, if ever, occur whereas nonspecific high intensity abnormalities in the brain are not uncommon, especially with aging. By performing both brain and spinal cord imaging, clinical presentations in patients with MS may be thoroughly and properly evaluated. Negative brain and spinal MR imaging, with contemporary hardware and software, almost certainly (but nothing is perfect so don't bet your baseball card collection—but how about your preferred dot com stocks) rules out MS.

Clinical differential diagnosis of Spinal Cord MS When confronted with a clinical condition that is suggestive of MS and you see high intensity lesions enhancing spinal cord lesions, what is the differential diagnosis? It should include vascular lesions, particularly dural arteriovenous malformation producing venous hypertension and subsequent venous infarction, as well as other vascular malformations and arterial lesions. In addition, collagen vascular diseases, such as lupus, can produce myelitis, and other inflammatory diseases, such as sarcoid and acute disseminated encephalomyelitis also involve the spinal cord. Other considerations also include intrinsic spinal cord neoplasms and infections, both viral (including HIV) and bacterial, which can all masquerade as spinal MS. An appropriate history, cerebrospinal fluid analysis, and careful examination of the MR are important in differentiating these lesions (also see Differential Diagnosis of MS Lesions on MR). Subacute combined degeneration of the spinal cord caused by vitamin B12 deficiency involves the spinal cord posterior columns symmetrically and is associated with a peripheral neuropathy. Box 7-2 lists the differential diagnosis of an enlarged spinal cord.

MS syndromes Many syndromes are associated with MS. Devic's disease or neuromyelitis optica (Fig. 7-8) represents either an acute variant of MS or a separate demyelinating disease. Experts cannot agree on its classification, but as we are dilettantes, it is an MS syndrome. The disease consists of both transverse myelitis and bilateral optic neuritis (Fig. 7-9). Symptoms may occur simultaneously or be separated by days or weeks. The clinical manifestations can be severe.

Box 7-2 Differential Diagnosis of Enlarged Spinal Cord

Transverse myelitis from MS, ADEM
Spinal cord tumor (primary or metastatic)
Syringohydromyelia
Acute infarction
Vascular lesions including dural arteriovenous
   malformation, infarction
Infectious processes (toxoplasmosis, vacuolar
   myelopathy in AIDS, herpes zoster)
Lupus
Trauma (hematomyelia)
Diffuse leptomeningeal coating of the
   spinal cord from sarcoid, lymphoma,
   or other tumors.

ADEM, Acute disseminated encephalomyelitis

Balo's disease (concentric sclerosis) represents a histologic MS lesion with alternating concentric regions of demyelination and normal brain (Fig. 7-10). Rarely, a similar pattern may be observed on T2WI. Diffuse sclerosis (Schilder's disease) is an acute, rapidly progressive form of MS with bilateral relatively symmetric demyelination. It is seen in childhood and rarely after the age of 40 years. It is characterized by large areas of demyelination that are well circumscribed, often involving the centrum semiovale and occipital lobes. Marburg variant of MS is defined as repeated relapses with rapidly accumulating disability producing immobility, lack of protective pharyngeal reflexes and bladder involvement.

New Methods

Magnetic resonance spectroscopy N-acetyl aspartate (NAA) is decreased in MS. This indicates that MS is more than a white matter disease. Axonal-neuronal loss occurs both early and often. It is suggested that the neuronal loss is associated with irreversible neurologic impairment. Choline (CHO) is increased and is associated with membrane (Myelin) breakdown, inflammation, and remyelination. Creative (Cr) may also be decreased. Lipid resonances have been observed in acute lesions using short echo-times (TE $\leq$ 30 ms). Myo-inositol and lactate have also been reported to be present in some lesions.

Magnetization transfer (MT) MT results from the transfer of magnetization from protons attached to rigid macromolecules (such as myelin) to free water protons. The effect is observed by noting a decrease in intensity on MR images (particularly PD weighted) performed with an off resonance pulse (MT). Injury resulting in demyelination causes a decrease in MT. Usually, MT effects are noted as one minus the ratio of the image intensity with a saturation pulse on divided by the intensity with the saturation pulse off ($1 -$ MTs/MTo). This is termed the magnetization transfer ratio (MTR). Thus, (for the physically challenged) low MTR equates with myelin loss. Remember, physically challenged, we are not referring to MT in the setting of enhancement. Rather we are attempting to look at tissue specificity.

There is decreased MT in MS, including in plaques and in NAWM, MTR is highest in homogeneously enhancing lesions, lower in nonenhancing lesions, and lowest in the central portion of ring-enhancing lesions, suggesting possible evolutionary patterns for lesions. Correlation with clinical disability has been found using MT. Histogram analysis using MT enables interrogation of the entire brain. Combined with techniques that segment the brain into gray and white matter one can tease out the effect of disease on specific brain components.

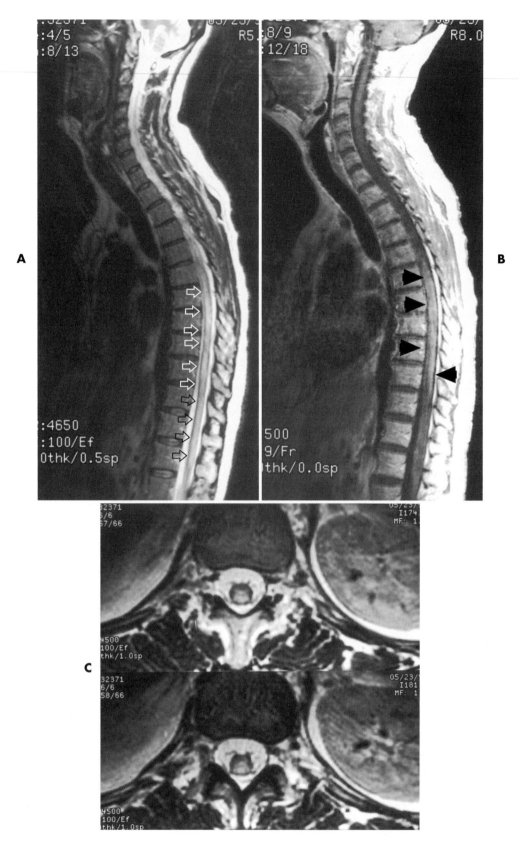

Fig. 7-8   Devic's disease (brain and batteries not included). **A,** High intensity on T2W sagittal image involving more than 7 vertebral body segments *(arrows).* **B,** Enhancement throughout the upper area of abnormality. **C,** Axial T2WI with central hyperintensity.

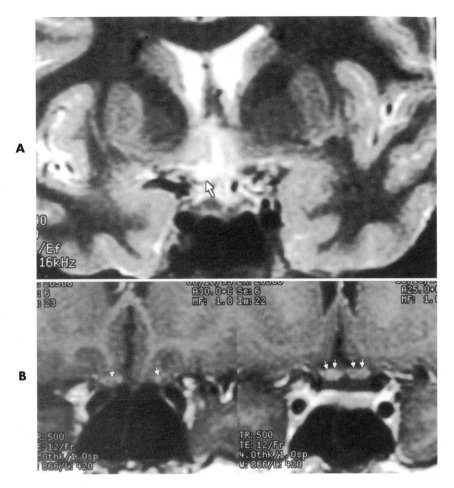

Fig. 7-9   Optic neuritis. **A,** Coronal T2WI with high intensity in the intracranial right optic nerve *(arrow)*. **B,** Enhanced image of intracranial optic nerves with bilateral enhancement *(arrows)*.

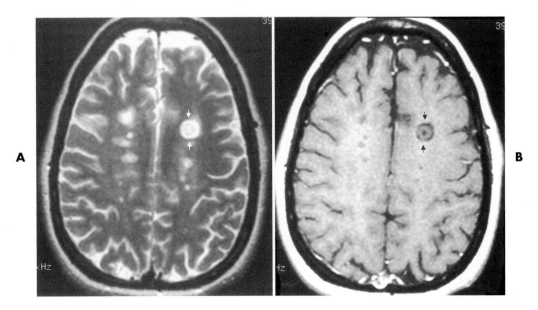

Fig. 7-10   Balo sclerosis. **A,** Left frontal high intensity lesion. There are alternating rings of different intensities *(arrows)*. **B,** Note the rings of intensity on this postgadolinium T1WI *(arrows)*.

Diffusion Diffusion is higher in MS plaques compared with normal-appearing white matter, and higher in acute plaques when compared with chronic. There is elevated ADC in acute plaques, and it is also increased in the NAWM. This finding is probably due to an increase in the extracellular space with edema and demyelination.

Differential Diagnosis of MS Lesions on MR

The following lesions are truly not primary demyelinating processes but may simulate MS in their MR appearance. These conditions manifest lesions with or without enhancement and occur in a similar patient population to that with MS. They include a veritable delicatessen of diseases.

Lyme disease An important infection that may produce symptoms similar to MS is Lyme disease. It is discussed thoroughly in the infection chapter; however, Lyme disease can have high intensity lesions on T2WI that enhance (Fig. 7-11). The cranial nerves may also demonstrate enhancement. It can present with acute CNS manifestations including transverse myelitis.

Vasculitides Vasculitides (see Chapters 4 and 6) including primary angiitis of the central nervous system, polyarteritis nodosa, Behçet's disease, syphilis, Wegener's granulomatosis, Sjogren syndrome, and lupus should be in the differential diagnosis of MS both clinically and radiographically.

Hypertension and ischemic white matter lesions High intensity abnormalities on T2WI generally increase as one ages and have been associated with hypertension (Fig. 7-12). In patients with malignant hypertension, high intensity abnormalities in the brain may be observed, most likely representing regions of cerebral edema (Fig. 7-13). When appropriate treatment is rendered, these areas of abnormality may decrease in size or resolve.

Ischemic white matter lesions may be of two varieties: (1) lesions involving the watershed distributions of the major cerebral arteries (anterior, middle, and posterior cerebral arteries) or (2) lesions caused by intrinsic disease of the small penetrating medullary arteries (arteriolar sclerosis). The term leukoaraiosis has also been applied to symmetric patchy or diffuse bilateral periventricular white matter changes in these regions. Leukoaraiosis is associated with increasing age and the presence of small vessel disease manifested by the presence of lacunar infarction. High signal on T2WI in the elderly is identified in the periependymal region and is thought to be related to ischemia with a histopathologic substrate of myelin pallor (weak staining of myelin with luxol fast blue, gliosis, and dilated perivascular spaces. Focal high signal abnormalities separate from the ventricular surface in elderly persons have been termed deep white matter infarctions. The high signal of T2WI is larger than the area of infarction and this may relate to increased water and protein content in reactive, swollen astrocytes

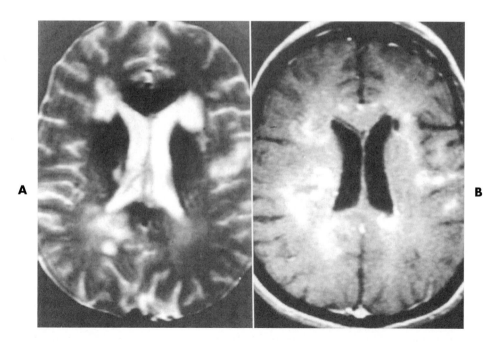

Fig. 7-11 Lyme disease. **A,** T2WI demonstrates multiple high intensity lesions throughout the brain parenchyma. No arrows are needed for this finding. (If this is not the case, we suggest you come to one of our postgraduate seminars.) **B,** Many of these areas are noted to enhance.

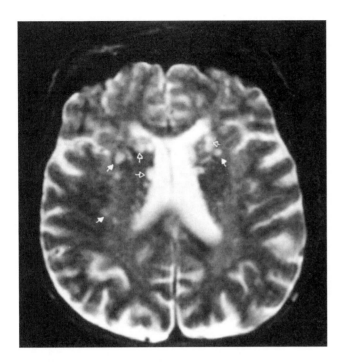

Fig. 7-12 Unidentified bright object (UBO). *Arrows* demonstrate multiple high intensity abnormalities on this T2WI in a patient with hypertension. The exact nature of these lesions is unknown. The presence of lesions in the caudate nucleus *(open arrows)* makes the diagnosis of MS unlikely, not to mention the fact that the patient was 85.

oriented along the path of the myelin sheaths (isomorphic gliosis).

Virchow-Robin spaces The Virchow-Robin spaces are invaginations of the subarachnoid space into the

brain associated with leptomeningeal vessels (Fig. 7-14). Dilated perivascular spaces occur in rather characteristic locations, typically in the basal ganglia, around the atria, near the anterior commissure, in the corona radiata, centrum semiovale, periinsular region, and in the middle of the brain stem, medial and posterior to the reticular portion of the substantia nigra. Usually, they follow the intensity of CSF, being hypointense to brain on T1WI and PDWI, and hyperintense on T2WI. The FLAIR/PDWI are best at discriminating perivascular spaces from white matter lesions because the perivascular spaces remain isointense to CSF, whereas MS and other lesions are hyperintense on these pulse sequences. Note that both brain lesions and perivascular spaces are hypointense on T1WI and hyperintense on T2WI. Occasionally, gliosis may be associated with these spaces, causing a perivascular space to be bright on PDWI. Conversely, a vacuolated lacune may simulate a Virchow-Robin space on FLAIR/PDWI. These spaces have linear courses when the section is along the long axis of the structure but appear as a punctate regions when the imaging slice is perpendicular to the long axis of the perivascular space.

Virchow-Robin spaces tend to enlarge with age and hypertension as the vessels within the space become more ectatic. This has been termed état criblé. État criblé is defined as dilatation of these perivascular spaces, usually with thinning and pallor of the perivascular myelin associated with shrinkage, atrophy, and isomorphic gliosis around the vessel. If this sounds familiar, "you're cookin' with gas," because this is similar to the description of hypertensive white matter changes. These are probably normal changes associated with arteriolar ag-

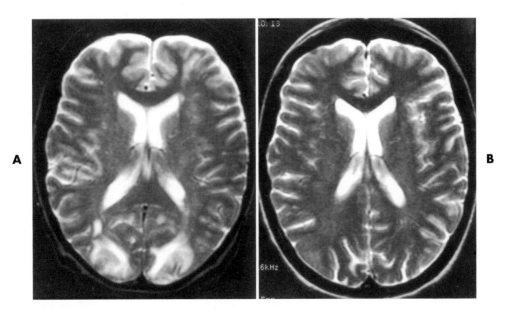

Fig. 7-13 Patient with eclampsia. **A,** Bilateral occipital high intensity regions on T2WI, which are characteristic. These lesions are transient. **B,** T2WI 1 month later at approximately the same level. There is resolution of these abnormalities.

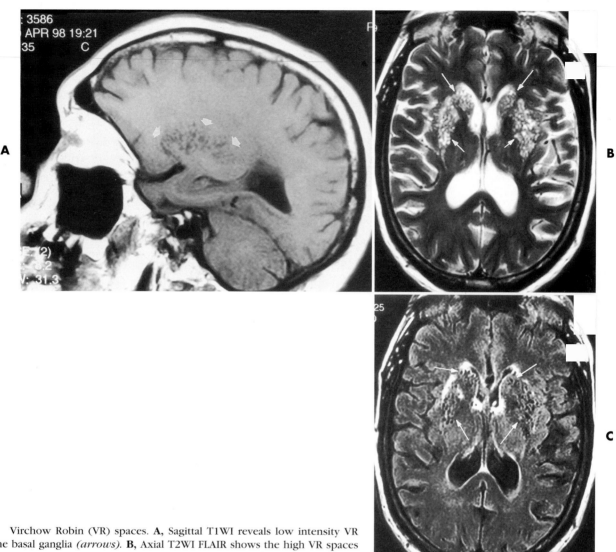

Fig. 7-14   Virchow Robin (VR) spaces. **A,** Sagittal T1WI reveals low intensity VR spaces in the basal ganglia *(arrows)*. **B,** Axial T2WI FLAIR shows the high VR spaces *(arrows)* in the caudate, globus pallidus, and putamen bilaterally. **C,** FLAIR image showing VR spaces have similar intensity to CSF *(arrows)*.

ing. The term *état lacunaire* refers to old cavitary infarcts in the basal ganglia and thalamus.

Migraine   Migraine should also be considered in the differential diagnosis of white matter abnormalities. Persons less than 40 years of age with migraine can have high-signal abnormalities predominantly in the centrum semiovale and the frontal subcortical white matter, which can extend into the deeper white matter at the level of the basal ganglia. The cause of these high signal abnormalities remains a mystery, although platelet aggregation is increased during attacks and some investigators hypothesize that these lesions could be the result of microemboli. They could also be the consequence of primary neuronal damage related to the migraine pathophysiology. These high intensity abnormalities are not transient, are seen in young patients, and appear to be a diffuse process.

Trauma   Diffuse axonal injuries (see Chapter 5 Diffuse Axonal Injuries [DAI]) induce high signal abnormalities on T2WI at the gray-white junctions, brain stem, corpus callosum, and internal capsules but should have an appropriate history.

Uncommon situations   There are a number of other conditions which have been reported associated with white matter abnormalities on T2WI. It is not clear if there really is indeed a relationship but we thought we'd throw them at the wall and see if any of them stick. These include lightning injury, chronic fatigue syndrome, asymptomatic alcoholics, and amyotrophic lateral sclerosis (in addition to the high intensity in the motor pathways).

Unidentified bright objects (UBOs)—Last words of caution   The final common pathway with respect to high intensity on T2WI is increased water content. Unfortunately, although MR is sensitive, it lacks specificity, particularly when interpreted without pertinent clinical information (Of course, if the diagnosis is known, then we would call such abnormalities BOs, but somehow this may be too descriptive.) There are pathologic studies of these small white matter lesions in "healthy" patients and the results are controversial. These may be areas of perivascular demyelination around arteriosclerotic vessels or areas of myelin pallor and dilated perivascular spaces, or small lacunar infarcts. Bottom line is that there is no agreement. Say whatever you think when asked what do these UBOs represent—it's all good!

Final Thoughts

It is critical for the radiologist to understand that the diagnosis of MS is based on the clinical signs and symptoms of the patient. The principal role of imaging is still (1) to confirm or not to confirm the clinical suspicion of MS and (2) to suggest plausible alternative diagnoses for the patient's neurologic complaints. MR alone cannot make the diagnosis of MS, so neurologists can still bring home the baguettes; although managed care has made it a day-old loaf. MR can suggest this disease, but without supporting clinical data other diagnoses may be more likely. A little knowledge here can be very dangerous. Think about a young patient who gets an MR for headache or some other unrelated symptom, and a few scattered high signal abnormalities are observed. A report that labels this appearance as MS is misleading and can do great harm to this individual's insurance eligibility, career, and life. Caution is urged when an interpretation of isolated high intensity abnormalities is made that may not be consistent with clinical information.

SECONDARY DEMYELINATING DISEASES

Allergic

Acute disseminated encephalomyelitis Acute disseminated encephalomyelitis (ADEM) is generally considered a monophasic demyelinating disease. There are reports of occasional recurrent bouts of the disease, and the question of a recurrent bout of ADEM versus the beginning of MS. The usual history is of a recent viral infection, vaccination, respiratory infection, or exanthematous disease of childhood. ADEM has been identified most frequently with antecedent measles, varicella, mumps, and rubella infection, but is not limited to these viruses. Today Epstein-Barr virus, cytomegalovirus, or *Mycoplasma pneumoniae* respiratory infections are the most common precipitants, but others include myxoviruses, herpes group, and HIV. It may also be idiopathic. The suspected etiology is based on an allergic or auto-

immune (cell-mediated immune response against myelin basic protein) cross-reaction with a viral protein. Symptoms are similar to a single episode of acute MS. These lesions, which may be multiple and large, are high intensity on T2WI and may enhance in a nodular or ring pattern (Fig. 7-15). No new lesions should appear on MR after approximately 6 months from the start of the disease. There may, however, be incomplete resolution of lesions. ADEM can enlarge the spinal cord or brain stem (and appear as a mass lesion), but it usually is seen in the cerebrum. Clinical syndromes of acute transverse myelitis, cranial nerve palsy, acute cerebellar ataxia (acute cerebellitis), or optic neuritis are well described. Gray matter lesions can also be identified. The diagnosis is usually made by history and CSF, which may demonstrate increase in white cells with a lymphocytic predominance and increased myelin basic protein. ADEM may have a mortality rate of up to 30%, and steroid therapy is commonly rendered.

Although rare, at the fulminant end of the spectrum of ADEM is acute hemorrhagic leukoencephalitis (Hurst's disease) associated with diffuse multifocal perivascular demyelination and hemorrhage confined to the cerebral white matter with strict sparing of the subcortical U-fibers (Fig. 7-16). The disease develops 3 to 14 days after a respiratory tract infection and progresses rapidly from confusion to stupor and coma. Death occurs an average of 6 days after the onset of symptoms following the development of cerebral edema and acute herniation. Histopathologically, there is a necrotizing angitis with petechiae and perivascular ring and ball hemorrhages. These hemorrhages (despite the name) may not be evident on CT or conventional MR but are seen at autopsy. On MR, there is massive brain swelling and evidence of high intensity on T2WI. Enhancement may not be prominent. As noted, hemorrhage may or may not be demonstrated.

Viral

Progressive multifocal leukoencephalopathy Progressive multifocal leukoencephalopathy (PML) is a demyelinating disease with a known viral etiology. It is caused by a JC virus infecting the oligodendrocyte and is associated with the immunosuppressed state. Box 7-3 lists the conditions that have been associated with PML. Although originally described as having a propensity for the parietooccipital region, PML can occur anywhere in the brain (including the posterior fossa), particularly in patients with AIDS, and may be solitary or multifocal with eventual widespread confluence. PML may present on MR as a focal region of low intensity on T1WI with high intensity on T2WI, most often without enhancement (so, what else is new?) (Fig. 7-17). Histologically, there are multifocal demyelinating plaques involving the subcortical U-fibers with sparing of the cortical ribbon and the deep gray matter. In a patient with HIV and sub-

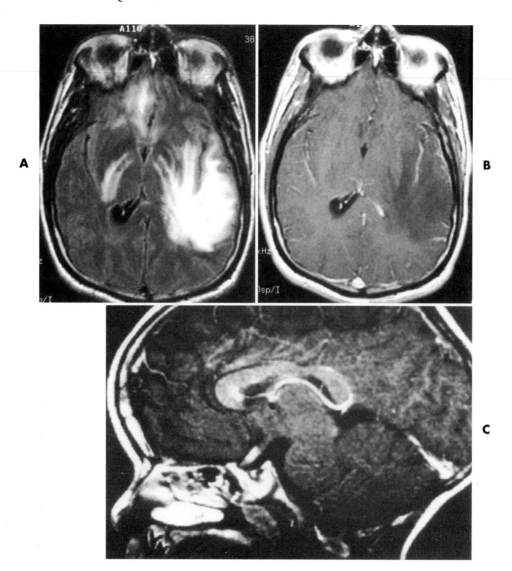

Fig. 7-15 ADEM. **A,** FLAIR image with high intensity in right frontal, internal capsule, and left temporal regions. **B,** Enhanced T1WI with significant mass effect but no enhancement. **C,** ADEM may occasionaly present with an optic neuritis picture. Enhancement is identified in the region of the optic chiasm on this sagittal T1WI. Although the latter presentations are somewhat uncommon, one should be aware that ADEM is probably more common that the average tire-kicking radiologist thinks.

Illustration continued on following page

cortical white matter abnormality, favor PML over other HIV related diseases. This disease is becoming more common in the face of the AIDS epidemic, with 2% to 7% of AIDS patients acquiring PML. MT ratios (MTR) are much lower in PML compared to normal white matter (40% less), and white matter in patients with HIV without PML, most likely secondary to the JC infection of the oligodendrocyte. Although less well recognized, PML may present as a mass lesion. It may demonstrate enhancement, atrophy, may involve gray matter including the deep gray matter, and produce widespread punctate abnormalities (Fig. 7-18). Angiographic abnormalities identified are a parenchymal blush in the early to mid-

arterial phase with persistence into the venous stage associated with arteriovenous shunting. This correlates with neoangiogenesis associated with microvascular inflammatory disease.

PML is usually a fatal infection, with death occurring 6 months to 1 year after onset of the disease. However, there are now a few early reports suggesting that highly active antiretroviral therapy may improve the prognosis. PML must be considered in the differential diagnosis of white matter lesions in immunosuppressed patients or in those with AIDS.

HIV (See Chapter 6.) The patient with AIDS has a propensity for multiple CNS infections as well as changes

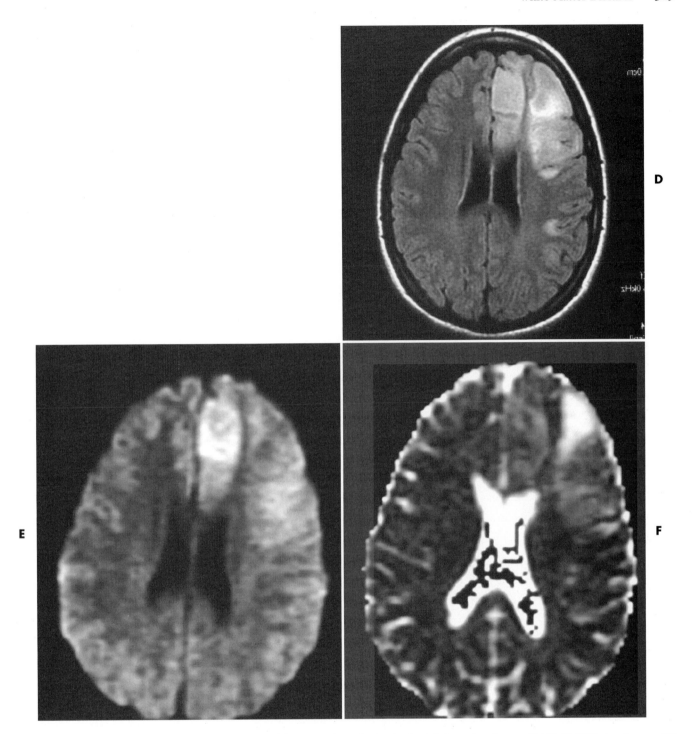

Fig. 7-15 *Continued.* **D,** Another example of ADEM showing a large lesion in the left frontal region on FLAIR. **E,** Diffusion image of **D** showing high intensity. This can be either T2 shine through or cytotoxic edema. **F,** The apparent diffusion coefficient (ADC) map clearly demonstrates brightness. Thus, the high intensity on the diffusion image **D** is T2-shine through.

related to intrinsic HIV infection. This situation is further confounded by the propensity of this population to develop neoplasms and PML. Patients with the AIDS dementia complex (ADC) develop atrophy and regions of demyelination in the white matter. This most commonly affects the supratentorial compartment particularly the deep gray and white matter.

Subacute sclerosing panencephalitis Subacute sclerosing panencephalitis is discussed fully in Chapter 6. It is caused by measles virus, but it is not known how

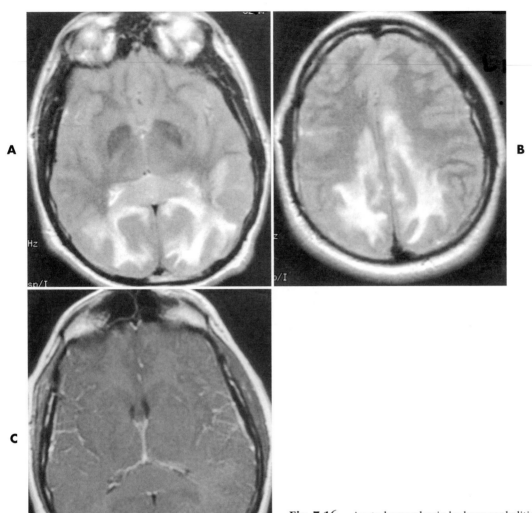

Fig. 7-16 Acute hemorrhagic leukoencephalitis (in another setting this could be called posterior reversible leukoencephalopathy syndrome—PRES). **A,** Axial T2WI with bilateral lesion involving the splenium of the corpus callosum. **B,** Axial T2WI at a higher level with involvement of the parietal and medial posterior frontal lobes. **C,** Postgadolinium image shows no enhancement but a markedly thickened corpus callosum.

Box 7-3   Conditions Associated with PML
AIDS
Autoimmune disease
Cancer
Immunosuppressive therapy
Lymphoproliferative disorders
Myeloproliferative disorders
Nontropical sprue
Sarcoid
Transplantation
Tuberculosis
Whipple disease

the intracellular viral particles produce this chronic infection. The white matter is predominantly affected with patchy demyelination and sparing the subcortical U fibers. Generalized atrophy is present with the severity related to the duration of disease. On MR, asymmetrical gray matter and adjacent subcortical white matter high intensity is seen in the parietooccipital region. Within the first year of the disease, periventricular white matter and basal ganglia lesions may also be seen (minority of cases). In the second year, cortical/subcortical lesions regress and asymmetrical periventricular white matter high intensity is identified. After the second year, atrophy is prominent as well as extensive symmetrical diffuse periventricular white matter changes. The diagnosis is made by finding intranuclear inclusions (Cowdry type A) on brain biopsy or autopsy.

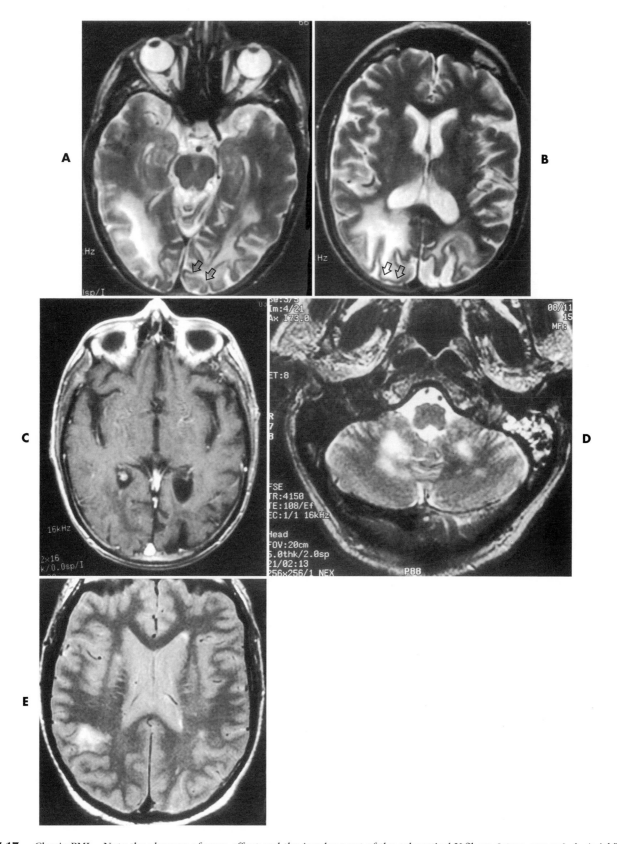

Fig. 7-17   Classic PML—Note the absence of mass effect and the involvement of the subcortical U-fibers *(open arrows)*. **A,** Axial T2WI with high intensity in the parieto-occipital white matter. **B,** Higher section. **C,** T1 enhanced axial image with no enhancement. **D,** Another patient T2WI with posterior fossa involvement and supratentorial subcortical lesions **(E).**

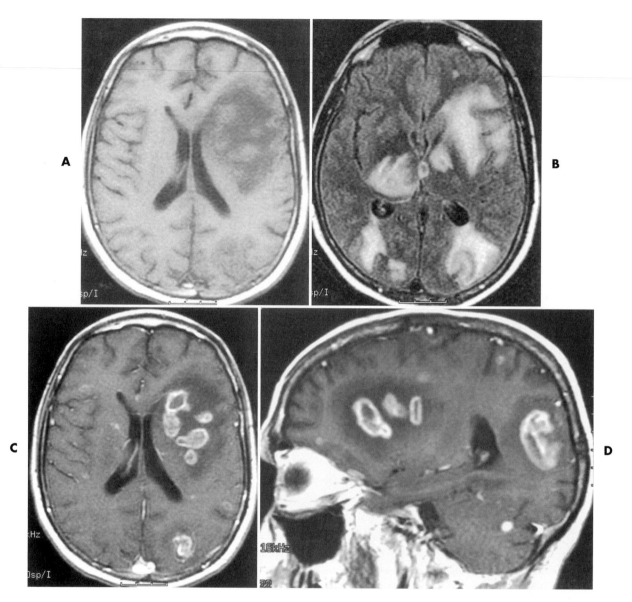

Fig. 7-18 Atypical PML in an HIV positive patient—Note mass effect, enhancement, and edema. **A,** Axial T1WI with left sided hypointense mass compressing the lateral ventricle. **B,** Axial FLAIR image with multiple high intensity lesions. **C,** Axial postcontrast T1WI with multiple ring enhancing lesions. **D,** Sagittal enhanced T1WI again demonstrating ring enhanced lesions.

Congenital rubella Adult survivors of congenital rubella with schizophrenic-like symptoms have been reported to have focal high signal abnormalities on T2WI predominantly in the parietal and frontal lobes. These lesions are thought to represent ischemic sequela of perivascular degeneration in the deep white matter from the initial infection.

Vascular

You should appreciate that the elderly (65+) accumulate white matter abnormalities that result, at some level, from ischemia secondary to injury to the long penetrating arteries of the brain. They have been correlated

with several clinical factors including silent stroke, hypertension (especially systolic blood pressure), depression, spirometry, and income (the poor shall inherit the earth, but they might have to hire the rich to run it). The greater the amount of white matter abnormality, the more likely the individual is to have impaired cognitive function and gait. However, mild periventricular white matter abnormality probably has little clinical equivalents. There has been some histopathologic correlations: (1) small patchy T2WI hyperintensities not attached to the ventricles were associated with myelin pallor, decreased numbers of myelinated fibers and an increased number of reactive glial cells. Small vessels were thickened, but no cerebral infarction was identified; (2)

"caps" hyperintense regions on T2WI around the anterior or posterior poles of the lateral ventricles were associated with myelin pallor, dilated perivascular spaces, and vascular changes similar to the small patchy lesions; (3) "rims" thin linear T2 hyperintense lesions along the body of the lateral ventricles were associated with subependymal gliosis and partial disruption of the ependymal lining.

Binswanger disease (subcortical arteriosclerotic encephalopathy) Binswanger disease, described in 1894, is a demyelinating disease equally affecting men and women generally more than 55 years old. It is associated with hypertension (approximately 98% of patients) and lacunar infarction. These features distinguish it from MS. Patients may have acute stroke followed by declining mental status or slower insidious mental status changes with decreased levels of mentation, dementia, psychiatric disturbances, seizures, urinary incontinence, and gait disturbance. MR reveals broad regions of high intensity abnormalities in the white matter of the frontal-parietal-occipital regions into the centrum semiovale (Fig. 7-19). It is interesting that the MT ratios in this abnormal white matter are significantly lower in Binswanger disease than in age matched nondemented patients, but not as low as infarcted tissue. This suggests that the tissue damage in Binswanger disease is more severe than in the high intensity regions in the nondemented patient, but not as severe as in infarction.

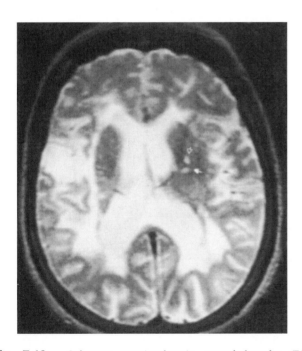

Fig. 7-19 Subacute arteriosclerotic encephalopathy (Binswanger Disease). Note the appearance of significant white matter involvement throughout the brain. On this slice also note the focal areas of lacunar infarction *(arrows)* in the basal ganglia and a focal right MCA stroke. This patient had a subacute onset of psychosis, a single seizure, and memory loss.

Histopathology in Binswanger disease usually displays demyelination with relative axonal sparing, and in association with arteriosclerosis, narrowing of white matter arteries and arterioles. Lacunar infarction is present in more than 90% of cases. The subcortical U fibers, which have a dual blood supply from the involved medullary arteries and uninvolved cortical arteries implicating an ischemic etiology, are spared. Binswanger disease differs from multi-infarct dementia because of its distinctive white matter involvement and the absence of consistent focal stroke syndromes. This again is a disease that needs the appropriate history to aid in focusing on the correct diagnosis.

Cerebral autosomal dominant arteriopathy with subcortical infarcts and leukoencephalopathy (CADASIL) CADASIL is an inherited arterial disease caused by mutations of Notch 3 gene on chromosome 19. Its onset is in the fourth decade of life, with a mean age of death at 59. The disease is characterized by recurrent TIAs, strokes, dementia, depression, pseudobulbar palsy, and hemi- or quadriplegia. It affects the frontal lobes, temporal lobes, and insula. Hyperintensity on T2WI is observed in the white matter, particularly periventricular and deep white matter, basal ganglia, and brain stem. Recently subcortical lacunar lesions representing distended perivascular spaces at the gray/white junction and adjacent spongiosis have been identified in the subinsular region in CADASIL. Hypointense lesions are seen on T1WI (Fig. 7-20). The regions affected by deep perforating arteries are most affected. CADASIL typically involves the subcortical U-fibers and anterior inferior temporal lobes and inferior frontal lobes. The frequency of MR lesions increases dramatically with the age of the patient. Both symptomatic and asymptomatic (but with Notch 3 mutation) have MR lesions. Diffusion tensor measurements have revealed increased diffusivity and concomitant loss of diffusion anisotropy in CADASIL patients that can be correlated with clinical impairment. This diffusional abnormality is hypothesized to be the result of neuronal loss and demyelination.

Postanoxic Encephalopathy

Postanoxic encephalopathy occurs after an anoxic episode severe enough to produce coma. The patient recovers in 24 to 48 hours and then precipitously declines within a 2-week period, progressing from confusion to coma and death. This is most likely an allergic demyelination caused by exposure to a myelin antigen during the hypoxic period. Pathologic changes are most prominent in the white matter with demyelination and necrosis.

MR demonstrates high signal on T2WI throughout the white matter particularly involving the corpus callosum, subcortical U-fibers, and internal/external capsules. Low intensity on T2WI has also been observed in the thala-

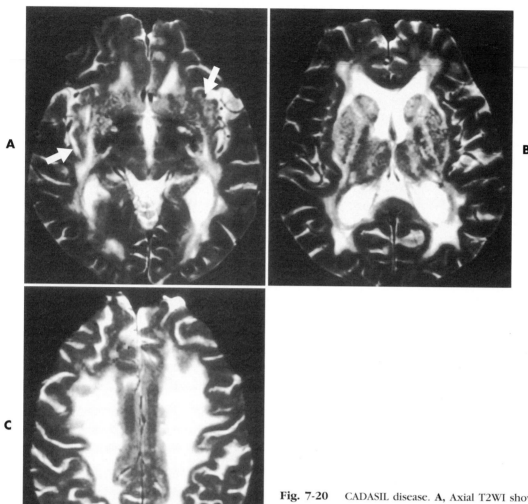

Fig. 7-20   CADASIL disease. **A,** Axial T2WI showing diffuse high intensity in the white matter and particularly in the insular region. Subcortical lacunar lesion is identified *(arrows)* and thought to increase specificity for CADASIL disease. **B,** Higher image with involvement of the striatal-capsular region. **C,** Note the diffuse high intensity throughout the white matter with sparing of the subcortical U-fibers.

mus and putamen. Diffusion images are positive (Fig. 7-21). Carbon monoxide exposure can produce a similar MR and clinical picture. In carbon monoxide poisoning, however, there is a propensity for symmetric globus pallidus lesions. The differential diagnosis of bilateral basal ganglionic lesions is provided in Box 7-4.

Reversible Posterior Leukoencephalopathy or Posterior Reversible Encephalopathy Syndrome (PRES) (Box 7-5)

The syndrome is controversial not only in name (PRES; RPL), but also in etiology. There are a diverse group of etiologies that produce high intensity abnormality on T2WI primarily in the cortex and subcortical white matter of occipital parietal region (Fig. 7-22). The abnormality is usually reversible, and can extend into other regions including the temporal and frontal lobes, pons, and

cerebellum. Enhancement may or may not be present and the pattern is variable. The most likely underlying problem is the inability of the posterior circulation (sparsely innervated by sympathetic nerves) to auto-regulate in response to acute changes in blood pressure. This leads to hyperperfusion and blood-brain barrier disruption with escape of fluid from the intravascular compartment into the interstitium (subcortical edema) but without infarction of the brain (classical explanation).

In preeclampsia-eclampsia there is data to suggest that the brain edema was associated with abnormalities in red blood cell morphology and elevated LDH and not with hypertension level. These findings signify microangiopathic hemolysis resulting from endothelial damage. The cause of the endothelial damage is thought to be from circulating endothelial toxins or antibodies against the endothelium. Indeed, in many of the conditions listed in Box 7-5, there is evidence of endothelial dysfunction or damage.

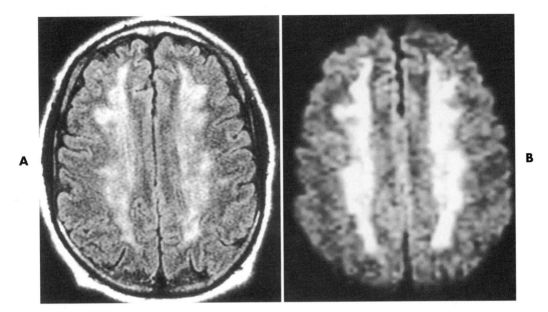

Fig. 7-21   Postanoxic encephalopathy. **A,** FLAIR image with diffuse high intensity throughout the centrum semiovale. **B,** Corresponding DWI image with high intensity (ADC was low) representing cytotoxic edema.

Patients have a variety of symptoms including headache, seizures, confusion, drowsiness, and visual disturbances. Most of the patients have a recent history of elevated blood pressure. Diffusion imaging can distinguish reversible changes from early ischemia. Conditions associated with this syndrome include malignant hypertension, toxemia of pregnancy, renal disease, immunosuppressive drugs, antiphospholipid antibody syndrome, and porphyria.

Osmotic Demyelination or Central Pontine Myelinolysis

Central pontine myelinolysis is a demyelinating disorder recognized in alcoholic, debilitated, or malnourished persons with rapid correction of hyponatremia. It has been also associated with chronic renal failure, liver disease, diabetes mellitus, dysequilibrium syndrome (complication to rapid dialysis), and the syndrome of inappropriate antidiuretic hormone secretion. In the pediatric population, it has been associated with orthotopic liver transplantation, acute myelogenous leukemia, Hodgkin disease, Wilson disease, and craniopharyngioma. The usual scenario is that the patient is admitted to a Veterans Administration hospital with a low serum sodium

---

Box 7-4   Bilateral Basal Ganglionic Lesions

AIDS
Aminoacidopathies
Andyia
Calcium phosphate dysmetabolism
Canavan disease
Cockayne syndrome
Fahr disease
Hallervorden-Spatz syndrome
Hepatic Encephalopathy
Huntington disease
Hypoglycemia
Hypothyroidism
Infarction (CO, H_2S)
Ischemia
   Artery of Percheron
   Vein of Galen thrombosis
Lead
Methanol poisoning (putamen)
Mitochondrial encephalopathies
Multisystem atrophy
Neoplasms (lymphoma, multicentric glioma)
Neurofibromatosis
Toluene abuse
TORCH
Wilson disease

Box 7-5   PRES

1. Hypertension
2. Cyclosporine
3. ARA-A/ARA-C
4. FK 506 (tacrolimus)
5. DMSO
6. Eclampsia/Preeclampsia
7. SLE, cryoglobulinema, hemolytic uremic syndrome
8. Cis-platinum

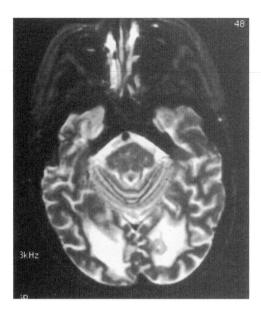

Fig. 7-22 PRES. T2WI in a patient on cyclosporine. Note the high intensity in the occipital region. (Also see Fig. 7-13.)

level, which is enthusiastically corrected by the overzealous intern looking to be rewarded by the attending staff for prompt attention to the numbers. Unfortunately, the patient deteriorates subacutely (usually within a few days) to coma, quadriparesis, pseudobulbar palsy, and extrapyramidal motor symptoms. The intern decides to go into radiology. This condition can be fatal, although with increasing awareness of this diagnosis, persons may survive, often with significant neurologic impairment.

What is most interesting is that the disease may involve extrapontine structures including the thalamus; putamen; caudate nuclei; internal, external, and extreme capsules; claustrum; amygdala; and cerebellum (Fig. 7-23). The deep gray matter structures can be involved bilaterally out to the insular cortex (see Fig. 7-23B). The cortex and subcortical regions may also be involved. Demyelination is noted without an inflammatory response, with sparing of the blood vessels, most nerve cells, and axons. In the pons, the T2WI exhibits high intensity with sparing of the outermost tegmentum and a peripheral rim of ventral pontine tissue. Many times, two central symmetric isointense structures encircled by the abnormal high intensity may be observed. These are the descending corticospinal tracts, which may be spared. The lesions are not associated with mass effect or enhancement. There is a single case report documenting the reversibility of the pontine lesion in a child—here's to case reports! The propensity of extrapontine involvement suggests that a more appropriate term, osmotic demyelination, be used to describe this process.

Alcoholism

Alcoholic patients and others with nutritional deficiencies may sustain demyelination of the corpus callosum. This may be considered a variant of extrapontine myelinolysis and has the eponym of Marchiafava-Bignami syndrome. (The Italian wine industry took offense to this eponym and so Fig. 7-24 is from France.) It may also be extensive and involve other brain regions. It should be considered in cases of sudden encephalopathy in alco-

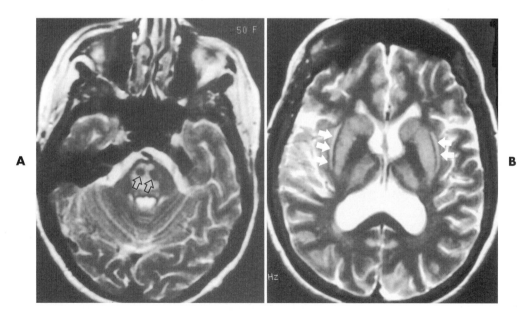

Fig. 7-23 Osmotic demyelination. **A,** T2WI with high intensity in the pons with sparing of the periphery and the descending corticospinal tracts *(open arrows)*. **B,** T2WI with involvement of the caudate nuclei, putamen, thalami, and claustrum *(arrows)*.

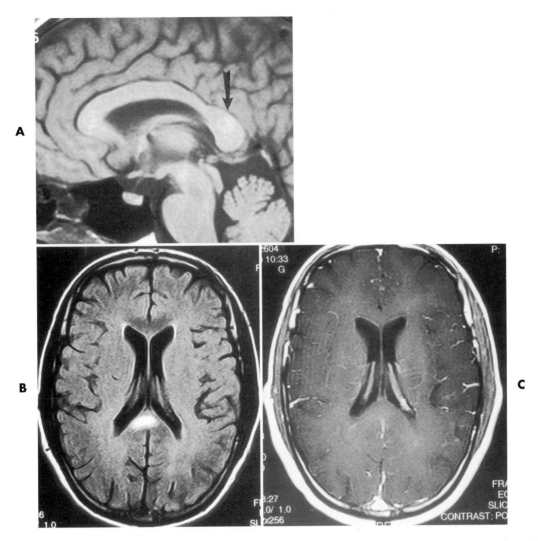

Fig. 7-24 Marchiafava-Bignami. **A,** T1 sagittal image with swollen splenium of corpus callosum *(arrow).* **B,** Axial FLAIR with high intensity in the splenium. **C,** Postgadolinium T1WI show no enhancement.

Illustration continued on following page

holic patients. Typically occurring in severe alcoholics, it is characterized by demyelination and central necrosis of the corpus callosum. Hemorrhage and hemosiderin deposition have also been reported. The acute form presents with seizures, neurologic dysfunction (muteness, diffuse muscular hypertonia with dysphagia), and coma and is usually fatal. Other forms of the disease exist. A subacute form displays the sudden onset of dementia progressing to the chronic vegetative state. The chronic form is distinguished by progressive dementia and a disconnection syndrome. The genu and splenium are involved more in the acute form and the body in the chronic category. This is depicted as a low-signal abnormality on T1WI (particularly in the sagittal plane) (edema and cystic changes) and high signal on the T2WI (see Fig. 7-24E). Diffusion images are positive in the acute form. The acute variety may reveal swelling and en-

hancement whereas the chronic variety demonstrates atrophy.

Wernicke's Encephalopathy

This results from thiamine deficiency. The hallmark is severe memory impairment with anterograde amnesia. There is atrophy of the mamillary bodies and there may be high intensity in the mamillothalamic tracts.

Toxic Lesions (Box 7-6)

Toxins can produce white matter abnormalities. Methanol poisoning causes optic nerve atrophy with necrosis of the putamen and subcortical white matter. The caudate and hypothalamus are less commonly involved. Methanol can produce hemorrhage as well as pe-

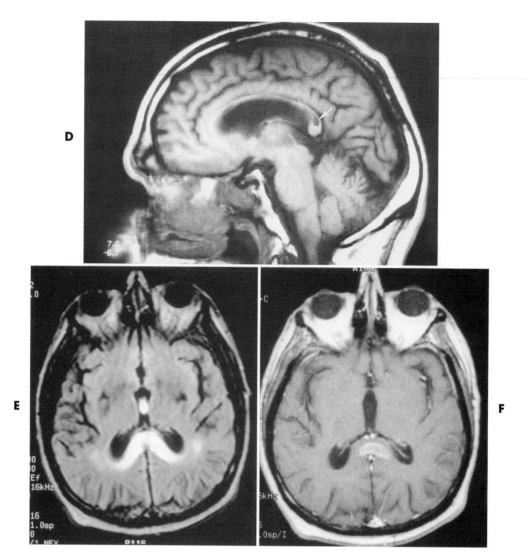

Fig. 7-24 *Continued.* **D,** Sagittal T1WI in a patient with chronic Marchiafava-Bignami disease shows low intensity in the splenium (*arrow*) of an atrophic corpus callosum in this Frenchman who had a long history of *vin ordinaire* intoxication. **E,** FLAIR image in another case with high intensity in the splenium of the corpus callosum. **F,** Observe the enhancement in the splenium following gadolinium.

ripheral white matter lesions. Ethylene glycol toxicity affects the thalamus and pons. Toluene affects include atrophy of the cerebrum, corpus callosum, and cerebellar vermis. It is associated with high signal on T2WI in the white matter, poor gray-white differentiation, and low signal in the basal ganglia and thalamus. Carbon monoxide poisoning produces low or high intensity on the T1WI and high intensity on T2WI in the globus pallidus. It also affects the white matter and hippocampus.

Organic mercury poisoning (Minamata disease) affects the calcarine area, cerebellum, and postcentral gyri on MR and these regions are responsible for the characteristic manifestation of the disease including constriction of the visual fields, ataxia, and sensory disturbance.

A fellow asks why are different regions affected by different toxins? We suggested the fellow learn the ap-

pearance of these lesions and then write his Ph.D. thesis on why. He remarked that he would do that if the authors supported his wife and children while he washed the test tubes.

Wallerian Degeneration

Wallerian degeneration can result in high signal abnormalities and atrophy in the white matter and is defined as antegrade destruction of axons and their myelin sheaths secondary to injury of the proximal axon or cell body. It has many causes including infarction, hemorrhage, white matter disease, trauma, MS, and neoplasia. On MR, it is relatively easy to demonstrate wallerian degeneration by noting high intensity on PDWI/ T2WI that follows a particular white matter pathway (Fig. 7-25).

Box 7-6 Drugs, Toxins, and Conditions Associated with White Matter Abnormalities

DRUGS

IV drug abuse
   Methamphetamine
   Cocaine
   Heroin
Isoniazid
Chemotherapeutic agents
   Actinomycin D
   Cis-platinum
   Cytosine arabinoside
   Adenine arabinoside
   Cyclosporine
   Methotrexate

TOXINS

Occupational exposure to compressed-air tunnels
Triethyl tin
Hexachlorophene
Lead intoxication
Methanol
Mercury
Toluene

OTHER

Hypertensive encephalopathy
Eclampsia
Radiation

Radiation Changes

MR is particularly sensitive to radiation changes in the brain. (Radiation changes are also covered in Chapter 3.) Commonly found in the irradiated fields are high signal abnormalities on T2WI and atrophy, both of which conform to the radiation portal.

Radiation alone can produce demyelination. It can also generate, usually when associated with chemotherapy (particularly methotrexate), a mineralizing microangiopathy. This is best characterized on CT, where calcification is identified as high density in the basal ganglionic region, the anterior cerebral—middle cerebral and middle cerebral—posterior cerebral watershed zones, and the cerebellum. On MR, this calcification usually displays low intensity on T2WI and particularly on T2*WI. Other radiation-induced findings include hemosiderin deposition, telangiectasia, and BBB disruption.

Disseminated Necrotizing Leukoencephalopathy and Chemotherapy

Disseminated necrotizing leukoencephalopathy (DNL) is a demyelinating disease first described in children undergoing cranial and/or spinal radiation in combination with intrathecal methotrexate for leukemia. Subsequently, it has been reported after combination radiation and chemotherapy in adult leukemia, bone and soft-tissue sarcoma, and small-cell carcinoma of the lung.

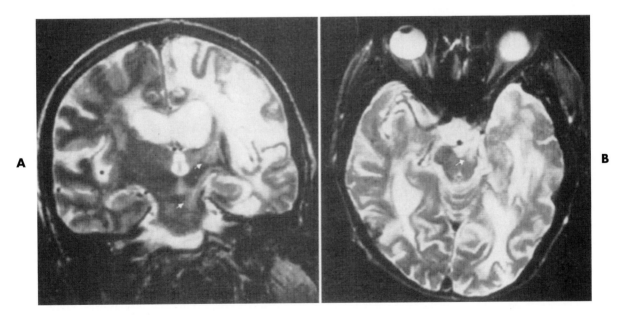

Fig. 7-25 Wallerian degeneration after left hemispheric infarction. **A,** High signal on coronal T2WI in the left internal capsule *(arrow)*. **B,** This high signal extends into the atrophic left cerebral peduncle *(arrow)* as part of the wallerian degeneration.

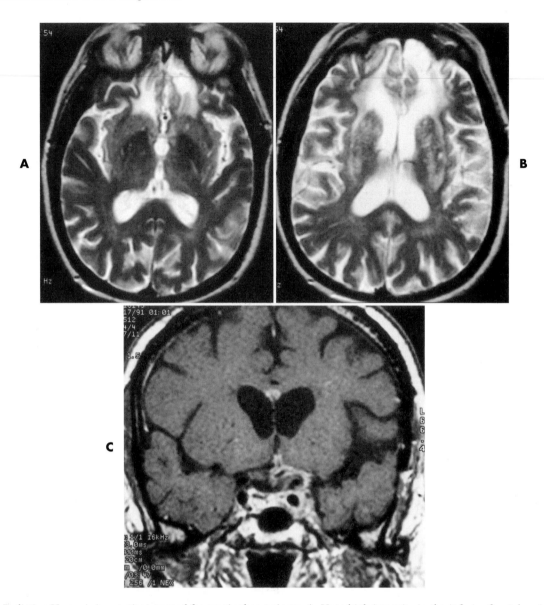

Fig. 7-26 Radiation Necrosis in a patient treated for craniopharyngioma. **A,** Note high intensity in the inferior frontal region on this axial image. **B,** Slightly superior section. **C,** Coronal T1 with enhancement in the corpus callosum.

In these patients, a progressive neurologic disorder develops. It is characterized by decreasing mental status and neurologic changes including seizures, usually progressing to coma and death. Associated with this neurologic syndrome is the appearance of marked low density in the white matter. Pathologic findings of DNL include axonal swelling, multifocal demyelination, coagulation necrosis, and gliosis. These changes have a predilection for the periventricular region and centrum semiovale with sparing of the U-fibers. On MR, diffuse regions of high intensity on T2WI may be visualized throughout the white matter (Fig. 7-26). There have been reports of enhancement in the lesion.

Chemotherapeutic white matter injury has been reported more frequently in children. It can cause white matter changes that are indistinguishable from radiation. Transient white matter high signal abnormalities that are not precursors of DNL may also develop in children undergoing chemotherapy for acute lymphocytic leukemia, but may resolve with cessation of chemotherapy. This is well described with methotrexate therapy. A special form of this injury occurs when chemotherapy is instilled directly into the brain by an indwelling ventricular catheter, resulting in the production of focal necrosis. In such instances, high intensity on T2WI MR or low density with focal enhancement can be seen adjacent to the catheter. Thus, chemotherapy and/or radiation therapy can result in white matter changes characterized by high intensity on T2WI. Focal mass lesions produced by radiation and/or chemotherapy may enhance.

Dysmyelinating diseases are much rarer than the previously described conditions. How rare are they? As rare as the truth from your used car dealer (or a former President with Peyronie's disease). Their appearance, particularly on MR, is usually much more bizarre. One often notes diffuse high intensity on T2WI throughout the white matter.

DYSMYELINATING DISEASES

Metachromatic Leukodystrophy

Metachromatic leukodystrophy (MLD) is the most common of these uncommon dysmyelinating diseases. It is an autosomal recessive disease that results from a deficiency of the enzyme arylsulfatase A, which hydrolyzes sulfatides to cerebrosides. There is a failure of myelin to be degraded and then reused with accumulation of ceramide sulfatide within macrophages and Schwann cells. Metachromatic-staining lipid granules (sulfatides) are found within neurons, and diffuse myelin loss is observed in central and peripheral nerves. There is symmetrical demyelination with characteristic sparing of the subcortical U-fibers.

Several varieties of MLD are characterized by age at onset (late infantile, juvenile, and adult), which probably relates to the degree of enzyme deficiency. The diagnosis is confirmed by documenting decreased arylsulfatase activity in peripheral leukocytes or urine. Clinical findings include peripheral neuropathy, psychosis, hallucinations, delusions, impaired gait, hypotonia, and dementia. There is symmetric diffuse high signal on T2WI throughout the white matter and the cerebellum (Fig. 7-27). Enhancement is the exception. In the adult form, multifocal lesions in the white matter with a propensity for the frontal lobes, and atrophy with ventricular dilatation have been noted.

Adrenoleukodystrophy

Adrenoleukodystrophy is a x-linked or autosomal recessive (neonatal) peroxisomal disorder associated with cerebral degeneration and adrenal cortical insufficiency (which may be clinically inapparent). It is caused by a deficiency of acyl-CoA synthetase preventing breakdown of very long-chain fatty acids with accumulation of these fatty acids in the white matter, adrenal cortex, as well as in plasma and red blood cells. This disease possesses some characteristics of a demyelinating disease with prominent perivascular inflammation and extensive demyelination, although it is classified as a dysmyelinating disease. Impaired hearing and vision, abnormal skin pigmentation, hypotonia, difficulty in swallowing, behavioral difficulties, and seizures are the most common clinical manifestations of the disease. There have been several phenotypes of this disease and variations in the imaging characteristics of adrenoleukodystrophy. One type starts in the parietooccipital region and progresses anteriorly to involve the temporal and frontal lobes together with the corpus callosum. The disease can also progress from anterior to posterior. The advancing edge of the lesion represents the region of active demyelination and enhances, whereas the nonenhanced regions are gliotic (Fig. 7-28). Patients have been described with enhancement of major white matter tracts including the corticospinal, spinothalamic, visual (including the lateral geniculate body), auditory, and dentatorubral pathways. Other findings include calcifications in the trigone or around the frontal horns, mass effect in the advancing region of demyelination, and isolated frontal lobe involvement. On MR, there may be relative sparing of the subcortical U fibers. Spinal cord disease can be seen with degeneration of the entire length of the corticospinal tracts and cord atrophy.

Alexander Disease

Alexander disease is a nonneoplastic disease of astrocytes characterized by fibrinoid degeneration of astrocytes and diffuse Rosenthal fibers in the subependymal, subpial, and perivascular regions. It has been divided into three clinical subgroups. The infantile group has seizures, spasticity, psychomotor retardation, and megalencephaly (not a constant feature) associated with extensive demyelination. The juvenile group (7 to 14 years old) demonstrates progressive bulbar symptoms with spasticity, and the adult group may have similar clinical appearance to MS or may be asymptomatic. The latter two groups have preservation of neurons and less myelin loss. On CT, hyperdensity has been described in the caudate nucleus and diffuse hypodensity in the white matter and in the internal and external capsules. Enhancement has been observed early in the course of the disease. On T1WI, hypointensity may be in the white matter and associated with subtle hyperintensity on T2WI. Brain stem atrophy and decreased intensity in the basal ganglia have also been reported.

Canavan Disease

Canavan disease (spongiform degeneration) is an autosomal recessive leukodystrophy resulting from a deficiency in the enzyme N-acetylaspartoacylase. The age at disease onset is from 2 to 4 months. Hallmarks including a large brain, hypotonia, and failure to thrive are followed by seizures, optic atrophy, and spasticity. Death usually occurs by the age of 5 years. Proton spectroscopy has shown high levels of NAA, which is synthesized in the mitochondria, and may be the carrier for acetyl

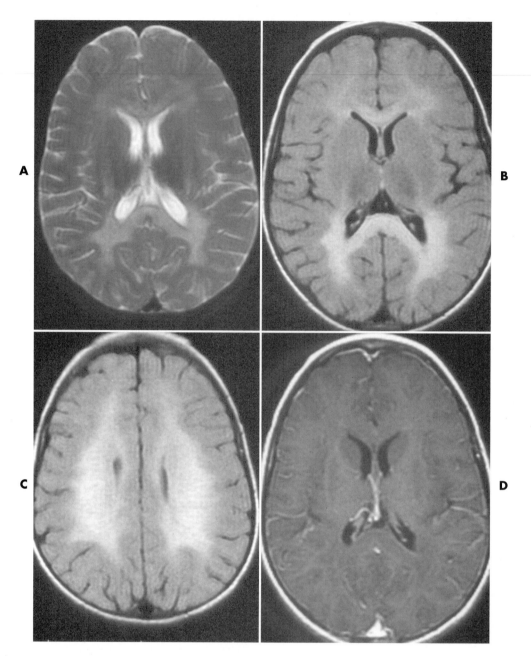

Fig. 7-27 Metachromatic leukodystrophy. **A,** T2WI revealing widespread symmetrical high intensity throughout the white matter with sparring of the U-fibers. **B,** FLAIR image revealing abnormal white matter in the corpus callosum. **C,** Higher axial FLAIR with diffuse white matter abnormality without U-fiber involvement. **D,** No contrast enhancement is identified.

Illustration continued on following page

groups across the mitochondrial membrane. *N*-acetylas-partoacylase cleaves NAA into acetate and aspartate in the cytosol, and deficiencies in this enzyme can interfere with the supply of acetate for fatty acid synthesis and myelination. This is one of the few diseases that spectroscopy has made a contribution to and thus is included for those minutiae-hungry persons. The deep gray matter and adjacent subcortical white matter are most involved. Symmetric involvement of white matter (high signal on T2WI) and ventriculomegaly have been de-scribed (Fig. 7-29). Alexander and Canavan diseases should also be considered in the differential diagnosis of macrocephaly (see Chapter 9).

Krabbe Disease (Globoid Cell Leukodystrophy)

This obscure entity (1 in 100,000 to 200,000 live births) hardly warrants discussion in two chapters (7 and 8), but we believe it is appropriate for those who will skip one

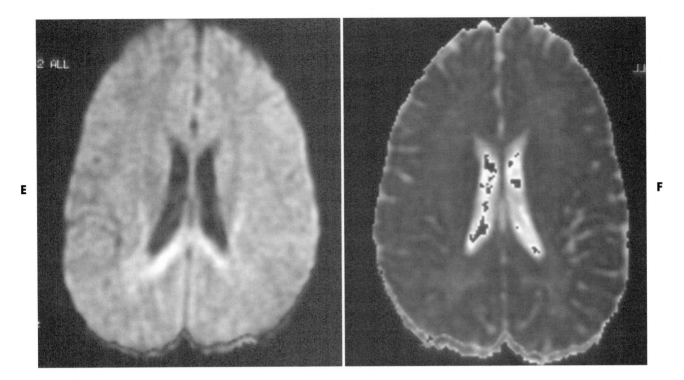

Fig. 7-27 *Continued.* **E,** Abnormal diffusion is seen in the splenium of the corpus callosum. **F,** ADC map reveals that the DWI high intensity is not cytotoxic edema.

of these two chapters in favor of a night out. Krabbe disease is caused by a deficiency of a lysosomal enzyme (beta-galactocerebrosidase) normally present in white and gray matter and involved in the metabolism of galactosylcerebroside-beta-galactosidase, hydrolyzing the galactose moiety from the galactocerebroside. Clinically, the leukodys-

trophy has been classified into an early infantile, late infantile (early childhood), late childhood, and even possibly an adolescent or adult onset group who had galactosylceramide deficiency. The infantile form is the most frequent with age at onset within the first 6 months of life. These patients have seizures, spasticity, and pro-

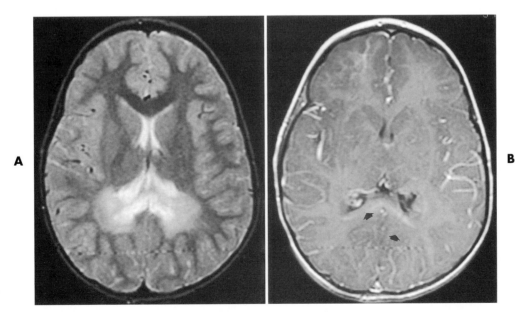

Fig. 7-28 Adrenoleukodystrophy. **A,** T2WI showing high intensity in the splenium of the corpus callosum. **B,** Enhancement is seen in this area *(arrows).*

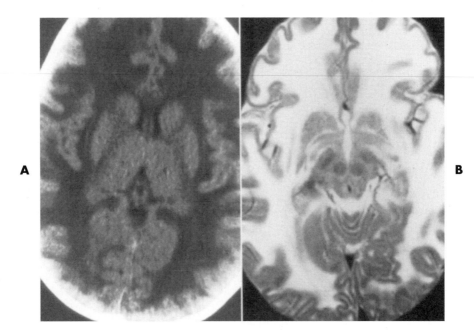

Fig. 7-29 Canavan disease. **A,** CT with diffuse low density throughout the white matter. **B,** On T2WI virtually all the white matter is abnormal. This patient also had an enlarged head (our secretary performed spectroscopy and told us there were elevated levels of *N*-acetyl aspartate). (After the diagnosis of Canavan disease was made, the secretary turned down admission to the first-year medical school class for a more lucrative job offer—bureaucrat in an HMO.)

gressive psychomotor retardation. It is characterized by globoid cell infiltration and demyelination. Increased density on CT (some of which represents calcification) in the basal ganglia, thalami, corona radiata, and cerebellar cortex, and hyperintensity on T2WI throughout the cerebral (parietal lobe) and cerebellar white matter have been noted. Late in the disease atrophy and high density in the corona radiata have been identified. Enlargement of the optic nerves in association with patchy high intensity in the white matter on T2WI has been reported. The differential diagnosis of bilateral symmetric thalamic lesions is provided in Box 7-7. Symmetric linear signal abnormalities on T1WI and T2WI have been reported from the periventricular to subcortical regions in the centrum semiovale. This represents demyelination with axon preservation associated with globoid cell infiltration and gliosis.

Sudanophilic Leukodystrophy

Sudanophilic leukodystrophy is a degenerative myelin disorder distinguished by accumulation of sudanophilic material in the brain. On CT, atrophy, low density in the white matter, and pinpoint periventricular calcifications have been reported. Pelizaeus-Merzbacher disease is a form of sudanophilic leukodystrophy. It is an x-linked recessive dysmyelinating disease with variable age at onset, usually within the first months of life (but can be seen from neonatal to late infancy), and slow progression. The disease is divided into three groups, classic

(slowly progressive with death in young adulthood), connatal (more severe, with death in the first decade of life), and transitional (less severe than connatal, with average age at death of 8 years). These differ in their onset and clinical severity. There appears to be failure of myelin maturation. This may be related to a deficiency of proteolipid apoprotein and reduced amount of other myelin

Box 7-7 Bilateral Symmetric Thalamic Lesions

Acute febrile encephalopathy
Artery of Percheron infarction (single trunk that supplies paramedian thalamic arteries)
Cytoplasmically inherited striatal degeneration
Deep venous occlusion, infarction
Glioma
Hypotic ischemic encephalopathy
Krabbe disease
Kernicterus
Leigh disease
Measles encephalitis
Molybdenum deficiency
Near-drowning
Reye syndrome
Sandhoff's disease (GM_2 gangliosidosis)
Wernicke-Korsakoff syndrome
Wilson disease

proteins (necessary for oligodendrocyte differentiation). Clinical findings include bizarre eye movements associated with head shaking, psychomotor retardation, and cerebellar ataxia. The disease should be considered in the differential diagnosis of male patients with cerebral palsy, especially if there is more than one case in the family. MR may be useful in defining carrier states of this disease if "normal" members of the affected family have abnormal scans. MR may be normal early on, but later they reveal cerebral, cerebellar, brain stem, and upper cervical cord atrophy. On MR, diffuse symmetric increased signal in the white matter (more or less complete lack of myelination) associated with low intensity on T2WI in the lentiform nucleus, substantia nigra, dentate nuclei, and thalamus has been described and is probably related to increased iron deposition. A "tigroid" pattern has been noted that corresponds to histopathologic findings in which small regions of normal neurons and myelin sheaths are scattered in the diffusely abnormal white matter. The corpus callosum is atrophic and undulating.

Vanishing White Matter Disease

This recently described disease (van der Knapp, 1997) is seen in children and teenagers. The clinical findings consist of prominent ataxia, spasticity, optic atrophy, and relatively preserved mental capabilities. The disease follows a chronic progressive course with decline being associated with episodes of minor infections and head trauma. The cortex is relatively normal. However, beneath the cortex the white matter is largely destroyed with the exception of some sparing of the U-fibers. There is cystic degeneration from the frontal to the occipital region with the temporal lobe being least involved. In noncystic regions of the brain, there was diffuse and severe myelin loss. MR demonstrates regions of white matter that have a signal intensity similar to CSF on all pulse sequences, and the brain has a swollen appearance with cystic degeneration around the periventricular region. Cerebellar atrophy is present and may be severe particularly in the vermis. Symmetric high intensity in the pontine tegmentum on T2WI has also been observed. MRS findings included decreased NAA, normal or slightly elevated Cho, and the presence of lactate. The features of Alexander's disease that differentiate it from vanishing white matter disease include macrocephaly, unremitting course, fronto-occipital gradient, and Rosenthal fibers on histologic examination.

SUGGESTED READINGS

Abe K, Fujimura H, Nishikawa Y, et al: Marked reduction in CSF lactate and pyruvate levels after CoQ therapy in a patient with mitochondrial myopathy, encephalopathy, lactic acidosis and stroke-like episodes (MELAS), *Acta Neurol Scand* 83:356-359, 1991.

Adams CWM: Perivascular iron deposition and other vascular damage in multiple sclerosis, *J Neurol Neurosurg Psychiatry* 51:260-265, 1988.

Atlas SW, Grossman RI, Golberg HI, et al: MR diagnosis of acute disseminated encephalomyelitis, *J Comput Assist Tomogr* 10:798-801, 1986.

Aubourg P, Blanche S, Jambaque I, et al: Reversal of early neurologic and neuroradiologic manifestations of X-linked adrenoleukodystrophy by bone marrow transplantation, *Neurology* 42:85-91, 1992.

Austin SJ, Connelly A, Gadian DG, et al: Localized 1H NMR spectroscopy in Canavan's disease: a report of two cases, *Magn Res Med:* 19:439-445, 1991.

Ay H, Furie K, Yamada K, et al: Diffusion-weighted MRI characterizes the ischemic lesion in transient global amnesia, *Neurology* 51(3): 901-903, 1998.

Baker LJ, Stevenson DK, Enzmann DR: End-stage periventricular leukomalacia: MR evaluation, *Radiology* 168:809-815, 1988.

Berger JR, Kaszovitz B, Post JD, et al: Progressive multifocal leukoencephalopathy associated with human immunodeficiency virus infection, *Ann Intern Med* 107:78-87, 1987.

Bewermeyer H, Bamborschke S, Ebhardt G, et al: MR imaging in adrenoleukomyeloneuropathy, *J Comput Assist Tomogr* 9:793-796, 1985.

Boon AP, Potter AE: Extensive extrapontine and central pontine myelinolysis associated with correction of profound hyponatraemia, *Neuropathol Appl Neurobiol* 13:1-9, 1987.

Brismar J, Brismar G, Gascon G, et al: Canavan disease: CT and MR imaging of the brain, *AJNR* 11:805-810, 1990.

Brooks BS, Gammal TE: An additional case of adrenoleukodystrophy with both type I and type II CT features, *J Comput Assist Tomogr* 6:385-388, 1982.

Brunberg JA, Kanal E, Hirsch W, et al: Chronic acquired hepatic failure: MR imaging of the brain at 1.5T, *AJNR* 12:157, 909-914, 1991.

Chabriat H, Mrissa R, Levy C, et al: Brain stem MRI signal abnormalities in CADASIL, *Stroke* 30(2):457-459, 1999.

Chabriat H, Pappata S, Poupon C, et al: Clinical severity in CADASIL related to ultrastructural damage in white matter: in vivo study with diffusion tensor MRI, *Stroke* 30(12):2637-2643, 1999.

Challa VR, Moody DM: White-matter lesions in MR imaging of elderly subjects, *Radiology* 164:3, 1987.

Chen JC, Schneiderman JF, Wortzman G: Methanol poisoning: bilateral putaminal and cerebellar cortical lesions on CT and MR, *J Comput Assist Tomogr* 15:522-524, 1991.

Clavier E, Thiebot J, Delangre T, et al: Marchiafa-Bignami disease, *Neuroradiology* 28:376, 1986.

Coker SB: The diagnosis of childhood neurodegenerative disorders presenting as dementia in adults, *Neurology* 41:794-798, 1991.

Di Chiro G, Eiben RM, Manz JH, et al: A new CT pattern in adrenoleukodystrophy, *Radiology* 137:687-692, 1980.

Dietemann JL, Beigelman C, Rumbach L, et al: Multiple sclerosis and corpus callosum atrophy: relationship of MRI findings to clinical data, *Neuroradiology* 30:478-480, 1988.

Dietrich RB, Bradley WG, Zaragoza EJ, et al: MR evaluation of early myelination patterns in normal and developmentally delayed infants, *AJNR* 9:69-76, 1988.

Drayer B, Burger P, Hurwitz B, et al: Reduced signal intensity on MR images of thalamus and putamen in multiple sclerosis: increased iron content? *AJNR* 8:413-419, 1987.

Dubois PJ, Freemark M, Lewis D, et al: Atypical findings in adrenoleukodystrophy, *J Comput Assist Tomogr* 5:888-891, 1981.

Flodmark O, Lupton B, Li D, et al: MR imaging of periventricular leukomalacia in childhood, *AJNR* 10:111-118, 1989.

Furuse M, Obayashi T, Tsuji S, et al: Adrenoleukodystrophy: a correlative analysis of computed tomography and radionuclide studies, *Radiology* 126:707-710, 1978.

Gallassi R, Morreale A, Montagna P, et al: Binswanger's disease and normal-pressure hydrocephalus, *Arch Neurol* 48:1156-1159, 1991.

Gaul HP, Wallace CJ, Fong TC, et al: MR findings in methanol intoxication, *AJNR* 16(9):1783-1786, 1995.

Gean-Marton AD, Venzina G, Peyster RG, et al: Abnormal corpus callosum: sensitive and specific indicator of multiple sclerosis, Presented at 75th RSNA, November 27,1989.

Gebarski SS, Babrielsen TO, Knake JE, et al: Cerebral CT findings in methylmalonic and propionic acidemias, *AJNR* 4:955-957, 1983.

Gebarski SS, Gabrielsen TO, Gilman S, et al: The initial diagnosis of multiple sclerosis: clinical impact of magnetic resonance imaging, *Ann Neurol* 17:469-474, 1985.

Geis JR, Hendrick RE, Lee S, et al: White matter lesions: role of spin density in MR imaging, *Radiology* 170:863-868, 1989.

George AE, de Leon MJ, Gentes CI, et al: Leukoencephalopathy in normal and pathologic aging: 1. CT of brain lucencies, *AJNR* 7:561-566, 1986.

Gerard E, Healy ME, Hesselink JR: MR demonstration of mesencephalic lesions in osmotic demyelination syndrome (central pontine myelinolysis), *Neuroradiology* 29:582-584, 1987.

Geyer CA, Sartor KJ, Prensky AJ, et al: Leigh disease (subacute necrotizing encephalomyelopathy): CT and MR in five cases, *J Comput Assist Tomogr* 12:40-44, 1988.

Gillams AR, Allen E, Hrieb K, et al: Cerebral infarction in patients with AIDS, *Am J Neuroradiol* 18:1581–1585, 1997.

Grossman RI, Gonzalez-Scarano F, Atlas S, et al: Multiple sclerosis: gadolinium enhancement in MR imaging. *Radiology* 161:721-725, 1986.

Grossman RI, Braffman BH, Brorson JR, et al: Multiple sclerosis: serial study of gadolinium-enhanced MR imaging, *Radiology* 169:117-122, 1988.

Hanyu H, Asano T, Sakurai H, et al: Diffusion-weighted and magnetization transfer imaging of the corpus callosum in Alzheimer's disease, *J Neurolog Sci* 167(1):37-44, 1999.

Hanyu H, Asano T, Sakurai H, et al: Magnetization transfer ratio in cerebral white matter lesions of Binswanger's disease, *J Neurolog Sci* 166(2):85-90, 1999.

Hausegger KA, Millner MM, Ebner F, et al: Mitochondrial encephalomyopathy: two years follow-up by MR, *Pediatr Radiol* 21:231-233, 1991.

Heier LA, Bauer CJ, Schwart L, et al: Large Virchow-Robin spaces: MR-clinical correlation, *AJNR* 10:929-936, 1989.

Holman RC, Janssen RS, Buehler JW, et al: Epidemiology of progressive multifocal leukoencephalopathy in the United States: analysis of national mortality and AIDS surveillance data, *Neurology* 41:1733-1736, 1991.

Hong-Magno ET, Muraki AS, Huttenlocher PR: Atypical CT scans in adrenoleukodystrophy, *J Comput Assist Tomogr* 11:333-336, 1987.

Horowitz AL, Kaplan RD, Grewe G, et al: The ovoid lesion: a new MR observation in patients with multiple sclerosis, *AJNR* 10:303-305, 1989.

Igarashi H, Sakai F, Kan S, et al: Magnetic resonance imaging of the brain in patients with migraine, *Cephalalgia* 11:69-74, 1991.

Illowsky BP, Laureno R: Encephalopathy and myelinolysis after rapid correction of hyponatraemia, *Brain* 110:855-867, 1987.

Inoue E, Hori S, Narumi Y, et al: Portal-systemic encephalopathy: presence of basal ganglia lesions with high signal intensity on MR images, *Radiology* 179:551-555, 1991.

Inui K, Miyagawa H, Sashihara J, et al: Remission of progressive multifocal leukoencephalopathy following highly active antiretroviral therapy in a patient with HIV infection, *Brain & Development* 21(6):416-419, 1999.

Inzitari D, Giordano GP, Ancona A, et al: Leukoaraiosis, intracerebral hemorrhage, and arterial hypertension, *Stroke* 21:1419-1423, 1990.

Kiel MK, Greenspun B, Grossman RI: Magnetic resonance imaging and degree of disability in multiple sclerosis, *Arch Phys Med Rehabil* 69:11-13, 1988.

Kingsley DPE, Kendall BE: Review: CT of the adverse effects of therapeutic radiation of the central nervous system, *AJNR* 2:453-460, 1981.

Knapp MSV, Valk J: MR imaging of the various stages of normal myelination during the first year of life, *Neuroradiology* 31:459-470, 1990.

Koci TM, Chiang F, Chow P, et al: Thalamic extrapontine lesions in central pontine myelinolysis, *AJNR* 11:1229-1233, 1990.

Korogi Y, Takahashi M, Shinzato J, et al: MR findings in seven patients with organic mercury poisoning (Minamata disease), *AJNR* 15(8):1575-1578, 1994.

Kumar AJ, Rosenbaum AE, Naidu S, et al: Adrenoleukodystrophy: correlating MR imaging with CT, *Radiology* 165:497-504, 1987.

Lane B, Sullivan EV, Lim KO, et al: White matter MR hyperintensities in adult patients with congenital rubella, *AJNR* 17(1):99-103, 1996.

Laureno R: Central pontine myelinolysis following rapid correction of hyponatremia, *Ann Neurol* 13:232-242, 1983.

Lebow S, Anderson DC, Mastri A, et al: Acute multiple sclerosis with contrast-enhancing plaques, *Arch Neurol* 35:435-439, 1978.

Longstreth WT, Jr, Manolio TA, Arnold A, et al: Clinical correlates of white matter findings on cranial magnetic resonance imaging of 3301 elderly people. The Cardiovascular Health Study [see comments], *Stroke* 27(8):1274-1282, 1996.

Mark AS, Atlas SW: Progressive multifocal leukoencephalopathy in patients with AIDS: appearance on MR images, *Radiology* 173:517-520, 1989.

Mayer PL, Kier EL: The controversy of the periventricular white matter circulation: a review of the anatomic literature, *AJNR* 12:223-228, 1991.

Miller GM, Baker HL, Okazaki H, et al: Central pontine myelinolysis and its imitators: MR findings, *Radiology* 168:795-802, 1988.

Moody DM, Bell MA, Challa VR: The corpus callosum, a unique white-matter tract: anatomic features that may explain sparing in Binswanger disease and resistance to flow of fluid masses, *AJNR* 9:1051-1059, 1988.

Nelson PK, Masters LT, Zagzag D, et al: Angiographic abnormalities in progressive multifocal leukoencephalopathy: an explanation based on neuropathologic findings, *AJNR* 20(3):487-494, 1999.

Nowell MA, Grossman RI, Hackney DB, et al: MR imaging of white matter disease in children, *AJNR* 9:503-509, 1988.

Okeda R, Kitano M, Sawabe M, et al: Distribution of demyelinating lesions in pontine and extrapontine myelinolysis: three autopsy cases including one case devoid of central pontine myelinolysis, *Acta Neuropathol* 69:259-266, 1986.

Olsen WL, Longo FM, Mills CM, et al: White matter disease in AIDS: findings at MR imaging, *Radiology* 169:445-448, 1988.

Paltiel HJ, O'Gorman AM, Meagher-Villemure K, et al: Subacute necrotizing encephalomyelopathy (Leigh disease): CT study, *Radiology* 162:115-118, 1987.

Penner MW, Li KC, Gebarski SS, et al: MR imaging of Pelizaeus-Mezbacher disease, *J Comput Assist Tomogr* 11:591-593, 1987.

Pfister HW, Einhaupl KM, Brandt T: Mild central pontine myelinolysis: a frequently undetected syndrome, *Eur Arch Psychiatr Neurol Sci* 235:134-139, 1985.

Post MJD, Tate LG, Quencer RM, et al: CT, MR and pathology in HIV encephalitis and meningitis, *AJNR* 9: 469-476, 1988.

Richardson EP: Progressive multifocal leukoencephalopathy, *N Engl J Med* 265:17, 1961.

Rieth KG, DiChiro G, Cromwell LD, et al: Primary demyelinating disease simulating glioma of the corpus callosum, *J Neurosurg* 55:620-624, 1981.

Rolfs A, Schumacher HC: Cyclosporine-related central nervous system toxicity in cardiac transplantation, *N Engl J Med* 323:6, 1990.

Romain GC: White matter lesions and normal-pressure hydrocephalus: Binswanger disease or Hakim syndrome, *AJNR* 12: 40-41, 1991.

Rubinstein D, Escott E, Kelly JP, et al: Methanol intoxication with putaminal and white matter necrosis: MR and CT findings, *AJNR* 16(7):1492-1494, 1995.

Sandhu FS, Dillon WP: MR demonstration of leukoencephalopathy associated with mitochondrial encephalomyopathy: case report, *AJNR* 12:375-379, 1991.

Schipper HI, Seidel D: Computed tomography in late-onset metachromatic leukodystrophy, *Neuroradiology* 26:39-44, 1984.

Schwartz R, Feske S, et al: Preeclampsia-eclampsia:clinical and neuroradiographic correlates and insights into the pathogenesis of hypertensive encephalopathy, *Radiology* 217(2): 371-376, 2000.

Seales D, Greer M: Acute hemorrhagic leukoencephalitis: a successful recovery, *Arch Neurol* 48:1086-1088, 1991.

Shah M, Ross JS: Infantile Alexander disease: MR appearance of a biopsy-proved case, *AJNR* 11:1105-1106, 1990.

Silverstein AM, Hirsh DK, Trobe JD, et al: MR imaging of the brain in five members of a family with Pelizaeus-Merzbacher disease, *AJNR* 11:495-499, 1990.

Smith AS, Meisler DM, Weinstein MA, et al: High-signal periventricular lesions in patients with sarcoidosis: neurosarcoidosis or multiple sclerosis, *AJNR* 10:485-490, 1989.

Takao M, Koto A, Tanahashi N, et al: Pathologic findings of silent hyperintense white matter lesions on MRI, *J Neurolog Sci* 167(2):127-131, 1999.

Truwit CL, Denaro CP, Lake JR, et al: MR imaging of reversible cyclosporin A-induced neurotoxicity, *AJNR* 12:157, 651-659, 1991.

van der Knaap M, Barth P, Gabreels FJ, et al: A new leukoencephalopathy with vanishing white matter, *Neurology* 48(4): 845-855, 1997.

Zeiss J, Velasco ME, Coombs RJ, et al: Cerebral CT of lethal ethylene glycol intoxication with pathologic correlation, *AJNR* 10(2):440-442, 1989.

CHAPTER 8

Neurodegenerative Diseases and Hydrocephalus

The debate over whether a patient has atrophy or hydrocephalus has consumed an enormous number of pages in the neuroradiologic literature and whole sessions of national meetings. Why the fuss? Well, the implications as far as prognosis and treatment are vastly different between the two, so accurate distinction is essential. So naturally, if a lot of attention has been paid to it, it must be because we ain't so good at it! Here is the condensed and succinct treatise on the issue.

Let us start with the basics. Atrophy reflects the loss of brain tissue, be it cortical, subcortical, or deep. With the loss of cell bodies in the cortex (gray matter), axonal wallerian degeneration occurs with white matter atrophy or demyelination. Selective atrophy of the white matter may also occur with perivascular small-vessel insults. Generally, there is no treatment for atrophy; what's gone is gone. Therefore, beware of overcalling atrophy. Remember that certain drugs (steroids) or metabolic states (dehydration, alcoholism) may cause an appearance of increased cerebrovascular fluid (CSF) spaces (suggesting atrophy) but

are potentially reversible (Box 8-1). Marijuana has also been implicated as a cause of reversible atrophy (but only if you inhale).

Until you have a good sense of what the normal brain looks like at all ages, be hesitant to label a brain "atrophic." You should use the terms, *age-related changes* or *volume loss appropriate for age.* Normally functioning elderly persons may get offended (if not litigious) at the neuroradiologist who labels their brains "atrophic." There is a spectrum of normal brain parenchymal volume for any age, and you will be surprised at how well an atrophic brain in an NYU department chair can function (Fig. 8-1). Remember also that men have more prominent sulci at most ages than women, a fact wives like to emphasize to their spouses. Of course this may be an effect a woman has on her husband and vice versa. Also remember Yousem's first axiom: The sum of the intelligence on the planet remains a constant; the population however continues to grow. This means there will be more and more cerebral atrophy with time.

Hydrocephalus reflects expansion of the ventricular system from increased intraventricular pressure, which is in most cases caused by abnormal cerebrospinal fluid (CSF) hydrostatic mechanics. Hydrocephalus may be due to three presumed causes: (1) overproduction of CSF; (2) obstruction at the ventricular outlet level; or (3) obstruction at the arachnoid villi level, leading to poor resorption of CSF back into the intravascular space. Although atrophy and hydrocephalus often share the finding of dilatation of the ventricular system, the prognostic and therapeutic implications of the two are markedly different. Hydrocephalus can often be treated with well-placed ventricular or subarachnoid space shunts and/or removal of the obstructing or overproducing lesion. There may be hope for hydrocephalic patients, but a truly atrophic brain is usually gone for good. "Hasta la vista, baby!"

Computed tomographic (CT) or magnetic resonance (MR) imaging findings that suggest hydrocephalus over at-

Box 8-1   Causes of Reversible Atrophy

Alcoholism
Anorexia
Chemotherapeutics
Dehydration
Marijuana (Mary-Jane, pot, weed, grass, like M-J dude)
Radiation injury
Starvation
Steroid use

rophy are summarized in Table 8-1 (Fig. 8-2). At a first glance level, the presence of dilatation of the chiasmatic, infundibular and suprapineal recesses of the third ventricle, rounding of the frontal horns, convexity to the third ventricle, expansion of the temporal horns, effacement of sulci, enlargement of ventricles out of proportion to sul-

cal dilatation, periventricular smooth high signal representing transependymal CSF exudation (best seen on FLAIR), marked accentuation of the aqueductal signal void, narrowing of mamillopontine distances, and associated papilledema are indicative of hydrocephalus (Fig. 8-3).

The corpus callosum may be compressed against the rigid falx in long-standing hydrocephalus. Clefts of abnormal signal in the body of the corpus callosum, scalloping of its dorsal surface, and tethering of pericallosal vessels can be seen in cases of hydrocephalus due to aqueductal stenosis possibly owing to the impact of the towering corpus callosum against the falx. The damage may be due to arterial or venous vascular compromise.

These criteria seem simple enough. Why the confusion? Long-standing hydrocephalus may simulate atrophy on occasion, and the presence of hydrocephalus does not preclude concomitant atrophy (and vice versa). The distinction may become blurred. Let us explore some of the entities in greater depth, chére etudiante.

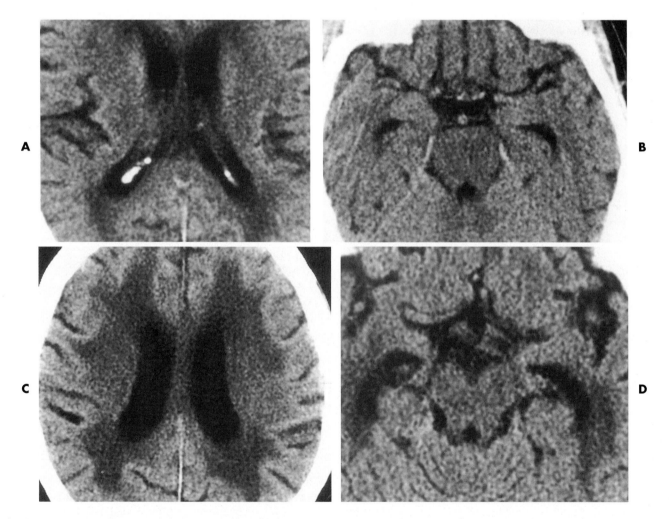

Fig. 8-1   Atrophy or hydrocephalus? Bob's brain in Philadelphia versus New York. **A,** This is Bob's brain while working in Philadelphia. Note the small temporal horns **(B). C,** Although there is periventricular low density and large ventricles, the sulci are somewhat prominent. Is this bad white matter disease from arteriosclerosis or are the ventricles obstructed? In this case it is a difficult call, but the diagnosis was progressive dementia inherent to all New York department chairmen. **D,** The smallish temporal horns and the change from 2 years before argue in favor of a frontotemporal dementia.

Table 8-1 Differentiation of hydrocephalus and atrophy

Characteristic	Hydrocephalus	Atrophy
Temporal horns	Enlarged	Normal except in Alzheimer's disease
3rd ventricle	Convex	Concave
	Distended anterior recesses	Normal anterior recesses
4th ventricle	Normal or enlarged	Normal except with cerebellar atrophy
Ventricular angle of frontal horns on axial scan	More acute	More obtuse
Mamillopontine distance	<1 cm	>1 cm
Corpus callosum	Thin, distended, rounded elevation	Normal or atrophied
	Increased distance between corpus callosum and fornix	Normal fornix–corpus callosum distance
Transependymal migration of CSF	Present acutely	Absent (rule out ischemia)
Sulci	Flattened	Enlarged out of proportion to age
Aqueductal flow void	Accentuated in normal pressure hydrocephalus	Normal
Choroidal-hippocampal fissures	Normal to mildly enlarged	Markedly enlarged in Alzheimer's disease
Sellar changes	Erosion of floor and ballooning of sella	None

HYDROCEPHALUS

Overproduction of Cerebrospinal Fluid

Classically, it was stated that patients with choroid plexus papillomas and choroid plexus carcinomas have hydrocephalus based on the overproduction of CSF (see Fig. 3-24). Increasingly, this hypothesis has come into question because it is believed that some cases of hydrocephalus may in fact be due to obstruction of the arachnoid villi or other CSF channels secondary to adhesions from tumoral hemorrhage, high protein levels, or intraventricular debris. This is particularly true with fourth ventricular choroid plexus papillomas, which generally tend to obstruct the sites of egress of the CSF in the foramina of Luschka and Magendie. In the cases

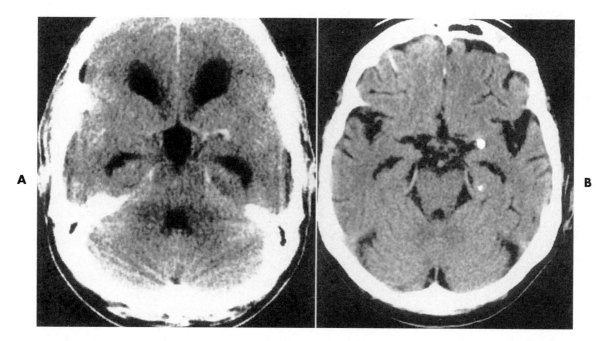

Fig. 8-2 Hydrocephalus versus atrophy. **A,** Hydrocephalus. Appearance of hydrocephalus with dilatation of the frontal horns of the lateral ventricles, the temporal horns of the lateral ventricles, and the third ventricle, but a normal-appearing fourth ventricle. The angle of the frontal horns of the lateral ventricles is more acute than seen in atrophy. No sulcal dilatation exists. **B,** Atrophy. CT demonstrates sulcal prominence and mildly enlarged temporal horns. In comparison with the patient in **A,** the temporal horns, although enlarged, are not enlarged to the same degree. Furthermore, there is obvious sulcal prominence with atrophy; this is not demonstrated with communicating hydrocephalus.

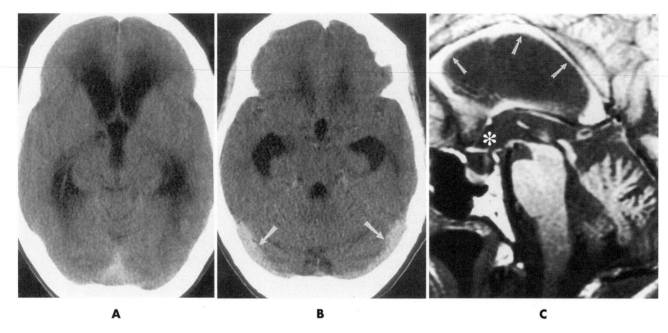

A **B** **C**

Fig. 8-3 Hydrocephalus. **A,** Transependymal CSF flow and the ballooned out nature of the frontal horns implies hydrocephalus. The sulci are inapparent. **B,** Note the markedly enlarged temporal horns and the rounded inferior third ventricle. Slow flow and polycythemia account for the high density of the transverse sinus and torcula *(arrows)* in this child, but good pick-up. **C,** The third ventricle is enlarged *(*)* and the high arching lateral ventricles with thinned corpus callosum *(arrows)* implies hydrocephalus.

of lateral ventricle choroid plexus papillomas (particularly in the pediatric population), the overproduction of CSF may be the cause of hydrocephalus.

Noncommunicating Hydrocephalus

Obstructive hydrocephalus may be separated into noncommunicating and communicating forms. Noncommunicating forms are due to abnormalities at the ventricular outflow levels (see Box 8-2). Communicating hydrocephalus is due to abnormalities at the level of the arachnoid villi or blockage at the incisura of the foramen magnum. Noncommunicating types often need brain surgery to remove offending agents; communicating types respond best to shunts. This is also how women categorize men. Hydrocephalus, like a man, is better when it communicates. Brain surgery (among other therapies) has often been recommended by women for men who do not communicate. Food for thought: Communist columnists who do not communicate or co-mingle are likely to be excommunicated (Say that 3 times fast).

Causes of Obstructive Hydrocephalus

Colloid cyst The classic cause of obstruction at the foramina of Monro (no relation to another classic—Marilyn) is the colloid cyst (see Fig. 3-69). This is typically located in the anterior region of the third ventricle. On CT, the lesion is high in density before enhancement. MR often shows a lesion that is high intensity on T1WI

and T2WI. The signal of colloid cysts is variable, depending on the protein concentration, hemorrhage, and other paramagnetic ion effects.

Congenital aqueductal stenosis The cerebral aqueduct is one of the narrowest channels through which the CSF in the ventricles must flow. (Let us sue the architect who designed to have all that CSF pass through such a narrow channel—there is no room for error.) Congenital aqueductal stenosis is just one of the obstructors of the aqueduct. This is most commonly an X-linked recessive disorder seen in early childhood, although it can present at any age. Children typically have enlarging head circumferences and dilatation of the lateral and third ventricles, but with a normal-appearing fourth ventricle. Gliosis of the aqueduct or forking, where the duct divides into blind-ending sacs, may cause the stenosis. Aqueductal webs, septa, or diaphragms may also obstruct the exit from the third ventricle. Aqueductal stenosis may be seen in neurofibromatosis (NF) type 1 and as a complication of inflammatory and neoplastic disorders (see following section).

CRASH syndrome refers to corpus callosum hypoplasia, retardation, adducted thumbs, spastic paraparesis, and hydrocephalus secondary to aqueductal stenosis. This is an X-linked disorder.

Sagittal MR is essential for distinguishing extrinsic mass compression from an intrinsic aqueductal abnormality (Fig. 8-4). Aqueductal stenosis may also be diagnosed on CSF flow imaging. The normal aqueductal signal in this case should be bright, signifying CSF flow. With aqueductal obstruction, a dark signal is seen on the

Box 8-2   Causes of Noncommunicating Hydrocephalus

Obstruction of lateral ventricles
  Colloid cyst
  Tumors
    Choroid plexus papilloma (children)
    Ependymoma
    Meningioma
    Neurocytoma
    Other
    Subependymal giant cell astrocytoma
Obstruction of 3rd ventricle
  Aqueductal webs, fenestrations, diaphragms
  Congenital aqueductal stenosis (autosomal recessive)
  Tumors
    Craniopharyngiomas
    Ependymomas
    Hypothalamic gliomas
    Pineal neoplasms
    Vein of Galen aneurysm
Obstruction of 4th ventricle
  Tumors
    Astrocytomas
    Choroid plexus papillomas (adults)
    Ependymomas
    Medulloblastoma (PNET)
Obstruction of any site
  Arachnoid cysts
  Complications of hemorrhage, infection, synechiae
  Cysticercosis
  Hematomas
  Meningiomas
  Other tumors with mass effect

PNET, Primitive neuroectodermal tumors.

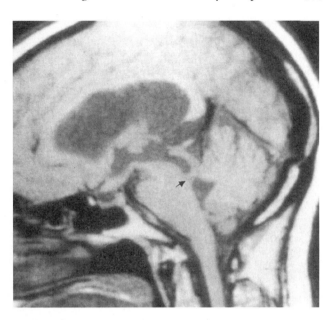

Fig. 8-4   Aqueductal web. Sagittal T1WI shows a web *(arrow)* along the inferior aspect of the aqueduct, causing hydrocephalus.

flow scan (Fig. 8-5). Phase contrast MR with a velocity encoding set to 10–15 ml/sec may be the best way to assess aqueductal patency. Interstitial edema, bright on a FLAIR scan, will also be present in the periventricular zone.

Clots or synechiae   Other intrinsic causes of aqueductal obstruction include clots or synechiae resulting from trauma or chronic infection. Patients with a large amount of subarachnoid hemorrhage may demonstrate obstruction caused by clot formation in the aqueduct or in the foramina of the fourth ventricle. Synechiae may be due to fibrous adhesions of the third ventricle after ventriculitis or meningitis. A rare infectious cause of aqueductal obstruction is cysticercosis.

Masses or tumors   Masses of the pineal gland are the most common causes of extrinsic obstruction of the aqueduct. These generally compress the aqueduct from posteriorly and cause dilatation of the lateral and third ventricular system. Tectal gliomas also obstruct the aque-

duct early in their course (Fig. 8-6). Occult cerebrovascular malformations may occur there as well. The base of the aqueduct may be obstructed by tumors of the posterior fossa such as medulloblastomas (PNETs) or ependymomas. In a child, a vein of Galen "aneurysm" (a true arteriovenous malformation or fistula) could compress the aqueduct. This is controversial because some investigators believe that veins cannot significantly compress structures such as this. Furthermore, the hydrocephalus associated with vein of Galen malformations may be the result of venous hypertension rather than aqueductal obstruction.

Any of the pediatric and adult posterior fossa tumors may obstruct the fourth ventricle and/or lower portion of the aqueduct. Ependymomas are one of the classic intraventricular tumors to infiltrate the foramina of Magendie and Luschka and may cause hydrocephalus from outflow obstruction. Cerebellar astrocytomas, medulloblastomas, or hemangioblastomas may compress the fourth ventricle extrinsically.

Intraventricular tumors besides choroid plexus papillomas and ependymomas may obstruct parts of the ventricular system. The masses that can arise intraventricularly include meningiomas, neurocytomas, astrocytomas, choroid plexus papillomas, oligodendrogliomas, subependymal giant cell tumors, arachnoid ependymal cysts, craniopharyngiomas, and dermoids.

Hematomas and infarcts   A well-placed hematoma can compress the ventricles and lead to occlusion at the foramen of Monro, aqueduct, or fourth ventricle. We have seen this in the settings of trauma, acute subdural and/or epidural posterior fossa hematomas, and with hy-

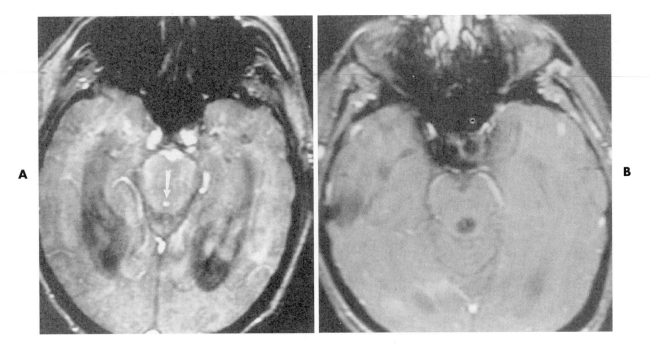

Fig. 8-5 Aqueductal gradient echo study. **A,** Axial gradient echo scan with gradient moment nulling applied shows high signal intensity within the aqueduct *(arrow)*, representing patent flow. A potential pitfall in this diagnosis would be a high signal intensity thrombus simulating flow. **B,** Aqueductal obstruction caused by an occult cerebrovascular malformation shows absence of the high signal intensity of flow within the aqueduct.

pertensive bleeds. Posterior fossa strokes are notorious for bringing about the downfall of the patient by eliciting acute hydrocephalus as the fourth ventricle is compressed and obliterated by mass effect.

Trapped ventricles So called "trapping of the temporal horn" may occur when the egress of CSF from this

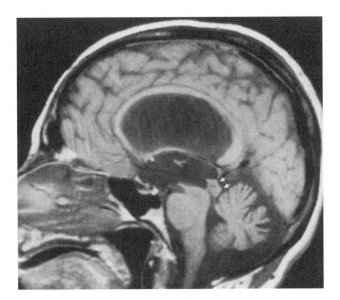

Fig. 8-6 Tectal glioma. A mass in the quadrigeminal plate of the tectum *(arrows)* occludes the aqueduct and causes hydrocephalus seen as bowing of the corpus callosum and dilatation of the third ventricle's anterior recesses.

anteroinferior extension of the lateral ventricle is obstructed. This usually occurs because of a blockage at the atrium, either from intrinsic or extrinsic masses.

Selective enlargement of the third ventricle can be confusing. This must be distinguished from the presence of an ependymal/arachnoid cyst and third ventricle squamopapillary craniopharyngiomas. Trapping of the third ventricle is uncommon.

Isolation of the fourth ventricle may occur when the aqueduct of Sylvius, foramina of Magendie, and Luschka are occluded. The fourth becomes "trapped" and will expand as CSF production by the choroid plexus continues unabated (Fig. 8-7). This expansion may compress the cerebellum and brain stem and lead to posterior fossa symptoms.

Now we have given you all the necessary trappings—for this book.

Communicating Hydrocephalus

Infection, hemorrhage, tumors The arachnoid villi are sensitive, delicate structures that may get gummed up by insults of several causes, resulting in communicating hydrocephalus (Box 8-3). Think of them as the little fenestrations in your bathtub drain: the whole tub will overflow if these tiny conduits are obstructed (usually by hair from members of the more hirsute sex). The most common causes of obstruction include infectious meningitis, ventriculitis, ependymitis, subarachnoid hemorrhage, and car-

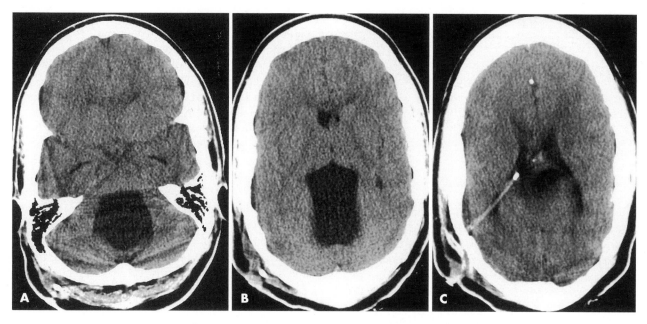

Fig 8-7   Trapped fourth ventricle. **A,** The fourth ventricle is markedly enlarged with effacement of cerebellar sulci. Note however how small the temporal horns and frontal horns are. **B,** A more superior cut shows the ballooning upward of the fourth. Did you catch the edge of the skull film finding? **C,** Yes there was a shunt present that decompressed the ventricles above, but the aqueductal obstruction coupled with Magendie and Luschka outflow occlusion trapped the fourth.

cinomatous meningitis. As the CSF becomes more viscous with a higher protein concentration, the arachnoid villi lose their ability to reabsorb the fluid. This causes hydrocephalus with dilatation of the ventricular system.

Box 8-3   Causes of Communicating Hydrocephalus

Obstruction of arachnoid villi
  Carcinomatous meningitis
  Chemical meningitis (fat, arachnoiditis, intrathecal
    medications)
  Hemorrhage
    Subarachnoid hemorrhage from aneurysm
    Traumatic intraventricular, subarachnoid hemorrhage
  High-protein level in tumors (acoustic schwannomas)
  Increased venous pressure from AV shunt,
    vein of Galen malformation
  Infectious meningitis
  Mucopolysarcoidosis
  Noninfectious inflammatory (sarcoidosis)
  Venous thrombosis
Obstruction at skull base
  Achondroplasia
  Chiari II, III
  Dandy Walker
Unknown cause
  External hydrocephalus
  Normal-pressure hydrocephalus

Do not let a normal appearance to the fourth ventricle dissuade you from considering communicating hydrocephalus or obstruction distal to the fourth ventricle. The fourth ventricle is the last ventricle to dilate, possibly because of its relatively confined location in the posterior fossa, surrounded as it is by the thick calvarium and sturdy petrous bones. Thus, it is not uncommon to see dilated lateral and third ventricles but a normal-sized fourth ventricle and have communicating hydrocephalus. Still the most sensitive indicator will be the enlargement of the temporal horns and/or anterior recesses of the third ventricle—without that you probably do not have hydrocephalus. The hunt for a source of the ventricular dilatation should not stop at the aqueductal level with this pattern.

As with any cause of hydrocephalus, there may be periventricular high signal intensity on MR, very nicely demonstrated with FLAIR scanning. This is due to transependymal CSF migration into the adjacent white matter leading to interstitial edema (dark on DWI). This is most commonly seen at the angles of the lateral ventricles and, because of its smooth and diffuse nature, can usually be distinguished from the focal periventricular white matter abnormalities associated with atherosclerotic small vessel ischemic disease. Be aware that there may normally be mild high intensity at the angles of the ventricle (ependymitis granulosa) in middle-aged patients.

Normal-pressure hydrocephalus Normal-pressure hydrocephalus (NPH) has a classic triad of clinical findings; the recent onset of gait apraxia, dementia, and urinary incontinence (Box 8-4). We like to think of NPH as a treatable cause of a nontraumatic DAI (dementia, ataxia, and incontinence). Although NPH was initially described as being idiopathic, patients with a remote (cryptic) history of infection or hemorrhage are still lumped into this category when they have the clinical triad. This probably accounts for 50% of NPH cases. The patients have enlarged ventricles from communicating hydrocephalus with particular enlargement of the temporal horns. They may show evidence of transependymal CSF leakage on MR or CT. MR often shows accentuation of the cerebral aqueduct flow void (Fig. 8-8). These patients may respond to shunting procedures with amelioration of their clinical symptoms. The most accurate predictors of a positive response to shunting are (1) absence of central atrophy or ischemia, (2) gait apraxia as the dominant clinical symptom, (3) upward bowing of the corpus callosum with flattened gyri and ballooned third ventricular recesses, (4) prominent CSF flow void, and (5) a known history of intracranial infection or bleeding (nonidiopathic NPH). It is important to entertain this diagnosis because there is a chance at the possibility of return of function with a shunt. The alternative is to consign the patient to a lifetime of dementia based on inexplicable atrophy. Make their day—shunt these patients—and the neurosurgeons will like you too.

In patients with suspected NPH, an indium 111-DTPA (diethylenepentaacetic acid) study is sometimes ordered. The agent is instilled in the CSF through a lumbar puncture. Normally, the tracer is resorbed over the convexities without ventricular reflux within 2 to 24 hours. In cases of communicating hydrocephalus and NPH, reflux of the tracer into the ventricles is seen with lack of tracer accumulation over the convexities 24 to 48 hours after instillation (Fig. 8-9). Patients who demonstrate this scintigraphic appearance allegedly have a better response to shunting than patients with normal or equivocal indium findings.

The rate of clinical improvement after shunting of patients with NPH is still only 50%. Prominence of the CSF flow void in patients with this condition has led some investigators to use phase contrast MR techniques to measure the flow through the cerebral aqueduct. A

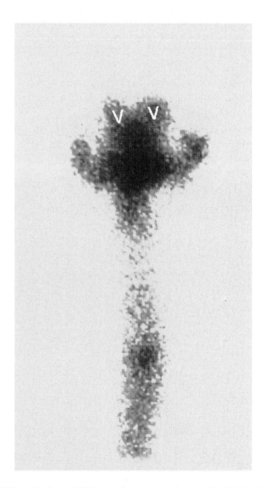

Fig. 8-9   Indium-DTPA study in a patient with NPH. Coronal indium-labeled study shows lack of ascension of the radiotracer over the convexities with reflux of the tracer into the lateral ventricles (V). This study was taken 48 hours after intrathecal tracer insertion.

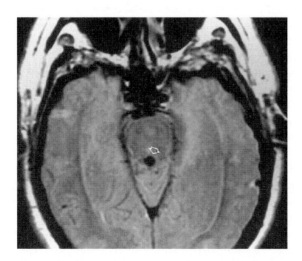

Fig. 8-8   NPH with accentuation of aqueductal flow void. Note the very low signal intensity of the aqueduct (open arrow) due to accelerated flow on this PDWI.

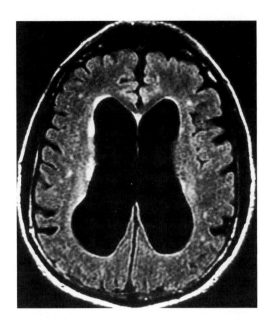

Fig. 8-10   Normal pressure hydrocephalus. Ventricular enlargement out of proportion to sulcal dilatation without an obstructing lesion is the *sine qua non* of NPH. Minimal periventricular high signal on this FLAIR scan is of limited differentiating value as in this age group small vessel ischemic changes abound.

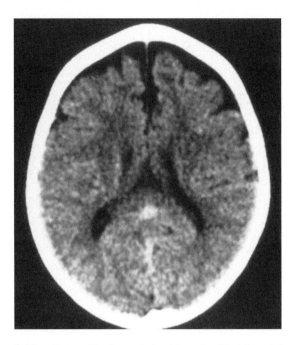

Fig. 8-11   External hydrocephalus. Note the dilatation of the interhemispheric fissure and the frontal cortical sulci in this infant with external hydrocephalus. Often the ventricles are not dilated.

stroke volume of greater than 42 μL was predictive of better response to shunting. The specific parameters inherent in this measurement are related to scanner field strength and pulse sequences, so they are not necessarily transferrable to your own scanner, but the point made is that greater flow through the aqueduct means a better chance for shunt improvement. The rationale for this is that the brain is pushed centrifugally in NPH from enlarged ventricles (Fig. 8-10). As systole occurs, the blood being pumped into the closed space of the cranium forces CSF out of the lateral ventricles and into the aqueduct. Expansion of the lateral ventricles leads to shearing strains on the white matter and clinical symptoms.

External hydrocephalus   Another benign cause of hydrocephalus from arachnoid villi malfunction is "external hydrocephalus," also referred to as "benign enlargement of the subarachnoid spaces in infants," "benign extra-axial collections of infancy," "extraventricular obstructive hydrocephalus," "benign subdural effusions of infancy," and "benign macrocephaly of infancy." This may be due to immaturity of the arachnoid villi with a decreased capacity to absorb CSF. External hydrocephalus is typically seen in children less than 2 years old who have a rapidly enlarging head circumference, going off the scale on the pediatrician's graph. Neurologically, the bigheaded kids are as normal as these bigheaded authors—but what does that tell you? Prematurity (immaturity), a history of intraventricular hemorrhage, and some genetic syndromes predispose to external hydrocephalus and co-authorship. CT or MR shows dilatation of the CSF spaces over the frontal lobes and along the interhemispheric fissure but with relatively normal-sized ventricles (Fig. 8-11). The disorder usually resolves by the time the child is 3 to 4 years old and the head circumference returns to normal. The ventricles are usually normal in size (64% of cases); thus the term *external hydrocephalus;* it is the CSF spaces external to the ventricles that are dilated. Why do the ventricles fail to dilate? Presumably because the cranial sutures are open, so the head enlarges instead. The differential diagnosis includes chronic subdural hygromas and atrophy caused by previous injury. When one sees sulcal dilatation and vessels coursing through the CSF collection, chronic subdural hygromas are much less likely (see Fig. 6-1). Atrophy is not usually associated with an enlarged head circumference.

The Almighty Failed Shunt

Shunt failure accounts for a large number of unenhanced CT scans in pediatric neuroradiology and ruins the evening plans of many a pediatric neurosurgeon. The typical scenario is a child with a ventriculoperitoneal shunt in place who presents with nausea, vomiting, and a fever. Now you and me, we've got the flu. A child with a shunt—it could be due to shunt failure. This occurs in 30% of individuals in their first year with a shunt and in 50% of subjects within the first 6 years after shunt placement. Shunt infection occurs at a rate of about 10% in the first year. Hence, the unenhanced CT scan and the desperate search through the film vaults for the dusty old comparison EMI films (often never to be found). On the other hand, if you are a modern radiologist you will query the PACS system for the old study and find nothing but a network hiccup.

First and foremost, compare ventricular size, stressing changes in temporal horn and third ventricular size over the rest. Next, contemplate the principal mechanisms responsible for shunt failure; (1) obstruction of the catheter end in the ventricular system, (2) malfunction of the valve, (3) kinks in the tubing, (4) obstruction at the peritoneal or atrial end, and (5) component disconnection. The valves come in a variety of pressure settings for various resistances. Shuntograms in which 2 to 3 cc of nonionic contrast are injected into the shunt reservoir may be revealing. Normally, the contrast clears from the shunt tube within 3 to 10 minutes. In adults, it may take 10 to 15 minutes to clear.

The first step in the evaluation is withdrawing CSF from the shunt valve. If CSF cannot be withdrawn the ventricular catheter is obstructed or the valve is faulty. If contrast refluxes from valve to ventricle the valve is faulty as this is supposed to be a one-way valve to prevent "dreck" from the peritoneal cavity flowing backwards to the ventricles. If the contrast does not flow freely out but after pumping the valve it seems to work, there is probably incomplete obstruction of the shunt system and/or a malfunctioning valve-pressure system. If there is no spillage intraperitoneally even after pumping the valve, or if what spills gets loculated, clearly, there is a problem with the peritoneal end of the shunt system. Ventricular catheter obstruction, valve malfunction, and distal obstruction are the most commonly seen phenomena.

Third ventriculostomies, where a small hole is made that allows communication between the floor of the third ventricle and the suprasellar cistern, has proven to be effective in relieving hydrocephalus. This is most useful for those obstructions distal to the third ventricle as it bypasses the obstructed region. These are often placed through the use of a fiberoptic endoscope and/or 3D reconstructions with image-guided navigation. Expect the reduction in ventricular size to appear within a couple of weeks of the procedure—not as rapidly as with lateral ventricular shunts. Flow through the third ventriculostomy may be visualized with phase contrast flow studies at a velocity encoded at 5 cc/min.

Slit ventricle syndrome Sometimes shunted patients are symptomatic but have tiny ventricles. These are usually patients who have had long-term shunt problems. The thought here is that the ventricles and/or brain loses their compliance and cannot expand despite the fact that they are under high pressure. This is probably due to the decreased compliance in the lateral ventricular walls owing to fibrosis in chronically shunted patients. Alternatively, they may be small owing to marked reduc-

tion in the pressure because of chronic overdrainage or leakage. The calvarium will thicken due to the overdrainage of the CSF. Then, if the cranial sutures close early, the brain has nowhere to go as it grows, being confined by the calvarium. This in turn leads to small ventricles and no capacity to accommodate normal variations in intracranial pressure. In this way, you can have small ventricles yet high pressure. The flow out the shunt will be limited.

Pseudotumor Cerebri

Pseudotumor cerebri, or idiopathic benign intracranial hypertension or idiopathic intracranial hypertension, is appropriately included in a chapter on atrophy and hydrocephalus because it is also a disease of abnormal CSF mechanics. The abnormality may be due to decreased absorption of CSF at the arachnoid villi, increased water content in the brain, or increased resistance to drainage because of venous obstruction. Patients with this disorder are typically obese (95% of patients), black (62%), young or middle-aged women. They have frequent headaches, cranial nerve VI palsies, papilledema, or visual field deficits on examination. The disease may occur in association with pregnancy, endocrine abnormalities, medications, or intracranial venoocclusive disease. One should exclude a dural venous malformation or venous thrombosis as potential causes for the elevated pressure. On physical examination, the patients may have other signs of increased intracranial pressure. The lumbar puncture (LP) demonstrates extreme elevations of CSF pressure (up to 600 mm Hg). This LP is often performed under fluoroscopy (and duress) by the neuroradiology fellow as he calls for a 7 cm harpoon and a shield to prevent the CSF geyser from "facing" him. It is still better than being a colonoscopist!

The ventricles are either normal in size or slightly small. The cerebral subarachnoid space volume is larger in patients with pseudotumor cerebri compared with age-matched control subjects. Most MR studies in patients with pseudotumor cerebri are normal, but calculated measurements of white matter intensity on T2WI may show subtle increases over normal control subjects. The venous sinuses and veins may be small and may enlarge after spinal fluid drainage. If an orbital study is performed, reverse cupping of the optic disk corresponding to the papilledema may be noted, and this finding correlates well with the degree of vision loss. The optic nerve sheath complex is also enlarged and more tortuous in pseudotumor cerebri. The posterior sclera may be flattened as well. The patients have a higher rate of expanded, empty sellas (greater than the 30% rate of partially empty sellas seen in the normal population). Treatment consists of repetitive LP to drain CSF (performed by the same unfortunate fellow), but often the disease remits spontaneously. Occasionally, CSF shunting or lumbar drain placement is required for those patients with intractable headaches and visual impairment. Diuretics and carbonic anhydrase inhibitors may reduce CSF pressures as well. The prognosis is generally good when the disorder is treated expediently.

Migraines As pseudotumor cerebri often presents with severe headache, this is an appropriate time to write a few words about migraines. One of the authors has published contradictory articles as to whether or not there are "UBOs" associated with migraines so he has recused himself from this discussion. Suffice it to say that the smarter of the two authors believes that punctate white matter high intensity foci do occur in migraineurs, usually in the subcortical white matter (though this migraineur author has one in the anterior limb of his internal capsule). They do not arise in the periventricular zones and hence should not be confused with multiple sclerosis. Remember that migraines are vascular in etiology—usually due to hypersensitivity of meningeal vessels.

A transient enhancement of the cisternal segment of the third nerve has also been reported in patients with ophthalmoplegic migraines.

ATROPHY

As the authors grow older and not much wiser, the issues of atrophy become more pressing.

Cerebral Atrophy

The disorders that demonstrate gross supratentorial atrophy are often associated with dementia (Table 8-2).

Alzheimer disease Of the disorders in Table 8-2, Alzheimer disease (dementia Alzheimer type, or DAT) is one of the most notorious and common, accounting for 60% to 90% of the dementing disorders with progressive memory loss. DAT affects 2 to 4 million Americans and 8% of the population older than 65 and 30% of those over 85 years old. Women are more commonly affected by a 2:1 margin. With DAT, life can be fascinating or petrifying, because memory is severely affected. Although some of us would love to erase some bad memories in life, this is not the way to do it! DAT usually occurs in the late middle-aged adult, with the major dysfunction noted in memory, personality, and thought. Olfaction is one of the first senses to show some effects of the disease, but this is rarely tested. The patient's social skills, personality, and speech pattern are also affected early. Depression often coexists. Late in the course the patient becomes severely impaired, myoclonic, vegetative, and weak. Current treatment consists of antioxidants, vitamin E, and cholinesterase inhibitors, but the results are not uniformly positive. Rest assured that hundreds of bril-

liant minds sponsored by the National Institutes of Health are working furiously on ways to prevent or treat DAT so there is still hope for those of our readers of residency and fellowship age. For those older, what are you doing reading our book anyway! With the numbers of persons projected to have this disease as the population ages, a breakthrough is critical or else the national health care system will implode from the cost of caring for them.

Senile plaques, seen as amorphous material in the cerebral cortex, and neurofibrillary tangles in the nerve cells in the form of tangled loops of cytoplasmic fibers, are the diagnostic pathologic features of DAT. Disease progression from the entorhinal cortex to the hippocampus to the neo cortex is the rule. Curiously, these same pathologic findings are seen in adult patients with Down syndrome, Parkinson disease, and "punch-drunk" fighters.

The main finding on CT and MR scanning of DAT is diffuse cortical atrophy, often more prominent in the temporal lobes. Temporal horn dilatation more than 3 mm in diameter is seen in more than 65% of patients with DAT. Increases in ventricular size, sulcal size, sylvian fissure size, and total CSF volume are noted in patients with DAT compared with age-matched control subjects. On longitudinal studies, the rate of atrophic change in patients with DAT is much faster than in normal persons. Atrophy (and entropy) increases over time. The subiculum of the parahippocampal region appears to be most severely affected in DAT.

One study found that the measure with the best sensitivity in discriminating DAT patients from control subjects was the width of the temporal horn. If one combines the measure of width of the temporal horn, width of the choroid fissure, height of the hippocampus, and the interuncal distance into a compound factor one can discriminate patients with mild DAT from control subjects with 86% sensitivity. There may, in fact be a continuum of progressive hippocampal atrophy between normal elderly, those with mild cognitive impairment (MCI) and DAT. The substantia innominata, located between the globus pallidus and the anterior perforated substance is also thinned in patients with Alzheimer disease.

Even more selective studies have shown hippocampal-parahippocampal atrophy in DAT patients, causing dilatation of the choroidal-hippocampal fissure complex and temporal horns of the lateral ventricle (Fig. 8-12). The third ventricle also dilates. Other investigators have reported finding gyral bands of low intensity in the parietal lobes on T2WI, thought to represent lipofuscin deposition. The money spent on DAT research is enormous, but the radiographic features are nonspecific and imaging studies are not the primary diagnostic test. Usually one is attempting to exclude treatable conditions with the im-

Table 8-2   Neurodegenerative causes of atrophy

Entity	Distinguishing imaging findings	MRS features	Distinguishing clinical findings
Alzheimer's disease	Temporal lobe predominance Increased hippocampal-choroidal fissure size Hippocampal and amygdala atrophy, global atrophy	Decreased NAA Increased mI, increased phosphomonoester	Severe memory loss Speech and olfaction affected early No early myoclonus or gait disturbance Course in years
Frontotemporal dementia	Semantic variant has temporal lobe atrophy including polar regions and parahippocampal regions, hemispheric asymmetry Frontal variant has anterior temporal and frontal atrophy, hemispheric asymmetry Progressive nonfluent aphasia variant has perisylvian and insular atrophy especially of superior temporal gyrus	No data on proton MRS—at least not that we can remember	Semantic: Speech issues in naming, word comprehension, and personality disorders Age of onset, inheritance Frontal variant has greater personality disorder Progressive nonfluent aphasia has word finding difficulties and less cognitive deficit
Pick's disease	Severe frontal and mild temporal lobe predominance Caudate atrophy, sparing of parietal cortex	Increased PME, PDE NKY	Cognition, personality severely affected Abulia and apathy
Creutzfedt-Jakob disease	Frontal predominance Abnormal intensity basal ganglia and thalami	Normal early, late reduction in NAA and increased mI (in hamsters)	Transmission of prion Rigidity Myoclonus Course in months
Parkinson's disease	Substantia nigra decreased in size Basal ganglia intensity changes	Normal spectrum or decreased NAA and elevated lactate in demented patients	Rigidity, bradykinesia, tremor
Multisystem atrophy	Variants include olivopontocerebellar degeneration with olive, pons, cerebellar and putaminal atrophy, striatonigral degeneration with smaller midbrain	NKY	Parkinsonism, autonomic dysfunction, cerebellar gait disorders
Progressive supranuclear palsy	Midbrain, collicular atrophy, periaqueductal abnormal signal, increased putaminal iron	Decreased NAA/Cr	Ophthalmoplegia, pseudobulbar palsy, rigidity
Cortical-basal ganglionic degeneration	Atrophy of the paracentral structures, superior parietal lobule knife blade atrophy, dilated central sulcus asymmetry characteristic	NKY	Rigidity of limbs, alien limb phenomenon, personality disorders, myoclonus
Lewy body dementia	Brainstem, substantia nigra cortical atrophy	NKY	Visual difficulties, hallucinations, early symptoms

Table continued on following page

Table 8-2   Neurodegenerative causes of atrophy (*Continued*)

Entity	Distinguishing imaging findings	MRS features	Distinguishing clinical findings
AIDS	Atrophy	Decreased NAA/Cho	Young age
	High intensity in basal ganglia	Decreased NAA/Cr	Risk factors
	Superimposed infection PML, and lymphoma	Increased Cho/Cr	Positive HIV
		Increased mI/Cr	
		All P levels lower	
Multi-infarct dementia	White matter and deep gray lacunae	Decreased NAA	Stuttering course with discrete events
	Stokes of different ages		Stroke risk factors
	Central pontine infarcts		Early gait disturbance
Amyotrophic lateral sclerosis (ALS)	Hypointensity motor cortex (T2WI)	Decreased NAA/Cr	Weakness
	Hyperintensity in cortical spinal tract (T2WI)	Decreased NAA/Cho	Atrophy
		Decrease PCr/Pi	Spasticity
	Anterior horn cell atrophy		Preserved cognition

NAA, N-acetyl aspartate

Cho, Choline

CR, Creatine

P, Phosphorous

mI, Myo-inositol

NKY, Not known yet

Pi, Inorganic phosphate

aging studies, such as anterior cranial fossa meningiomas or strokes.

There has been considerable investigation concerning the presence of deep white matter and periventricular white matter areas of high signal intensity on the T2WIs in patients with DAT. In the absence of cardiovascular risk factors, these white matter changes are not seen with a statistical significance in patients with DAT more than in normal age-matched patients. However, there is a nonstatistical trend toward more small foci of white matter abnormality in patients with clinically diagnosed probable DAT.

On MR spectroscopy reduced levels of *N*-acetyl aspartate (NAA) and increased levels of myoinositol characterize DAT. The NAA levels are significantly reduced in frontal, temporal, and occipital cortex of DAT patients, presumably due to neuronal loss. Being able to distinguish between normal aging and DAT with MRS runs at the mid 80% range; distinguishing between DAT and other dementias drops the accuracy to the mid 70% range. Myoinositol elevation has also been reported in AIDS-related dementia and Pick disease.

Positron emission tomographic scanning has demonstrated decreased oxygen utilization and decreased regional cerebral blood flow in frontal, parietal, and temporal lobes in patients with DAT. The findings are most striking in the posterior temporoparietal lobes. On single-photon emission computed tomography (SPECT)

brain studies, patients with DAT have reduced cerebral blood flow as measured by parietal-to-cerebellar and parietal-to-mean cortical activity. The severity of symptoms may correspond to the reduction in uptake of technetium hexa-methyl propylene amine oxime (HMPAO).

Recently, some investigators have used dynamic susceptibility contrast-enhanced MR perfusion imaging to try to duplicate the nuclear medicine flow studies and triplicate the patient's bill. Indeed, they have found that relative values of temporoparietal regional cerebral blood volume (as a percentage of cerebellar rCBV) were reduced by a factor of 20% bilaterally in the patients with DAT compared with normals. Using left and right temporoparietal rCBV as index measures, specificity was 96% and sensitivity was 95% in moderate DAT and 88% in mild DAT.

There is a dose-related association between apolipoprotein E-4 (APOE-4) allelic frequency on chromosome 19 and the development of DAT. One or more APOE-4 alleles occur in 66% of patients whereas they occur in only 27% of control subjects and two alleles produce the highest risk and more rapid disease progression (a tenfold increase in dementia). This risk is modulated by APOE allelle 2, which actually may confer protection. Recent studies have shown a decline in resting parietal, temporal, and prefrontal PET glucose metabolism in cognitively intact patients with APOE-4. It remains to be seen whether this, and/or an analogous fMRI study, may serve to be a predictor of development of DAT.

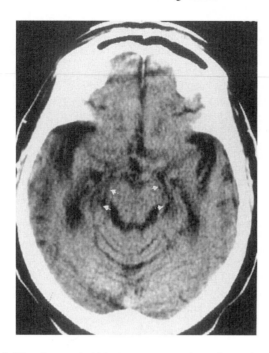

Fig. 8-12   Dementia Alzheimer type. Axial unenhanced CT scan shows dilatation of the choroidal-hippocampal fissure complex *(arrows)* with dilatation of the adjacent temporal horns caused by temporal lobe atrophy.

Other genes that are associated with DAT include amyloid precurson protein (APP) on chromosome 21, presenilin 1 on chromosome 1, and presenilin 2 on chromosome 14. These genes may code for malfunctioning secretases that lyse intracellular proteins in an inappropriate fashion. The abnormal secretases influence the development of the alpha and beta amyloid and amyloid precursor proteins, which are deposited in the brains of demented patients. In addition, the tau protein, which is excessively cross-linked and phosphorylated, may be the source of neurofibrillary tangles histopathologically. The theme that the dementing disorders may be due to abnormal protein processing has been advanced in recent publications. The misprocessed protein deposits in different locations, interferes with different neurons, and manifests different phenotypes for each disease. Tauopathies are commonly separated by the number of repeats of the microtubule-binding domain of the tau gene on chromosome 17. DAT, and Pick's disease have three repeats whereas progressive supranuclear palsy and cortical-basal ganglionic degeneration have four repeats. The characterization of the relationship of taugenetics and frontotemporal dementia remains inconclusive but is a source of research. Therapies of the future may be directed at inhibiting the bad (beta and gamma) secretases, augmenting the good (alpha) secretases, or clearing the bad proteins (beta amyloid) through vaccines or anti-inflammatory agents.

Frontotemporal dementia (FTD)   The term "frontotemporal dementia" is used to classify patients with fo-

cal cortical atrophy affecting the frontal and/or temporal lobes. The FTDs are usually separated into 3 varieties: (1) the frontal variant (dementia of frontal type) (40%), (2) semantic dementia (40%), and (3) progressive nonfluent aphasia (20%). Each of these variants may be associated with motor neuron disease (i.e. amyotrophic lateral sclerosis). Clinically, patients with FTD have peculiar behaviors (hyperorality, hypersexuality, lack of personal awareness, apathy, and perseverations) with personality shifts, inappropriate social conduct, and psychiatric overtones. This entity is thought to represent a constellation of diseases that lead to widespread cortical atrophy. Some people include Pick disease in this category. The differentiation with DAT is difficult, however, in general the frontal and anterior temporal lobes are more atrophic in frontal variant FTD than in DAT. Technetium HMPAO SPECT scans will show hypoperfusion (and hypometabolism) in the ventromedial frontal lobes with frontal variant FTD. DAT shows reduced temporoparietal activity.

Semantic dementia (temporal lobe variant FTD) shows difficulties with naming, word comprehension, object recognition, semantic relatedness of objects, and interrelations between words and meanings. Like, you know, whatchamacallits and their dooflinguses. The working vocabulary of the patient keeps shrinking to simple terms—kind of the way we've written this book—for our FTD readers. Syntax, executive functioning, and phonology is spared. Short-term memory is usually intact—longer term memory is affected worse in a pattern opposite that of DAT. The technetium SPECT scans show hypoperfusion of one or both temporal lobes. Temporal lobe atrophy is more dramatic with semantic FTD than with frontal variant FTD. The temporal pole and inferolateral gyri (including the parahippocampal gyri) are more affected than the hippocampi, marking a distinction from DAT. The left temporal lobe is more often affected than the right with hemispheric asymmetry not unusual.

Progressive nonfluent aphasia is the least well understood variant of FTD. In nonfluent progressive aphasia one sees cognitive diminution over a period of years with word finding difficulties leading over time to mutism. Phonologic competence is impaired. Behaviorial changes (as in frontal variant FTD) are less prominent. Atrophy is seen in a perisylvian location rather than the hippocampal region. "Knife blade shaped gyri" (knife blade atrophy) are described in the anterior aspect of the superior temporal gyrus with a widened sylvian fissure and insular atrophy. This seems, histopathologically, to represent a disease that combines features of Pick disease and Alzheimer disease.

The tau protein has been implicated in the frontotemporal dementias and studies as to the role of the tau gene in this subset of demented patients are ongoing.

Pick disease Pick disease is another cause of cerebral atrophy manifested by memory loss, confusion, cognitive and speech dysfunction, apathy, and abulia. In some classifications this is included in frontotemporal dementias, frontal variant. As in DAT, there is an anterior temporal lobe predominance to the atrophy; however, inferior frontal lobe changes are also present, sometimes focally (Fig. 8-13). The posterior cortex and parietal lobe (as opposed to cortical basal ganglionic degeneration described below) in general is spared. Pathologically, there is severe atrophy of the anterior frontal and temporal lobes with swollen nerve cells and spherical intracytoplasmic inclusions (Pick bodies). Pick bodies may represent the abnormally synthesized protein in this dementing disorder. Some studies have shown concomitant caudate atrophy. No treatment is available, and so the patient's cognition spirals downward within months to years. Fortunately, Pick disease is uncommon.

Pick syndrome, bilateral temporal lobectomies, and herpes encephalitis can cause Kluver-Bucy syndrome—the association of psychic blindness, oral infatuation, increased appetite, placidity, and heightened sexual activity (sounds like Bob's son, a typical college student). The common denominator appears to be decreased flow or atrophy to the temporal lobes.

Creutzfeldt-Jakob disease Creutzfeldt-Jakob disease (CJD) is a rare dementing disorder that often affects a younger population than DAT. It is thought to be due to a prion (a small proteinaceous infectious agent devoid of DNA and RNA) and is related to diseases that occur in New Guinea; when seen in brain-eating cannibals the disease is called *kuru*, but it is called *scrapie* in New Guinea sheep. Prion diseases result from the conversion of the protein molecule PrP^C to PrP^{SC}. Scrapie in European sheep has been thought to be responsible for the spread to cattle in the form of bovine spongiform encephalopathy. CJD is a human disease that occurs as a rapidly progressive dementing disorder, usually in indi-

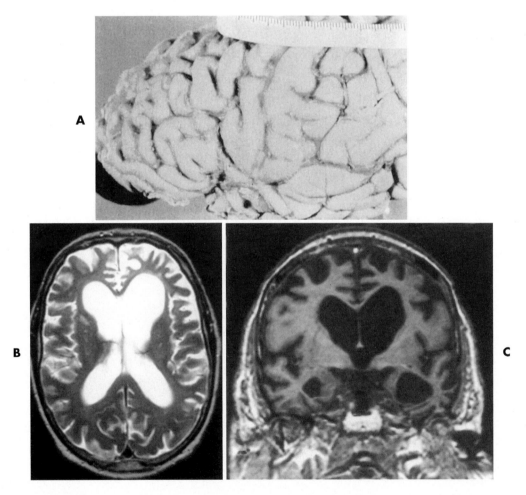

Fig. 8-13 Pick disease. **A,** Gross specimen from a volunteer with Pick disease demonstrates severe frontal lobe atrophy characteristic of the disease. This entity is sufficiently uncommon that even finding a case in a teaching file for publication is difficult. **B,** Axial T2WI is remarkable for the dilated subarachnoid space over the frontal lobes signifying atrophy. The frontal horns of the lateral ventricle enlarge to fill the void. The atrophy is striking in its frontal predominance (age 102 frontally, but age 48 occipitally by our guess). This is typical of Pick disease. **C,** The coronal T1WI again shows the striking frontal and anterior temporal atrophy. The patient was in his late 50s.

viduals in the seventh decade of life. CT studies may be normal (80%) or may show rapidly progressive atrophic changes (20%) in the brain. On MR, 80% of the cases are abnormal (GO MR! BLOW CT AWAY!)—with moderate to marked bilateral, symmetrical increased signal intensity in the putamen and caudate nuclei on long TR scans. With time, cerebral atrophy and symmetric high signal intensity foci in all of the basal ganglia, thalami, occipital cortex (the Heidenhain variant), and white matter may develop (Fig. 8-14). Diffusion weighted scans may be positive in the basal ganglia. Microscopically, the frontal and temporal lobes are most commonly affected, with neuronal loss, gliosis, and spongiform neuronal vacuolation. The lesson to be learned from this disease is to be polite but to forgo any dishes containing human brains when you travel in the Far East. Disease transmission to normal persons via corneal transplantation from affected patients has also been implicated. Fatal insomnia is another form of PrP gene dis-ZZZZZZ. Still another disease that may be related in part to CJD but manifesting with severe cerebellar dysfunction, is termed Gerstmann-Straussler-Scheinker disease.

Fludeoxyglucose F 18 and positron emission tomography may show marked cerebral hypometabolism corresponding to clinical deterioration in early CJD even when no parenchymal abnormalities are present on MR imaging.

Mad cow disease Mad cow disease (bovine spongiform encephalopathy) was first recognized in 1986 and is characterized by the cows being apprehensive, hyperesthetic, and uncoordinated (sounds like my wedding night). They develop mental status deterioration and are difficult to handle (sounds like my first year of marriage) and in some cases go into a frenzy (second year), hence the name "mad cow disease" (Maybe I married a cow, [sorry Honey! Anything for a laugh]). The brains of these cattle revealed spongiform encephalopathy. It was caused by feeding cattle with infected awful offal (animal tissue discarded by slaughterhouses), which contained the prions from sheep with scrapie. The transmission to humans led to new variant CJD. As opposed to CJD where one often sees bilateral globus pallidus and putaminal and caudate region hyperintensities on long TR sequences, with bovine spongiform encephalopathy the MR abnormalities are usually limited to bilateral thalamic pulvinar hyperintensity. New variant CJD (NvCJD) differs from CJD in that psychiatric and painful sensory symptoms are evident at presentation. EEG and CSF analysis for 14-3-3 protein is useful to assist in suggesting the diagnosis. The MR finding of bilateral high signal in the pulvinar and dorsal medial nucleus of the thalami has also been described in over 70% of pathologically proven cases. So add NvCJD to thalamic infarcts (artery of Percheron), venous thromboses, venous congestion, hemochromatosis, Wilson disease, lymphoma, astrocytoma, hemolytic uremia syndrome, encephalitis, osmotic demyelination, Tay-Sach disease, Sandhoff disease, and methanol poisoning to your list of bilateral thalamic lesions.

Parkinson disease Parkinson disease (PD) is characterized by progressive dementia, bradykinesia, shuffling gait, rigidity, and involuntary tremors. It is the disease that has reduced the most famous boxer of all time, Muhammed Ali, from "floating like a butterfly" to shuf-

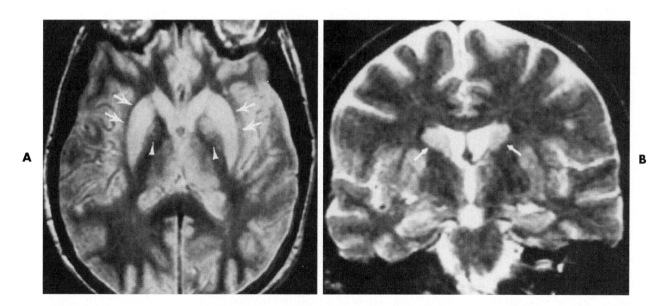

Fig. 8-14 Creutzfeldt-Jakob disease. **A,** Axial PDWI through the basal ganglia shows bilateral increased signal intensity to the putamina *(arrows)* and the globus pallidus *(arrowheads),* particularly on the left side. **B,** Coronal T2WI reveals abnormal intensity to the caudate nuclei bilaterally *(arrows)* and cortical sulcal enlargement throughout the brain. DWI scans are often positive, too.

fling like a man many years his senior. CT scans show nonspecific atrophy with enlarged ventricles and sulci. The lesion in PD has been localized to the dopaminergic cells of the pars compacta of the substantia nigra. Treatment consists of dopamine stimulation therapy (levodopa), bromocriptine, anticholinergics (benztropine), piperidyl compounds (trihexyphenidyl), and/or tricyclic antidepressants. Research into surgical implantation of fetal substantia nigra or stem cells has shown some promise (under Democratic presidential administrations) but remains experimental at this time.

Although no statistically significant differences in signal intensity or size of the substantia nigra's pars compacta have been identified on MR, a trend toward a decreased width of the pars compacta has been noted (Fig. 8-15). There is a lateral to medial gradient of loss of the normal signal of the pars compacta as well as volume loss in PD patients. The disease affects the lateral segment earliest and proceeds medially. On spectroscopy, one sees a diminution in NAA (what else?) and a significant increase in the ratio of lactate to NAA especially in those PD patients with dementia.

PD may be mediated by the Parkin and alpha synuclein genes. These genes are believed to be responsible for the accumulation of the pathologic protein (in the form of Lewy bodies seen histologically) in this disease. Catch the theme?

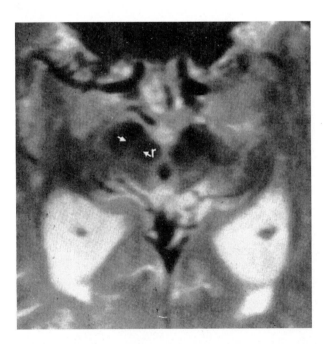

Fig. 8-15 Parkinson's disease. Note the relatively normal pars compacta (between *arrows*) on the right side, lying between the darker pars reticularis of the substantia nigra and the red nucleus (*r*). On the left side the width of the pars compacta is decreased. This patient had Parkinson's disease. (BH Braffman et al: MR imaging of Parkinson disease with spin echo and gradient-echo sequences, *AJNR,* 9, 1093-1099, 1988. copyright by *ASNR.*)

More and more neurosurgeons are employing image guidance for stereotactic pallidotomy for patients with PD and/or dystonia. The surgeons combine our ability to provide anatomic 3D guidance with microelectrode electrophysiologic recording to identify the ventral internal globus pallidus. Then they burn a 100 to 200 mm³ hole in the brain and when the smoke clears, voila, less rigidity and less bradykinesia. It is not uncommon to see hemorrhage and edema after this procedure, even extending into the optic tract or internal capsule (structures in proximity to the posterolateral internal globus pallidus), but this is usually asymptomatic when done right. Oh the wonders of modern science—and shish-kabob. The GPi (globus pallidus internus) can be targeted for barbecuing or for stimulator implantation and is usually found 2 to 3 mm anterior, 20 to 22 mm lateral, and 4 to 6 mm inferior to the midpoint of the line connecting the anterior commissure and posterior commissure (AC-PC line). However, with good quality phase sensitive inversion recovery sequences anatomic coordinates may be replaced with actual visualization of this structure. This is then corroborated intraoperatively by microelectrode identification of movement-related kinesthetic cell firing. This is scary business—the target is within 2 mm of the optic tract and the accuracy of MR guidance is quoted as being 0.3 mm +/− 1.35 mm. Two standard deviations away and—thank goodness for microelectrode guidance. Otherwise . . . Bzzzzzzz. Sorry. Field cut.

The subthalamic nucleus may also be targeted. It is found on coronal T2WI 15 to 17 mm posterior to the anterior commissure, 1.5 to 3 mm anterior to the red nucleus and just above and lateral to the pars reticulata of the substantia nigra. One can also find the subthalamic nucleus 4 mm posterior, 12 mm lateral, and 4 mm inferior to the midpoint of the AC-PC line. Chronic stimulation of the subthalamic nucleus can reduce parkinsonian movement disorders.

Still others are using the gamma knife radiosurgical technique to perform thalamotomies and pallidotomies for movement disorders. One should expect to see abnormal signal in the target (globus pallidus interna or ventralis intermedius thalamic nucleus). A ring-enhancing focus with vasogenic edema is typically seen at the 3-month mark after the radiosurgery, but therapeutic benefit usually begins at 1 month.

The Parkinson Plus syndromes include the entities of multisystem atrophy, progressive supranuclear palsy, cortical-basal ganglionic degeneration, and dementia with Lewy bodies. In each of these entities there is a movement disorder.

Dementia with Lewy bodies   Dementia with Lewy bodies is an entity probably related to Parkinson disease in which Lewy bodies are found not only in deep gray matter structures, but diffusely in the brain, including the cortex. While dementia may be primarily associated with Parkinson disease, the clinicians distinguish these entities based on the fact Parkinson disease dementia shows parkinsonism preceding the dementia by one year or more. Dementia preceding or accompanying parkinsonism is DLB (dementia with Lewy bodies). PD dementia is termed "subcortical" (psychomotor slowing, difficulty concentrating, impaired retrieval), but DLB is a cortical dementia (aphasia, anomia, apraxia, visuospatial problems, memory deficits). Histopathologically, they may look the same. Clinically patients with DLB show fluctuating cognitive impairment, visual hallucinations, and parkinsonism. DLB presents in older subjects than PD and accounts for 25% of dementing disorders. Cognitive deficits are usually in memory, attention, executive function, and visuospatial and visuoconstructional abilities. Brain stem and substantia nigra atrophy may be evident and only a greater degree of cortical atrophy distinguishes DLB from DLB—not (too subtle). SPECT scans show occipital hypoperfusion in DLB.

Multiple system atrophy (Shy-Drager disease, multisystem atrophy) Shy-Drager syndrome, olivopontocerebellar atrophy (described below), and striatonigral degeneration can be lumped into the disorder known as multisystem atrophy (MSA). MSA is associated with autonomic system dysfunction that presents in middle age and simulates PD (tremors, cogwheel rigidity, bradykinesia, and ataxia) in some aspects. MSA-striatonigral type displays more parkinsonian features (rigidity, bradykinesia, postural instability) and autonomic dysfunction (impotence, incontinence, orthostatic hypotension), whereas MSA-olivopontocerebellar atrophy type is char-

acterized by dominance of cerebellar dysfunction. Patients may have autonomic abnormalities of temperature regulation, sweat gland function, and maintenance of the blood pressure (orthostatic hypotension). Brain stem, putaminal, and cerebellar atrophy may be associated, and the posterolateral putamina may show iron-related decreased signal intensity on T2WI. T1 and T2 shortening may also be found in the cortex and globus pallidus. Neuromelanin may also account for some signal changes in the putamina. Often the symptoms do not respond to levo dopa. Dementia is usually not a prominent component of MSA.

The "hot cross buns" sign (Fig. 8-16) has recently been described in this disorder in which there is a cruciform linear area of high signal on T2WI in the pons with tiny round darker areas within the checkerboard of the cross. This is relatively specific for multisystem atrophy, though the cause of this finding has yet to be determined.

Progressive supranuclear palsy Progressive supranuclear palsy (PSP) (Steele-Richardson-Olszewski syndrome) resembles PD in its manifestations (rigidity, bradykinesia) but also expresses a severe supranuclear ophthalmoplegia (impaired downward gaze), gait disorder, dysarthria, postural instability and pseudobulbar palsy a few years after the onset of parkinsonian symptoms. Patients present with hyperextension of the neck and contracted facial muscles giving a "surprised look" to the face. PSP is another dementing disorder associated with personality changes of uncontrolled emotions, social withdrawal, and depression (sounds like what the two of us are going through the galleys on this book!). On CT and MR there are dilatation of the third ventricle, atrophy of the

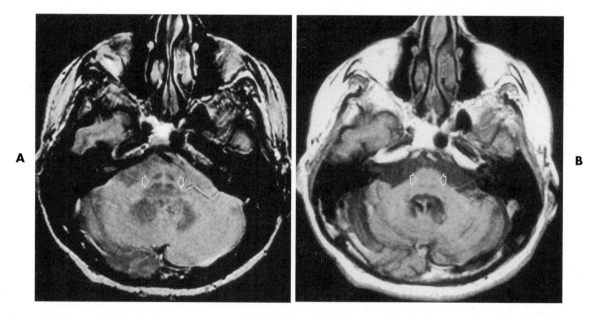

Fig. 8-16 Hot cross buns sign. Note the four areas of dark signal that make up the "hot cross buns sign" in the pontine region in this patient with multisystem atrophy. This term has been coined by Claudia Kirsch and associates and can be seen on PDWI **(A)**, T1WI **(B)**, or T2WI. (Case courtesy of Devang Gor, D. Sklar, and Claudia Kirsch, University of Medicine and Dentistry in New Jersey.)

midbrain, and enlargement of the interpeduncular cistern. MR may show decreased width of the pars compacta of the substantia nigra, atrophy of the superior colliculi, and high intensity to the periaqueductal gray matter. Increased iron may be found in the putamen so that it appears more hypointense than the globus pallidus on T2WI (the opposite of normal patients). This disorder, like cortical-basal ganglionic degeneration, frontotemporal dementia, and Pick's disease is a tauopathy with tau protein expressed histopathologically.

Cortical-basal ganglionic degeneration Cortical-basal ganglionic degeneration (CBGD) presents with postural instability, dystonia, akinesia, apraxia, myoclonus, bradykinesia, and limb rigidity. This disease demonstrates neuronal loss in substantia nigra, frontoparietal cortex, and striatum. MR will demonstrate symmetric or asymmetric thinning of pre- and post-central gyri with central sulcus dilatation. The superior parietal lobule and superior frontal gyrus seem to be at particular risk for volume loss (knife-blade atrophy) as well, whereas the

temporal and occipital lobes are less involved. Parasagittal involvement is prominent. These features clearly distinguish this dementing disorder from DAT or FTD. Atrophy of the basal ganglia may be subtle. Subcortical gliosis seen as high intensity on T2WI may be a clue to this diagnosis. One feature typical of CBGD is the asymmetry in the parasaggital and paracentral atrophy from one hemisphere to the next. This also is not a common feature of DAT, PD, MSA, DLB, or PSP. FTD does show asymmetry, but the anterior frontal and temporal lobe involvement is more distinctive.

AIDS dementia complex dementia The acquired immunodeficiency syndrome dementia complex (ADC) has become a more and more common source of dementia. Although the overall manifestations of AIDS are best described in the chapter on inflammation it is important to note that a young patient with cerebral atrophy and mild to marked white matter hyperintensity without mass effect may well have ADC (Fig. 8-17). One need not invoke other opportunistic infections or PML

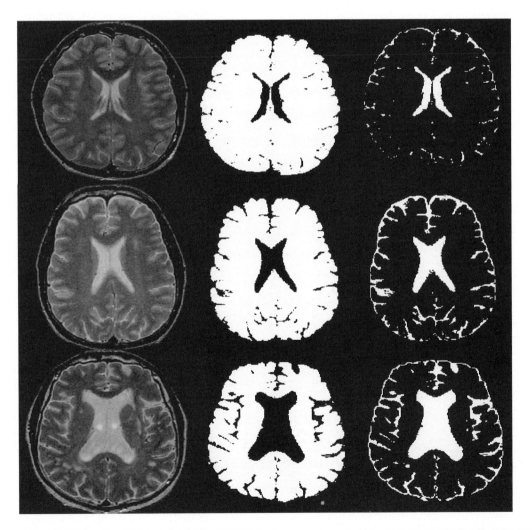

Fig. 8-17   Spectrum of HIV brain with top row normal T2WI, brain parenchymal segmentation, and CSF segmentation *(from left to right)*. Middle row is in asymptomatic HIV patient and lower row is in AIDS dementia complex. Observe how the CSF spaces increase and the parenchyma volume decreases.

in this population to account for the findings. MR spectroscopic imaging often reveals diffuse decreases in NAA and elevated choline in ADC. These spectroscopic findings may precede mental status deterioration and are present in children and adults with AIDS.

Myoinositol/creatine ratios may actually rise (similar findings to DAT). Once a superimposed CMV infection occurs, the patient may develop a more fulminant decline in mentation. The magnetization transfer ratios of HIV related white matter disease are higher than those of PML. As the viral load in HIV positive individuals increases the water diffusivity increases as well and the white matter anisotropy decreases. Protease inhibitors may cause reversal in the cognitive decline associated with HIV encephalopathy and may also result in the regression of periventricular white matter and basal ganglia signal intensity abnormalities. However, the MR imaging response to the "highly active antiretroviral therapy (HAART)," is often delayed compared with the clinical response. In fact, the MR findings may progress for the first 6 months before regressing or stabilizing with time. Basal ganglia and brain stem manifestations seem to respond to the greatest degree.

The vascular dementias Multiinfarct dementia (MID) is an entity seen in patients with long-standing hypertension and/or other risk factors for atherosclerotic disease. The patients are demented and manifest unusual personalities, pseudobulbar affect and/or palsies, incontinence (watch the BVDs with MID!), and ataxia. MID is characterized on imaging studies by multiple areas of white matter infarction accompanied by severe deep gray matter lacunar disease caused by atherosclerosis of deep penetrating arteries (Fig. 8-18). MID is characterized clinically by a progressive, episodic, stepwise downward course. There may be intervals of clinical stabilization or even limited recovery. Overall, cerebral blood flow is diminished. People have also called this disease Binswanger disease or subcortical arteriosclerotic encephalopathy, but some neurologists distinguish the stepwise gray and white matter disease (MID) from Binswanger (see Chapter 7), which they claim is slowly progressive and exclusively involves white matter. Try to envision the vascular dementias in terms of a continuum of multi-infarct dementia, deep gray infarcts and white matter disease, severe white matter disease only, Binswanger disease, and CADASIL (see below). Even if there really is a clinical difference between Binswanger disease and MID, pathophysiologically, the mechanism is the same—arteriolosclerosis. Lacunar infarcts and central pontine ischemic foci (in 61% of cases) may coexist. Histologically, one sees myelin and axonal loss, astrocytosis, and areas of infarction in deep white matter.

Cerebral autosomal dominant arteriopathy with subcortical infarcts and lekoencephalopathy (CADASIL), discussed in the white matter chapter, is another source of

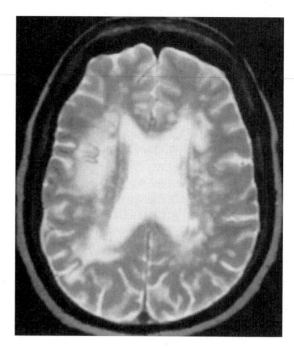

Fig. 8-18 Multiinfarct dementia. Multiple white matter ischemic foci and a right MCA cortical infarct can be found on T2WI in this demented patient with hypertension and diabetes.

vascular dementia. As you will recall, this disorder, linked to a gene on chromosome 19, presents with severe lacunar disease and subcortical white matter ischemic changes and reduced perfusion to affected areas. Clinically, the patients present with presenile dementia and migraine headaches in the third to fourth decade of life.

Subcortical ischemic vascular dementia shows lacunes and white matter infarctions. Cortical hypometabolism is present out of proportion to the degree of tissue loss, thought to be due to loss of connecting axons. Neuronal loss and laminar necrosis may be present on pathologic examination owing to retrograde effects. De-afferentation may occur from striatocapsular lacunar disease.

Amyotrophic lateral sclerosis Amyotrophic lateral sclerosis (ALS; also known as Lou Gehrig's disease) is a degenerative disease of upper motor neurons, generally manifested in the spine, but also affecting the full extent of the corticospinal tract. The disease causes relentless loss of motor strength in facial, limb, and diaphragmatic musculature with atrophy and hyperreflexia. Death usually occurs from pulmonary infections as airway competency and respiratory muscle integrity are lost. The most common finding seen on brain MR is high signal intensity of the corticospinal tract at the level of the internal capsules. Occasionally, one sees extension of the atrophy or wallerian degeneration along the full length of the corticospinal or bulbospinal tract into the brain stem, cerebral peduncles, internal capsule, corona radiata, and Betz cells of the cortex (Fig. 8-19). This is best

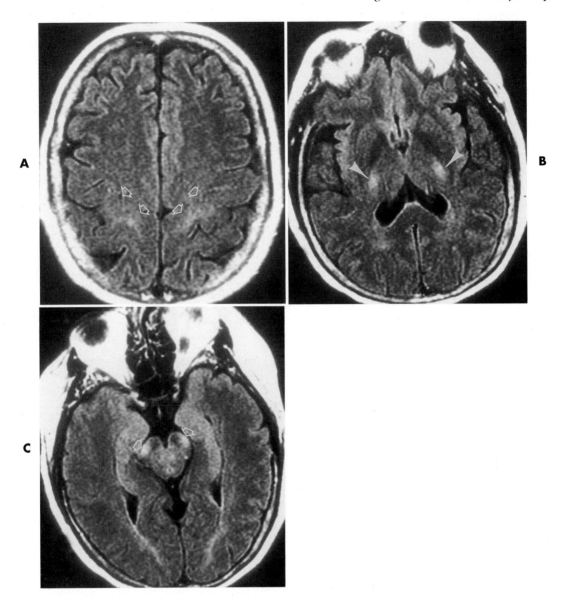

Fig. 8-19   ALS. Follow the high signal on these FLAIR scans from the white matter of the motor strip anterior to the central sulcus bilaterally *(arrows)* **(A)**, to the posterior limb of the internal capsule *(arrowheads)* **(B)**, to the cerebral peduncles *(arrows)* **(C)** in this patient with amyotrophic lateral sclerosis.

seen on coronal FLAIR scans. The more severe the MR findings the more rapid the progression and severe the disease. Sometimes, (around 40% to 60% of cases) the signal intensity of the precentral gyrus is decreased on T2WI, thought to be due to iron deposition. This finding correlates positively with disease severity, but is nonspecific, being seen in some normal controls as well. Atrophy of the anterior horn cell region of the spinal cord may be evident. This disease spares the patient from dementia, which may be more tragic because the patient is cognizant of the deadly downward course, which occurs over 3 to 6 years.

A recent spectroscopic study of the precentral gyrus region revealed a strong correlation between reductions in NAA and glutamate levels and increases in choline and myoinositol levels with increasing ALS disease severity.

Rett syndrome   Rett syndrome occurs in girls almost exclusively and is associated with atrophy. Despite apparent normal development in the first 6 to 18 months of life, there is deceleration of head growth from the second to fourth months of life (stage 1). Arrest in motor and cognitive development is followed by a period of behavioral regression with irritability and inability to communicate, and apraxia that is often mistaken for autism (stage 2). After 2 to 3 years of age, there is reduction in the irritability and improvement of the autistic-like features. Language skills do not recover, and the girls exhibit stereotyped behaviors, the most prominent of which is hand wringing or clapping. Recently, the disorder has been mapped to the Xq28 region. Frontotemporal regions and the caudate show reduced gray matter by volumetric MRI analyses.

Cerebrotendinous xanthomatosis Cerebrotendinous xanthomatosis is also associated with cerebral and cerebellar atrophy. There may be secondary effects of brain stem and corpus callosum atrophy. This is a rare autosomal recessive disorder affecting the bile acid synthesis pathway characterized by a defective sterol 26-hydroxylase (yes, you will be asked this question at the boards) in cholesterol metabolism. The enzyme deficiency causes elevated blood cholestanol levels, tendinous xanthomas, early cataracts, diarrhea, osteoporosis, early atherosclerosis, mental retardation, epilepsy, polyneuropathy, and spasticity. This is an autosomal recessive lipid storage disease that occurs in childhood. Deep gray matter (globus pallidus) and supratentorial white matter structures (corticospinal tracts especially in the cerebral peduncles) may demonstrate focal areas of T2 high signal and there may be dentate nuclei microcalcifications visible on CT. Enlargement of Virchow-Robin spaces may be seen. In the spine, the posterior and lateral columns may be selectively affected.

Cerebellar involvement typically starts in the dentate nucleus but can extend throughout the white matter of the cerebellar hemispheres. Pathologically, one sees neuronal loss, demyelination, fibrosis, focal calcifications, and deposition of hemosiderin. Perivascular macrophage infiltration is present. Thus, when one has a consolation of cataracts in a young individual with deep gray matter (particularly globus pallidus and dentate nucleus) lesions in a symmetric pattern, which may involve the posterior columns of the spinal cord, one should suggest a diagnosis of cerebrotendinous xanthomatosis.

Dyke-Davidoff-Masson syndrome In Dyke-Davidoff-Masson syndrome, hemiatrophy of one hemisphere is present. The calvarium may be thickened on that side, the petrous ridge and sphenoid wing elevated, and the frontal sinus may be grossly enlarged on the side of the atrophy (Fig. 8-20). This denotes a cerebral injury that occurred early in life or in utero. Usually, a middle cerebral vascular-ischemic cause is invoked. Dyke-Davidoff-Masson syndrome is also seen with Sturge-Weber syndrome (see Chapter 12). Are there enough eponyms to go around?

Porencephaly Porencephaly refers to an area of focal encephalomalacia that communicates with the ventricular system, causing what appears to be a focally dilated ventricle (Fig. 8-21). When the dilated ventricle abuts the inner cortex of the skull without significant brain tissue superficially, the CSF pulsations within the ventricle may cause remodeling of the bone. Sometimes synechiae may actually be within the ventricle, creating a ball-valve effect that leads to progressive enlargement

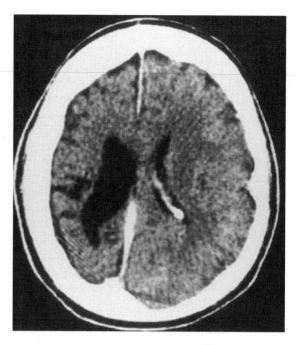

Fig. 8-20 Dyke-Davidoff-Masson syndrome. CT of a patient with Dyke-Davidoff-Masson syndrome shows enlargement of the cortical sulci on the right side with a smaller right hemisphere. Note that the ventricle and the cortex of the bone are larger on the right. Often one sees petrous ridge and sphenoid wing elevation with sinus enlargement ipsilateral to the hemiatrophy.

of the ventricle and expansion of the skull. Alternatively, when there is intervening brain tissue and CSF pulses are not transmitted to underlying structures, the skull may thicken in a Dyke-Davidoff-Masson fashion. The causes of porencephaly are manifold and include trauma, infection, and perinatal ischemic injury.

Miscellaneous causes Atrophy may also be caused by previous infections, long-standing multiple sclerosis, and extensive traumatic injury to the brain. Schizophrenic patients tend to have smaller hippocampi than matched controls.

A word on dementia (from people who have an intimate knowledge of the topic) It should be stated that progressive dementia and delirium need not be associated with brain atrophy (present company included). In other words, you do not need a brain shaped like a walnut to have dementia. A case in point; numerous examples of dementia associated with the venous congestion (venous hypertensive encephalopathy) induced by posterior fossa dural vascular malformations. Treatment of these AVMs by relieving the venous obstruction can "cure" the dementia. In these patients, the sulci, if anything, are smaller than usual because of the increased pressure. Note that mental status changes are a frequent accompaniment to sagittal sinus thrombosis even without dural fistulae.

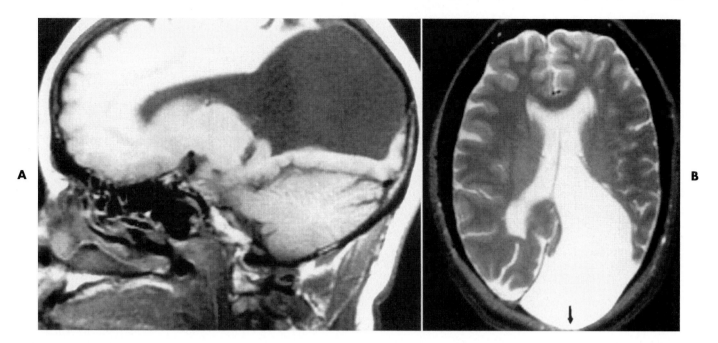

Fig. 8-21   Porencephaly. **A,** Sagittal T1WI shows a CSF intensity collection communicating with the lateral ventricle with no significant overlying cortical tissue. **B,** On the axial T2WI you should note that the bone at the edge of the film *(arrow)* is remodeled because of the long-term transmission of CSF pulsations.

Deep Gray Nuclei Disorders

The diseases that affect the deep gray matter nuclei (Table 8-3) are fascinating because of the movement disorders they produce. If you ever wonder what role the caudate nucleus or globus pallidus has in coordination, observe a patient with a degenerative deep gray matter disease. Smooth motor control is dependent on these structures; it is a wonder that larger blood vessels were not devoted to their supply.

Huntington chorea   Huntington chorea is a dementing disorder manifested by selective atrophy of the caudate nuclei. The patients have involuntary choreoathetoid movements and severe memory impairment. The Huntington gene on the short arm of chromosome 4 has been identified and there are genetic tests available for this disorder. This gene may affect the processing of the Huntington protein, which may be the mediator of this basal ganglionic disease. Histochemical analysis may show increased deposition of iron in the caudate and putamen. The disorder has an autosomal dominant inheritance pattern and is expressed in young adulthood. Considerable research has been performed concerning the deficiencies in the γ-aminobutyric acid inhibitory neurotransmitter and/or choline acetyltransferase in this disorder. On imaging studies, the frontal horns of the lateral ventricles are dilated and rounded as a result of caudate atrophy. Increased signal intensity in the putamen and globus pallidus has been described in

the juvenile form of Huntington disease, and frontal atrophy is usually present (Fig. 8-22). Hypometabolism in the caudates on PET and hypoperfusion on SPECT have been reported.

Hallervorden-Spatz syndrome   Hallervorden-Spatz syndrome is significant for its unusual MR findings. This familial autosomal recessive disorder is associated with abnormal involuntary movements, spasticity, and progressive dementia. Characteristic accumulation of iron-containing compounds is present in the globus pallidus, red nuclei, and substantia nigra pathologically. This is seen on MR as decreased intensity on T2WI. Reports of high signal intensity in the globus pallidus and white matter have also been reported on T2WI, presumably caused by gliosis and/or demyelination with axonal swelling. In addition, cortical and sometimes caudate atrophy is present. Unfortunately, the variability in iron deposition of the basal ganglia can be striking in normal persons depending on age. However, in the presence of a young adult with bradykinesia, muscle rigidity, and choreoathetoid movements of the body with ataxia, the presence of dramatic iron deposition within the basal ganglia with a central spot of high signal in the globus pallidus seen on T2W MR should suggest the diagnosis of Hallervorden-Spatz syndrome (Fig. 8-23). This pattern is that of the "eye of the tiger" though this has a limited differential diagnosis (see Box 8-5).

Although an uncommon disease, Hallervorden-Spatz syndrome is a pet entity for board reviewers and intel-

Table 8-3   Deep gray nuclei disorders

Deep gray matter disease	Distinguishing imaging features	MRS features	Distinguishing clinical features
Huntington's chorea	Caudate atrophy Abnormal signal in lentiform nuclei	Increased lactate	Familial transmission autosomal dominant Choreiform movements
Wilson's disease	Abnormal intensity in basal ganglia Cerebellar atrophy	Decreased NAA/Cho Increased Lactate/NAA	Kayser-Fleischer copper rings in globes Coexistent liver disease Ataxia, dysarthria
Hallervorden-Spatz syndrome	Basal ganglia, red nuclei low intensity Globus pallidus atrophy	Increased glutamate-glutamine/creatine Decreased PME Increased PCR/Pi	Dementia in young adults Rigidity, bradykinesia, toe-walking, hyperreflexia Familial transmission autosomal recessive
Leigh syndrome	Favors putamen, other basal ganglia, brain stem tegmentum	Increased lactate	Childhood onset Failure to thrive Lactic acidosis

lectual discussion: is the lentiform nucleus dark or bright, and at what field strength? It is typically dark on high field strength magnets.

Wilson disease Wilson disease (hepatolenticular degeneration) is an autosomal recessive disorder caused by abnormal ceruloplasmin metabolism with deposition of copper in the liver and brain. Patients are seen in early adulthood with dysarthria, dystonia, and tremors. Rigidity and ataxia may follow. Copper deposition in the cornea accounts for the classic Kayser-Fleischer rings seen on slit-

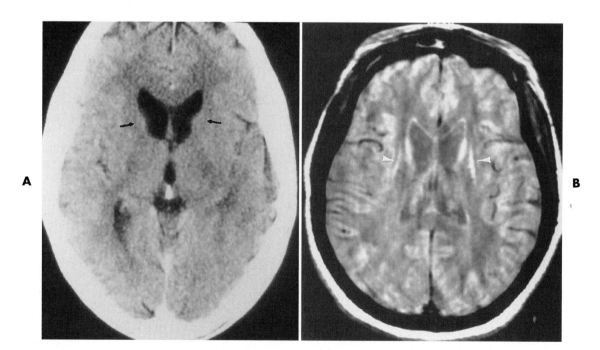

Fig. 8-22   Huntington disease. **A,** Axial unenhanced CT demonstrates caudate atrophy *(arrows)* with ballooning of the frontal horns of the lateral ventricles. **B,** PDWI has high signal intensity in the caudate nuclei bilaterally and in the putamen *(arrowheads).* Again seen is frontal horn dilatation caused by the atrophy of the caudate nuclei.

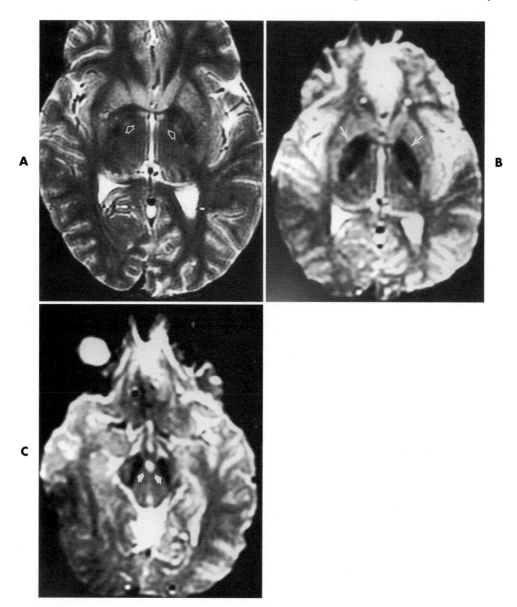

Fig. 8-23   Hallervorden-Spatz disease. **A,** The eye-of-the-tiger sign is seen in this 8-year-old-child who has an area of linear high signal *(arrow)* amidst a dark globus pallidus on this T2W1. The increased iron content *(arrows)* of the globus pallidus **(B)** and substantia nigra **(C)** in typical of Hallervorden-Spatz disease and is particularly well seen on this diffusion-weighted B=0 image.

lamp ophthalmologic examination. On CT, the patients have atrophy involving the caudate nuclei and brain stem, with nonenhancing foci of hypodensity in the basal ganglia and thalami. MR findings in Wilson disease include hypointensity in the lentiform nucleus and thalami, possibly caused by a paramagnetic form of copper and/or associated iron deposition. Still others have noted bilateral and symmetric deep gray areas of abnormally increased signal on T2WI, in the outer rim of the putamen (Fig. 8-24), ventral nuclear mass of the thalami, and the globus pallidus. In cases of copper toxicosis, one may also see bright hypothalami and bright anterior pituitary glands on T1WI. Scattered areas of abnormality may also be seen in

---

Box 8-5 Differential Diagnosis of "Eye of the Tiger" Sign

Carbon monoxide poisoning
Corticobasal ganglionic degeneration
Hallervorden-Spatz disease
Leigh syndrome
Neurofibromatosis
Parkinson disease
Progressive supranuclear palsy
Shy-Drager syndrome
Toxins

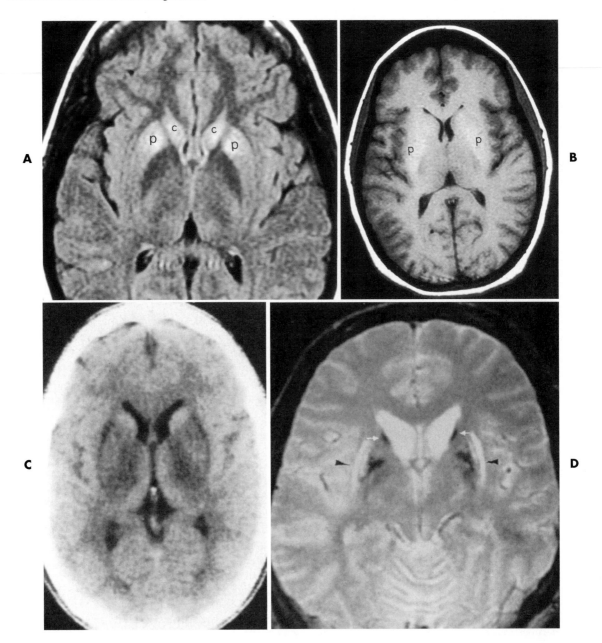

Fig. 8-24   Wilson disease. **A,** FLAIR images are particularly valuable in showing the bright signal in the caudate heads *(c)* and putamina *(p)* in this patient with Wilson disease. **B,** The T1 weighted scan also shows high signal intensity in the putamen *(p)*. Although the differential diagnosis is quite broad, the presence of Kayser-Fleisher rings in this individual clinched the diagnosis of Wilson disease. **C,** Hypodensity in the basal ganglia and thalami is seen on this CT of a patient with Wilson disease. **D,** T2WI shows abnormally low intensity in the caudate nuclei bilaterally *(arrows)* and in the putamina bilaterally. Mild caudate atrophy is evidenced by the dilatation of the frontal horns of the lateral ventricles. High signal intensity in the external capsule *(arrowheads)* is also present and has been reported in this disease.

the brain stem, particularly the tegmentum of the midbrain, the red nuclei, and pons. Atrophy is common, especially in the caudate nuclei. Scattered high signal intensity foci in the white matter, pathologically correlating to demyelination, may be present as well. These high intensity foci tend to occur in the corticospinal tract, dentatorubrothalamic tract, and pontocerebellar tract. Bringing structure and function together, some investigators have shown that abnormalities of the basal ganglia and

pontocerebellar tracts depicted on MR images correlated with pseudoparkinsonian signs whereas abnormal dentatothalamic tracts correlate with cerebellar signs.

Leigh disease   This entity, also referred to as necrotizing encephalomyelopathy, affects the putamina bilaterally but may involve other deep gray matter structures. The disease is due to pyruvate carboxylase/dehydrogenase deficiencies. It is more thoroughly discussed under metabolic disorders below. Other mitochondrial disorders such as Kearns-Sayre syndrome and MELAS syndrome will often affect the basal ganglia.

As noted above CJD is often associated with basal ganglionic lesions.

Metabolic and toxic disorders High signal intensity in the basal ganglia on T1WI has also been described in patients with hepatic encephalopathy, portosystemic shunting without hepatic encephalopathy, and disorders of calcium-phosphate regulation, and in those patients receiving parenteral nutrition therapy (Fig. 8-25). With hepatic failure, one may see increased signal intensity in the globus pallidus and putamina, the midbrain, and the anterior pituitary gland. T2 values as well as T1 values are shortened in cases of hepatic encephalopathy, particularly in the globus pallidus. Atrophy is usually seen elsewhere as well, especially affecting the cerebellum. Deposition of manganese, which bypasses the detoxification in the liver, has been postulated as the source of the high signal intensity in the globus pallidus. The high signal finding is reversible after correction of the underlying hepatic disorder and/or a return to peroral alimentation. Do not forget that children can have liver failure too. You may see a bright hypothalamus and pituitary gland in childhood hepatic disease owing to Crigler-Najjar disease, copper toxicosis, Byler disease, biliary atresia, Alagille syndrome and so on.

With short echo time STEAM sequences on MRS, patients with hepatic encephalopathy have decreased myoinositol (mI) to creatine (CR) and choline to creatine

ratios and elevated glutamine-glutamate to creatine ratios compared with normals. These ratios will normalize or even overshoot the other way with correction of the hepatic dysfunction. The mI/CR ratio seems to be the most sensitive (80% to 85%) indicator of hepatic encephalopathy. The MRS (and clinical) response return toward normal before reversal of the bright basal ganglia sign, which is delayed 3 to 6 months. With liver transplantation, the bright basal ganglia on T1WI return to normal intensity within one year postoperatively.

Hyperintense basal ganglia have been reported in cases of AIDS (due to a microangiopathy and infarcts), Langerhans cell histiocytosis, and in the unusual bright lesions associated with neurofibromatosis type 1 (NF-1). NF-1 may be associated with symmetric nonenhancing hypodensities in the dentate nuclei region of the cerebellum, which are hypointense on T1WI and hyperintense on T2WI. Other causes of bilateral increased signal intensity on T1WI of the basal ganglia are found in Box 8-6 (Fig. 8-26).

Drugs and toxins Several toxic substances have been implicated in basal ganglionic and diffuse white matter lesions. These are enumerated in Table 8-4 (Fig. 8-27). Recent reports have noted that abuse of "ecstasy," a popular recreational party drug, also known as 3,4 methylenedioxymethamphetamine (MDMA) to the nonparty goers, can cause bilateral globus pallidus necrosis, possibly due to prolonged vasospasm. The relative cerebral blood volume of the globus pallidus is reduced in chronic ecstasy abusers. This drug releases serotonin-like substances from neurons and the globus pallidus has

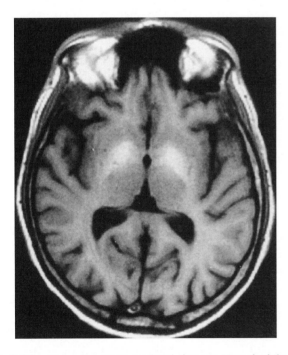

Fig. 8-25 Hyperalimentation-related changes. Note the bilateral increased signal intensity in the globus pallidus on this T1WI. The apparent cause of the hyperintensity is thought to be related to manganese metabolism, which is abnormal in patients undergoing hyperalimentation.

Box 8-6   Causes of Hyperintense Basal Ganglia on T1WI

AIDS (due to microinfarcts)
Carbon monoxide poisoning
Fucosidosis
Hallervorden-Spatz syndrome
Hemorrhage
Hepatic encephalopathy
Hyperalimentation therapy
Hyperparathyroidism
Hypoxic-ischemic encephalopathy
Idiopathic calcification
Japanese encephalitis
Kernicterus
Langerhans cell histiocytosis
Neurofibromatosis Type I
Pseudohypoparathyroidism, pseudopseudohypo-
    parathyroidism, hypoparathyroidism
Wilson's disease
Lai, *AJR* 172:1109-1115, 1999.

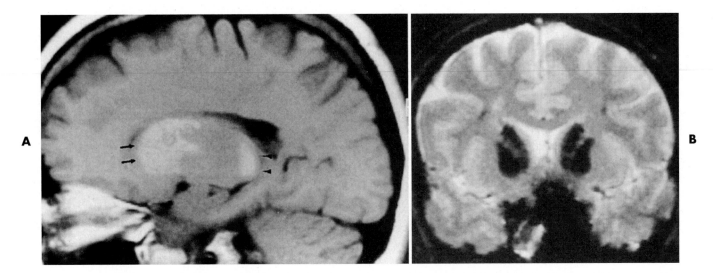

Fig. 8-26   Basal ganglia changes in a patient with pseudohypoparathyroidism. **A,** Sagittal T1WI shows bright signal intensity in the head of the caudate *(arrows),* with similar changes in the posterior portion of the thalamus *(arrowheads).* **B,** On a gradient echo T2WI the striking hypointensity in the basal ganglia is caused by the paramagnetic accumulation.

high concentrations of these nerve terminals. With excessive release of serotonin, the brain down-regulates the receptor density in the cortex to reduce the overwhelming effects of the drug. Death of serotonergic neurons does occur at high levels of abuse. Yes, Virginia, you can have too much ecstasy—but we have tried to keep it to a limit in this book.

In a similar vein (or is it artery), cocaine can induce ischemia, vasoconstriction, vasculitis, hypertensive white matter changes, intraparenchymal hematomas, subarachnoid hemorrhage, and even moya-moya vasculopathy. "Crack" cocaine has an even higher rate of drug-induced ischemic strokes, secondary to vasoconstriction, platelet dysmetabolism, and episodic hypertension.

Basal ganglionic calcification   The basal ganglia need not be atrophic to show manifestations of diseases. Although basal ganglionic calcification may be a normal senescent process, there are endocrinologic/metabolic (hyperparathyroidism [Fig. 8-28], hypoparathyroidism, pseudohypoparathyroidism, pseudopseudohypoparathyroidism, and hypothyroidism) mitochondrial (Kearns-Sayre, MELAS, and MERRF), idiopathic (Fahr disease), congenital (Cockayne syndrome, Down syndrome, trisomy 13), phakomatoses (neurofibromatosis and tuberous sclerosis), inflammatory (TORCH infections, cysticercosis, and AIDS), traumatic (dystrophic calcifications), ischemic (anoxia, carbon monoxide poisoning), and iatrogenic (radiation therapy, methotrexate therapy, foreign body reaction to retained shunt catheters) sources of this finding.

Ninety percent of the aforementioned cerebral/cerebellar atrophic diseases have no cure or have limited recovery with medication. As stated earlier, once the brain has been insulted and important structures are lost, it is hard to get function to return. In this regard,

the brain is like your favorite old car in an accident—hard to fix if the damage to it is too severe.

Cerebellar Atrophy

Atrophy of the cerebellum has many causes (Box 8-7).

Alcohol abuse   Chronic ingestion of excessive amounts of alcohol is probably the most common cause of cerebellar atrophy. The vermis appears to be more commonly involved than other parts of the brain with alcohol abuse, but the whole cerebellum suffers (Fig. 8-29). When one adds poor nutrition to the alcohol abuse, the brain stem and basal ganglia are damaged. This condition is known as Wernicke encephalopathy. By that point, the patient has tremors, delusions, confabulation, ophthalmoparesis, ataxia, and confusion. When severe amnesia accompanies Wernicke's encephalopathy, Korsakoff syndrome is invoked, although the two diseases are caused by the same factors. *(Neuroradiologists, eat healthfully and restrict your Lafite-Rothschild wine. Tremors, amnesia, and cerebral angiography do not mix well.)*

Wernicke encephalopathy is thought to be due to thiamine deficiency and is usually caused by chronic alcoholism. Other possible etiologies include hyperemesis gravidarum, prolonged infectious-febrile conditions, carcinoma, anorexia nervosa, and prolonged voluntary starvation. In addition to generalized cortical and cerebellar vermian atrophy seen on CT and MR, recent reports have noted the presence of high signal intensity areas in the periaqueductal gray matter of the midbrain (40%), the paraventricular thalamic regions (46%), the mamillothalamic tract, and in the tissue surrounding the third ventricle on T2WI (Fig. 8-30). Reversible thalamic/pulvinar lesions in the dorsal medial nuclei have also been re-

Table 8-4   Manifestations of toxic insults to the basal ganglia

Toxin	Basal ganglia findings	Other imaging findings
Alcohol	Limited until portosystemic shunts, then hyperintense lentiform nucleus	Cerebellar (superior vermis) and cortical atrophy, Wernicke's changes in periaqueductal gray matter, hypothalamus
Carbon monoxide	Bilateral globus pallidus injury	Diffuse anoxic ischemia to brain, white matter injury sparing subcortical fibers, injury to the hippocampus and cerebellum
MDMA	Globus pallidus necrosis	
Methanol	Putaminal necrosis	Edema of brain, petechial hemorrhages
Mercury	None	Cerebellar, calcarine cortex atrophy
Manganese (see total parenteral nutrition, portosystemic shunts)	Hyperintense globus pallidus	Diffuse injury when severe
Lead	Late basal ganglia calcification	Swelling, then atrophy of cerebrum (favoring limbic system) and cerebellum
Cyanide	Globus pallidus infarctions	Diffuse swelling of cerebrum early after ingestion, demyelination
Reye's syndrome (aspirin)	Abnormal basal ganglionic signal	Diffuse swelling, increased gray-white differentiation
Hydrogen sulfide	Basal ganglia infarction	Diffuse swelling
Anorexia nervosa (what is this doing here?)	None described yet (are you hungry for the diagnosis?)	Reversible enlargement of CSF spaces
Trytophan (eosinophilic myalgia syndrome)	Atrophy	Subcortical focal lesions, focal lesions in deep white matter, cortical atrophy, ventricular dilatation, and diffuse and periventricular white matter abnormalities Elevated glutamine and decreased myoinositol residues on spectroscopy
Toluene	Basal ganglia increased intensity	White matter disease in infratentorial (brain stem and cerebellum) and supratentorial compartments, diffuse white matter change showed obvious brain atrophy, including hippocampal atrophy and thinning of the corpus callosum
Typewriter correction fluid (trichloroethane)	Lesions in basal ganglia and cortex similar to those observed in patients with methanol and carbon monoxide poisoning	Lesions in basal ganglia and cortex similar to those observed in patients with methanol and carbon monoxide poisoning

ported. These areas may or may not enhance (in some cases the enhancement may be dramatic, almost sarcoid-like), and may be associated with mamillary body atrophy. Mamillary body enhancement or abnormal signal may be the sole manifestation of Wernicke encephalopathy. Myelin degeneration, mamillary body volume loss, intracellular edema, and microglial proliferation are seen pathologically (but may be present in alcoholics without Wernicke).

Long-term drug use   Infratentorial atrophy is also a common finding after long-term use of certain drugs. Phenytoin (Dilantin) and phenobarbital are the classic drugs that produce cerebellar atrophy. Patients may have reversible nystagmus, ataxia, peripheral neuropathies, and slurred speech. The cerebellar degeneration becomes irreversible after long-term administration. It is

manifested by dilatation of the fourth ventricle and cerebellar sulci, with the cerebellar folia seeming to float amid the CSF like delicate fronds of ferns on a crystal lake. Phenytoin may also cause thickening of the skull when used early in life for a long period.

Olivopontocerebellar degeneration   Several diseases with a congenital or degenerative basis may cause cerebellar atrophy. As discussed above, olivopontocerebellar degeneration is a disease that occurs in young adults and is associated with cerebellar and brain stem atrophy. The pons and inferior olives are strikingly small, as are the cerebellar peduncles (Fig. 8-31). Cerebellar atrophy, particularly of the vermis, is marked. Patients generally have truncal and limb ataxia. Problems with speech, tremors, nystagmus, rigidity, brain stem dysfunction, and mild mental impairment may ensue. The disease may oc-

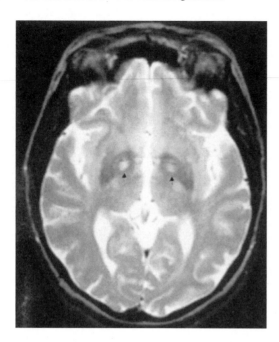

Fig. 8-27   Toxic basal ganglia lesion. Axial T2WI shows bilateral high signal foci in the globus pallidus *(arrows)*. The differential diagnosis includes ischemic foci, carbon monoxide poisoning, cyanide toxicity, or anoxic injury. This patient had tried to commit suicide by carbon monoxide inhalation.

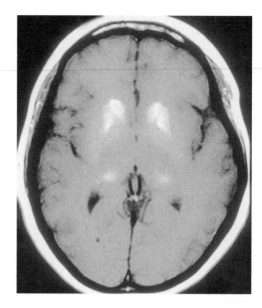

Fig. 8-28   Hyperparathyroidism. The caudate heads, putamina, and thalami are bright on this T1WI. One should consider causes of calcium-phosphorous dysmetabolism, especially given the absence of globus pallidus involvement. The corollary on CT would be calcification. How does calcification cause T1-shortening—back to Chapter 1 you go. Do not pass go, do not get a refund for this book.

cur sporadically or may be transmitted in an autosomal dominant inheritance.

Cerebellar olivary degeneration   Cortical cerebellar degeneration shows selective atrophy of the lateral cerebellum (fish-mouth deformity), superior vermis, especially the declive, folium, and tuber (but not the chives, endives, and pimentos). The fourth ventricle and the primary semilunar fissure are markedly enlarged. The olives are secondarily reduced in size—the primary defect is in the cerebellar cortex.

Friedreich ataxia   Friedreich ataxia is an autosomal disorder associated with cerebellar atrophy that presents in the second decade of life. It has autosomal dominant and recessive forms (FRDA gene mutation leading to frataxin mitochondrial protein defect) related to chromosome 9 abnormalities. Cardiac anomalies may co-exist, particularly affecting the conduction pathways. Patients are usually seen in late childhood with lower extremity ataxia, kyphoscoliosis, and tremors of the upper extremity. Areflexia in the lower extremeties, scoliosis, deafness, optic atrophy, and dysarthria may occur, but one variant (Friedreich ataxia with retained reflexes-FARR), does not show reflex abnormality. Atrophy of the cervicomedullary junction with a decreased anteroposterior diameter of the upper part of the cervical cord has been reported. Signal intensity in the cerebellum and cord is normal.

Hereditary cerebellar atrophy   Dramatic cerebellar atrophy is identified in cases of hereditary cerebellar de-

Box 8-7   Causes of Cerebellar Atrophy

Toxic
   Alcohol abuse
   Long-term use of phenytoin (Dilantin), phenobarbital,
     high dose cytosine arabinoside
   Mercury poisoning
   Poor nutrition without alcoholism
   Thallium poisoning
Hereditary/degenerative
   Ataxia telangiectasia
   Creutzfeldt-Jakob disease
   Friedreich's ataxia
   Hereditary ataxia
   Menkes' kinky hair syndrome
   Olivopontocerebellar degeneration
     Cerebellar-olivary degenerate
     Dandy Walker syndrome
     Infantile cerebellar ataxia
     Joubert syndrome
   Shy-Drager syndrome
Vascular
   Vertebrobasilar insufficiency
Neoplastic
   Paraneoplastic syndromes
Radiation to posterior fossa
CMV, rubella infections
Multiple sclerosis

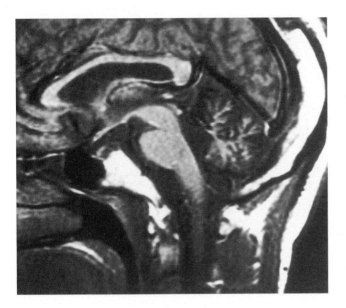

Fig. 8-29   Cerebellar atrophy caused by alcohol abuse. Sagittal T1WI shows enlargement of the cerebellar sulci and decrease in the size of the cerebellum.

generation described by Marie in 1893, distinct from Friedreich ataxia. This disorder is seen in middle-aged patients, with severe superior vermian atrophy and lesser involvement of the rest of the cerebellar cortex. Patients have lower extremity gait ataxia, optic atrophy, and ophthalmoparesis in later life. The disorder progresses slowly but relentlessly in a setting of otherwise good

health. Dentatorubral-pallidoluysian atrophy is another tongue twister of a hereditary disorder that exemplifies cerebellar atrophy, and falls within this category.

Patients with Marinesco-Sjögren syndrome have hypoplastic cerebellar hemispheres and a hypoplastic vermis in a small posterior fossa. There may be associated midline posterior fossa cysts and agenesis of the corpus callosum.

Other autosomal recessive hereditary ataxias include ataxia with vitamin E deficiency (AVED), infantile onset spinocerebellar ataxia, autosomal recessive spastic ataxia of Charlevoix-Saguenay (ARSACS), and ataxia telangiectasia. Autosomal dominant ataxias include episodic ataxai, spinocerebellar degeneration, polyQ ataxias, myotonic dystrophy, and oculopharyngeal dystrophy.

Ataxia telangiectasia   Ataxia telangiectasia (Louis-Bar syndrome) is an autosomal recessive disorder characterized by cerebellar vermian and hemispheric atrophy and telangiectatic lesions on the face, mucosa, and conjunctiva. It occurs in 1 in 20,000 to 100,000 live births and has been mapped to chromosome 11. An associated abnormality of the immune system (predominantly affecting immunoglobulin A) causes recurrent sinus and lung infections. Leukemia or non-Hodgkin lymphoma may develop, and the patients usually die of the disease in childhood. If the patients survive in adulthood, they may be besieged by breast, gastric, CNS, skin, and liver malignancies. Increased sensitivity to radiation effects, possibly leading to progeria, precludes these individuals from careers in interventional neuroradiology.

The typical findings of this atypical disorder are

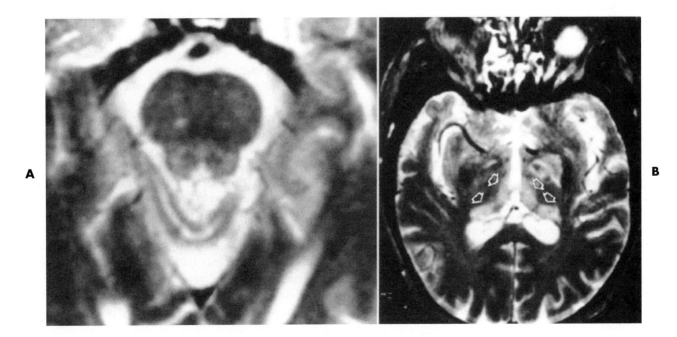

Fig. 8-30   Wernicke encephalopathy. **A,** There is periaqueductal high signal abnormality. on this T2WI. **B,** Evidence of high signal abnormality *(arrows)* is noted in the mamillothalamic tract in this alcoholic patient with acute encephalopathy.

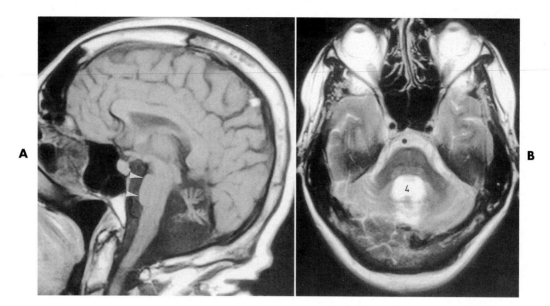

Fig. 8-31 Olivopontocerebellar degeneration. **A,** Sagittal T1WI shows marked cerebellar atrophy with flattening of the belly *(arrowheads)* of the pons and the enlarged inferior cerebellar cistern. **B,** Axial T2WI reveals atrophy of the pons as it swims in the prepontine cistern. Also note the enlarged fourth ventricle *(4).*

vermian/holocerebellar atrophy and white matter signal intensity increases. Rarely, intracranial occult cerebrovascular malformations may be present. These are manifest as dark dots of hemosiderin on T2* scans of the brain and may be due to perivascular hemorrhages.

Ischemia Chronic vertebrobasilar atherosclerotic disease may cause what appears to be cerebellar atrophy resulting from multiple small foci of white matter dropout from ischemia. Usually supratentorial manifestations of atherosclerotic ischemic disease (lacunar infarctions, white matter gliosis) coexist and are the tip-off to the disease.

Hypertrophic olivary degeneration (HOD) HOD may be caused by an ischemic, traumatic, neoplastic, or vascular insult to the components of the "triangle of Guillain and Mollaret," that is, the dentate nucleus, red nucleus, and inferior olivary nucleus. These structures are connected by the superior cerebellar peduncle (dentate to red nucleus), the central tegmental tract (red nucleus to inferior olivary nucleus), and the inferior cerebellar peduncle (inferior olivary nucleus to dentate nucleus—the olivodentate tract). Lesions in the first two tracts can lead to de-afferentation of the inferior olivary nucleus. Initially this leads to high T2W signal (first 2 months) and then hypertrophy (6 months to 3 to 4 years) of the inferior olivary nucleus of the medulla. In the later stages, contralateral cerebellar atrophy can occur although this is more commonly seen with involvement of the olivo-dentate fibers. Patients typically present with a palatal tremor, "palatal myoclonus."

Paraneoplastic syndromes Cerebellar atrophy is one of the manifestations of paraneoplastic syndromes. These may be associated with neuroblastoma, Hodgkin disease, and ovarian, gastrointestinal, lung, and breast cancers. An autoimmune mechanism (anti-Yo antigen syndrome) is implicated because antibodies to cerebellar antigens (predominantly directed against Purkinje cells) may be identified. The cerebellar degeneration precedes discovery of the primary tumor in up to 60% of cases. As if having the primary tumor itself is not enough bad luck.

Palatal myoclonus There is a syndrome of patients with palatal myoclonus in which the inferior olivary nuclei enlarge. The dentate nuclei opposite enlarged inferior olivary nuclei may shrink and have high signal intensity on T2WI. The cerebellar cortex may show atrophy ipsilateral to the dentate changes.

Toxic exposure Minamata disease, which represents methylmercury poisoning, usually from seafood, causes severe atrophy of the cerebellar vermis. The visual cortex, cerebellar hemispheres, and postcentral cortex may also atrophy and become bright on T2WI.

The literature is replete with a dispute as to whether autistic children have vermian cerebellar atrophy. Pack that one away.

METABOLIC DISORDERS

The number of metabolic disorders that affect the brain is probably in the hundreds. Worse, each one has an eponym with the names of two MDs and one PhD attached to it. Forget trying to remember every one of them and instead try to get a feel for their effects on the brain. Remember, the brain has a limited way it responds to insults. Basically, it swells, it atrophies, and it does not myelinate correctly. Consult the tables included here for more specific information.

Mucopolysaccharidoses

Clinically, the mucopolysaccharidoses (MPS) are characterized by mental retardation, peculiar facies, and musculoskeletal deformities. The mucopolysaccharidoses (Table 8-5) are associated with brain atrophy and abnormalities of the white matter on imaging. The diagnoses of these disorders are usually based on biochemical and/or chromosomal evaluation. The mucopolysaccharidoses are usually manifested on MR as diffuse cribriform or cystic-appearing areas of abnormal signal intensity in the white matter (low on T1WI, high on T2WI) and hypodensity in the white matter on CT (Fig. 8-32). At the foramen magnum, thickening of the dura (Fig. 8-33) (or mucopolysaccharide deposition) may cause medullary compression in some of the mucopolysaccharidoses. Some of these disorders are associated with enlarged heads and thickened skulls (I know a co-author who fits that bill). MPS III, Sanfilippo disease is unique among the mucopolysaccharidoses in that the non-CNS

abnormalities are relatively minor. Several reports of the intracranial findings with MPS III and other MPS disorders have included arachnoid cysts. It is presumed that build-up of glycosaminoglycans in the leptomeninges account for the arachnoid membrane obstruction and ball valve effect that can lead to such cysts (as well as optic nerve sheath dilation—see Fig. 8-33B).

Lipidoses and Other Storage Diseases

The gangliosidoses are diseases that manifest white matter abnormalities and cortical atrophy. Lacunar and white matter small vessel infarctions may occur in Fabry and Gaucher disease. Of the lipidoses (Table 8-6), cerebellar ataxia and cerebellar atrophy are more common in Tay-Sachs disease and Niemann-Pick disease (Fig. 8-34). Bilateral thalamic abnormalities with hyperdensity on CT is characteristic of Sandhoff disease, but may also be seen with toxic exposures (Fig. 8-35).

Mitochondrial Defects

Leigh disease (subacute necrotizing encephalomyelopathy) Leigh disease, (not to be confused with

Table 8-5   Imaging findings in mucopolysaccharidoses

Eponym	Deficient enzyme	Inheritance	CNS findings
Hurler (MPS I)	α-L-Iduronidase	AR	Thickened meninges, atrophy, kyphosis, atlantoaxial subluxation, ligamentous thickening causing cord compression, cribriform or cystic areas within white matter and/or basal ganglia, delayed myelination, hydrocephalus, vertebra plana
Scheie (MPS IS)*	α-L-Iduronidase	AR	Pigmentary retinopathy
Hunter (MPS II)	Iduronate sulfatase	XR	Macrocrania, enlarged Virchow-Robin spaces, cribriform or cystic areas within white matter, corpus callosum and/or basal ganglia, delayed myelination, thickening of dura matter especially in the spine, communicating hydrocephalus
Sanfilippo (MPS III)	Sulfamidase	AR	Atrophy, cribriform or cystic areas within white matter and/or basal ganglia, delayed myelination, retinal degeneration
Morquio (MPS IV)	Galactosamine-6-sulfate sulfatase	AR	Ligamentous thickening leading to cord compression, odontoid hypoplasia, atlantoaxial subluxation, vertebra plana, white matter high intensity
Maroteaux-Lamy (MPS VI)	N-Acetylgalactosamine-sulfatase B	AR	Meningeal thickening, hydrocephalus, perivascular gliosis, cord compression from ligamentous thickening, atlantoaxial subluxation
Sly (MPS VII)	Glucuronidase	AR	None or hydrocephalus, white matter high intensity
DiFerrante (MPS VIII)	N-Acetyl glucosamine-6-sulfate-sulfatase	?	Odontoid hypoplasia

MPS, Mucopolysaccharidosis.

AR, autosomal recessive.

XR, X-linked recessive

*Initially classified as MPS V.

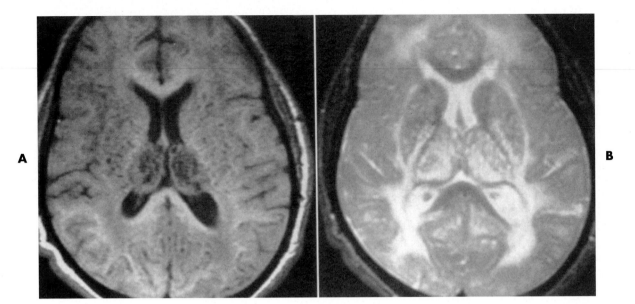

Fig. 8-32 Hunter mucopolysaccharidosis. **A,** Axial T1WI demonstrates the cribriform appearance to the thalami, basal ganglia, and central white matter. **B,** On T2WI abnormal signal intensity is seen within the internal and external capsules and in the frontal and occipital white matter.

"Leighsy" disease seen in some of our fellows) may be the prototype of the mitochondrial enzymatic disorders (Table 8-7). It is manifested clinically by motor system abnormalities, ataxia, nystagmus, ophthalmoplegia, spasticity, psychomotor retardation, cranial palsies, and metabolic acidosis. Leigh disease is a neurodegenerative disorder seen in children under 2 years old and expressed on MR by abnormally high signal intensity of the putamina bilaterally on T2WI (Fig. 8-36). Other areas may also show abnormal intensity including the caudate nuclei, globus pallidi, thalami, and brain stem. A classification of disease in which (1) basal ganglia lesions predate brain stem ones, (2) brain stem lesions appear with or without basal ganglia or white matter lesions, and (3) white matter lesions are followed by brain stem lesions has been used to describe risk for fatal complications of Leigh disease. Lower brain stem involvement correlates with loss of respiratory control, a potentially fatal complication of the disease. Diffuse supratentorial white matter T2 hyperintensity may accompany the deep gray matter findings. These areas do not enhance. MR may also detect midbrain and spinal cord atrophy in this disorder. The telltale laboratory finding is metabolic acidosis with increased lactate levels; the lactate may be detectable with proton or phosphorous MR spectroscopic examination. The disease is thought to be due to a deficiency in the enzymes associated with pyruvate breakdown; its accumulation leads to lactic acid build-up.

MELAS (*m*itochondrial *e*ncephalomyopathy, *l*actic *a*cidosis, and *s*trokelike episodes) syndrome represents an unusual form of mitochondrial dysmetabolism. Imaging studies demonstrate multiple areas of cortical high signal intensity abnormality on T2WI, which often crosses a traditional cerebral artery distribution (Fig. 8-37). Although the lesions may be bright on DWI scans, they do NOT show reduced ADC values and are therefore not acute infarcts. The patients may have cortical blindness. Strangely enough, these lesions may disappear with time, leaving only minimal sulcal dilatation in their place. The abnormality is associated with serologic and spectroscopic evidence of elevated lactic acid levels. The lesions associated with MELAS have also been reported in the putamen, caudate nuclei, and thalami. Contrast enhancement may be present. Although resolution of the lesions is the expected course, one may see new lesions appearing as well. Ultimately, atrophy favoring the posterior cerebrum is expected.

Other mitochondrial encephalomyopathies include Kearns-Sayre syndrome (which also affects the basal ganglia), mitochondrial cytopathies, and MERRF (*m*yoclonus, *e*pilepsy, *r*agged *r*ed muscle *f*ibers) syndrome. MERRF has a higher rate of brain stem focal lesions than MELAS or Kearnes Sayre.

Kearns-Sayre syndrome affects the orbits with retinitis pigmentosa, ophthalmoplegia, extraocular muscle weakness (and possible atrophy), and affects the heart, resulting in cardiac conduction deficits and a cardiomyopathy. Basal ganglia calcification occurs in Kearns-Sayre syndrome more frequently than in MELAS or MERRF syndrome. Hyperintense basal ganglia, cerebral and cerebellar atrophy, and diffuse white matter hyperintensity are the most common MR findings in Kearns-Sayre syndrome

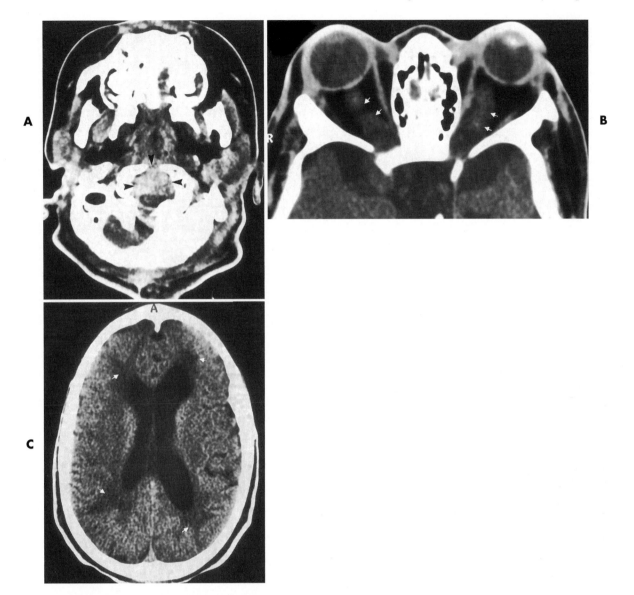

Fig. 8-33   Maroteaux-Lamy (MPS VI). **A,** CT of base of skull with compression of subarachnoid space by thickened dura *(arrowheads)* infiltrated with glycosoaminoglycans (mucopolysaccharide). **B,** CT with dilated subarachnoid spaces around optic nerves *(arrows)* from increase intracranial pressure as a result of obstruction to the flow of CSF at the base of the brain from glycosoaminoglycans. **C,** CT with hydrocephalus and low density in the white matter *(arrows)*, which can be the result of intrinsic white matter changes from the disease itself or subependymal migration of CSF from the hydrocephalus.

and chronic progressive external ophthalmoplegia. Microcephaly, cerebellar hypoplasia, and white matter demyelination may occur as well. Progressive cytochrome C oxidase deficiency may cause the syndrome.

MERRF, MELAS, and Kearns-Sayre syndromes all may cause dementia and myopathy in the second and third decades of life. Distinguishing features are the strokelike episodes in MELAS and the myoclonus in MERRF.

Zellweger syndrome is characterized by hypomyelination, microgyric and pachygyric cortical malformations that are most severe in the perisylvian and perirolandic regions, and caudothalamic groove cysts.

This is an autosomal recessive disorder with the defective gene on chromosome 8. Soft-tissue calcifications may be present. Dolichocephaly and sutural widening and macrocephaly are seen. A marked decrease in NAA is found at MRS.

Aminoacidopathies and Other Enzyme Deficiencies

As a group, the amino acid metabolic disorders (Table 8-8) are usually seen in children and are manifested neurologically by developmental delay, mental retardation,

Table 8-6 Imaging findings in lipidoses, gangliosidoses, and other storage diseases

Disorder	Deficient enzyme	Inheritance	CNS findings
Ceroid lipofuscinosis (Batten disease)	Unknown	A-R	Cerebellar or less often cortical atrophy, periventricular gliosis, optic atrophy, thickened dura, thick skull
Fabry's disease	α-Galactosidase A	X-R	Multiple infarcts, vascular stenoses, and thromboses basal ganglia lacunae
Farber's disease (lipogranulomatosis)	Acid ceramidase	A-R	Atrophy, hydrocephalus
Fucosidosis	α-L-Fucosidase	A-R	Demyelination, gliosis, atrophy, high intensity TI in basal ganglia, thickened skull, craniostenosis, poorly developed sinus, short odontoid, platyspondyly, anterior beaking, scoliosis, vacuum disk, square vertebrae
Gaucher's disease	Acid β-glucosidase	A-R	Minimal to no atrophy, vertebral body collapse, dementia, infarcts
GM₁ gangliosidosis	β-Galactosidase	A-R	White matter disease, late atrophy, macroglossia, organomegaly, dementia (1–3 yr), seizures, gibbus, beaked vertebrae, bright putamen caudate atrophy, on T2WI
Krabbe's disease (Globoid cell leukodystropy)	Galactocerebroside β-galactosidase	A-R	Increased CT attenuation in cerebellum, thalami, caudate nuclei, decreased signal on T2WI of cerebellum, optic atrophy, small atrophic brain, demyelination, and intracranial optic nerve enlargement
Mannosidosis	α-Mannosidase	A-R	Low density in parietooccipital white matter, atrophy, thickened skull, lenticular opacities, brachycephaly, craniostenosis
Niemann-Pick disease	Sphingomyelinase	A-R	Normal vs areas of demyelination, gliosis, slight atrophy, small corpus callosum
Pompe's disease	Acid maltase	A-R	Gliosis, macroglossia
Sandhoff's disease	Hexosaminidase A and B (gangliosidase)	A-R	Atrophy, thalamic hyperdensity on CT possibly caused by calcification; diffuse white matter disease
Tay-Sachs disease (GM₂ gangliosidosis)	Hexosaminidase A (gangliosidase)	A-R	Megalencephaly early; atrophy late, especially of optic nerves and cerebellum; demyelination; high-density thalami, deep gray abnormal signal, large caudate

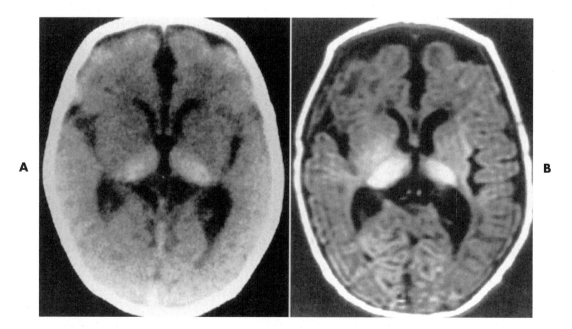

Fig. 8-34 Tay-Sachs disease. **A,** Axial unenhanced CT shows bilateral thalamic hyperdensity presumably caused by calcification, which is seen in some cases of Tay-Sachs and Sandhoff disease. **B,** T1WI shows hyperintensity to the thalami bilaterally and diffuse cortical atrophy in the same patient. Cerebellar atrophy is another common manifestation of Tay-Sachs disease.

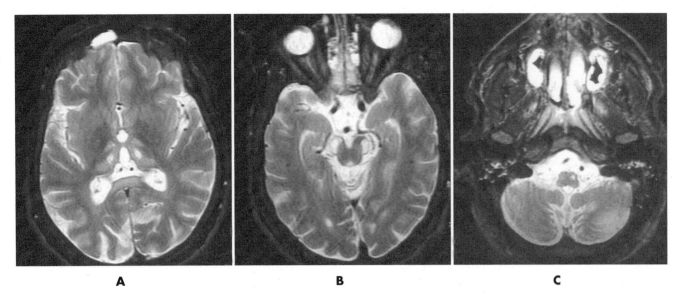

Fig. 8-35   Degenerative unspecified disorder, but if you have a clue we will let you author the third edition: Probable gangliosidosis. **A,** Thalamic high intensity, coupled with splenial bright signal, yet without atrophy in this child. **B,** The cerebral peduncles are bright bilaterally implying corticospinal tract degeneration yet the volume is maintained. **C,** The process extends into the medulla.

seizures, and vomiting (when not diagnosed early by screening tests). The normal maturation of the brain is often delayed, and myelination may be affected. Same old story: swelling first, then atrophy with abnormal myelination. Usually dietary manipulations and/or replacement therapies are effective in some return of function and control of the disease.

Krabbe disease   Krabbe disease, also referred to as globoid cell leukodystrophy (GLD), is due to galacto-cerebroside–beta-galactocerebrosidase deficiency. The gene for this disease has been mapped to chromosome 14. Cerebrosides from catabolized myelin cannot be degraded to galactose and ceramide in this condition and leads to harmful build-up of galactosylsphingosine

Table 8-7   Imaging findings in the mitochondrial disorders

Disorder	Inheritance	Deficient enzyme	CNS findings
MELAS syndrome	NK		Pseudostrokes, demyelination in cord
MERRF syndrome	NK		White matter demyelination, esp. superior cerebellar peduncles, posterior columns, gliosis
Kearns-Sayre syndrome	NK		Diffuse white matter disease, calcified basal ganglia, more cerebellar than cortical atrophy, retinopathy, ophthalmoplegia, microcephaly
Alpers' disease	AR	Cytochrome *c*-oxidase	Microcephaly, posterior cortical encephalomalacia, atrophy
Leigh's disease	AR	Pyruvate dehydrogenase	Periaqueductal gray and putaminal abnormal signal intensity, swollen caudate, low density in putamina on CT, demyelination, lactate MRS
Menkes' kinky hair disease	XR	Copper metabolism	Subdural effusions, irregular vascular lumina, atrophy, gliosis, increased wormian bones, infarcts, tortuous dilated vessels
Zellweger syndrome (cerebrohepatorenal syndrome)	AR		Abnormal neuronal migration (polymicrogyria, heterotopias, pachygyria), white matter disease, optic atrophy, decreased *N*-acetylaspartate level macrocephaly, open sutures, ventricular dilatation
Refsum's disease	AR	Phytanic acid-2-hydroxylase	Demyelination of spinal cord tracts, of the atrophy, abnormal signal intensity dentate nucleus

NK, not known.

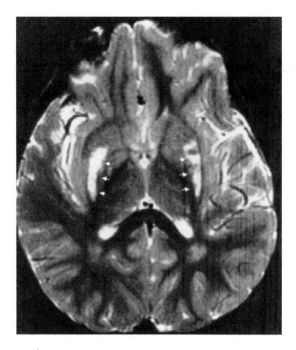

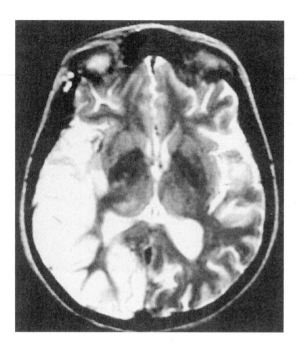

Fig. 8-36   Leigh disease. T2WI demonstrates bilateral symmetric putaminal high signal intensity *(arrows)*, which is characteristic of this disorder.

Fig. 8-37   MELAS syndrome. Observe the abnormally high signal intensity in the massively swollen cortex on the right side. Note that the area of abnormality spans the right middle cerebral artery and posterior cerebral artery distributions without affecting the basal ganglia.

cerebroside and psychosine in the brain parenchyma. When the disease presents before age 2 (the infantile form) the pyramidal tracts, cerebellar white matter, deep gray matter, posterior corpus callosum, and parietooccipital white matter are usually involved (as they are the first areas to myelinate). The U-fibers are gen-

erally spared. Hyperdensity of the thalami may be seen on CT. MRS findings include abnormally elevated choline and myoinositol (thought to be secondary to myelin breakdown products or phospholipid membrane metabolism). Atrophy will develop. There is a

Table 8-8   Imaging findings in amino acid disorders

Disorder	Inheritance	Deficient enzyme	Brain findings
Hyperglycinemia		Glycine metabolism	Microcephaly, atrophy, dysmyelination, corpus callosum anomalies
Maple syrup urine disease	AR	Branch-chain amino acid decarboxylase	Abnormal neuronal migration, acute edema after birth followed by atrophy at few months, demyelination of posterior white matter, dorsal midbrain edema, deep gray matter swelling, deep cerebellum, edema, MRS shows branch chain amino acids
Methylmalonic acidemia	AR	CoA carboxylase and/or mutase	Early swelling then atrophy, decreased density in white matter, basal ganglia (especially globus pallidus) injury, delayed myelination
Phenylketonuria	AR	Phenylalanine hydroxylase	White matter demyelination posteriorly (often optic radiations), neuronal migrational abnormalities, atrophy, cerebellar and brain stem high signal foci, basal ganglia calcification, atrophy
Proprionic acidemia	AR	CoA carboxylase	Atrophy, decreased density in white matter
Glutaric acidemia type II	AR	Acyl CoA dehydrogenase	Globus pallidus and white matter hyperintensities on T2WI, macrocephaly, atrophy (frontal/temporal) hydrodense basal ganglia, bat-wing dilatation of sylvian fissures, temporal arachnoid cysts

marked decrease in relative anisotropy of the affected white matter tracts identified on diffusion-weighted scans.

In the late-onset group, the same locations may be involved except for the cerebellar white matter and deep gray matter. The corticospinal tract is involved consistently (as it is in the infantile form). Splenial disease is also common in this form. The upper motor tract, corresponding to the lower extremity region, is affected to a greater extent than the regions that subserve the face and arms. Cerebral atrophy is present in early but not late disease. Optic atrophy is present in both varieties, although a report of optic nerve hypertrophy has also been published in a child with Krabbe disease. (Isn't it bad enough to have a neurodegenerative disorder, but to also have one with such a demeaning name? Double insult.) Treatment trials of stem cell transplantation have been encouraging. Successful treatment has corresponded with a trend toward increased relative anisotropy.

Patients with 3-hydroxy-3-methylglutaryl-coenzyme A lyase deficiency have a problem with leucine metabolism. They present with infantile hypoglycemia, acidosis, hepatomegaly, and mental status changes. A leukodystrophy with preferential involvement of the deeper arcuate fibers is seen on MR, which may simulate Canavan disease. Atrophy may coexist.

Glutaric acidemia may be suggested when one finds macrocephaly with open opercula and abnormally high signal in the basal ganglia especially the globus pallidus. Patients may present with encephalitis. Other imaging findings include atrophy, subarachnoid space dilatation anterior to the temporal lobes and basal ganglia volume loss.

Patients with methylenetetrahydrofolate reductase deficiency (a cause of hyperhomocystinemia) may show MR evidence of severe atrophy and hypomyelination. Proton MR spectroscopy reveals reduction of NAA. Treatment with betaine may reverse these findings. Homocystinuria is a different disease caused by cystathionine beta synthase deficiency, mapped to chromosome 21. The resultant high plasma levels of homocysteine result in multiple thrombotic events, including strokes. Premature atherosclerosis occurs. The thromboses may be either arterial or venous. The presence of lens subluxations might suggest a diagnosis of Marfan syndrome but those with homocystinuria are up and in and those with Marfan disease are down and out. Other neuroradiologic findings may include optic atrophy, osteoporosis, cata-racts, scoliosis, and biconcave vertebral bodies.

In maple syrup urine disease (secondary to abnormal decarboxylation of branched chain amino acids) an ultrasound study may show symmetric increase of echogenicity of periventricular white matter, basal ganglia (mainly pallidi), and thalami. CT and MR show diffuse edema in similar locations as well as in the cerebellum and capsular regions. Delayed myelination is present. MRS may show a peak at 0.9 ppm representing the branched chain amino acid peaks.

Propionic acidemia (PPA) and methylmalonic acidemia (MMA) are inherited disorders of the tricarboxylic cycle caused by enzymatic defects, which can lead to metabolic acidosis. These diseases are detected within the first month of life as babies have feeding difficulties, muscular hypotonia, choreoathetosis, microcephaly, and seizures. The disease occurs more frequently in patients from Saudi Arabia where it is transmitted as an autosomal recessive disorder (though can be seen with biotin and/or cobalamin deficiency also). Atrophy and abnormal white matter signal with delayed myelination are seen at conventional MRI. Basal ganglionic lesions (typically in the globus pallidus in MMA and in globus pallidus, caudates, and putamina in PPA) after one year of age may appear. The etiology is unclear, probably on a demyelinationstatus spongiosus basis, and sometimes they resolve (Fig. 8-38). Lactate peaks may be seen on proton MRS. Children who have methylmalonic or propionic acidemia may evidence widening of sulci and fissures in the first year of life. These two entities look alike except that low-density white matter is present in PPA but not in MMA. Delays in myelination are more evident in MMA.

Patients with 3-hydroxy-3-methylglutaryl coenzyme A lyase deficiency may show a diffuse mild abnormality in signal intensity of the cerebral white matter.

L-Carnitine deficiency is a rare metabolic disorder leading to cerebral infarctions in children, associated with hypoglycemia and myopathy.

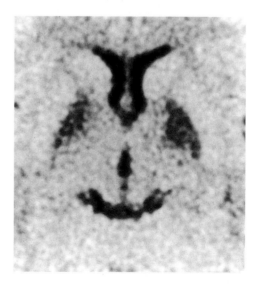

Fig. 8-38   Methylmalonic acidemia. Low density in the globus pallidus bilaterally is seen on this CT. Although one might have suspected carbon monoxide poisoning, in fact, this patient had methylmalonic acidemia.

Lysosomal Disorders

In Salla disease, a lysosomal storage disease process, cerebral myelination process is defective and may show centrifugally progressive destruction. The corpus callosum is thinned.

Juvenile neuronal ceroid lipofuscinosis is a lysosomal neurodegenerative disorder caused by the accumulation of lipopigment in neurons. Volume loss of the CNS, most prominently in the cerebellum, hypointense thalami and hyperintense periventricular white matter on T2WI, and proton MRS spectra revealing reduced NAA and increased myoinositol and glutamate/glutamine characterize this disorder. The neonatal form of this disease is associated with microcephaly, visual deficits, atrophy after the first year of life, hyperdense thalami on CT, and hypointense thalami on T2WI. Periventricular high-signal rims are seen after one year of life. Hypointensity of the thalami and basal ganglia and peritrigonal CSF-like hyperintensities on T2W scans are also seen.

When evaluating a patient's vents
See if the third looks tense
When the sulci are small
Give your surgeon a call
Place a shunt or prepare your legal defense.

The neurologist was in a fright
DAT was such a plight
But the gait was apraxic
ETOH made him ataxic
And MR provided no further insight.

A single nip of gin
Is certainly worth the sin
Since it keeps our sulci thin
But used to nimiety
It causes global atrophy
And affects our present company.

SUGGESTED READINGS

Aisen AM, Martel W, Gabrielsen TO, et al: Wilson disease of the brain: MR imaging, *Radiology* 157:137-141, 1985.

Bradley WG Jr, Whittemore AR, Kortman KE, et al: Marked CSF flow void: an indicator of successful shunting in patients with suspected normal pressure hydrocephalus, *Radiology* 178:459-466, 1991.

Brismar J, Gascon GG, von Steyern KV, Bohlega S: Subacute sclerosing panencephalitis: evaluation with CT and MR, *AJNR* 17:761-772, 1996.

Brismar J, Ozand PT: CT and MR of the brain in disorders of the propionate and methylmalonate metabolism, *AJNR* 15:1459-1473, 1994.

Brismar J, Ozand PT: CT and MR of the brain in glutaric acidemia type I: a review of 59 published cases and a report of 5 new patients, *AJNR* 16:675-683, 1995.

Brunberg JA: Hyperintense basal ganglia on T1-Weighted MR in a patient with Langerhans cell histiocytosis [letter; comment], *AJNR* 17:1193-1194, 1996.

Cohn MC, Hudgins PA, Sheppard SK, et al: Pre- and postoperative MR evaluation of stereotactic pallidotomy [see comments], *AJNR* 19:1075-1080, 1998.

De Haan J, Grossman RI, Civitello L, et al: High-field magnetic resonance imaging of Wilson's disease, *J Comput Tomogr* 11:132-135, 1987.

Dotti MT, Federico A, Signorini E, et al: Cerebrotendinous xanthomatosis (van Bogaert-Scherer-Epstein disease): CT and MR findings, *AJNR* 15:1721-1726, 1994.

Engelbrecht V, Rassek M, Huismann J, Wendel U: MR and proton MR spectroscopy of the brain in hyperhomocysteinemia caused by methylenetetrahydrofolate reductase deficiency, *AJNR* 18:536-539, 1997.

Engelbrecht V, Rassek M, Preiss S, et al: Age-dependent changes in magnetization transfer contrast of white matter in the pediatric brain, *AJNR* 19:1923-1929, 1998.

Falcone S, Quencer RM, Bowen B, et al: Creutzfeldt-Jakob disease: focal symmetrical cortical involvement demonstrated by MR imaging, *AJNR* 13:403-406, 1992.

Fariello G, Dionisi-Vici C, Orazi C, et al: Cranial ultrasonography in maple syrup urine disease, *AJNR* 17:311-315, 1996.

Frisoni GB, Beltramello A, Bianchetti A, Trabucchi M: Hippocampal atrophy as detected by width of the temporal horn is greater in Alzheimer dementia than in nondementing cognitive impairment [letter], *AJNR* 18:1192-1193; discussion 1193-1195, 1997.

Frisoni GB, Beltramello A, Weiss C, et al: Linear measures of atrophy in mild Alzheimer disease, *AJNR* 17:913-923, 1996.

Frisoni GB, Bianchetti A, Trabucchi M, Beltramello A: The added value of neuroimaging for diagnosing dementia [letter], *AJNR* 20:947-949, 1999.

Frisoni GB, Pizzolato G, Geroldi C, et al: Dementia of the frontal type: neuropsychological and [99Tc]-HM-PAO SPET features, *J Geriatric Psychiatr Neurol* 8:42-48, 1995.

Gallucci M, Bozzao A. Splendiani A, et al: Wernicke encephalopathy: MR findings in five patients, *AJNR* 11:887-892, 1990.

Gaul HP, Wallace CJ, Auer RN, Fong TC: MR findings in methanol intoxication, *AJNR* 16:1783-1786, 1995.

George AE, de Leon MJ, Golomb J, et al: Imaging the brain in dementia: expensive and futile? *AJNR* 18:1847-1850,1997.

George AE, DeLeon MJ, Stylopoulos LA, et al: CT diagnostic features of Alzheimer's disease: importance of the choroidal/hippocampal fissure complex, *AJNR* 11:101-107, 1990.

Georgy BA, Snow RD, Brogdon BG, Wertelecki W: Neuroradiologic findings in Marinesco-Sjögren syndrome, *AJNR* 19:281-283, 1998.

Harris GJ, Aylward EH, Peyser CE, et al: Single photon emission computed tomographic blood flow and magnetic resonance volume imaging of basal ganglia in Huntington's disease, *Arch Neurol* 53:316-324, 1996.

Harris GJ, Lewis RF, Satlin A, et al: Dynamic susceptibility contrast MR imaging of regional cerebral blood volume in

Alzheimer disease: a promising alternative to nuclear medicine, *AJNR* 19:1727-1732, 1998.

Harris GJ, Schlaepfer TE, Peng LW, et al: Magnetic resonance imaging evaluation of the effects of ageing on grey-white ratio in the human brain, *Neuropathol Appl Neurobiol* 20:290-293, 1994.

Inoue E, Hori S, Narumi Y, et al: Portal-systemic encephalopathy: presence of basal ganglia lesions with high signal intensity on MR images, *Radiology* 179:551-555, 1991.

Jinkins JR: Clinical manifestations of hydrocephalus caused by impingement of the corpus callosum on the fax: an MR study in 40 patients, *AJNR* 12:331-340, 1991.

Mirowitz SA, Westrich TJ, Hirsch JD: Hyperintense basal ganglia on T1 weighted MR images in patients receiving parenteral nutrition, *Radiology* 181:117-120, 1991.

Pearsen KD, Jean-Marton AD, Levy HL, et al: Phenylketonuria: MR imaging of the brain with clinical correlation, *Radiology* 177:437-440, 1990.

Petrella JR, Coleman RE, Doraiswamy PM: Neuroimaging and early diagnosis of Alzheimer disease: A look to the future, *Radiology* 226:315–336, 2003.

Rusinek H, de Leon MJ, George AE, et al: Alzheimer disease: measuring loss of cerebral gray matter with MR imaging, *Radiology* 178:109-114, 1991.

Seitz D, Grodd W, Schwab A, et al: MR imaging and localized proton MR spectroscopy in late infantile neuronal ceroid lipofuscinosis, *AJNR* 19:1373-1377, 1998.

Sonninen P, Autti T, Varho T, et al: Brain involvement in Salla disease, *AJNR* 20:433-443, 1999.

Thompson JE, Castillo M, Kwock L, et al: Usefulness of proton MR spectroscopy in the evaluation of temporal lobe epilepsy, *AJR* 170:771-776, 1998.

Thompson JE, Smith M, Castillo M, et al: MR in children with L-carnitine deficiency, *AJNR* 17:1585-1588, 1996.

van der Knaap MS, Bakker HD, Valk J: MR imaging and proton spectroscopy in 3-hydroxy-3-methylglutaryl coenzyme A lyase deficiency, *AJNR* 19:378-382, 1998.

van der Knaap MS, van Wezel-Meijler G, Barth PG, et al: Normal gyration and sulcation in preterm and term neonates: appearance on MR images, *Radiology* 200:389-396, 1996.

van Wassenaer-van Hall HN, van den Heuvel AG, Algra A, et al: Wilson disease: findings at MR imaging and CT of the brain with clinical correlation, *Radiology* 198:531-536, 1996.

van Wassenaer-van Hall HN, van den Heuvel AG, Jansen GH, et al: Cranial MR in Wilson disease: abnormal white matter in extrapyramidal and pyramidal tracts, *AJNR* 16:2021-2027, 1995.

Wippold FJ II, Gado MH, Morris JC, et al: Senile dementia and healthy aging: a longitudinal CT study, *Radiology* 179:215-219, 1991.

Yamaji S, Ishii K, Sasaki M, et al: Changes in cerebral blood flow and oxygen metabolism related to magnetic resonance imaging white matter hyperintensities in Alzheimer's disease, *J Nucl Med* 38:1471-1474, 1997.

Yamamoto T: Subthalamus versus substantia nigra [letter; comment], *AJNR* 16:613, 1995.

Yamanouchi N, Okada S, Kodama K, et al: White matter changes caused by chronic solvent abuse, *AJNR* 16:1643-1649, 1995.

CHAPTER 9

Congenital Disorders of the Brain and Spine

TIMING OF FORMATION OF CONGENITAL LESIONS

It is very important to understand the timing of congenital lesions in the brain and spine and how it is that one can get multiple spinal, supratentorial, and infratentorial anomalies all in the same individual. To put things very simply, the central nervous system (CNS) goes through a five stage process that includes dorsal induction (3 to 4 weeks), ventral induction (5 to 8 weeks), neuronal proliferation/differentiation/histogenesis (8 to 18 weeks), migration (12 to 22 weeks), and myelination (5 months fetal age to 2 years postnatal age).

Dorsal Induction

Under the rubric of dorsal induction, the brain undergoes primary and secondary neurulation, that is, turning a flat bed of cells into a round piece of brain and spinal cord.

Disorders of primary neurulation predominantly affect the spinal cord and include those due to adhesions between the inwardly oriented endoderm and the outer ectoderm. This is the presumed etiology for neurenteric cysts and diastematomyelia. If there is premature separation of the neuroectoderm and the cutaneous ectoderm, it is usually the fat that is left behind and fuses with the neuroectoderm. This produces the lipomyelocele, lipomyelomeningocele, and the intradural lipoma. If the separation never occurs, one gets persistent communication of the CNS with internal or external structures, hence cephaloceles, myeloceles, meningomyeloceles, anencephaly, exencephaly (brain outside the skull), craniorachischisis, (congenital fissure of the skull and spine) and dermal sinus tracts. These entities may be associated with the Chiari II malformation because the posterior fossa calvarium is developing at the same time.

Disorders of secondary neurulation generally affect the conus medullaris, filum terminale, and cauda equina. Lipomas of the filum, short thickened tethered fila and tethered cords, and caudal regression syndrome with sacral agenesis are usually listed under this category.

Ventral Induction

Holoprosencephaly represents the signature anomaly associated with failure of ventral induction. Because the premaxillary facial structures are formed in association with ventral induction, it is not uncommon to see cyclopia and probosci in patients with ventral induction failures (please do not comment on the authors' four eyes and large nose in this context!). Septooptic dysplasia and pituitary anomalies are also disorders of ventral induction.

Cerebellar development also occurs at the 5 to 15 week period of fetal development. Just as there is cerebral hemispheric development from neural tissue derived from the germinal matrix around the lateral ventricles, so too is cerebellar development dependent on the germinal matrix about the fourth ventricle. Because hemispheric development occurs before vermian devel-

opment, and the superior vermis forms before the inferior vermis, it is rare to see hemispheric anomalies without vermian maldevelopments and superior vermian lesions without associated inferior vermian anomalies. Inferior vermian hypoplasia may be seen in isolation. Those entities associated with vermian dysgenesis include the Dandy-Walker complex lesions (Dandy-Walker malformation, Dandy-Walker variant, and giant cisterna magna), rhombenencephalosynapsis, and Joubert syndrome.

Disorders of hemispheric development include hemispheric hypoplasia, but this is a rare bird more commonly seen with other supratentorial and vermian anomalies.

Neuronal Proliferation, Differentiation, and Histogenesis

Disorders of neuronal proliferation, differentiation, and histogenesis are disorders that occur because of abnormal proliferation such as microencephaly, macroencephaly, neurocutaneous syndromes, and aqueductal stenosis. Microencephaly occurs because of less brain tissue. In megalencephaly, one has marked overproduction of neurons. Primary causes include achondroplasia, Soto syndrome, and Beckwith-Wiedemann syndrome.

Neuronal Migration

Neuronal migrational anomalies are based on the centrifugal movement of neuroblasts and glioblasts. From the periventricular region, the neuroblasts are first to migrate and they take up residence in the molecular layer of cortical zone 1, the most peripheral of the gray matter zones. Cells (glioblasts and neuroblasts) from the intermediate zone then migrate in fanlike waves along radial glial fibers out to the periphery and then double back on themselves to first fill the sixth deepest layer of the cortex, followed by zones 5, 4, 3, and 2. You can imagine that this can get hectic with cells going this way and that passing each other in as close quarters as the Tokyo subway. Somehow, this is supposed to result in cortical organization, creating the many layers of the brain and mind. When this gets mixed up, one has pachygyria, polymicrogyria, schizencephaly, and the like.

Myelination

White matter, when myelinated, is bright on a T1WI and dark on a T2WI. The development of myelination is a complicated process but proceeds from posterior to anterior and from central to peripheral (Tables 9-1, 9-2). Barkovitch has done a good job in mapping normal myelination dates in term babies. In general, the white matter is seen to be myelinated earlier on T1 weighted images than on T2 weighted images for reasons that have to do with water content versus lipid content. It then

Table 9-1   Timing of myelination

Structure	T1-weighted scans	T2-weighted scans	FLAIR scans
Posterior limb internal capsule (posterior portion)	Birth	Birth–2 mo	3 mo
Dorsal brainstem	Birth	2–4 mo	3–5 mo
Cerebellar peduncles	Birth	Birth–2 mo	1–3 mo
Pre- and postcentral gyrus	Birth	2–3 mo	
Posterior limb internal capsule (anterior portion)	Birth–1 mo	4–7 mo	3–8 mo
Anterior limb internal capsule	2–3 mo	5–11 mo	8–11 mo
Cerebellar white matter	3 mo	3–5 mo	
Splenium	3–4 mo	4–6 mo	5 mo
Genu callosum	4–6 mo	5–8 mo	5 mo
Occipital white matter (central)	3–5 mo	9–14 mo	1, 12 mo
Frontal white matter (central)	4–6 mo	11–16 mo	2, 14 mo
Occipital white matter (peripheral)	6 mo	11–15 mo	
Frontal white matter (peripheral)	7–11 mo	13–18 mo	
Normal maturation	8–11 mo	14–18 mo	24 mo

takes a bit of wizardry to apply this to the premature infant. The chart attached is a good start for determining if there is delayed myelination.

Then along came fluid-attenuated inversion recovery (FLAIR) imaging to drive us insane. The signal intensity of white matter on FLAIR initially is dark because of the marked water content, turns brighter as the "watery brain" of infancy resolves, than again becomes dark as the white matter myelinates. The timing of these stages, summarized in Table 9-1, varies from structure to structure. The cerebellar peduncle and the posterior limb of the internal capsule, show high signal intensity relative to gray matter at birth. Thereafter, the white matter loses signal intensity with time and shows low signal intensity at 50 weeks and beyond. The unmyelinated white matter, including the frontal deep white matter, the occipital deep white matter, and the centrum semiovale, shows low signal intensity at birth, converts to high signal intensity at 20 to 30 weeks, and back to low signal intensity after 2 to 3 years of age.

It is useful to separate congenital disorders of the brain into those involving the supratentorial structures and those involving the infratentorial structures, because radiologists think in terms of anatomy rather than embryology. We synthesize information based on imaging findings and then think about developmental issues later.

Naturally, disorders can affect both spaces, but as an initial classification scheme, this may be helpful. In addition, in a newborn infant, separating the lesions into those that are cystic and those that are solid is of some help in arriving at a differential diagnosis. Clinical information is also useful in distinguishing among various congenital abnormalities, because several disorders also have associated cutaneous, ocular, or metabolic abnormalities.

Congenital anomalies strike fear in parents both prenatally and postnatally. Parents wonder, "Is my child normal?" from the first sonogram to postgraduate school and beyond. Therefore, it is important to consider the prognostic implications of each entity and the potential for correction. We do not have the luxury of sending the product back to the factory for replacement parts, an upgrade, or a second printing (needed in our case).

Table 9-2   Trends in myelination—for future general radiologists

Posterior to anterior
Central to peripheral
Motor to sensory
Inferior to superior
T1WI to T2WI
Immature to mature

SUPRATENTORIAL CONGENITAL LESIONS

Arachnoid Cysts

If you had to have a congenital lesion in the brain, this would be the lesion of choice. The arachnoid cyst is the most common congenital cystic abnormality in the brain. It consists of a cerebrospinal fluid (CSF) collection within layers of the arachnoid, which may distort the normal brain parenchyma.

The arachnoid cyst is typically a serendipitous finding and may not be symptomatic. The most common supratentorial locations for an arachnoid cyst are (in decreasing order of frequency) (1) the middle cranial fossa,

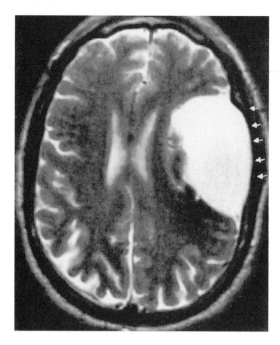

Fig. 9-1   Arachnoid cyst. T2WI at the level of the top of the lateral ventricle shows a CSF intensity collection that remodels the bone *(arrows)* and causes mild midline shift.

(2) perisellar cisterns, and (3) the subarachnoid space over the convexities (Fig. 9-1). Infratentorially (see discussion later in this chapter), arachnoid cysts commonly occur in the (1) retrocerebellar cistern, (2) cerebellopontine angle cistern, and (3) quadrigeminal plate cistern. Intraventricular cysts are rare (Fig. 9-2).

Computed tomographic (CT) scans demonstrate a CSF density mass that typically effaces the adjacent sulci and may remodel bone. The mass measures from 0 to 20 Hounsfield units (HU) and shows no enhancement. In those difficult cases where an arachnoid cyst and a dilated subarachnoid space must be distinguished, one can instill intrathecal contrast to differentiate the cyst (which does not immediately fill with contrast) from the subarachnoid space (which immediately fills) (Fig. 9-3). Be careful though. In time, the arachnoid cyst will imbibe contrast.

On magnetic resonance (MR) imaging the most common appearance is that of an extraaxial mass that has signal intensity identical to CSF on most pulse sequences. Occasionally, the signal intensity may be greater than that of CSF on the proton density-weighted images (PDWI) because of the stasis of fluid within the cyst as opposed to the pulsatile CSF of the ventricular system and subarachnoid space. FLAIR and DWI scans usually show a dark mass similar in intensity to CSF (again pulsation effects may cause some higher intensity). Rarely, the fluid within the arachnoid cyst may be of higher protein content than that of the CSF, accounting for the difference in the signal intensity.

The differential diagnosis of an arachnoid cyst is limited and generally revolves around three other diagnoses: a subdural hygroma, dilatation of normal subarachnoid space secondary to underlying atrophy or encephalomalacia, and epidermoid (Fig. 6-1, Fig. 9-4, and Table 9-3). Although subdural hygromas have been thought to be due to chronic CSF leaks through traumatized lep-

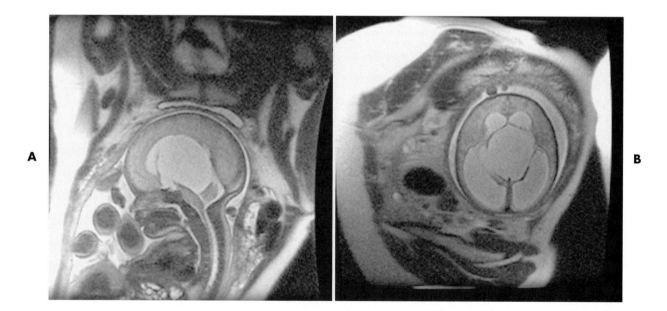

Fig. 9-2   Fetal imaging of an arachnoid cyst. **A,** The in utero MR defined an arachnoid cyst of the third ventricle, which was misinterpreted by our Sonar operators as hydrocephalus or scud missiles in the Kuwaiti desert. Treated intrauterine and baby did well. **B,** There was hydrocephalus but the ballooning of the third ventricle was the cyst itself.

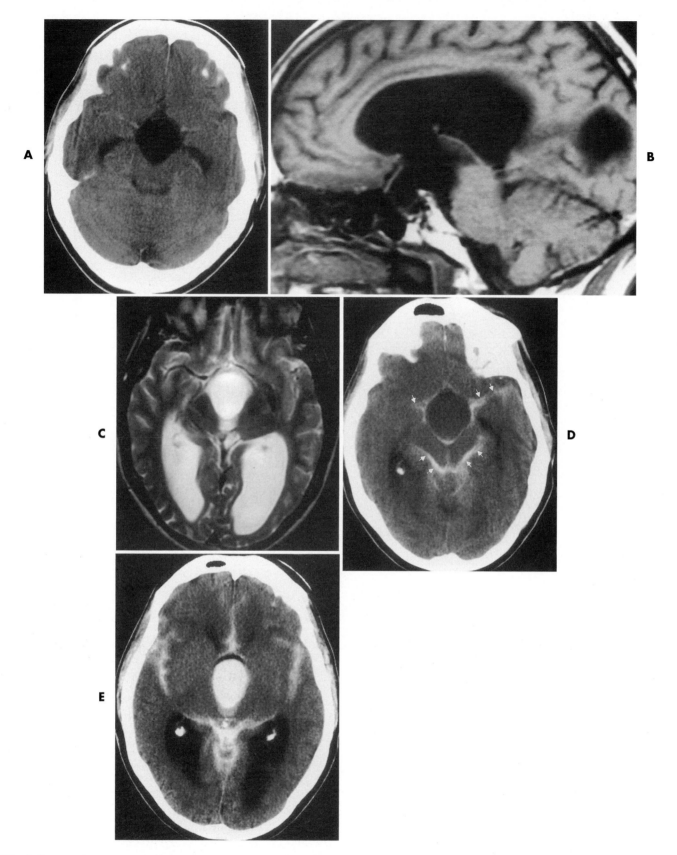

Fig. 9-3 Arachnoid cyst of third ventricle. **A,** Initial unenhanced CT scan showed a cystic mass widening the third ventricle. The sagittal T1WI **(B)** showed a mass with the same intensity as cerebrospinal fluid that appears to communicate with the lateral ventricular system and extend into the sella. T2W scan **(C)** showed the lesion to have the same signal intensity as CSF. **D,** Intrathecal contrast was administered from a lumbar approach and the contrast was allowed to flow superiorly to the intracranial compartment. The initial CT scan showed minimal filling of the cyst (only apparent to the Professor). Contrast material is in the subarachnoid space *(arrows).* **E,** On delayed axial scans the cyst filled with contrast. This is characteristic of an arachnoid cyst.

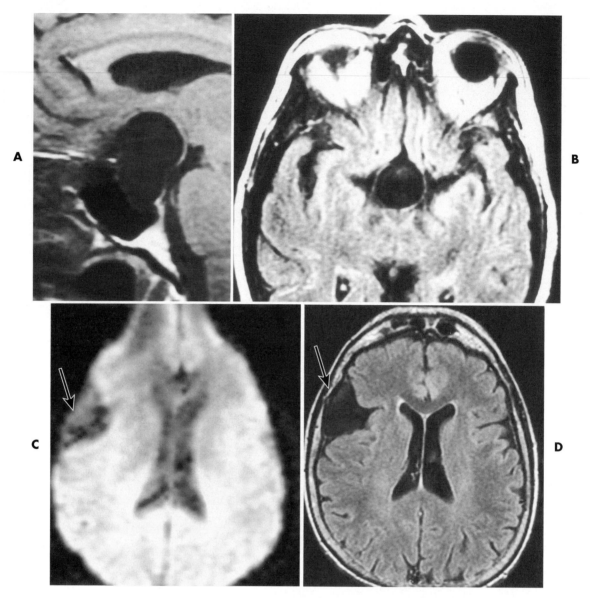

Fig. 9-4   Arachnoid cyst. This collection has the same intensity as CSF on sagittal T1WI **(A)** and axial FLAIR **(B)** scans. Diffusion weighted **(C)** and FLAIR **(D)** scans in a different case has the lesion *(arrow)* with the same isointensity to CSF.

tomeninges, in most cases the trauma results in sufficient blood deposited within the "hygroma" so that the signal intensity on T1WI and FLAIR is different from that of CSF. In addition, subdural hygromas are typically crescentic in shape whereas arachnoid cysts tend to have convex borders. Both efface sulci and show mass effect. In contradistinction, dilatation of the subarachnoid space secondary to underlying encephalomalacia does not demonstrate mass effect and the adjacent sulci are enlarged. Another distinguishing feature is the fact that the cerebral veins in the subarachnoid space are seen to course through the CSF in the case of underlying encephalomalacia, as opposed to the subdural hygroma and arachnoid cyst, where the veins are displaced inward. An epidermoid may simulate an arachnoid cyst on CT

and T2WI, however FLAIR scanning and diffusion weighted imaging (DWI) nicely shows higher signal intensity than CSF. In fact, the T1WI will often also be brighter than CSF and will be obvious to those who are not "neuroradiologically challenged."

A feature, often seen in association with arachnoid cysts, that may suggest the diagnosis is bony scalloping. The bone may be thinned or remodeled, probably because of transmitted pulsations and/or slow growth. This would not be seen with hygromatous collections or atrophy. However, the finding may be seen occasionally in epidermoids or porencephaly, where the ventricular pulsations are transmitted through the porencephalic cavity to the inner table of the skull (Fig. 8-21). When arachnoid cysts are seen in the middle cranial fossa, the

Table 9-3   Arachnoid cyst vs. subdural hygroma, epidermoid, encephalomalacia

Feature	Arachnoid cyst	Subdural hygroma	Epidermoid	Widened CSF spaces as result of atrophy*
Intensity	Isointense to CSF on all sequences	Hyperintense to CSF on T1WI	Hyperintense on FLAIR, slightly hyperintense to CSF on T1	Isointense to CSF on all sequences
Vein location	Pushed inward	Pushed inward	Nondisplaced; epidermoids envelop vascular structures	Coursing through CSF
Mass effect	Positive	Positive	Positive	Negative
Bone remodeling	Present	Absent	Intradural epidermoids slowly remodel bone; intradiploic epidermoids have beveled edges	Absent
Sulci	Flattened	Flattened	Grows into sulcal space	Enlarged
Intrathecal contrast	Delayed opacification	Does not opacify	Outlines mass	Immediate opacification
DWI	Dark	Variable	Bright	Dark
Ca++/FAT	(−/−)	(+/−)	(+−/+−)	(−/−)

*Includes large cisterna magna.

temporal lobe may be hypoplastic (Fig. 9-5). In fact, it is unclear which came first, the hypoplastic temporal lobe or the arachnoid cyst or the chicken or the egg (get the yolk?). To recapitulate, absence of soft-tissue intensity or density, calcification, or fat distinguishes these cysts from those of the dermoid-epidermoid line.

Pineal cysts are discussed in Chapter 3.

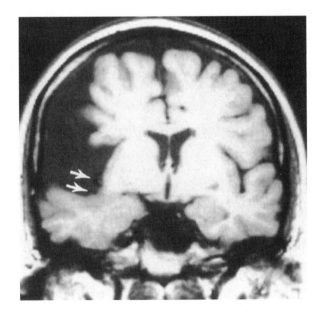

Fig. 9-5   Arachnoid cyst and temporal lobe hypoplasia. Coronal T1WI shows a right-sided arachnoid cyst that displaces the blood vessels inward *(arrows)* and that is associated with hypoplasia of the right temporal lobe.

Rathke Cleft Cysts

Rathke cleft cysts are embryologic remnants of Rathke's pouch, the neuroectoderm that ascends from the oral cavity to the sellar region to form the pituitary anterior lobe and pars intermedia. These cysts are lined with a single layer of cuboidal or columnar cells and may arise within the sella, the suprasellar region, or most commonly both. They occur in up to 13% of autopsy studies of the sella. The cysts can compress normal posterior or anterior pituitary tissue to cause symptoms of hypopituitarism, diabetes insipidus, headache, and visual field deficits but are usually asymptomatic. The cysts are well-defined masses that on MR may have high or low signal intensity on T1WI and high signal intensity on T2WI, and on CT are hypodense and most often nonenhancing (Fig. 11-31). Intracystic, yellow waxy solid nodules have recently been reported in Rathke cysts containing cholesterol and/or mucinous proteins probably accounting for the bright signal on T1WI in some cysts. The differential diagnosis is a craniopharyngioma or hemorrhagic pituitary gland; the presence of calcification, soft-tissue mass, and/or areas of enhancement would lead one away from Rathke cleft cyst as the diagnosis (see Chapter 11). Treatment is cyst aspiration and/or removal with little chance of recurrence.

Meningoencephaloceles

A meningocele is a congenital malformation in which the meninges protrude through the bony confines. As

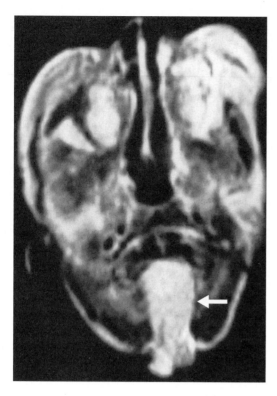

Fig. 9-6 Occipital encephalocele. Axial T2WI shows protrusion of meninges *(arrow)* at the foramen magnum-C1 region. Patient had this lesion at birth.

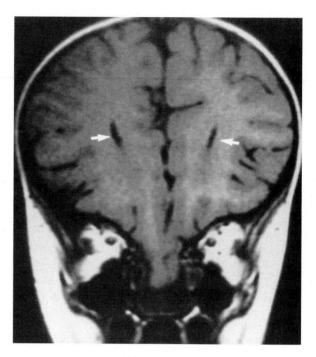

Fig. 9-7 Anterior basal encephalocele. Coronal T1WI demonstrates inferior misplacement of the medial frontal lobes and gyrus rectus into the nasal cavity with hypertelorism. Wide frontal horns *(arrows)* suggest corpus callosum agenesis.

opposed to encephaloceles, meningoceles do not include brain tissue within the protrusion. Usually, an encephalocele also contains meninges, so it should really be called a meningoencephalocele, but that is too many syllables for most neurosurgeons. In fact, they have become resigned to use the shortened noun cephalocele. The terms are used interchangeably in this chapter for confusion's sake. Meningoceles are rarer than encephaloceles. The most common location for meningoencephaloceles associated with Chiari III malformations is the occipital region. These may also be associated with holoprosencephaly, and aqueductal stenosis (Fig. 9-6). In the United States, parietal (10%) and frontal (9%) meningoencephaloceles are the next most common locations for this abnormality. Vietnamese and Southeast Asian women have a propensity for nasofrontal or sphenoethmoidal meningoencephaloceles (Fig. 9-7). The diagnosis of meningoencephalocele is often made clinically when the protrusion is through the occipital, parietal, or frontal region. On the other hand, nasofrontal or sphenoethmoidal encephaloceles may be clinically occult and may have a wide clinical differential diagnosis when seen through a nasoscope. Otorhinolaryngologists will love you if you let them know that the polyp they plan to remove from the nasal vault is actually the *frontal lobe.* Brownie points. The anterior meningoencephaloceles have a higher rate of associated anomalies such as

agenesis of the corpus callosum, colobomas, and cleft lips.

Encephaloceles may also be suspected when one sees enlargement of a basal neural foramen. An MR study will usually discern that there is herniated brain and/or CSF in the hole (Fig. 9-8). There often is a distortion of the adjacent brain tissue with maloriented white matter tracts.

On CT the meningocele is seen as a CSF-density protrusion through a bony defect in the calvarium (Fig. 9-9). MR scans demonstrate continuity of the meningocele with the underlying leptomeninges. The critical task is to find the abnormality; secondarily one should tell the surgeons whether brain tissue is protruding through the defect. For this reason MR, with its superior soft-tissue resolution, is the primary study in this evaluation. The brain tissue within the meningoencephalocele typically has the signal intensity of normal brain. However, occasionally one may see heterotopic or disorganized brain tissue, which has a more heterogeneous signal intensity.

Neuroepithelial Cysts

Neuroepithelial cysts may arise within the ependyma of the ventricular system. Although lateral ventricular cysts are most common, often associated with the glomus of the trigone, they may also occur in the other ventricles. Typically, they follow CSF intensity, however,

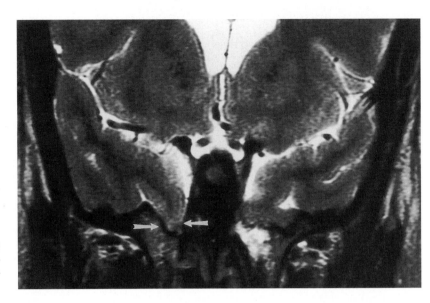

Fig. 9-8   Basal cephalocele. Seizures were the presenting symptom in this patient with a right temporal encephalocele, which was herniating *(arrows)* into the basisphenoid.

they may be bright on T1WI owing to high protein, mucin, cholesterol, or viscous content. The lining of this cyst is epithelial (duh-uh) and they are thought to arise from ectoderm. Differential diagnoses might include epidermoid cysts, cysticercosis, or echinococcal cysts.

Anencephaly

Anencephaly means no brain. In the course of your daily life you probably will run into several people you believe to be adult anencephalics—this is a misdiagnosis; these persons are probably just pneumocephalics (airheads) or have cranio-rectal inversion (anusencephaly). Other pejorative terms are usually applied; however, our editors have restrained us.

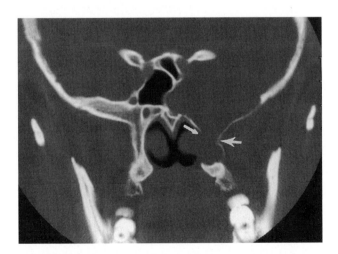

Fig. 9-9   Meningocele. Coronal CT scan image demonstrates a defect in the skull base on the right side *(arrows)* with remodeling of the bone indicative of a long-standing process. This represented a meningocele coming from the floor of the right middle cranial fossa.

Anencephaly should now be a diagnosis made prenatally because most women are screened relatively early in pregnancy for elevated levels of serum α-fetoprotein, a marker of neural tube defects. The diagnosis by obstetric ultrasound (US) is made when the cranial vault is seen to be small, with only the fetus's face and posterior fossa well seen (Fig. 9-10). Only a nubbin of tissue is seen at the skull base on ultrasound, and amniotic fluid α-fetoprotein levels are elevated. These babies do not do well and may be allowed to die if the diagnosis is not made prenatally. An association with spinal dysraphism exists.

Hydranencephaly

Hydranencephaly has the appearance of absence of that part of the brain supplied by anterior and middle cerebral arteries. The parts of the brain supplied by the posterior circulation are preserved, so the posterior temporal lobes, occipital lobes, thalami, and infratentorial structures are well formed. The brain stops there. In place of the remainder of the brain is a CSF-contained space (Fig. 9-11). The chief differential diagnosis is termed "maximal" hydrocephalus (severe hydrocephalus with a thin cortical mantle plastered against the sides of the calvarium) (Fig. 9-12). This will also usually affect the occipital region as opposed to hydranencephaly. To detect this thin rim of cortical tissue, MR is probably more accurate than CT. Shunting is the treatment for maximal hydrocephalus; some return of function may occur with shunting. With hydranencephaly, no treatment is effective. Bad brain: bad prognosis.

Holoprosencephaly

Holoprosencephaly (Table 9-4) refers to a constellation of congenital abnormalities where separation of the

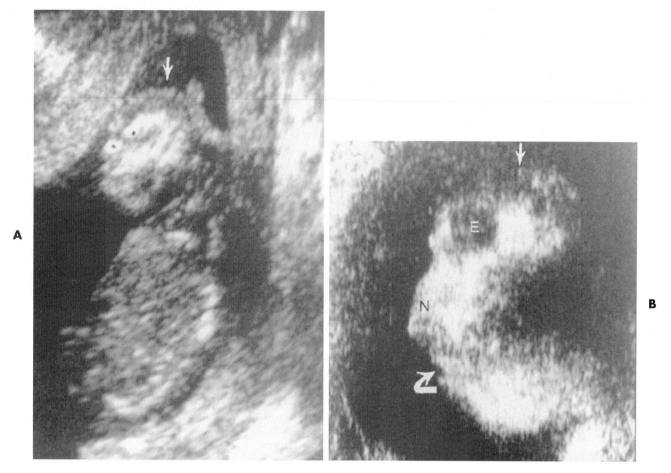

Fig. 9-10   Anencephaly. **A,** Obstetric US shows lack of development of the cranial vault *(arrow)* in this fetus. Eyes are marked by *asterisks.* **B,** Profile view of the face of the fetus shows nondevelopment of the skull *(arrow)* above the eye *(E). N,* nose; *(curved arrow),* mouth. (Compliments of Peggy Brennecke, M.D.)

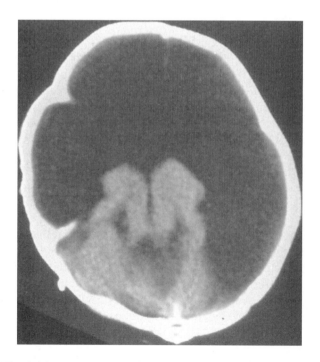

Fig. 9-11   Hydranencephaly. Axial CT shows absence of brain tissue in the anterior and middle cerebral artery distributions with preservation of the brain stem and cerebellum.

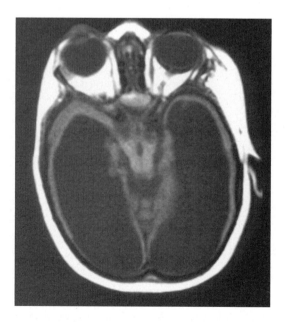

Fig. 9-12   Maximal hydrocephalus. The presence of a cortical mantle peripherally and bilaterally suggests that this case represents maximal hydrocephalus and NOT hydranencephaly.

Table 9-4   Holoprosencephaly variants

Feature	Lobar	Semilobar	Alobar
Facial deformities (cyclopia)	None	None to minimal	Yes
Falx cerebri posteriorly	Anterior tip missing or dysplastic	Absent	Present
Thalami	Separated	Partially fused	Fused
Interhemispheric fissure	Formed	Present posteriorly	Absent
Dorsal cyst	No	No	Yes
Frontal horns	Yes, but unseparated	No	No
Septum pellucidum	Absent	Absent	Absent
Vascular	Normal	Normal except rudimentary deep veins	Azygous ant. cerebral artery, absent venous sinuses and deep veins
Splenium	Present	Posterior may be present w/o genu or body	Absent
3rd ventricle	Normal	Small	Absent
Occipital horns	Normal	Partially formed	Absent

right and left cerebral hemispheres is incomplete (Fig. 9-13). The range of this disorder includes a minor form, lobar holoprosencephaly, in which separation of the cerebral hemispheres and lateral ventricles is near normal but formation of an interhemispheric fissure and cerebral falx is incomplete. Even in the mildest of forms you may see fusion of the hypothalamus, cingulum, and caudate nuclei. The frontal horns are closely apposed to each other, with partial fusion of frontal lobes. The most severe form is designated alobar holoprosencephaly, which demonstrates almost no separation of the cerebral hemispheres and ventricles. One is left with a single large ventricle with a horseshoe-shaped appearance (monoventricle) (Fig. 9-14). No interhemispheric fissure,

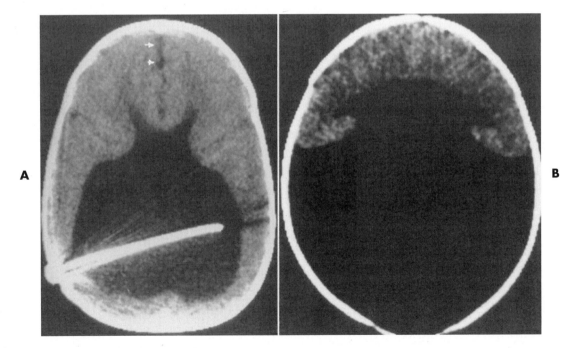

Fig. 9-13   Holoprosencephaly. **A,** Interhemispheric fissure anteriorly is well formed; however, posteriorly the ventricles expand into a monoventricle with a shunt tube within it. Although we asked the surgeon to remove the drainage tube for the figure, more level heads (scaphocephalics) prevailed. Relatively well-developed anterior hemispheric fissure *(arrows)* suggests lobar holoprosencephaly. Note that no falx is seen. **B,** Monoventricle with no septum pellucidum or interhemispheric separation in a patient with alobar holoprosencephaly.

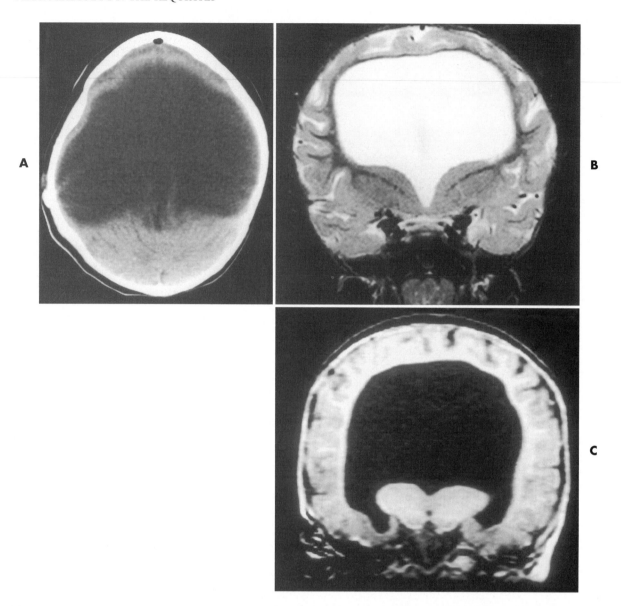

Fig. 9-14   Alobar holoprosencephaly. **A,** The monoventricle is seen on CT with a small cortical mantle peripherally. No falx or hemispheric separation is evident. **B,** Coronal T2WI shows the absence of hemispheric separation except at the lamina terminalis level. **C,** Fusion of the thalami more posteriorly.

falx, or significant separation of the hemispheric structures is identified. The basal ganglia and thalami are fused, and the septum pellucidum and corpus callosum are absent. Because one needs an interhemispheric fissure to form the corpus callosum, it is not surprising that this is commonly absent in patients with holoprosencephaly. Similarly, a dorsal cyst will interfere with callosal formation in holoprosencephaly. Between the two extremes of lobar and alobar holoprosencephaly is semilobar holoprosencephaly (like ex-president Clinton who hugged the center . . . among other things), in which there is partial development of the falx and the interhemispheric fissure (with partial separation of the lateral

ventricles) (Fig. 9-15). The basal ganglia and thalami are still fused. These abnormalities are associated with rather severe mental retardation, microencephaly, hypotelorism, and abnormal facies. The finding of a solitary median maxillary central incisor is also indicative of holoprosencephaly.

The CT findings in cases of holoprosencephaly include the absence or partial formation of the falx, interhemispheric fissure, and lateral ventricles. Patients typically have absence of the corpus callosum and an abnormally formed third ventricle. MR is a useful first study to examine patients with holoprosencephaly, because the evaluation of the corpus callosum, third ventricle, venous si-

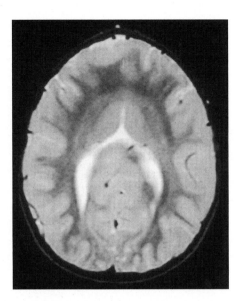

Fig. 9-15   Semilobar holoprosencephaly. The posterior hemispheres are separated and the falx is implied to be present. The posterior ventricles look nearly normal but there is no development of the frontal horns. Fusion across the midline is seen anteriorly.

nuses, vascular abnormalities, and septum pellucidum are better evaluated with MR. The olfactory bulbs and tracts are usually absent with lack of development of olfactory sulci and flat gyri recti. Associations with holoprosencephaly are listed in the Box 9-1

Often you must distinguish alobar holoprosencephaly from hydranencephaly and "maximal" hydrocephalus. If no cortical mantle is discernible around the dilated CSF space centrally, the diagnosis is hydranencephaly, especially if all that can be seen is a nubbin of occipital or posterior temporal cortex remaining with a falx present. If you see a well-formed falx, cortical mantle, and separated ventricles with a septum pellucidum, suggest maximal hydrocephalus. If the thalami are fused, septum pellucidum, or falx is absent, a cortical mantle is seen, and the ventricles have lost their usual shape, diagnose alobar holoprosencephaly.

A pearl: Holoprosencephaly is the one lesion where the splenium and posterior portions of the corpus cal-

Box 9-1   Associations with Holoprosencephaly
Caudal agenesis
DiGeorge syndrome
Fetal alcohol syndrome
Kallmann syndrome
Maternal diabetes
Trisomy 13, 15, 18

losum may be formed, but the anterior corpus callosum is absent. Exception to this exceptional rule: the rostrum normally forms after the splenium.

Septooptic Dysplasia (de Morsier Syndrome)

Septooptic dysplasia is best considered as part of the spectrum of holoprosencephaly. As such, it represents a minor form of holoprosencephaly. The septum pellucidum is either absent (64%) or partially absent (36%), causing a squared-off appearance to the frontal horns of the lateral ventricles (Fig. 9-16). When the septum pellucidum is partially absent, usually the anterior portion is present. This is best seen on coronal MR. Agenesis of the corpus callosum and white matter hypoplasia may be associated with this abnormality. In general, patients with septooptic dysplasia demonstrate small hypoplastic optic nerves and a small optic chiasm resulting from the dysplastic optic pathways. In some cases that dysplasia may be limited to the optic disk and the nerves/chiasm may not be small. Patients often (60%) have hormonal abnormalities (usually diminished levels of growth hormone) related to the hypothalamic-pituitary axis abnormality. Check for pituitary gland hypoplasia. Seizures coexist. Effects on the visual pathway may range from blindness to normal vision, nystagmus to normal eye movements.

Schizencephaly (see section below) and neuronal migrational disorders may accompany septooptic dysplasia in 50% of cases. Patients with schizencephaly and septooptic dysplasia are more likely to have normal-sized ventricles, portions of the septum pellucidum spared, normal optic radiations, and seizures as a presentation. If schizencephaly does not coexist, hypoplasia of the white matter (evidenced by corpus callosum thinning

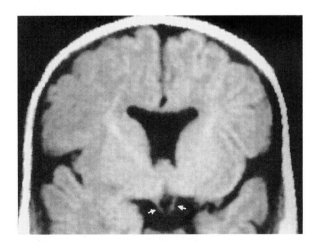

Fig. 9-16   Septooptic dysplasia. Coronal T1WI shows absence of the septum pellucidum with small optic tracts *(arrows).*

and ventricular enlargement), complete absence of the septum pellucidum, and worse hypothalamic-pituitary dysfunction usually are present.

Congenital Optic Nerve Hypoplasia

Congenital optic nerve hypoplasia commonly accompanies isolated growth hormone deficiency and multiple pituitary hormone deficiency syndromes. The absence of an anterior pituitary gland, a truncated pituitary stalk, and ectopic or absent posterior pituitary bright spot may also be found in this condition. Small optic nerves are a mandatory feature.

Schizencephaly

Schizencephaly refers to an abnormality of neuronal migration at the fifth to seventh week of gestation in which a cleft is seen coursing from the ventricular ependyma to the pial surface of the brain. This cleft has a gray matter lining (usually from polymicrogyric brain) and is usually seen in the supratentorial space (near the sylvian fissure) coursing to the lateral ventricles. The lips of the cleft may be apposed ("closed lipped") (Fig. 9-17) or gaping ("open lipped"). (As you would expect, the open-lipped variety is more interesting to the authors.) The closed-lipped variety may be missed if the clefts are tightly apposed, but a dimple at the ventricle-cleft interface should suggest the diagnosis. The cause of this disorder is thought to be an ischemic watershed insult in utero that leads to infarction of the germinal matrix and radial glial fibers near the ventricles. If there is failure of the germinal matrix to form, there will be fusion of the pia and the ependymal lining of the ventricles. Normal migration to the cortex is impeded. Other theories espoused as to etiology include toxin exposure, viral infections, and genetic factors. Schizencephaly is often associated with focal cortical dysplasia (polymicrogyria), gray matter heterotopias, agenesis of the septum pellucidum (80% to 90%), and pachygyria (see following sections). Some believe that focal cortical dysplasias are a form of schizencephaly or vice versa—just that the "cleft" never reaches the ventricle in the former. The lining of the cleft with gray matter, best seen on MR, is the differential point in this lesion and distinguishes it from encephalomalacic abnormalities (porencephaly), which are usually lined by white matter (Fig. 9-18). The inner surface of the cleft is pia-lined and communicates with the ependyma of the ventricle, which differentiates the lesion from an enlarged sylvian fissure seen in premature infants.

Schizencephaly occurs most commonly in the frontal (44%), frontoparietal (30%), and occipital (19%) lobes. Bilateral involvement (35% to 67%) is associated with seizures, worse developmental delay, and developmen-

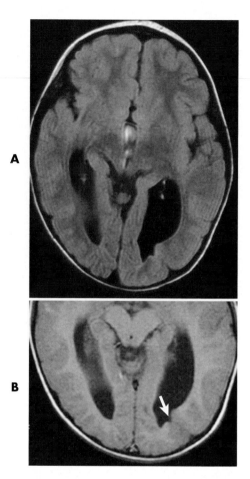

Fig. 9-17 Schizencephaly. **A,** Can you find the evidence of the closed lip schizencephaly on this FLAIR scan? **B,** The nipple at the ventricular surface *(arrow)* on the T1WI should eliminate any doubt.

tal dysphasia. Motor dysfunction is more common with frontal lobe schizencephaly, open-lipped varieties, and wider gaps in the open lips. Anomalous venous drainage may also be associated with schizencephalic brain.

Agenesis of the Corpus Callosum

Agenesis of the corpus callosum is one of the more common congenital abnormalities (occurring in 0.7% of all births). Patients with this anomaly often present with refractile seizures or mental retardation. The corpus callosum develops from anterior genu to posterior splenium, accounting for splenial absence in partial agenesis of the corpus callosum. The rostrum is the last portion of the corpus callosum to form, so the combination of absence of the splenium with rostrum agenesis should not put the neoneuroradiologist into a quandary. MR is ideal for the visualization of the corpus callosum because a midline sagittal image demonstrates all the portions of the corpus callosum (Box 9-2). Various degrees of corpus callosum agenesis may occur after complete agene-

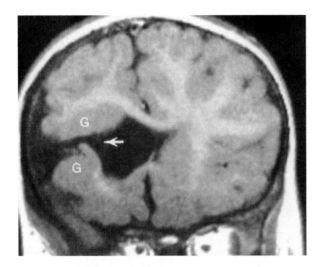

Fig. 9-18   Schizencephaly. Coronal T1WI reveals an open-lipped schizencephaly *(arrow)* connecting to the lateral ventricle. Note the gray matter-lined lips *(G)* of the cleft.

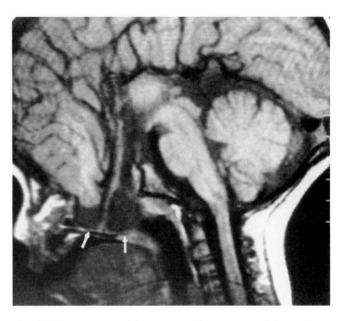

Fig. 9-19   Agenesis of the corpus callosum. Sagittal T1WI shows complete absence of the corpus callosum. Associated encephalocele in the nasofrontal region is identified by *arrows.*

sis, loss of the splenium is the next most common manifestation of this disorder (Fig. 9-19). If the splenium is absent, colpocephaly, dilatation of the occipital horns of the lateral ventricles caused by a decrease in the posterior white matter mass, is seen. With complete agenesis a high-riding, posteriorly oriented dilated third ventricle, parallel and widely spaced orientation of the lateral ventricles, and impression on the medial aspect of the lateral ventricles because of Probst bundles are seen. The longitudinal Probst bundle is a parallel track of white matter that runs anteroposteriorly and is due to the alternative white matter tract development when the corpus callosum (CC) is absent (Fig. 9-20). As the fibers can not cross, they redirect. (If the CC is not there, Probst beware.) The lateral ventricles (especially the occipital horns) are usually moderately dilated and concave medially, as is the third ventricle. Eversion of the cingulate

gyrus is also present and the cingulate sulci are therefore not formed. This leads to a picture on the sagittal midline image where the medical hemispheric sulci extend down to the third ventricle. The third ventricle, in turn, extends into the interhemispheric fissure.

Other midline abnormalities may be associated with agenesis of the corpus callosum (see Box 9-2) such as an interhemispheric arachnoid cyst in the expected location of the corpus callosum or a pericallosal lipoma. A cyst would have low density on CT and signal intensity comparable to CSF on T1WI and T2WI. This can be distinguished from a lipoma (Fig. 9-21), which has less than −30 HU on the CT and a density paralleling that of subcutaneous fat. On MR, a lipoma is bright on T1WI, with a decrease in the signal intensity on the conventional T2WI. Look for the chemical shift artifact at the fat-CSF-brain interface. Calcification around the borders of the lipoma may be identified on CT.

Associated congenital abnormalities include agyria, pachygyria, heterotopias, Dandy-Walker syndrome, holoprosencephaly, septooptic dysplasia, cephaloceles, and Chiari I and II malformations. Trisomy 13, 15, and 18, fetal alcohol syndrome, Meckel syndrome (occipital encephalocele, microcephaly, polycystic kidneys, polydactyly) are also associated with agenesis of the corpus callosum (and also with holoprosencephaly).

Aicardi syndrome is seen in female patients and consists of the triad of agenesis of the corpus callosum, epilepsy, and choroidal abnormalities. Abnormal myelination, neuronal migrational abnormalities, colobomas, posterior fossa cysts, and microphthalmia may coexist.

Box 9-2   Findings in Agenesis of Corpus Callosum

Colpocephaly
High-riding enlarged 3rd ventricle
Incomplete development of hippocampal formation
Interhemispheric cyst or lipoma
Medial impingement of Probst bundle on ventricles
Missing portions of corpus callosum
No cingulate sulcus with radially oriented fissures
   (eversion of cingulate gyrus) into the high riding
   3rd ventricle
Pointed crescent-shaped frontal horns
Septum pellucidum absent or widely separated

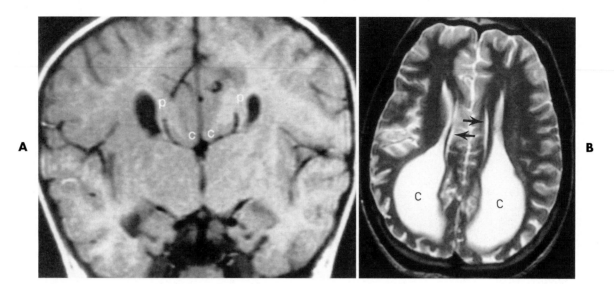

Fig. 9-20   Agenesis of the corpus callosum. **A,** Probst bundle in agenesis of corpus callosum. Coronal T1WI shows the Probst bundle *(P)* causing lateral displacement of the frontal horns of the lateral ventricles. Cingulate gyri *(C)* are malformed. **B,** The shape of the ventricles suggests agenesis of the corpus callosum with colpocephaly *(c)*. Probst bundles account for the inward bowing of the lateral wall of the lateral ventricle. Evagination of the cingulate sulcus *(arrows)* accounts for the high signal intensity medial to the lateral ventricles.

Hamartomas

Hamartomas represent an abnormal proliferation of normal brain tissue in an abnormal location. Whereas the heterotopias are due to anomalous neuronal migration, hamartomas are a nonneoplastic proliferation of well-organized brain tissue. There is a propensity for hamar-

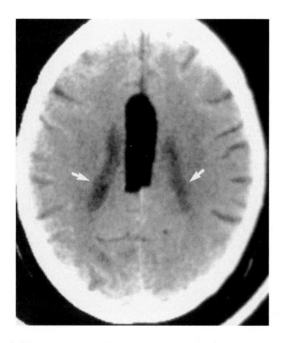

Fig. 9-21   Agenesis of the corpus callosum with a fatty lipoma. Axial CT reveals a low density lipoma in the midline associated with agenesis of the corpus callosum. Lateral splaying of the lateral ventricles *(arrows)* is the tip-off to the agenesis.

tomatous formation in the hypothalamus (Fig. 11-39). The patients typically present with precocious puberty; however, occasionally, visual disturbances may be present, because the hypothalamic hamartoma involves the optic pathways. Boys are more commonly affected than girls and symptoms may also include seizures and/or laughing spells (gelastic seizures). Because the tissue that makes up a hamartoma is essentially normal brain substance, the hamartoma is isodense with gray matter on CT. On MR, the hamartoma is isointense to gray matter on T1WI and variable on T2WI. The abnormality is identified as a bulbous protrusion of the hypothalamic region in the midline. The hamartomas do not have an abnormal blood-brain barrier and are not expected to show enhancement on either CT or MR. Occasionally, mass effect may be associated with the hamartoma as evidenced by displacement of the inferior portion of the third ventricle.

Hamartomas may occur in other locations. After the hypothalamic region, the next most common location for hamartomas is the cerebral cortex-subcortical region. Occasionally hamartomas may be seen in a periventricular location.

Fetus in fetu refers to duplication of brain structures, usually seen as an extraaxial frontal region mass. The signal intensity approaches that of normal brain. Case studies of ectopic brain in the nasopharynx or pterygopalatine fossa have also been reported.

There is some dispute about the cause of the abnormal areas of signal intensity that are seen on T2WI of the brain in patients with neurofibromatosis Type 1. These areas of abnormal signal are generally located in the deep gray matter structures, brain stem, and cerebellar peduncles. Although some people believe these lesions are heterotopias, others believe the areas of abnormality to be hamartomas. One study with pathologic "proof" even called these lesions "vacuolar or spongiotic change." Barkovich's text *Pediatric Neuroimaging*, 3rd edition refers to these lesions as myelin vacuolization in areas of dysplastic white matter. They appear in the first decade of life and regress in the second and third decades in patients with NF-1. Occasionally, growth or enhancement of one of these high intensity foci is detected, and when this occurs one must be concerned about the possibility of an astrocytoma instead. Patients with neurofibromatosis types 1 and 2 have increased incidences of gliomas in the brain (see discussion later in this chapter).

ABNORMALITIES OF NEURONAL MIGRATION

Heterotopias

Heterotopic brain is disorganized brain tissue, usually gray matter, that is located in the wrong place because of a premature arrest in neuronal migration from the germinal matrix to the cerebral cortex (Fig. 9-22). Patients usually have seizures, weakness, spasticity, hyperreflexia, or developmental delay. Heterotopias form as a result of an abnormality in neuronal migration at the seventh to sixteenth week of gestation, when migration of the neuroblasts from the periventricular region to the pia is thwarted, possibly because of damage to the radial glial fibers, which orient migrating neurons. The classification of heterotopias

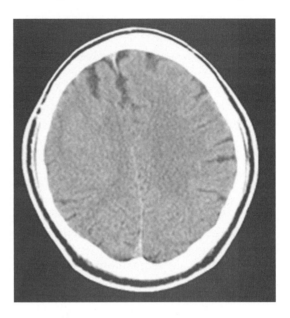

Fig. 9-22   Brain tumor...NOT! The first year fellow read the case as a low-grade glioma. No wonder our program is a two year fellowship. The absence of edema and the isodensity to gray matter should have suggested a gray matter heterotopia. That is an OK miss in August (1 month into fellowship), but a May reprimand for a first year fellow, and a "see you next year" at the CAQ's.

is usually divided into two varieties; nodular and band types. Under nodular types, you will find subependymal and subcortical variants. A subependymal location is very common, and these gray matter heterotopias are usually truly nodular in appearance (Fig. 9-23). Hyperintensity on

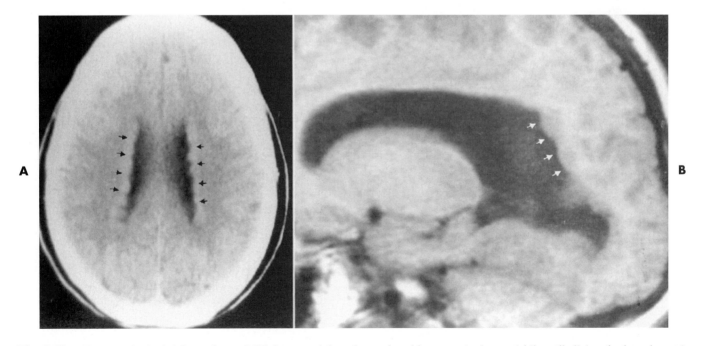

Fig. 9-23   Heterotopia. **A,** Axial unenhanced CT shows nodular subependymal heterotopia *(arrows)* bilaterally lining the lateral ventricle. This patient did not have tuberous sclerosis. **B,** Sagittal T1WI shows indentation of the lateral ventricle by gray matter nodules *(arrows)* from subependymal heterotopia. Tuberous sclerosis nodules have intensity similar to white matter.

T1WI may be due to dystrophic microcalcifications and these may show hyperdensity at CT. They may occur as an isolated anomaly or in association with other congenital lesions. A gene, responsible for the protein filamin-1, on the long arm of the X chromosome, has recently been implicated in some cases of nodular subependymal heterotopia.

Patients with subcortical heterotopias often have abnormal sulcation patterns superficial to the heterotopia. The hemisphere ipsilateral to the site of the subcortical heterotopia may be smaller with thinning of the overlying cortex. Subcortical heterotopias may be nodular or curvilinear in shape. The nodular variety of subcortical heterotopias are usually identified in a periventricular or subcortical location, whereas the diffuse (or laminar) heterotopias are seen more commonly in or close to the cortex. These lesions do not enhance and do not elicit edema.

The "band" type of heterotopias is associated with severe developmental delay and earlier onset of seizures than the focal type (Fig. 9-24). Once again that bloody X chromosome seems to be the source of the gene "doublecortin (XLIS)" which predisposes to lissencephaly in men (with our solitary X chromosome), but band heterotopia in women (protected by two X chromosomes). Band heterotopias are isointense with cortical gray matter with well-defined smooth margins. A thin interface of white matter is located between the band (laminar) heterotopia and the cortex creating the "double cortex" sign. The heterotopic tissue may demonstrate mass effect and distort deep gray or white matter structures. The overlying cortex may be abnormal as well due to abnormal sulcation/gyration/and migration. Band heterotopias are explained as anomalies arising because of arrest of neuronal migration in the intermediate zone between the germinal matrix and the outer cortex (where the cells belong)—such as getting caught behind the front lines in a remote mountainess region in Eastern Afghanistan.

The abnormality is difficult to diagnose by CT but may be suggested when one identifies an island of higher density, nonenhancing tissue suggestive of gray matter in a white matter location. These abnormalities are much better demonstrated with MR where one can distinguish the gray matter from the white matter on a T2WI with a high degree of accuracy. Within the dark myelinated white matter, one typically finds a higher signal intensity island of irregular tissue representing the heterotopia. Look for gray, white, gray, white, ventricle as the pattern for band heterotopias—it is the second gray that is the rub.

Encephaloceles, holoprosencephaly, schizencephaly, Chiari malformations, and agenesis of the corpus callosum may coexist with gray matter heterotopias.

Pachygyria

Pachygyria (incomplete lissencephaly) is a condition of short, broad, fat gyri caused by abnormal sulcation and gyration of the cortical mantle. It is a congenital abnormality that occurs relatively late in gestation, at 12 to 24 weeks, because of neuroblastic migration not proceeding completely to the superficial layers of the cortex (Fig. 9-25). At its most extreme, no sulcation at all may occur,

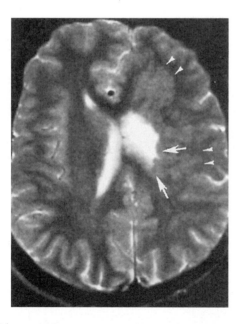

Fig. 9-24 Band heterotopia. Axial T2WI delineates gray matter signal intensity within the centrum semiovale and corona radiata on the left side *(arrowheads)*. Note the distortion of the left lateral ventricle at the interface with heterotopic gray matter *(arrows)*.

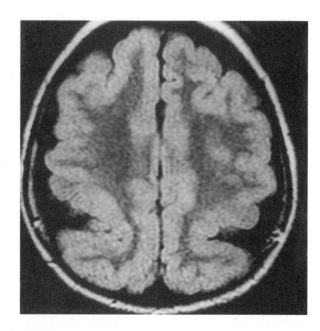

Fig. 9-25 Pachygyria. Bilateral symmetric pachygyric brain is seen in the parietal lobes on this FLAIR study. The white matter does not arborize in these regions.

creating a smoothly outlined hourglass configuration to the brain. No sylvian fissures are formed. This condition is termed agyria or complete lissencephaly and is due to abnormal formation of the superficial cortex of the brain where incomplete neuroblastic migration to the six-layered cortex has occurred possibly from cortical laminar necrosis of the third cortical layer (Fig. 9-26). A bright rim around the cortex may be seen on T2WI because of this laminar necrosis in the "cell-sparse layer" of the cortex. Patients with congenital cytomegalovirus (CMV) infection have high rates of pachygyria. As opposed to hemimegalencephaly, white matter volume will be decreased; in both, gray matter appears thicker because of poor sulcation. Abnormal myelination may coexist.

Two chromosomes have been associated with lissencephaly. With those from the X chromosome, you tend to see a more severe involvment with a frontal lobe predominance, predominating in men. Lissencephaly associated with chromosome #17 affects the parietal lobe more than the frontal lobe. Cobblestone lissencephaly is seen in association with Fukuyama muscular dystrophy and Walker-Warburg syndrome.

Polymicrogyria

It is believed that polymicrogyria is due to ischemic laminar necrosis of the fifth cortical layer after the twentieth week of gestation, by which time the neurons have reached the cortical surface. CMV infection has been implicated as a cause, but other infections or vascular insults in utero may also lead to polymicrogyria. This disorder is frequently seen in patients with the Chiari malformation and schizencephaly. Patients usually have developmental delay, spasticity, and/or seizures.

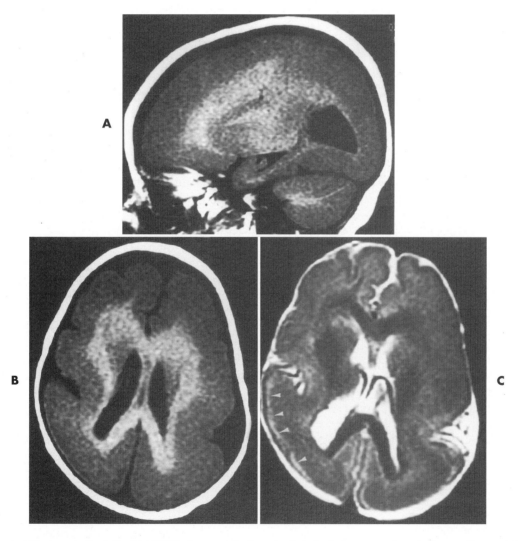

Fig. 9-26   Classical lissencephaly. **A,** Sagittal T1W1: Incomplete lissencephaly includes areas of agyria (more often parieto-occipital) and pachygyria (frontotemporal). **B,** Axial T1W1: The sylvian fissures are shallow and maloriented, causing a figure-eight appearance (in this case a bit topheavy—the Pamela Anderson sign). **C,** On this T2WI, one can identify posteriorly the unmyelinated white matter of the cell sparse layer *(arrowheads)* that separates the thin cortex from the deeper thickened gray matter in lissencephaly.

Grossly, one can see excessive numbers of small, disorganized cortical convolutions. The cortex appears thickened. The white matter thickness is normal (remember that it is increased in hemimegalencephaly and smaller in agyria). On MR, one is unable to distinguish pachygyria from polymicrogyria, but the cortex is less thick with polymicrogyria (5 to 7 mm) than with true pachygyria (>8 mm thick). On thin section images polymicrogyria is "bumpier" than pachygyria. Another distinguishing feature between pachygyria and polymicrogyria is the possible presence of abnormal white matter deep to the latter. An association with developmental venous anomalies (anomalous venous drainage) is noted with polymicrogyria. When focal some people use the term cortical dysplasia for polymicrogyria.

Congenital bilateral perisylvian (opercular) syndrome is recognized as an entity in which there is polymicrogyria involving the opercular cortex associated with abnormal sylvian fissure sulcation. Patients with congenital bilateral perisylvian syndrome disorder have seizures, congenital pseudobulbar paresis, and developmental delay. The abnormal sylvian fissure may have cortical thickening on either side of it. Schizencephaly may also be present.

Cerebellar polymicrogyria, lissencephaly, and clusters of intraparenchymal cerebellar cysts may occur in Fukuyama-type muscular dystrophy (are you out of your Fukuyama mind?). When one sees disordered cerebellar folia and small cysts in the cerebellum in a Japanese patient one should consider this diagnosis. The cysts may predominate in the semilunar lobule. Cerebral polymicrogyria or pachygyria, absent or delayed myelination, thickened meninges, vermian hypoplasia, fused folia, and hydrocephalus may coexist. The polymicrogyria tends to involve the frontal and parietotemporal lobe whereas pachygyria involves the temporooccipital lobes. The polymicrogyria, sometimes called cobblestone lissencephaly, can affect the frontoparietal regions with a smooth lissencephaly of the temporo-occipital zone. Other forms of congenital muscular dystrophy are also associated with polymicrogyria and cortical dysplasias.

In contrast to Fukuyama-type muscular dystrophy above, classic muscular dystrophy associated with merosin deficiency (a molecular component in the basement membrane of muscle fiber) leads to diffuse periventricular and subcortical white matter high signal with sparing of the corpus callosum and internal capsule.

Focal Cortical Dysplasia (Without Balloon Cells)

Cortical dysplasia may be a source of seizures both for the patient and for the unwary neuroradiologist trying to find the entity. It is said that such developmental anomalies are present in 11% to 23% of specimens from surgical procedures performed for epilepsy. The findings may be very subtle, manifested as thickening of cortex, abnormal sulcation, and/or blurring of cortical margins, without signal intensity variation from gray matter.

Bronen and colleagues have described the CSF cleft overlying a cortical dimple as a specific sign of cortical dysgenesis. The cortex buckles inward away from the brain surface leading to a dilated subarachnoid space overlying it. This is seen in more than 80% of patients with nonballoon cell focal cortical dysplasia, 100% of cases of polymicrogyria, and all cases of schizencephaly.

Other MR findings suggesting dysplasia rather than tumor include the presence of homogeneous hyperintense T2WI signal in the subcortical white matter that tapers as it extends to the lateral ventricle. This signal may be due to hypomyelination or wallerian degeneration. A frontal lobe location favors a balloon cell dysplasia, whereas a temporal lobe (especially medial temporal lobe) location is more suggestive of a neoplasm. Most clinical manifestations are motor, with spastic hemiplegia.

Balloon Cell Focal Cortical Dysplasia of Taylor

Disorders of abnormal neuronal proliferation include balloon cell focal cortical dysplasia of Taylor. This entity manifests cortical thickening, hyperintense subcortical white matter on T2W scans, and radial bands from the ventricle to the cortex. These bands may be of white or gray matter intensity. The gray-white junction is blurred. The appearance is similar to a cortical tuber. In focal gray transmantle dysplasia gray matter extends from the subependymal zone to the cortex with associated pachygyria, heterotopia, polymicrogyria, and schizencephalic defects. Clinical presentation is that of seizures and sensor motor deficits.

Rarely, one may see anomalous venous drainage from areas of cortical dysplasia. Other associations include dysembryoplastic neuroepithelial tumors, gangliogliomas, gangliocytomas, and mesial temporal sclerosis.

Megalencephaly

Megalencephaly is defined as enlargement of all or part of the cerebral hemisphere. (Large heads associated with hypoplasias of other organs have been reported in low level academicians.) Bilateral causes (Box 9-3) and unilateral causes (Box 9-4) may have some overlap and account for various head shapes. Often polymicrogyria (associated with increased hemispheric size) or agyria (associated with less severe hemispheric enlargement) is found on the affected side. MR demonstrates a distorted, thickened cortex with ipsilateral ventricular dilatation

Box 9-3   Bilateral Megalencephaly

Achondroplasia
Acromegaly
Alexander's disease
Canavan's disease
Co-authors of REQUISITES
Congenital neuronal migrational anomaly
Mucopolysaccharidoses
Neurofibromatosis
Proteus syndrome
Tay-Sachs disease
Tuberous sclerosis

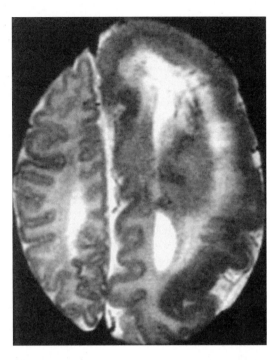

Fig. 9-27   Hemimegalencephaly. Axial T2WI discloses enlargement of the left hemisphere with disorganized brain tissue and a neuronal migrational anomaly. Note the lack of sulcation and the abnormal white matter formation in this child. Big brain, big ventricle.

(Fig. 9-27). This unique feature, that of ventricular dilatation on the side of the enlarged hemisphere, separates congenital hemimegalencephaly from other infiltrative lesions. In some cases, it may be due to an enlarged fornix obstructing the foramen of Monro. Heterotopias and cortical thickening are characteristic. Myelination is delayed but overall white matter volume is increased. If lissencephaly is present, a high-intensity (on T2W) cortical rim of laminar necrosis may be seen. Alternatively, megalencephaly may be an isolated finding. Patients have seizures, hemiplegia, developmental delay, and abnormal skull configurations.

Interestingly, a patient with hemimegalencephaly of one hemisphere in infancy may actually show hemimicrocephaly of the hemisphere in later life as there may be retarded growth of the dysmorphic brain, causing the contralateral hemisphere to seem larger. (Ooh what a concept, think about it.) Hemimegalencephaly may occur in a variety of syndromes including neurofibromatosis, Soto syndrome, tuberous sclerosis secondary to complex cortical malformations, Klippel-Trenaunay-Weber syndrome, or as an isolated lesion.

Proteus syndrome, which has cutaneous manifestations similar to neurofibromatosis and encephalocraniocutaneous lipomatosis, may present with hemimegalencephaly, subependymal calcified nodules, and

Box 9-4   Unilateral Cranial Enlargement

Dyke-Davidoff-Masson syndrome/Sturge Weber
    association
Epidermal nevus syndrome
Hemimegalencephaly (neuronal migrational anomaly)
Klippel-Trenaunay syndrome
McCune Albright syndrome (fibrous dysplasia)
Neurofibromatosis
Proteus syndrome
Tuberous sclerosis

periventricular cysts. Irregularly shaped vertebrae may accompany the intracranial findings. Macrocephaly, macrodactyly, hemihypertrophy, cutaneous nevi, soft-tissue tumors, and lipomatosis may make for one unusual looking patient.

Lipomas

It is now generally accepted that most intracranial lipomas represent congenital abnormalities rather than neoplasms. Lipomas occur because of persistence or maldevelopment of the meninx primitiva, the neural crest tissue that ultimately forms the neural tube. The most common sites of lipomas are the interhemispheric fissure (50%), the quadrigeminal plate cistern, the pineal region, hypothalamic region, and the cerebellopontine angle cistern. These lesions do not grow and are symptomatic only because of other associated congenital anomalies and/or mass effect on neighboring structures. Many (up to 50%) are associated with agenesis of the corpus callosum. Treatment tends to be conservative because vessels often course through the lipoma, making surgical removal that much harder.

Lipomas have attenuation values on CT that are in the negative range, usually −30 to −100 HU, and are isodense to subcutaneous fat (see Fig. 9-21). High in intensity on T1WI and intermediate to low on conventional T2WI and bright on fast spin echo T2WI, the fat of the lipoma can be corroborated by the presence of a chemical shift artifact along the frequency encoding direction. This causes one edge of the lesion to be highlighted as very bright on T2WI and the other edge along the frequency-encoded axis to be darkened. Alternatively, a fat-suppression pulse sequence can verify the fat by demonstrating signal diminution after it is applied. Calcification may be seen.

Aqueductal Stenosis

Aqueductal stenosis, causing lateral and third ventricular enlargement without fourth ventricular dilatation, is usually seen in boys as part of an X-linked recessive hereditary disorder. This is thought to be due to an abnormality of proliferation and differentiation of the periaqueductal gray matter of the mesencephalon, leading to the stenosis. Acquired causes of aqueductal stenosis are numerous and include clots from subarachnoid hemorrhage and fibrosis after bleeds or infections. The congenital causes occur in the setting of enlarged head circumference in infant boys and may be due to webs, septa, or membranes. This entity is covered in greater depth in Chapter 8.

INFRATENTORIAL ABNORMALITIES

Dandy-Walker Syndrome

People keep adding layers onto the Dandy-Walker syndrome (DWS), so that now nearly every posterior fossa congenital anomaly can somehow tie into the Dandy-Walker complex (Table 9-5). Terminology was clearer when DWS stood alone as an entity. Classically, the Dandy-Walker malformation was described as partial or complete absence of the vermis, dilatation of the fourth ventricle into a large cystic mass in an enlarged posterior fossa, hydrocephalus, and torcular-lambdoid inversion (elevation of the torcular above the lambdoid suture) (Fig. 9-28). (Please note that the authors thought the word was "torcula," whereas the more erudite editors insisted "torcular" was the proper term. They have Dorland's, Stedman's, and Gray's on their side. We have our secretary on ours.) The etiology that has been proposed for the Dandy-Walker malformation is obstruction of outward flow of the CSF at the foramina of Magendie and Luschka. This leads to ballooning upward of the fourth ventricle between the cerebellar hemispheres, preventing their fusion to form the cerebellar vermis and changing the osseoanatomic configuration of the posterior fossa. The cerebellar vermis is the missing part in the picture of DWS anomalies. Patients with Dandy-Walker malformation have a high incidence (68%) of other syndromes (Box 9-5) and other congenital CNS abnormalities, including agenesis of the corpus callosum, holoprosencephaly, schizencephaly, polymicrogyria, meningoencephaloceles, lipomas, infundibular hamartomas, malformed olives (the pits), hydromyelia, and cerebral heterotopia. Patient's functional status is more directly correlated with these supratentorial anomalies.

The CT findings in patients with manifestations of Dandy-Walker malformation include (1) a large cystic structure in the posterior fossa, which represents the ballooned-out fourth ventricle; (2) hydrocephalus; (3) torcular-lambdoid inversion; and (4) inferior vermian hypoplasia or aplasia.

Again, because of the prevalence of midline abnormalities, MR is the ideal study for examining patients with DWS (whereas a breathalyzer is the ideal study to test for DWI and a coroner to test for DOA). With this technique, one can identify the communication of the posterior fossa cyst with the fourth ventricle. In addition, one may identify the straight sinus entering the torcular in a high location. The posterior fossa cyst typically has signal intensity exactly that of CSF elsewhere. In the midline MR section you should appreciate the degree of vermian hypoplasia and the presence of concomitant agenesis or lipoma of the corpus callosum.

Table 9-5 Dandy-Walker complex			
Feature	**Dandy-Walker malformation**	**Dandy-Walker variant**	**Giant cisterna magna**
Posterior fossa size	Enlarged	Normal	Normal or enlarged
Vermis	Absent or very hypoplastic	Hypoplastic	Normal
Hydrocephalus	75%	25%	Unusual
Supratentorial anomalies	Common (68%)	Uncommon (20%)	Rare (6%)
Torcular-lambdoid inversion	Yes	No	No
Hypoplastic cerebellar hemisphere	Yes	Rare	No
Prognosis	Poor	Good	Good
Falx cerebelli	Absent	Present in 32%	Present in 63%
4th Ventricle	Opens into cyst	Cyst dilatation	Normal

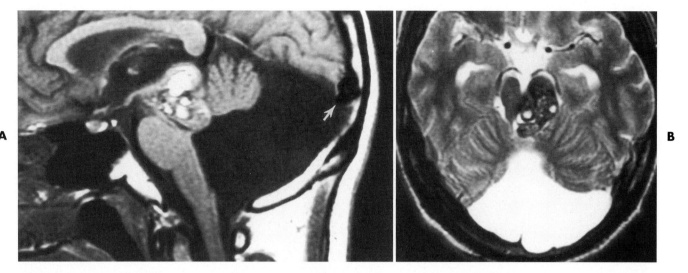

Fig. 9-28   DWS and OCVM. **A,** Classic sagittal T1W showing the cystic expansion of the fourth ventricle, lifting of the torcular *(arrow)*, inferior vermian absence, enlarged posterior fossa. But wait, what is going on at the collicular plate (extra credit for this one!) **B,** The axial T2W scan shows the ballooned-out fourth ventricle and the heterogeneous hemorrhagic mass in the posterior midbrain. The absence of edema associated with the brain stem lesion and its signal intensity leads to the diagnosis of a cavernous hemangioma or occult cerebrovascular malformation (OCVM).

The Dandy-Walker variant is a less severe form of the Dandy-Walker complex in which there is better development of the vermis and the fourth ventricle posterior fossa cyst is smaller. Neither significant enlargement of the posterior fossa nor torcular-lambdoid inversion is present (Fig. 9-29). Hydrocephalus is variably present since one or more foramina from the fourth ventricle are presumed to be open. Heterotopias and callosal dysgenesis occur in about 20% of cases of Dandy-Walker variant.

In recent literature, all cases of hypoplasia of the vermis have now been termed forms of the Dandy-Walker complex (Fig. 9-30). This type of classification has not become uniformly accepted. The Dandy-Walker malformation should be differentiated from the arachnoid cyst of the posterior fossa, which is located behind the cerebellum, does not communicate with the fourth ventricle, and is not generally associated with hydrocephalus or vermian hypoplasia (Fig. 9-31). In addition, the giant cisterna magna is a normal variation, with dilatation of the subarachnoid space posterior to the cerebellum. It is not associated with fourth ventricular abnormalities, hydrocephalus, or torcular-lambdoid inversion. The vermis is usually normal. As opposed to DWS, patients with a giant cisterna magna or arachnoid cyst of the posterior fossa have a normal (giant cisterna magna) or compressed (arachnoid cyst) cerebellum and fourth ventricle. Compression of the fourth ventricle by the cyst may lead to hydrocephalus, further confusing the picture. You may identify vessels coursing through the subarachnoid space of the giant cisterna magna. The arachnoid cyst demonstrates displacement of those vessels but without associated congenital malformations as described in the DWS. Septations within the subarachnoid space of the cisterna magna and infoldings of the meninges are frequently seen. The falx cerebelli may be bifid and show infoldings as well. Because of this, one may see stranding fibers normally within the posterior fossa CSF spaces even with a giant cisterna magna.

Box 9-5   Associations with Dandy-Walker Syndrome

Aicardi
Ellis van Creveld
Facial hemangiomas
Fetal alcohol syndrome
Fetal TORCH infection
Klippel-Feil syndrome
Meckel-Gruber (occipital encephalocele, microcephaly, polycystic kidneys, polydactyly)
Trisomy 9, 13, 18
Walker-Warburg
Warfarin embryopathy
X-linked cerebellar hypoplasia

Joubert Syndrome

The imaging findings in Joubert syndrome are virtually pathognomonic. One sees parallel, enlarged, horizontally oriented superior cerebellar peduncles, which,

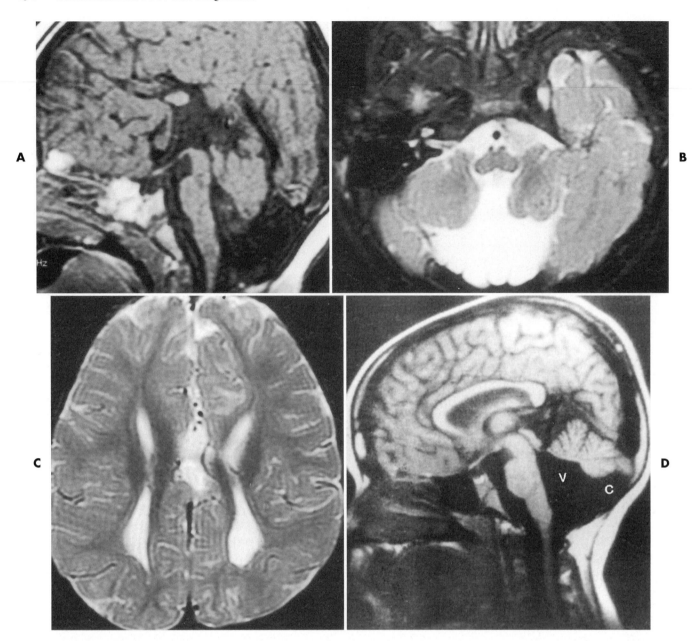

Fig. 9-29 Dandy-Walker variant. **A,** There is a large cystic structure in the posterior fossa that communicates with the fourth ventricle, but the posterior fossa is not particularly enlarged, nor is there hydrocephalus judging from the appearance of the third ventricle. Agenesis of the corpus callosum coexists. **B,** There is little inferior vermis left on this axial T2WI, but the cyst replaces the space. **C,** The shape of the ventricles is indicative of agenesis of the corpus callosum, not hydrocephalus. **D,** Dandy-Walker variant. A large cyst *(c)* communicating with the fourth ventricle *(v)* and causing partial inferior vermian hypoplasia is seen on this sagittal T1WI. Note that there is no hydrocephalus and the torcular Herophili is not elevated. These findings suggest Dandy-Walker variant. (Courtesy of NR Altman et al, Posterior fossa malformations, figure 19, *AJNR,* 13, March–April, 691-724, 1992, © *AJNR.*)

coupled with the elongated pontine-midbrain junction have the appearance of a molar tooth (Fig. 9-32). Hypoplasia of the vermis brings the two cerebellar hemispheres in virtual contact with each other and a nodulus is not seen. The fourth ventricle develops a "bat wing" appearance from middle cerebellar peduncle, superior cerebellar peduncle, and pyramidal decussation maldevelopment. Associations including dysgenesis of the corpus callosum, retinal dysplasia, and cystic renal disease coexist and lead to a poor prognosis.

Clinically, the patients have developmental delay, poor visual development with oculomotor disturbances, colobomas, and abnormal respirations (neonatal tachypnea or apnea). Inheritance is autosomal recessive.

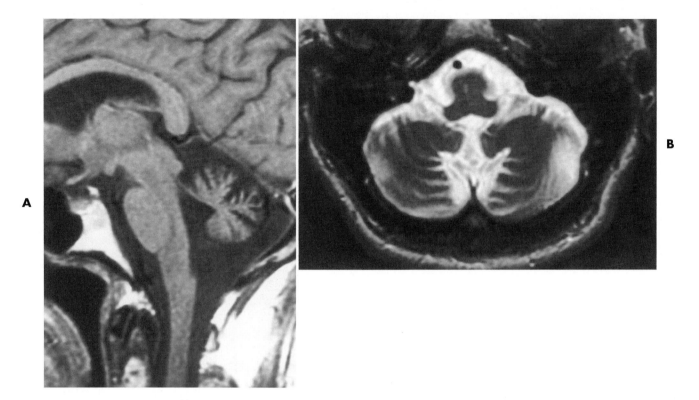

Fig. 9-30   Vermian hypoplasia. Whether this is developmental, toxic, congenital, or environmental is not clear. Nonetheless this case of inferior vermian hypoplasia on sagittal T1WI **(A)** and axial T2WI **(B)** reflects a spectrum of disease that are classified as posterior fossa anomalies.

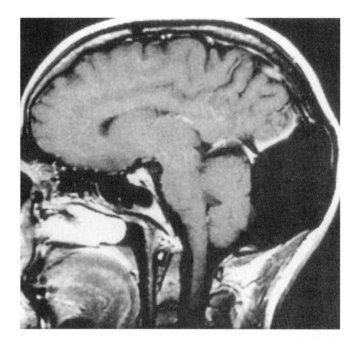

Fig. 9-31   Retrocerebellar arachnoid cyst. Enhanced sagittal T1WI shows a large arachnoid cyst behind the cerebellum. Note that, although the straight sinus is elevated, this CSF collection does not communicate with the fourth ventricle and no hydrocephalus is present.

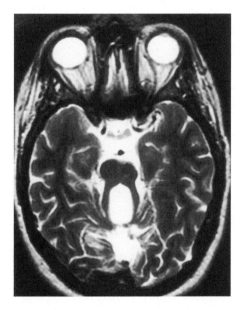

Fig. 9-32   The molar tooth sign. Note how the brain stem and the elongated superior cerebellar peduncles simulate a molar tooth. Couple this with the vermian hypoplasia evident by the dilated subarachnoid space posteriorly and it will make Aunt Minnie cry out, "Joubert, Whazzup?"

Vermian Dysgenesis/Hypoplasia

The number of entities associated with vermian hypoplasia or dysgenesis warrants a whole separate paragraph and/or box devoted to it. In fact, the role of the vermis in development and physiology should be studied more carefully because of the wide range of diseases that can affect it. Inferior vermian hypoplasia may occur in isolation and in patients with congenital ocular motor apraxia syndrome. Patients with Walker-Warburg syndrome have vermian hypoplasia, diffuse cerebral cobblestone cortex, absence of cerebral and cerebellar myelin, cerebellar polymicrogyria (with or without cysts), hydrocephalus, and variable callosal hypogenesis. There are many metabolic and drug causes of vermian atrophy. Although we discuss metabolic and toxic lesions that cause cerebellar atrophy in the neurodegenerative chapter it behooves us to remind our dedicated readers that Dandy-Walker malformations, Chiari malformations, and Down syndrome are associated with vermian dysgenesis. These and other more obscure entities for the connoisseur de cerebellae may be found in Box 9-6.

Rhombencephalosynapsis

Rhombencephalosynapsis is a rare entity in which the cerebellar hemispheric separation is lost and there is fusion across midline of the cerebellum. There appears to be an absence of the anterior vermis, fusion of the dentate nuclei and middle cerebellar peduncles, and a deficiency of the posterior vermis. Agenesis of the septum pellucidum may coexist.

Arachnoid Cysts

As described previously, arachnoid cysts are common in the infratentorial space. The posterior fosa sites of the arachnoid cyst are the regions of the cisterna magna and the cerebellopontine angle cistern. The signal intensity within the posterior fossa arachnoid cysts duplicates that of CSF in most cases. One should be cognizant of the association of the arachnoid cyst with acoustic schwannomas in the cerebellopontine angle cistern. Arachnoid cysts occasionally cause hydrocephalus, leading to a clinical presentation.

Differential diagnosis includes cysticercosis, epidermoids, porencephaly, and dilated CSF spaces (repeated just for those who slept through the previous few pages).

Chiari Malformations

The spectrum of congenital anomalies labeled the Chiari malformation spans a wide range. The fundamental problem appears to be underdevelopment of the posterior fossa from para-axial mesoderm that forms the occipital somites (a cranial base dysplasia). CSF and posterior cranial fossa volumes are decreased compared with controls but overall brain volumes are the same. Chiari I malformations are diagnosed when the cerebellar tonsils alone are below the foramen magnum. How low can they go? (Sounds like the limbo song!) Tonsils less than 5 mm below the foramen magnum are very common but that is the current lower limit of normal most people cite in the literature. Are all these asymptomatic patients a forme fruste of the malformation? Only the *Great Neuroradiologist in the Sky* knows for sure. In its pure form, a Chiari I malformation shows tonsils down to the C1—C2 region but with normal brain stem location. The incidence of cervical syringohydromyelia in these flagrant cases has been reported to be between 20% and 73% (Fig. 9-33) but the incidence of syringomyelia in *symptomatic* patients with Chiari I malformations and tonsillar herniation greater than 5 mm is reported to be 53% in the surgical literature. No hydrocephalus is present, and the fourth ventricle is normal in location. There is an association with Klippel-Feil syndrome (C2—C3 fusion), short clivus, and odontoid or C1 abnormalities. Compression of CSF spaces posterior and lateral to the cerebellum and reduced height of the supraocciput have also been commented on.

The symptoms that are most commonly reported in patients with Chiari I malformations are suboccipital headaches, retroorbital pressure or pain, clumsiness, dizziness, vertigo, tinnitus, paresthesias, muscle weakness, and lower cranial nerve symptoms (i.e., dysphagia, dysarthria, sleep apnea, tremors). The entity usually presents in the second or third decade of life (mean age of 25 years +/−14 years) and women outnumber men by a 3:1 ratio.

There has been a lot of focus lately on the issue of CSF, spinal cord, and medullary movement in patients with Chiari malformations. Foramen magnum obstruction may lead to increased systolic spinal cord motion, impaired spinal cord recoil, and impaired diastolic CSF motion anteriorly at the C2—C3 level. Impaired systolic

---

Box 9-6   Causes of Vermian Dysgenesis

Chiari malformations
Congenital ocular motor apraxia syndrome
Dandy-Walker syndrome
Down syndrome
Joubert syndrome
Meckel-Gruber syndrome
Olivopontocerebellar degeneration
Retrocerebellar cysts (Blake pouch cyst)
Walker-Warburg syndrome
X-linked hypoplasia of vermis

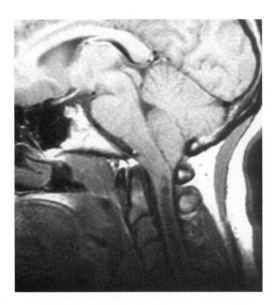

Fig. 9-33   Chiari malformation with a syrinx. The sagittal T1WI shows the low tonsils, the low cervicomedullary junction and the cervical syrinx (fading into the distance). It is our policy that, even with a classic congenital syrinx, the first study of a syrinx should include an enhanced study to exclude a neoplastic cause, rare though that may be. Ockham's razor be damned! (Ockham's Razor is "non sunt multiplicanda entia praeter necessitatem" [entities are not to be multiplied beyond necessity] credited to William of Ockham, 1285-1347/49). It is also called the "Law of Economy" and the "Law of Parsimony.")

and unimpaired diastolic flow may also be seen just below the foramen magnum. Some neurosurgeons have been performing suboccipital decompression procedures on patients with a variety of clinical symptoms including headaches, vertigo, weakness, and fibromyalgia who have imaging findings of abnormal CSF motion with or without tonsillar ectopia. Frankly, we still have a lot to learn about CSF motion and neurosurgical motivations. It is true that one will often see reduced CSF flow posteriorly at the foramen magnum with low tonsils. Others have reported hyperdynamic movement of the tonsils with posterior movement of the medulla in patients with Chiari malformations. However, in our anecdotal experience, there are many patients we see with no evidence of crowding at the foramen magnum who still have "funny" CSF flow patterns. Just as fibromyalgia and chronic fatigue syndrome are poorly understood diseases, so are the imaging findings associated (or not associated) with these entities.

Dramatic tonsillar herniation through the foramen magnum may be present in patients with osteopetrosis owing to decreased intracranial volume secondary to the thickened calvarium and increased intracranial pressure. This forces the tonsils down, down, down.

Chiari II (the original Arnold-Chiari malformation) anomalies occur in 0.02% of births and affect girls twice as often as boys. The cerebellar tonsils, vermis,

fourth ventricle, and brain stem are herniated through the foramen magnum, and the egress from the fourth ventricle is obstructed (Box 9-7, Fig. 9-34). A kink may be present at the cervicomedullary junction. Hydrocephalus occurs. The frontal horns of the lateral ventricles are squared off, the fourth ventricle is compressed, and the aqueduct is stretched inferiorly. The tectum of the midbrain is beaked, and the massa intermedia is abnormally enlarged (Fig. 9-35). The superior cerebellum towers superiorly through a widened tentorial incisura because the whole posterior fossa is too small. The rest of the cerebellum may literally wrap around the brain stem. Associated complete agenesis of the corpus callosum occurs in one third of cases, and partial abnormalities occur in 75% to 90%, predominantly affecting the splenium. Heterotopias and abnormal gyral patterns are common.

A tethered cord with a lumbosacral myelocele (Fig. 9-36) or meningomyelocele protruding through the skin is seen in nearly all patients with Chiari II malformations. A lipoma of the filum may coexist. The anchoring of the

---

Box 9-7   Findings in Chiari II Malformation

INFRATENTORIAL FINDINGS

1. Tonsils and medulla below foramen magnum
2. Beaking of tectum
3. Bullet-shaped towering cerebellum
4. Cerebellum wrapped around brain stem
5. Petrous bone scalloping
6. Myelomeningocele, syringohydromyelia
7. Fourth ventricle compressed, elongated, trapped, and low
8. Enlarged foramen magnum
9. Cervicomedullary kinking
10. Small posterior fossa
11. Low torcular
12. Dysplastic tentorium
13. Scalloping of clivus posterior
14. Absent hypoplastic arch of C1

SUPRATENTORIAL FINDINGS

1. Falx hypoplasia
2. Hydrocephalus
3. Callosal hypogenesis
4. Fused, enlarged massa intermedia
5. Colpocephaly
6. Abnormal gyral patterns
7. Caudate hypertrophy, bat-wing lateral ventricles
8. Interdigitation of gyri along widened interhemispheric fissure
9. Lückenschädel
10. Biconcave 3rd ventricle

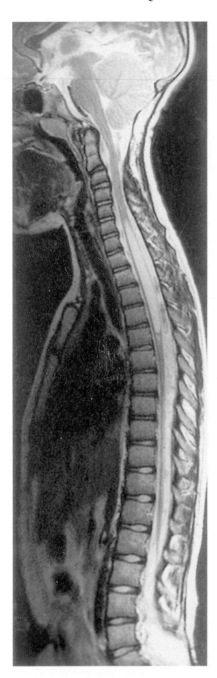

Fig. 9-34   The whole Sh'bang. This patient has the Chiari II malformation, cord syrinx, and a treated myelomeningocele, all shown on this 48 FOV T2WI. Is that great tectal beaking, or what?

malformations. Nearly all Chiari III encephaloceles contain brain tissue, usually cerebellum, although even the brain stem can herniate outward (Fig. 9-37). Heterotopias, agenesis of the corpus callosum, anomalies of venous drainage, and syringohydromyelia are commonly associated. It's like Yousem's seventh corollary to Murphy's law—if multiple things can go wrong, they all will.

Symptomatic patients with Chiari II and III malformations are seen with ataxia, vertical nystagmus, headache, cranial nerve VI through XII findings, and occasionally, central canal syndromes caused by syringohydromyelia. At autopsy, disordered neuronal tissue is present in the brain stem and cerebellum. Thus, it is not clear whether the symptoms are entirely due to compression at the foramen magnum or due to dysplastic neurons. Decompression of the foramen magnum often does not improve symptoms in most individuals with Chiari II, suggesting that disorganized medullary tissue may be etiologic in some cases.

SKULL ANOMALIES

Craniostenosis

At birth the sagittal, coronal, lambdoid, and metopic sutures are open. Occasionally, one will see a suture, which crosses from one lambdoid suture to the other, as the persistent mendosa suture. Craniostenosis, or craniosynostosis, refers to abnormal early fusion of one or more of the sutures of the skull. In 75% of the cases, only one suture or part of a suture is fused; in 25% of cases, more than one suture is affected. This leads to abnormal head shapes and a palpable ridge at the site of fusion. Males are affected much more often than females. These disorders, if severe and early in development, can cause abnormal growth of the brain. Microcephaly may occur. Syndromes associated with early sutural closure include Crouzon disease, Apert syndrome, hypophosphatasia, and Carpenter syndrome. Endocrinologic abnormalities including rickets, hyperthyroidism, and hypophosphatasia can cause craniosynostosis. Sagittal suture premature closure, the most common variety, produces a head that cannot grow side to side, so the head looks long and thin, or scaphocephalic, also termed dolichocephalic (Table 9-6). The incidence of sagittal synostosis is approximately 1 in 4200 births. If the coronal suture fuses early, the head is short and fat, or brachycephalic. Sometimes only one portion of a coronal or lambdoid suture fuses too early, leading to an asymmetric skull with plagiocephaly. The forehead and orbital rim (eyebrow) have a flattened appearance on that side. This gives a harlequin "winking" eye. Lambdoid suture closure can lead to turricephaly, with a high-riding vertex (Fig. 9-38). Unilateral lambdoid suture fusion results

distal portion of the craniospinal axis may account for the downward herniation of intracranial contents in this disorder. Rarely the tonsils may necrose secondary to vascular compression at the foramen magnum. The evidence of this crime is fragments of cerebellar tissue floating in a sea of cervical CSF (the Teddy Kennedy sign).

Chiari III malformations are associated with herniation of posterior fossa contents in an occipital or high cervical encephalocele with other features of Chiari II

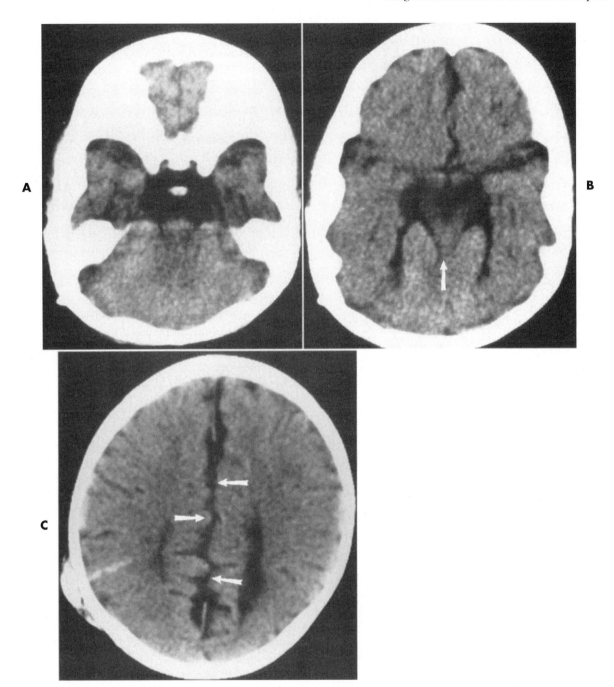

Fig. 9-35   Imaging findings with Chiari II malformation. **A,** Axial CT through the posterior fossa shows absence of the fourth ventricle. Posterior fossa seems small. **B,** Axial scan through the level of the midbrain reveals tectal beaking *(arrow)* with the cerebellum wrapping around the posterior lateral aspect of the midbrain. Cerebellum is towering between the leaves of the tentorium. **C,** Axial CT through the supraventricular region shows interdigitation of the gyri *(arrows)* with hypoplasia of the falx. This patient has a right shunt tube in place. Do you think the corpus callosum is present? Are those ventricles parallel?

in a posterior flattered plagiocephaly. Metopic sutural closure causes trigonocephaly with a ridge that runs down the forehead like a triceratops.

Surgery is attempted when elevations of intracranial pressure are dangerous secondary to the growth of the brain against the noncompliant calvarium. The elevated

ICP may lead to reduction in brain perfusion. If brain growth is stunted because of craniostenosis operative intervention is also indicated. Aesthetic reasons may also dictate earlier intervention.

Chronic venous hypertension due to jugular foramen stenosis has been proposed as an etiology for the in-

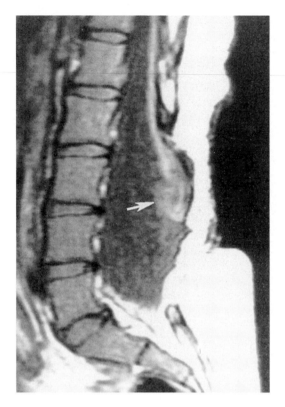

Fig. 9-36   Myelomeningocele. Sagittal T1WI shows spinal dysraphism with herniation of the spinal cord, neural placode *(arrow)*, and CSF through the gap of the bony anomaly.

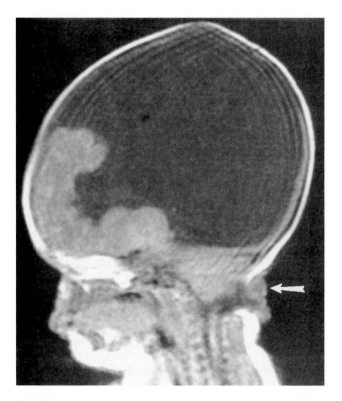

Fig. 9-37   Chiari III abnormality. Sagittal T1WI shows downward herniation of the cerebellar tonsils associated with an occipital encephalocele *(arrow)*. Patient has associated agenesis of the corpus callosum and maximal hydrocephalus.

Table 9-6   Craniostenosis

Type	Suture involved	Head shape
Dolichocephaly	Sagittal	Long and thin
Brachycephaly	Coronal	Round and foreshortened
Turricephaly	Lambdoid	High-riding top
Plagiocephaly	Any unilateral suture	Asymmetric
Trigonocephaly	Metopic	Anteriorly pointed head
"Harlequin eye"	Unilateral coronal	One eye points upward

creased intracranial pressure, communicating hydrocephalus, and tonsillar herniation seen in some patients with complex craniosynostosis. This can be seen with Crouzon syndrome. Stenosis of the jugular foramen may also be found in achondroplasia, which can lead to hydrocephalus.

Osteopetrosis

Osteopetrosis may be inherited as an autosomal dominant or recessive condition with the latter being the more virulent form. Calvarial involvement is frequent in both types with clinical manifestations mostly relating to involvement of skull base foramina. Therefore, cranial nerve palsies, optic atrophy, and stenoses of the carotid

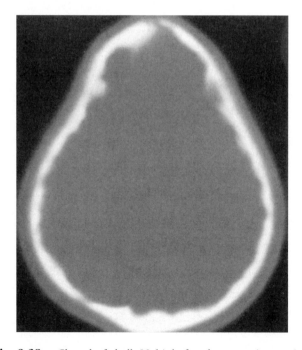

Fig. 9-38   Cloverleaf skull. Multiple fused sutures, in a patient with Crouzon syndrome, produced anterior beaking and a cloverleaf shape.

and jugular vessels may be present. One may see diffuse bone thickening and increased density (or decreased intensity) on imaging studies. MR may depict optic nerve sheath dilatation, tonsillar herniation, ventriculomegaly, and meningoencephaloceles (especially through craniotomy sites).

Achondroplasia

Achondroplasia is the most common cause of dwarfism and is characterized by a small foramen magnum but a large head. The macrocephaly may be secondary to hydrocephalus. The hydrocephalus may be due to venous outflow obstruction at the jugular foramen level leading to elevated venous pressure and reduced flow in the superior sagittal sinus. The lack of resorption in the arachnoid villi because of these pressure effects produces larger CSF volume in the ventricles, increased intracranial pressure, maintenance of widened calvarial sutures, and an enlarged head.

Other features of achondroplasia include a short clivus, platybasia, and a J-shaped sella. Spinal stenosis due to short pedicles is another feature of this disease.

Increased Wormian Bones

Increased wormian bones (secondary ossification centers within sutural lines) are seen in osteogenesis imperfecta, cleidocranial dysplasia, cretinism, pyknodysostosis, Down syndrome, hypothyroidism, progeria, and hypophosphatasia.

Basilar Invagination and Platybasia

Basilar invagination refers to upward protrusion of the odontoid process into the infratentorial space. Two lines must be memorized: (1) McGregor's line, extending from the posterior margin of the hard palate to the undersurface of the occiput, and (2) Chamberlain's line, from the hard palate to the opisthion (the midportion of the posterior margin of the foramen magnum) (Fig. 9-39). If the dens extends more than 5 mm (or half its height) above these lines, basilar invagination is present. Paget disease, rickets, fibrous dysplasia, osteogenesis imperfecta, hyperparathyroidism osteomalacia, achondroplasia, cleidocranial dysplasia, and Morquio syndrome are among the causes of this finding. In adults think rheumatoid arthritis (Fig. 9-40)

Basilar invagination should not be confused with platybasia. *Platybasia* literally means "flattening of the base of the skull" and is said to be present when the basal angle formed by intersecting lines from the nasion to the tuberculum sellae and from the tuberculum along the clivus to the anterior aspect of the foramen magnum (basion) is greater than 143 degrees (see Fig. 9-39). Platybasia is seen with Klippel-Feil anomalies, cleidocranial dysplasia, and achondroplasia.

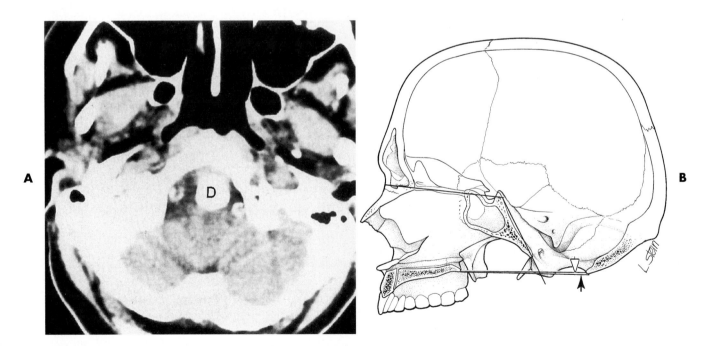

Fig. 9-39   Basilar invagination. **A,** CT demonstrates basilar invagination with dens *(D)* impinging on medulla. This has been likened to the pumpkin rotting on a fence post. **B,** Diagram of McGregor's *(black arrow)* and Chamberlain's *(open arrow)* lines. Note the basal angle from the nasion to tuberculum sellae to basion.

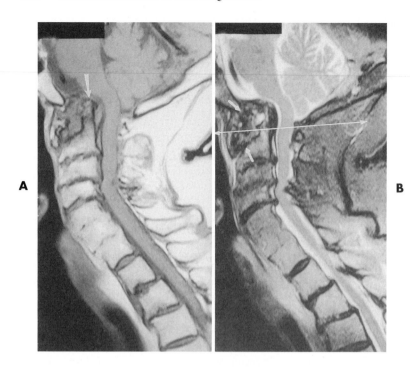

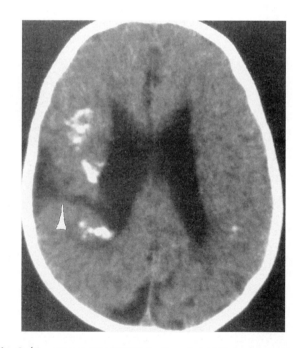

Fig. 9-40 Rheumatoid arthritis producing basilar invagination. **A,** T1WI sagittal showing penciling *(arrow)* of the odontoid process and pannus formation around it. **B,** Pannus is dark on T2WI *(arrows)*. Observe that there is no high intensity within the spinal cord, however, the foramen magnum and high cervical region do appear to be compressed. Obvious basilar invagination is present by eyeball (and criteria).

CONGENITAL INFECTIONS

In utero infections with *to*xoplasmosis, *r*ubella, *c*yto megalovirus (CMV) and *h*erpes simplex (TORCH infections) can cause brain injury (Fig. 9-41). Congenital syphilis is also frequently included with this group. In many instances, where the infection is transmitted hematogenously from the mother or ascends from the vagina through the cervix to the placenta, these infections lead to in utero death. Other infants are seen in the perinatal period with failure to thrive, hydrocephalus, and/or seizures (Table 9-7) The transmission may be at the time of passage through the vaginal canal during delivery.

On CT, these infections most commonly manifest as periventricular calcifications and leukomalacia with cerebral atrophy. CMV is the most common of the TORCH infections and is usually transmitted hematogenously from maternal infection. In addition to periventricular calcifications, porencephaly, delayed myelination, polymicrogyria, and pachygyria may also be seen with CMV infection. Microcephaly caused by atrophy is common with CMV infections. Periventricular cysts, usually around the occipital poles, may also be present. Echogenic basal ganglia vasculature has been reported on sonograms of infants with CMV and rubella infections.

Toxoplasmosis calcifies most frequently of the congenital infections (71% of the time in one series). With treatment of congenital toxoplasmosis 75% of cases show diminution or resolution of the intracranial calcifications by 1 year of age. If treatment does not occur,

is delayed, or inadequate the intracranial calcifications may increase. The status of the calcifications often mirrors neurologic function. On MR, periventricular and subcortical white matter injury is seen as high signal intensity on T2WI. Obstruction of the ventricular system

Fig. 9-41 Congenital CMV infection. Axial CT demonstrates calcifications in a periventricular location and in the cortex. Note that the patient also has ventricular dilatation and what appears to be a schizencephalic cleft *(arrowhead)*. Pachygyria is also associated with CMV infections.

Table 9-7 In utero infections

	Rubella	Herpes simplex virus (Type 2 > 1)	Toxoplasmosis	CMV	HIV
Frequency	0.0001% of neonates	0.02% of neonates	0.05% of neonates	Most common, 1% of neonates	Growing exponentially
Clinical manifestations	Hearing loss, MR, autism, speech defects	Skin lesions	Usually fetal death, developmental delay, seizures	Hearing loss, psychomotor retardation, visual defects, seizures, optic atrophy	Asymptomatic *at birth, later* presentation, developmental delay, late spastic paraparesis, ataxia
Ocular changes	Cataracts, glaucoma, pigmentary retinopathy	Chorioretinitis, microphthalmos	Chorioretinitis	Chorioretinitis	
Neuronal migrational anomaly	Rare	None	None	Frequent (polymicrogyria, heterotopia, hydranencephaly, lissencephaly, pachygyria), cerebellar hypoplasia	
Head size	Microcephaly	Microcephaly unless hydrocephalus	Microcephaly unless hydrocephalus	Microcephaly	Microcephaly
Parenchymal changes	Necrotic foci, delayed myelination	Hydranencephaly, patchy areas of low density in cortex, WM, vast encephalomalacia, cortical laminar necrosis, NO PREDILECTION FOR TEMPORAL LOBE	Hydrocephalus from aqueductal stenosis, intracranial calcifications	Hemorrhage esp. at germinal matrix, loss of white matter, delayed myelination, cortex, subependymal cysts around occipital horns, cerebellar hypoplasia, atrophy	Glial, microglial nodules in basal ganglia, brainstem, WM, demyelination, atrophy, corticospinal tract degeneration
Vessels	Vasculopathy	Can infect endothelial cells		Infarctions	Vasculopathy, vasculitis with calcifications
Calcifications	Basal ganglia, cortex		71%, periventricular, basal ganglia, parenchyma	Frequent (40%), periventricular, can have cortical calcifications	Perivascular in basal ganglia, cerebellum
Non-CNS	Patent ductus arteriosus, pulmonic stenosis, rash, hepatosplenomegaly		Hepatosplenomegaly rash	Hepatosplenomegaly	Neck adenopathy, oral candidiasis

443

with resultant hydrocephalus may occur because of synechiae at the aqueduct or foramina of Monro, Magendie, or Luschka.

Herpes simplex may have a similar appearance to CMV, but microcephaly and microphthalmia are more prevalent. Marked cystic encephalomalacia is the finding in end-stage herpes infection. Hemorrhagic foci may be present in the basal ganglia and cortical laminar necrosis may be seen as high signal on T1WI. This virus is usually transmitted during delivery from mothers with genital herpes.

Rubella infection may lead to cataracts, chorioretinitis, glaucoma, and cardiac myopathies. Deafness caused by sensorineural injury is very common. Microcephaly and seizures may lead to medical attention. Calcifications in the periventricular white matter and basal ganglia can develop on CT, as a sequela to the ischemia from vasculopathy.

Congenital acquired immunodeficiency syndrome (AIDS) infection can cause a diffuse pattern of calcification throughout the brain, not limited to the periventricular region or the basal ganglia. Microcephaly may develop. More often, the disease manifests in early childhood with hemorrhagic diathesis caused by thrombocytopenia, severe nonopportunistic infections, and seizures. On imaging, the findings include intracranial hemorrhages, infections, atrophy, arterial ectasias, and calcifications.

Congenital HIV infection is associated with arteritis, fusiform aneurysms, and arterial sclerosis with vascular occlusion. One can see diffuse dilatation of circle of Willis vessels in these children. Ninety percent of HIV-infected infants get AIDS within the second year of life and thus, they may develop AIDS encephalitis, infections, and lymphoma at early age. The AIDS encephalitis is characterized by atrophy, diffuse white matter hyperintensity on T2WI, and basal ganglia vascular calcification. Progressive multifocal leukoencephalopathy (PML), toxoplasmosis, and tuberculosis are rare in kids with AIDS.

Congenital syphilis leads to seizures and cranial nerve palsies in infancy. Radiological manifestations include optic atrophy, tabes dorsalis, meningitis, and vasculitis with enhancing meninges and perivasular spaces. Vasculitis may lead to infarctions.

See also Chapter 6, Infectious and Noninfectious Inflammatory Diseases of the Brain, for more information on congenital infections.

VASCULAR DISEASES OF INFANCY

Hypoxic-Ischemic Encephalopathy

Hypoxic-ischemic disease in neonates is often found in the setting of fetal distress leading to or from placen-tal abruption, meconium stained amniotic fluid, prolapsed umbilical cords, uterine rupture, or severe placenta previa. Apgar scores are diminished at birth with neonatal acidosis, hypotonia, lethargy, and seizures. One can find a variety of patterns of injury in neonates who experience hypoxic-ischemic injury. Four patterns of injury: (1) deep gray matter involvement; (2) cortical involvement in watershed zones or the peri-Rolandic region; (3) periventricular white matter injury without cortical extension; and (4) a mixed injury pattern with or without hemorrhage have been described. These findings are usually bilateral and symmetrical.

In the first 24 hours, edema may affect posterior cortical, hippocampal, and basal ganglionic regions. High signal in the thalami, basal ganglia, and central sulcus region on T1WI may then develop followed by subsequent T2 shortening. DWI scans and ADC maps may suggest restricted diffusion in the posterior limbs of the internal capsules and thalami. A second pattern with diffuse white matter restricted diffusion in the corona radiata and parietal zones can be seen. The basal ganglia injury is more evident in early life because of its high metabolic rate. These findings may be very subtle the first couple of days of life, so, if possible, find a reason to defer scanning until the end of the first week, early second week. Otherwise you will be calling many normal brains on asphyxiated children—it is very hard to see edema in a watery neonatal brain without myelin. On follow-up studies, loss of the normal cortical T2 hypointensity may suggest the diagnosis of anoxic brain injury.

Echoplanar DWI images reveal the true extent of and number of hypoxic ischemic abnormalities compared with FLAIR or fast spin echo T2W images in most neonates. This is in part due to the watery brain of the infant, which leads to high signal on T2W that obscures vasogenic and cytotoxic edema. The DWI extent of disease correlates well with short-term neurologic prognosis in these patients.

Patterns of Injury Based on Fetal Age and Degree of Asphyxia

Profound asphyxia from cardiopulmonary arrest or hypotension before 32 weeks gestational age shows dramatic and often bilateral injury to the thalami, subcortical white matter, basal ganglia, and posterior brain stem. Posterior circulation structures seem to fare more poorly than anterior circulation structures in this scenario. The deep gray structures become hypodense on CT and show increased echogenicity on US. The same areas, especially the thalami early on, are bright on T1WI. If contrast enhancement of the basal ganglia or brain stem is present, the children seem to do worse on follow-up.

Partial (less severe than above) asphyxia in *premature* infants usually produces the classical pattern of periventricular leukomalacia. The term *periventricular leukomalacia* (PVL) is now being used generically to signify the nonspecific white matter small vessel ischemic foci seen in elderly patients in the corona radiata and centrum semiovale. In the pediatric population, PVL refers to a white matter insult usually seen in premature infants because of watershed ischemia in the perforating arteries. Cystic cavitation and necrotic areas in a periventricular location may be striking. Classically, there is a posterior predominance with the most severe changes seen around the trigone of the lateral ventricle. There is a decrease in the width of white matter between the atria and the parietooccipital cortex, resulting in gliosis (Fig. 9-42). These findings may be seen on transcranial US, CT, or MR. The ventricles enlarge and are irregular in shape. Clinically the patients have spastic diplegia and visual field deficits.

On US, increased echogenicity of the periventricular white matter is seen in the first 2 days after the hypoxic-ischemic insult, being as echogenic as the normal choroid plexus. After a few weeks this pattern is replaced by cystic cavitated areas amidst the echogenic background. Subsequently, the lateral ventricles expand, volume loss is evident, and the intervening tissue is diminished in size but of normal echotexture. The grading of PVL by US consists of grade 1, evanescent periventricular echogenicity lasting less than 7 days; grade 2, prolonged periventricular echogenicities lasting greater than 7 days; grade 3, periventricular lesions evolving into small cysts; grade 4, periventricular lesions evolving into extensive periventricular cysts; and grade 5, periventricular lesions involving the subcortical white matter and creating extensive periventricular and subcortical cysts.

The MRs of patients with sonographic evidence of PVL may show more extensive hemorrhagic foci in the periventricular and subcortical regions, even when only periventricular echogenicity is evident on US. MR also demonstrates more extensive cyst formation than US. The more areas of hemorrhage, the more likely cyst formation and the worse the long-term outcome. The MR findings of PVL correlate well with clinical evidence of visual loss and spastic paraparesis. Volumetric reduction and signal hyperintensity of the peritrigonal white matter and atrophy of the calcarine cortex correspond to the finding of visual impairment in children. One may even see secondary degeneration of the lateral geniculate bodies.

Partial asphyxia in *term* infants causes cortical watershed distribution lesions between cerebral arteries. The long-term consequences of partial asphyxia in the term infant is a peculiar-shaped atrophy of the cortex in para-sagittal locations termed ulegyria (mushroom shaped). The cortex at the depth of the sulci suffers more profound cortical loss than those more superficial in the infant leading to this unusual shape. This pattern of injury seems to differ from that of partial asphyxia in premature infants (where the damage is predominantly periventricular) and of profound asphyxia in term infants.

Term infants with *profound* asphyxia have greater involvement of the lateral thalami, corpus striatum, hippocampus, and dentate nuclei of the cerebellum. The cortex is spared except around the central sulcus region. Again, the key to the detection is to note the low density of the deep gray matter structures on CT and high signal on T1WI 2 to 3 days post partum.

Cerebral Palsy

The development of cerebral palsy in premature infants is most closely related to early MR findings of subependymal hemorrhage associated with parenchymal destruction, periventricular signal alteration with irregularity of the ventricular wall, and widespread cerebral infarction (usually middle cerebral artery distribution). In term asphyxiated infants, deep gray matter and/or diffuse involvement of the hemispheres are predictive of a poor prognosis. Parenchymal periventricular encephaloclastic cysts also bodes poorly for outcome in premature infants, whereas focal parenchymal damage is less debilitating (perhaps because of the plasticity of the brain). In term asphyxiated infants, T2 signal alterations of the deep gray matter rather than T1 shortening and diffuse involvement of the hemispheres are predictive of long-term deficits. Focal hemispheric parenchymal lesions alone are not predictive of cerebral palsy.

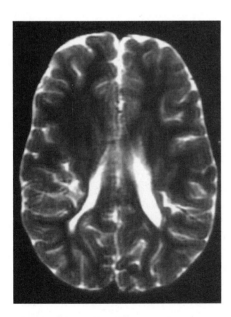

Fig. 9-42 PVL. This child, who was born prematurely, shows the diminution in white matter volume and abnormal configuration of the ventricles indicative of periventricular leukomalacia of prematurity. Note how deep the sulci dive on this T2WI.

Grade	Location of hemorrhage, findings
1	Limited to germinal matrix
2	Germinal matrix and intraventricular
3	Germinal matrix and intraventricular with hydrocephalus
4	Germinal matrix, intraventricular, and intraparenchymal

Table 9-8   Grading of Germinal Matrix Hemorrhage

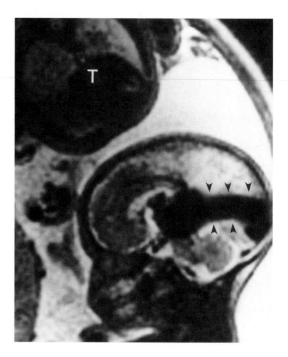

Fig. 9-43   In utero demonstration of vein of Galen malformation on MR. Note the very large flow void *(arrowheads)* in the expected location of the vein of Galen in this fetus. The large size portends a bad prognosis. Shhhhhhh! Don't wake up the twin *(T)* seen sharing the sac.

Germinal Matrix Hemorrhages

Germinal matrix and caudate-thalamic junction hemorrhages are also seen in premature infants (usually those that are 32 weeks gestation or less). Ninety percent of hemorrhages in premature infants occur in the first week of life, hence the screening US that are often ordered. The hemorrhages are thought to be venous in origin. The hemorrhage may track along the venous perivascular space and rupture into the parenchyma. Hydrocephalus caused by intraventricular blood, clots in the aqueduct, or arachnoid villi plugging occurs in 70% of premature infants with intraventricular hemorrhage (Table 9-8). Grade IV hemorrhages may actually be bleeds into venous infarctions secondary to occlusions of thalamostriate veins.

Arteriovenous Anomalies

The arteriovenous malformations are described fully in Chapter 4. The only "congenital" malformation that presents in infancy is the so-called vein of Galen aneurysm. This is really a central arteriovenous malformation or fistula. The tremendous arteriovenous shunting may lead to congestive heart failure in a newborn infant. To make matters worse, congenital cardiac anomalies may coexist. We are able to make this diagnosis in utero by US and/or MR (Fig. 9-43) and plan for treatment immediately after birth. Intrauterine therapy has not been contemplated by neuroradiologists just yet, but may be described in the third edition of this book, no doubt.

Miscellaneous Insults

Parry-Romberg syndrome

In Parry-Romberg syndrome, aka progressive facial hemiatrophy, one can find unilateral focal infarctions in the corpus callosum, diffuse deep and subcortical white matter signal changes, mild cortical thickening, and lep-

tomeningeal enhancement with dense mineral deposition. The pathogenesis of this process is thought to be a chronic vasomotor/ischemic one related to sympathetic nervous system inflammation.

Maternal cocaine abuse

Another scenario where neonatal ischemia may be present is in children of women abusing cocaine. "Normal" neonates with a maternal history of cocaine use are more likely to have focal infarctions in their basal ganglia. They also have a higher rate of neural tube closure defects. The mechanism for these abnormalities is probably due to vasospasm caused by cocaine when used in pregnancy. Bad mommy!

Neonatal hypoglycemia

Neonatal hypoglycemia (glucose <30 mg/dL) secondary to hyperinsulinemia can cause seizures and altered mental status. The cause may range from maternal diabetes to hypoxic-ischemic injury, to sepsis, gestational immaturity or malnutrition, or glucose dysmetabolism (Beckwith-Wiedemann syndrome, endocrinopathies). Brain damage in the parietal-occipital region is most common. High signal on T2WI is understandable but high signal on T1WI may coexist, secondary to hemorrhage, calcification, or myelin breakdown.

Kernicterus

Kernicterus (bilirubin encephalopathy) is associated with high signal intensity in the globus pallidus, which resolves with normalization of the bilirubinemia.

Attention deficit hyperactivity disorder (ADHD)

No definite structural lesions have been identified in ADHD patients though some interesting functional work has been done. ADHD is thought to represent dopamine dysfunction localized to the frontal lobes and striatum. Medications that increase the availability of dopamine receptor sites affect the core behaviors that define ADHD. Functional brain imaging shows that frontal lobe abnormalities in children with ADHD worsen with concentration exercise and are reversible following stimulant administration. Children with ADHD show frontal lobe deactivation during concentration tasks. They show decreased left prefrontal lobe and dorsal frontal lobe activity at rest compared with controls as well as with concentration.

MESIAL TEMPORAL SCLEROSIS

The search for mesial temporal sclerosis (MTS) is like the Holy Grail of neuroimaging as this entity is a common source for seizures in adolescents and young adults. How good you are at finding MTS may depend on your LSD levels and your ability to hallucinate or visualize subtleties in the size of the hippocampi, parahippocampi, temporal horns, and the cortices of the inferomedial temporal lobe.

How we have gotten through a combined 40 years of neuroradiology attendinghood without learning this anatomy well is amazing, but we shall not allow you to fall into the same trap (Fig. 9-44). Going from the superomedial to inferolateral surface of the hippocampus one passes from the fimbria to the alveus to the dentate fascia and then Ammon horn (zones 1 to 4) region. Once passing around the hippocampal fissure one proceeds into the subiculum (the superomedial border) to the parahippocampal gyrus medially and the entorhinal and piriform cortex inferiorly. The collateral sulcus separates the parahippocampus above from the occipitotemporal gyrus below. We hope that we learn this by the next edition (due out in 2030, however, 3 strikes and we're out). Ammons horn or cornu ammonis has four zones of granular cells. CA1 is also called the vulnerable sector because it is the most sensitive area of the brain (with the globus pallidus) to anoxia. CA2 (dorsal resistant zone) and CA3 (resistant Spielmeyer sector) are thought to be more resistant to anoxic damage. CA4 (end folium) is partially affected by anoxia. Sclerosis of CA1, and to a lesser extent CA4 is the etiology of mesial temporal sclerosis or hippocampal atrophy and has been linked to cerebral ischemia and febrile seizures. The selective vulnerability of

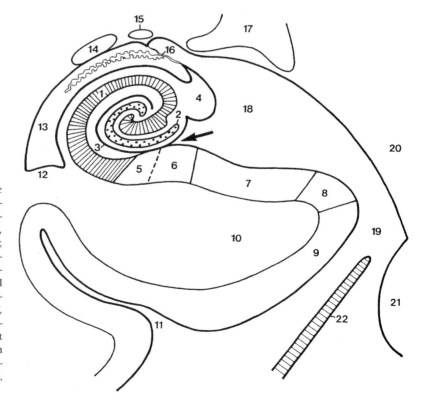

Fig. 9-44   Hippocampal anatomy. *Arrows* indicate the hippocampal sulcus (superficial part). *1,* cornu Ammonis (Ammon's horn); *2,* gyrus dentatus; *3,* hippocampal sulcus (deep or vestigial part); *4,* fimbria; *5,* prosubiculum; *6,* subiculum proper; *7,* presubiculum; *8,* parasubiculum; *9,* entorhinal area; *10,* parahippocampal gyrus; *11,* collateral sulcus; *12,* collateral eminence; *13,* temporal (inferior) horn of the lateral ventricle; *14,* tail of the caudate nucleus; *15,* stria terminalis; *16,* choroid fissure and choroid plexuses; *17,* lateral geniculate body; *18,* lateral part of the transverse fissure (wing of ambient cistern); *19,* ambient cistern; *20,* mesencephalon; *21,* pons; *22,* tentorium cerebelli. (Modified after Williams, 1995.) (From Duvernoy HM: *The Human Hippocampus.* New York, Springer-Verlag, 1998, p 18. Used with permission.)

CA1 may be due to overactivity of glutamate receptors and increased concentration of intracellular calcium ions in these granular cells. Hypoglycemia and kanic acid toxicity could also injure hippocampal structures.

Mesial temporal sclerosis accounts for as much as 50% of subjects undergoing temporal lobe surgery. However the causes of temporal lobe seizures are manifold (see Box 9-8). In those patients with ipsilateral hippocampal atrophy, surgical removal of MTS is 90% effective in eliminating seizures. In adults with temporal lobe epilepsy who have resection of their temporal lobe, 65% of the time, the pathology shows MTS. Pretty good odds. Twenty percent of cases show normal MRI structural scans—hence the potential for MRS to rear its opportunistic head (see below).

Although most cases present after or in adolescence, the roots of MTS may reside in febrile seizures in infancy. Multiple seizures in early childhood are associated with hippocampal atrophy. Nonetheless, MTS is considered a progressive disease and the imaging findings of selective atrophy may progress with age.

Atrophy of the mesial temporal lobe may affect the amygdala (12%), hippocampal head (51%), hippocampal body (88%), and hippocampal tail (61%) (Fig. 9-45). Hyperintense signal on T2W scans may involve the amygdala (4%), hippocampal head (39%), hippocampal body (81%), and hippocampal tail (49%) and/or the entire ipsilateral hippocampus (44%). Bilateral involvement occurs in approximately 20% of cases. Another finding in the spectrum of mesial temporal sclerosis is the loss of the normal cortical interdigitations of the hippocampal head. The sensitivity of this finding is approximately 90% and may be present even when atrophy and signal intensity changes are absent in the medial temporal lobe. Histopathologically, one sees neuronal loss and gliosis in the patients. The mechanism for congenital, nonfebrile development of MTS is MySTerious, but may be due to a perinatal ischemic event due to compression of arteries during delivery, intrauterine hypoxia, hypoxia secondary to status epilepticus, neurotoxic effects of excessive glutamate production, and/or hypoglycemia. Please feel free to add your own hypothesis here. Sky's the limit.

One can obtain greater and greater layers of sophistication in the analysis of the temporal lobes using quantitative volumetry, T2 relaxometry, MRS (decreased NAA, what else? Also reported as NAA/Cho <0.8 and NAA/Cr <1.0), PET, SPECT, and gross vomitry (where you have emesis from data overload). If you scan the patients during or within 24 hours of acute temporal lobe seizures, one finds lactic acid build-up and/or lipid peaks on the proton MRS studies of the affected temporal lobe—and bumps on the patient's heads as they bang the sides of the scanner during the seizures. The bottom line is that simple 512 × 512 matrix FLAIR or T2WI for signal intensity changes and 512 × 512 resolution inversion re-

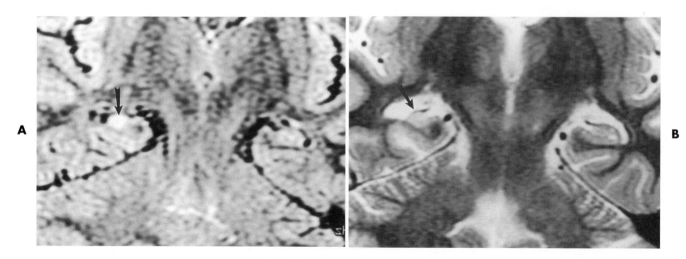

Fig. 9-45   Mesial temporal sclerosis. **A,** Note the focal area of high signal in the right hippocampus *(arrow)* on the FLAIR study. **B,** Atrophy of the hippocampus and high signal is also apparent on the T2WI. Compare with Fig. 9-44 to show Ammon's horn hyperintensity.

covery T1W scans (phase sensitive inversion recovery) for the presence of hippocampal atrophy will tell you which temporal lobe is abnormal in the vast majority of cases. Or you can call for the electroencephalograph (EEG) results and be done with it. For those cases with equivocal EEGs and/or bilateral disease careful scrutiny of the images will stand you in good stead. There is a whole cottage industry of volumetric programs that will determine which hippocampus is smaller—they can be extremely accurate.

The fornix and mamillary body ipsilateral to the side of mesial temporal sclerosis may be atrophic secondary to the decreased input to crossing fibers and limbic contributions. These findings may also be present in cases of temporal lobe resections, strokes, and tumors.

When the localization of a seizure focus is problematic, the neurosurgeons may place stainless steel or platinum alloy subdural grid contact arrays. This is a last resort when ictal scalp recordings have failed and when functional cortical mapping is required before surgery. The placement of these grids is not without risk; be wary of the reported complications of extraaxial hematomas or effusions, venous thromboses, subfalcine or transtentorial herniations, tension pneumocephalus, intraparenchymal hemorrhage, and cerebral infections.

One potential obstacle associated with the work-up for seizures should be recognized. If you image the patient immediately after a seizure or even during status epilepticus that is inapparent to the clinicians (yes this can happen with some temporal lobe cases—do not blame the neurologist) you may see meningeal enhancement and high signal intensity in the seizing temporal lobe. This may imply a more diffuse process than is actually there (encephalitis and/or gliomatosis) and in fact, this "abnormality" may resolve completely on MR in a few days. This is probably due to the increased blood flow to the seizing temporal lobe, that is, a perfusion effect. Even DWI scans may be transiently positive.

Other sources of seizure foci include (in the young patient) neoplasms, vascular malformations, gliotic abnormalities, and malformations of cortical development. Add strokes to this list for older adults. Occipital lobe epileptogenic foci are most often due to developmental abnormalities (e.g., focal cortical dysplasia, heterotopias, hamartomas, migrational anomalies) or tumors (usually gliomas).

PHAKOMATOSES

The phakomatoses refer to a group of hereditary diseases of the neuroectoderm characterized by cutaneous manifestations and sometimes called neurocutaneous disorders. Phakos is Greek for mother-spot, probably reflecting the cutaneous manifestation. These disorders in-clude neurofibromatosis, tuberous sclerosis, von Hippel-Lindau disease, and Sturge-Weber syndrome. The quintessential leasion is the neurogenic tumor, the tuber, the hemangioblastoma, and the angiomatosis respectively. Hereditary hemorrhagic telangiectasia, ataxia-telangiectasia, neurocutaneous melanosis, basal cell nevus syndrome, Wyburn-Mason syndrome, and Parry-Rombery syndrome are also classified as phakomatoses. Read on, tender student.

Neurofibromatosis

Neurofibromatosis type 1 Neurofibromatosis type 1 (von Recklinghausen disease, or NF-1) (Table 9-9) is a disease of childhood that occurs in a hereditary form transmitted by autosomal dominance in 50% of cases and sporadically in the other 50%. Overall, the incidence of neurofibromatosis is approximately 1 in 2000 to 6000 live births. NF-1 is diagnosed if there are two or more of the following findings: (1) six or more café-au-lait spots, (2) two or more Lisch nodules (hamartomas) of the iris, (3) two or more neurofibromas or one or more plexiform neurofibromas, (4) axillary/inguinal freckling, (5) one or more bone dysplasias or pseudarthrosis of a long bone, (6) optic pathway glioma, or (7) a first-degree relative with the diagnosis of NF-1.

NF-1 appears to be transmitted on the long arm of chromosome 17 (17q11) and occurs in 1 in 2500 to 4000 live births. In NF-1 the patients have many café-au-lait spots and have a preponderance of optic pathway pilocytic astrocytomas. These optic gliomas present in childhood yet may have little effect on vision until they are large. Ten percent to 38% of patients with optic gliomas have NF-1, and 15% to 40% of patients with NF-1 have optic pathway gliomas (Fig. 9-46). Cerebellar, brain stem, and cerebral astrocytomas are also seen with NF-1. In addition, as noted on MR, the patients have high signal intensity foci that appear in the peduncles or deep gray matter of the cerebellum, the brain stem (especially the pons), the basal ganglia (especially the globus pallidus), and the white matter of the supratentorial space (Fig. 9-47). There is considerable debate concerning what these areas of high signal intensity on T2WI represent, as described earlier under hamartomas. At this time most people believe that they are due to myelin vacuolization or hamartomas, focal areas of gliosis, wallerian degeneration, dysplastic white matter, or, less likely, pre-neoplastic lesions. (How helpful—really narrows the differential, eh?). These basal ganglia foci may also be bright on T1W scans.

Follow-up studies of these high intensity foci in NF patients suggest that, though present in the basal ganglia and brain stem in the younger decades with relatively high frequency, they often decrease in size with age. Lesions in the cerebellar white matter and dentate

Table 9-9   NF-1 versus NF-2

Feature	NF-1	NF-2
Chromosome involved	17	22
Optic gliomas	Yes	No
Acoustic schwannomas	No	Yes
Meningiomas	No	Yes
UBOs in deep gray matter, cerebellum	Yes	No
Incidence	1/4,000	1/50,000
Skin findings	Many	Few
Spinal gliomas	Astrocytoma	Ependymoma
Skeletal dysplasias	Yes	No
Lisch nodules (iris hamartomas)	Yes	No, but sublenticular cataracts
Dural ectasia	Yes	No
Age at presentation (yr)	<10	10–30
Vascular stenoses	Yes	No
Plexiform neurofibromas	Yes	No
Malignant change	Yes	No
Sphenoid wing absence	Yes	No
Hydrocephalus	Yes, obstructed/stenotic aqueduct	No
CNS hamartomas	Yes	No
Paraspinal necrofibromas	Yes	Yes
Meningocele	Yes, lateral thoracic	No

UBOs. Unidentified bright objects.

nuclei are found in younger patients and are rare after the third decade. Rarely they may enlarge in adulthood.

Astrocytomas may arise within the previously described locations in the basal ganglia, optic radiations, cerebellar gray or white matter, or brain stem. When the high intensity foci enhance or grow after adolescence, the specter of neoplasm must be raised (pretty graphic, da?). Short follow-up scans are indicated. Patients with NF-1 also have increased incidence of astrocytomas of the spinal cord.

On imaging one may see enlargement of the optic nerves or chiasm. These tumors are generally low-grade pilocytic astrocytomas and slow growing and are usually watched; treatment is withheld until the patients

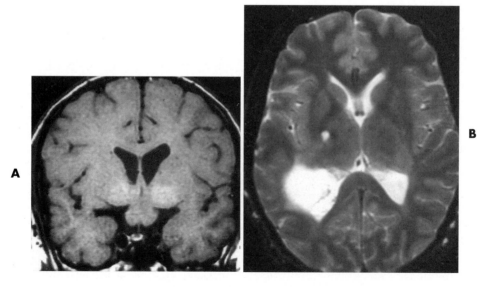

Fig. 9-46   Optic pathway glioma. **A,** There is marked enlargement of the optic chiasm in this individual. **B,** The optic fibers adjacent to the right occipital horn of the lateral ventricle are involved. The tiny deep gray matter focus is indicative of NF-1.

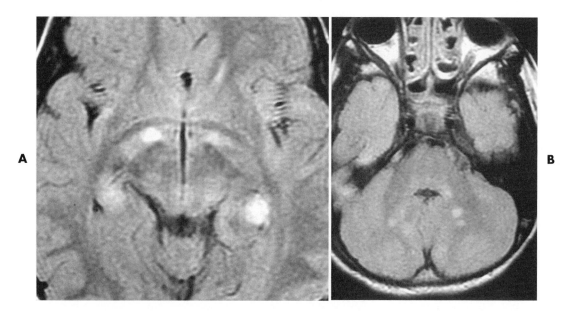

Fig. 9-47   UBOs of NF-I. **A,** This FLAIR scan epitomizes the vexing lesions of the basal ganglia in patients with NF-1. Histopathologically, these UBOs have yet to be well-characterized. **B,** They are also seen in the thalami and the cerebellar white matter tracts.

become progressively symptomatic. Enhancement is variable.

The presence of a plexiform neurofibroma strongly suggests NF-1. A plexiform neurofibroma consists of sheets of collagen and Schwann cells that spread in an aggressive manner, insinuating themselves in a cylindrical fashion around a nerve. These lesions tend to involve the scalp, neck, mediastinum, retroperitoneum, cranial nerve V, and orbit (Fig. 9-48). The lesions are soft and elastic, and probably account for the "elephantiasis" of neurofibromatosis.

Sarcomatous degeneration of neurofibromas occurs in about 5% of patients with peripheral nerve sheath neural tumors. The more neurofibromas one has, the higher the likelihood of malignant degeneration, but this usually occurs in midadulthood (small consolation, eh?). Plexiform neurofibromas have a higher rate of malignant change, much more so than schwannomas.

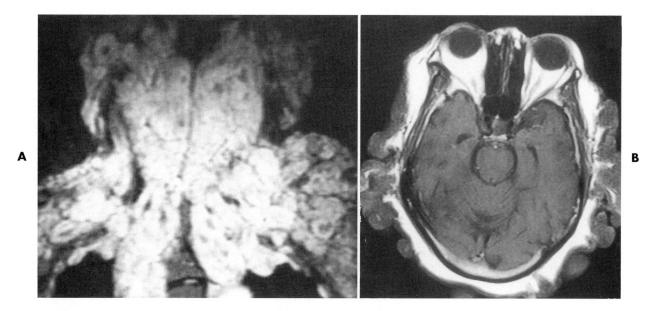

Fig. 9-48   Plexiform neurofibroma. **A,** Coronal MR depicts an enormous plexiform neurofibroma of the spine, shoulders, and neck. **B,** Multiple cutaneous neurofibromas: Despite the numerous cutaneous neurofibromas, which extended into the subcutaneous tissue bilaterally, this patient's brain was normal. Which would you rather have, the cosmetic deformity of multiple cutaneous neurofibromas or the potential danger of intracranial (optic pathway) manifestations? (Case courtesy of Stuart Bobman.)

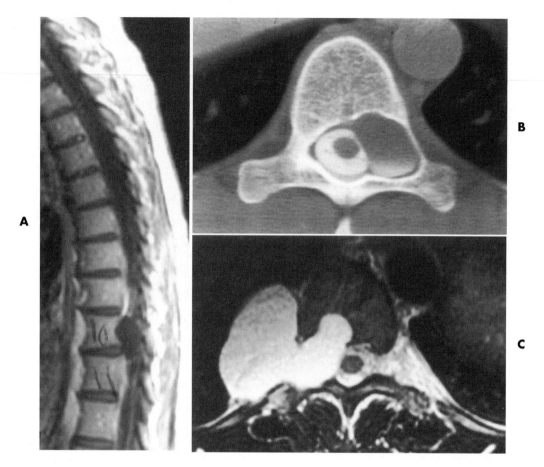

Fig. 9-49   NF-1. **A,** Sagittal T1WI with posterior scalloping of the T10 vertebral body. **B,** After intrathecal contrast a fluid level is observed in the lateral meningocele. The pedicle is thinned and the left posterior margin of the vertebral body is scalloped. **C,** T2WI in another patient demonstrating a large lateral thoracic meningocele. Marked scalloping is noted in the posterior aspect of the vertebral body.

Additional findings that one might see in patients with neurofibromatosis include spinal dural ectasia (Fig. 9-49), lateral thoracic meningoceles, posterior vertebral body scalloping, aqueductal stenosis, pachygyria, polymicrogyria, syringomyelia, and other heterotopias. Neuroradiologists can have a field day with neurofibromatosis (note: this, too, is a favored topic for board examinations).

Neurofibromatosis type 2   Neurofibromatosis type 2 (NF-2) appears to be transmitted on chromosome 22q12 and is approximately one tenth as common as NF-1. The patients have fewer skin lesions, but the pathognomonic sign of NF-2 is bilateral (2 is the unlucky number) cranial nerve VIII vestibular schwannomas (Fig. 9-50). Diagnosis is made if the patient has one of the following features: (1) bilateral vestibular acoustic schwannomas; (2) a first-degree relative with NF-2 and either a single acoustic schwannoma or any two of the following: schwannomas, neurofibromas, meningiomas or gliomas. A posterior sublenticular capsular cataract in a young patient is also typical of this disorder. Cranial nerve V is the second most common site of schwannomas in NF-2. Sensory roots are affected more commonly than motor roots. The patients also have increased incidence of meningiomas and rarely

have other glial tumors (ependymomas). The nickname MISME (multiple inherited schwannomas, meningiomas, and ependymomas) attests to the fact that *neurofibromas* are not a feature of NF-2.

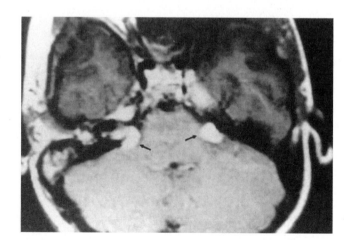

Fig. 9-50   Neurofibromatosis type 2. Axial enhanced T1WI shows bilateral acoustic schwannomas *(arrows)*. This finding is the *sine qua non* of NF-2. Forget it and you fail your boards.

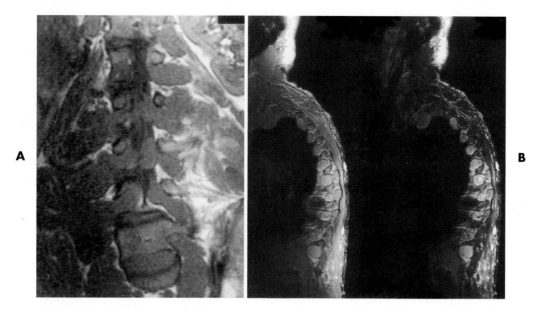

Fig. 9-51 Extensive neurofibromatosis. **A,** T1W scan shows multiple lumbar spine neurofibromas extending both intrathecally as well as extradurally bilaterally. Parasagittal PDWI and T2WI **(B)** show numerous neurofibromas extending through the neural foramina and into the paraspinal soft tissues.

Spinal manifestations of NF-2 can be seen in 63% to 90% of cases. Patients with nonsense or frame shift mutations had a higher rate of spinal tumors than those with splice-shift and all other types of genetic mutations. In one report 53% of patients had intramedullary lesions, 55% intradural extramedullary tumors (88% were nerve sheath tumors and 12% meningiomas), and 45% both intramedullary and extramedullary masses (Fig. 9-51). Of those with intramedullary masses, over half had multiple ones. Multiple nerve sheath tumors (both schwannomas [75%] and neurofibromas [25%]) are usually seen in the cauda equina and may be intradural and/or extradural. Of intramedullary tumors, ependymomas predominate, but astrocytomas and intramedullary schwannomas may occur.

The patients with NF-2 demonstrate enhancing masses located in and around the cerebellopontine angle or extending into the internal auditory canal. The lesions generally are slightly hyperintense on T2WI. (Please see Chapter 3 for typical and atypical features of vestibular schwannomas.) Occasionally, dural ectasia of cranial nerve VIII root sleeve can enlarge the internal auditory canal, producing the same type of bony flaring seen with acoustic schwannomas. Arachnoid cysts may accompany the vestibular schwannomas. In addition, meningiomas may occur at this location, although the parasagittal regions predominate.

Tuberous Sclerosis

Tuberous sclerosis (Bourneville disease) (Box 9-9) is a disease that most commonly occurs spontaneously (60%) but is also seen in an autosomal dominant form transmitted on the long arm of chromosome 9 (9q34) and/or 16 (16p13). It arises in 1 in 6000 to 15,000 live births. The characteristic findings with tuberous sclerosis are adenoma sebaceum (60% to 90% of cases), mental retardation (50%), and seizures (60% to 80%). All three findings occur in only one third of cases. Patients also may have retinal hamartomas (50%), shagreen patches (20% to 40%), ungual fibromas (20% to 30%), rhabdomyomas of the heart (25% to 50%), angiomyolipomas of the kidney (50% to 90%), cystic skeletal lesions, and the intracranial manifestations. Tuberous sclerosis is like a shotgun blast: it can hit all parts of the body.

The intracranial manifestations include periventricular subependymal nodules (candle gutterings) (90% to 100%), cortical and subcortical peripheral tubers (94% of patients on MR), white matter hamartomatous lesions, and subependymal giant cell astrocytomas (6% to 16%) (Fig. 9-52). Patients may have cortical heterotopias and ventriculomegaly as well. Eighty-eight percent of periventricular subependymal nodules are calcified, whereas only 50% of the parenchymal hamartomas are calcified. The frequency of cortical tubers and white matter lesions is highest in the frontal lobes followed by the parietal, occipital, temporal, and cerebellar regions. Tubers may expand gyri or show central umbilication and are bright on long TR sequences. Patients with cerebellar tubers are older than those with cerebral tubers, have more extensive disease, and may have focal cerebellar atrophy associated with those tubers. White matter lesions may appear on MR as curvilinear or straight thin bands radiating from the ventricles (88%), wedge-shaped

Box 9-9 Tuberous Sclerosis Findings

CLINICAL

1. Adenoma sebaceum
2. Ash-leaf spot
3. Cafe au lait spots
4. Mental retardation
5. Retinal hamartomas
6. Retinal phatoma
7. Seizures
8. Shagreen patches
9. Subungual fibromas

RADIOGRAPHIC CNS

1. Atrophy
2. Calcified optic nerve head drusen
3. Cortical tubers
4. Giant cell astrocytomas
5. Intracranial calcifications
6. Neuronal migrational anomalies
7. Periependymal nodules
8. Radial glial fiber hyperintensity

RADIOGRAPHIC NON-CNS

1. Angiomyolipomas of kidneys
2. Aortic aneurysm
3. Hepatic adenomas
4. Pulmonary lymphangiomyomatosis
5. Rhabdomyomas of heart
6. Renal cell carcinoma
7. Renal cysts
8. Skeletal cysts, sclerotic densities, periosteal thickening
9. Upper lobe interstitial fibrosis, blebs, pneumothorax, chylothorax
10. Vascular stenosis

lesions with apices near the ventricle (31%), or tumefactive foci of abnormal intensity (14%). Subependymal nodules (31%), cortical tubers (3%), and white matter lesions (12%) may show enhancement on MR. FLAIR imaging is particularly good at spotting subcortical small tubers, even more so than T2W scans. It should be noted, however, that the number, size, and location of tubers seems to be unrelated to the neurologic symptoms in adults. A greater number of tubers occur in children with infantile spasms, seizures before 1 year of age, and mental disability. The pathogenesis of the various lesions of tuberous sclerosis is thought to be due to abnormal radial-glial migration of dysgenetic giant cells that are capable of astrocytic or neuronal differentiation. Multipotential cells with multiproblems.

In infants, the subependymal nodules of tuberous sclerosis are hyperintense on T1WI and hypointense on T2WI, the opposite of what is seen in adults. They are not isointense to gray matter and therefore should not be confused with subependymal nodular heterotopias in Louisville. White matter anomalies are more visible in infants. However, cortical tubers are more difficult to identify in infants. In utero demonstration of periventricular subependymal nodules and cardiac rhabdomyomas has been reported in a fetus of 28 weeks gestational age.

Tuberous sclerosis has an association with subependymal giant cell astrocytomas (SGCA) that generally occur around the foramina of Monro (see Chapter 3) (Fig. 9-53). As opposed to subependymal tubers, these lesions enhance commonly and uniformly, are large, grow with time, cause obstructive hydrocephalus, and have a lower rate of calcification. Nonetheless, it is believed that these tumors arise from subependymal nodules. They occur in approximately 1.7% to 15% of patients who have tuberous sclerosis. Their malignant potential is small.

On CT, the periventricular calcified nodules are seen easily; however, the more peripheral tubers are harder to detect. Calcification obviously would be difficult to detect on MR without gradient-echo scans. Nonetheless, the tubers are well seen by MR, showing up as increasing intensity on T2WI. The subependymal tubers may be better seen on T1WI. The subependymal giant cell astrocytomas are increased in signal intensity on the T2WI and demonstrate moderate enhancement. CT may be more specific than MR for SGCA because enhancement on CT implies a SGCA whereas enhancement on MR (because of the sensitivity) may be seen with tubers and subependymal nodules.

Sturge-Weber Syndrome

Sturge-Weber syndrome (encephalotrigeminal angiomatosis) (Box 9-10) is associated with facial port wine stain (nevus flammeus) with hemiplegia and a seizure disorder. Other manifestations include congenital glaucoma and buphthalmos, choroidal or scleral hemangiomas, and mental retardation. This disease usually occurs sporadically with equal male and female incidence. The cutaneous vascular nevus in the face is usually in the V-1 distribution. There are rare cases reported where the patient has Sturge-Weber without the facial nevus. Ipsilateral to the vascular angioma within the brain, one often identifies enlargement and enhancement of the choroid plexus, suggesting an angioma.

Leptomeningial capillary-venous angiomatosis is also seen in Sturge-Weber syndrome. On CT Sturge-Weber syndrome is usually detected by cortical calcification (tram-line) in the ipsilateral occipital, parietal, or temporal lobe underlying the leptomeningeal vascular malformation with associated hemiatrophy (Fig. 9-54). The abnormality is truly a pial vascular abnormality, which demonstrates underlying patchy gliosis and demyelination. Patients usually have a homonymous hemianopsia,

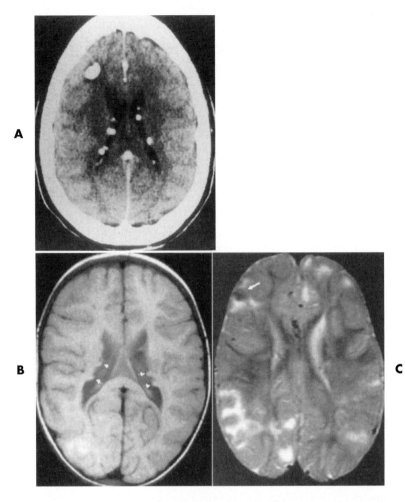

Fig. 9-52 Tuberous sclerosis. **A,** Note the periventricular calcified subependymal nodules on this CT. Cortical calcified tuber is also located in the right frontal region. **B,** Axial T1WI shows the subependymal nodules *(small arrows)* lining the lateral ventricles bilaterally isointense to white matter. **C,** Axial T2WI demonstrates foci of abnormal signal intensity throughout the subcortical white matter and in the cortex corresponding to areas of abnormal myelination and cortical tubers. Right frontal cortical tuber *(arrow)* is probably calcified (because it is very low in intensity on T2WI). Calcified subependymal nodules are present; find them.

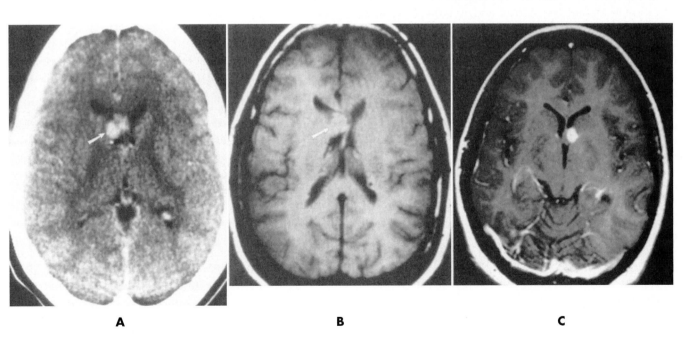

Fig. 9-53 Subependymal giant cell astrocytoma in tuberous sclerosis. **A,** Enhanced CT demonstrates high density in this patient with tuberous sclerosis. On the basis of the CT we cannot tell whether the lesion enhances or is calcified. This would be important because on CT subependymal giant cell tumors enhance, whereas tubers usually do not. **B,** T1WI without contrast also shows the isointense subependymal mass. Unfortunately, the patient left before contrast could be given to go to an Ozzy Osborne reunion. However, on MR this does not help in distinguishing subependymal giant cell tumor from a subependymal nodule because both have been reported to enhance. **C,** Another case shows enhancement on T1WI of a subependymal giant cell astrocytoma.

455

Box 9-10 Findings in Sturge-Weber Syndrome

CLINICAL

1. Accelerated myelination
2. Choroidal angioma
3. Glaucoma-buphthalmos
4. Hemiparesis, hemiplegia
5. Mental retardation
6. Scleral telangiectasia
7. Seizures
8. Trigeminal angioma (capillary telangiectasia); port wine nevus in V-1 distribution
9. Visceral angioma

RADIOGRAPHIC

1. Anomalous venous drainage to deep veins
2. Choroid plexus angioma or hypertrophy ipsilateral to angiomatosis
3. Dyke-Davidoff-Masson syndrome
   a. Elevated petrous ridge, sphenoid wing
   b. Enlarged frontal sinuses
   c. Hemihypertrophied skull
4. Hemiatrophy
5. Intracranial calcification (tram-tracks)
6. Pial angioma

contralateral hemiplegia, and hemisensory loss. The calcification is within the cortex and not the meninges, arises in the fourth layer of the cortex, and is thought to be due to anoxia from stasis of flow within the meninges. Calcification, however, is not seen until about the second year of life. CT demonstrates the cortical calcification to best advantage. Atrophy is present on the ipsilateral side, as is enlargement of the choroid of the lateral ventricles. In fact, the size of the choroid plexus and extent of leptomeningeal involvement in children with Sturge-Weber syndrome correlates well.

MR detects a greater extent of disease than CT, particularly on enhanced T1WI. In this instance the pia enhances dramatically, giving a true demonstration of the degree of the vascular abnormality (Fig. 9-55). Cortical enhancement caused by ischemic injury may also be present. Abnormally low signal intensity within the white matter on T2WI is probably related to abnormal myelination from ischemia. Bilaterality of the vascular lesion is often seen on MR.

On angiography an increase in the number and size of the medullary veins with decreased cortical veins (anomalous venous drainage) and a capillary stain are usually seen in the parietal and occipital lobes. There is slow cerebral blood flow, and the ipsilateral cerebral arteries are generally small.

Keep your eyes on your patients' eyes! In nearly 50% of patients with Sturge-Weber syndrome you will find abnormal ocular enhancement, be it due to choroidal hemangiomas or inflammation from glaucoma. (Sorry to steal from the orbit chapter). Visualization of ocular hemangiomata is increased with bilateral intracranial disease, extensive facial nevi, and ocular glaucoma.

The Wyburn-Mason syndrome may be a forme fruste of Sturge-Weber syndrome. Patients have a facial vascular nevus in nerve V distribution, retinal angioma, and a midbrain arteriovenous malformation. The differential diagnosis also includes Klippel-Trenaunay-Weber syndrome (hemihypertrophy, cutaneous angiomas, varices, and/or anomalous venous drainage).

von Hippel-Lindau Disease

CNS hemangioblastomas combine with retinal hemangioblastomas (67%), cysts of the kidney, pancreas, and liver, renal cell carcinomas, islet cell tumors and adenomas to form von Hippel-Lindau disease (VHL). Diagnosis is based on a capillary hemangioblastoma of the CNS or retina and the presence of one VHL associated-tumor or a previous family history. Pheochromocytomas of the adrenal gland may also be present, linking the multiple endocrine neoplasia syndromes with VHL. Endolymphatic sac tumors have also been described with this entity. There also appears to be a link to neurofibromatosis.

Multiple CNS hemangioblastomas are the *sine qua non* of this syndrome, and they may arise in the cerebellum (most commonly), the medulla, the spinal cord, or less commonly, supratentorially. The lesions may be cystic, solid, or combined (see Chapter 3, Figs. 3-38, 3-39). The classic description is a highly vascular, enhancing mural nodule associated with a predominantly cystic mass in the lateral cerebellum.

Spinal hemangioblastomas represent about 3% of spinal cord tumors. One-third are associated with von Hippel Lindau disease. Of all spinal hemangioblastomas 80% are single, 20% multiple (almost all associated with VHL), 60% intramedullary, 11% intra and extramedullary, 21% intradural but purely extramedullary, and 8% extradural. Their location is usually characterized by the surgeons as "sub-pial." They are more commonly found in the thoracic cord than the cervical cord. Most hemangioblastomas seen with VHL are 10 mm or less in size and may be intramedullary or along the dorsal nerve roots. If you are expecting to see vascular flow voids to make the diagnosis of spinal hemangioblastoma, you had better wait for our third edition—it is extremely rare to see flow voids on MR in hemangioblastomas under 15 mm in size—you will have to wait for the tumors to grow. On the other hand, a syrinx may be present in 40% to 60% of cases (often out of proportion to the small size of the tumor).

The disorder appears to be transmitted through autosomal dominant inheritance in 20% of cases on chro-

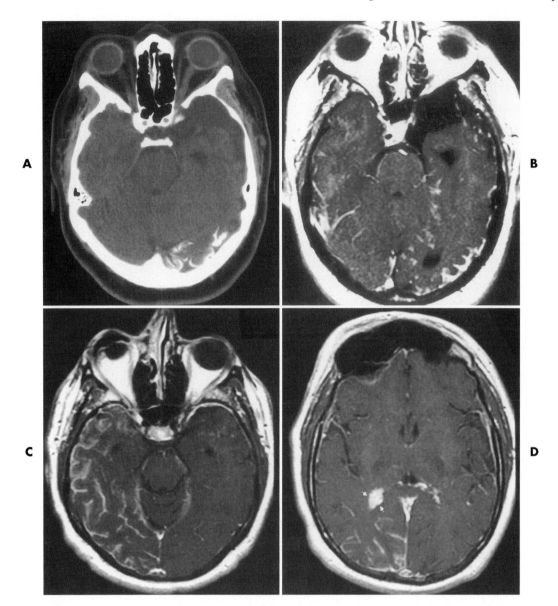

Fig. 9-54   Sturge-Weber. **A,** This CT scan is filmed at intermediate windows to bring out the cortical calcification of the Sturge-Weber malformation. Hemiatrophy of the left temporal lobe is suggested by the dilatation of the subarachnoid space anteriorly. **B,** Corresponding enhanced MR shows the leptomeningeal angiomatosis of the occipital lobe with pial enhancement. **C,** This enhanced scan in another case shows diffuse meningeal and pial enhancement in the right temporal lobe. The observant grasshopper will note that the patient has had an enucleation on the right side secondary to a large angioma of the choroid of the right globe. **D,** The ancillary finding of enlargement of the choroid of the right lateral ventricle supports the diagnosis. Is the right frontal sinus enlarged suggestive of Dyke-Davidoff-Masson syndrome?

mosome 3p25. Twenty percent of patients with hemangioblastomas of the cerebellum have VHL. Cerebellar hemangioblastomas ultimately develop in 83% of patients with VHL.

Meningiomatosis

Meningiomatosis, or meningioangiomatosis, refers to a disorder in which there is hamartomatous proliferation of meningeal cells via the intraparenchymal blood vessels into the cerebral cortex. The leptomeninges are thick and infiltrated with fibrous tissue, and may be calcified. Cor-

tical meningovascular fibroblastic proliferation along the Virchow-Robin spaces is also present with psammomatous calcification, causing a tram-track appearance. The lesion resembles Sturge-Weber syndrome, but no vascular abnormalities are present. Meningioangiomatosis may be considered a forme fruste of neurofibromatosis.

Neurocutaneous Melanosis

Another relatively obscure syndrome put in the classification of the phakomatoses is neurocutaneous melanosis. Melanoblasts from neural crest cells are present in

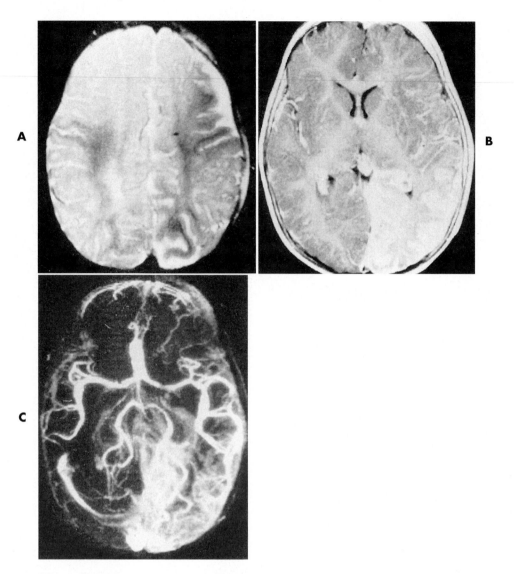

Fig. 9-55 Sturge-Weber on MR. **A**, T2WI demonstrates atrophic changes in the left hemisphere. Hypointensity is noted in the left occipital, posterior temporal region. There is also hypointensity on the contralateral side, although the atrophic changes are not as marked. **B**, Enhanced T1WI illustrates dense gyriform enhancement in the occipital, posterior temporal region. **C**, Enhanced time-of-flight MR angiogram outlines dense vascularity in the lesion.

the globes, skin, inner ear, sinonasal cavity, and leptomeninges and are the source of this disorder. It is characterized by cutaneous nevi and melanotic thickening of the meninges. Diffuse enhancement of the meninges of the brain and spine (20%) is seen; the melanin may (Fig. 9-56) or may not be detected on the preenhanced T1WI image. Hydrocephalus, cranial neuropathies, and syringohydromyelia may develop.

Although malignant degeneration of the skin lesions is very uncommon, malignant transformation of CNS melanosis occurs in up to 50% of cases. When this occurs, parenchymal or intramedullary infiltration is the hallmark.

Neurocutaneous melanocytosis is usually a sporadic disease discovered in children due to hydrocephalus

from gummed up arachnoid villi. Multiple cranial neuropathies may develop.

Hereditary Hemorrhagic Telangiectasia

Hereditary hemorrhagic telangiectasia also known as HHT or Osler-Weber-Rendu syndrome is an entity consisting of mucocutaneous telangiectasias and visceral arteriovenous malformations. One of the many presenting symptoms may be epistaxis secondary to sinonasal mucocutaneous telangiectasias. However, one should not forget that 5% of patients with HHT have a cerebral arteriovenous malformation (AVM) and 2% of AVMs are associated with HHT. When a patient with HHT has one cerebral AVM, there is a 50% chance of a second AVM

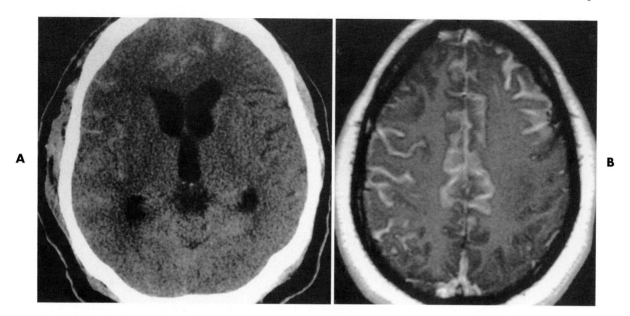

Fig. 9-56   Neurocutaneous melanosis. **A,** This CT scan shows hyperintensity to the sulci. First diagnosis is subarachnoid hemorrhage but there was no blood in the basal cisterns. Next thought—meningitis? **B,** Precontrast T1WI showed high intensity to the pia arachnoid. Hemorrhagic meningitis? No, neurocutaneous melanosis!

of the brain elsewhere. The AVMs may have a nidus (seen more frequently in adults) or may actually represent a fistula (more common in kids)

CONGENITAL SPINAL ANOMALIES

Bony Disorders

Many bony disorders are associated with spinal anomalies. Hypoplasia and/or incomplete development of the C1 arch and/or odontoid process is a common occurrence and may be asymptomatic. Occipitalization of the C1 vertebral body may be associated with atlantoaxial destabilization, however.

The Klippel-Feil anomaly refers to fusion of multiple cervical spine bodies. It may be associated with the Chiari malformations and syringohydromyelia. The C2—C3 and C5—C6 levels are the most common sites of fusion.

Meningoceles, Myeloceles, and Meningomyeloceles

The mechanism for development of spinal dysraphic conditions is a lack of folding of the primordial neural tissue into a tube. Thus, the skin remains lateral to the unfolded superficial neural ectoderm, leaving a midline defect. Although no bone is induced directly over the neural tissue, it may develop laterally where skin ectoderm and neural ectoderm are in continuity. The neural

ectoderm is uncovered at birth. The size of the pia-arachnoid and CSF over the neural tissue is variable. Many of these disorders will be detected prenatally by serologic or ammocentesis tests (elevated α-fetoprotein level) and US (Fig. 9-57).

Meningocele, myelocele, myelomeningocele, and lipo(myelo)meningocele are terms used to describe the tissue extending through the bony spinal canal defect in a person with spinal dysraphism (Fig. 9-58). Together with the bony defect in the spine (usually seen in the lower lumbar or sacral region), there may be an opening in the skin, a dimple at the skin surface, or a hairy patch on the back. (Do not get out the mirror—it is usually detectable at birth.) A meningocele refers to herniation of meninges alone without spinal cord or nerve roots into the defect in the bony spinal canal. This is an uncommon type of spinal anomaly (Fig. 9-59). Even rarer is the anterior sacral meningocele, where the mass protrudes into the pelvis, causing compression on the rectum and/or bladder. The anterior meningocele may be inapparent at the skin surface. Currarino's triad refers to (1) anorectal malformation, (2) bony sacral defect, and (3) presacral mass (e.g., anterior sacral meningocele). These meningoceles are more common in NF-1 and Marfan's.

A myelocele refers to herniation of the neural placode (a flat plate of unneurulated neural tissue) through the bony defect such that it lies flush with the surface of the skin of the back (see Fig. 9-36). The neural placode may also be evident with myelomeningoceles and is the "working part" of the now-opened lower spinal cord.

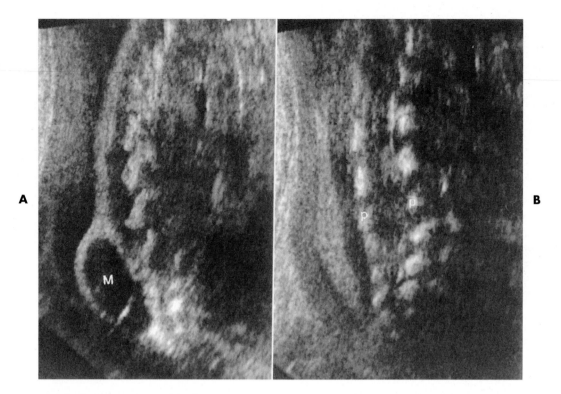

Fig. 9-57   Meningocele. **A,** US reveals a CSF collection *(M)* herniating through the spinal canal in this 20-week fetus. **B,** Coronal US through the spinal canal shows widening of the interpediculate distance *(P)* from the meningocele. (Compliments of Peggy Brennecke, MD)

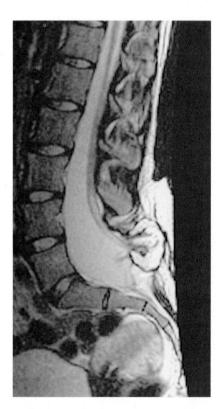

Fig. 9-58   Myelomeningocele. It is rare to actually obtain an MR image in an infant with a myelomeningocele because the child is usually sent right to surgery. Note the neural placode, enlarged spinal canal, and spinal dysraphism. Can you see the distal syrinx? Could that be the terminal ventricle (ventriculus terminalis) in a tethered, low conus?

Very little CSF is evident, and only a layer of arachnoid is present over the myelocele. A myelomeningocele contains meninges and either spinal cord or nerve root structures. The myelocele and the myelomeningocele are the most common forms of dysraphism; these entities are usually associated with Chiari II malformations and with syringohydromyelia. Myelomeningoceles are repaired quickly after birth, often without any pre-op imaging since the dang thing is hanging there in the breeze of the incubator, open for inspection.

Meningoceles are one tenth as common as myelomeningoceles. When meninges, cord, roots, and fat (usually associated with the filum terminale or neural placode) protrude through the bony defect, the term used is *lipomyelomeningocele.* All these entities are usually associated with a low-lying, tethered conus medullaris below the L2—L3 disk (Fig. 9-60). The normal termination of the conus after age 3 months is above the L2–3 disk level; less than 2% of normal humans have a conus below the L2–3 disk level. The clinical presentation of myelomeningoceles, meningoceles, or lipomyelomeningoceles that are not detected at birth includes hyperreflexia, bladder and bowel difficulties, and spasticity.

The goal of therapy is to (1) enclose the defect into the intraspinal structures so that infection is prevented and (2) free up the distal end of the neural tube so that tethering does not occur as the patient grows. If tethering does occur, then downward herniation of intracranial contents through the foramen magnum is a pos-

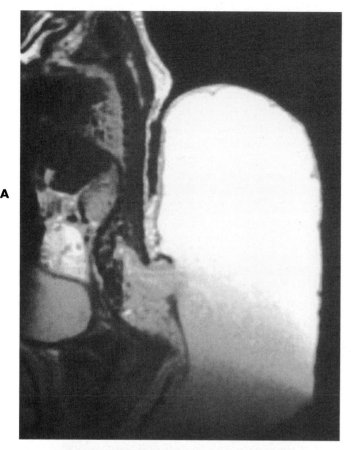

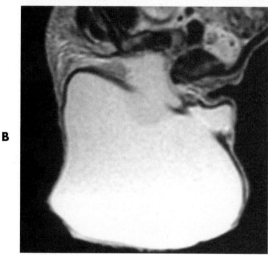

Fig. 9-59 Meningocele. **A,** Huge collection of CSF spills out of a defect in the spinal canal. **B,** Axial T2WI through the lumbosacral region shows no solid material in the fluid herniating through the dysraphic spine.

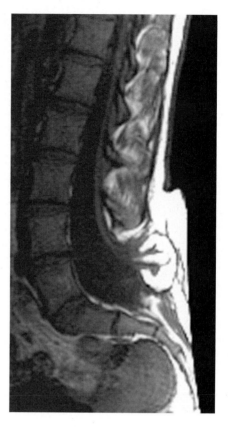

Fig. 9-60 Lipomyelomeningocele. Sagittal T1WI shows fat and thickened cord with abnormality of the bony canal compatible with the lipomeningocele. Note that we tricked you. This is the same case as Fig. 9-58, except T1WI.

provement usually occurs even with no change in the site of the bottom of the cord. Presumably CSF pulsations return to normal and the cord and hindbrain can move again. Still, the surgeon hates to see the lack of change on postoperative MR. Be a hedgehog.

Recall that, as opposed to meningoceles, myeloceles, and meningomyeloceles, which are lesions of absence of separation between cutaneous and neural ectoderm and are associated with Chiari malformations, lipomyeloceles and intradural lipomas are lesions due to premature separation of these two types of ectoderm. They are NOT associated with Chiari malformations. Lipomyelomeningoceles have skin covering the dysraphism. The fat may insert into the conus or along the dorsal surface of the conus with nerve roots anterior to the lipoma.

Spina Bifida Occulta

With isolated spinal bifida occulta the skin surface of the back is normal; however, a cleft in the posterior elements of the vertebrae is seen. No myelomeningocele is present; however, this defect may be seen with tethered cords and/or diastematomyelia. Rarely one may have a skin-covered myelocystocele in which dura,

sibility. One of the complications of the surgery is production of fibrous tissue, which may retether the dysraphic tissue (Fig. 9-61). On postoperative examination, you may not see a difference in the location of the conus medullaris from the preoperative location, a fact that infuriates the surgeon. Nonetheless, symptomatic im-

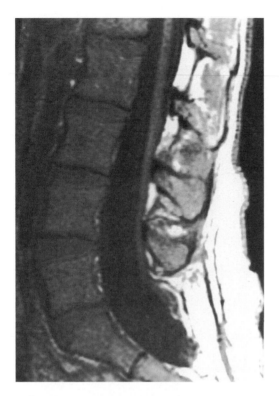

Fig. 9-61   Postoperative meningocele repair, now an adult. The sagittal T1WI shows the postoperative defect from the myelomeningocele repair. The thickened filum extends to the operative defect and the conus termination is probably at the L3—L4 disk level, a bit low. The patient had spasticity and was losing bladder function. Could this be a normal postoperative appearance? The answer is yes, unfortunately.

der the skin. This entity is seen in patients with cloacal exstrophy.

Diastematomyelia

Diastematomyelia refers to a longitudinal split in the cord. The split may also involve the dura so that there may be two dural sacs, or, more commonly, two hemicords within one enlarged sac. In this case, two is not better than one. Usually this abnormality occurs in the lower thoracic-upper lumbar region and is associated with bony abnormalities 85% of the time including spina bifida, widened interpediculate distances, hemivertebrae, and scoliosis. Hairy skin patches occur in 75% of cases. The separation of the spinal cord into two hemicords may be due to a bony spur, cartilaginous separation, or fibrous bands (Fig. 9-62). When this occurs, generally the cord reunites below the cleft. There often is some asymmetry in the size of the hemicords. A bony spur causing the diastematomyelia is more commonly associated with two separate dural sacs than a fibrous split. The cleft is between T8–T12 25% of the time; 60% of the time it is in the lumbar region. Associated tethering of the conus medullaris, Chiari II malformations, myelomeningoceles (31–46%), and hydrosyringomyelia are common.

All these neural tube defects are best evaluated with MR in conjunction with CT. Although CT is useful in detecting the bony canal abnormalities and the bony spur between the diastematomyelia, MR is superior in locat-

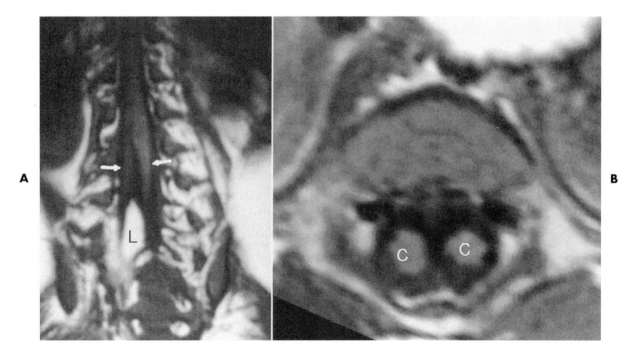

Fig. 9-62   Diastematomyelia. **A,** Separation of two hemicords *(arrows)* with intervening CSF is seen on coronal T1WI. Note the lipoma *(L)* below the level of the split. Spinal canal is markedly widened at the level of the diastematomyelia. **B,** Axial T1WI shows the two cords *(C)* with an enlarged thecal sac. A thin bony separation or fibrous band would not be readily detectable on MR and might be better seen with intrathecal contrast and axial CT.

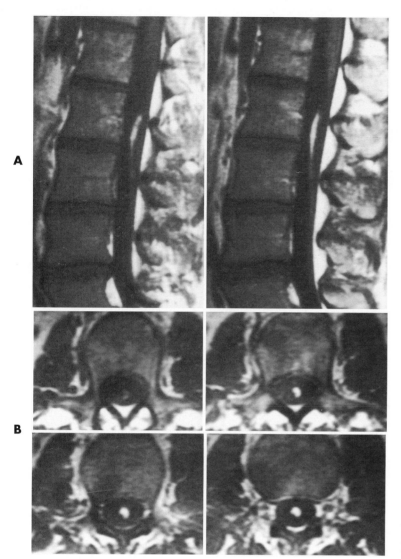

Fig. 9-63   Lipoma of the filum. These T1W unenhanced scans (**A,** sagittal and **B,** axial) show a fatty streak not in a vessel but along the filum terminale. Although the former may be dangerous, the latter, given an untethered cord, is usually asymptomatic.

ing the distal portion of the conus medullaris and identifying the thickening of the filum terminale, the fatty component to the dysraphic state, and the presence of hemicords. Obviously, the presence or absence of a hydromyelic cavity within the spinal cord is better identified with MR than with CT (see Chapter 17). A full examination of the patient who has spinal dysraphism should include MR evaluation of the skull base to assess for a Chiari malformation, the cervical spine to detect the hydromyelic cavity, the thoracolumbar portion of the spine to evaluate for the position of the conus medullaris and the identity of the structures protruding through the bony defect, and CT or plain films of the spine to evaluate for block-vertebrae or hemivertebrae in other locations.

An extremely rare condition is diplomyelia, which in the strictest sense is a duplication of the spinal cord with a full set of motor and sensory roots emanating from each cord. Thus, two ventral and two dorsal roots are at each affected level. Most cases reported as diplomyelia are in fact cases of diastematomyelia where the two hemicords

together provide a single set of nerve roots. Now you will never make that mistake.

Abnormalities of the Filum Terminale

Lipomas of the filum terminale are another form of spinal dysraphism that may cause tethering of the cord. These lesions are identified as having fat density on CT or intensity on MR. (Fig. 9-63). Small amounts of fat in the filum are usually asymptomatic in kids and may be termed "fibrolipomas." As adults a small percentage do result in tethering. Thoracic lipomas outnumber lumbosacral ones. Alternatively the filum terminale may be markedly thickened and tethered without fatty infiltration (the adult tethered spinal cord syndrome) (Fig. 9-64). The conus medullaris may be dragged downward by the thick filum. The normal filum is less than 2 mm in cross-sectional diameter. Associated findings with a taut filum terminale (adult tetheral cord syndrome) are kyphoscoliosis, midline bony defects in the lumbosacral

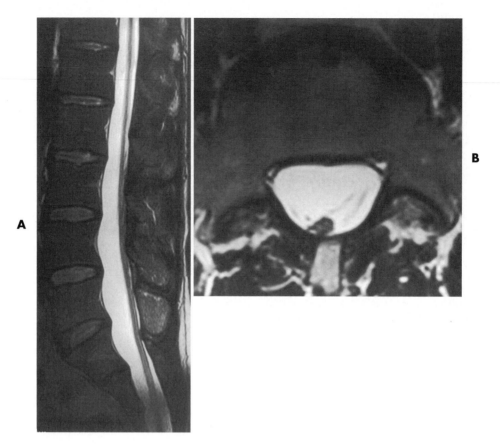

Fig. 9-64   Adult tethered cord. Note the thickened filum and tethered cord with the filum going off the screen **(A)**. The filum can be well outlined on the T2W axial scan **(B)** at the L5 level on this patient. The thecal sac seems somewhat "empty." (Case courtesy of Stuart Bobman.)

part of the spine, and fatty infiltration of the filum. Patients may develop conus ischemia, the dreaded sphincteric dysfunction (that sphinks!), foot deformities, and abnormal gait.

Caudal Regression Syndrome

In caudal regression syndrome you may see a trunculated, blunt spinal cord in the lower thoracic level associated with incomplete formation of the sacrum, let alone the genitourinary-rectal tract. This entity is most commonly seen in children of diabetic mothers. Variable amounts of vertebral body fusion and stenoses may be seen but the Aunt Minnie is the wedged-shaped distal cord terminating at the T–12 region (Fig. 9-65). The cord may be tethered despite being high. The filum is thick. One can have myelocystoceles also.

Pilonidal Cysts

Pilonidal cysts are the most benign form of spinal dysraphism. The cord and thecal sac and vertebral column are normal. A tuft of hair with a small subcutaneous cyst is seen at the level of the coccyx. When a dermal sinus coexists, it is usually seen at a higher level. A dermal sinus has the potential to communicate with the thecal sac (Fig. 9-66). This is a nidus for spread of infection and must be removed in its entirety. It is caused by failure of separation of cutaneous ectoderm from neuroectoderm. Lumbosacral dermal sinus tracts outnumber occipital, thoracic, and cervical in that order. The tract may be seen on MR and dimpling of the thecal sac at the site of entry may be present. A dermoid or epidermoid tumor may co-exist, and may be intra- or extramedullary. Tethering may occur.

Marfan syndrome   Dural ectasias can be seen in Marfan syndrome. If one measures the diameter of the dural sac and corrects for vertebral body diameters one finds that the dural sac ratios in patients with Marfan syndrome are increased compared with controls, particularly at L3 and S1. The sensitivity and specificity of dural ectasia for Marfan syndrome at either of these levels is 95% and 98% respectively using cut-off values of 0.47 for L3 and 0.57 for S1. Dural ectasia, after excluding neurofibromatosis as a cause, is considered a principal criterion for Marfan syndrome. Associated findings include

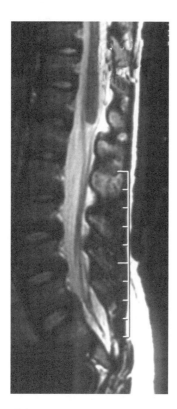

Fig. 9-65   Caudal regression syndrome. Note the truncated appearance to the cord; rounded off like a pencil eraser. This, in association with sacral dysplasia suggests caudal regression syndrome. Remember, nothing is ever so bad that it can't get worse.

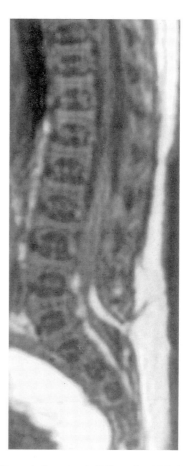

Fig. 9-66   Dermal sinus tract. Follow the high intensity fat on the T1WI from the subcutaneous region into the spinal canal in this patient with a patient dermal sinus tract. The lumbosacral spine is dysraphic.

widening of the canal, thinning of adjacent bone, enlargement of neural foramina, increased interpediculate distance, scalloping of the posterior vertebral body, and meningocele formation.

Genetic mutations associated with Marfan syndrome have been mapped to chromosome 15's long arm (fibrillin-1 gene). Other manifestations include aortic dilatation, dissection, or coarctation, lens dislocation (up and out), arachnodactyly, pectus excavatum, tall stature, osteopenia, dolichocephaly, pes planus, scoliosis, ligamentous laxity, glaucoma, mitral valve regurgitation, pulmonary cysts, and blue sclerae.

Lateral thoracic meningoceles are most commonly seen with neurofibromatosis type 2, but can be seen in Marfan syndrome. Lehman's syndrome includes wormian bones, hypoplastic atlas, and malar hypoplasia with lateral meningoceles. Ehlers-Danlos can also be associated.

Syringohydromyelia

A cavity in the cord may be due to central canal dilatation (hydromyelia) or a cavity eccentric to the central canal (syrinx). Because the resolution of most CT and some MR studies is not sufficient to distinguish these two entities, most neuroradiologists hedge and call the cavities syringohydromyelia. Most hydromyelic cavities are associated with congenital spinal and hindbrain anomalies such as Chiari malformations and myelomeningoceles. Most syringes are also congenital but may arise as a result of spinal cord trauma, ischemia, adhesions, or neoplasms (see Chapter 17). Be aware that at the conus medullaris level in neonates one may see the "fifth ventricle" also called the ventriculus terminalis. This appears as an ovoid, nonenhancing, smooth dilation of the central canal with the signal intensity of cerebrospinal fluid on all pulse sequences. This is a normal variant and is asymptomatic.

Although it used to be thought that syringomyelic cavities form in association with Chiari malformations due to transmitted pressures down the central canal from the fourth ventricle, most researchers now believe that the obstruction of CSF flow at the foramen magnum is to blame. The pulsatile systolic CSF flow from the spinal canal is driven into perivascular and interstitial spaces of the cord and then into the central canal.

Well, you've come to the terminal ventricle and the terminal portion of this chapter. We hope you are asymptomatic and ready to tackle more adult, mature problems—so why are you reading this book?

SUGGESTED READINGS

Aida N, Nishimura G, Hachiya Y, et al: MR imaging of perinatal brain damage: comparison of clinical outcome with initial and follow-up MR findings [see comments], *AJNR* 19:1909-1921, 1998.

Aida N, Tamagawa K, Takada K, et al: Brain MR in Fukuyama congenital muscular dystrophy [see comments], *AJNR* 17:605-613, 1996.

Aida N, Yagishita A, Takada K, Katsumata Y: Cerebellar MR in Fukuyama congenital muscular dystrophy: polymicrogyria with cystic lesions, *AJNR* 15:1755-1759, 1994.

Aizpuru RN, Quencer RM, Norenberg M, et al: Meningioangiomatosis: clinical, radiologic and histopathologic correlation, *Radiology* 179:819-821, 1991.

Altman NR, Naidich PP, Braffman BH: Posterior fossa malformations, *AJNR* 13:619-624, 1992.

Aoki S, Barkovich AJ, Nishimura K, et al: Neurofibromatosis types 1 and 2: cranial MR findings, *Radiology* 172:527-534, 1989.

Ashikaga R, Araki Y, Ono Y, et al: Appearance of normal brain maturation on fluid-attenuated inversion-recovery (FLAIR) MR images, *AJNR* 20:427-431, 1999.

Barkovich AJ: *Pediatric Neuroimaging*, 3rd ed, 2000, Philadelphia, Lippincott Williams & Wilkins.

Barkovich AJ, Ali FA, Rowley HA, Bass N: Imaging patterns of neonatal hypoglycemia [see comments], *AJNR* 19:523-528, 1998.

Barkovich AJ, Edwards MSB, Cogen PH: MR evaluation of spinal dermal sinus tracts in children, *AJNR* 12:123-129, 1991.

Barkovich AJ, Ferriero DM, Bass N, Boyer R: Involvement of the pontomedullary corticospinal tracts: a useful finding in the diagnosis of X-linked adrenoleukodystrophy, *AJNR* 18:95-100, 1997.

Barkovich AJ, Fram EK, Norman D: Septo-optic dysplasia: MR imaging, *Radiology* 151:189-192, 1991.

Barkovich AJ, Gressens P, Evrard P: Formation, maturation, and disorders of brain neocortex, *AJNR* 13:423-446, 1992.

Barkovich AJ, Hajnal BL, Vigneron D, et al: Prediction of neuromotor outcome in perinatal asphyxia: evaluation of MR scoring systems, *AJNR* 19:143-149, 1998.

Barkovich AJ, Kjos BO, Norman D, et al: Revised classification of posterior fossa cysts and cystlike malformations based on the results of multiplanar MR imaging, *AJR* 153:1289-1300, 1989.

Barkovich AJ, Kjos BO: Nonlissencephalic cortical dysplasias: correlation of imaging findings with clinical deficits [see comments] *AJNR* 13:95-103, 1992.

Barkovich AJ, Kjos BO: Gray matter heterotopias: MR characteristics and correlation with developmental and neurologic manifestations, *Radiology* 182:493-499, 1992.

Barkovich AJ, Latal-Hajnal B, Partridge JC, et al: MR contrast enhancement of the normal neonatal brain, *AJNR* 18:1713-1717, 1997.

Barkovich AJ, Peck WW: MR of Zellweger syndrome, *AJNR* 18:1163-1170, 1997.

Barkovich AJ, Rowley H, Bollen A: Correlation of prenatal events with the development of polymicrogyria, *AJNR* 16:822-827, 1995.

Barkovich AJ, Rowley HA, Andermann F: MR in partial epilepsy: value of high-resolution volumetric techniques, *AJNR* 16:339-343, 1995.

Barkovich AJ, Sargent SK: Profound asphyxia in the premature infant: imaging findings, *AJNR* 16:1837-1846, 1995.

Barkovich AJ, Westmark K, Partridge C, et al: Perinatal asphyxia: MR findings in the first 10 days, *AJNR* 16:427-438, 1995.

Barkovich AJ: Analyzing the corpus callosum [comment], *AJNR* 17:1643-1645, 1996.

Barkovich AJ: Imaging of the cobblestone lissencephalies [comment], *AJNR* 17:615-618, 1996.

Barkovich AJ: MR of the normal neonatal brain: assessment of deep structures, *AJNR* 19:1397-1403, 1998.

Barkovich AJ: Neuroimaging manifestations and classification of congenital muscular dystrophies [see comments], *AJNR* 19:1389-1396, 1998.

Barkovich AJ: Subcortical heterotopia: a distinct clinicoradiologic entity, *AJNR* 17:1315-1322, 1996.

Barkovich AJ: The encephalopathic neonate: choosing the proper imaging technique, *AJNR* 18:1816-1820, 1997.

Barnes PD, Lester PD, Yamanashi WS, et al: Magnetic resonance imaging in infants and children with spinal dysraphism, *AJNR* 7:465-572, 1986.

Becker LE: Infections of the developing brain, *AJNR* 13:537-550, 1992.

Becker LE: Lysosomes, perioxisomes, and mitochondria; function and disorder, *AJNR* 13:609-620, 1992.

Braffman BH, Bilaniuk LT, Naidich TP, et al: MR imaging of tuberous sclerosis: pathogenesis of this phakomatosis, use of gadopentetate dimeglumine, and literature review, *Radiology* 183:227-238, 1992.

Bronen RA, Spencer DD, Fulbright RK: Cerebrospinal fluid cleft with cortical dimple: MR imaging marker for focal cortical dysgenesis, *Radiology* 214:657-663, 2000.

Castillo M, Quencer RM, Dominguez R: Chiari III malformation: imaging features, *AJNR* 13:107-113, 1992.

Chu B-C, Terae S, Hida K, et al: MR findings in spinal hemangioblastomas: correlation with symptoms and with angiographic and surgical findings, *AJNR* 22:206-217, 2001.

Cox JE, Mathews VP, Santos CC, Elster AD: Seizure-induced transient hippocampal abnormalities on MR: correlation with positron emission tomography and electroencephalography, *AJNR* 16:1736-1738, 1995.

Davis PC, Hoffman JC Jr, Ball TI, et al: Spinal abnormalities in pediatric patient: MR imaging findings compared with clinical, myelographic, and surgical findings, *Radiology* 166:679-685, 1988.

Dietrich RB, Glidden DE, Roth GM, et al: The Proteus syndrome: CNS manifestations, *AJNR* 19:987-990, 1998.

Dietrich RB, Lis LE, Greensite FS, Pitt D: Normal MR appearance of the pituitary gland in the first 2 years of life, *AJNR* 16:1413-1419, 1995.

Flodmark O: Neuroradiology of selective disorders of the meninges, calvarium and venous sinuses, *AJNR* 13:483-492, 1992.

Ghazi-Birry HS, Brown WR, Moody DM, et al: Human germinal matrix: venous origin of hemorrhage and vascular characteristics [see comments], *AJNR* 18:219-229, 1997.

Hamilton J, Blaser S, Daneman D: MR imaging in idiopathic growth hormone deficiency, *AJNR* 19:1609-1615, 1998.

Han JS, Benson JE, Kaufman B, et al: MRI imaging of pediatric cerebral abnormalities, *J Comput Assist Tomogr* 9:103-114, 1985.

Lee BCP, Lipper E, Nass R, et al: MR of the central nervous system in neonates and young children, *AJNR* 7:605-616, 1986.

Milhorat TH, Chou MW, Trinidad EM, et al: Chiari I malformation redefined: clinical and radiographic findings in 364 symptomatic patients, *Neurosurgery* 44:1005-1014, 1999.

Oosterhof T, Groenink M, Hulsmans F-J, et al: Quantitative assessment of dural ectasia as a marker for Marfan's syndrome, *Radiology* 220:514-518, 2001.

Patronis NJ, Courcoutsakis N, Bromley CM, et al: Intramedullary and spinal canal tumors in patients with neurofibromatosis 2: MR imaging findings and correlation with genotype, *Radiology* 218:434-442, 2001.

Raghavan N, Barkovich AJ, Edwards M, et al: MR imaging in the tethered spinal cord syndrome, *AJR* 152:843-852, 1989.

Samuelsson L, Bergstrom K, Thuomas K-A, et al: MR imaging of syringohydromyelia and Chiari malformations in myelomeningocele patients with scoliosis, *AJNR* 8:539-546, 1987.

Shah SS, Zimmerman RA, Rorke LB, Vezina LG: Cerebrovascular complications of HIV in children, *AJNR* 17:1913-1917, 1996.

Shaw DWW, Cohen WA: Viral infections of the CNS in children: imaging features, *AJR* 160:125-133, 1993.

Silberbusch MA, Rothman MI, Bergey GK, et al: Subdural grid implantation for intracranial EEG recording: CT and MR appearance, *AJNR* 19:1089-1093, 1998.

Smirniotopoulos JG, Murphy FM: Phakomatoses, *AJNR* 13:725-746, 1992.

Thompson JE, Castillo M, Thomas D, et al: Radiologic-pathologic correlation polymicrogyria, *AJNR* 18:307-312, 1997.

Truwit CL, Barkovich AJ: Pathogenesis of intracranial lipoma: an MR study in 42 patients, *AJNR* 11:665-674, 1990.

Utsunomiya H, Takano K, Ogasawara T, et al: Rhombencephalosynapsis: cerebellar embryogenesis, *AJNR* 19:547-549, 1998.

Utsunomiya H, Takano K, Okazaki M, Mitsudome A: Development of the temporal lobe in infants and children: analysis by MR-based volumetry, *AJNR* 20:717-723, 1999.

Walker HS, Lufkin RB, Dietrich R, et al: Magnetic resonance imaging of the pediatric spine, *Radiographics* 7:1129-1152, 1987.

Wolf RL, Zimmerman RA, Clancy R, Haselgrove JH: Quantitative apparent diffusion coefficient measurements in term neonates for early detection of hypoxic ischemic brain injury: initial experience, *Radiology* 218:825-833, 2001.

CHAPTER 10

Orbit

This chapter takes you to the big dance—the eyeball—so grab your coat and take your hat, we are going to start by fox globe trotting through the anatomy. The orbit is a pear-shaped structure made up of seven bones (Fig. 10-1). The roof is formed by the orbital plate of the frontal bone anteriorly and the lesser wing of the sphenoid bone posteriorly. The lateral wall of the orbit is composed of the zygomatic bone anteriorly and the greater wing of the sphenoid posteriorly. The orbital floor consists primarily of the orbital plate of the maxillary bone; however, the zygoma forms part of the anterolateral floor, whereas the palatine bone is at the pos-

terior aspect of the floor. The bones of the medial wall are the lacrimal (anterior), lamina papyracea (ethmoid), and sphenoid (posterior). The orbit is bordered superiorly by the anterior cranial fossa, medially by the ethmoid sinus, inferiorly by the maxillary sinus, posteriorly by the middle cranial fossa, and laterally by the temporal fossa. Fortunately, the supreme neuroradiologist has decided not to change the anatomy for this second edition. She also told us to place orbital trauma in Chapter 5 (Trauma).

ANATOMY

Globe

The globe usually approaches a sphere in shape with a diameter of approximately 2.5 cm, containing three lamellae: (1) sclera, (2) uvea, and (3) retina. The most peripheral outer layer is the sclera, composed of collagen-elastic tissue. Covering the sclera anteriorly is the conjunctiva, a clear mucous membrane. The sclera is continuous with the cornea, with the boundary between the opaque sclera and the transparent cornea termed the limbus. Beneath the sclera is the vascular pigmented layer termed the uveal tract, composed of the choroid, ciliary body, and the iris. The inner layer of the globe is the retina, which is continuous with the optic nerve. It can be further separated into an inner sensory layer containing photoreceptors, ganglion cells, and neuroglial elements, and an outer layer of retinal pigment epithelium, which is adjacent to the basal lamina of the choroid (Bruchs membrane)

The anterior segment lies between the cornea and the lens and is separated into an anterior chamber and a posterior chamber by the iris. The lens consists of a central part, the nucleus, and a peripheral component, the cor-

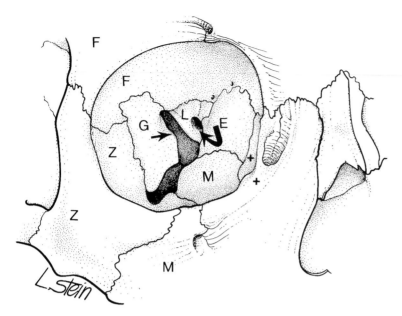

Fig.10-1   Bones of the orbit. A diagram of the bony orbit as seen from the front. The bones of the medial wall are the lacrimal *(+)*, ethmoid (lamina papyracea *[E]*), and sphenoid (lesser wing *[L]*). The orbital roof is formed by the orbital plate of the frontal bone *(F)* anteriorly and the lesser wing *(L)* of the sphenoid bone posteriorly. The lateral wall of the orbit is composed of the zygomatic bone *(Z)* anteriorly and the greater wing of the sphenoid *(G)* posteriorly. The orbital floor consists primarily of the orbital plate of the maxillary bone *(M)*; however, the zygoma *(Z)* forms part of the anterolateral floor while the palatine bone (not seen) is at the most posterior aspect of the floor. The superior orbital fissure is identified *(straight arrow)* as well as the optic canal *(curved arrow)*.

tex. Clear aqueous humor circulates from the posterior to the anterior chamber. The ciliary body lies between the iris and choroid, contains muscles attached to the lens by the suspensory ligament that control the curvature of the lens, and secretes aqueous humor. Posterior to the lens is the posterior segment filled with a jelly-like substance the vitreous body (humor). What would the eye or this book be without its humor?

There are four potential spaces for bad humors to accrue. The space between the base of the vitreous and the sensory retina is the posterior hyaloid space. The space between the layers of the retina (sensory retina and retinal pigment epithelium) is the subretinal space, and between the choroid and the sclera is the suprachoroidal space. When the posterior hyaloid membrane separates from the sensory retina it is termed a posterior vitreous detachment. It is curvilinear in shape and anterior to the retina and separate from the optic disc. Total retinal detachments are V shaped with the apex pointing to the optic disc and the arms at the ora serrata (the anterior aspect of the retina). In fact, retinal separation is probably a better term as the two layers of the retina, neurosensory and retinal pigment epithelium, separate. Choroidal detachments are generally limited by the vortex veins or posterior ciliary arteries and usually do not reach the optic disc. In addition, choroidal detachments can extend anteriorly beyond the ora serrata to the ciliary body occasionally detaching it. Subtenon space is located between the sclera and the fibrous membrane (Tenon capsule) adjacent to the orbital fat extending from the ciliary body to the optic nerve. Hemorrhages in this space, most often from trauma, conform to the curvilinear shape of the eyeball (Fig. 10-2)

Hemorrhage may occur within different compart-ments—hyphema within the anterior chamber and posterior chamber (eight-ball hyphema).

Foramina

Three major foramina are in the orbit: (1) the optic canal, (2) the superior orbital fissure, and (3) the inferior orbital fissure (see Fig. 10-1). Table 10-1 lists the structures that traverse these foramina. The optic canal is formed by the lesser wing of the sphenoid bone and is oriented inferiorly and laterally (from proximal [intracranial] to distal [intraorbital] end). The shape of the canal is horizontally oval at its intracranial entrance (4.5 × 6 mm), round at its midportion (5 × 5 mm), and vertically oval (5 × 6 mm) at its orbital end. The superior orbital fissure is formed from the greater and lesser wings of the sphenoid and is separated from the optic canal by a thin strip of bone, the optic strut. The inferior orbital fissure lies between the orbital plate of the maxilla and palatine bones, and the greater wing of the sphenoid. The fissure communicates with the pterygopalatine fossa. A few other foramina are in the orbit, including the anterior and posterior ethmoidal foramina just medial to the optic canal. These transmit the anterior and posterior ethmoidal arteries. Trivia buffs will appreciate Hyrtl canal, which is an inconstant aperture in the greater wing of the sphenoid through which the meningolacrimal artery may run. The nasolacrimal duct on the inferomedial surface of the orbit communicates with the inferior meatus and can serve as a pathway for nasal tumors to extend directly into the orbit. The soft tissues of the orbit are principally composed of the lacrimal gland, six extraocular muscles, optic nerve, orbital fat, and many vascular structures. Very dry!

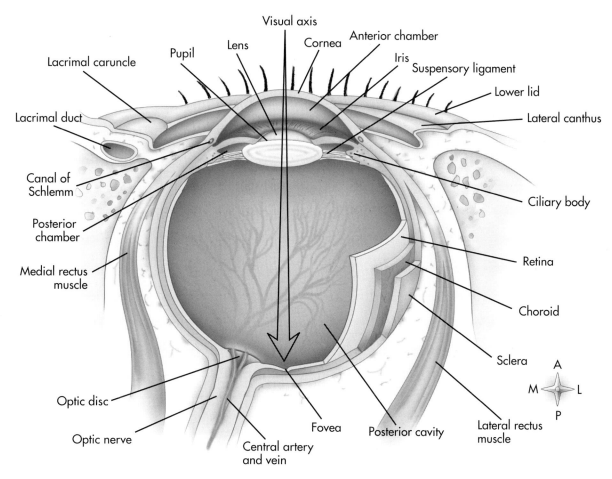

Fig. 10-2   Horizontal section through left eyeball, viewed from above. (From Thibodeau GA, Patton KT: *Anatomy and Physiology,* ed 4. St. Louis, Mosby, 1999, p 462. Used with permission.)

Extraocular Muscles

The extraocular muscles include the medial, superior, inferior, and lateral rectus, which originate from the annulus of Zinn at the optic foramen and insert on the globe. The superior oblique and inferior oblique muscles

Table 10-1	Contents of major orbital foramina
Orbital foramen	**Contents**
Optical canal	Optic nerve, sympathetic fibers, ophthalmic artery
Superior orbital fissure	Cranial nerves III, IV, 1st division of V, and VI; superior ophthalmic vein; sympathetic fibers; orbital branch of middle meningeal artery
Inferior orbital fissure	2nd division of cranial nerve V, infraorbital artery and vein, inferior ophthalmic vein

have separate origins (superomedial to the optic foramen and orbital plate of the maxilla, respectively). The levator palpebra superioris muscle arises above the superior rectus and inserts into the upper lid. The four rectus muscles are classically thought to be connected by an intramuscular fibrous membrane creating the so-called intraconal space (Fig. 10-3). This anatomic concept may not truly exist beyond the globe. However, for radiologic purposes this boundary serves as a useful landmark in categorizing and diagnosing orbital lesions. Thus, intraconal lesions are associated with the optic nerve, its vessels, and orbital fat; conal lesions involve the muscles; and extraconal disease includes the bony orbit and peripheral fat.

Optic Nerve

The optic nerve is a white matter tract that is sheathed by the leptomeninges and dura mater. The subarachnoid space of the optic nerve sheath is continuous with the intracranial subarachnoid space. The thickness of the intraorbital segment of the optic nerve measured from

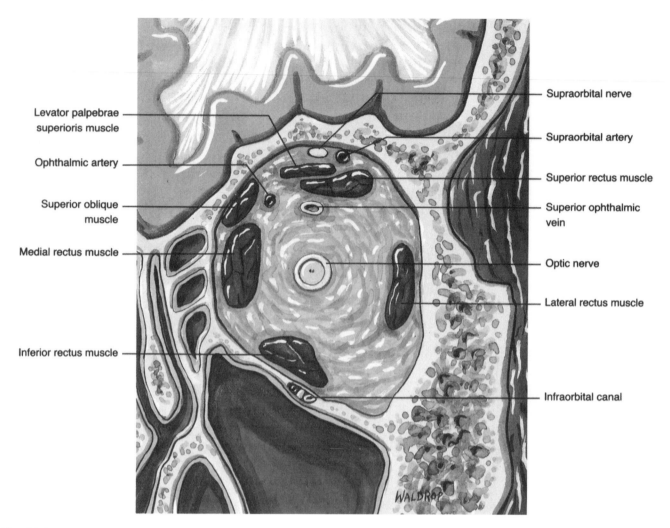

Fig. 10-3   Muscles, nerves and vessels of the orbit are identified on this coronal drawing. (From Dutton JJ: *Atlas of Clinical and Surgical Orbital Anatomy*. Philadelphia, WB Saunders, 1994, p 224. Used with permission.)

oblique coronal MR images ranges between 3.2mm (anteriorly) and 2.6mm (posteriorly), whereas the mean dural diameter measures between 5.2 (anteriorly) and 3.9 mm (posteriorly). The subarachnoid space between the pial and dural sheath of the optic nerve is 0.5 to 0.6 mm wide and may be wider at the optic nerve head (Fig. 10-4). This communicates freely with the subarachnoid space and provides a pathway for spread of infection, inflammation, tumors, or hemorrhage. After intrathecal contrast, enhancement is noted around the optic nerve in the subarachnoid space encircling the nerve. However, this is not always the case. The subarachnoid space may be attenuated on one side. This may explain cases of unilateral filling of the optic nerve subarachnoid space by intrathecal contrast or blood. This has also been hypothesized to explain the finding of unilateral papilledema in certain clinical situations. With the advent of MR, intrathecal contrast with CT is seldom used for the evaluation of the subarachnoid space.

The course of the optic nerve may be divided into four segments: intraocular, intraorbital, intracanalicular, and intracranial. The intraorbital nerve has a sinuous course in both horizontal and vertical planes. After the optic nerves leave the canals, they ascend at an angle of approximately 45 degrees and meet to form the chiasm beneath the floor of the third ventricle. The chiasm is approximately 10 mm above the diaphragma sellae.

The imaging appearance of the nerve depends on the plane and thickness of the section. In thick (8 mm) axial computed tomography (CT) slices the optic nerve appears uniform in density and straight in course. This is due to volume averaging. If thin slices (1.5 mm) are used, the nerve may appear to have a hypodense portion caused by volume averaging of orbital fat or cerebrospinal fluid (CSF) in the subarachnoid space surrounding the nerve. The caveat that should be kept in mind when the optic nerve is evaluated, particularly in the setting of trauma (e.g., optic nerve avulsion), hypo-

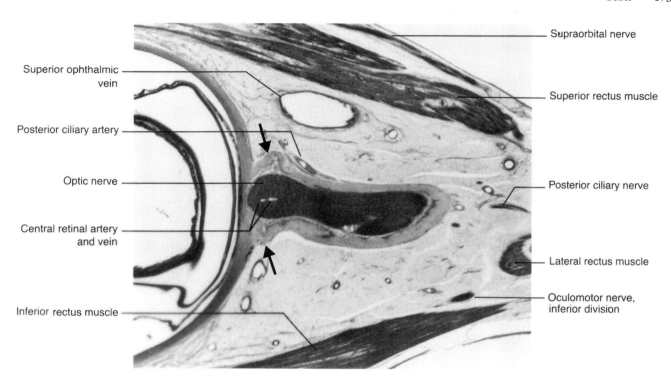

Fig. 10-4   Optic nerve sheath anatomy. Sagittal histologic section demonstrating optic nerve sheath enlargement *(arrows)* at the head of the optic nerve. (From Dutton JJ: *Atlas of Clinical and Surgical Orbital Anatomy.* Philadelphia, WB Saunders, 1994. Used with permission).

density or thinning of segments of the optic nerve must be demonstrated on reformatted or true oblique views parallel to the segment in question before the finding is considered pathologic. The best way to study the optic nerve on CT is to take sections with the patient looking upward, at a −20 degree angulation to the orbitomeatal line and at 1.5 mm thickness (do as we write not as we scan). On magnetic resonance (MR) imaging this is less of a problem because of its multiplanar capability.

Vascular Structures

The important vascular structures in the orbit are the ophthalmic artery and its branches, and the superior and inferior ophthalmic veins. The ophthalmic artery usually arises from the internal carotid artery just after emerging from the cavernous sinus. On entering the orbit, the ophthalmic artery is initially inferolateral to the nerve. It may cross over (72% to 95%) or under (5% to 28%) the nerve to then run on its superomedial side. The orbital arteries radiate from the apex and diverge through the orbital fat to pierce the orbital septa. The main trunk of the ophthalmic artery divides into two relatively independent systems: the retinal vascular system, which supplies the optic nerve and inner aspect of the sensory retina, and the ciliary vascular system.

The ophthalmic artery constitutes a major anastomotic pathway between the internal and external carotid

artery. These anastomoses are listed in Box 10-1 and are particularly important in extracranial occlusive vascular disease. The choroidal plexus of the eye, supplied by the short posterior ciliary arteries, is seen on the lateral arteriogram as a thin crescent (choroidal crescent) with an anterior concavity. In patients older than 30 years, delay in appearance of the choroidal blush (>6 seconds) should suggest hemodynamically significant disease of

Box 10-1   External Carotid-Ophthalmic Artery Anastomoses

SUPERFICIAL TEMPORAL ARTERY BRANCHES

1. Supratrochlear artery
2. Supraorbital artery
3. Internal palpebral artery

INTERNAL MAXILLARY BRANCHES

1. Anterior deep temporal artery
2. Middle meningeal artery (anterior division)
3. Infraorbital artery
4. Sphenopalatine artery

FACIAL ARTERY BRANCHES

1. Angular artery
2. Lateral nasal artery

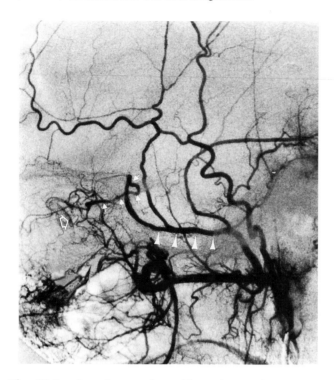

Fig. 10-5   Lateral external carotid arteriogram demonstrating middle meningeal artery *(arrowheads)* going through superior orbital fissure to become meningolacrimal artery *(arrows)*. Note the presence of the choroidal blush *(open arrow)*. For those of you who are expert angiographers, at the corner of the film is a meningioma supplied by the posterior division of the middle meningeal artery. Guess which corner?

the internal carotid artery. Anatomic variations of the ophthalmic artery are important when embolizations and carotid surgery are planned (Fig. 10-5). The ophthalmic artery can originate from the middle meningeal artery (meningolacrimal artery), or branches of the meningeal artery may connect with the ophthalmic artery. Occlusion of the external carotid during carotid endarterectomy or embolization of the middle meningeal artery could result in visual loss when these vascular anomalies are present.

There is an extensive venous network throughout the orbit arranged in a circular fashion following the fibrous septa of the orbital connective tissue. The superior ophthalmic vein is formed by the angular, nasofrontal, and supraorbital veins, which converge at the superolateral aspect of the nose. The superior ophthalmic vein (1.5 to 3 mm in diameter on MR) runs under the orbital roof in its anterior and posterior segments. Its middle segment pierces the muscle cone to course under the superior rectus in a connective tissue septum (superior ophthalmic vein hammock) and over the ophthalmic artery. Posteriorly, it enters the superior orbital fissure and then drains into the cavernous sinus. Its position may cause it to be obstructed by an enlarged inflamed superior rectus muscle (from Graves or pseudotumor). The inferior ophthalmic vein starts as a plexus of small veins beneath the globe and courses posteriorly above the inferior rectus muscle to join the superior ophthalmic vein or to enter the cavernous sinus directly. Inferiorly, a second branch passes through the inferior orbital fissure to drain into the pterygoid venous plexus. A medial ophthalmic vein, observed in about 40% of cases, runs in the nasal extraconal space and joins the superior ophthalmic vein near the superior orbital fissure. These veins are all valveless with numerous anastomoses, which can serve as a conduit for facial infections (zit-popper syndrome) to proceed intraorbitally, into the cavernous sinus, and intracranially. These veins can be ignored except when the patient has a dural malformation or carotid cavernous fistula, when they can become engorged and relate to the symptom complex.

Fat

The orbit is fortuitously lined with adipose tissue that is well organized and divided by fibrovascular septa. This fat produces the contrast, enabling orbital structures to stand out on MR or CT, and of course decreases the conspicuity of enhancing lesions on MR unless fat-saturation MR techniques are used. The orbital septum is a reflection of orbital periosteum (periorbita) inserting on the tarsal plate of the eyelids. The periorbita is an excellent barrier to neoplastic or inflammatory disease emanating from the sinuses. The lacrimal gland is an almond-shaped structure in the anterosuperolateral portion of the orbit lying in the lacrimal fossa at the level of the zygomatic process of the frontal bone. The fat functions as a shock absorber for squash balls and other orbit-seeking foreign bodies.

Lacrimal System

Tears produced by the lacrimal system track medially and flow through the lacrimal puncta in each lid margin. Nasolacrimal drainage follows superior and inferior canaliculi, which are situated along the medial part of the lids and drain via the sinus of Maier into the lacrimal sac (Fig. 10-6). The lacrimal sac is a membranous tissue situated in the medial inferior wall of the orbit (lacrimal fossa) and drains via the valve of Krause into the nasolacrimal duct and through the valve of Hasner into the nasal cavity beneath the inferior turbinate (more trivia). Obstruction of this drainage system results in epiphora and sometimes dacryocystitis (infection of the nasolacrimal sac).

Visual Pathway

Just a brief word concerning the visual pathway (see Chapter 2 for more detail). Lesions of the prechiasmatic optic nerve generally produce monocular visual loss, those involving the optic chiasm cause bitemporal or heterony-

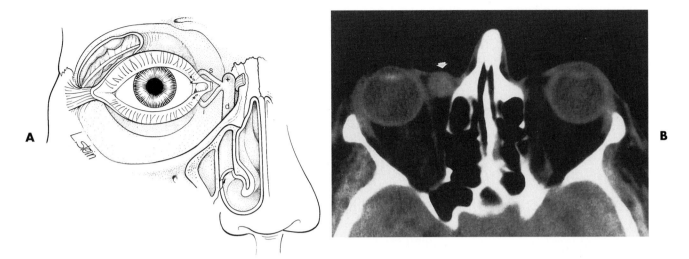

Fig. 10-6   Diagram of lacrimal system. **A,** The lacrimal puncta in the medial aspect of the lid margin *(small arrows)* drains via the superior *(s)* and inferior *(i)* canaliculi into the lacrimal sac *(+)* via the sinus of Maier. The lacrimal sac lies in the medial inferior wall of the orbit (lacrimal fossa) and drains via the valve of Krause into the nasolacrimal duct *(d)* through the valve of Hasner into the nasal cavity beneath the inferior turbinate *(squiggly arrow).* **B,** CT of dacryocele. Round lesion in region of nasolacrimal duct representing a dacryocele *(arrow).* This is in a classic location representing dilatation of the lacrimal sac from a distal obstruction secondary to trauma.

mous field defects, and those behind the chiasm result in visual loss restricted to one side of the visual field (homonymous hemianopsia).

IMAGING CONSIDERATIONS: INDICATIONS FOR MR, CT, AND ORBITAL ULTRASOUND

Orbital imaging has dramatically changed with the advent of MR. Although CT provided an excellent window into pathologic processes involving the globe and retrobulbar structures, it lacks certain features that are furnished by MR. These include (1) true multiplanar imaging; (2) tissue differentiation based on signal intensity characteristics; (3) absence of artifacts from fillings in the teeth; (4) absence of beam-hardening artifact from bone, particularly in the optic nerve canal; (5) excellent anatomic resolution especially of the optic nerve and orbital apex; (6) the ability to detect blood flow as well as its cessation; (7) the diagnosis of all stages of hemorrhage; and (8) the ability to identify lesions containing melanin (paramagnetic). There are, however, significant indications for CT. It is very fast and much less cumbersome than MR. In addition, the patient does not need to be as cooperative as in MR. It is the initial imaging modality of choice for most traumatic situations involving the orbit. Fractures are easier to detect with CT, and bone lesions are usually better visualized with CT. Furthermore, orbital metallic foreign bodies are a contraindication to MR. One of the most important attributes of CT is its ability to detect calcium and calcification. This is particularly crucial in the diagnosis of retinoblastoma, where calcification appears to be a hallmark of the tumor (but many other lesions may calcify).

> Friends, Californians, and country club men
> Lend me your ears eyes?
> We have come to praise CT
> Not to bury it!
> —*Anonymous*

MR is our first choice in the diagnosis of most orbital lesions except in patients with trauma, foreign bodies, sinus disease with orbital infection, or suspected retinoblastoma.

A word (and only a word) about ultrasonography. It is useful to determine the integrity of the globe following trauma, to look for retained foreign bodies, to demonstrate choroidal rupture, retinal detachment, flow dynamics in the orbit, that is, carotid cavernous fistula, vascular disease, to separate vascular tumors from melanoma, to rule out retinal detachment or mass when opaque media prevents visualization (so we lied).

A Few Technical Points

With a fundamental understanding of anatomy, radiologic diagnosis is greatly facilitated. CT imaging in axial and coronal planes, encompassing the eye, results in a radiation dose to the lens of 50 mGy, and overlapping images significantly increase that dose. CT is an excellent method for detection and localization of intraocular and intraorbital foreign bodies (Fig. 10-7) The minimum detectable intraocular particle size for steel is 0.06 mm³, and 1.82 mm³ for auto window glass. Helical CT particularly with reformatted images may be more sensitive than conventional scanning for detection of metallic foreign bodies.

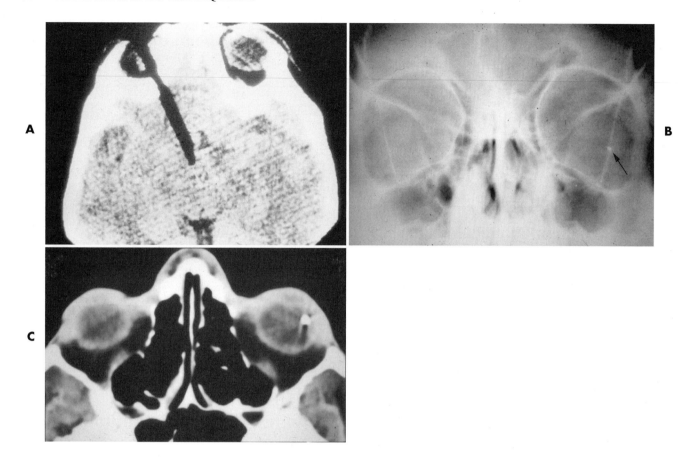

Fig. 10-7 A, Wooden branch has punctured the orbit and is seen in the brain. Density of the wood is close to that of air. **B,** AP skull film at barely shows metallic foreign body *(arrow)* over left innominate line. **C,** CT is superior in revealing presence and location of foreign body. (Anybody see an antibody?)

Interestingly, small fragments of wood (a source of orbital infection) may not detected by CT. Freshly cut wood has a high water content and may be difficult to distinguish from orbital soft tissues on CT or MR. Hardwoods such as oak also have higher CT attenuation values than do softwoods like balsa wood. When wood dries out or is cut the water content is replaced by gas content, and the CT values can appear more like air or fat. Extremely dry wood looks like air on CT; on T1WI, dry wood is hypointense.[3] Wide bone window settings can show the reticulated matrix of wood. On soft-tissue windows wood may be mistaken for air. Wood with lead paint appears high density. "Woodeyes" are bad, "Woodies" are great.

MR of the globe and orbit has the potential for superb delineation of anatomic structures. Surface coils are particularly useful in imaging the eye. T1-weighted images (T1WI) provide excellent anatomic detail. The use of fast spin-echo techniques with increased matrix size (512 × 512) can provide beautiful T2-weighted images (T2WI) of the optic nerve and demonstrate intrinsic lesions such as optic neuritis. These images enable differentiation of the nerve and sheath. The major problem with conventional spin-echo T2WI is related to the longer scan duration and concomitant image degradation from motion.

Now to the standard of care (for all the lawyers attempting to feast on some unfortunate radiologist). Due diligence must be used in obtaining a history of ocular foreign body (iron filings, shrapnel), particularly in lathe operators, sheet metal workers, or military personnel exposed to metallic fragments. Such ferromagnetic particles may torque or move in a magnetic field, potentially producing ocular hemorrhage and blindness. Orbital foreign body screening before MR examination in HMO, cost effective, decreased reimbursement, contemporary practice is controversial. The authors will provide the standard disclaimers, however, one should remember that the recommendation to perform orbital screening before MR is the result of a single case report (at 0.35 T) where a patient sustained an ocular injury from a retained ferromagnetic foreign body after it moved and produce an ocular hemorrhage with complete visual loss. This was truly the multimillion-dollar man. Recently, it has been suggested that radiographic orbital screening is not mandated by occupational history alone. Rather, the history of removal of the foreign body would be a more appropriate rationale to precipitate a pre-MR radiographic screen to look for retained fragments. If there is a suggestion of a metallic foreign body, we presently use two anteroposterior plain films of the orbits, taken with two different cassettes, to rule out the presence of a metallic foreign body. CT in the axial plane, through the orbits with 3-mm sections, is slightly more accurate (0.12 mm versus 0.07 mm) but much less cost effective (and for the extra 0.05 mm, take the risk and educate your kids). Particular attention should be paid to streak artifact from metal, which may be better appreciated on bone windows.

Artifacts

One may encounter many MR artifacts in the course of the examination. Motion of the globes is a serious problem and produces significant image degradation. This obviously increases with increasing scan length and becomes a major deterrent to using surface coils with long TR images. This can be improved with fast scanning techniques (CT or MR). The phase-encoding axis is the most sensitive direction for motion, and the artifacts may appear as blurring, ghosting (aliasing), and/or mottled bands. The motion-induced noise produces increased or decreased intensity around the orbit, rendering diagnosis very difficult. To compensate for this, have your patients stare at something (appropriate centerfold) in the bore of the magnet. You can also phase encode left to right on the axial images to avoid ghosting over the posterior globe.

Chemical shift artifact results from the fact that the molecular environment of fat protons is different from water protons, and thus fat and water protons precess at slightly different rates (Larmor frequency). The Larmor frequency must be uniform throughout the slice section for the proper function of the gradients and correct spatial localization. Because of the slight differences in Larmor frequency, both species of protons are excited by the radiofrequency pulse but precess at different rates (fat proton precession rate is slower than that of water protons). The position of the fat protons relative to the water protons is altered during frequency encoding because its signal is assumed to be originating from an incorrect location. This effect is seen in the orbit at the fat-tissue interfaces. The chemical shift increases with increasing field strength and occurs along the frequency-encoding gradient. It appears as high and low intensity bands at the interface between orbital fat and soft tissue. Silicone, which is used for retinal detachments, resonates slower than both fat and water. Try fat suppression to eliminate this artifact.

Eye makeup (e.g., mascara) is cobalt based, which produces susceptibility artifacts such as other metallic foreign bodies, resulting in signal loss over the lids (Fig. 10-8). Eyelid tattoos contain ferromagnetic iron oxide pigments.

Other effects that ruin your image include susceptibility from air in the sinuses, dental prostheses, and signal drop off with the use of surface coils (see following discussion).

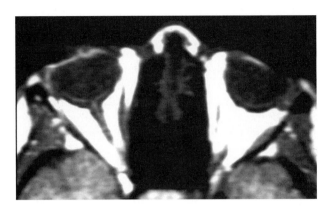

Fig. 10-8   MR in a femme fatale who overdosed with mascara. Note the artifact from susceptibility obscuring the anterior globes.

Remember CT is not without artifact. In the orbit, partial volume averaging, motion artifact, and beam hardening/metallic artifact do occur. Beam hardening, from dental amalgam or hardware, can particularly affect coronal images. Angulation to avoid the amalgam diminishes this problem.

Hydroxyapatite orbital implants   These are used after enucleation. The porous nature enables fibrovascular ingrowth. When placed in the orbit the implant is intermediate intensity on all MR pulse sequences and enhances variably. Enhancement is hypothesized to represent vascularization of the implant. Fibrovascular ingrowth (weeks to months) is a prerequisite for drilling and pegging of the hydroxyapatite sphere required to translate the ocular motion to the prosthesis. Nodular or infiltrating areas of enhancement around the implant may suggest recurrent tumor or inflammation.

Prosthetic intraocular lens   Contemporary cataract surgery usually includes placement of an intraocular lens. These can be identified on CT or T2WI. This becomes an issue in orbital trauma when concern is raised regarding the position of the lens or about whether the patient has one.

The crystalline lens can be dislocated in a variety of different medical conditions. Box 10-2 provides a list of these conditions as well as the common position of these dislocations.

Box 10-2   Lens Dislocations

Marfan—up and out
Homocystinuria—down and in
Ehlers Danlos
GEMSS syndrome (glaucoma, lens ectopia, microspherophakia, stiffness, and shortness)
Weill-Marchesani syndrome
Trauma

Surface coils

Surface coil imaging of the orbit, although the optimal technique for studying the orbit, sometimes has signal loss at the orbital apex and beyond. The depth sensitivity of the surface coil falls off with distance from the coil. The sensitivity of the surface coil should match the region of interest. The depth sensitivity (for a loop coil) is slightly greater than the coil diameter. Signal drop off from surface coils is another factor that affects image quality. This is a major problem when lesions are traced to the chiasm. The diagnosis of lesions beyond the orbital apex or along the visual pathways necessitates supplemental images with the head coil.

Contrast enhancement   The orbit contains considerable fat, which is high intensity on T1WI and low intensity on conventional T2WI and high intensity on fast spin echo images. Gadolinium produces enhancement that also causes shortening of T1 and T2, and high intensity on the T1WI. Thus, an enhancing lesion in the orbit lacks conspicuity because the lesion and the surrounding fat are all of high intensity. Fat suppression techniques nullify the high intensity of fat and demonstrate high intensity of enhancement on T1WI and fast spin echo T2 against a dark fat background. Contrast provides information about whether a particular lesion enhances, the morphologic characteristics of the enhancement, and the degree of enhancement. These may be useful in constructing a differential diagnosis. Gadolinium is also effective in demonstrating active intrinsic lesions of the optic nerve/sheath such as optic neuritis and can assess intracranial extension of orbital lesions. The extraocular muscles enhance more intensely than skeletal muscle because of their vascularity and large extravascular spaces.

For diagnostic purposes, it is convenient to divide orbital disease into ocular and retrobulbar components. The latter region is subdivided into intraconal, conal, and extraconal lesions. We will consider each location and develop a differential diagnosis based on anatomic region.

"So [said the doctor].
Now vee may perhaps to begin. Yes?"
—*Philip Roth, Portnoy's Complaint*

OCULAR LESIONS

CT is somewhat limited in the diagnosis of ocular lesions because of its present inability to resolve the retina, choroid, and sclera. It is exquisitely sensitive to ocular calcification. Box 10-3 lists the causes of ocular calcification (Fig. 10-9). It should be appreciated that the lens appears dense on CT because of its high protein content. On T1WI and T2WI, most pure calcifications (with-

---

Box 10-3   Causes of Ocular Calcification

DEGENERATIVE

Cataracts
Optic nerve drusen
Phthisis bulbi
Retinal detachment
Retrolental fibroplasia
Senile calcification of insertion of muscle tendons
   in the globe

NEOPLASMS

Astrocytic hamartoma
   Neurofibromatosis
   Tuberous sclerosis
   von Hippel-Lindau syndrome
Choroidal osteoma
Retinoblastoma

INFECTION

Cytomegalovirus
Herpes simplex
Rubella
Syphilis
Toxoplasmosis
Tuberculosis

HYPERCALCEMIC STATES

Chronic renal failure
Hyperparathyroidism
Hypervitaminosis D
Milk-alkali syndrome
Sarcoidosis

---

out paramagnetic ions) are hypointense and do not change in intensity as one increases the echo time. This is caused by the lack of mobile protons. In some instances calcification may be high intensity on T1WI. Most of these situations occur in the basal ganglia but potentially could occur in other areas. Rapidly flowing blood also appears hypointense on T1WI and T2WI. On gradient echo images emphasizing flow (relatively T1 weighted), flowing blood appears as high intensity. Exceptions to this include turbulent and in-plane flow as well as very slow flow, which all appear as low-intensity regions. Another gradient echo imaging sequence can be employed that emphasizes T2* effects (see Chapter 1). In this case, susceptibility differences produce hypointensity so that calcium, which has altered diamagnetic susceptibility compared with tissue, would appear hypointense. This is sometimes useful in detecting calcium on an MR of a patient with retinoblastoma. This hypointensity is not specific for calcium and other entities including blood products (deoxyhemoglobin, intra-

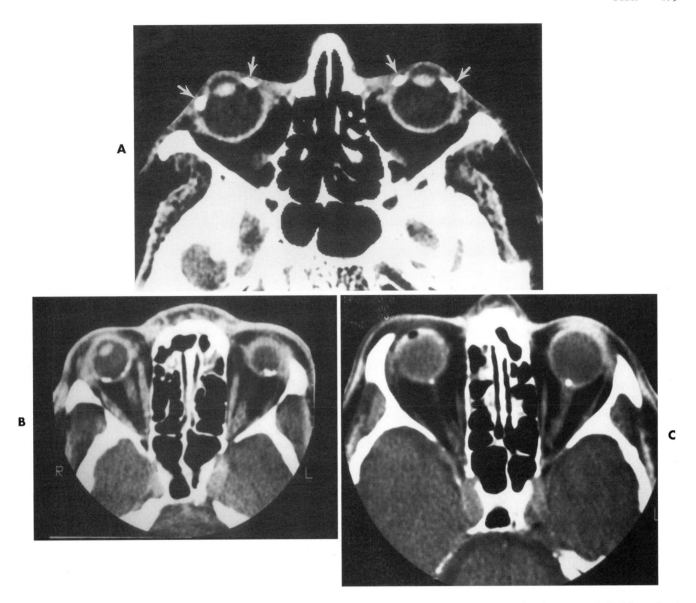

Fig. 10-9   Orbital calcification. **A,** CT with exuberant senescent calcifications in insertions of tendon sheaths *(arrows).* **B,** Bilateral retinal calcifications in a patient with previous rubella retinitis. **C,** Bilateral punctate calcifications on CT at the junction of the head of the optic nerve and globe. These are drusen bodies.

cellular methemoglobin, hemosiderin), and paramagnetics are hypointense on gradient echo images.

Neoplasia and Related Lesions

The majority of primary and metastatic ocular neoplasms involve the choroid. The radiologist can play an important role in the diagnosis of ocular neoplasms and in recognizing some of the nonneoplastic mimics of these conditions. Imaging is essential in detection of episcleral spread of tumor or for showing lesions spreading posteriorly along the nerve. Furthermore, there are circumstances in which the ophthalmologist may have a limited view of contents of the globe and retina because of cataract formation and/or corneal opacities.

Leukokoria

Leukokoria (white pupil) is due to the inability of light to be reflected off the retina, and it is caused by any opaque tissue that interferes with the passage of light through the globe. Thus, leukokoria itself is a nonspecific sign with many causes including retinoblastoma (a little less than half of all comers with leukokoria), congenital cataract, retinopathy of prematurity, chronic retinal detachment associated with retrolental fibroplasia, choroidal hemangioma, retinal astrocytoma, persistent hyperplastic primary vitreous, Coats disease, and *Toxocara canis* infection. Only the most radiologically relevant lesions are considered.

Retinoblastoma   Retinoblastoma is the most common intraocular tumor of childhood. It usually presents before the age of 3 years with leukokoria, strabismus, decreased vision (particularly in bilateral lesions), retinal detachment, glaucoma, ocular pain, or signs of ocular inflammation. The vast majority of lesions occur as sporadic mutations (90%) whereas approximately 10% are familial. Ninety-eight percent occur in children less than 3 years of age.

Accurate radiologic diagnosis is crucial for timely treatment and survival. Familial retinoblastoma is an autosomal dominant trait, with variable penetrance and a propensity for bilaterality and multifocality (same globe) (30% of cases). The retinoblastoma gene has been localized on chromosome 13 at the q14 locus. Absence or inactivation of both alleles of the gene within immature retinal cells is required for retinoblastoma to develop. In cases with heritable retinoblastoma inactivation or absence of one allele is present in all cells. Only one mutation resulting in inactivation or loss of the remaining allele in the developing retinal cells is all that is needed to develop clinical retinoblastoma.

Retinoblastoma may also occur sporadically as a somatic mutation, and these lesions are unilateral, occurring later than the inherited form. Children with monocular disease are more likely to have a single tumor and negative family history. In the nonheritable retinoblastoma, both alleles of the retinoblastoma gene are present and functioning. Thus, two separate mutations affecting both retinoblastoma alleles are required to produce clinical retinoblastoma.

There is also a rare (1.4% of all retinoblastoma) histologic form of retinoblastoma characterized by diffuse infiltration of the retina without a tumor mass. It presents at 6 years (range 1 to 11 years). It is unilateral with frequent vitreous dissemination. On MR, retinal detachment is present with thickening, irregularity, and nodularity of the leaflets. Calcification is absent in the majority of cases (making it difficult to differentiate from Coats disease) and diagnosis is frequently delayed.

Although ophthalmoscopy is usually able to visualize the ocular abnormalities, imaging is of critical importance in revealing retrobulbar disease including other tumors, metastasis, and invasion of the optic nerve posterior to the lamina cribrosa where the meninges insert on the optic nerve (associated with a poor prognosis). Retinoblastoma may spread directly into the subarachnoid space via the optic nerve (occasionally producing spinal implants), hematogenously, or via lymphatics and has a propensity to hemorrhage. Metastases from retinoblastoma occur within the first 2 years after treatment. There is a high incidence of nonocular tumors in the hereditary form (the "oncogene") with this predisposition for cancer leading to a 59% 35-year mortality rate. These include midline, primitive neuroectodermal, pineal tumors, osteogenic sarcoma, soft-tissue sarcoma, malig-

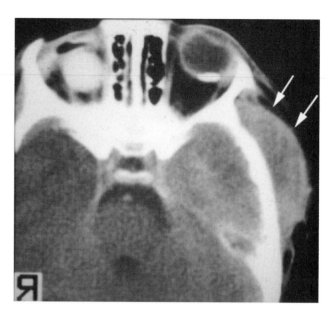

Fig. 10-10   CT of bilateral retinoblastoma with enucleation of the right globe. Note the fibrosarcoma in the left temporal region *(arrows)*.

nant melanoma, basal cell carcinoma, and rhabdomyosarcoma (Fig. 10-10). Pineoblastoma, although usually associated with bilateral retinoblastoma, has been noted with unilateral retinoblastoma and may be detected simultaneously with, after, or even before the ocular lesion. Ectopic retinoblastoma has also been reported in the parasellar or suprasellar regions. The pineal gland in lower animals contains photoreceptors and has been

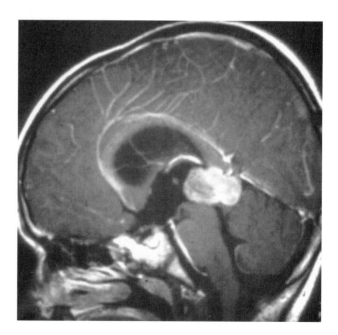

Fig. 10-11   Trilateral retinoblastoma—Note the pineoblastoma in a patient with bilateral retinoblastoma.

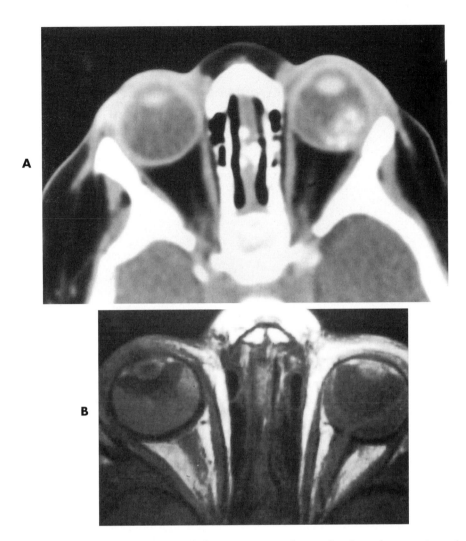

Fig. 10-12 Retinoblastoma. **A,** On CT retinoblastoma calcifications are noted extending from the posterior retina into the vitreous on the left. **B,** T1WI of bilateral retinoblastoma. Notice that one cannot discern evidence of calcification, thus making the diagnosis of retinoblastoma problematic in this situation. Also, observe the bilateral retinal detachments.

termed the "third eye," so that pineal tumors (usually pineoblastoma) associated with bilateral retinoblastoma have been named "trilateral" retinoblastoma (Fig. 10-11). For those erudite readers the pineal gland is also considered the "third testicle" because of the origin of germ cell tumors.

The CT findings are those of calcifications in the posterior portion of the globe with extension into the vitreous, (Fig. 10-12). The calcification may be homogeneous or irregular and occurs in 95% of patients. Noncalcified retinoblastoma has been reported in infants with a family history, under close observation. In children less than 3 years of age, ocular calcification is highly suggestive of retinoblastoma; conversely, its absence in this same group makes the diagnosis of retinoblastoma highly unlikely. These lesions minimally enhance; how-

ever, contrast is useful to appreciate the intracranial extension. With orbital involvement, proptosis may be seen. Coronal imaging is useful in assessing enlargement of the optic nerve secondary to invasion by the tumor.

MR findings in retinoblastoma include moderately high intensity on T1WI and hypointensity on T2WI, with the noncalcified portion of the lesion less hypointense than the calcification. We speculate that the high intensity on T1WI may be caused by calcium or by some coexistent paramagnetic, tumor protein, or hemorrhagic component. Associated retinal detachment may be high intensity on T1WI and of variable intensity on T2WI, depending on the protein content and whether there is associated hemorrhage in the subretinal fluid. The hypointensity in retinoblastoma on T2WI is related in part to calcification in the lesion. In patients with suspected retinoblastoma CT and MR are complementary examinations. CT detects calcification better whereas MR is more sensitive to tumoral extension into the nerve and intracranial space, and to secondary lesions.

A number of conditions can occasionally simulate retinoblastoma and should be distinguished from it. Most of these lesions can be differentiated by history, clinical presentation, and examination. These lesions have been termed pseudoglioma or pseudoretinoblastoma. The more common ones are considered.

Persistent hyperplastic primary vitreous Persistent hyperplastic primary vitreous (PHPV) is caused by persistence of various portions of the primary vitreous (embryonic hyaloid vascular system) with hyperplasia of the associated embryonic connective tissue, and may present as leukokoria in the neonate. The globe usually demonstrates microophthalmia, although this can be minimal, and the lens can be small with flattening of the anterior chamber. Initially, a funnel-shaped mass of fibrovascular tissue (including the hyaloid artery) is present in the retrolental space and runs in an S-shaped course (termed Cloquet canal) between the back of the lens and the head of the optic nerve. PHPV is vascular, prone to repeated hemorrhages, and may vary in size. CT demonstrates generalized increased density in the globe and enhancement of the intravitreal tissue after intravenous contrast. Unlike retinoblastoma, PHPV does not calcify (this is key!). The CT diagnosis is facilitated by observing the S-shaped tubular fetal tissue between the lens and head of the optic nerve (Fig. 10-13). A blood-vitreous layer may be seen as a result of posterior hyaloid detachment. On MR, vitreal intensity is variable; however, the visualization of Cloquet canal makes the diagnosis. Norrie disease is an inherited form of PHPV with similar ocular findings associated with seizures, mental retardation, and cataracts.

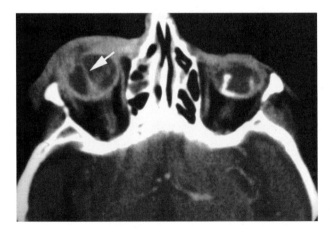

Fig. 10-13 PHPV. Note the presence of Cloquet canal in the right globe *(arrow)*. There is a calcified retinal detachment (chronic) in the left globe.

Coats disease Coats disease is a vascular anomaly of the retina that may be clinically difficult to distinguish from retinoblastoma. This lesion is usually unilateral. These telangiectatic vessels leak serum and lipid into the retina (lipoproteinaceous effusion) and subretinal space. Patients are usually seen when retinal detachment occurs. It is common for patients to become symptomatic in the first 2 years of life, although the age at discovery is usually 6 to 8 years with approximately two thirds of cases in boys. The CT appearance is of high density in the vitreous related to the exudate. Calcification is rare, again distinguishing it on CT from retinoblastoma, however, it cannot be distinguished from the noncalcifying variant of retinoblastoma, or when there is calcification, from calcified retinoblastoma. On MR, Coats disease is hyperintense on T1 and T2WI whereas retinoblastoma tends to be high intensity on T1WI but low intensity on T2WI. Coats disease enhances along the leaves of the detached retina and at the sites where the retina reinserts whereas retinoblastoma enhances in a masslike fashion. MR spectroscopy has been reported to show a large peak at 1 to 1.6 ppm that is thought to correspond to lipids and/or complex proteolipids.

Toxocara canis infection *Toxocara canis* infection begins when a child ingests soil contaminated with dog feces containing the ova of the nematode *T. canis* (the definition of a dirt ball). The ova hatch in the gastrointestinal tract and then migrate throughout the body. The ocular *T. canis* infection results when larvae of *T. canis* within the eye die, producing an inflammatory reaction (just like cysticercosis in the brain) with vitrous opacification and retinal detachment. Antibody titers for *Toxocara* are helpful in confirming the diagnosis and should be drawn when there is any suspicion of pica.

Ocular lesions occur months to years after initial infection. This chronic endophthalmitis causes unilateral leukokoria. Your children should ask the waiter for their dirt sans worms. On CT, diffuse high density is identified within the globe without calcification. Thick enhancement of the sclera has been observed. On MR, these lesions are reported to be high intensity on T1WI and T2WI. This is somewhat different from the appearance of retinoblastoma, which is generally of lower intensity on T2WI. The intensity patterns are related to the protein content and/or associated hemorrhage in the globes. With the small number of reports, one should not take these intensity patterns as "classic."

Retrolental fibroplasia Retrolental fibroplasia is the result of prolonged oxygen therapy in premature infants. The severity of the condition is related to the birth weight, amount of oxygen used, and extent of prematurity. Retrolental fibroplasia can in extreme cases present as bilateral leukokoria because of traction retinal detachments. CT findings are of increased density in the posterior portion of the globe, which may represent calcification. Occasionally, a thin line representing the detached retina can be identified beneath the high density.

Melanoma

Melanomas of the uveal tract are the most common intraocular malignancy in adults and have a characteristic intensity pattern on MR. They are rare in blacks but when they occur tend to be larger, more pigmented, and more necrotic. Conditions predisposing to uveal melanoma include congenital melanosis, ocular melanocytosis, oculodermal melanocytosis, and uveal nevi. Unlike most other tumors, melanotic melanomas are hyperintense on T1WI and hypointense on T2WI. Free radicals known to exist in melanin are responsible for the associated T1 and T2 shortening by the proton-electron dipole-dipole proton relaxation enhancement mechanism (Fig. 10-14). The degree of T1 and T2 shortening appears to be related to the melanin content. Amelanotic melanomas have MR characteristics similar to those of other tumors (hypointense on T1WI and hyperintense on PDWI/T2WI). Other lesions with similar intensity patterns that could be confused with melanoma include fat and subacute hemorrhage in the intracellular methemoglobin state. Use of fat saturation images can easily separate fat from melanotic tumor. There have been reports of mucin-secreting adenocarcinoma metastatic to the choroid and other carcinomas having similar signal characteristics to a choroidal melanotic melanoma. (Nothing is perfect!) Associated with the melanoma may be retinal detachments, with subretinal proteinaceous effusions, that appear as high intensity on T2WI. To differentiate melanoma from other lesions, both T1WI and T2WI must be used. Senile macular degeneration results from arteriosclerosis. It is associated with retinal detachment, hemorrhage, and gliotic scar in the macular region, which can appear as a masslike lesion and be mistaken for melanoma.

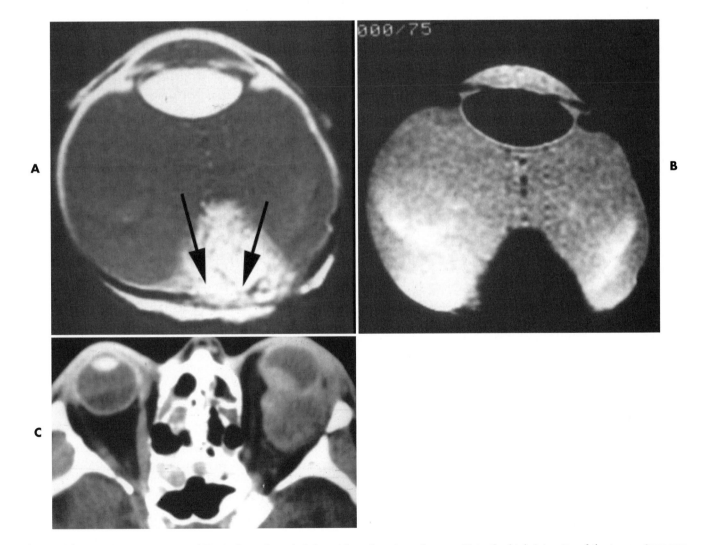

Fig. 10-14   Ocular melanoma. **A,** T1WI of enucleated globe with melanotic melanoma. Note the high intensity of the tumor (paramagnetic effect of melanin) and the episcleral extension *(arrows).* **B,** T2WI with marked hypointensity. **C,** CT of melanoma with posterior episcleral/orbital extension.

On CT, uveal melanomas are high density on non-contrast images and enhance. MR is superior to CT in visualizing retinal detachment, for noting associated vitreous changes, and for differentiating uveal melanoma from choroidal hemangioma (based on intensity characteristics) and choroidal detachment (based on enhancement). Extraocular invasion is important to detect as it is associated with a poorer prognosis and has different therapeutic implications. Ocular ultrasound and CT may be particularly useful here. Choroidal melanoma has a propensity for metastasis to the liver and lung. Melanoma is a bad actor. It is a good reason not to show off your body at the beach.

Melanoma may also arise in the orbit from native orbital melanocytes located along ciliary nerves, optic nerve leptomeninges, and scleral emissary vessels. These lesions tend to be associated with pigmentary disorders including nevus of Ota, ocular melanocytosis, and blue nevi.

Choroidal hemangioma This is a vascular hamartoma detected in middle-aged and elderly individuals. There are two varieties—a circumscribed or solitary form, unassociated with other abnormalities and a diffuse angiomatous lesion associated with Sturge-Weber or facial nevus flammeus. The solitary lesion has been mistaken for choroidal melanoma. On MR, these lesions are iso to slightly high intensity and hyperintense on T2WI. They enhance avidly.

Medulloepithelioma This tumor, formally termed dictyoma (we will pass on this joke), arises from the primitive unpigmented epithelium lining of the ciliary body. It occurs in pediatric as well as adult patients. Its MR appearance is similar to melanoma. In children it is in the differential diagnosis of retinoblastoma whereas in adults think melanoma. These tumors are benign or locally invasive. Rarely, distal metastasis occurs.

Metastases

Metastatic breast and lung cancer, lymphoma, and leukemia are common ocular malignancies seen in adults. Many metastatic neoplasms of the globe can have eccentric thickening of the uveoscleral rim and retrobulbar extension, which can be detected on CT and MR, and may not be clinically apparent (Fig. 10-15). Choroidal lymphoma and leukemia can appear on MR to be similar to uveal melanoma, may cause retinal detachment and may be bilateral (rare for melanoma) (Fig. 10-16).

Choroidal osteoma

Choroidal osteoma is a benign tumor seen in young women. These lesions are usually unifocal, demonstrate ossification, and are juxtapapillary in location. CT is the imaging modality of choice in this situation. Punctate calcification in the posterior pole of the globe, usually on the temporal side of the optic nerve, may be easily

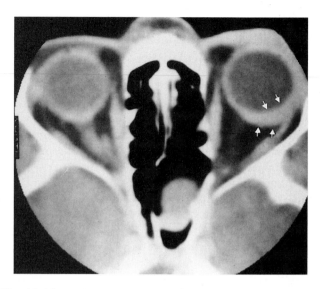

Fig. 10-15 CT of lymphoma with uveoscleral thickening. Note the uveoscleral thickening in the left globe *(arrows)* representing lymphoma.

identified. The differential diagnosis of choroidal osteoma includes amelanotic melanoma and choroidal hemangioma (which do not ossify), metastatic carcinoma, mucinous adenocarcinoma, leukemic or lymphomatous infiltrates, macular choroidal scars, and resolving subretinal hemorrhage. An astrocytic hamartoma could look identical (Fig. 10-17). CT is the modality of choice for imaging calcification (how many more times should we say this?). MR is complementary in separating hemorrhagic and nonhemorrhagic entities.

Other Ocular Issues

Vogt-Koyanagi-Harada syndrome This is an interesting systemic disorder with bilateral panuveitis, exudative retinal detachment, and optic nerve hyperemia associated with cutaneous and neurologic findings including vitiligo, alopecia, meningismus, and dysacusis. MR findings include diffuse choroidal thickening with sparing of the sclera. This finding separates the syndrome from posterior scleritis, which involves both the choroid and the sclera. CT cannot separate the choroid (and retina) from the sclera.

Intraocular hemorrhage following subarachnoid hemorrhage Retinal hemorrhage occurs in 18% to 41% of adults with subarachnoid hemorrhage and may be as high as 70% in children. If vitreous hemorrhage also occurs the condition is termed Terson syndrome. Fundal hemorrhage is believed to be caused by a sudden rise in intracranial pressure transmitted into the distal optic nerve sheath. This pressure may compress the central retinal vein and cause the intraocular hemorrhage. Intraocular hemorrhage has also been seen in HIV patients with CMV retinitis.

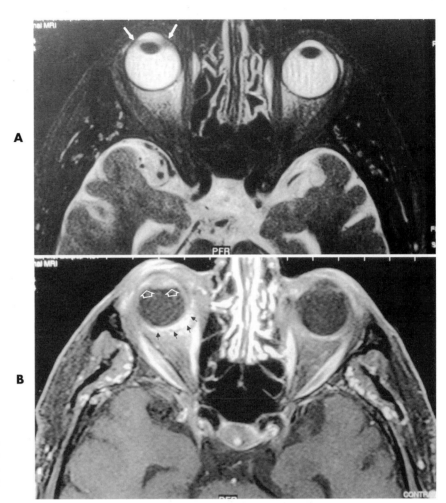

Fig. 10-16 Uveal tract (ciliary body) lymphoma. **A,** T2WI with thickening of ciliary body of right globe *(arrows).* **B,** T1WI with enhancement in the ciliary body *(open arrows)* and black arrows on enhancing choroid.

Ocular Hypotony and Choroidal Detachments

Ocular hypotony is defined as low tension in the globe secondary to surgery, trauma, or glaucoma therapy, and may be observed on CT as uveoscleral infolding also re-

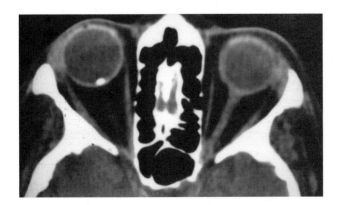

Fig. 10-17 Astrocytic hamartoma. Note the calcification.

ferred to as the "flat tire" or "umbrella" sign (Fig. 10-18). This is most often seen after perforation and can be reversed by instillation of saline, silicone oil, or sodium hyaluronate (Healon), which expand the globe. Just two more words: double perforation. This term is used by ophthalmologists and means a perforation through the anterior and posterior portions of the globe. The posterior perforation is one reason to perform an imaging study; it usually cannot be repaired (poor outcome). The most common cause of the double perforation is the BB sized shot.

Ocular hypotonia, either from inflammatory diseases (uveitis or scleritis), medication, or from traumatic perforation of the globe, is the cause of serous choroidal detachments. Table 10-2 compares the various ocular detachments radiologist commonly encounter (Fig. 10-19). Hemorrhagic choroidal detachment may be observed after penetrating injury or intraocular surgery and has a lenticular morphology. This is bad news because it means that you have had a rupture of a choroidal vessel, which has an associated poor prognosis. Serous choroidal detachment (benign prognosis) is crescentic

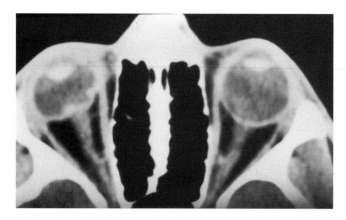

Fig. 10-18   Ocular hypotony. CT following perforation of the right globe. The globe has the appearance of an umbrella or a flat tire, which is characteristic of this condition.

or ring shaped, and the curvilinear choroid can be identified. Serous choroidal effusions beneath the detached choroid appear as convex regions of low density outlined by the detached choroid. Hemorrhagic choroidal effusions are high density and do not change with position. Inflammatory choroidal effusions secondary to uveitis and posterior scleritis, are high density but may change in location with changes in head position. Uveoscleral thickening and enhancement can be seen in inflammatory choroidal detachment.

MR is beneficial in distinguishing hemorrhagic choroidal detachment from serous choroidal detachments. On MR, hemorrhagic choroidal detachment can display a variety of intensity patterns related to age of the hemorrhage (see Chapter 4). Serous choroidal detachment has been noted to be high intensity on T1WI and T2WI.

Globe Tenting

Globe tenting occurs when the posterior globe configuration changes so that it appears as a conical or tented structure. It is caused by an intraorbital mass lesion, either acute or subacute, producing proptosis with tethering of the globe by the stretched optic nerve. Ocular tenting has been reported in acute trauma, inflammatory processes, carotid cavernous fistula, subperiosteal abscess, hemorrhage into lymphangioma, and varix. Tenting with acute proptosis is an indication for emergent surgical decompression.

Ocular Infections

We again perseverated here. Should *T. canis* be placed in this subsection or under Leukokoria? We left it in the Leukokoria subsection so that this subsection really should be entitled "Nonnematodal Infections." Both CT and MR are nonspecific in identifying particular ocular infections. Imaging is useful in ocular pseudomonas infections to rule out posterior scleritis, which demonstrates posterior scleral thickening and enhancement. In

Table 10-2 **Types of ocular detachments**				
Detachment	**Separated layers**	**Shape**	**Extent**	**Association**
Retinal	Sensory retina from retinal pigment epithelium—subretinal space	V shaped with apex at optic disk (total)	To ora serrata	Retinoblastoma, Coats disease, *Toxocara* endopthalmitis, diabetes, melanoma, choroidal hemangiomas, following subretinal hemorrhage from trauma, senile macular degeneration, or PHPV
Choroidal-Serous or hemorrhagic	Between choroid and sclera—Suprachoroidal space	Linear, cresentic, or ring-shaped -serous Convex-hemorrhagic	Leaves do not extend to the optic disc because the posterior choroids is anchored by short posterior ciliary arteries and nerves	Ocular hypotony, trauma, surgery, inflammatory choroidal lesions, melanoma
Posterior hyaloid space	Between posterior hyaloid membrane and sensory retina	Thin, semilunar, gravitational layering	Variable	Macular degeneration, PHPV Posterior vitreous detachment (PVD)

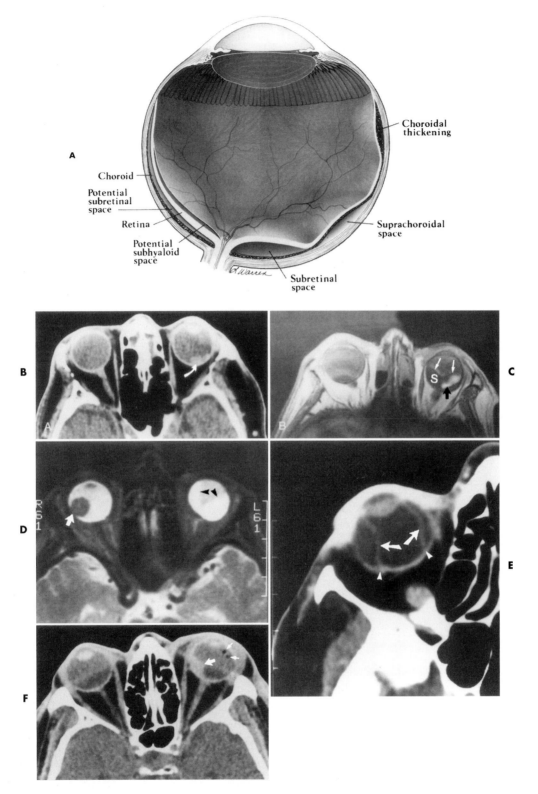

Fig. 10-19   **A,** Artist's rendition of various types of retinal detachments. **B** and **C,** Macular degeneration associated with subretinal hemorrhage and posterior hyaloid detachment. **B,** CT scan shows an area of increased density *(arrow).* **C,** T1-weighted image in same patient shows detachment of the posterior hyaloid membrane *(white arrows)* and fluid (acute hemorrhage) in the subhyaloid (S). Notice a hyperintense mass *(black arrow)* compatible with subacute blood in the subretinal space. On CT scan (B), only the subretinal blood is visualized. **D,** Retinal detachment. T2-weighted MR image shows total retinal detachment of the left eye *(arrowheads).* Notice a large choroidal melanoma *(arrow)* involving right eye without retinal detachment. **E,** Serous choroidal detachment. Axial CT scan shows the detached choroid *(arrows).* Owing to the anchoring effect of the vorticose veins, the detached choroid stops at the expected location of the vorticose veins *(arrowheads).* **F,** Hemorrhagic choroidal detachment CT scan shows post-traumatic choroidal hematomas *(large arrow).* Notice intravitreal air bubbles *(small arrows).* (B–F from Mafee, Neuroimaging Clinics, Philadelphia, WB Saunders, 1998.)

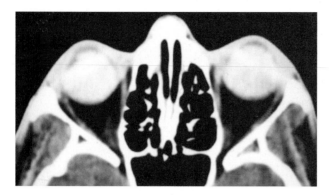

Fig. 10-20   Hemorrhagic CMV. CT reveals bilateral hemorrhages in a patient with AIDS.

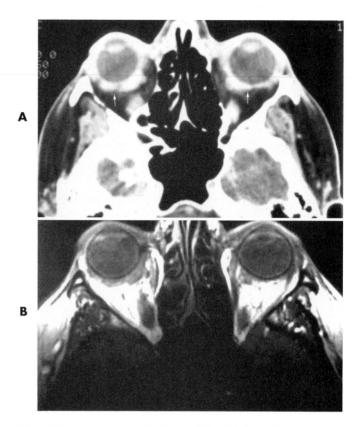

Fig. 10-21   Posterior scleritis. **A,** CT with bilateral posterior enhancement of episcleral region *(arrows).* **B,** T1WI with shaggy posterior margins of both globes representing episcleritis.

patients positive for human immunodeficiency virus, cytomegalovirus (CMV) infection-related arcuate retinal enhancement can be seen.

CMV is the most common opportunistic infection of the retina and choroid. Up to one fourth of patients with AIDS have cytomegalovirus. It is hemorrhagic and can produce high density on CT or various MR appearances depending upon the stage of blood (Fig. 10-20). Other infectious pathogens affecting the retina in AIDS include toxoplasmosis, herpes simplex, and herpes zoster. Orbital infections are discussed later in the chapter.

Posterior Scleritis

This can be infectious (bacterial, fungal, or viral) or autoimmune (collagen vascular diseases) in origin. It is separated into acute and chronic categories. Findings include thickening and enhancement of the posterior sclera and uveal layers (Fig. 10-21). The thickening may be nodular or diffuse. The nodular variety can be mistaken for melanoma; the diffuse type can mimic lymphoma.

Staphyloma

Posterior staphyloma and coloboma may be detected by CT or MR and are superficially similar (Fig. 10-22). Staphylomas are acquired defects in the sclera or cornea. They are lined with uveal tissue. Posterior staphyloma is associated with increasing globe size in patients with axial myopia and is usually on the temporal side of the optic disc. With posterior staphyloma one may demonstrate outward bulging (which is more diffuse than the cone-shaped deformity in coloboma) of the posterior portion of the globe with uveoscleral thinning and lack of enhancement. Posterior staphyloma can be a cause of proptosis.

Coloboma

A coloboma of the eye is a congenital defect in any ocular structure. It is classified as typical or atypical de-

pending on location and derivation. Atypical colobomas occur in the iris. The typical coloboma is a cone-shaped or notch deformity that occurs in the inferior medial portion of the globe. It is caused by incomplete closure of the choroidal fissure. This can result in an abnormal elon-

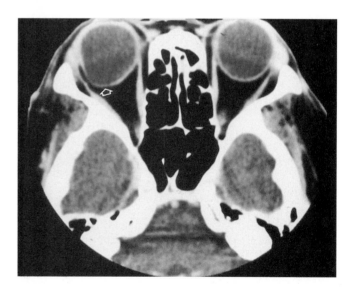

Fig. 10-22   CT of posterior staphyloma. Notice the uveoscleral thinning in the posterior lateral margin of the globe *(open arrow)* in this patient with axial myopia.

gated or malformed globe or ocular cyst at the site of the fetal optic fissure closure. It may be associated with orbital cysts, midline craniocerebrofacial clefting including sphenoidal encephalocele, agenesis of the corpus callosum, and olfactory hypoplasia, as well as cardiac abnormalities, retardation, genital hypoplasia, and ear anomalies. It is a part of the CHARGE syndrome (coloboma, heart defects, atresia of the choana, retarded growth and development, and ear anomalies). Other syndromes having coloboma include Len's microphthalmia syndrome, Meckel syndrome, trisomy 13, Goldenhar syndrome, Rubinstein-Taybi syndrome, Aicardi syndrome, and Waardenburg anophthalmia syndrome.

On imaging there is a cone- or notch-shaped deformity, usually of the posterior globe, that may involve the optic nerve, with eversion of a portion of the posterior globe (Fig. 10-23). Other structures including retina, choroid, iris, and lens can be affected. The sclera is normal. Colobomas usually arise sporadically and are unilateral, although rarely an autosomal dominant form can exist, with about 60% of those affected having bilateral coloboma.

Phakomatoses

Astrocytic (glial) hamartomas (see Fig. 10-17) are observed in cases of tuberous sclerosis, neurofibromatosis, and rarely von Hippel-Lindau disease (see Chapters 3 and 9). On CT, a focal region of calcification is noted in the retina. This can potentially be confused with retinoblastoma. These hamartomas grow slowly and do not metastasize. A hallmark of von Hippel-Lindau disease is retinal angiomatosis (which is not identified angiographically). Hemangioblastomas of the retrobulbar optic nerve and

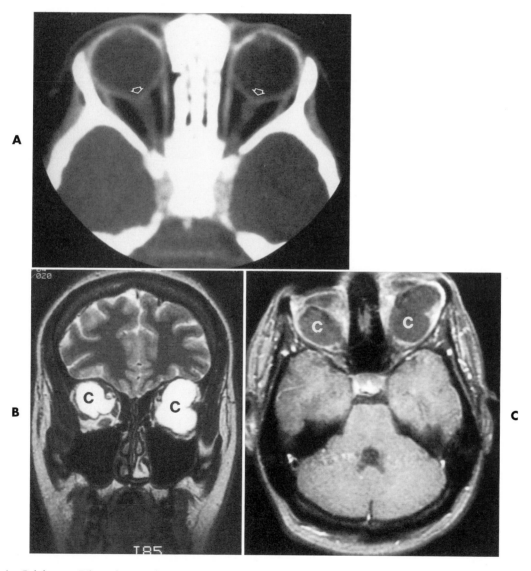

Fig. 10-23   **A,** Coloboma. Bilateral cone-shaped deformities at the junction of the optic nerve head and globe *(open arrows)*. **B,** Bilateral orbital cysts *(c)* coronal T2WI, and **(C)** axial enhanced T1WI in a patient with colobomas.

orbit have been reported in von Hippel-Lindau disease. The primary differential diagnosis of such optic nerve lesions is angioblastic meningioma and optic nerve glioma. Half the patients with optic nerve hemangioblastoma have other associated lesions of von Hippel-Lindau disease. Choroidal hemangiomas are reported in Sturge-Weber syndrome (tomato ketchup retina).

The Big or Small Globe (Box 10-4)

Occasionally, one is confronted with an image of an enlarged globe. The most common cause of this is axial myopia. The most common cause of axial myopia is reading too many books in your training, so throw out your other neuroradiology texts and protect yourself. Other conditions causing enlarged globes include congenital glaucoma (buphthalmos), collagen disorders (e.g., Marfan's syndrome), posterior staphyloma, coloboma, juvenile glaucoma in patients with Sturge-Weber syndrome, Proteus syndrome, and neurofibromatosis.

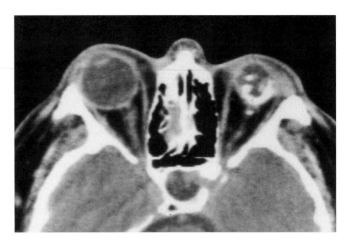

Fig. 10-24   Phthisis bulbi. A shrunken calcified globe is seen in this patient long after orbital trauma.

Small globes (microophthalmia) have been reported as an isolated event or may be associated with conditions such as craniofacial anomalies, congenital rubella, persistent hyperplastic primary vitreous, retinopathy of prematurity, and phthisis bulbi (a small shrunken calcified globe, usually the result of a traumatic injury) (Fig. 10-24 and also see 10-22). Anophthalmia represents complete absence of ocular tissue.

RETROBULBAR LESIONS

Retrobulbar lesions may be conveniently divided into intraconal, conal, and extraconal locations. The differential diagnosis of lesions by virtue of their anatomic origin is provided in Boxes 10-5 to 10-8. MR, by virtue of its superior anatomic and multiplanar imaging, is the imaging modality of choice for localizing orbital lesions.

Intraconal Lesions

Lesions of the optic nerve (Box 10-6)
Enlarged CSF space An enlarged perioptic subarachnoid space is easily detected by MR and may occur

---

Box 10-4   Causes of Macro-ophthalmia and Micro-ophthalmia

Macro-ophthalmia	Micro-ophthalmia
Axial myopia	Trisomy 13 (Patau syndrome)
Aniridia	PHPV
Lowe syndrome	Retinopathy of Prematurity
Sturge-Weber	Lowe syndrome (Oculocerebrorenal syndrome: small orbits, small globe, hypotonia, retardation, rickets, pathologic fractures, periventricular white matter lesions)
Intraocular masses	Phthisis bulbi
Congenital glaucoma	Surgery
Marfan	Radiation
Neurofibromatosis 1	CHARGE syndrome
Proteus	Infant of diabetic mother
Weill-Marchesani syndrome (short stature, short limbs, stiff joints, brachycephaly, lens ectopia)	Pseudohypoparathyroidism
Ehlers Danlos	Fetal rubella, varicella, herpes simplex, infection
Homocystinuria	Holoprosencephaly
Staphyloma	Fetal alcohol syndrome

Box 10-5   Intraconal Lesions

Lymphangioma
Lymphoma
Hematoma
Metastasis
Optic nerve lesions: Glioma, meningioma, hemangioblastoma, schwannoma, neuritis, sarcoid
Orbital pseudotumor
Rhabdomyosarcoma
Schwannoma
Vascular: Cavernous hemangioma, varix

Box 10-6 Causes of Optic Nerve Complex Enlargement

TUMORS

Leukemia, lymphoma
Hemangioblastoma
Meningioma
Metastasis
Optic nerve glioma
Schwannoma

NONNEOPLASTIC CAUSES

Central retinal vein occlusion
Cysticercosis
Graves' disease
Increased intracranial pressure
Normal variant with enlarged subarachnoid space
Optic neuritis
Orbital pseudotumor
Sarcoidosis
Toxoplasmosis
Traumatic hematoma of optic nerve
Tuberculosis

Table 10-3 Benign intracranial hypertension

Primary Forms
  Idiopathic
  Precipitating Factors Associated with
  Metabolic disorders
    Galactosemia,
      Maple syrup disease and other enzyme deficiencies
  Nutritional Disease
    Vitamin A deficiency
    Vitamin D deficiency
  Deprivation dwarfism
    Cystic fibrosis
  Endocrine Disorders
    Corticosteroid deficiency
    Cushing disease
  Thyroid disease
  Parathyroid disorders
    Pituitary disorders
  Hematological disorders
    Anemias
    Polycythemia vera
  Infections
    ENT infections
    Viral infections
    Lyme disease
    Diphtheria
    Tetanus
  Drugs
    Antibiotics
    Steroids
    Psychiatric drugs
    Indomethacin
  Traumatic head injury
Obesity
  Secondary form
    Cerebral vein or sagittal sinus thrombosis
    Post-meningitis syndromes

(Giuseffi V, et al: *Neurology* 41: 239-244, 1991.)

congenitally, as a result of optic atrophy, or in situations where raised intracranial pressure exists (such as benign intracranial hypertension, also known as pseudotumor cerebri). Symptoms include headaches, transient visual obscuration, and intracranial noises. This condition may be further divided into a primary and secondary forms listed in Table 10-3. In cases of raised intracranial pressure the globe at its junction with the optic nerve can be indented (reverse cupping) by the transmitted raised intracranial pressure (Fig. 10-25). Marked enhancement of the optic nerve heads has also been observed and thought to be secondary to breakdown of the blood retinal barrier following sudden rise in intracranial CSF pressure.

Optic nerve atrophy The end result of a variety of insults to the optic nerve is optic atrophy. The nerve loses both function and its pink color from loss of vascular supply. On MR, the nerve looks atrophic (Fig. 10-26). Causes of optic nerve atrophy include congenital optic nerve hypoplasia, macrophthalmos, compression lesions including pituitary tumors and craniopharyngioma, herpes zoster, multiple sclerosis, trauma, glaucoma, ischemic optic neuropathy, and toxic and nutritional.

When you see optic nerve hypoplasia in children think De Morsier (septooptic dysplasia) syndrome, which has associated poor vision, hypotelorism, absence of the septum pellucidum, and hypopituitarism.

Optic nerve drusen Drusen are composed of a mucoprotein matrix with significant quantities of acid mucopolysaccharides together with small quantities of ri-

bonucleic acid and, occasionally, iron. They are laminated calcareous deposits located in the substance of the optic nerve anterior to the lamina cribrosa. They may form when partially calcified extracellular mitochondria from disrupted axons serve as the substrated for calcium deposition. There is evidence to suggest that in the normal course of drusen there is progressive enlargement over years. This condition has an incidence of up to 2% of the population. Drusen may be familial (typically bilateral) or may be associated with other conditions such as retinitis pigmentosa. They may be unilateral or bilateral and are located at the junction of the optic nerve and globe.

CT demonstrates punctate calcifications at the junction of the nerve and the globe (see Fig. 10-9C). MR has difficulty detecting this condition because of its relative insensitivity to calcium. The clinical issue for the radiologist is that if the drusen is buried below the surface of the nerve head it is not seen by the ophthalmologist and

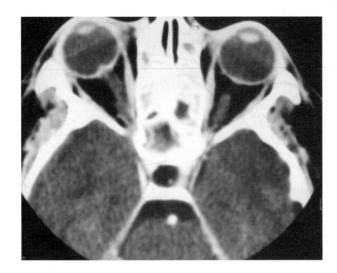

Fig. 10-25   Reversal of optic nerve head. CT reveals inversion of the right optic nerve head secondary to pseudotumor cerebri with raised intracranial pressure.

the patient may be referred for workup of what appears to be papilledema. The radiologist can thus be a hero—announcing the diagnosis of drusen, rather than optic nerve gruesome, and preventing the surgeon from doing some.

Optic neuritis   Optic neuritis is an inflammatory lesion of the optic nerve clinically associated with pain, decreased visual acuity, abnormal color vision, and afferent pupillary defect. Optic neuritis occurs in up to 87% of patients with multiple sclerosis (MS) and may be the first clinical manifestation of MS. In patients with their first attack of optic neuritis, up to 65% have asymptomatic white matter abnormalities in the brain on MR. Other less common diseases associated with optic neuritis include ischemia, vasculitis, sarcoid, systemic lupus erythematosus, syphilis, Lyme disease, viral infection, toxoplasmosis, tuberculosis, chemotherapy (cis-Platinum), and radiation therapy (Fig. 10-27). MR is the best

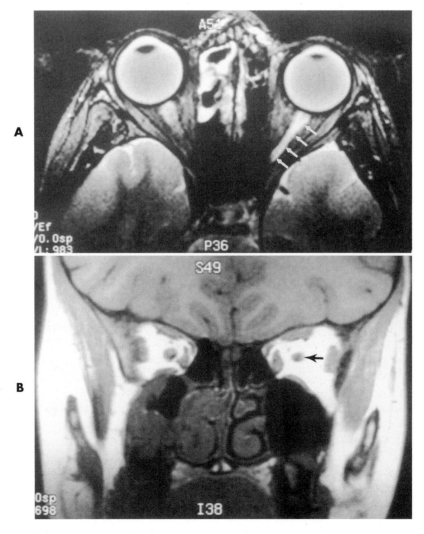

Fig. 10-26   Left optic nerve atrophy. **A,** Axial T2WI with small nerve *(arrows).* **B,** Coronal T1WI clearly reveal just how small the optic nerve is *(arrow).*

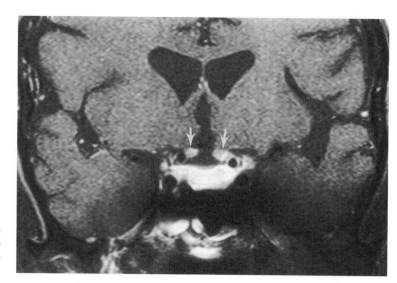

Fig. 10-27   Radiation induced optic neuritis. Observe the bilateral enhancement of the prechiasmatic segments of the optic nerves on T1WI in a patient radiated for adenocarcinoma of the ethmoid sinus *(arrows).*

imaging modality for optic neuritis (Fig. 10-28). Visualization is quite technique dependent. T2WI occasionally reveals high intensity of the involved nerve; however, motion and volume averaging of the CSF surrounding the nerve makes this pulse sequence less than adequate. Coronal imaging will minimize volume averaging. With the advent of fast spin-echo pulse sequences (with fat suppression), use of 3-mm sections, and 256 × 256 matrix coronal images, high intensity optic nerve lesions are readily imaged. A short TR inversion recovery pulse sequence has also been reported to be helpful, again demonstrating high signal intensity in the abnormal nerve with low signal from CSF. The nerve is almost always normal in size. The use of enhancement is particularly useful, especially with fat saturation for the orbital portion of the nerve. Perivenous inflammation is responsible for the enhancement, which can be seen in approximately 50% of patients with acute optic neuritis. Enhancement can also be observed in the intracranial portion of the optic nerve.

Devic disease (see Fig. 7-8) (neuromyelitis optica) is characterized by demyelination in the optic nerves and chiasm as well as lesions in the spinal cord. Most of the patients with this presentation ultimately have MS, however, there are cases where individuals do not progress to MS. Whether to classify this disease as MS or a separate disorder is open to debate, nevertheless, the radiologist should be aware of the presentation of optic neuritis associated with transverse myelitis as the entity of Devic disease.

Optic nerve and visual pathway glioma   Optic glioma is classified as a juvenile pilocytic astrocytoma and represents about two thirds of all primary optic nerve tumors, 1.5% to 3% of all orbital tumors, and up to 1.5% of all intracranial tumors. Optic gliomas have a mean age at presentation of 8.5 years (5 years old in neurofibromatosis type 1 and 12 years old in the absence of

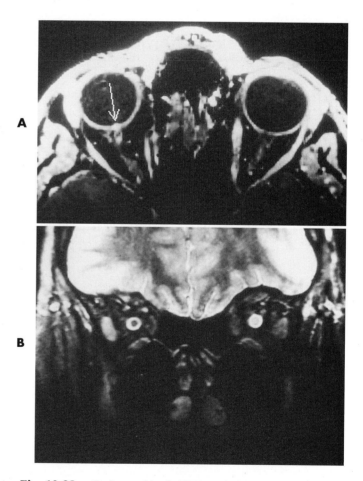

Fig. 10-28   Optic neuritis. **A,** T1WI with fat saturation demonstrates enhancement in the head of the optic nerve in this patient with papillitis. **B,** Coronal T2 fast spin echo image demonstrates high intensity in the left optic nerve in a patient with optic neuritis. Compare this intensity with that of the normal right optic nerve.

neurofibromatosis), with more than 80% occurring before 20 years of age. Optic nerve lesions tend to occur more often in females whereas chiasmal tumors are present equally in males and females. These lesions have a growth phase during childhood and become symptomatic. Most of the tumors then stabilize with indolent progression in about 40% of children. Patients may be asymptomatic and those with symptoms tend to have strabismus, visual loss, and afferent pupillary defect followed by proptosis. Decreased visual acuity is an early finding in meningioma but occurs late in the course of optic nerve glioma. In 10% to 38% of cases (25% average) there is an association with neurofibromatosis type 1 (von Recklinghausen's disease, NF-1), in which case the optic nerve glioma may be bilateral. In children with NF1 a negative initial imaging study does not rule out future development of optic glioma.

Approximately one fourth of visual pathway gliomas are confined to the intraorbital optic nerve. The rest occur in the intracranial portions of the optic nerve, the chiasm, or along the remainder of the visual pathway. Optic nerve gliomas tend not to extend intracranially, although there are exceptions. Prepubertal children have a higher incidence of glioma restricted to the optic nerve. Forty percent of chiasmatic gliomas extend into the hypothalamus, which significantly increases the morbidity and mortality rate. As opposed to children, in whom the lesions are slow growing and benign, the rare optic nerve glioma in the adult is commonly malignant, often extending intracranially, and is associated with a very poor prognosis (Fig. 10-29). The differential diagnosis in the adult includes multiple sclerosis, sarcoid, meningioma, hemangioblastoma, lymphoma, leukemia, and metastatic disease.

MR is the imaging modality of choice for this lesion (Fig. 10-30). It beautifully defines the tortuous enlarged

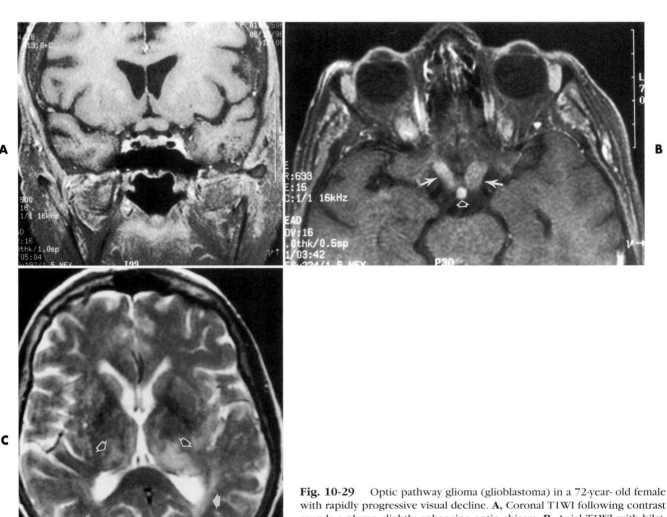

Fig. 10-29 Optic pathway glioma (glioblastoma) in a 72-year-old female with rapidly progressive visual decline. **A,** Coronal T1WI following contrast reveals a plump slightly enhancing optic chiasm. **B,** Axial T1WI with bilateral enhancement of both intracranial optic nerves *(arrows)*. *Open arrow* shows pituitary stalk enhancement (normal). **C,** Axial T2WI revealing extensive neoplastic involvement of the thalami *(open arrows)* and left optic radiations *(arrow)*.

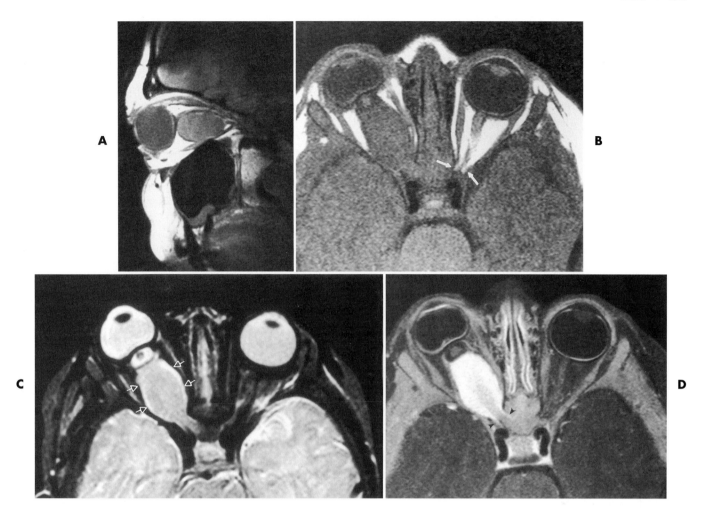

Fig. 10-30   Optic pathway gliomas. **A,** Sagittal T1WI demonstrates a large optic nerve glioma. Note that one cannot separate the nerve from the tumor. **B,** Axial T1WI with fusiform enlargement of the optic nerve. Note that the orbital apex has been remodeled and the normal fat *(arrows* on the normal left side) is missing from the right apex. The tumor mass produces proptosis and indents the globe. **C,** Axial T2WI. Tumor in this patient with neurofibromatosis appears low intensity whereas peripherally there is surrounding high intensity *(open arrows).* This has been termed arachnoidal gliomatosis. **D,** T1 enhanced image with enhancement of the tumor, which appears to be going through the optic foramen *(arrowheads).*

nerve that usually appears isointense on T1WI and of isointensity to high intensity on T2WI. MR is especially advantageous for lesions at the orbital apex and in the optic canal. Prominent CSF spaces around a normal nerve are differentiated from tumor in that they follow the intensity of CSF whereas tumor may be higher intensity on PD and lower intensity on T2WI. These lesions demonstrate variable enhancement. In a patient with neurofibromatosis, the low intensity on T2WI has been reported in the tumor to be surrounded by a fusiform region of higher signal intensity. This peripheral zone corresponds histopathologically to perineural glial proliferation intermixed with reactive proliferation of the fibrovascular arachnoidal trabeculae ("arachnoidal gliomatosis"), a feature of orbital optic gliomas in neurofibromatosis. The central low intensity core represents the optic nerve glioma, which contains dense fibrous tis-

sue, perhaps accounting for its lower intensity. Because this surrounding region has somewhat similar characteristics to CSF, it can be confused with dilated subarachnoid space. MR not only depicts the orbital lesion but is also very useful in discerning the associated cerebral abnormalities. These include enlargement and abnormal signal in the intracranial portion of the optic nerves, chiasm, and optic tracts.

CT reveals an enlarged optic nerve and canal (if the lesion extends through the optic canal). The nerve enlargement may be fusiform or nodular. Enhancement is variable, and calcification is rare unless the patient has been previously treated with radiation. The mass usually cannot be radiographically separated from the optic nerve, as opposed to optic nerve meningioma, in which the tumor can be separated from the nerve. Optic nerve gliomas may have cystic components associated with them. These result from ischemia, radiation therapy, or mucin deposition. The nerve-tumor complex may display kinks or buckling, perhaps secondary to the mucin content of the tumor (which would make it more pliant) and perineural axial growth.

Optic nerve sheath meningioma Meningiomas may arise primarily from the meninges of the orbital optic nerve or extend secondarily from the cranial meninges. They originate from meningothelial cells within the meninges. Orbital optic nerve sheath meningiomas present with the insidious onset of visual loss, optic atrophy, mild proptosis, and opticociliary shunts (dilated veins from the optic nerve head, observed in 32% of cases). These lesions have a predominance for middle-aged women but may also be seen in children with neurofibromatosis. Patterns of optic nerve enlargement may include diffuse tubular appearance, fusiform mass, or globular perioptic enlargement. In many cases, the nerve may be visualized as a separate entity in the mass of tumor. This helps differentiate the nerve sheath meningioma from the optic nerve glioma, where in most instances the nerve cannot be separated from the tumor. Bilateral optic nerve sheath meningiomas are rare lesions that most often arise from the region of the tuberculum sellae or planum sphenoidale and grow forward along both optic nerves. Bilateral tumors are found in patients with neurofibromatosis type 1 or 2. Associated findings in this situation include pneumosinus dilatans of the sphenoid sinus and blistering of the planum sphenoidale. As opposed to optic nerve gliomas, which do not calcify, optic nerve sheath meningiomas may demonstrate calcification (20% to 50% of cases).

CT findings include a high density mass that demonstrates enhancement. Bony changes may be present in the region of the optic nerve canal with bone erosion and occasionally hyperostosis. The optic canal is commonly normal, although it may be large or small. Thin CT sections (1.5 to 3 mm) are useful in evaluating the nerve. On axial CT the appearance after contrast has been termed the "sandwich sign" (also called the "tram track" sign) with the nerve (the "bologna") sandwiched between the "bread" of the meningioma. Calcified meningiomas can have a similar appearance on unenhanced images. The enhancement on axial MR has been analogized to tram tracks in the axial image or a doughnut in the coronal plane. The differential diagnoses of axial tram-tracking include pseudotumor, sarcoid, metastatic disease, lymphoma, leukemia, and (how's this for a pearl?) Erdheim-Chester disease (systemic xanthogranulomatosis with bilateral granulomatous involvement of the orbit). Other lesions that simulate the appearance of optic sheath meningioma include hemangioblastoma of the optic nerve in von Hippel-Lindau disease, cavernous hemangioma, and rarely, optic nerve glioma.

MR reveals isointensity/or slight hypointensity on T1WI and slightly high intensity on T2WI (Fig. 10-31). Optic nerve sheath meningiomas enhance, and such enhancement is particularly evident with fat saturation techniques. MR is exceptionally useful for orbital apex and intracanalicular lesions, whereas detection on CT might be difficult in this region because of the high-density values of bone.

Other intraconal lesions

Cavernous and capillary hemangioma Vascular intraconal masses include capillary and cavernous hemangiomas, venous angiomas, and varices. The cavernous hemangioma is the most common primary orbital tumor, consisting of dilated endothelial lined vascular channels encompassed by a fibrous pseudocapsule. It occurs in females more commonly than males and presents in the second to fifth decade of life with the slow onset of proptosis (which commonly goes unnoticed) and visual disturbance. Growth can be exceedingly slow and may stop after a certain time period; however, rapid growth has been observed during pregnancy. The CT shows a smoothly marginated high density round or oval intraconal mass that densely enhances. Commonly, there is evidence of orbital bone expansion. In one study, calcification was not observed in 66 pathologic specimens, although it may uncommonly be seen on CT. MR depicts a smoothly marginated, intraconal mass that has no flow voids and demonstrates marked enhancement. Cavernous hemangiomas are isointense to muscle and hypointense to fat on T1WI and high intensity on T2WI (Fig. 10-32). On early postcontrast images they enhance in a patchy fashion but totally fill in within 30 minutes. A chemical shift effect may be seen at the periphery of the lesion. Infrequently, cavernous angiomas may be extraconal. Hemangiopericytoma has a similar CT appearance to cavernous hemangioma. It is a rare lesion with signs of slowly developing unilateral proptosis. Other lesions to consider include neurofibroma, schwannoma, hemangiopericytoma, or benign mesenchymal tumor (Fig. 10-33).

Capillary hemangiomas are seldom seen after the age of 3 years. They are usually not well circumscribed and are not intraconal lesions. MR is the imaging modality of choice for diagnosis of these lesions. Use of multiplanar imaging helps localize the lesion to the appropriate anatomic region. Capillary hemangiomas may have many small vessels containing flowing blood. These appear as punctate hypointensities (flow voids) on MR.

Orbital venous anomalies These anomalies may be divided into those with a venous connection (varices) and those without (lymphangiomas). No arterial supply is demonstrated angiographically and there is low intensity on MR in the vascular channels intermixed with high intensity for areas of thrombosis, phleboliths, or hemorrhage. There is no difference in the incidence of

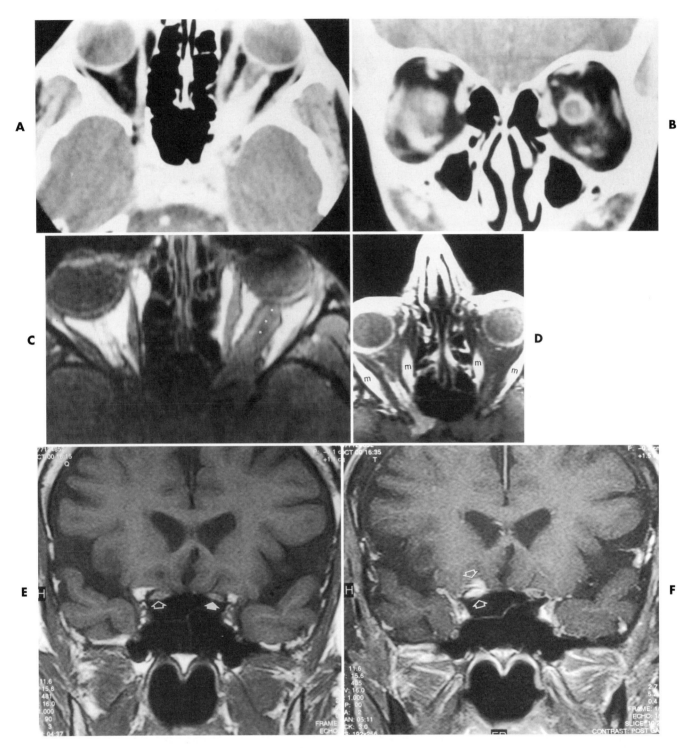

Fig. 10-31   Optic nerve meningiomas. **A,** This CT demonstrates high density around the optic nerve in a tram-track pattern. **B,** Coronal CT of left optic nerve demonstrating a doughnut sign (of meningioma) around the optic nerve. **C,** T1WI of an optic nerve meningioma. Nerve *(asterisk)* can be separated from the tumor. This is usually not possible with optic nerve glioma. **D,** Enhanced T1WI fat-suppressed image demonstrates enhancement along the nerve and through the optic canal to the intracranial portion of the optic nerve. Note that on this fat-suppressed image the extraocular muscles *(m)* enhance. This is normal. **E,** Meningioma of the intracranial optic nerve. *Open arrow* on coronal T1WI demonstrates a subtly enlarged optic nerve. Compare it to the normal right intracranial optic nerve *(closed arrow)*. **F,** Following contrast the you can visualize the not so subtle enhancement of the meningioma of the optic nerve.

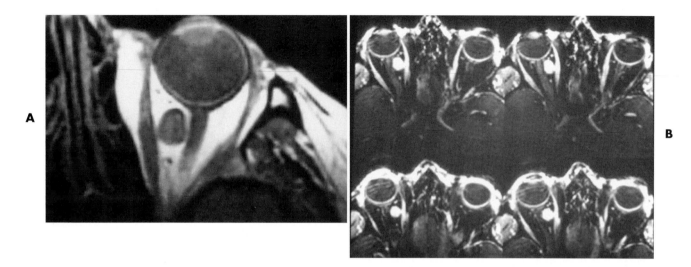

Fig. 10-32. **A,** Axial T1WI of a cavernous hemangioma. Note that it is a smooth, well-marginated intraconal mass that can be separated from the optic nerve, which is slightly indented by the mass. **B,** Axial T1W fat sat postgadolinium image with avid enhancement is cavernous hemangioma.

hemorrhage between lesions with a venous connection and those without. In addition, histopathologic differentiation between lymphatic and venous channels is extremely difficult. Thus, venous anomaly may be a more appropriate term than lymphangioma. There may also be another type of lesion termed the combined venous lymphatic malformation of the orbit, which has both venous and lymphatic components. There has been a reported association of these lesions with intracranial vascular malformations. Nevertheless, we will still use the "classic" terms as we remember what happened when Coke tried to modernize its approach—we can't afford failure

and neither can our readers. Imagine the board examiner's response when the examinee blurts out venous anomaly rather than lymphangioma. See you next year says the examiner. The examinee sues the publisher, the publisher cuts the royalty, and our kids are excommunicated from the Trustafarians.

Orbital varix   The orbital varix is a venous malformation in which there is dilatation of an otherwise normal venous system or abnormal venous channels affecting the superior and/or inferior ophthalmic veins, resulting in intermittent proptosis associated with retrobulbar pain. The spectrum can range from a single di-

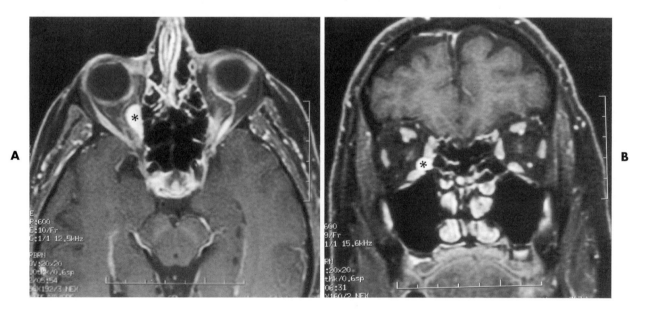

Fig. 10-33   Orbital Schwannoma of the Fifth Nerve. **A,** T1 postcontrast image shows a smoothly marginated mass in the medial posterior region of the orbit (*). The mass enhances and is extraconal. **B,** Postcontrast T1 coronal of the same lesion (*).

lated venous structure to multiple varicosities. Varices are associated with a history of proptosis in conjunction with maneuvers, such as straining (this can be a bathroom diagnosis) or coughing, that increase venous pressure. This increase is transmitted through the valveless jugular veins to the dilated intraorbital venous network. These lesions are considered congenital venous vascular malformations but can also be related to orbital trauma or associated with orbital or intracranial arteriovenous malformations or carotid-cavernous fistula. Plain CT reveals a high density intraconal mass. Enhanced CT of the patient in the prone position with Valsalva maneuver often results in significant change in the size of orbital mass (Fig. 10-34). In the past, diagnosis was confirmed by orbital venography or intravenous digital angiography. Presently, MR is the method of choice. Flow in the varix is detected as low intensity on spin echo sequences in a vascular-shaped structure. With cessation of blood flow

and thrombosis, the appearance is variable, depending on the stage of the clot. MR is the best noninvasive imaging modality for detecting flow and the cessation of flow. Superior ophthalmic vein thrombosis is likewise diagnosed by lack of a flow void.

Lymphangioma Lymphangiomas consist of dysplastic vascular channels (lymphatic or venous), loose connective tissue, and smooth muscle bundles. They are most likely vascular hamartomas that arise from an anlage of vascular mesenchyme. Lymphangioma of the orbit is generally an extraconal mass that may be located anteriorly or posteriorly, however, lymphangiomas may occur in any orbital space. These tumors are not well encapsulated. The mean age at presentation in one series was 23 years but lymphangiomas can be seen in the newborn to adult patient. These tumors have a tendency to hemorrhage with the acute onset of symptoms. CT exhibits orbital expansion, irregular margins crossing

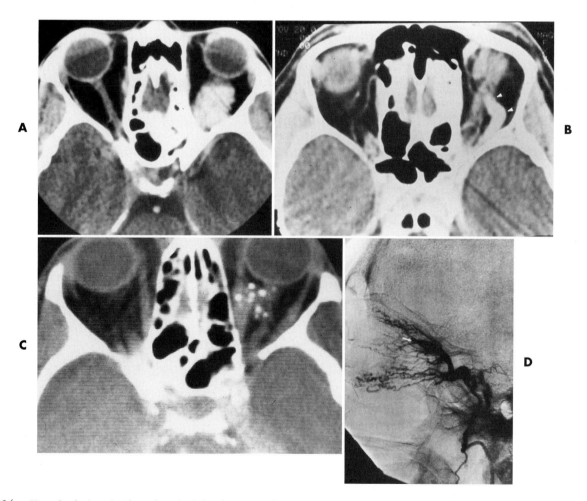

Fig. 10-34   Vascular lesions in the orbit. **A,** Orbital varix in the prone position. Notice the contrast level in an orbital *varix.* There is slight proptosis here. **B,** Enlargement of the left superior ophthalmic vein *(arrowheads)* in a patient with a carotid-cavernous fistula. **C,** CT of a patient with an arteriovenous malformation of the orbit demonstrates calcified phleboliths. **D,** Lateral angiogram of a selective accessory meningeal artery in a patient with a dural fistula. Notice significant orbital varices secondary to obstruction *(arrow)* of the distal superior ophthalmic vein.

Illustration continued on following page

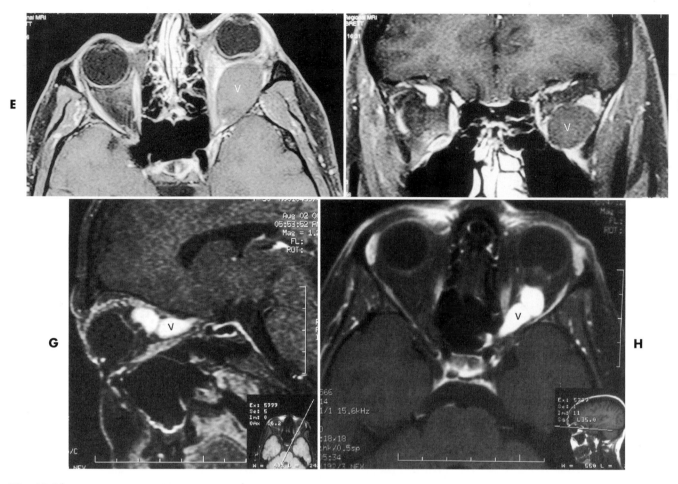

Fig. 10-34 *Continued.* **E** and **F,** Axial and coronal postcontrast T1WI of a thrombosed orbital varix *(v).* **G** and **H,** Sagittal and axial postcontrast T1WI shows enhancement in a dilated superior ophthalmic vein which has become a varix *(v).* Observe that the ipsilateral cavernous sinus is not enlarged.

anatomic boundaries and increased density on plain scan but variable enhancement. Peripheral enhancement can be demonstrated in cystic regions of the lesion. Calcified phleboliths have been noted. In addition to the morphologic characteristics, MR can show evidence of hemorrhage into multiple or single cysts (Fig. 10-35). These appear as high signal intensities on T1WI, and fluid levels are identified.

Carotid-cavernous fistula and dural vascular malformation Carotid-cavernous fistula is a direct communication between the intracavernous portion of the carotid artery and the venous cavernous sinus. These most often result from significant trauma, either nonpenetrating or penetrating. Another cause is the spontaneous rupture of a cavernous carotid aneurysm, usually in an elderly patient. The clinical presentation is of pulsating exophthalmos, orbital bruit, and motility disturbance with dilated conjunctival vessels, and glaucoma. Carotid-cavernous fistula causes enlargement of the extraocular muscles, proptosis, and dilatation of the

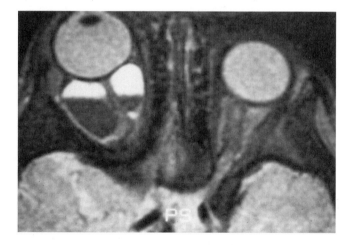

Fig. 10-35 Lymphangioma. Axial PDWI in a young man who had acute proptosis demonstrates hemorrhagic fluid levels. This case is somewhat unusual because the lesion appears to be intraconal.

superior ophthalmic vein secondary to congestion and edema from orbital venous hypertension (see Fig. 10-34D). CT nicely shows these findings with enlargement of the superior ophthalmic vein (see Fig. 10-34B). Irregularity or absence of superior ophthalmic vein enhancement suggests partial or complete thrombosis. The superior ophthalmic veins can also be enlarged in patients with diffuse cerebral swelling. In such cases the veins are enlarged bilaterally as opposed to carotid cavernous fistula where they are usually unilaterally enlarged. Periorbital swelling and blurring of the globe's margin related to conjunctival edema or pulsations can be observed on CT. The cavernous sinus may be distended and bowed convex to the middle cranial fossa. MR shows similar findings and can indicate, with flow techniques, either flow or its absence in the superior and inferior ophthalmic veins. Cavernous carotid artery aneurysms as a potential source of the fistula can be visualized with MR. Ultrasound is also useful and demonstrates reversal of blood flow.

Carotid angiography exhibits direct communication between the cavernous carotid artery and the cavernous sinus. There may be filling of other venous structures including ophthalmic veins (superior and inferior), the petrosal sinuses, at times cortical veins, and other veins that communicate with the cavernous sinus. Filling may be bilateral due to intercavernous venous connections. One easy way to think about this lesion is that arterial flow is being pumped into the cavernous sinus and that it must be decompressed. This occurs with retrograde filling of the orbital veins and with filling of any other veins that drain into the cavernous sinus. Fistulas with cortical venous drainage are prone to intracranial hemorrhage. The ipsilateral carotid injection displays the site of the fistula, the extent of steal, and cortical venous drainage. The contralateral carotid injection is important in determining the extent of collateral flow, particularly if the ipsilateral carotid artery must be sacrificed to close the fistula. At times, it is very difficult to visualize the exact site of the fistula because of its rapid filling on the ipsilateral carotid injection. A useful technique for finding the opening of the fistula is to inject the vertebral artery, with compression in the neck of the ipsilateral carotid artery during the injection. Contrast will flow across the posterior communicating artery into the carotid and then flow retrograde from the supraclinoid carotid into the cavernous carotid through the opening of the fistula. Spontaneous carotid cavernous fistula has been reported in osteogenesis imperfecta (even more imperfecta than you knew), Ehlers-Danlos, and pseudoxanthoma elasticum. This subject is also briefly discussed in Chapter 5.

Dural malformations involving the cavernous sinus are different from direct carotid-cavernous fistula in many ways. They are not usually associated with a traumatic event. Venous thrombosis has been linked to the development of these malformations. Symptoms are generally not as fulminant as the direct carotid-cavernous fistula, although if venous pressure is increased, periocular pain, third, fourth, and sixth nerve palsies, and visual loss (secondary to acute glaucoma) can rapidly occur. If the venous drainage is posterior, that is, out the inferior petrosal sinus (see Chapter 11 for your anatomic refresher of this area) you may have a "white-eyed" cavernous shunt. The sixth nerve palsy may result from venous compression in Dorello canal. Supply is from branches of the meningohypophyseal artery, ascending pharyngeal artery, middle meningeal artery, accessory meningeal artery, artery of the foramen rotundum, or other meningeal tributaries, and supply can be bilateral in patients with unilateral symptoms. If there is partial or complete thrombosis of the venous drainage of the orbit including the superior ophthalmic vein, patient's symptoms could be temporarily paradoxically worsened although this is ultimately therapeutic.

Both lesions are amenable to interventional embolization. The preferred treatment of direct carotid-cavernous fistula is the use detachable coils or detachable balloons flow-directed through the fistula into the cavernous sinus, tamponading the hole in the carotid. Another approach, reserved for cases in which the balloon cannot be placed safely through the fistula, involves trapping of the fistula above and below its origin with balloons and/or surgical intervention. Dural fistulas respond to particulate or liquid embolic material. The trick here is to promote venous thrombosis so that the fistula occludes. At times these fistulas spontaneously thrombose, although other therapies include angiography and carotid massage (spa therapy). Partial embolization can also result in complete thrombosis at times. However, dural malformations can recur and may be difficult to cure. Emergency intervention is required for acute visual deterioration, thrombosis of the superior ophthamic vein with increased collateral orbital blood flow, or the presence of cortical venous drainage.

Neurogenic tumors   These lesions can arise from orbital branches of cranial nerves III, IV, V, VI, sympathetic and parasympathetic nerves, and the ciliary ganglion. They include Schwannomas (neurolemmomas), neurofibromas, and amputation neuromas. Schwannomas appear similar to those in other locations with cystic and solid components and a propensity to contain blood products (Fig. 10-36). Neurofibromas may be localized, diffuse or plexiform, all three associated with neurofibromatosis with plexiform being pathognomic. Amputation neuromas arise after trauma or surgery.

Metastases and lymphoma   Metastases and lymphoma can involve any part of the orbit, presenting as

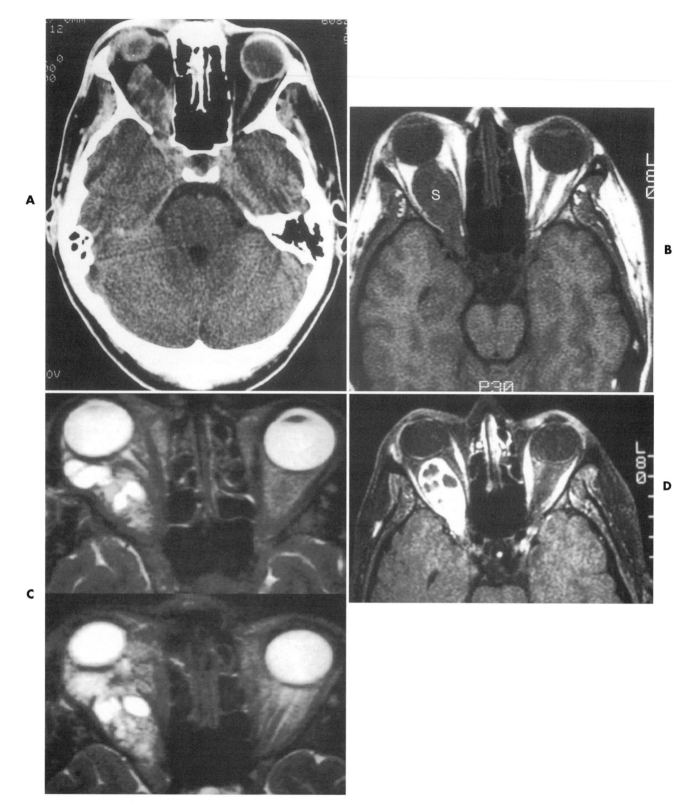

Fig. 10-36   Schwannoma of orbit (nerve unknown). **A,** Unenhanced CT show large mass in right orbit. No calcifications, however, there is a suggestion of solid and cystic components. **B,** T1W axial MR shows mass *(s)*. **C,** T2WI axial MR. Note the multiple high intensity cysts. T2WI axial MR. Note the multiple high intensity cysts in the lesion. **D,** T1WI with contrast shows inhomogeneous enhancement of the lesion. The cysts are obvious.

Box 10-7   Conal Lesions

Acromegaly
Carotid-cavernous fistula, thrombosis, or dural
  malformation
Cellulitis
Hematoma or swelling from trauma
Lymphoma, leukemia
Metastasis
Myositis
Orbital pseudotumor
Rhabdomyosarcoma
Sarcoid
Thyroid ophthalmopathy
Wegener

intraconal, conal, or extraconal lesions. Metastatic scirrhous breast carcinoma and neuroblastoma in children have a propensity for the latter and are discussed in the extraconal lesion section.

Conal Lesions

Box 10-7 enumerates lesions that primarily involve the muscles (conal lesions).

Thyroid ophthalmopathy. (Graves orbitopathy)

The term "orbitopathy" has been suggested to replace ophthalmopathy because of the presence of optic neuropathy. The authors are thoroughly neuropathic fence sitters and so we will use both terms. Graves ophthalmopathy is usually asymptomatic and can be present in euthyroid or hyperthyroid persons. Women have a 4:1 predominance over men. It may occur before, during, or after treatment and has a subacute onset, extending for months. CT exhibits prominent extraocular muscle enlargement and proptosis. There are normal muscle insertions on the globe, fusiform enlargement of the muscle belly, and protrusion of the orbital fat. In patients with clinical thyroid ophthalmopathy 85% have bilateral involvement, 5% have unilateral involvement, and 10% have normal muscles. The most frequently affected muscles are the inferior and medial rectus, although the most common single pattern is enlargement of all muscles. The lateral rectus muscle is rarely if ever involved alone and is the last to be affected when all muscles are involved. Try this mnemonic for remembering the frequency of muscle involvement in Graves—"I'm sol"—inferior, medial, superior, oblique muscle involvement.

There are muscle fibers in the superolateral intermuscular orbital septum that extend from the lateral rectus to the levator palpebrae superioris. Anatomically, the anterior part of the septum becomes significantly thicker than other orbital septa that form compartments within the orbit. Anteriorly, the septum fuses with the aponeurosis of the levator palpebra muscle to form the lateral part of the levator aponeurosis, and within this septum, are circumferentially oriented striated muscle fibers that have been termed the tensor intermuscularis muscle. This muscle also enlarges in Graves. It may function to help stabilize the lateral position of the globe against the pull of the oblique muscles or it may control opening of the upper lid. This may explain the greater degree of lateral eyelid retraction in Graves. Coronal scanning is the method of choice for assessing muscle thickness. Orbital fat may be increased alone in 8% of cases with forward displacement of the orbital septum, whereas approximately 46% of cases involve both muscle and fat. The lacrimal glands and eyelids may be swollen. Increased orbital fat, producing exophthalmos, also has been reported to be caused by exogenous steroids and Cushing disease. The eyebrow fat pad can be involved producing bulky eyebrows. The superior ophthalmic vein can be distended. Progressive optic neuropathy is a serious complication of Graves orbitopathy and is seen in 5% of patients. There is an association of optic neuropathy and intracranial prolapse of orbital fat through the superior orbital fissure. Other features of the neuropathy include increased volume of orbital contents with severe proptosis and lacrimal gland displacement or apical crowding with dilatation of the superior ophthalmic vein and optic nerve sheath (just eyeball it). Optic nerve thickening and bony erosion occur in the late stages of Graves disease. At present, MR may not add much more useful information than CT (Fig. 10-37). It has not been able to distinguish changes in the orbital fat. Although the MR intensity changes of the muscles do not permit one to distinguish pseudotumor from thyroid ophthalmopathy, it can precisely define the anatomic boundaries involved.

Many of the signs and symptoms of Graves orbitopathy including lid lag, diplopia, limited extraocular muscle movements, proptosis, and optic nerve compression result from the periorbital fibrosis that develops when the inflammation resolves. Orbital fat volume may actually be decreased relative to the total orbital volume in some patients with optic neuropathy. The T2 relaxation times of the extraocular muscles in Graves have been reported to be prolonged most likely secondary to increased water content as a manifestation of inflammation. Potentially, this can be used to distinguish patients with inflammatory changes (long T2) from those of fibrosis (shorter T2). This can have therapeutic implications, that is, treatment of inflammation versus no treatment for fibrosis.

Multiplanar MR or CT is important in assessing the degree of optic nerve compression by the enlarged muscles at the orbital apex. It is easy to appreciate the ex-

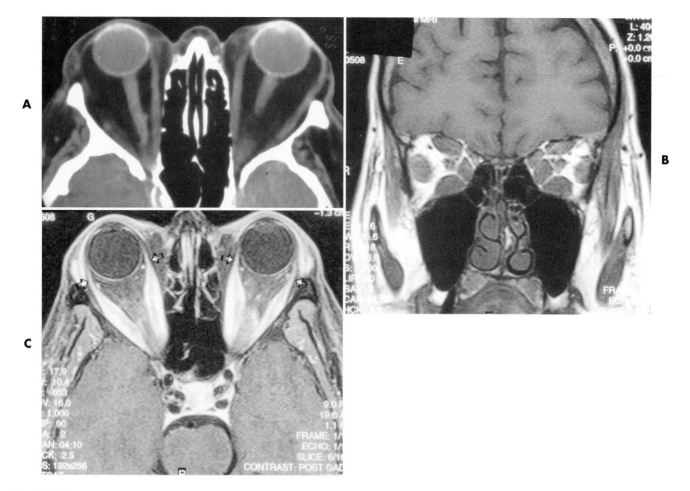

Fig. 10-37   Thyroid ophthalmopathy. **A,** CT with bilateral exophthalmos with marked increased orbital fat. **B,** T1WI with bilateral asymmetric muscle involvement. **C,** Postcontrast T1WI axial with sparing of the tendinous insertions *(arrows)* characteristic of thyroid disease and avid muscular enhancement.

tent of optic nerve compression, particularly on the coronal image. In extreme cases where vision is threatened, orbital decompression is performed with partial removal of the floor or medial wall of the orbit.

The differential diagnosis of enlarged muscles is similar to that of conal lesions (obviously).

Orbital pseudotumor

Orbital pseudotumor may mimic a variety of pathologic states so that the appropriate history (rarely found on radiology request slips) is essential for making the correct diagnosis. It is a common cause of unilateral exophthalmos (as opposed to Graves disease, which is often bilateral). Other clinical features include restriction of ocular motility, chemosis, lid swelling, and pain. These findings usually have a rapid onset and respond to steroids, although there is also a chronic form with progressive fibrosis and a mild or poor response to steroids. In such cases, chemotherapy or radiation therapy is used. Acute orbital pseudotumor is an inflammatory condition that may be the result of an autoimmune condition in-

volving the lacrimal gland (dacryoadenitis), lacrimal sac, the extraocular muscles, the connective tissue surrounding the dura of the optic nerve, the orbital fat—lids, the epibulbar connective tissue, and the sclera. In fact, orbital pseudotumor may show intracranial extension. In contrast to Graves disease the contour of the enlarged muscles may not be smooth and the insertions may be affected. Unfortunately, this is not true for all orbital pseudotumors! Indeed, some pseudotumors may have smooth muscles with uninvolved tendons. At times pseudotumor may be bilateral.

Pseudotumor may present as a lacrimal mass, a diffuse, ill-defined retrobulbar enhancing mass obscuring fascial planes, or simply as thickened muscles and/or their tendons and sheaths. Over 70% of cases display proptosis. There may be a subtle increase in the density of orbital fat (dirty fat) or optic nerve thickening. Systemic diseases associated with orbital pseudotumor (<10% of cases) include Wegener granulomatosis, polyarteritis nodosa, sarcoidosis, as well as autoimmune conditions such as lupus erythematosus, dermatomyositis, and rheumatoid arthritis. Related and associated fibrotic processes include retroperitoneal fibrosis, sclerosing cholangitis, Riedel thyroiditis, and mediastinal fibrosis. The term "multifocal fibrosclerosis" is used as a collective description of these disorders.

On T1 and T2WI pseudotumor has a tendency to be low intensity whereas metastatic lesions have a longer T2 (high intensity) (Fig. 10-38).

Tolosa-Hunt

Tolosa-Hunt syndrome is an idiopathic inflammatory condition similar to orbital pseudotumor that involves the cavernous sinus and orbital apex. It presents with painful ophthalmoplegia. With respect to the orbit, inflammatory tissue can be identified in the orbital apex in the majority of cases. Pathologically lymphocytes and plasma cells infiltrate the involved region and there is thickening of the dura matter. On CT, the low density of orbital fat is replaced by soft tissue. This is a subtle but important finding in lesions of the orbital apex. On MR, soft tissue isointense to muscle can be recognized at the orbital apex (Fig. 10-39). This tissue enhances. Tolosa-Hunt syndrome is discussed further in Chapter 11.

Sarcoidosis

Sarcoidosis commonly involves the orbit. Up to 25% of all patients with sarcoid have ophthalmic involvement. Isolated orbital disease is rare and is usually limited to the lacrimal glands (Fig. 10-40). Uveitis is the most common manifestation with other lesions involving the lacrimal gland, optic nerve/sheath, chiasm, muscles, and retrobulbar tissue producing proptosis.

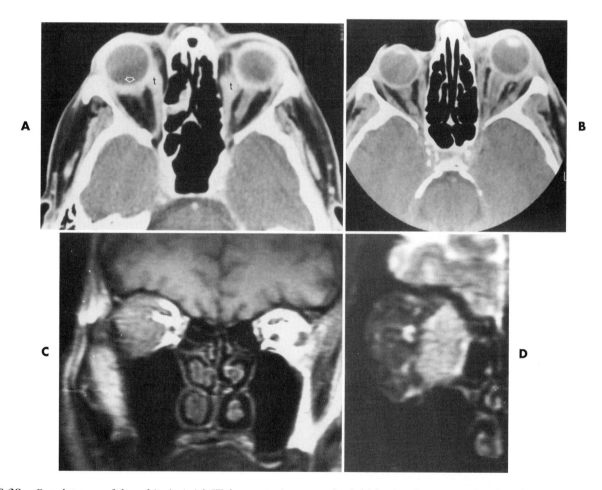

Fig. 10-38   Pseudotumor of the orbit. **A,** Axial CT demonstrating uveoscleral thickening *(open arrow)* and tendinous involvement *(see the t and A)* by the pseudotumor process. In this case, the orbital pseudotumor was bilateral. **B,** Tram-tracking in a patient with pseudotumor. Axial CT demonstrates the appearance of tram tracking in the left orbit. This could be mistaken for meningioma with the exception of the anterior soft-tissue thickening around the globe. **C,** Coronal T1WI in another patient with pseudotumor demonstrates the mass that encompasses the superior, lateral, and medial rectus as well as the optic nerve. **D,** T2WI of a patient with pseudotumor demonstrates high intensity compared with orbital muscle but low intensity compared with brain. Oops, we made a mistake! This is actually lymphoma. Now you can appreciate how difficult this differential diagnosis is.

Illustration continued on following page

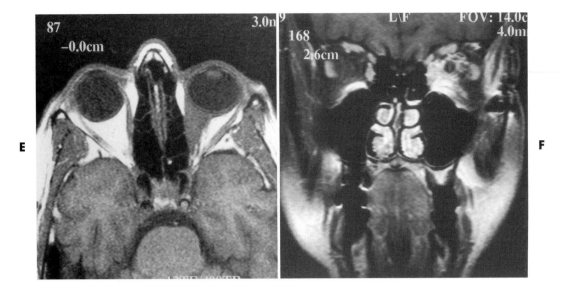

Fig. 10-38 *Continued.* **E,** Another case of pseudotumor with involvement of insertion of left medial rectus. **F,** Postcontrast coronal T1WI with perioptic enhancement and infiltration of medial and inferior rectus muscles.

Wegener's granulomatosis

Wegener's granulomatosis is characterized by granulomatous inflammation, tissue necrosis, and vasculitis that involve arteries, veins, and capillaries. It may involve the orbit secondarily from the paranasal sinuses, or may demonstrate primary orbital disease. Up to 54% of all patients with Wegener have neurologic involvement and half have disease in the orbit. The most common ocular manifestations (15% of Wegener's) are keratitis and scleritis, whereas the orbital involvement (initially present in only 2% of cases but the most common form later in the course of the disease) produces pain, proptosis, erythematous eyelid edema, and limitation of extraocular movements. The ocular and orbital processes may coexist. Antineutrophil cytoplasmic antibodies are highly sensitive indicators of the disease. On MR, Wegener's has been reported to be hypointense relative to orbital fat on T2WI and enhance homogeneously. The classic lesion is a homogeneously enhancing mass with associated sinus disease and bone destruction, but if everything were classic—radiology would be pretty dull and you wouldn't rate the big bucks.

The anterior segment is usually involved more than the posterior segment. Orbital inflammation may cause painful swelling, proptosis, nasal-lacrimal obstruction, or dacryocystitis. The most common neurologic manifestation is a peripheral neuropathy, particularly, mononeuropathy multiplex. Other manifestations include cranial neuropathies, ophthalmoplegia, Horner syndrome, papilledema, hearing loss, headache, meningitis, meningeal thickening, myelopathy, myopathy, cerebritis, strokes, and seizures. The differential diagnosis includes polyarteritis nodosa and lymphomatoid granulomatosis, Beçhet's disease, primary CNS vasculitis, lymphoproliferative disorders, sarcoidosis, Churg-Strauss syndrome, Erdheim-Chester disease, and infectious/inflammatory or neoplastic meningeal infiltration. Bottom line here is that Wegener granulomatoses should be in the differential diagnosis of leptomeningeal enhancement associated with ophthalmic and neurologic signs and symptoms.

Kimura disease

Kimura Disease (for our Asian customers)—This is probably an allergic or autoimmune disease usually, but not always, seen in young Asian males. It has a propensity for the skin of the head and neck region. In the orbit, patients present with exophthalmos, palpable orbital and/or eyelid lesions, and eyelid edema. The mass lesions on CT appear similar to orbital pseudotumor.

Orbital lymphoma

Lymphoma may occur as a primary orbital tumor or may be associated with systemic lymphoma. It is generally seen in older persons presenting with slowly progressive painless periorbital swelling and low-grade proptosis. CT reveals a diffuse infiltrative mass that destroys the normal orbital architecture so that anatomic struc-

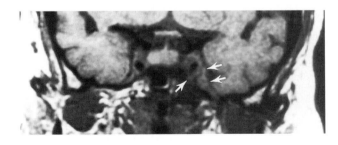

Fig. 10-39 Tolosa-Hunt syndrome. T1WI with soft tissue in an enlarged left cavernous sinus *(arrows)*. Patient had painful ophthalmoplegia.

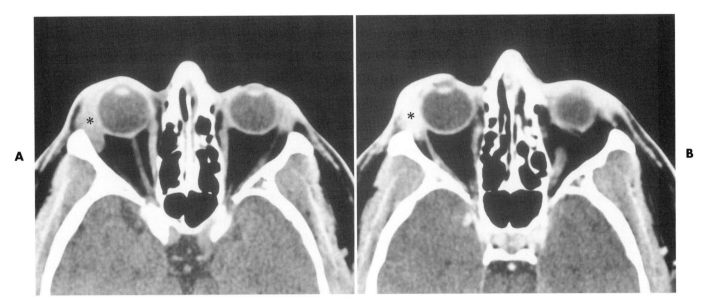

Fig. 10-40   **A** and **B,** Pre **(A)** and post **(B)** contrast CT of sarcoidosis affecting the right lacrimal gland *(*)*. Observe the mass and enhancement. Also, note that the bone is NOT remodeled and there is lid thickening.

tures cannot be defined. If the globe is invaded, one may see increased density on the precontrast scan. This disease can often appear similar to diffuse orbital pseudotumor. Tumors tend to be superior in location, but extension beyond the orbit is unusual. The lesions can extensively infiltrate muscles and/or the lacrimal gland. Lymphoma molds to the contour of the orbit and its structures. Bone destruction is rare. The superior rectus is the extraocular muscle most often involved. Distinguishing lymphoma from orbital pseudotumor on MR is problematic because signal intensities and location are similar (Figure 10-38D) (history is useful).

Posttransplantation lymphoproliferative disorder (PTLD)   This problem occurs in approximately 2% to 3% of patients undergoing organ transplantation and is usually seen within the first year after transplantation. It is defined by Epstein-Barr virus-induced B-cell proliferation uncontrolled by T cell mediated processes. The orbit is a common location for this lesion. There is a soft-tissue mass with a propensity for the lacrimal region that demonstrates contrast enhancement (Fig. 10-41). As opposed to lymphoma, which molds around the orbit, PTLD can appear aggressive with destruction of orbital bones.

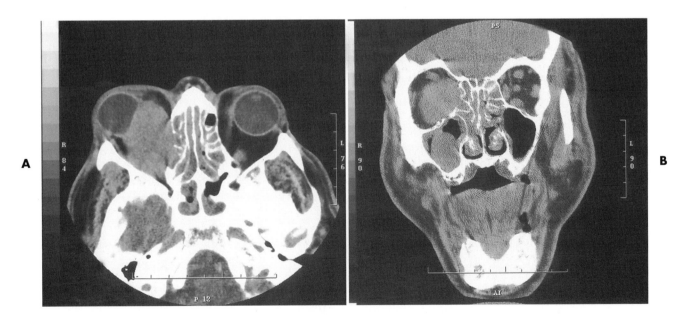

Fig. 10-41   PTLD. **A,** axial and **B,** coronal CT. Observe the aggressive nature of the lesion destroying the medial ethmoid sinuses (unlike lymphoma). The presence of sinusitis in an immunosuppressed host is also of clinical significance.

Box 10-8 Extraconal Lesions

Bone lesions including fibrous dysplasia, Langerhans histiocytones
Capillary hemangioma
Cellulitis, abscess
Dermoid, epidermoid/terratoma
Fractures, hematoma
Granulomatous disease
Lacrimal gland tumor
Lacrimal sac abnormalities
Lymphangioma
Lymphoma/leukemia
Meningioma
Metastases
Mucocele
Orbital cyst
Pseudotumor
Rhadomyosarcoma
Schwannoma/plexiform neurofibroma
Sinus carcinoma

Extraconal Lesions

The extraconal lesions (Box 10-8) arise from structures outside the muscle cone such as the lacrimal gland, peripheral fat, sinuses, or adjacent bony orbit. Bilateral orbital masses suggest the diagnosis of inflammatory, leukemic, lymphoproliferative, histiocytic, or metastatic diseases.

Orbital infection

The periorbita (periosteum), which lines the orbit, is reflected anteriorly on the tarsal preseptal (anterior to septum) space and globe proper. The orbital septum is a fibrous barrier, attached to the outer bony orbital periphery continuous with the orbital periosteum, that acts as a barrier to the spread of infection, and can be seen on high resolution MR. The superior aspect can be observed descending from the superior orbital rim and fusing with the levator aponeurosis before reaching the superior aspect of the tarsus. The inferior aspect of the septum ascends from the inferior orbital rim towards the lower lid tarsus. It divides the orbit into the superficial anterior preseptal space and the deep postseptal space. The clinical manifestations of preseptal cellulitis are painless swelling and erythema of the skin and subcutaneous tissues of the eyelids. There is no evidence of proptosis, disturbances of ocular motility, or chemosis. CT/MR demonstrates no abnormalities posterior to the orbital septum and these are treated medically.

Orbital (postseptal) cellulitis is located within the bony orbit and beneath the orbital septum. It presents with painful ophthalmoplegia, proptosis, chemosis, and decreasing visual acuity. There is edema and inflammation without discrete abscess formation within the orbit. The causes of orbital inflammatory disease include sinus infection, bacteremia, skin infection (secondary to trauma, insect bite, and impetigo), or foreign body. CT has an advantage over MR in the diagnosis of orbital cellulitis because of its ability to visualize the air-filled sinuses and demonstrate foreign bodies. CT can distinguish between preseptal cellulitis, orbital cellulitis, and subperiosteal infection. CT in preseptal cellulitis shows swelling and obliteration of the preseptal soft tissues without extension deep to the orbital septum (Fig. 10-42). In orbital (postseptal) cellulitis, the orbital tissue planes are poorly defined and there may be either an intraconal or an extraconal soft-tissue mass. On fat-saturated T1WI MR, one can detect enhancement in the pre and postseptal tissue.

Nodular coalescence or focal gas collection with ring enhancement suggests discrete abscess. A soft-tissue mass extending from the bony wall of the orbit with displacement of muscle and preservation of a thin strip of extraconal fat implies subperiosteal infection, a known complication of rhinosinusitis. There is marked swelling, chemosis, proptosis, and limitation of motility particularly to the side of the subperiosteal abscess. The common location of these lesions is in the medial orbit subjacent to the ethmoid air cells. Most often, this requires surgical intervention.

Orbital infection can produce venous thrombosis of the orbital veins with extension into the cavernous sinus. It is important to image the brain in cases of orbital cellulitis and abscess and of subperiosteal infection. Occasionally foci of infection are seen as a frontal epidural abscess, subdural empyema, or an intraparenchymal abscess. Intracranial complications are associated with a 50% to 80% mortality rate. Specific infectious agents are discussed in Chapter 6.

Opportunistic infections, a hallmark of AIDS, often involve the anterior and posterior segments of the eye. Rarely do they involve the orbit. Spread from contiguous sinusitis, usually the ethmoid and maxillary sinuses, is the most common source of orbital cellulitis. Think orbital aspergillosis in HIV patients with proptosis, pain, visual loss, and ophthalmoplegia.

Herpes zoster ophthalmicus, a grouped vesicular eruption, occurring along the first division of cranial nerve V. It is observed in both immunosuppressed and nonimmunosuppressed (usually elderly) individuals. When seen in patients less than 45 years old think about HIV. This can be a virulent infection where the virus grows along the optic nerve and vessels producing infarction of the optic nerve and large vessel vasculitis in the brain.

Rhinoscleroma is a granulomatous disease endemic in Africa, Asia, South America, and Eastern Europe caused by *Klebsiella rhinoscleromatis*. It initially involves the sinuses but can invade the lacrimal sac and orbits. It is

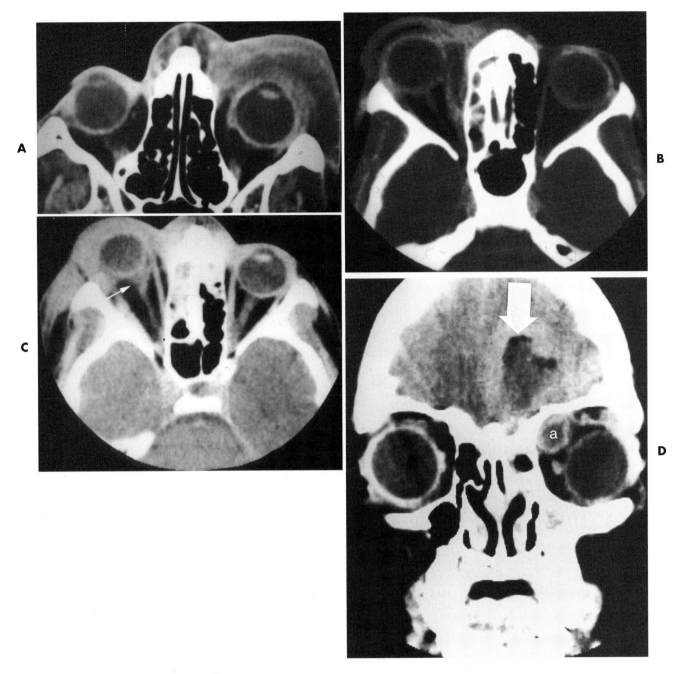

Fig. 10-42   Manifestations of orbital infection. **A,** Preseptal cellulitis. CT shows large preseptal mass. Observe that there is no soft tissue behind the globe. **B,** Subperiosteal abscess. Appreciate the lateral extension of the ethmoid sinusitis into the subperiosteal region with lateral displacement of the medial rectus muscle and orbital fat. There is also significant preseptal swelling. **C,** Orbital cellulitis with abscess *(arrow)*. This patient had sinusitis. **D,** Orbital cellulitis developed and coalesced into an abscess *(a)*. Careful attention should be given to observing intracranial extension as in this patient who has a gas-forming organism producing an intraparenchymal brain abscess *(arrow)*. (From Grossman RI, Lynch RM: Neuroimaging in Neuro-Ophthalmology, *Neurol Clin* 4:831-858, 1983.)

intermediate intensity on T1WI, low intensity on T2WI, and enhances. These radiologic features are similar to malignant tumors and fungal sinusitis.

Lacrimal sac lesions

The anatomy of the lacrimal sac region was briefly discussed at the beginning of this chapter. The lacrimal sac is a preseptal structure lying anterior to the medial or-bital septum. Obstruction of the sac or the nasolacrimal duct may lead to dilatation and inflammation (dacryocystitis). Trauma can interrupt the normal lacrimal drainage, producing epiphora and dacryocystitis. Lacrimal sac dilatation is observed on CT or MR, and preseptal swelling, and/or cellulitis can be noted (Fig. 10-43). Enhancement is seen in the walls of the dilated sac, producing a ring configuration on axial images. Tumors of the lacrimal sac

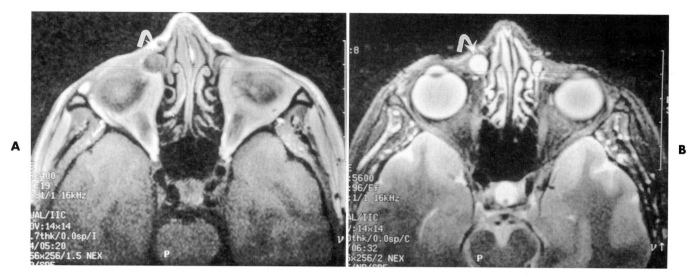

Fig. 10-43   MR of lacrimal sac cyst. **A,** T1WI and **B,** T2WI show low and high intensity respectively of the cyst fluid in the lacrimal sac *(curved arrow).*

are uncommon, with the most common malignancy being transitional cell carcinoma. Bone erosion with a mass lesion occurs with this unusual lesion. The most common benign tumor is the papilloma, which has a distinct incidence of malignant degeneration.

Mucoceles

Mucoceles are expansile extraconal masses occurring after obstruction of sinus ostia and presenting clinically with diplopia and proptosis. The common locations are the frontal and ethmoidal sinuses. Patients have a history of sinusitis, allergy, or trauma. CT manifests an isodense smooth mass (with an enhancing rim) with its epicenter in the sinus. Bowing and thinning of the bony margins can be seen. MR shows the anatomic limits of the lesion (Fig. 10-44). Mucoceles have variable intensities depending on the protein concentration and viscosity but

commonly are observed to be high intensity on T1WI and T2WI. They demonstrate peripheral enhancement as opposed to neoplasms, which have solid enhancement. These are discussed further in Chapter 13.

Lacrimal gland lesions

The lacrimal gland is histologically similar to the salivary gland and can be involved by a comparable spectrum of pathologic entities. Inflammatory conditions (dacryoadenitis) such as Mikulicz (nonspecific swelling of the lacrimal and salivary glands in association with conditions such as sarcoid, tuberculosis, and leukemia) and Sjögren's (lymphocytic infiltration and enlargement of the lacrimal and salivary glands associated with connective tissue diseases) syndromes, lymphoid hyperplasia, and acute dacryoadenitis have well-defined margins with a homogeneous density on CT. The first two conditions moderately enhance. Sarcoid can commonly involve the associated lacrimal gland and is associated with enlargement and enhancement (see Fig. 10-40). Dacryoadenitis may be caused by viral infections and has been reported in 1 out of 300 patients with infectious mononucleosis.

Box 10-9 provides a list of lacrimal gland masses. Lymphoid and inflammatory lesions comprise about 50% of lacrimal masses whereas epithelial tumors represent the other 50% (Fig. 10-45). Common presentations of patients with lacrimal gland tumors include a palpable lacrimal fossa mass or proptosis. These epithelial tumors include the benign pleomorphic adenoma (most common benign tumor), which develops during the course of a year or more and is well tolerated. Pleomorphic adenomas may have cystic spaces without lytic destruction of adjacent bone. With long-standing lesions, remodeling or excavation of bone may be present. Minimal or moderate enhancement can be observed. Malignant ade-

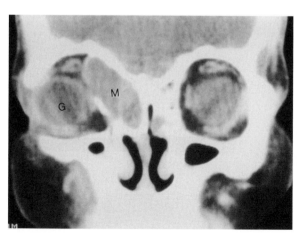

Fig. 10-44   CT of mucocele. Frontoethmoidal mucocele *(M)* with thinning of the bony wall of the sinus, and displacement of the globe *(G)* laterally.

Box 10-9   Lacrimal Gland Enlargement

INFLAMMATION

Collagen vascular lesions
Dacryoadenitis
Mikulicz/Sjogrens
Other granulomatous disorders
Pseudotumor
Sarcoidosis
Wegener's granulomatosis

NEOPLASMS

Germ cell tumors: Dermoid, epidermoid
Lymphoma, leukemia
Metastasis
Minor salivary gland (epithelial) tumors
Sarcoma

noid cystic carcinoma (most common epithelial malignant tumor) presents with pain, diplopia, and visual loss during a 3- to 6-month period. Bone involvement is common. The overall 5-year survival is 21% and death is usually secondary to intracranial spread. This tumor has a propensity for perineural spread proceeding into the cavernous sinus. Lytic bone destruction can be identified. Calcifications may be seen on CT. Other tumors involving the lacrimal gland include lymphoma, mucoepidermoid carcinoma, adenocarcinoma, malignant mixed cell tumors, squamous cell carcinoma, undifferentiated (anaplastic carcinoma, sebaceous carcinoma, and metastasis. Mucoepidermoid carcinoma displays high density on plain CT that markedly enhances. Along with sebaceous carcinoma, it may reveal high intensity on T1WI. The other lesions have variable CT/MR characteristics.

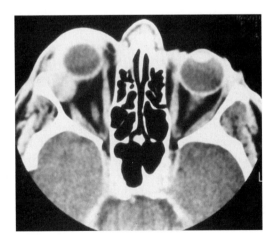

Fig. 10-45   CT of right lacrimal gland tumor. A smoothly marginated mass in the right lacrimal fossa is demonstrated. Because very few characteristics distinguish tumors in this region, we will call this a pleomorphic adenoma. Scalloping from the tumor in the lacrimal fossa suggests that this lesion has been there for sometime.

A mass lesion in the lacrimal fossa that does not produce bony erosion is most likely lymphoid (lymphoma or benign pseudolymphoma) or inflammatory whereas epithelial neoplasms generally involve bone. Lymphoma demonstrates diffuse homogeneous involvement of the lacrimal gland that molds to the bony orbit or globe. MR appearances of these lesions are nonspecific.

Dermoids

Dermoid cysts are the most common benign congenital lesion of the orbit, accounting for 1% to 2% of all orbital masses. They usually present in the first decade of life but can be subclinical until adulthood, where they may present by rupturing, inducing granulomatous inflammation, and scar formation. They arise from epithelial rests, most often in the superolateral portion of the orbit at the frontozygomatic suture near the lacrimal fossa, but are not true lacrimal gland tumors. They can also arise medially, inferiorly, or posteriorly. These lesions are extraconal and displace the globe medially and inferiorly. CT exhibits either no enhancement or a well-defined enhancing margin with a low-density center (fat). Bony scalloping is present, and partial marginal calcification can sometimes be identified. On MR, the diagnosis is clinched by high signal on T1WI in this region, which suppresses with fat saturation techniques (Fig. 10-46). Fat may be seen floating in cystic fluid on T1WI. The differential diagnosis of orbital cysts is provided in Box 10-10.

Orbital rhabdomyosarcoma

Orbital rhabdomyosarcoma is the most common primary malignant orbital tumor of childhood as well as the most common site of head and neck rhabdomyosarcomas. Mean age is 7 to 8 years with 90% occurring before the age of 16. Children present with rapidly progressive painless exophthalmos although about 10% may have headache or periorbital discomfort. On examination, a mass may be palpable and ecchymosis, conjunctival chemosis, and ophthalmoplegia may be present. Primary orbital tumor arises from primitive orbital mesenchymal elements whereas secondary involvement occurs from the extraocular muscles, nasopharynx, or paranasal sinuses. It is isodense or slightly high density and uniformly enhances. It is usually seen behind the globe (50%), although other locations—above the globe (25%), below the globe (12%) are common. Bone destruction has been reported with intraorbital extension of paranasal rhabdomyosarcoma. The tumor appears as a homogeneous well-defined enhancing mass without definite density/intensity characteristics. MR reveals the extent of tumor spread, and this has important prognostic implications.

Lymphangioma

Lymphangioma is discussed under venous anomalies but you should appreciate that it can occur as an extraconal or a diffuse process.

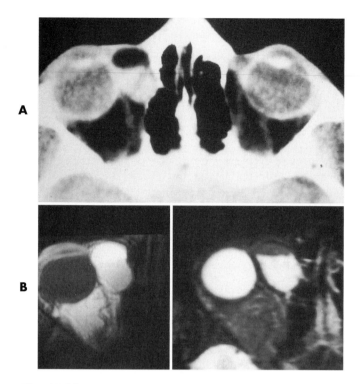

Fig. 10-46   CT and MR of dermoid. **A,** Medial orbital mass is seen on this axial CT with a fluid level. Uppermost portion of the level is low density, indicating that this is most likely fat. **B,** T1WI *(left)* and T2WI *(right)* confirm that the upper portion of this cyst contains fat and that the lower portion contains proteinaceous debris.

Fibrous Histiocytoma

Although less than 1% of all primary orbital tumors, fibrous histiocytoma is the most common primary orbital mesenchymal tumor in adults. They are mostly benign or locally aggressive, however, malignant forms also occur. Histologically, the lesions are combinations of histiocytes and fibroblasts. The clinical presentation includes proptosis, diplopia, and a palpable mass. The tumor is seen in patients in their 40s and 50s. These le-

---

Box 10-10   Differential Diagnosis of Orbital Cysts
Epidermal inclusion cysts
Lymphangioma
Hematic cyst
Dermoid cyst
Teratoma
Encephalocele
Meningocele
Mucocele
Dacryocystocele
Easter-cele

---

sions may be discrete, smooth masses that can be intra or extraconal and usually enhance. They may also display an infiltrating pattern, however, the behavior of the lesion is not necessarily related to its appearance. Other rare mesenchymal orbital tumors include fibroma, fibromatosis, fibrosarcoma, solitary fibrous tumor, leiomyoma, leiomyosarcoma, lipoma, liposarcoma, and mesenchymal chondrosarcoma.

Metastases

The majority of retrobulbar metastases are extraconal; however, as they enlarge, the intraconal compartment may also be affected. They account for approximately 10% of orbital neoplasms with an average survival after detection of approximately 9 months. Patients complain of diplopia, ptosis, proptosis, eyelid swelling, pain, and visual loss. The greater wing of the sphenoid is the most common site of bone metastasis. CT depicts the orbital and cranial soft-tissue components of the lesion. Metastatic lesions are isodense or high density on unenhanced scan and may enhance. Most lesions have associated bone involvement. Although CT is generally nonspecific for histologic findings, a picture of an infiltrative retrobulbar mass and enophthalmos is characteristic of scirrhous breast carcinoma (Fig. 10-47). Breast and lung cancers account for over 50% of orbital metastases. Breast is thought to initially involve orbital fat whereas prostate goes to bone. Most metastatic lesions with time produce diffuse lesions, however, thyroid, carcinoid, and renal cell may remain as discrete nodules. Metastatic disease may account for 7% of cases of extraocular muscle enlargement found on CT. Isolated enlargement of the lateral rectus should be thought to be secondary to metastasis or orbital pseudotumor as it does not occur in Graves.

Metastatic neuroblastoma is second to rhabdomyosarcoma as the most frequent malignant orbital tumor in childhood with 8% presenting initially with orbital lesions. Metastasis to the bone displaces or elevates the periosteum, producing a smooth extraconal mass. These lesions can be high density on CT or display MR characteristics of blood secondary to intratumoral hemorrhage. Neuroblastoma can be distinguished from rhabdomyosarcoma by its high-density values and its lack of preseptal extension (which is much more common in rhabdomyosarcoma). In children, also think of Ewing sarcoma (especially with sudden proptosis and orbital hemorrhage), which commonly involves the sphenoid wing and has extensive soft-tissue multicompartmental components involving the middle cranial fossa, the posterior lateral portion of the orbit, and the soft tissues of the temporal region.

Sphenoid wing meningioma

Sphenoid wing meningioma presents as a hyperostotic mass displacing the muscles and causing proptosis.

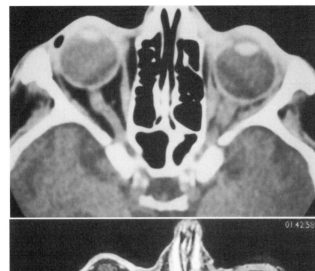

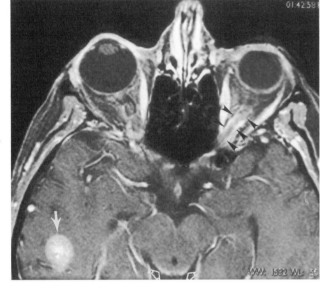

Fig. 10-47 **A,** Breast carcinoma with enophthalmos of the left globe secondary to the tumor desmoplastic reaction. **B,** Axial post contrast fat sat images showing subarachnoid seeding along the optic nerve *(arrowheads)* and in the posterior midbrain *(open arrows).* Also note the large mass in the right temporal region *(arrow).*

It can have a sizable component both in the orbit and intracranially. A number of fibroosseous lesions also give a somewhat similar radiologic appearance including ossifying fibroma (which has discrete bony margins and is monostotic), osteoma, sclerotic metastases such as prostate, and fibrous dysplasia (which has poorly defined margins and may be polyostotic).

Primary bone lesions

Fibrous dysplasia In fibrous dysplasia, normal bone is replaced by immature bone and osteoid in a cellular fibrous matrix. Pain, swelling, and disfigurement occur. Malignant transformation is rare and is associated with previous radiation. In about 20% of cases, craniofacial bones are involved. Most orbital lesions are monoostotic but frequently involve multiple skull bones and cross

suture lines. This disease can occur in adults as well as adolescents and children. The typical appearance is that of "ground glass" on plain films. It can produce significant dysfunction and disfigurement. Orbital symptoms include decreased visual acuity, proptosis, and orbital mass. Differential diagnosis includes Paget's disease and meningioma, which produces homogeneous thickening of bone, and often displays soft-tissue involvement rarely seen in fibrous dysplasia.

Primary bone lesions of the orbital walls include eosinophilic granuloma and fibro-osseous lesions of the orbit including osteoma, ossifying fibroma, osteoblastoma, osteosarcoma, osteoclastoma, brown tumor of hyperparathyroidism, aneurysmal bone, and cyst giant cell reparative granuloma. The giant cell reparative granuloma can be locally aggressive and result in bone destruction. It is hypothesized to be a reaction to intraosseous hemorrhage, however, a history of trauma may not be elicited in all cases. The mass may contain heterogenous internal structure and fluid levels. It generally presents within the first two decades of life. Careful windowing on CT demonstrates a mass with significant bony involvement. Excuse the superficial treatment of bone tumors—what do you expect from neuroradiologists?

SUGGESTED READINGS

Adam G, Brab M, Bohndorf K, et al: Gadolinium-DTPA-enhanced MRI of intraocular tumors, *Magn Res Imaging* 8:683-689, 1990.

Ahmadi J, Teal JS, Segall HD, et al: Computed tomography of carotid-cavernous fistula, *AJNR* 4:131-136, 1983.

Albert A, Lee BCP, Saint-Louis L, et al: MRI of optic chiasm and optic pathways, *AJNR* 7:255-258, 1986.

Anderson RL, Epstein GA, Dauer EA: Computed tomographic diagnosis of posterior ocular staphyloma, *AJNR* 4:90-91, 1983.

Atlas SW, Grossman RI, Savino PJ, et al: Surface-coil MR of orbital pseudotumor, *AJNR* 8:141-146, 1987.

Barrett L, Glatt HJ, Burde RM, et al: Optic nerve dysfunction in thyroid eye disease, *Radiology* 167:503-507, 1988.

Bernardino ME, Danziger J, Young SE, et al: Computed tomography in ocular neoplastic disease, *AJR* 131:111-113, 1978.

Boyce SW, Platia EV, Green WR: Drusen of the optic nerve head, *Ann Ophthalmol* 10:695-704, 1978.

Brant-Zawadzki B, Enzmann DR: Orbital computed tomography: calcific densities of the posterior globe, *J Comput Assist Tomogr* 3:503-505, 1979.

Brodey PA, Andel S, Lane B, et al: Computed tomography of axial myopia, *J Comput Assist Tomogr* 7:484-485, 1983.

Bryan RN, Lewis RA, Miller SL: Choroidal osteoma, *AJNR* 4:491-494, 1983.

Chacko JG, Figueroa RE, et al: Detection and localization of steel intraocular foreign bodies using computed tomography. A comparison of helical and conventional axial scanning, *Ophthalmology* 104(2):319-323, 1997.

Char DH, Hedges TR, Norman D: Retinoblastoma, CT diagnosis, *Ophthalmology* 91:1347-1350, 1984.

Clark CW, Theofilos CS, Fleming JC: Primary optic nerve sheath meningiomas, *J Neurosurg* 70:37-40, 1989.

Curtin HD, Wolfe P, Schramm V: Orbital roof blowout fractures, *AJNR* 3:531-534, 1982.

Davidorf FH, Chambers RB, Gresak P: False-positive magnetic resonance imaging of a metastatic carcinoma simulating a malignant melanoma, *Ann Ophthalmol* 24:391-394, 1992.

Dilenge D, Ascherl GF: Variations of the ophthalmic and middle meningeal arteries: relation to the embryonic stapedial artery, *AJNR* 1:45-53, 1980.

Dolan K, Jacoby C, Smoker W: The radiology of facial fractures, *Radiographics* 4:4, 1984.

Dresner SC, Rothfus WE, Slamovits TL, et al: Computed tomography of orbital myositis, *AJNR* 5:351-354, 1984.

Dutton J: *Atlas of Clinical and Surgical Orbital Anatomy.* Philadelphia, WB Saunders, 1994.

Edwards MG, Pordell GR: Ocular toxocariasis studied by CT scanning, *Radiology* 157:685-686, 1985.

Flanders AE, Mafee MF, Rao VM, et al: CT characteristics of orbital pseudotumors and other orbital inflammatory processes, *J Comput Assist Tomogr* 13:40-47, 1989.

Fries PD, Char DH, Norman D: MR imaging of orbital cavernous hemangioma, *J Comput Assist Tomogr* 11:418-421, 1987.

Gardner TW, Zaparackas AG, Naidich TP: Congenital optic nerve colobomas: CT demonstration, *J Comput Assist Tomogr* 8:95-102, 1984.

Giuseffi V, Wall M, et al: Symptoms and disease associations in idiopathic intracranial hypertension (pseudotumor cerebri): a case-control study." *Neurology* 41(2):239-244, 1991.

Goldberg MF, Mafee M: Computed tomography for diagnosis of persistent hyperplastic primary vitreous (PHPV), *Ophthalmology* 90:442-451, 1983.

Goldberger S, Sarraf D, et al: Involvement of the eyebrow fat pad in Graves' orbitopathy, *Ophthal Plast Reconstr Surg* 10(2):80-82, 1994.

Gomori JM, Grossman RI, Shields JA, et al: Choroidal melanomas: correlation of NMR spectroscopy and MR imaging, *Radiology* 158:443-445, 1986.

Gomori JM, Grossman RI, Shields JA, et al: Ocular MR imaging and spectroscopy: an ex vivo study, *Radiology* 160:201-205, 1986.

Graeb DA, Rootman J, Robertson WD, et al: Orbital lymphangiomas: clinical, radiologic, and pathologic characteristics, *Radiology* 175:417-421, 1990.

Grossman RI, Lynch RM: Neuroimaging in neuro-ophthalmology: symposium on neuro-ophthalmology, *Neurol Clin* 1:4, 1983.

Hedges TR, Mucelli RP, Char DH, et al: Computed tomographic demonstration of ocular calcification: correlations with clinical and pathological findings, *Neuroradiology* 23:15-21, 1982.

Hesselink JR, Davis DK, Dallow RL, et al: Computed tomography of masses in the lacrimal gland region, *Radiology* 131:143-147, 1979.

Holman RE, Grimson BS, Drayer BP, et al: Magnetic resonance imaging of optic gliomas, *Am J Ophthalmol* 100:596-601, 1985.

Hopper KD, Katz NNK, Dorwart RH, et al: Childhood leukokoria: computed tomographic appearance and differential diagnosis with histopathologic correlation, *Radiographics* 5:377-395, 1985.

Hoyt WF, Baghdassarian SA: Optic glioma of childhood: natural history and rationale for conservative management, *Br J Ophthalmol* 53:793, 1969.

Imes RK, Hoyt WF: Magnetic resonance imaging signs of optic nerve gliomas in neurofibromatosis I, *Am J Ophthalmol* 111:729-734, 1991.

In S, Miyagi J, Kojho N, et al: Intraorbital optic nerve hemangioblastoma with von Hippel-Lindau disease, *J Neurosurg* 56:426-429, 1982.

Jakobiec FA, Depot MJ, Kennerdell JS, et al: Combined clinical and computed tomographic diagnosis of orbital glioma and meningioma, *Ophthalmology* 91:137-155, 1984.

Jend HH, Jend-Rossmann I: Sphenotemporal buttress fractures, *Neuroradiology* 26:411-413, 1984.

Johns TT, Citrin CM, Black J, et al: CT evaluation of perineural orbital lesions: evaluation of the "tram-track" sign, *AJNR* 5:587-590, 1984.

Katz BJ, Nerad JA: Ophthalmic manifestations of fibrous dysplasia: a disease of children and adults [see comments], *Ophthalmology* 105(12):2207-2215, 1998.

Kuboto T, Kuroda E, Fujii T, et al: Orbital varix with a pearly phlebolith, *J Neurosurg* 73:291-295, 1990.

Lallemand DP, Brasch RC, Char DH, et al: Orbital tumors in children, *Radiology* 151:85-88, 1984.

Lewis T, Kingsley D, Moseley I: Do bilateral optic nerve sheath meningiomas exist? *Br J Neurosurg* 5:13-18, 1991.

Lund E, Halaburt H: Irradiation dose to the lens of the eye during CT of the head, *Neuroradiology* 22:181-184, 1982.

Mafee MF, Goldberg MF, Cohen SB, et al: Magnetic resonance imaging versus computed tomography of leukocoric eyes and use of in vitro proton magnetic resonance spectroscopy of retinoblastoma, *Ophthalmology* 96:965-976, 1989.

Mafee MF, Goldberg MF, Valvassori GE, et al: Computed tomography in the evaluation of patients with persistent hyperplastic primary vitreous (PHPV), *Radiology* 145:713-717, 1982.

Mafee MF, Linder B, Peyman GA, et al: Choroidal hematoma and effusion: evaluation with MR imaging, *Radiology* 168:781-786, 1988.

Mafee MF, Peyman GA: Choroidal detachment and ocular hypotony: CT evaluation, *Radiology* 153:697-703, 1984.

Merandi SF, Kudryk BT, Murtagh FR, et al: Contrast-enhanced MR imaging of optic nerve lesions in patients with acute optic neuritis, *AJNR* 12:923-926, 1991.

Nerad JA, Kersten RC, Anderson RL: Hemangioblastoma of the optic nerve: report of a case and review of literature, *Ophthalmology* 95:398-402, 1988.

Nugent RA, Belkin RI, Neigel JM, et al: Graves orbitopathy: correlation of CT and clinical findings, *Radiology* 177:675-682, 1990.

Nugent RA, Lapointe JS, Rootman J, et al: Orbital dermoids: features on CT, *Radiology* 165:475-478, 1987.

Nugent RA, Rootman J, Robertson WD, et al: Acute orbital pseudotumors: classification and CT features, *AJR* 137:957-962, 1981.

Raymond WR, Char DH, Norman D, et al: Magnetic resonance imaging evaluation of uveal tumors, *Am J Ophthalmol* 111:633-641, 1991.

Rootman J, Nugent R: The classification and management of acute orbital pseudotumors, *Ophthalmology* 89:1040-1048, 1982.

Rothfus WE, Curtin HD: Extraocular muscle enlargement: a CT review, *Radiology* 151:677-681, 1984.

Rothfus WE, Curtin HD, Slamovits TL, et al: Optic nerve/sheath enlargement: a differential approach based on high-resolution CT morphology, *Radiology* 150:409-415, 1984.

Rush JA, Younge BR, Campbell RJ, et al: Optic glioma: long-term follow-up of 85 histopathologically verified cases, *Am Acad Ophthalmol* 89:1213-1219, 1982.

Russell EJ, Czervionke L, Huckman M, et al: CT of the inferomedial orbit and the lacrimal drainage apparatus: normal and pathologic anatomy, *AJNR* 6:759-766, 1985.

Seiff SR, Brodsky MC, MacDonald G, et al: Orbital optic glioma in neurofibromatosis: magnetic resonance diagnosis of perineural arachnoidal gliomatosis, *Arch Ophthalmol* 105:1689-1692, 1987.

Sevel D, Krausz H, Ponder T, et al: Value of computed tomography for the diagnosis of a ruptured eye, *J Comput Assist Tomogr* 7:870-875, 1983.

Sherman JL, McLean IW, Brallier DR: Coats' disease: CT-pathologic correlation in two cases, *Radiology* 146:77-78, 1983.

Shnier R, Parker GD, Hallinan JM, et al: Orbital varices: a new technique for noninvasive diagnosis, *AJNR* 12:717-718, 1991.

Siatkowski R, Sanchez J, et al: The clinical, neuroradiographic, and endocrinologic profile of patients with bilateral optic nerve hypoplasia, *Ophthalmology* 104(3):493-496, 1997.

Sibony PA, Krauss HR, Kennerdell JS, et al: Optic nerve sheath meningiomas: clinical manifestations, *Ophthalmology* 91:1313-1326, 1984.

Simmons JD, LaMasters D, Char D: Computed tomography of ocular colobomas, *AJNR* 4:1049-1052, 1983.

Spencer WH: Drusen of the optic disk and aberrant axoplasmic transport, *Am J Ophthalmol* 85:1-12, 1978.

Swayne LC, Garfinkle WB, Bennett RH: CT of posterior ocular staphyloma in axial myopia, *Neuroradiology* 26:241-243, 1984.

Turner RM, Gutman I, Hilal SK, et al: CT of drusen bodies and other calcific lesions of the optic nerve: case report and differential diagnosis, *AJNR* 4:175-178, 1983.

Wright JE, McNab AA, McDonald WI: Primary optic nerve sheath meningioma. *Br J Ophthalmol* 73:960-966, 1989.

Yeo JH, Jakobiec FA, Abbott GF, et al: Combined clinical and computed tomographic diagnosis of orbital lymphoid tumors, *Am J Ophthalmol* 94:235-245, 1982.

Zimmerman CF, Schatz NJ, Glaser JS: Magnetic resonance imaging of optic nerve meningiomas, *Ophthalmology* 97:585-591, 1990.

Zimmerman RA, Bilaniuk LT: CT of orbital infection and its cerebral complications, *AJR* 134:45-50, 1980.

REFERENCES

Lam BL, Glasier CM, Fever WJ, et al: Subarachnoid fluid of the optic nerve in normal adults, *Ophthalmology* 104(10):1629-1633, 1997.

Ettl A, Kramer J, et al: High resolution magnetic resonance imaging of neurovascular orbital anatomy, *Ophthalmology* 104(5):869-877, 1997.

Dalley RW: Intraorbital wood foreign bodies on CT: use of wide bone window settings to distinguish wood from air, *AJR* 164(2):434-435, 1995.

Seidenwurm DJ, McDonnell CH, 3rd, et al: Cost utility analysis of radiographic screening for an orbital foreign body before MR imaging [see comments], *AJNR* 21(2):426-433, 2000.

Flanders AE, De Potter P, et al: MRI of orbital hydroxyapatite implants, *Neuroradiology* 38(3):273-277, 1996.

Kuo MD, Hayman LA, et al: In vivo CT and MR appearance of prosthetic intraocular lens, *AJNR* 19(4):749-753, 1998.

Brisse H, Lumbroso L, et al: Sonographic, ct, and mr imaging findings in diffuse infiltrative retinoblastoma: report of two cases with histologic comparison *AJNR* 22(3):499-504, 2001.

Eisenberg L, Castillo M, et al: Proton MR spectroscopy in Coats disease, *AJNR* 18(4): 727-729, 1997.

Mafee M: Uveal melanoma, choroidal hemangioma, and simulating lesions. Role of MR Imaging, *Radiol Clin North Am* 36(6):1083-1099, 1998.

Scott IU, Murray TG, et al: Evaluation of imaging techniques for detection of extraocular extension of choroidal melanoma, *Arch Ophthalmol* 116(7):897-899, 1998.

Ibanez HE, Grand MG, et al: Magnetic resonance imaging findings in Vogt-Koyanagi-Harada syndrome, *Retina* 14(2):164-168, 1994.

Kuhn F, Morris R, et al: Terson syndrome. Results of vitrectomy and the significance of vitreous hemorrhage in patients with subarachnoid hemorrhage [see comments], *Ophthalmology* 105(3):472-477, 1998.

Kiriakopoulos ET, Gorn RA, et al: Small retinal hemorrhages as the only sign of an intracranial aneurysm [see comments], *Am J Ophthalmol* 125(3):401-403, 1998.

Hunyor AP, Harper CA, et al: Ocular-central nervous system lymphoma mimicking posterior scleritis with exudative retinal detachment, *Ophthalmology* 107(10):1955-1959, 2000.

Manfre L, Lagalla R, et al: Idiopathic intracranial hypertension: orbital MRI, *Neuroradiology* 37(6):459-461, 1995.

Mansfield SH, Castillo M: MR of cis-platinum-induced optic neuritis, *AJNR* 15(6):1178-1180, 1994.

Sklar EM, Schatz NJ, et al: MR of vasculitis-induced optic neuropathy, *AJNR* 17(1):121-128, 1996.

Massry GG, Morgan CF, et al: Evidence of optic pathway gliomas after previously negative neuroimaging, *Ophthalmology* 104(6):930-935, 1997.

Miller W, Tartaglino L, Sergott RC, et al: MR of malignant optic glioma of adulthood, *AJNR* 16:1673-1676, 1995.

Wilms G, Raat H, et al: Orbital cavernous hemangioma: findings on sequential Gd-enhanced MRI, *J Computer Assist Tomogr* 19(4):548-551, 1995.

Wright JE, Sullivan TJ, et al: Orbital venous anomalies [see comments], *Ophthalmology* 104(6):905-913, 1997.

Katz SE, Rootman J, et al: Combined venous lymphatic malformations of the orbit (so-called lymphangiomas). Association with noncontiguous intracranial vascular anomalies *Ophthalmology* 105(1):176-184, 1998.

Khanna RK, Pham CJ, et al: Bilateral superior ophthalmic vein enlargement associated with diffuse cerebral swelling. Report of 11 cases, *J Neurosurgery* 86(5):893-897, 1997.

Acierno MD, Trobe JD, et al: Painful oculomotor palsy caused by posterior-draining dural carotid cavernous fistulas, *Arch Ophthalmol* 113(8):1045-1049, 1995.

Goodall KL, Jackson A, et al: Enlargement of the tensor intermuscularis muscle in Graves' ophthalmopathy. A computed tomographic and magnetic resonance imaging study." *Arch Ophthalmol* 113(10):1286-1289, 1995.

Birchall D, Goodall KL, et al: Graves ophthalmopathy: intracranial fat prolapse on CT images as an indicator of optic nerve compression [see comments], *Radiology* 200(1):123-127, 1996.

Ohnishi T, Noguchi S, et al: Extraocular muscles in Graves ophthalmopathy: usefulness of T2 relaxation time measurements *Radiology* 190(3):857-862, 1994.

Hardman JA, Halpin SF, et al: MRI of idiopathic orbital inflammatory syndrome using fat saturation and Gd-DTPA, *Neuroradiology* 37(6):475-478, 1995.

Van Hoe L, Oyen R, et al: Case report: pseudotumoral pelvic retroperitoneal fibrosis associated with orbit fibrosis, *Br J Radiol* 68(808):421-423, 1995.

Simon EM, Zoarski GH, et al: Systemic sarcoidosis with bilateral orbital involvement: MR findings, *AJNR* 19(2):336-337, 1998.

Case records of the Massachusetts General Hospital. Weekly clinicopathologic exercises. Case 39, *N Engl J Med* 331(17):1143-1149, 1994.

Provenzale JM, Mukherji S, et al: Orbital involvement by Wegener's granulomatosis: imaging findings, *AJR* 166(4):929-934, 1996.

Pickhardt PJ, Wippold FJ, 2nd: Neuroimaging in posttransplantation lymphoproliferative disorder, *AJR* 172(4):1117-1121, 1999.

Hoffmann KT, Hosten N, et al: Septum orbitale: high-resolution MR in orbital anatomy, *AJNR* 19(1):91-94, 1998.

Eustis HS, Mafee MF, et al: MR imaging and CT of orbital infections and complications in acute rhinosinusitis, *Radiolog Clin North Am* 36(6):1165-1183, 1998.

Ormerod LD, Rhodes RH, et al: Ophthalmologic manifestations of acquired immune deficiency syndrome-associated progressive multifocal leukoencephalopathy, *Ophthalmology* 103(6):899-906, 1996.

Le Hir P, Marsot-Dupuch K, et al: Rhinoscleroma with orbital extension: CT and MRI, *Neuroradiology* 38(2):175-178, 1996.

Aburn NS, Sullivan TJ: Infectious mononucleosis presenting with dacryoadenitis, *Ophthalmology* 103(5):776-778 1996.

Goldberg R, Rootman J, et al: Tumors metastatic to the orbit: a changing picture, *Survey Ophthalmol* 35(1):1-24, 1990.

Rothfus WE, Curtin HD: Extraocular muscle enlargement: a CT review, *Radiology* 151(3):677-681, 1984.

Mercado GV, Shields CL, et al: Giant cell reparative granuloma of the orbit, *Am J Ophthalmol* 127(4):485-487, 1999.

CHAPTER 11

CNS Anatomy: Sella and Central Skull Base

Appreciation of the normal anatomy is the key to the radiologic evaluation of the sella and central skull base. It turns out that this property is in the "silk stocking district." Small lesions can have profound endocrinologic and neurologic manifestations. You want to make the diagnosis early because many lesions in this region are treatable and potentially curable. When the lesion gets to be the size of a baseball, even Barry Bonds can put it into the upper deck; however, the fat lady has already sung and she is playing the blues. The key is to find and localize the abnormality, define its imaging characteristics, and then arrive at a differential diagnosis—simple enough?

ANATOMY

We shall define the skull base as the region from the upper surface of the ethmoid bone and orbital plate of the frontal bone to the occipital bone. Central to the skull base is the sphenoid bone. The bone itself has the appearance of a bat with its wings extended (Fig. 11-1). The feet of the bat are the medial and lateral pterygoid processes, the head being the body of the sphenoid bone, and wings being the greater and lesser wings of the sphenoid. The body of the sphenoid bone is just behind the cribriform plate of the ethmoid bone. The medial anterior surface of the body of the sphenoid bone is flat and is termed the planum (jugum) sphenoidale. The planum sphenoidale is anterior to the sella turcica and connects the two lesser wings of the sphenoid, thus, forming a central portion of the anterior cranial fossa. The posterior aspect of the planum sphenoidale is

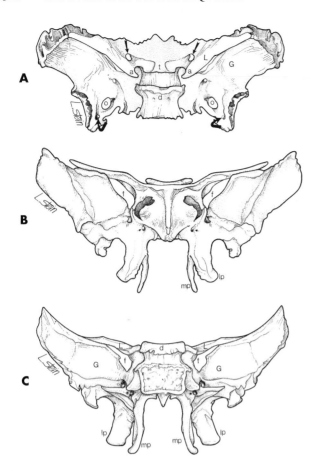

Fig. 11-1 Diagram of the sphenoid bone. **A,** Superior view. **B,** Anterior view. **C,** Posterior view. Anterior clinoid *(a),* tuberculum sellae *(t),* optic canal *(large arrows),* foramen spinosum *(curved arrows),* foramen ovale *(o),* foramen rotundum *(small open arrows),* dorsum sellae *(d),* lesser wing of sphenoid *(L),* greater wing of sphenoid *(G),* vidian canal *(small closed arrows),* medial pterygoid plates *(mp),* lateral pterygoid plates *(lp),* superior orbital fissure *(f).*

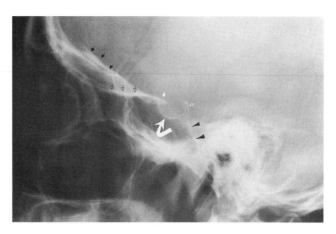

Fig. 11-2 Lateral radiograph of the sella. You can appreciate the floor of the anterior cranial fossa *(black arrows),* the planum sphenoidale *(open black arrows),* the anterior clinoid process *(white arrow),* the sella turcica *(curved arrow),* the dorsum sellae *(open white arrow),* and the clivus *(arrowheads).* In the days of the giants, this is almost all you had.

for the carotid artery can be quite thin normally. This contrasts to erosion or flattening of the vidian canal or foramen rotundum, which is suspicious for a lesion. The lateral recess air cells of the sphenoid sinus may extend outward from the main sinus cavities into the greater wing of the sphenoid bone. They pass above the vidian canal and below the foramen rotundum. A distance of 11.4 mm (between the vidian canal and foramen rotun-

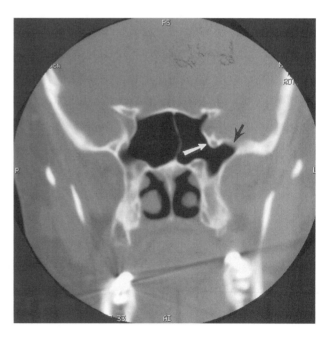

Fig. 11-3 Pteryoid extension of sphenoid. Lateral extension of the sphenoid sinus. Coronal CT showing lateral extension of the left portion of the sphenoid sinus *(arrow).* The sinus extends below and lateral to the foramen rotundum *(white arrow)* into the greater wing of the sphenoid.

termed the limbus of the planum sphenoidale. Just posterior to the limbus is the chiasmatic groove; then a bony prominence, the tuberculum sellae; and then the sella turcica (Fig. 11-2). The pituitary gland sits in the sella turcica, which (to reiterate) is bounded anteriorly by the chiasmatic groove (the optic chiasm is not located here; however, the lateral portions of the sulcus lead to the optic canals), the tuberculum sellae, and the anterior clinoid processes (part of the lesser wing of the sphenoid), onto which the tentorium cerebelli attaches. The posterior boundary of the sella is the dorsum sellae, from which arise the posterior clinoid processes, onto which the tentorium also inserts. Behind the dorsum is the clivus. Beneath the sella is the sphenoid sinus, which is usually separated asymmetrically by a vertical bony septum.

The sphenoid sinus displays a wide range of normal variations including asymmetric expansion of the lateral recess (Fig. 11-3). The sinus wall adjacent to the groove

dum) has been reported to be the top normal distance between these foramen based on coronal 3-mm CT. Having said that, lesions separating the two foramina would be obvious even to the cortically blind so put your ruler back and just read the film.

The lateral surface of the sphenoid body joins with the greater wings of the sphenoid and the medial pterygoid plates. The superior margin of the junction of the sphenoid body with the greater wings of the sphenoid is the carotid sulcus, over which the carotid artery runs. The inner surface of the greater wings of the sphenoid forms part of the floor of the middle cranial fossa and the posterior part of the lateral wall of the orbit. Behind the dorsum sellae is the clivus, which extends inferiorly to the foramen magnum. Anteriorly, the clivus merges with the sphenoid sinus and the (inferior third) of the nasopharynx. Its lateral margins are the petrooccipital fissure.

The pterygopalatine fossa (PPF) is an important conduit for the spread of tumor and infection in and around the skull base. This region can be easily recognized on axial CT (Fig. 11-4). The PPF is defined anteriorly by the maxillary bone, anterior medially by the perpendicular plate of the palatine bone, and posteriorly by the base of the pterygoid process. The PPF is shaped like a deflated balloon, narrower inferior and larger superior (Fig. 11-5). Anteriorly, the PPF communicates with the orbital apex, the inferior orbital fissure, and sphenopalatine foramen (entering the posterosuperior nasal fossa); laterally with the pterygomaxillary fissure (leading to the masticator space); superior posteriorly with the foramen rotundum (and therefore Meckel's cave and the cavernous sinus); inferior posteriorly with the vidian canal (which communicates with the region of the foramen lacerum); inferiorly with the greater and lesser palatine canals and foramina (to the palate).

> There was a small lesion of the skull base
> That was missed by a radiologist in some haste
> She neglected to look
> And forgot our book
> Her colleagues decided that she was a waste

Table 11-1 lists important foramina at the base of the skull and their contents. These need to be learned or relearned.

Let us start from below and work our way up.

The hypoglossal canal (anterior condyloid foramen) courses obliquely within the occipital bone (Fig. 11-6). Through it runs the hypoglossal nerve and, when present, the hypoglossal artery (a primitive connection between the proximal cervical internal carotid artery at approximately C1—C2 level and the proximal basilar artery). The meningeal branch of the ascending pharyngeal artery as well as a small emissary vein (anterior condyloid) arising from the inferior petrosal sinus may inconstantly also run through this foramen. The jugular tubercles separate the hypoglossal canal from the jugular foramen with the two regions being about 8 mm apart on the inner surface of the skull. Intracanalicular enhancement is always present representing multiple emissary venous radicles, and linear filling defects in the enhancement are the hypoglossal nerve rootlets. Occasionally these emissary veins can be prominent and have been reported to protrude into the cerebellomedullary cistern and mimic a nerve sheath tumor. The diagnosis can be confirmed by MRA and multiplanar images. In addition, dural enhancement can be seen along the margins of the entrance of the canal and anteriorly into the carotid space. Box 11-1 lists the lesions involving the hypoglossal canal.

The jugular foramen is demarcated by the petrous portion of the temporal bone anterolaterally and by the occipital bone posteromedially (Fig. 11-7). It is divided into two parts, the pars nervosa (anteromedial) and the pars vascularis (posterolateral), by a bony or fibrous septum (jugular spur). Cranial nerve IX runs lateral to the inferior petrosal sinus within the pars nervosa portion of the jugular foramen. The inferior petrosal sinus runs posterolaterally along the petrooccipital fissure to the pars nervosa and then into the jugular vein (within the pars vascularis). The pars vascularis is the larger of the two compartments and contains cranial nerves X and XI in a common sheath medial to the jugular bulb, which is also in the pars vascularis. The jugular bulb is the confluence between the sigmoid sinus and the jugular vein. It is usually larger on the right side. The petrous portion of the carotid artery is anterolateral to the pars nervosa.

The internal auditory canal is just superior to the jugular foramen. It contains cranial nerves VII and VIII. We have made an editorial decision to include lesions involving this region in Chapter 12 (Temporal Bone) rather than be repetitive, tedious, boring, irksome—ho hum.

The inferior petrosal sinus can be visualized on contrast CT or MR (Fig. 11-8). The basilar venous plexus connects the superior portions of the inferior petrosal sinuses. Dorello's canal (aka petroclival venous confluence, see below) is located just below the petrous apex and is a conduit for cranial nerve VI to reach the cavernous sinus (Fig. 11-9). The canal is located within the inferior petrosal sinus and can be observed on contrast enhanced axial MR as an unenhanced line crossing the enhanced sinus obliquely. There may be asymmetry and differences in size in this structure. The abducens nerve exits the pontomedullary sulcus, courses through the subarachnoid space and enters Dorello's canal and into the cavernous sinus running just lateral to the intracavernous internal carotid artery. Exiting the cavernous sinus it enters the orbit through the superior orbital fissure and terminates on the lateral rectus muscle. The dorsal

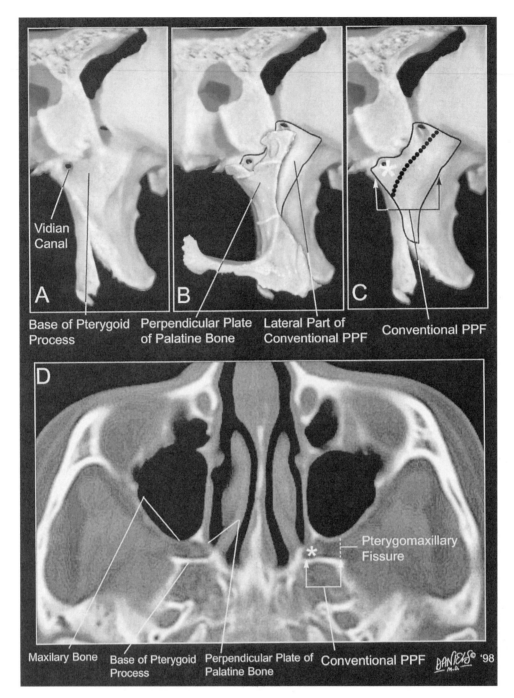

Fig. 11-4 Anatomy of pterygopalatine fossa. Frontal views **(A–C)** and axial CT scan **(D)** through the ptyergopalatine process. **B,** The palatine bone is in position and with the pterygoid process forms a small fossa that is hidden in this view. **C,** The palatine bone has been removed to show this small fossa *(asterisk)* that was probably called the PPF because it contains the pterygopalatine ganglion *(not shown),* which overlies the vidian canal, shown in A. However, by conventional usage, a larger fossa incorporating the small fossa and extending to the lateral edge of the base of the pterygoid process (as shown in B, C, and D) is designated the PPF. **D,** At this level, the margins of the PPF (consisting of the maxillary bone, angled upper part of the perpendicular plate of the palatine bone, and base of the pterygoid process) are shown with the latter two forming the small fossa. Also evident and by conventional usage is the lateral opening of the PPF, the pterygomaxillary fissure *(dotted line).* (From Daniels DL, Mark LP, Ulmer JL, et al: Osseous anatomy of the pterygopalatine fossa. *AJNR Am J Neuroradiol.* 1998 Sep;19(8):1423–32. Copyright © D. Daniels, 1998.)

meningeal artery (from the meningohypophyseal trunk), or a branch of it, may also run through Dorello's canal.

There is an opinion that old Dorello, rest his soul, while intoxicated on Chianti, described an area that was difficult to reliably identify. The term petroclival venous confluence (PVC) has been recently introduced to describe the region of Dorello's canal (see Fig. 11-9) and enable reliable identification. It is located between two

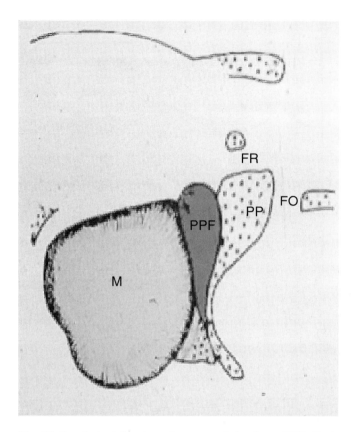

Fig. 11-5 Sagittal drawing of pterygopalatine fossa (PPF). Sagittal cartoon showing the deflated balloon shape of the PPF. Observe the maxillary sinus (M) anterior and the pterygoid process (PP) and feet posterially. FO, foramanovale; FR, foramen rotundum

Table 11-1	Major (and some minor) foramina at the base of the skull and their contents
Foramen	**Contents**
Superior orbital fissure	Cranial nerves III, IV. 1st division of V, VI; orbital branch of middle meningeal artery; sympathetic nerve; recurrent meningeal artery, superior ophthalmic vein
Optic canal	Optic nerve, ophthalmic artery
Inferior orbital fissure	Infraorbital artery, vein, and nerve (branch of 2nd division of cranial nerve V)
Foramen rotundum	2nd division of cranial nerve V, artery of foramen rotundum, emissary veins
Foramen ovale	3rd division of cranial nerve V, lesser petrosal nerve accessory meningeal artery, emissary veins
Foramen spinosum	Middle meningeal artery and vein, recurrent branch of 3rd division of cranial nerve V, lesser superficial petrosal nerve
Foramen lacerum	Meningeal branch of ascending pharyngel artery, nerve of pterygoid canal
Foramen of Vesalius	Emissary vein from cavernous sinus to pterygoid plexus
Vidian canal	Vidian artery and nerve
Jugular foramen	Pars nervosa: cranial nerve IX, inferior petrosal sinus
	Pars vascularis: Cranial nerves X, XI; jugular bulb
Hypoglossal canal	Cranial nerve XII, hypoglossal persistant artery (in rare instance when it is present)
Pterygopalatine fossa	Pterygopalatine ganglia (V-2) pterygopalatine plexus
Foramen magnum	Medulla oblongate, vertebral a, anterior spinal a, posterior spinal a

dural layers and demarcates an interdural venous confluens. The cranial nerve VI courses in this venous confluens and is separated from blood by a dural and/or arachnoidal sheath. The posterior portion of the cavernous sinus, the lateral basilar sinus along the clivus, and the superior petrosal sinus fill this region, which then forms the inferior petrosal sinus draining into the jugular bulb. Anatomically, the boundaries of the PVC are: (1) superiorly, the posterior petroclinoid fold, which inserts on the posterior clinoid process and continues posterolaterally to the petrous insertion of the tentorium; (2) anteroinferiorly, the posterosuperior aspect of the lateral border of the upper clivus and posterior clinoid process; (3) laterally, by the medial aspect of the petrous bone apex; (4) posteriorly, the cerebral layer of dura matter. After reading this description you might ask what the authors are smoking, but we really didn't inhale.

The PVC always contains the abducens nerve and is divided into two compartments by the petrosphenoidal ligament (or Gruber's ligament), which represents the largest of the fibrous trabeculations bridging the two dural layers limiting the PVC. The nerve usually runs below Gruber's ligament.

Who cares? Well, it turns out that this is more interesting than you think. There are conditions that produce abducens palsy precisely because of fixation of

the nerve in Dorello's canal. These include nerve injury caused by brain stem shifts from trauma or mass lesions, and Gradenigo's syndrome (cranial nerve VI palsy associated with inflammatory lesions of the petrous apex and facial pain caused by involvement of cranial nerve V as it crosses the petrous apex). Increased venous pressure in the PVC from carotid-cavernous fistula and dural malformations may compress and injure the nerve.

The foramen lacerum is not a true foramen and the carotid artery does not run through it. Rather, the carotid artery runs over the fibrocartilage (making up the endocranial floor of the foramen lacerum) on its way to the cavernous sinus.

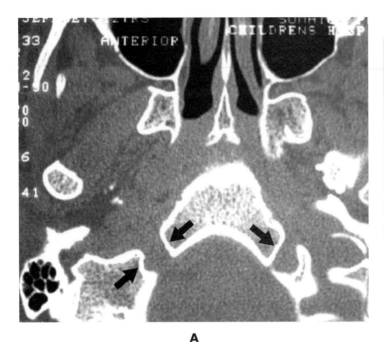

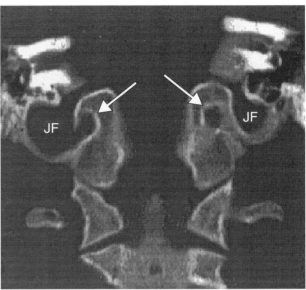

A

B

Fig. 11-6 **A,** The hypoglossal foramen is outlined by *arrows.* **B,** Coronal view. The hypoglossal foramen is indicated by *arrows.* It is separated from the jugular foramen (JF) by the jugular tubercles *(open arrows).*

The greater superficial petrosal nerve (GSPN) is a branch of the facial nerve that innervates the lacrimal glands and mucous membranes of the nasal cavity and palate. It is a mixed nerve containing sensory and parasympathetic fibers. The parasympathetic fibers exit the brain stem as the nervous intermedius. The GSPN courses anteromedially from the geniculate ganglion and exists the facial hiatus in the petrous bone. It passes under the gasserian ganglion in Meckel's cave and goes forward to the region of the foramen lacerum. Here it merges with the deep petrosal nerve from the sympathetic carotid plexus to form the vidian nerve. This nerve runs anteriorly in the vidian canal with the parasympathetic fibers synapsing in the pterygopalatine ganglia and the sensory fibers passing through the ganglion to the nasal cavity and palate. The vidian canal connects the pterygopalatine fossa anteriorly to the foramen lacerum posteriorly and transmits the vidian artery. The vidian artery, a branch of the maxillary artery, joins the carotid artery in its petrous segment.

The foramen of Vesalius is an inconstant emissary foramen that can be seen anterior and medial to foramen ovale. Besides the emissary vein, the ascending intracranial branch of the accessory meningeal artery can enter the middle cranial fossa through the foramen of Vesalius or the foramen ovale (Fig. 11-10).

On either side of the sella is the cavernous sinus (discussed later in this section), a trabeculated venous plexus containing cranial nerves III, IV, VI, and the first and second divisions of V. These are located in the lateral portion of the sinus. Cranial nerves III, IV, and the first and

second divisions of V are in the lateral wall of the cavernous sinus and maintain that order from superior to inferior in the coronal plane (Fig. 11-11). Cranial nerve VI is medial in the cavernous sinus but lateral to the cavernous carotid artery. Cranial nerve V exits the ventral pons as separate motor and sensory roots. The roots run forward together through the prepontine cistern and exit through the porus trigeminus of the petrous apex. These roots pass over the petrous apex, with the motor root exiting the foramen ovale without merging with the sensory root or gasserian ganglion (semilunar ganglion). The sensory root enters the trigeminal cistern (the space containing CSF), which is in Meckel's cave, a dural invagination at the posterior aspect of the cavernous sinus. The dural layers of Meckel's cave demonstrate thin peripheral enhancement. In addition, a discrete semilunar enhancing structure within the inferolateral aspect

---

Box 11-1 Lesions of the Hypoglossal Nerve and Canal

Large glomus jugulare neoplasms
Chordoma
Metastases
Myeloma
Schwannomas
Neuroma
Meningioma
Neurotropic spread of tumor

of Meckel's cave representing the gasserian ganglion has been observed to enhance suggesting the lack of a blood-nerve barrier. The gasserian ganglion is a meshwork of sensory neural fibers permeated by cerebrospinal fluid (CSF) from the trigeminal cistern. It is supplied from branches of the inferolateral trunk, the tentorial artery of the meningohypophyseal trunk, or the middle meningeal artery. On computed tomography (CT) or magnetic resonance imaging (MR) the CSF in the trigeminal cistern is obviously visualized, and with high resolution MR the nerve fibers can be seen. The three sensory divisions of the trigeminal nerve leave the gasserian ganglion, with the first and the second divisions running in the lateral wall of the cavernous sinus to exit the superior orbital fissure (along with cranial nerves III, IV, and VI and the superior ophthalmic vein) and foramen rotundum, respectively.

The superior and inferior ophthalmic veins drain into the cavernous sinus via the superior and inferior orbital fissures, respectively; however, there are many variations of this venous drainage pattern. The cavernous sinus is formed by two layers of dura mater. The periosteal layer forms the floor and most of the medial wall, and the meningeal layer (dura propria) forms its roof, lateral wall, and the upper part of its medial wall. The lateral wall may have two layers of dura: a deep layer, which ensheathes cranial nerves III and IV and first and second divisions of cranial nerve V, and a superficial dural layer. In addition, like most other venous structures in the body, the cavernous sinus has many variations and much

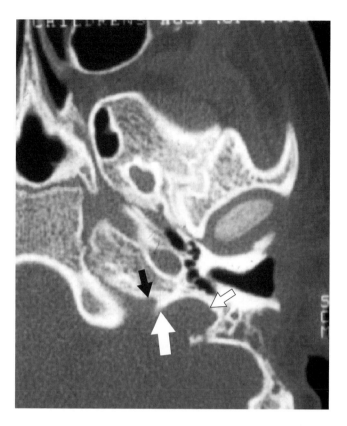

Fig. 11-7   Jugular foramen. Note the pars nervosa anteromedially *(arrow)*, and the pars vascularis posterolaterally *(open arrow)*. Between them is the jugular spur *(fat arrow)*.

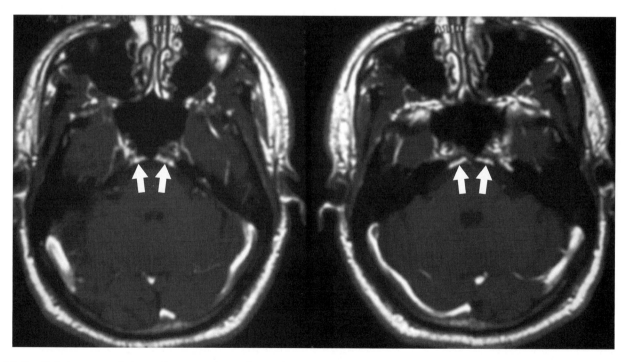

Fig. 11-8   Inferior petrosal sinus. Contrast enhanced MR, the inferior petrosal sinus is behind the clivus and enhances. The sixth cranial nerves can be seen coursing as an outline *(arrows)* in the enhancing inferior petrosal sinus.

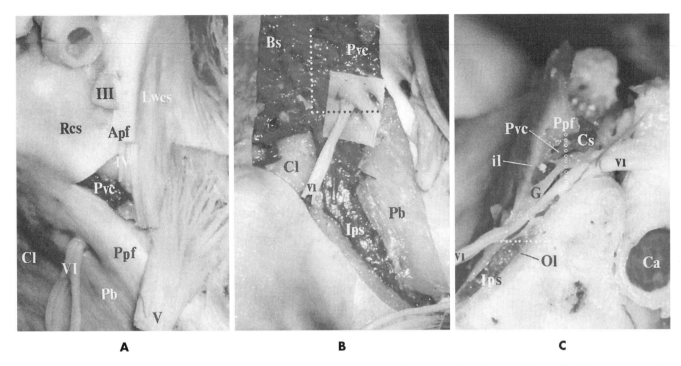

Fig. 11-9 **A,** Superior view of a right petroclival venous confluence (PVC). The posterolateral part of the roof of the cavernous sinus (Rcs), and the posterior part of the anterior petroclinoid fold (Apf) were removed. Posteriorly, the PVC was limited by the inner layer of the dura mater covering the clivus (Cl) and petrous bone (Pb). The abducent nerve (VI) pierced the dura mater and entered the PVC. The posterior petroclinoid fold (Ppf) was the superior limit of the PVC. The oculomotor (III) and trochlear (IV) nerves pierced the lateral part of the roof of the cavernous sinus and ran into the lateral wall of the cavernous sinus (Lwcs). The trigeminal nerve (V) was also partially embedded in this lateral wall. **B,** Posterior view of a right PVC. The dura covering the PVC, the basal sinus of the clivus (Bs), and the inferior petrosal sinus (Ips) was removed, except for a square around the abducent nerve. The PVC was limited inferiorly *(dots)* by the axial plane located below the dural foramen of the abducent nerve and medially by the sagittal plane extending upward from the medial limit of the inferior petrosal sinus. The PVC and inferior petrosal sinus were contained in a bone groove limited laterally by the medial aspect of the petrous bone apex and anteroinferiorly by the lateral border of the clivus. **C,** Transverse section of a right PVC after the roof of the cavernous sinus was removed. The PVC was quadrangular. Its four sides consisted of the inner layer (il) of dura mater posteriorly, the axial plane *(dots)* below the dural foramen of the abducent nerve inferiorly, the outer layer (Ol) of dura mater aneroinferiorly, and the vertical plane *(open dots)* containing the posterior petroclinoid fold anteriorly. The abducent nerve perforated the dura, coursed in the PVC below the petrosphenoidal ligament of Grüber (G), and reached the lateral wall of the intracavernous ICA (Cs). The PVC was continuous with the cavernous sinus (Cs) and the inferior petrosal sinus.

Illustration continued on following page

controversy about its exact internal venous anatomy. It has been reported that the true cavernous sinus (a large venous channel surrounding the internal carotid artery) exists in only 1% of patients. In the other instances the cavernous sinus is formed by numerous small veins including (1) the veins of the lateral wall, (2) the veins of the inferolateral group, (3) the medial vein, and (4) the vein of the carotid sulcus. For the purposes of simplicity, the authors, simple-minded as we are, will continue to use the cavernous sinus in its holistic sense (Fig. 11-12).

The cavernous sinus can be subdivided into an intracavernous and interdural compartments. Cavernous sinus tumors that arise interdurally (within the lateral wall) such as schwannomas of the cranial nerves, epidermoid tumors, melanomas, and cavernous angiomas have smooth contours, oval shape, and displace the intracavernous portion of the internal carotid without encasement or narrowing. Intracavernous lesions include meningiomas,

hemangiopericytomas, and ganglioneuroblastomas. These lesions tend to encase and narrow the internal carotid artery. The cavernous sinus may be compressed but not obliterated by interdural lesions whereas it may be obliterated by intracavernous tumors.

The cavernous sinus enhances dramatically within 30 seconds after contrast injection for CT or MR. After enhancement, cranial nerves are usually easy to identify on coronal CT. Dynamic coronal MR (rapid imaging of the same region repeated for a short time: six to eight thin sections every 30 seconds, for 3 to 5 minutes) has been advocated in pituitary adenomas to distinguish invasion of the medial wall of the cavernous sinus from tumor bulging along the medial wall. On a dynamic scan the venous spaces enhance before the tumor does, potentially demarcating the exact extent of the lesion. Dynamic imaging has also been advocated for the diagnosis of microadenomas by demon-

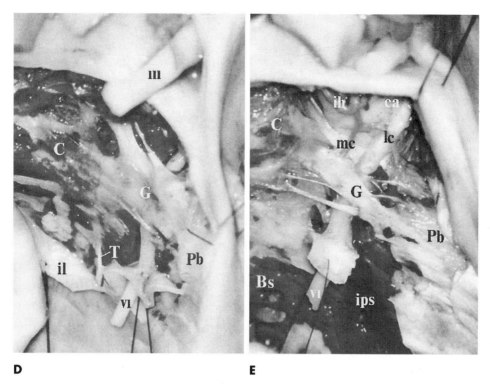

D **E**

Fig. 11-9 *Continued.* **D,** Posterior view of a right PVC after the inner layer of dura mater was removed. Fibrous trabeculations (T) were present between the inner and outer layers of dura mater, and the petrosphenoidal ligament of Grüber may be regarded as a larger trabeculation bridging the petrous bone apex (Pb), and the upper clivus. The abducent nerve was located below the petrosphenoidal ligament of Grüber. **E,** Posterior view of a right PVC after the inner layer of dura mater was removed. The petrosphenoidal ligament of Grüber was a thin trabeculation bridging the petrous bone apex and the upper clivus. The posterior bend of the intracavernous ICA (ca) gave rise to the so-called meningohypophyseal trunk vascularizing the posterior hypophysis (inferior hypophyseal artery [ih]), and the dura mater of the region (medial artery of the clivus [mc] and lateral artery of the clivus [lc]). The abducent nerve was surrounded by a dural sheath and was located below the petrosphenoidal ligament of Grüber. The PVC was continuous with the basal sinus of the clivus and the inferior petrosal sinus. (From Destrieux C, Velut S, Kakou MK, et al. A new concept in Dorello's canal microanatomy: the petroclival venous confluence: *J Neurosurg* 87:68, 70, 1997.)

strating greater conspicuity between the normally enhancing pituitary and the more slowly enhancing microadenoma (see discussion under Intrasellar Lesions). Some people think that cavernous sinus invasion of pituitary tumors is best visualized on unenhanced coronal MR.

The cavernous sinus drains into the superior and inferior petrosal sinuses. Many venous connections exist between the cavernous sinuses around the sella. The basilar venous plexus, the largest intercavernous connection, lies within the dura behind the clivus connecting the two cavernous sinuses and the superior and inferior petrosal sinuses. There are also venous communications between the cavernous sinus and the pterygoid plexus of veins via emissary veins in the foramen ovale and foramen rotundum, and through the inconstant foramen of Vesalius. These basilar foramina can be a path (and can demonstrate enlargement) for nasopharyngeal tumors coursing into the cavernous sinus.

The pituitary gland is surrounded by a dural bag with the medial wall of the cavernous sinus being the lateral extent of the dural bag. The gland may have a significant lateral extension normally making the diagnosis of cavernous sinus invasion difficult if the adenoma is in this lateral extension. The coronary sinus is located between the dural bag and the roof of the sphenoid sinus and joins the two cavernous sinuses.

The anterior lobe of the pituitary is divided into the pars tuberalis, pars intermedia, and the pars distalis. The pars tuberalis consists of thin anterior pituitary tissue along the median eminence and anterior infundibulum. Rarely, suprasellar adenomas and other suprasellar pituitary tumors may originate from this tissue, and it may function after hypophysectomy. The pars intermedia lies between the pars distalis and the posterior lobe of the pituitary. It is noted to contain small cysts (pars intermedia cysts, colloid cysts) and may be the origin of Rathke's cleft cysts. The pars distalis is the large intrasellar portion of the anterior pituitary. The adenohypophysis secretes prolactin (from lactotrophs), growth hormone (from somatotrophs), thyroid-stimulating hormone (from thyrotrophs), follicle-simulating hormone

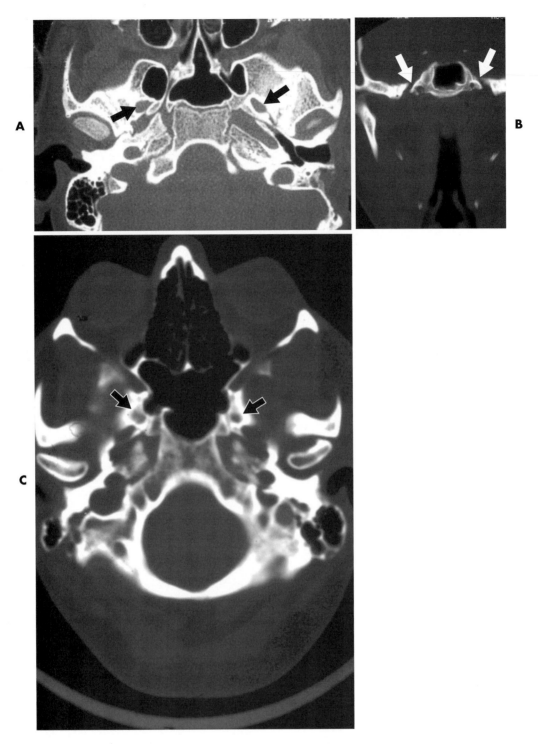

Fig. 11-10   Foramen ovale. **A,** Oxial CT of skull base with bone windows. *Arrows* point to foramen ovale. **B,** Coronal with *arrows* pointing to ovale. Note the medial to lateral slant in the foramen. **C,** *Arrows* point to foramen of Vesalius.

and luteinizing hormone (from gonadotrophs), and corticotropin (ACTH) precursor and melanocyte-stimulating hormone (from corticotrophs). The neurohypophysis is composed of the neural (posterior) lobe, the infundibular stem, and the median eminence. Besides storing antidiuretic hormone and oxytocin, the neural lobe also contains nonsecreting cells termed pituicytes. Their exact role is uncertain, but they may take up polypeptides and phospholipids released at the secretory terminals.

The posterior lobe of the pituitary has a direct blood supply from the inferior hypophyseal artery, a branch of the meningohypophyseal trunk arising from the cav-

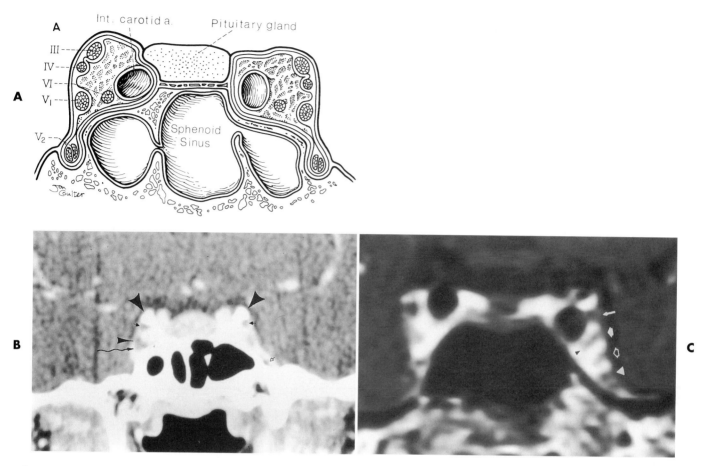

Fig. 11-11 **A,** Diagram of cranial nerves in the cavernous sinus. (From Latchaw RE: *MR and CT imaging of the head, neck, and spine,* ed 2, vol 2, St Louis, 1991, Mosby–Year Book.) **B,** Cranial nerves in cavernous sinus. Enhanced CT showing cranial nerves in cavernous sinus. Cranial nerve III *(black arrow)* is directly under the anterior clinoid process *(large arrowhead).* Also identified on the patient's left side are cranial nerves IV *(arrowhead)* and the first division of V *(squiggly arrow).* On the right side, the second division of V is marked *(open arrow).* **C,** MR with contrast outlines the cranial nerves in the cavernous sinus. *(Short skinny arrow* on III, *fat closed arrow* on IV, *open fat arrow* on V-1, *arrowhead* on V-2, and *black arrowhead* on VI) Note that VI is medial to IV and V-1 and is the closest to the carotid artery—in this case, those cranial nerves blur together.

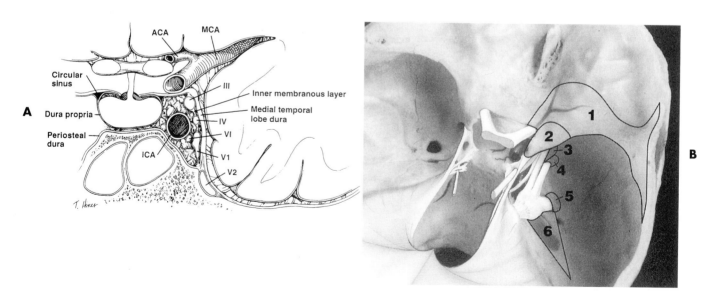

Fig. 11-12 Cavernous sinus diagram. **A,** Coronal of cavernous sinus. ACA, anterior cerebral artery; MCA, middle cerebral artery; ICA, internal carotid artery. Cranial nerves (III, IV, V1, V2). **B,** Base view, 1, greater wing of sphenoid; 2, anterior clinoid process; 3, superior orbital fissure; 4, foramen rotundum; 5, foramen ovale; 6, region of Meckel's cove.

ernous carotid. On lateral cerebral carotid angiography, a posterior pituitary blush can normally be seen from this supply. The superior hypophyseal arteries, arising from the supraclinoid internal carotid arteries and posterior communicating arteries (usually not visualized on angiography) supply a plexus around the base of the hypophyseal stalk and median eminence and then supply the anterior lobe of the pituitary indirectly through the pituitary portal system. McConnell's capsular arteries, small branches of the carotid artery (demonstrated in <30% of anatomic specimens) supply the floor and roof of the sella turcica. The implications of this quaint blood supply are that on dynamic imaging the posterior pituitary and infundibulum enhance immediately because of their direct blood supply, whereas the anterior pituitary is slightly delayed because of the portal system. The indirect blood supply to the anterior lobe of the pituitary makes it susceptible to ischemia, which can be seen in cases of autoinfarction of pituitary tumors and in postpartum pituitary necrosis (Sheehan syndrome). The venous drainage of the pituitary is into the cavernous sinuses.

The diaphragma sellae is the sheet of dura forming a roof over the sella turcica overlying the pituitary gland. The diaphragma has a central hiatus of variable size through which the infundibulum passes. The diameter of the diaphragmatic foramen is always more than twice the diameter of the infundibulum. The portion of the hypophysis located just below the diaphragma is concave superiorly like the region just around the stem of an apple and creates the hypophyseal cistern. This cistern is an expansion of the chiasmatic cistern and is separated from the interpeduncular and prepontine cisterns by the membrane of Liliequist.

> There once was an anatomist named Liliequist
> Students thought his membrane was silliquest
> If examiners should ask
> Wannabe Neuroradiologists would bask
> The remainder of the class didn't pass and graduated
>   in the rear of the class

The infundibulum arises from the tuber cinereum (a prominence of the inferior portion of the hypothalamus) and courses in an anterior inferior direction. It is an important landmark in pituitary anatomy, marking the anterior portion of the posterior pituitary gland. The anterior lobe of the pituitary is derived from Rathke's pouch, as are the pars intermedia and pars tuberalis. The posterior lobe develops as a downward projection of the neuroectoderm from the base of the brain.

The suprasellar cistern is superior to the diaphragma sellae. This cistern contains the circle of Willis with anterior cerebral arteries, anterior and posterior communicating arteries, and the tip of the basilar artery (Fig. 11-13). Anteriorly, the cistern is bounded by the inferior frontal lobes and the interhemispheric fissure, laterally by the medial portions of the temporal lobes, and posteriorly by the prepontine and interpeduncular cisterns. Lying central in the suprasellar cistern is the optic chiasm, which is anterior to the infundibular stalk. The normal chiasm is about 3 to 4 mm posterosuperior to the tuberculum sellae. In some circumstances the chiasm can overlie either the tuberculum sellae (prefixed optic chiasm, seen in 9% of cases) or the dorsum sellae (postfixed optic chiasm, seen in 11% of cases). Such anatomic anomalies are important with respect to visual symptoms and surgical approach to suprasellar lesions.

The hypothalamus forms the ventral and rostral part of the wall of the third ventricle. The chiasmatic and infundibular recesses of the third ventricle project inferiorly into these respective structures (chiasm and infundibulum). Posterior to the infundibular stalk is the anteroinferior third ventricle and mamillary bodies. The tuber cinereum is the lamina of gray substance from the

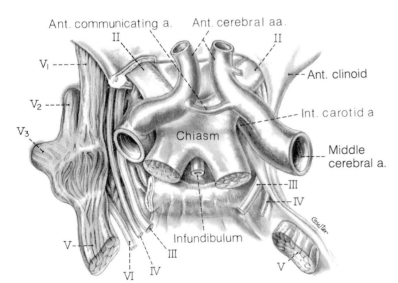

Fig. 11-13 Diagram of suprasellar cistern. (From Latchaw RE: *MR and CT imaging of the head, neck, and spine,* ed 2, vol. 2, St. Louis, Mosby-Year Book, 1991.)

floor of the third ventricle (hypothalamus) between the mamillary bodies and the optic chiasm. The infundibulum projects downward from the tuber cinereum. Inferior to the pituitary gland is the sphenoid sinus. The surgeons figured this out and designed the transsphenoidal hypophysectomy.

Are you still with us? If not, don't feel bad. There was a recent patient (NITWITPPP-neuroradiologist in training who intends to pursue private practice), whom the anesthesiologists had tremendous problems putting to sleep for an interventional neuroradiologic procedure. They stat-paged the authors, who proceeded to read the preceding pages, and with ease the patient was somnolent. He woke up when we started reading the "relevant" clinical material. Get your hippocampus humming—here we go!

IMAGING OF THE NORMAL PITUITARY GLAND AND THE PERISELLAR REGION

MR has several advantages over CT in imaging the sellar region; however, CT does have some use. MR can display pathologic lesions in three orthogonal planes without loss of information. It can demonstrate the relationship of pituitary lesions to the optic chiasm and cavernous sinuses. It has the capability of distinguishing solid, cystic, and hemorrhagic components of lesions. Calcification, although usually imaged as low intensity on T1-weighted images (T1WI) and T2-weighted images (T2WI), is better seen on CT. Bony septa in the sphenoid sinus are also better visualized on CT. This may be important if a transsphenoidal surgical approach is being considered. Rapidly flowing blood on spin-echo MR appears as absence of signal intensity from the vessel's lumen (flow void). This flow void can be observed in the cavernous and supraclinoid carotid arteries. Suprasellar aneurysms may be diagnosed without angiography, and old clotted blood in the wall of these aneurysms usually appears as high intensity.

In general, the coronal T1WI with thin sections (3 mm) is all that is necessary to image the pituitary gland. The T2WI can occasionally add additional information for the differential diagnosis by providing the intensity characteristics of a particular lesion. This is not usually the problem in cases of "rule out microadenoma." The normal pituitary gland has been measured on T1WI in several different studies. In women, the maximal height was 9 mm whereas in men it was 8 mm. In children less than 12 years of age, the gland should be 6 mm or less, with its upper surface flat or slightly concave. The gland may be increased in size and changes shape during puberty and pregnancy because of physiologic hypertrophy. For the obsessive-compulsive, the gland has been reported to increase linearly in height approximately

0.08 mm/week. During pregnancy, no gland was larger than 10 mm whereas in the immediate postpartum period the top height measured 11.8 mm. After the first postpartum week, the gland rapidly returns to normal. In teenaged girls it may measure up to 10 mm in height, and convex upper margins may be identified. This can be noted in teenaged boys but appears to be less striking. Convexity has been observed in children with precocious puberty. During pregnancy both the stalk and the gland can enlarge, with the latter growing to 10 mm or more and being convex superiorly. In the first week post partum the gland can be enlarged to 12 mm, with rapid shrinkage occurring thereafter. Like some other organs, the gland gradually decreases in size after the age of 50 years. The authors, for a variety of reasons and regions, think that size criteria are overrated. If the pituitary looks large, it probably is. Forget the measure, be a hedger, for pituitary treasure.

Intensity is important in MR diagnosis. The anterior lobe of the pituitary gland is isointense to brain on T1WI and T2WI. However, in children less than 2 months of age the pituitary is rounder, larger, and of higher intensity on T1WI than during the rest of infancy. This is most likely related to its high level of metabolic and hormonal function during early infancy, although it has been suggested that the high intensity results from an increase in the bound fraction of water molecules caused by hormone secretion. Hyperintensity on T1WI during pregnancy has also been noted. Reversible hyperintensity has been reported in patients receiving parenteral nutrition (as seen with the basal ganglia secondary to manganese deposition in liver disease). Iron can accumulate in the anterior lobe of the pituitary gland in patients with hemochromatosis and produce low intensity on T2WI and gradient echo T2* weighted images (Fig. 11-14).

The posterior pituitary gland is high intensity on the T1WI and of lower intensity on the T2WI (Fig. 11-15). The precise cause of the high signal in the posterior of the pituitary is unknown but is probably related to the carrier protein (neurophysin) stored in the neurosecretory granules of the posterior pituitary, intracellular lipid in glial cell pituicytes, water interactions with paramagnetic substances, or a low molecular weight molecule such as vasopressin or neurophysins (we have made a lot of progress since the last edition—NOT!). Posterior to the posterior pituitary is a rim of hypointensity, representing cortical bone of the dorsum. Posterior to this hypointense margin is the hyperintensity of fatty marrow in the clivus. High signal intensity has also been observed in the infundibular stalk on fluid-attenuated inversion recovery (FLAIR) images presumably related to the fluid rich component (prolonged T2) in the pituitary stalk.

The high intensity of the posterior pituitary gland has been noted to be absent in patients with diabetes in-

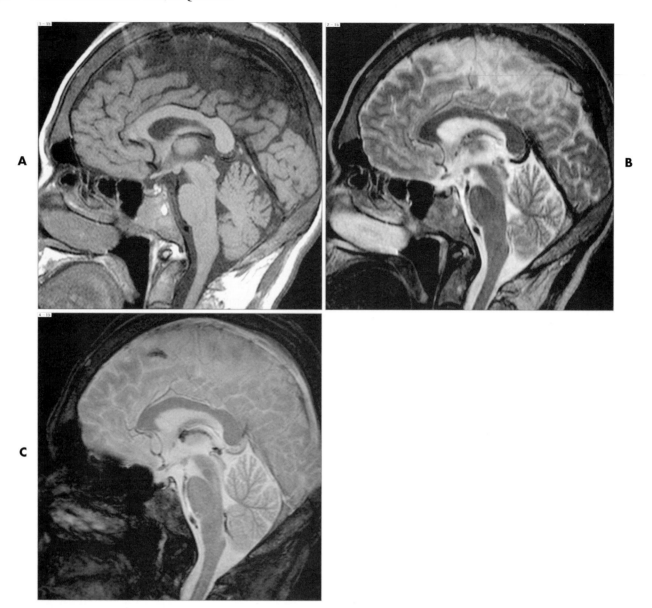

Fig. 11-14 Hemochromatosis affecting the pituitary. **A,** Sagittal T1WI of the pituitary. Note the posterior pituitary bright but the isointense anterior aspect. **B,** T2WI revealing marked anterior pituitary hypointensity representing iron deposition in the anterior pituitary. **C,** Gradient echo image emphasizing T2* shows increased susceptibility. (Courtesy of Y. Miki, M.D.)

sipidus but is identified in only about two thirds of healthy infants. In pituitary dwarfism, a high-intensity nodule on T1WI has been observed at the infundibular apex (Fig. 11-16).

After injection, enhancement is promptly noted on T1WI in the anterior pituitary gland, the infundibulum, and the cavernous sinuses. Remember that the posterior pituitary is already high intensity, so that any enhancement would be difficult to ascertain. The initial enhancement gradually fades in 20 to 30 minutes or more. The pituitary and cavernous sinuses generally enhance to a similar extent. The normal mucosa of the paranasal sinuses also enhances. Rapidly flowing blood such as in

the carotids does not demonstrate enhancement and appears hypointense on most imaging sequences. In the coronal plane the cranial nerves may occasionally be demonstrated on MR as soft-tissue structures or on enhanced CT as low density punctate structures in the lateral wall of the cavernous sinus.

CT of the pituitary gland has generally been replaced by MR. However, in cases and regions where this is not possible, it should be performed in the coronal plane with 1.5-mm sections after contrast. Dental amalgams and beam-hardening artifacts tend to degrade the image quality. Furthermore, patients have difficulty maintaining the coronal position. One concession given to CT

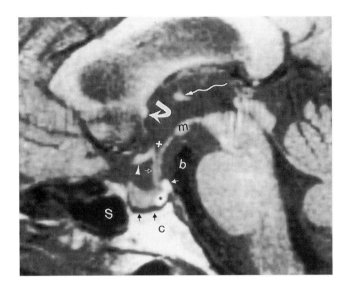

Fig. 11-15   Normal sellar anatomy. Sagittal T1WI with the posterior pituitary bright spot (*), fat in the dorsum *(white arrow)*, infundibular recess (+), infundibulum *(open white arrow)*, chiasm *(white arrowhead)*, mamillary body *(m)*, basilar artery *(b)*, clivus *(c)*, floor of sella *(black arrows)*, sphenoid sinus *(s)*, anterior commissure *(curved arrow)*, and massa intermedia *(squiggly arrow)*.

over MR is its ability to visualize bony sphenoid septa and nonpneumatization of the sphenoid sinus.

An important problem with CT is its difficulty in distinguishing vascular structures from other enhancing tissue. This is critical in the pituitary, where the question, "Are the carotid arteries medial, and could they be encountered in a transsphenoidal approach?" is often asked. The surgeon may need a stat asset transfer if he figures this out retrospectively. That is why you have a job; however, you will probably still be named in the suit.

INTRASELLAR LESIONS (Box 11-2)

Congenital Lesions of the Pituitary

The embryology of the pituitary gland has been reassessed. Classically, it was taught that the anterior lobe developed from Rathke's pouch, a diverticulum of the primitive buccal cavity (stomodeum). The posterior lobe originates from neuroectoderm and migrates inferiorly from the hypothalamus. Rathke's pouch starts growing toward the brain during the fourth week of gestation. By the eighth week, the connection with the oral cavity dis-

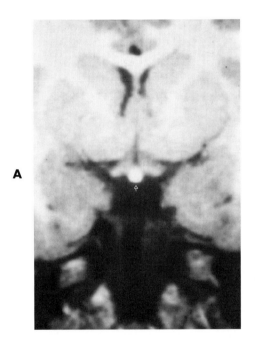

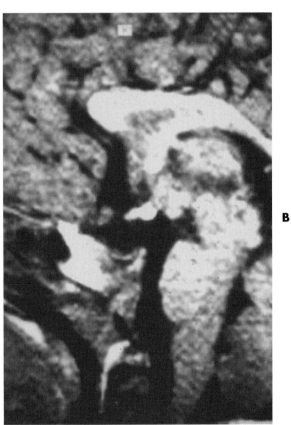

Fig. 11-16   Ectopic posterior pituitary. **A,** Noncontrast coronal T1WI in an intellectual political (oxymoron) dwarf showing high intensity in an ectopic posterior pituitary *(open arrow)*. The normal pituitary bright spot was missing, but for that matter there is probably nothing bright in the majority of politicians. **B,** Sagittal T1WI shows the ectopic posterior pituitary glands relationship to the adenohypophysis.

Box 11-2 Intrasellar Lesions

Abscess
Aneurysm
Arachnoid cyst
Chordoma
Choristoma
Craniopharyngioma
Empty sella
Granuloma (sarcoid, TB, EG, syphilis, Erdheim-Chester
    disease)
Lymphocytic adenohypophysitis
Meningioma
Metastasis
Parasitic infection
Pituitary adenoma
Pituitary apoplexy (infarct, hemorrhage)
Pituitary hyperplasia 2° to end organ failure
    (1° hypothyroidism)
Pituitary stone
Rathke's cleft cyst

appears and the pouch is in close contact with the infundibulum and posterior lobe of the pituitary. The remnants of this tract can persist in the form of the craniopharyngeal canal (which can be visualized on axial CT with bone windows as a small foramen in the sphenoid— 5% to 9% of children younger than 3 months and 0.42% to 0.5% of adults) or as ectopic pituitary tissue in the nasopharynx or sphenoid sinus. The craniopharyngeal canal extends from the floor of the sella through the sphenoidal septum into the vomer. Ectopic craniopharyngioma can therefore arise from the pharyngeal roof, sphenoid body, or floor of the sella. This nice little concept may not be entirely true. Rathke's pouch may not arise from the buccal cavity; rather, it may be of neuroectodermal origin derived from the ventral neural ridge.

The classic endocrinologic concepts have also been revised. A single pituitary cell type can secrete multiple hormones, and some hypothalamic releasing factors may act on more than one pituitary cell type. Furthermore, the traditional classification of pituitary tumors into basophilic, acidophilic, and chromophobe is also obsolete, having been replaced by a classification based on electron microscopic and immunohistochemical criteria. If you want classics, you are better off sticking with Mozart, the Beatles, and Coke.

Congenital abnormalities of the pituitary include aplasia, hypoplasia, or duplication. These have been observed to occur alone or with a variety of different developmental syndromes, including septooptic dysplasia; holoprosencephaly; anencephaly, sphenoidal encephalocele; Kallmann syndrome; Pallister-Hall syndrome; CHARGE syndrome (*c*oloboma, *h*eart disease, *a*tresia choanal, *re-*

tarded growth and development, *g*enital anomalies, and deformed *e*ars or deafness); and 17q, 18p, or 20p chromosomal deletions.

Pituitary Adenoma

Autopsy series indicate that the pituitary gland can be a reservoir for the "incidentaloma," including asymptomatic microadenomas (14% to 27% of cases), pars intermedia cysts (13% to 22%), and occult metastatic lesions (about 5% of patients with malignancy). This means that clinical input is critical in assessing small lesions of the pituitary because many "normal" patients may have small, insignificant abnormalities visualized on CT or MR. Serum prolactin levels of more than 200 ng/mL are highly specific for prolactin-secreting adenomas whereas markedly elevated prolactin levels (>1000 ng/mL) imply cavernous sinus invasion.

Pituitary microadenomas (<10 mm) are generally hypointense compared with the normal gland on T1WI and display a variable intensity on T2WI. On CT, the microadenoma is of low density compared with the normal gland with or without enhancement. In about 75% of cases, adenomas in general have associated hormonal abnormality, whereas nonhormonally active lesions become symptomatic because of their size, producing headache, visual disturbances (classically bitemporal hemianopsia), cranial nerve palsy, and CSF rhinorrhea. Secondary signs of an intrasellar mass lesion are most useful when CT images are obtained. These include focal erosion of the sellar floor, focal upward convexity of

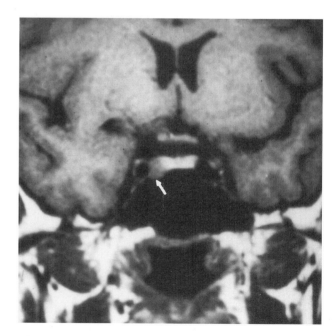

Fig. 11-17 Microadenoma. Unenhanced coronal MR shows lower intensity lesion *(arrow)* compared with normal pituitary.

the diaphragma sellae, and deviation of the stalk to the opposite side (this last sign is probably as overrated as the delta sign on CT for sinus thrombosis). Usually the diagnosis of pituitary microadenoma may be made without contrast (Fig. 11-17). The use of enhancement in the work-up of microadenoma is controversial. It may enable increased sensitivity in detecting those lesions that are not obviously hypointense on the unenhanced T1WI. Dynamic MR after contrast has been advocated not only for the detection of microadenomas but also for imaging what is left of the normal gland in cases of large tumor. The dynamic images obtained within the first minute appear to provide the greatest contrast between enhancing normal gland and pituitary tumor that does not initially enhance. However, if extrinsic causes of hyperprolactinemia have been excluded and the patient is considered likely to possess a microadenoma, then an unenhanced MR may be all that is necessary, particularly if the philosophy of the institution is to treat the tumor with drug therapy (bromocriptine). If, however, surgery is contemplated, then contrast is useful to direct the surgical approach to a particular side of the sella.

In most cases, on T1WI the microadenoma appears initially hypointense relative to the normally enhancing pituitary gland (Fig. 11-18). If a delayed scan (>20 minutes after the injection of contrast) is performed, the tumor may appear hyperintense relative to the gland. Enhancement can be helpful in determining whether the tumor has invaded the cavernous sinus. The cavernous sinus normally enhances immediately after contrast, whereas tumor is initially hypointense. Thus, lack of immediate enhancement in the cavernous sinus may imply invasion by tumor.

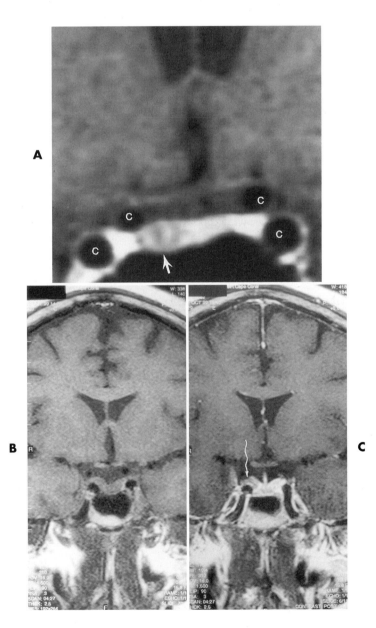

Fig. 11-18 Enhanced microadenoma. **A,** The normal pituitary gland enhances more than the microadenoma *(arrow)*. Note that the carotid arteries *(c)* have a flow void. **B,** Unenhanced MR of the pituitary. It is difficult (especially on this photograph) to see the lesion. However, after contrast **(C)** the basophilic adenoma *(squiggly arrow)* is obvious and the lesion even extends into the cavernous sinus.

Coronal MR beautifully shows the relationship of the tumor mass to the optic chiasm, third ventricle, and cavernous sinuses (Figs. 11-19 and Fig. 11-20). Pituitary adenomas have rarely been reported at extrasellar sites not in continuity with the sella, including the sphenoid sinus, nasal cavity, petrous bone, and third ventricle.

Enhancement is very useful in patients with Cushing disease (in the ancient vernacular, ACTH-secreting microadenoma, basophilic adenoma). It increases the examination's sensitivity significantly compared with the noncontrast MR images in the detection of these important lesions. Dynamic MR scanning with contrast and petrosal venous sampling has also been advocated to localize these lesions, which are generally the smallest of all pituitary adenomas, for surgical extirpation. Malignant pituitary adenomas have been reported in Cushing disease or Nelson syndrome (hyperpigmentation, elevated ACTH level, and an enlarged sella from an adenoma, after bilateral adrenalectomy).

Pituitary adenomas including those that secrete ACTH may originate in the infundibulum or extend into the infundibulum through the diaphragma sella.

Macroadenomas (>1 cm) are obvious abnormalities on unenhanced T1WI. They have roughly the same signal characteristics as microadenomas; however, they have a propensity for hemorrhage and infarction because of their marginal blood supply. Thus, these tumors can possess a variable intensity pattern. Treatment with bromocriptine increases the likelihood of hemorrhage, which has been reported in more than half of bromocriptine-treated adenomas. These hemorrhages may be asymptomatic or may be associated with the syndrome of pituitary apoplexy. Cystic regions in macroadenomas produce low intensity on T1WI and high intensity on T2WI.

Intracranial ectopic pituitary adenoma occurs most frequently in the suprasellar cistern most often continu-

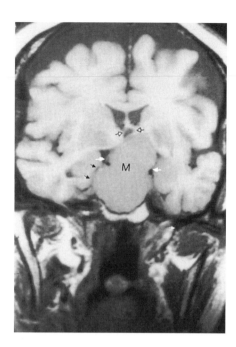

Fig. 11-20 Macroadenoma. Coronal T1WI of a large macroadenoma *(M)* extending from the sella superiorly to distort the third ventricle *(open arrows)*. Right cavernous sinus is bowed *(black arrows)*. When the tumor grows through the diaphragma sellae, it can be constricted by dural margins *(white arrows)* just above the flow voids in the carotids.

ous with the pituitary stalk. These lesions result from cells of the pars tuberalis located above the diaphragma sellae or from aberrant pituitary cells. Rarely, a connection with the stalk is not demonstrated and all that is observed is an enhancing mass in the suprasellar cistern.

Pituitary macroadenomas have been reported in the McCune-Albright syndrome (polyostotic fibrous dysplasia, hyperpigmented skin macules, and precocious puberty). Pituitary adenomas associated with hemorrhage occur in adolescence and can be confused with craniopharyngioma or Rathke's cyst on MR.

Pituitary Apoplexy

Pituitary apoplexy is a syndrome that appears suddenly with combinations of ophthalmoplegia, headache, visual loss, and/or vomiting. It should also be noted that pituitary apoplexy from pituitary infarction with little hemorrhage may be detected by MR (Fig. 11-21). In this case there is high intensity in the tumor on the T2WI. Pituitary hemorrhages follow the pattern of intraparenchymal hemorrhages, with acute hemorrhage revealing hypointensity on T2WI and subacute and chronic hemorrhages exhibiting high intensity on T1WI. As opposed to most simple intracranial hemorrhages, in which hemosiderin is deposited in the walls of the cavity, pituitary hemorrhage is not associated with hemosiderin deposition.

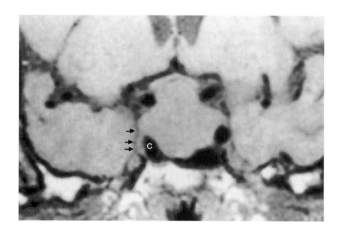

Fig. 11-19 Cavernous sinus invasion by a pituitary macroadenoma. Observe the extra soft tissue lateral to the cavernous carotid artery *(c)*. Lateral dural margin of the cavernous sinus *(arrows)* is bowed.

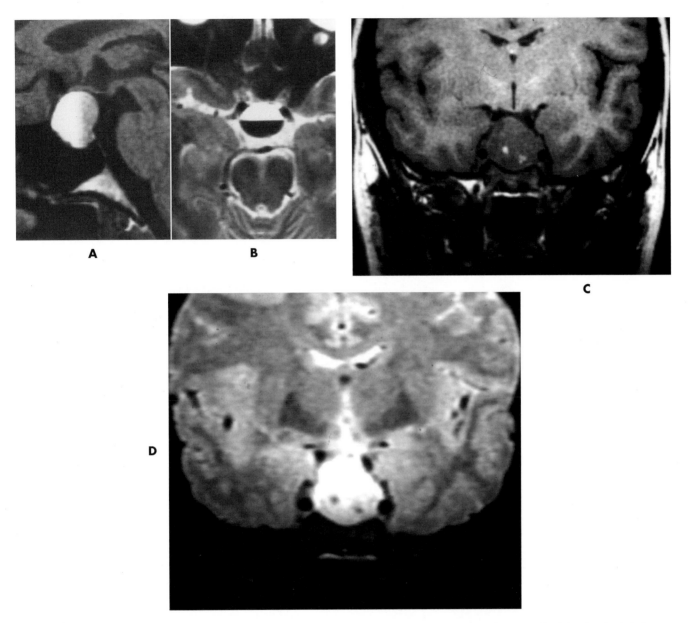

Fig. 11-21   Pituitary apoplexy. Sagittal T1WI **(A)** of large hemorrhage into a pituitary tumor. There is a fluid level, which is best appreciated on the axial **(B)** T2WI, with the hypointense lower level containing deoxyhemoglobin. **C,** The gland here is homogeneously dark except for two punctate areas representing hemorrhage. **D,** This pituitary gland has infarcted and is swollen and bright on T2WI.

Korean (epidemic) hemorrhagic fever caused by the Hantaan virus has been reported to produce pituitary necrosis (and atrophy in survivors) associated with visual field defects. The pathologic basis of this is postulated to be ischemic necrosis from disseminated intravascular coagulation. Sheehan syndrome is postpartum pituitary necrosis.

Metastatic Disease

Metastatic lesions can occur in the pituitary with a frequency reported from 1.8% to 12% of all pituitary lesions; the most common primary tumor is of the breast followed by gastrointestinal carcinoma. Usually, you cannot distinguish these metastatic lesions from nonmetastatic disease, although they should demonstrate increased enhancement compared with adenomas. These lesions can evoke an edematous response in the adjacent portion of the brain, whereas pituitary adenomas do not have this characteristic (Fig. 11-22). Metastases can, however, appear similar to macroadenomas with suprasellar extension and no brain reaction. Many pituitary metastases may be occult with respect to symptoms and found only by the compulsive pathologist. Obviously, multiplicity helps suggest this diagnosis.

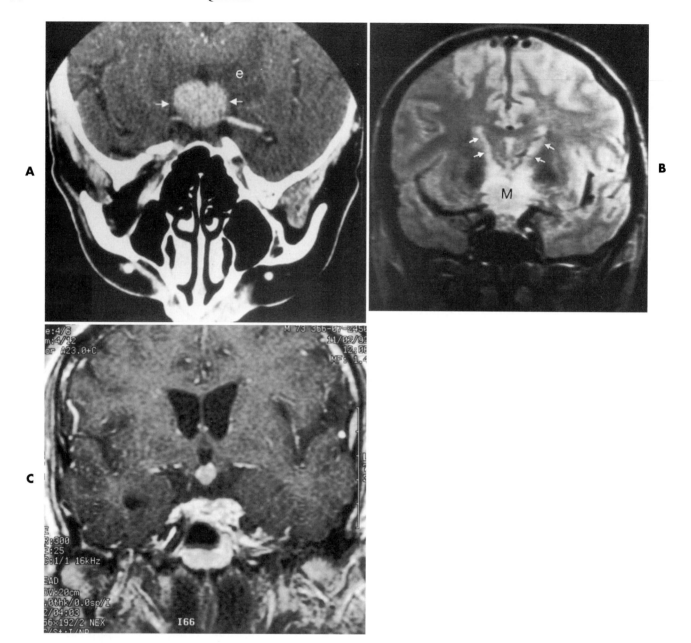

Fig. 11-22 Sellar and suprasellar breast metastasis. **A,** Enhanced coronal CT demonstrates mass *(arrows)* and associated edema *(e).* **B,** Coronal MR with mass *(M)* and edema tracking up the internal capsule *(arrows).* **C.** A coronal postcontrast T1WI in a patient with metastatic hepatocellular carcinoma shows enlargement and enhancement of the pituitary stalk in this patient who presented with diabetes insipidus.

Abscess

Abscess can form in the pituitary just as in other parts of the brain. This can occur after surgery but also in situations that predispose to infection, including sinusitis. These are uncommon lesions, and the patient is seen with symptoms such as fever and headache. The abscess produces compression of surrounding structures.

Granulomatous Disease

The pituitary gland can infrequently be affected by granulomatous diseases such as giant cell granuloma and sarcoidosis. In giant cell granuloma a pituitary mass is present with associated hypopituitarism and rarely diabetes insipidus. These lesions cannot be differentiated from other pituitary lesions; however, there is an association between giant cell granulomas and granulomas in the adrenal glands and liver. Sarcoidosis can produce intrasellar or suprasellar mass lesions that can masquerade as pituitary adenomas or as meningiomas.

Lymphocytic Hypophysitis

This is an uncommon inflammatory disease of the pituitary gland that can also involve the infundibulum. It is seen in young women during late pregnancy or in the postpartum period. However, it can also occur in nonpregnant women and men of all ages. The condition has also been termed lymphocytic infundibuloneurohypophysitis (if the neurohypophysis and infundibulum are involved). There is enlargement and enhancement of the pituitary gland and thickening of the stalk. (if involved) (Fig. 11-23). Endocrinologic abnormalities can include all anterior pituitary hormonal functions, and when the infundibulum and neurohypophysis are affected, diabetes insipidus. The inflammation has been reported to occasionally extend into the cavernous sinus. Dynamic enhanced MR studies indicate that the blood supply to the posterior pituitary is compromised by the inflammatory process. The enlargement may regress spontaneously or with steroids.

Posterior Pituitary Tumors

Although unusual, tumors of the posterior pituitary gland occur and can often be diagnosed without much difficulty on MR (Fig. 11-24). Choristoma (or granular cell tumor or myoblastoma of the posterior pituitary) may produce visual or endocrinologic disturbance. They

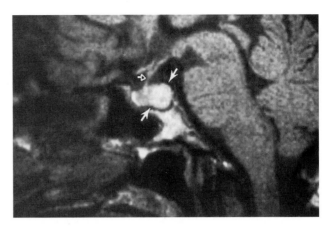

Fig. 11-24 Choristoma. Sagittal T1WI demonstrates this posterior pituitary tumor *(arrows)*. Observe that the mass is behind the infundibulum *(open arrow)* (and thus is located in the posterior pituitary) and is high intensity.

are of variable intensity on T1WI, proton density-weighted images (PDWI), and T2WI, and they enhance. However, some reports indicate a characteristic low intensity on T2WI. The key to the diagnosis is the sagittal MR, which localizes the lesion to the posterior pituitary. These tumors have also been reported in the suprasellar region and third ventricle. Choristoma may be vascular, so preoperative diagnosis is important.

Intrasellar Meningioma

Rarely an intrasellar meningioma can simulate the appearance of a pituitary tumor. These lesions are most

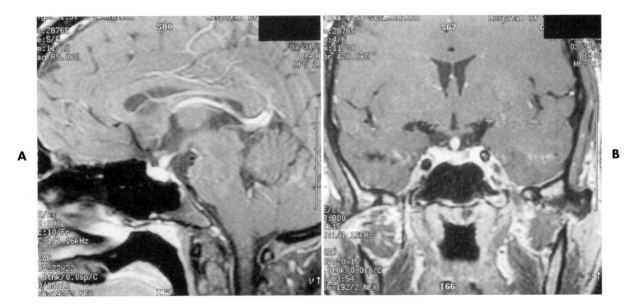

Fig. 11-23 Lymphocytic adenohypophysitis. Sagittal **(A)** and coronal **(B)** postcontrast T1WIs are remarkable for a prominent pituitary gland and vigorous enhancement with enlargement of the stalk. It should not be convex outward.

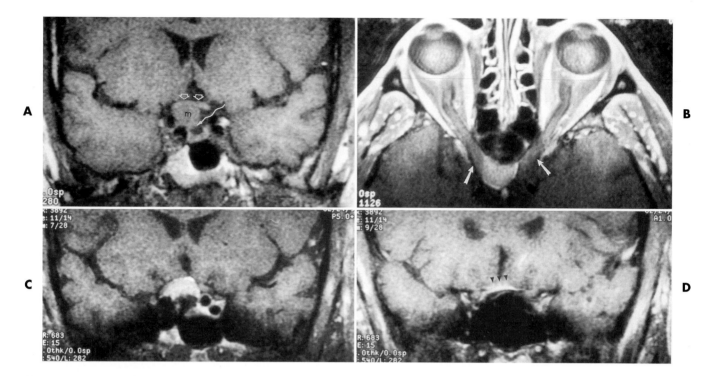

Fig. 11-25 Intrasellar meningioma. **A,** Unenhanced T1WI shows a mass *(m)* off the diaphragma sella *(squiggly arrow)*. The diaphragm is slightly depressed. Chiasmatic compression is present *(open arrows)*. **B,** The mass enhances. Its relationship to the two optic nerves *(arrows)* is worrisome on this axial scan. **C,** The bulk of the lesion enhances but so does the dural tail *(arrowheads)* extending anteriorly along the planum in **D.**

likely diaphragma sellae meningiomas (Fig. 11-25). The diagnosis can be suggested if the diaphragma sellae is visualized. In lesions originating in the suprasellar cistern the diaphragma should be depressed, whereas with intrasellar lesions the diaphragma is elevated. Careful observation also reveals slightly different intensity on MR between the meningioma and the inferior pituitary tissue. A dural tail and homogeneous enhancement may be visualized with meningioma, easily distinguishing it from pituitary adenoma.

Other Problems and Lesions of the Pituitary

Several other lesions and diagnostic dilemmas occur in the pituitary region. Rapid blood flow appears hypointense on MR, and it is the imaging modality of choice for vascular lesions or abnormalities in this area. Intrasellar carotid aneurysms or ectatic cavernous portions of the carotid arteries may produce sellar enlargement and mass effect (Fig. 11-26). About 50% of cases of persistent trigeminal artery (which arises from the carotid and courses posteriorly, penetrating the sella, before joining the basilar artery) have an intrasellar course (Fig. 11-27). Surgeons need to be informed and cognizant of these anatomic variations or else, after the transsphenoidal hypophysectomy, the radiologist may be on the

receiving end of an epistatic event. Rare primary intrasellar neoplasms include germinoma and melanoma. Infrequent inflammatory lesions occurring in the pituitary are cysticercosis, Erdheim-Chester disease (symmetric osteoblastic changes in the long bones, lipid-laden histiocytes and giant cells in bones and visceral organs, and rare suprasellar and/or sellar involvement), Langerhans cell histiocytosis (Histiocytosis X), Wegener granulomatosis, tuberculosis, and blastomycosis.

End-stage organ failure such as in hypothyroidism can produce pituitary gland enlargement. With its lack of a blood-brain barrier, the pituitary is susceptible to deposition diseases such as hemochromatosis, amyloidosis, and Hurler syndrome.

Empty sella syndrome CSF is easily noted in the empty or partially empty sella. This may be seen with aging and in women with pseudotumor cerebri (idiopathic intracranial hypertension). Other findings associated with pseudotumor include an enlarged optic nerve sheath, reversal of the optic nerve head (papilledema), small ventricles, enlarged or small extraventricular CSF spaces, and high intensity on T2WI within the white matter. Cases have been reported in which the appearance of the empty sella was observed to be reversible following treatment of the intracranial hypertension.

Secondary causes include pituitary infarction, surgery, and radiation therapy. Occasionally, the suprasellar

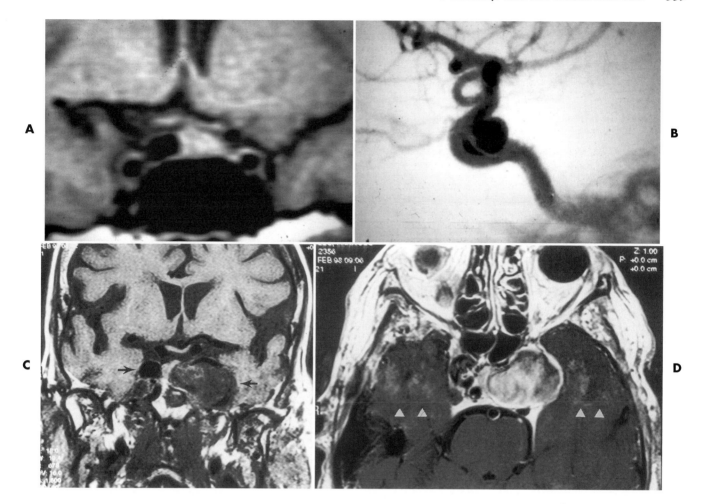

Fig. 11-26   Intrasellar aneurysms. **A,** Coronal T1WI shows a flow void along the pituitary gland on the right. **B,** Corresponding arteriogram confirms the aneurysm. **C,** Another patient with bilateral cavernous carotid aneurysms *(arrows)* had growth of the left one into the sella region. Who's doing transsphenoidal hypophysectomies today. Beware! **D,** Note the phase ghosting artifact *(arrowheads)* on the postcontrast axial scan confirming the vascular nature of the lesion for those of you who mistook the left-sided lesion in **C** for an epidermoid.

visual system is noted to herniate into the sella (Fig. 11-28). In fact, this results from traction from previous adhesions and from arachnoiditis. These patients seldom have symptoms. On coronal and sagittal images the herniated chiasm and floor of the third ventricle are noted in the sella. The partially empty sella is a normal variant and has virtually no clinical importance. The completely empty sella with secondary enlargement of the sellar floor is a secondary finding of previous disease. The completely empty sella may be associated with CSF rhinorrhea and distinguished from an arachnoid cyst. Even in cases of completely empty sellas, a remnant of pituitary tissue is squashed on the floor, so that these patients rarely have hypopituitarism.

Postoperative pituitary   The postoperative MR examination may reveal what appears to be persistent mass effect even though there is clinical evidence of chiasmatic decompression (Fig. 11-29). The effect of the surgery is best demonstrated by follow-up after 4 or more months. Additional postoperative changes include fat or other packing material in the sphenoid sinus and persistent enhancement in the operative tract (not to be confused with the optic tract).

Pituitary dwarfism   Pituitary dwarfism, produced by diminished levels of growth hormone, presents as delayed skeletal maturation, slow growth, short stature, and delayed dentition. More males than females have growth hormone deficiency, and isolated growth hormone deficiency can progress to multiple pituitary hormonal deficiencies. In most cases with only *isolated growth hormone deficiency* the infundibulum may be thin or truncated (most common), (rarely is it either normal or absent) and the adenohypophysis is either normal or small. Ectopic posterior pituitary glands are commonly seen. On the other hand patients with *multiple pituitary hormonal deficiencies* tend to have a small or absent anterior pituitary

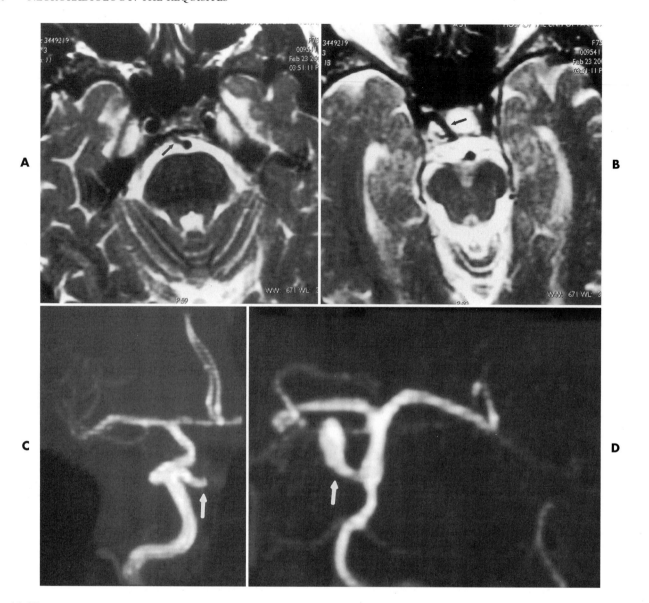

Fig. 11-27 Persistent trigeminal artery. **A** and **B,** T2WIs from pons **(A)** to midbrain **(B)** demonstrate a curious flow void *(arrows)* connecting the cavernous carotid artery with the basilar artery. The intrasellar course argues against an unusual PCOM. **C** and **D** from the MRA dramatically confirm the presence of a persistent trigeminal artery *(arrows)*.

and/or stalk, with the neurohypophysis being either ectopic or absent. The absent infundibulum and ectopic location of the normal posterior pituitary bright spot are identified on T1WI near the median eminence (ectopic posterior pituitary bright spot) (see Fig. 11-16). Thus, the presence of a thin stalk is very indicative of isolated growth hormone deficiency whereas its absence strongly suggests multiple pituitary hormonal abnormalities. To evaluate the pituitary stalk contrast enhancement is essential.

Finally, there is a subgroup of patients with hereditary isolated growth hormone deficiency due to a genetic defect that results in the inability to synthesize growth hormone. In this group of patients the pituitary hypothalamic region is normal.

The pituitary gland is smallest in dwarfs with an ectopic posterior pituitary but is also small in those dwarfs with a normal posterior lobe and growth hormone deficiency. The appearance of an ectopic posterior pituitary gland in a significant proportion of patients with pituitary dwarfism has been correlated with perinatal anoxic or ischemic episodes and breech delivery (although this is controversial).

Why do most patients with isolated growth hormone deficiency have normal posterior pituitary glands whereas multiple pituitary hormonal problems are associated with an ectopic posterior pituitary? The answer may be that the adenohypophysis does not function well in patients with an absent infundibulum. Disruption of the

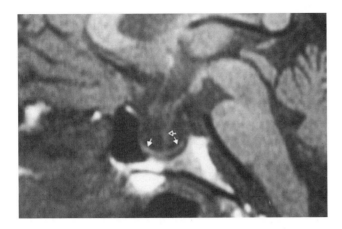

Fig. 11-28 Empty sella. Sella is expanded. Note the residual pituitary tissue *(arrows)* and infundibulum *(open arrow).*

infundibulum, which is distal to the ectopic neurohypophysis, interferes with the hypothalamohypophyseal portal system and anterior pituitary function. The neurohypophysis, which is ectopic and near the hypothalamus, functions normally. This is because communication still exists between the neurohypophysis and the hypothalamus, so that diabetes insipidus is not present. Isolated growth hormone deficiency may in some cases just be associated with abnormalities intrinsic to pituitary cells producing growth hormone or perhaps to partial transections of the infundibulum. Transections lead to bright signal above the cut, because of accumulations of neurosecretory granules.

The differential diagnosis of the ectopic posterior pituitary high signal includes tuber cinereum lipoma (look for chemical shift), Langerhans cell histiocytosis or other granulomatous processes (no high signal on T1WI), Rathke's cyst, craniopharyngioma, and fatty marrow in the tip of the dorsum.

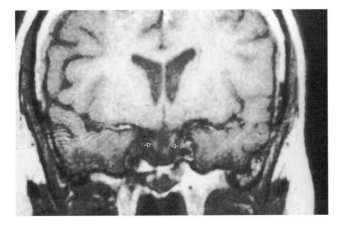

Fig. 11-29 Postoperative sella. Coronal T1WI shows the chiasm *(arrows)* tethered by adhesions into the postsurgical empty sella.

SUPRASELLAR LESIONS (Box 11-3)

The reader must be familiar with the appearance of the normal suprasellar cistern. On axial images at the level of the pons it has the configuration of a five-pointed star whereas just above, in the region of the midbrain, it is a six-pointed star (the brain has no religious preference). The hypothalamus and third ventricle mark its superior extent. The infundibulum runs through it, the optic chiasm lives in it, and the circle of Willis circumscribes its lateral margins. Make no mistake about it, this real estate is more expensive than anything in Tokyo (even before its real estate crash). Distortion of any aspect of this anatomy, or soft tissue replacing the normal CSF, should alert radiologists that this may be "the real thing," and they should study the images carefully so that the abnormality can be defined.

Infundibular Lesions (Box 11-4)

The infundibulum should generally not be larger than the basilar artery at the level of the clivus. Granulomatous diseases (Langerhans cell histiocytosis, sarcoid, tuberculosis, Erdheim-Chester disease) can enlarge the infundibulum. In many cases, these lesions involve the hypothalamus as well. Granulomas of the infundibular-hypothalamic region can be isointense to brain and enhance (Fig. 11-30). The differential diagnosis of this lesion is chiasmatic/hypothalamic glioma. Diabetes insipidus is a common finding in lesions affecting the stalk and hypothalamus. Other lesions that can involve

Box 11-3 Suprasellar Lesions

Aneurysm
Arachnoid cyst
Cavernous hemangioma
Chiasmatic or hypothalamic glioma
Craniopharyngioma
Cysticercosis or echinococcal cysts
Dermoid
Enlarged third ventricle extending into cistern
Epidermoid
Germinoma
Hamartoma of tuberculum
Infundibular lesions (see Box 11-4)
Lipoma
Lymphoma
Meningioma
Pituitary adenoma
Rathke's cleft cyst
Sarcoid and other granulomatous infections
Teratoma

Box 11-4 Infundibular Lesions

GRANULOMATOUS DISEASES

Sarcoid
Langerhans' cell histiocytosis
TB
Erdheim-Chester

TUMORS

Lymphoma
Metastases
Astrocytoma
Germinoma
Prolactinoma
Rathke's cleft cyst
Craniopharyngioma
Stalk transection

the infundibulum include metastasis, lymphoma, germinoma, craniopharyngioma, Rathke's cleft cyst, and prolactinoma.

An interesting but uncommon observation in prolactinoma is stalk enlargement, identified before surgery. If the lesion is subsequently "totally resected," then the stalk should return to normal size. Failure of this to occur suggests incomplete tumor resection.

Rathke's Cleft Cyst

Rathke's cleft cysts arise from Rathke's pouch and may be found in the anterior sellar and/or anterior suprasellar region. They are benign lesions lined with cuboidal or columnar epithelium, which may be ciliated and may contain goblet cells. The cysts may contain mucus. The difference between this lesion and craniopharyngioma is in the wall cell type. In craniopharyngioma, this is made of thick walls of squamous or basal cells. Rathke's cleft cysts may cause visual disturbances, pituitary insufficiency, or diabetes insipidus. These lesions have variable intensities on both T1WI and T2WI (Fig. 11-31). Their MR intensity is related to the contents of the cyst (e.g., protein, paramagnetic). The principal differential diagnosis of Rathke's cleft cyst is craniopharyngioma. CT may be useful here because of its sensitivity to calcification as compared with MR. In general, Rathke's cleft cysts do not calcify whereas a high percentage of craniopharyngiomas do. They have a smooth contour with homogeneous signal intensity within the lesion. Rathke's cleft cysts enhance much less consistently than craniopharyngioma, usually with just a rimlike configuration as opposed to solid or nodular enhancement in craniopharyngioma. This rim enhancement has been attributed in some cases to displaced pi-

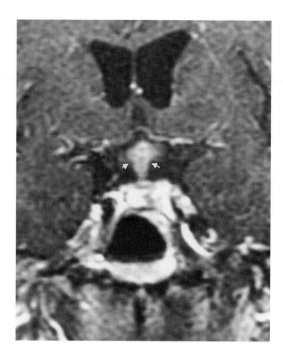

Fig. 11-30 Sarcoid involving the infundibulum. Coronal enhanced T1WI of an enlarged thickened infundibulum in a patient with intracranial sarcoid.

tuitary tissue and has not been associated with squamous metaplasia, hemosiderin, or cholesterol within the cyst wall. It also did not correlate with inflammation.

Arachnoid Cyst

Approximately 15% of all arachnoid cysts arise in the suprasellar region. It is hypothesized that they arise developmentally as a result of a lack of perforation of the membrane of Liliequist. If the membrane is imperforate, normal CSF flow anterior to the pons can produce a wind

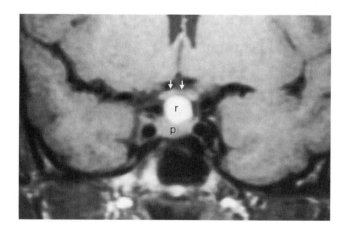

Fig. 11-31 Rathke's cleft cyst. Coronal T1WI of Rathke's cleft cyst *(r)*, which is in the suprasellar cistern. It is high intensity on T1WI. The pituitary *(p)* and optic chiasm *(arrows)* are identified.

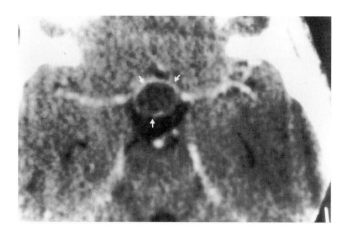

Fig. 11-32 Arachnoid cyst. Enhanced CT shows a smoothly marginated suprasellar mass *(arrows)*. Note the absence of enhancement in the mass. Arachnoid cyst displaces the normal vasculature around it. Density is slightly different from that of the rest of the suprasellar cistern. This can occasionally be seen in arachnoid cysts.

sock, which can subsequently close off and become a true cyst or may remain as an arachnoid pouch. Such a cyst produces mass effect on adjacent structures, including hypothalamus, chiasm, and brain stem (Fig. 11-32). These cysts can grow and produce hydrocephalus. Age at presentation is variable, from childhood to the second or third decade of life.

FLAIR and/or diffusion weighted images (DWI) easily separate these lesions from epidermoids (Fig. 11-33). The

density and intensity of these cysts are those of CSF. They are not associated with enhancement or calcification. However, if the arachnoid cyst invaginates into the third ventricle, it can be mistaken for an ependymal cyst (neuroepithelial cyst) of the third ventricle or an enlarged third ventricle on the basis of aqueductal stenosis (which you should see on the MR). The key here is to determine whether you can separate the third ventricle from the lesion (if you can, it is most likely an arachnoid cyst). Cisternography can be helpful in separating these lesions. Prompt filling with contrast indicates a dilated third ventricle as opposed to an arachnoid cyst. The sagittal MR is also particularly useful in trying to sort this out, but at times only the pathologist will know for sure.

Midline Developmental Lesions

Lipoma, teratoma, dermoid Dermoid, lipoma, teratoma, and epidermoid have already been discussed in Chapters 3 and 9. All can arise in the suprasellar cistern. On MR, high intensity on T1WI from fat is observed in lipomas, dermoids, and teratomas. Lipomas in this region are usually circumscribed (Fig. 11-34). Teratomas and dermoids can grow to be large, compressing the third ventricle and adjacent structures. Teratomas may contain dense calcification or ossification, which has been observed to be in the central portion of the lesion. Dermoids rarely arise in the suprasellar region (Fig. 11-35). They are midline lesions containing fat, squamous epithelium (as do epidermoids), hair follicles, sweat glands,

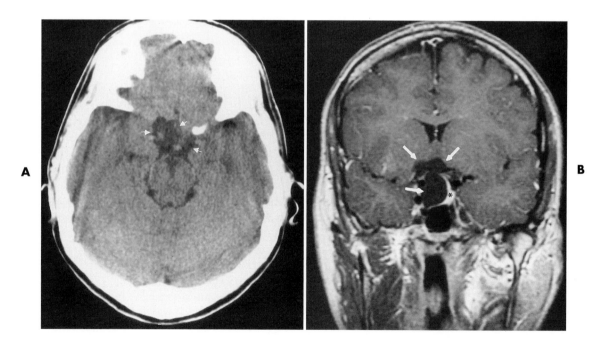

Fig. 11-33 Epidermoid. **A,** Unenhanced CT of a suprasellar epidermoid *(arrows)*. Lesion is irregular and distorts the suprasellar cistern. No calcification is seen. **B,** Coronal enhanced T1WI shows the extent of the lesion *(arrows)*, which actually distorts the pituitary gland *(*)* and infundibulum. It has the same intensity as CSF.   *Illustration continued on following page*

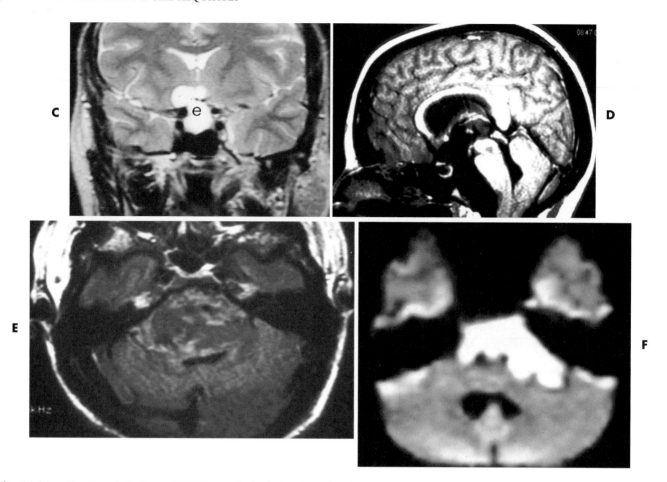

Fig. 11-33 *Continued.* **C,** Coronal T2W1 reveals the lesion (e) to be the same intensity as CSF. **D,** Sagittal t1W1 reveals a low-intensity mass extending along the clivus to the suprasellar region. **E,** On FLAIR, the mass is brighter than CSF. **F,** Babing. The DWI scan nails the diagnosis of an epidermoid.

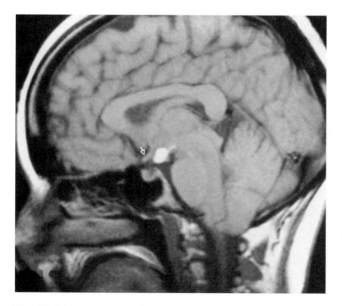

Fig. 11-34 Lipoma in the suprasellar cistern. A high intensity mass is seen on this sagittal T1WI, representing a lipoma in the suprasellar cistern. Optic chiasm *(arrow)* is anterior to the lipoma.

and sebaceous glands. Their capsules are thick with peripheral calcification.

Epidermoid The perisellar epidermoid is a much more difficult differential diagnosis. This lesion can have the same density and intensity on CT and MR as CSF. In the vast majority of cases it is of slightly higher density and intensity than CSF. It may be intradural or extradural, and can arise in the third ventricle and in the parasellar region around the gasserian ganglion, where it can erode the petrous apex. It can have a variegated appearance, which is best appreciated on CT after intrathecal contrast (with contrast accumulating in its interstices). Epidermoids insinuate throughout the suprasellar region and can grow behind the clivus, thereby pushing the brain stem posteriorly. Note the position of the basilar artery relative to the clivus (see Fig. 11-33). If there is more "CSF" space anterior to the basilar artery and the brain stem—guess what—it usually ain't CSF, it's epidermoid. Occasionally, epidermoids may have rim calcification. These lesions rarely if ever enhance. Fortunately, the diagnosis of these lesions has been made rather simple with the advent of FLAIR and difu$$ion weighted imaging.

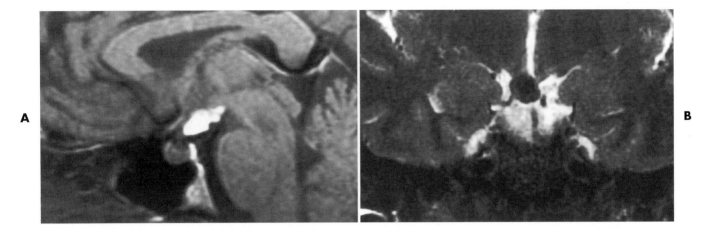

Fig. 11-35   Dermoid in suprasellar region. **A,** The fat of the dermoid looks very much like the lipoma in Fig. 11-34. **B,** Note decreased intensity of fat on this T2WI.

Here the lesion can be clearly separated from CSF being high intensity on both of the sequences. If you do not have these pulse sequences you need to be careful and spend some extra time while those who have them can generate more RVUs (to pay for the software).

Parasitic Infection

Cysticercosis or echinococcal parasitic cysts can be identified in this location. They are usually inhomogeneous and may be calcified. We threw in this caveat for the Third World radiologists who may not get the humor but are most familiar with these diseases. This one's for you!—Xie, Xie!

Craniopharyngioma

Craniopharyngiomas may be seen in children and adults. In children, they account for a greater percentage of tumor cases, but more than 50% of these lesions occur in adults. They comprise between 1.2% and 3% of all intracranial tumors. Their epicenter is usually in the suprasellar (90%), sellar, or infrasellar regions, but they can be extensive, including the anterior fossa, middle fossa, posterior fossa, retroclival region, and the lateral ventricles (Fig. 11-36). Other rare origins include the third ventricle (see following discussion), sphenoid bone, nasopharynx, cerebellopontine angle, and pineal gland. A good rule is that if the tumor looks bizarre and has a component at the base of the skull, think craniopharyngioma. They arise from metaplasia of squamous epithelial remnants (Rathke's pouch) of the adenohypophysis and anterior infundibulum, or from ectopic embryonic cell rests of enamel organs. Histologically, craniopharyngiomas are distinguished by palisading adamantinous epithelium, calcification, and keratin nodule formation. Another variety of craniopharyngioma,

termed squamous papillary craniopharyngioma, is a solid noncalcified tumor occurring predominantly in adults (see following discussion). Patients are seen with a variety of signs and symptoms including visual disturbances, endocrine abnormalities, mental changes, motor deficits, and raised intracranial pressure.

As with most issues in radiology, there is controversy here. Some groups do not find true distinct radiologic or histopathologic types of tumors (adamantinomatous versus squamous papillary) (Table 11-2). Other groups claim that craniopharyngiomas can be divided into these two clinical, histologic, and radiologic subtypes.

Three imaging hallmarks of craniopharyngioma have been identified (although an individual lesion may have from none to all these characteristics): (1) calcification, (2) cyst formation, and (3) enhancement (solid, nodular). Calcification may be nodular or rimlike, occurring in approximately 80% of cases. Cystic regions are observed in about 85% of cases. Because of its relative insensitivity to calcification, MR is not as specific as CT for the diagnosis of craniopharyngioma. Another plus for CT is that cyst formation is low density on CT, whereas cystic fluid can have a variable intensity on MR.

The intensity on T1WI ranges from hypointense to hyperintense and is usually high intensity on T2WI. The solid portion of the tumor enhances. The high intensity on T1WI appears not to be due to cholesterol or triglycerides but rather to methemoglobin and/or high protein (>9000 mg/dL). Some ultra-high-protein craniopharyngiomas are low intensity on T1WI. This has been attributed to the increased viscosity associated with such elevated protein levels.

The intraventricular variety of craniopharyngioma is unusual, probably originating from the pars tuberalis that extends to the tuber cinereum in the floor of the third ventricle (see Fig. 11-36). These lesions do not extend beneath the floor of the third ventricle (i.e., are not in

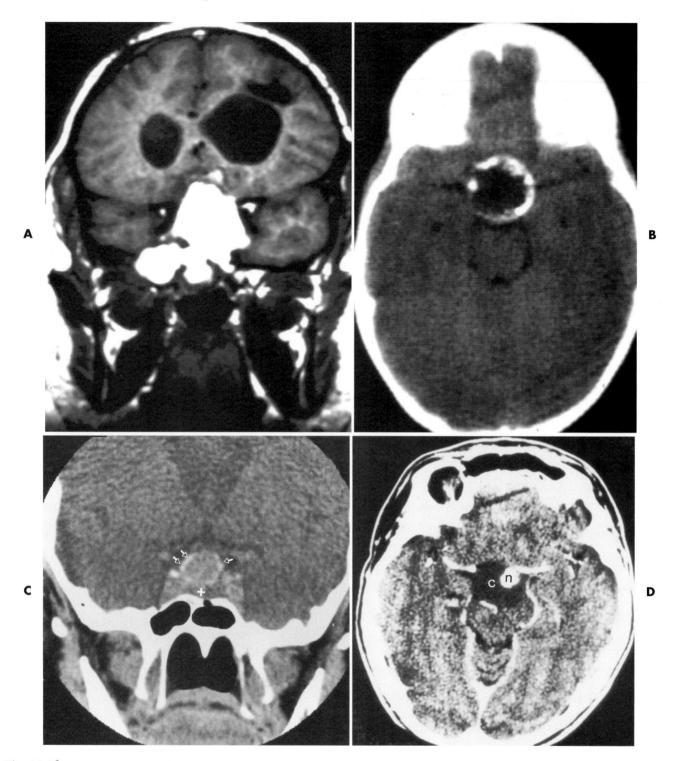

Fig. 11-36 Montage of craniopharyngiomas. **A,** Case 1. This postoperative study shows residual infrasellar and sellar high intensity mass with a focal area of signal void calcification characteristic of a craniopharyngioma. **B,** Case 2. Note the calcified rim around this cystic craniopharyngioma in the midline. **C to E,** Case 3. Multiple faces of craniopharyngioma. **C,** Coronal unenhanced CT demonstrates eggshell calcification in a suprasellar craniopharyngioma *(open arrows);* pituitary is identified *(+).* **D,** Axial enhanced CT depicts an enhancing nodule associated with a large cyst *(c)* in this noncalcified craniopharyngioma.

Illustration continued on following page

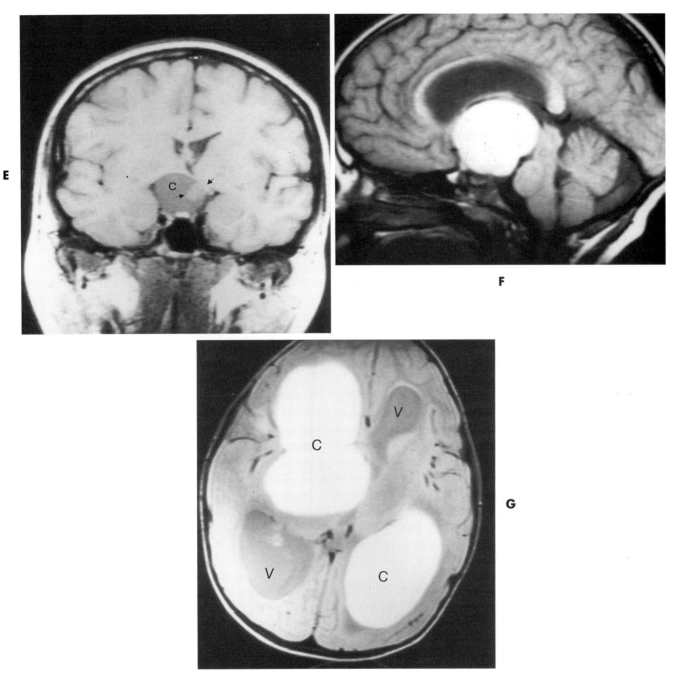

Fig. 11-36   *Continued.. **E,*** Coronal T1WI of the same lesion as in **D.** Note the tumor nodule *(arrows)* and the cyst *(c),* which has fluid that is hypointense to normal brain. **F,** Case 4. A sellar and suprasellar high intensity mass on T1WI (use powerpoint figure) has extension into the lateral ventricles in **G. G,** Axial PDWI shows the superior extension of the craniopharyngioma *(C)* into the lateral ventricles *(V).*

the suprasellar space). Other features distinguishing these lesions include their incidence in adults and their male preponderance. Hormonal and visual disturbances are rare, again because of their intraventricular location. There is a low incidence of calcification or cyst formation (as opposed to the run-of-the-mill craniopharyngioma), with uniform enhancement. This solid intraventricular lesion has no specific hallmarks. The differential

diagnosis of such third ventricular lesions besides the rare papillary craniopharyngioma is important and includes cavernous malformation of the third ventricle, choroid plexus papilloma, ependymoma, pilocytic astrocytoma, and meningioma.

Fusiform dilatation (pseudoaneurysm formation) of the supraclinoid carotid artery has been reported postoperatively in craniopharyngioma; however, to date no

Table 11-2   Histopathologic types of craniopharyngioma

	Adamatinous	Squamous-papillary
Location	Suprasellar	Intrasellar/suprasellar or suprasellar
Age	Children, occasionally adults	Adults
Tissue structure	Predominantly cystic	Predominantly solid
T1 without contrast	Hyperintense cysts typical	If ever hypointense cysts
Shape	Lobulated	Spherical
Encase vessels	yes	no
Tumor recurrence	+++	+
calcifications	+++	+

cases of subsequent subarachnoid hemorrhage have been reported.

Meningioma

Meningiomas in this region arise from the tuberculum sellae, anterior clinoid processes, diaphragma sellae, planum sphenoidale, and upper clivus. They tend to be challenging to diagnose and treat. Progressive visual loss is the most frequent complaint. As stated in Chapter 3, meningiomas have a heterogeneous texture, and are extraaxial in location, buckling the gray-white interface. CT can reveal hyperostosis, blistering of the tuberculum and planum sphenoidale, and erosion of the dorsum sellae.

On T1WI meningiomas are isointense to slightly hypointense and usually can be appreciated by a keen observer (who already knows the answer), who will notice some extra tissue in this region (Fig. 11-37). On T2WI, they are isointense to slightly hyperintense to brain. These lesions are generally not cystic. They enhance dramatically. On angiography, they have a characteristic stain from ophthalmic and carotid meningeal branches. Remember meningiomas commonly narrow the carotid artery. Careful imaging is critical because these tumors may be small and at times difficult to separate from normally enhancing pituitary tissue.

Chiasmatic and Hypothalamic Astrocytoma (Glioma)

Chiasmatic astrocytoma presents as a mass lesion in the suprasellar cistern. It is isointense to brain on T1WI and high intensity on T2WI. This high intensity may be noted throughout the visual pathway (Fig. 11-38). This is of uncertain significance. Enhancement is variable, and calcification in the nonirradiated tumor is rare. At times, a cystic component (high intensity on T2WI) is present with the tumor. Bilateral optic nerve astrocytomas are associated with neurofibromatosis. Hypothalamic astrocytomas and gangliogliomas may be difficult to distinguish from chiasmatic lesions because they may have similar intensity patterns. A normal chiasm, with an inhomogeneous mass in the floor of the third ventricle and suprasellar cistern, suggests a hypothalamic as opposed to a chiasmatic astrocytoma. The optic radiations are not involved in this lesion.

Hamartoma of the Tuber Cinereum

Hamartomas of the tuber cinereum are known to cause central precocious puberty and gelastic seizures (spasmodic laughter), an excuse for outbursts while you read this book. These lesions are congenital nonneoplastic heterotopias. The tuberoinfundibular tract probably carries releasing hormones that modulate gonadotropins. The mechanism for precocious puberty is neurosecretion by the hamartoma of luteinizing hormone–releasing hormone. Seizures may result from connections between the lesion and the limbic system or possibly, if present, associated brain abnormalities. It is odd that pituitary gland hypertrophy has not been reported in cases of precocious puberty associated with hamartomas of the tuber cinereum. Rarely, they coexist with other congenital anomalies, although there are some reports of associated abnormalities including callosal agenesis, optic malformation, heterotopias, and microgyria. These findings might indicate an insult in the first month of gestation. These tumors can be completely resected when they are pedunculated with amelioration of symptoms.

The anatomic location of these hamartomas (just anterior to the mamillary bodies) together with a signal intensity similar to gray matter on T1WI and most often higher intensity than gray matter on PDWI and particularly T2WI, strongly supports this diagnosis (Fig. 11-39). Morphologically, hamartomas may be pedunculated or broad based, from 0.4 to 4 cm in diameter. The run-of-the-mill hamartoma of the tuber cinereum does not cal-

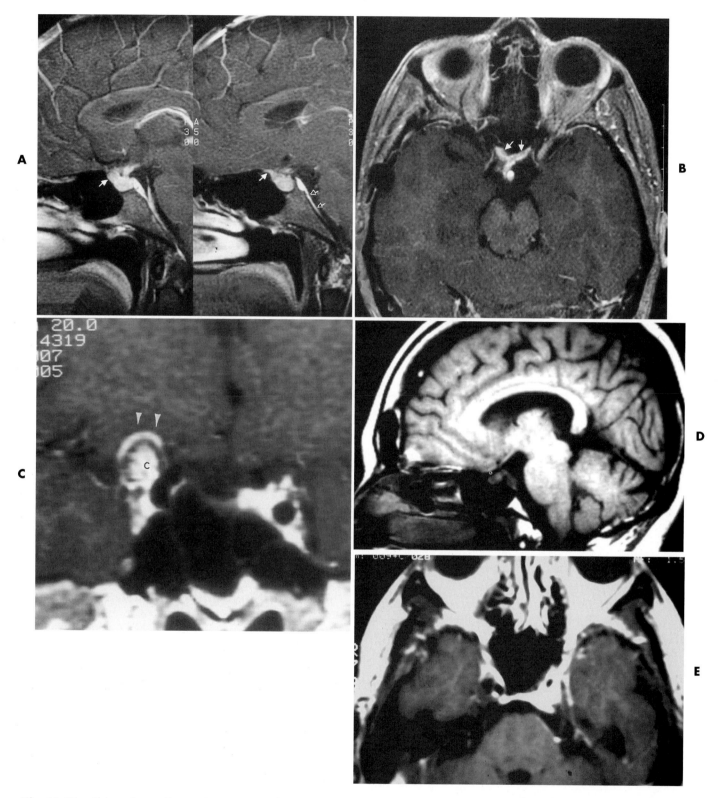

Fig. 11-37   Tuberculum sellae meningioma. **A,** Enhanced sagittal images reveal an extra bump *(arrow)* in the region of the tuberculum sellae. Figure at *right* demonstrates a dural tail *(closed arrow)* and basivertebral venous plexus *(open arrows)*. **B,** Meningioma has grown along both optic nerves, which are enhancing *(arrows)*. **C,** This meningioma *(arrowheads)* caused hyperostosis of the right anterior clinoid *(c)*. **D,** Sagittal T1WI shows a small soft-tissue mass along the superior portion of the clivus in a patient with an isolated sixth nerve palsy *(arrows)*. **E,** Axial image reveals enhancement of this dural-based mass. Dr. Dorello was paged to explain the sixth nerve palsy.

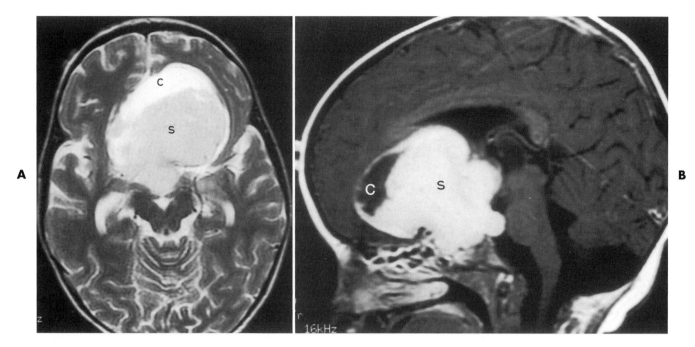

Fig. 11-38 Pilocytic astrocytoma of chiasm-hypothalamic origin. **A,** A huge mass with cystic *(c)* and solid *(s)* components infiltrates anteriorly from the suprasellar region. **B,** Enhancement of this degree is typical of pilocytic astrocytomas but does not imply high grade (see Chapter 3).

cify, enhance, contain fat, or have cysts (but there are exceptions to this and every other generalization in this book and in imaging). Histologically, they are composed of neurons supported by normal microglia. These lesions tend to be stable over time.

Can we distinguish this lesion from craniopharyngioma and hypothalamic glioma? It would be unusual for the latter to be isointense to brain on T1WI. CT is also more specific for calcification (craniopharyngioma). The hypothalamic glioma and the craniopharyngioma are

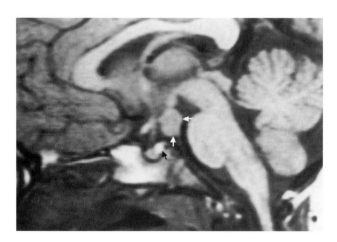

Fig. 11-39 Hamartoma of the tuber cinereum. Pedunculated mass extending from the tuber cinereum *(white arrows)* is isointense to brain. Note the high signal in the posterior pituitary gland *(black arrow).*

both heterogeneous lesions compared with the homogeneous appearance of the hamartoma. The absence of enhancement greatly favors hamartoma. Morphology, location, and clinical history usually make this a straightforward Aunt Minnie diagnosis.

Aneurysm

The diagnosis of aneurysm on MR has already been discussed and is elementary even for Dr. Watson, as long as there is no clot. Partially thrombosed giant aneurysms contain a flow void and signal intensities from the various stages of clot (see Fig. 11-26). Angiography is required to characterize the exact site of origin and identify the neck. Cavernous hemangiomas can also occur in the suprasellar region, and they have appearances similar to those in other locations in the brain (Fig. 11-40).

Germinoma

These lesions have a propensity for children and young adults. Presentation is variable, but common findings include diabetes insipidus, hypopituitarism, and optic chiasm compression. They arise from primitive germ cells in the suprasellar region. They appear as mass lesions, which may be locally invasive. On CT germinomas are high density on unenhanced scan and uniformly enhance (Fig. 11-41). The density is similar to lymphoma and probably the result of the increased tumor protein. These lesions do not calcify. Coexisting pineal masses

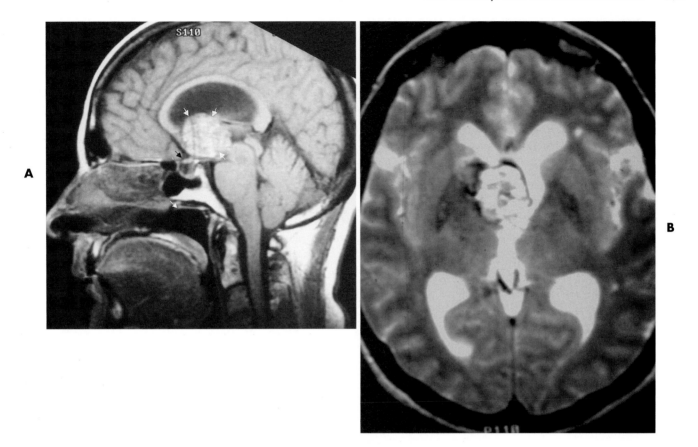

Fig. 11-40   **A,** Cavernous hemangioma. Sagittal T1WI shows a large, round, mottled high intensity suprasellar mass *(arrows)* above the chiasm *(black arrow).* **B,** The hemosiderin around the lesion is best seen on the long TR image.

may be identified. They can metastasize by subarachnoid seeding. On MR, there is less specificity between this lesion and other soft-tissue tumors in this region.

PARASELLAR LESIONS

Cavernous Sinus Lesions

The authors will try not to reiterate the imaging characteristics of lesions that have already been commented on earlier in this chapter and in other chapters in the book. Rather, we will focus on what other characteristics in this particular location aid in making the diagnosis. Lesions of the cavernous sinus (Box 11-5) tend to enlarge it by either focally bulging (aneurysms) or smoothly enlarging its lateral margin.

Vascular Lesions

Aneurysm and cavernous hemangioma Aneurysms may erode and undermine the anterior clinoid processes, and are associated with either obvious flow voids or layers of thrombus. You can make the diagnosis on the T1WI, and this can be supplemented by

magnetic resonance and conventional angiography. MR has in most cases taken the guesswork out of this lesion. Cavernous sinus aneurysms produce mass effect on the intracavernous cranial nerves. When they rupture, they create carotid-cavernous fistula as opposed to intradural aneurysms, which produce subarachnoid hemorrhage.

Cavernous hemangiomas have been reported in Meckel's cave and in the cavernous sinus. The limited reports of these lesions indicate that in contrast to the appearance of the typical intracranial cavernous hemangioma, the lesion lacks a hemosiderin rim, central large regions of hemorrhage, and calcification (thus it is probably an impossible diagnosis to make, but we threw it in at no extra cost for your reading pleasure).

Carotid-cavernous fistula or dural malformation Carotid-cavernous fistula or dural malformation can enlarge the cavernous sinus. Associated with a prominent sinus is usually an enlarged superior ophthalmic vein. Occasionally, dilated intercavernous sinus collateral veins can be identified. This can be seen on an angiogram when an ipsilateral carotid artery is injected and the contralateral cavernous sinus and its tributaries are opacified (Fig. 11-42; also see Fig. 10-34). These lesions have already been discussed in Chapters 5, 10, and 12.

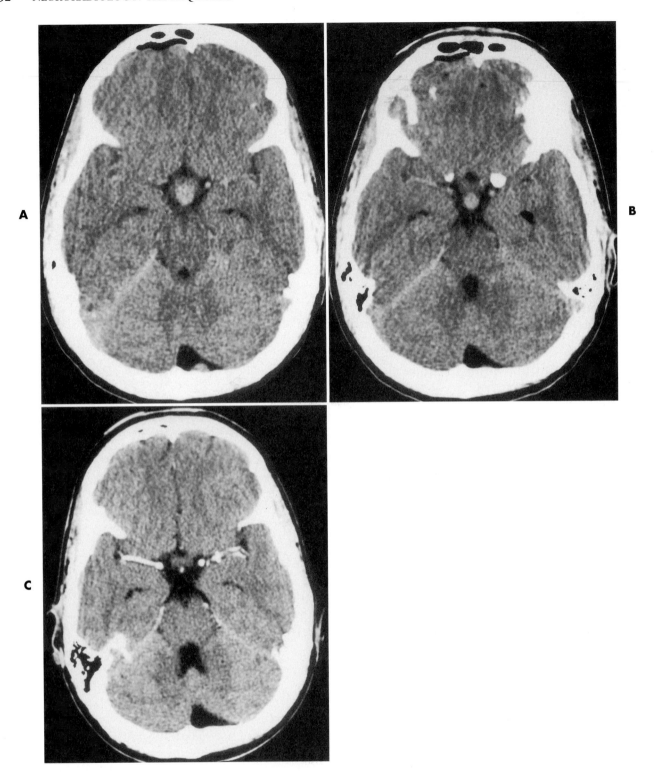

Fig. 11-41   Germinoma. **A,** Noncontrast CT demonstrates high density in a suprasellar mass representing a germinoma. **B,** Noncontrast CT inferior to A shows high density in a markedly enlarged infundibulum containing germinoma. **C,** Postcontrast CT following radiation therapy. Observe the normal infundibulum.

Box 11-5   Cavernous Sinus Lesions

Chondrosarcoma
Chordoma
Fat
Idiopathic inflammatory disease (Tolosa-Hunt syndrome)
Infection
Lymphoma
Meningioma
Metastasis (including perineural spread of tumor)
Pituitary adenoma
Plasmacytoma
Schwannoma (cranial nerves III, IV, V, and VI)
Vascular lesions (ectatic carotids, carotid-cavernous
    fistula, cavernous carotid aneurysm, cavernous he-
    mangioma, and cavernous sinus thrombosis)

Thrombosis of the cavernous sinus   Thrombosis of the cavernous sinus may occur as part of a septic process associated with spontaneous dural malformations or may result from an interventional or surgical procedure. The last situation most commonly occurs in conjunction with carotid-cavernous fistula or dural malformation. On MR without enhancement, high intensity may be seen in the occluded cavernous sinus. However, many times the sinus may be only partially occluded. Enhancement on MR is not very useful because nonthrombosed regions of the sinus enhance, and clot is also high intensity. On CT, irregularly enhancing sinus can be detected. An enlarged superior ophthalmic vein, periorbital swelling, or thickening of the extraocular muscles should send your eyes searching for clot in the cavernous sinus. Be careful not to confuse filling defects on CT or high intensity on T1WI in the cavernous sinus with fat seen in normal persons and in patients with Cushing's disease.

Intravascular papillary endothelial hyperplasia is an unusual form of thrombus organization with excessive papillary endothelial proliferation usually confined to the lumen of preexisting vessels. These lesions have been reported to occur in the cavernous sinus and extend into the sella and can mimic pituitary or cavernous sinus tumors.

Cavernous Sinus Meningioma

Cavernous sinus meningiomas are slightly different from other meningiomas. In general, they follow the lateral margin of the cavernous sinus and may extend posteriorly along the tentorial margin with a dove's tail appearance (Fig. 11-43). The lateral margin of the sinus is smoothly bulged. Meningiomas can encase or distort the cavernous portion of the internal carotid artery. Their intrinsic characteristics on CT, MR, or angiography are similar to those of meningiomas in other locations. Meningiomas in rare instances can extend through the base of the skull.

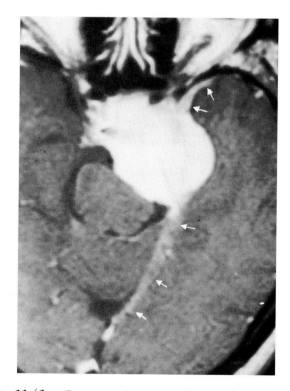

Fig. 11-43   Cavernous sinus meningioma. A large homogeneously enhancing cavernous sinus mass is identified. The lesion bulges the sinus laterally and presents with enhancement along its anterior and posterior (dove's tail) dural margins *(arrows)*.

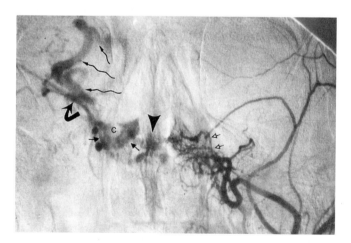

Fig. 11-42   Dural malformation with filling of contralateral superior ophthalmic vein and cavernous sinus. AP waters projection with injection of the left external carotid artery demonstrates filling of the ipsilateral cavernous sinus *(open arrows)* as well as filling via the coronary sinus *(arrowhead)* (intercavernous sinus) to the contralateral cavernous sinus *(arrows)*. Note the defect in the right cavernous sinus produced by the carotid artery *(c)*. The superior *(squiggly arrows)* and inferior *(curved arrow)* ophthalmic veins are identified.

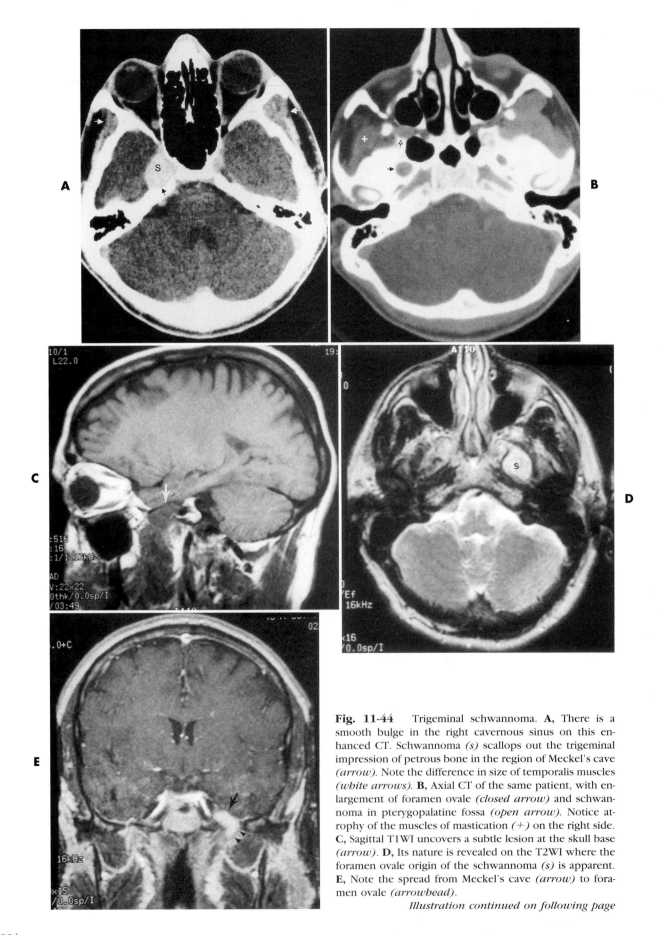

Fig. 11-44 Trigeminal schwannoma. **A,** There is a smooth bulge in the right cavernous sinus on this enhanced CT. Schwannoma *(s)* scallops out the trigeminal impression of petrous bone in the region of Meckel's cave *(arrow)*. Note the difference in size of temporalis muscles *(white arrows)*. **B,** Axial CT of the same patient, with enlargement of foramen ovale *(closed arrow)* and schwannoma in pterygopalatine fossa *(open arrow)*. Notice atrophy of the muscles of mastication *(+)* on the right side. **C,** Sagittal T1WI uncovers a subtle lesion at the skull base *(arrow)*. **D,** Its nature is revealed on the T2WI where the foramen ovale origin of the schwannoma *(s)* is apparent. **E,** Note the spread from Meckel's cave *(arrow)* to foramen ovale *(arrowhead)*.

Illustration continued on following page

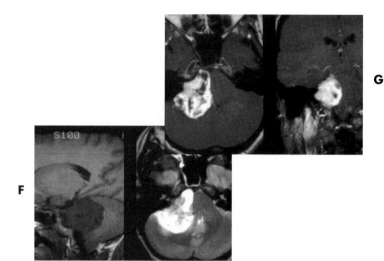

Fig. 11-44 *Continued.* **F** and **G.** The cystic and solid nature of this schwannoma is evident on the T2WI and the postcontrast scans. Cystic degeneration is more commonly seen in schwannomas than meningiomas.

Trigeminal Schwannoma

Trigeminal schwannomas are rare tumors (<0.4% of brain tumors) arising from the intracranial portion of the trigeminal nerve. They can be based predominantly in the middle cranial fossa, in the region of the gasserian ganglion (most common) or the posterior fossa (next most common), or may be dumbbell shaped (least common), involving both regions. The peak incidence of these tumors is in the fourth decade of life, with an equal prevalence between men and women. The most frequent symptom is trigeminal nerve dysfunction, including pain, numbness, and paresthesias.

On MR, they are smooth masses, isointense on T1WI and high intensity on T2WI, with avid enhancement (Fig. 11-44). Regions of "cystic" change may be observed in the enhancing mass. They may grow through neural foramina, producing smooth enlargement, and can be traced from the pons, prepontine cistern, and gasserian ganglia into the cavernous sinus. Sagittal MR is useful in following the course of the tumor along the nerve. On CT, particularly with bone windows, erosion can be appreciated at the petrous apex. The differential diagnosis of petrous apex erosion includes epidermoid tumor, giant petrous apex cholesterol cyst (granuloma), acoustic schwannoma, meningioma, mucocele, chordoma, metastasis, osteochondroma, and chondrosarcoma. Most of these lesions are readily distinguished from trigeminal schwannoma. Other findings associated with the slow growth of the tumor are erosion of the floor of the middle fossa and enlargement of the foramen ovale, foramen rotundum, and superior orbital fissure. Other lesions of Meckel's cave include meningioma, epidermoid, dermoid, lipoma, and metastases (see following subsection).

In general, schwannomas occur much more frequently on sensory nerves than they do on pure motor nerves. Thus, although they have been reported on cranial nerves III, IV, and VI, such lesions are zebras. Other rare lesions of the proximal portion of cranial nerve V include lipoma, epidermoid, metastasis (subarachnoid spread of tumor, breast, lymphoma), and inflammatory disease.

Imaging studies are performed in the workup of trigeminal neuralgia. In such cases the surgeons are looking for causes of tic douloureux, including (1) mass lesions such as a schwannoma, (2) vascular lesions (large looping vessels, arteriovenous malformations, cryptic malformations), and (3) other causes (such as multiple sclerosis). We cannot see the small vessels compressing the nerve; however, the other causes of this condition are well demonstrated by MR.

Melanocytoma

Primary melanocytomas are relatively benign lesions originating from the leptomeninges. These lesions are at one end of the spectrum that also includes primary or secondary meningeal melanoma. Primary melanocytoma has been reported to occur in the cavernous sinus, or in Meckel's cave. The tumor can be hyperdense on unenhanced CT and increased signal on T1 and hypointense on T2WI. These lesions have been reported not to enhance.

Perineural Spread of Tumor

The region of Meckel's cave including the gasserian ganglion is also a site for metastatic disease. Metastases occur via neurotropic, subarachnoid, and hematogenous spread. Such dissemination indicates a poor prognosis. Head and neck tumors may demonstrate perineural spread through the foramen at the skull base and into the brain. Adenoid cystic carcinoma, basal cell carcinoma, squamous cell carcinoma, lymphoma, mucoepi-

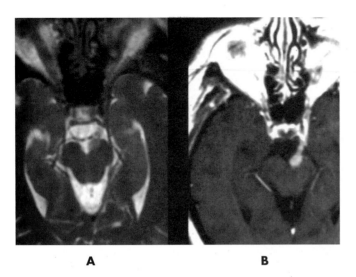

Fig. 11-45   Lymphoma of cranial nerve III. Infiltration of the third nerve is best viewed on the post contrast scan **(B)**, but the enlargement is even evident on the T2WI **(A)**.

dermoid carcinoma, melanoma, and schwannoma all have a propensity for this kind of infiltration (Fig. 11-45). Enlargement or asymmetry of any basal neural foramina in the appropriate clinical setting should alert you to this possibility. Infections such as actinomycosis, Lyme disease, and herpes zoster can also demonstrate perineural involvement. Rare reports of cranial nerve lesions include primary ependymoma, amyloidoma, glioblastoma multiforme, and eosinophilic granuloma.

The third division of cranial nerve V, because of its extensive neural network about the head and neck, is particularly prone to perineural spread of lesions. Such spread may be orthograde, such as in schwannoma or in metastasis beginning in Meckel's cave, or retrograde from peripheral involvement. The findings that can be noted with perineural invasion along the third division of cranial nerve V include (1) thickening of the nerve, (2) concentric enlargement of the foramen ovale, (3) replacement of the normal CSF density and intensity in the trigeminal cistern (region of Meckel's cave) by a soft-tissue mass, (4) mass in the cavernous sinus, and (5) atrophy of the ipsilateral masticator muscles (Fig. 11-46).

Tolosa-Hunt Syndrome

The Tolosa-Hunt syndrome is an idiopathic inflammatory disease of the cavernous sinus. It has been characterized clinically as (1) steady, gnawing, retroorbital pain; (2) defects in cranial nerves III, IV, and VI, and the first division of cranial nerve V; with less common involvement of the optic nerve or sympathetic fibers around the cavernous carotid artery; (3) symptoms lasting days to weeks; (4) occasional spontaneous remission; (5) recurrent attacks; and (6) prompt response to steroid therapy. Reports have demonstrated narrowing of the cavernous carotid on angiography and irregularity or thrombosis of the superior ophthalmic vein and thrombosis of the cavernous sinus on orbital venography. On MR, a spectrum of findings has been observed including (1) normal scan, (2) abnormal signal (isointense with muscle on T1WI and isointense with fat on T2WI) and/or mass lesions in the cavernous sinus (en-

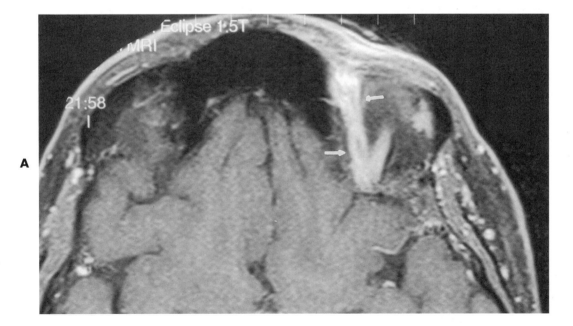

Fig. 11-46   This patient had a basal cell carcinoma of the skin above the left eyebrow. There was perineural spread *(arrows)* through the supraorbital foramen into the superior orbit and along the supraorbital nerve **(A)**.

Illustration continued on following page

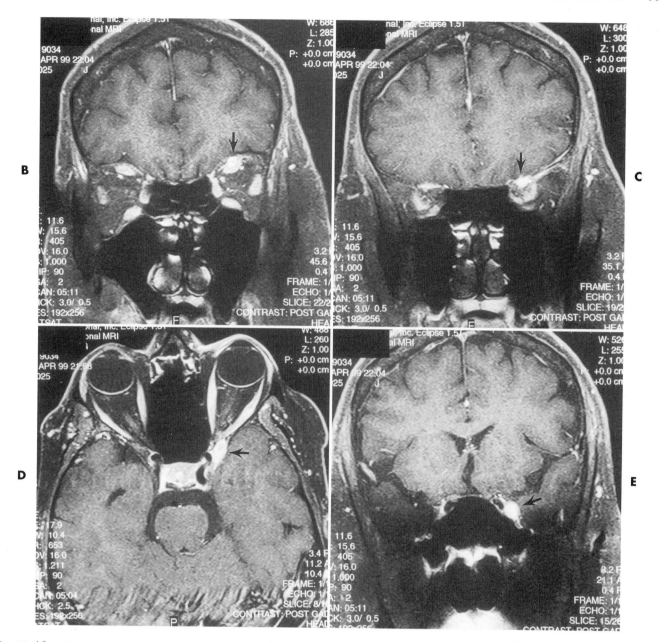

Fig. 11-46   *Continued.* This is also shown very well on coronal fat suppressed images **B** and **C** with *arrows*. From the orbit, the lesion *(arrows)* found its way to the cavernous sinus traveling along V-1 (**D** and **E**).

largement of the cavernous sinus), (3) extension of the lesion into the orbital apex, (4) thrombosis of the cavernous sinus and/or superior ophthalmic vein, and (5) enhancement that can extend into the orbital apex (identified with fat saturation techniques) and along the floor of the middle cranial fossa (see Fig. 11-47). The pathologic substrate of this syndrome is debated, with some investigators believing that it represents a granulomatous inflammation of the cavernous sinus and others finding no granulomas but rather nonspecific inflammatory changes. With a prompt response to steroid therapy, it is difficult in most cases, even for the sur-

geon with a large family to educate, to justify biopsy. This is analogous to the idiopathic inflammatory condition of orbital pseudotumor.

The differential diagnosis of Tolosa-Hunt syndrome includes (1) sarcoid, (2) meningioma, (3) lymphoma, (4) metastatic and neurotropic spread of tumor into the cavernous sinus, and (5) infections such as actinomycosis.

Chondrosarcoma

Chondrosarcoma is a rare neoplasm that is said to arise from embryonal rests, endochondral bone, or car-

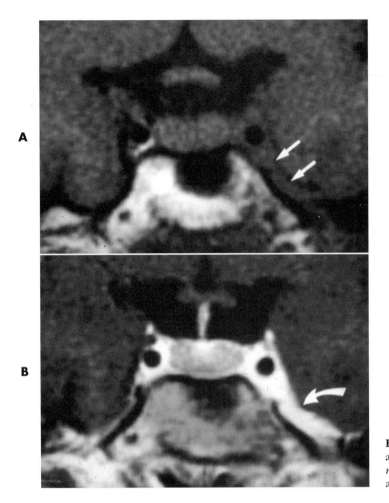

Fig. 11-47   Tolosa-Hunt syndrome. The unenhanced **(A)** and enhanced **(B)** scans show the infiltrative pseudotumor *(arrows)* entering the cavernous sinus. In many cases, an orbital apex component coexists.

tilage and is located at the skull base, in the meninges, or in the brain. Chondrosarcoma usually occurs in patients in their second to fourth decade of life. Signs and symptoms depend on the location of the lesion. Usually, patients have a long history of headache and cranial nerve problems (particularly cranial nerve VI), which are sometimes intermittent. In the days of the giants, plain films revealed calcification in approximately 60% of cases in a stippled, finely speckled, amorphous, or ringlike configuration. Pure lytic bone destruction may also occur. Locations for chondrosarcoma in decreasing order of frequency are the parasellar region, cerebellopontine angle, and the convexity. Maffucci syndrome has been associated with intracranial chondrosarcoma.

CT demonstrates the calcified mass and also reveals enhancing neoplastic tissue (Fig. 11-48). CT is probably more specific for this tumor because of its sensitivity to calcium. MR shows low to intermediate intensity on T1WI and high intensity on T2WI with heterogeneity. The lesions markedly enhance. The key here is appreciating whether there is calcification. Chondrosarcoma

should be in the differential diagnosis of calcified enhancing parasellar masses (Box 11-6).

INFRASELLAR AND BASE OF SKULL LESIONS (Box 11-7)

Developmental Lesions

Cephaloceles have already been described in Chapter 9. Basal cephaloceles comprise approximately 10% of all cephaloceles. They include sphenopharyngeal (through the sphenoid body), sphenoorbital (through the superior orbital fissure), sphenoethmoidal (through the sphenoid and ethmoid bones), transethmoidal (through the cribriform plate), and sphenomaxillary (through the maxillary sinus). These anomalies produce round, smooth erosion in the bone of the particular anatomic region. Their intensity on MR depends on the contents of the cephalocele, which include meninges, brain, and/or CSF. At the base, cephaloceles can present as a pharyngeal mass producing airway obstruction and CSF rhinorrhea, and can be a source for recurrent meningitis (Fig 11-49).

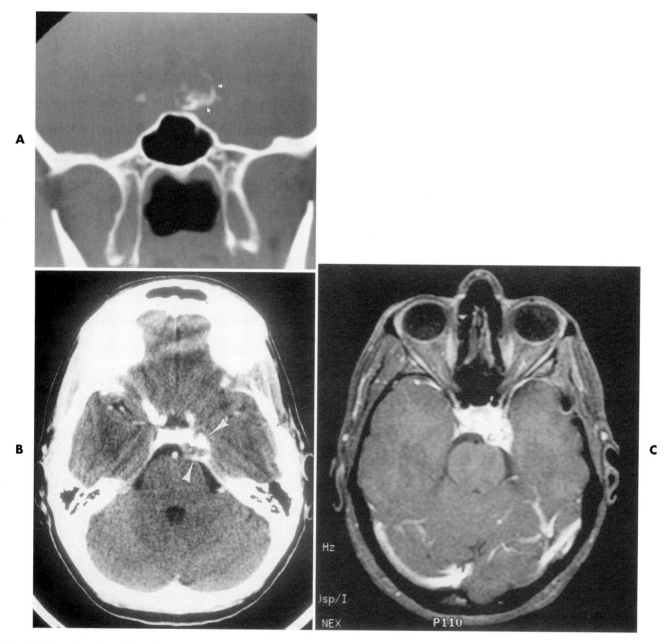

Fig. 11-48   Chondroid chordoma (low-grade chondrosarcoma). **A,** Coronal CT with bone windows demonstrates chondroid calcification in arcs *(arrows).* Differential diagnosis is chordoma, calcified aneurysm, and craniopharyngioma. **B,** A different patient also shows a left calcified parasellar mass *(arrowheads).* The calcification is seen as a low signal area amidst the enhancing mass on the postcontrast fat suppressed T1WI **(C).**

Juvenile Angiofibroma

Juvenile angiofibroma (also see Chapter 14) is seen in young male patients, accounts for approximately 0.5% of head and neck neoplasms, and is the most common benign tumor of the nasopharynx. These tumors may originate in the posterior lateral wall of the nasal cavity. Characteristically, they grow through the pterygopalatine foramina and may extend into the infratemporal fossa (Fig.

11-50). Other regions of spread include the sphenoid sinus, cavernous sinus, and paranasal sinuses. Unusual locations for these lesions include the parapharyngeal space and the pterygoid muscle region. The tumor can be seen with epistaxis, nasal obstruction, or facial deformity. These masses are extremely vascular. MR reveals the extent of the lesion. There are no specific intensity characteristics, although flow voids may be seen in highly vascular lesions. The tumor enhances. Angiography reveals a

Box 11-6   **Calcified Parasellar Lesions**
Aneurysm
Atherosclerosis-dolichoectasia
Chondrosarcoma
Chordoma
Craniopharyngioma
Epidermoid
Granuloma
Meningioma
Teratoma

dense tumor stain, and depending on its location, recruits blood vessels from around the base of the skull, including the inferolateral trunk and branches of the internal maxillary artery, including meningeal arteries. These lesions can become large. Preoperative embolization followed by surgery is the present approach to these lesions.

Chordoma

Chordomas (see also Chapters 15 and 17) occur at sites of notochordal remnants and constitute less than 1% of all intracranial tumors. Approximately 35% to 40% of chordomas are cranial (peak age between 20 and 40

Box 11-7   **Infrasellar and Base of the Skull Lesions**
Cholesterol granuloma
Chondrosarcoma
Chordoma
Craniopharyngioma
Developmental lesions (cephalocele)
Eosinophilic granuloma
Epidermoid
Fibrous dysplasia
Infection
Juvenile angiofibroma
Malignant otitis externa
Meningioma
Metastasis/perineural spread of tumor
Nasopharyngeal carcinoma
Paget's disease
Pituitary adenoma
Plasmacytoma/multiple myeloma
Sphenoid sinus carcinoma
Sphenoid sinus mucocele

years), 50% are in the sacrum (peak age 40 to 60 years, more commonly in men), and 15% are in the spine. Intracranially the most common site of origin is the clivus, near the sphenooccipital synchondrosis. Other sites of origin include the basioccipital and parasellar regions, and rarely the paranasal sinuses. Chordomas can be aggressive and extensive, spreading into the nasopharynx or the prepontine regions. Patients have headache, visual disturbances, and cranial nerve palsy. These signs and symptoms have a variable duration and can remit and recur spontaneously for months to years. Although most chordomas are histologically benign, they are locally invasive, with a poor overall prognosis. Complete surgical removal is rarely possible; thus, partial resection is performed followed by radiation therapy. Radiation with proton beam or linear accelerator therapy has been advocated because chordomas are resistant to standard radiation treatment protocols.

CT and MR are particularly complementary in imaging these lesions. CT demonstrates a soft-tissue mass, bone destruction, and calcification (approximately 50%). Chordomas can be very large, and multiplanar imaging is essential for delineation of tumor extent. MR reveals a mixed intensity pattern. On T1WI they are isointense to brain parenchyma, although some regions of low intensity (calcification) and high intensity can be identified. On T2WI, high intensity is the rule. Chordomas enhance. The key to the diagnosis is location, bone destruction, and calcification. Clival lesions can be tricky diagnostically. Assess the CT carefully for any attachment of the lesion to the clivus (Fig. 11-51). Sometimes this can be subtle; however, when identified, it favors chordoma. Similar-appearing lesions include chondroma, myelomas, osteochrondra, giant cell tumor, sphenoid sinus tumor, chondrosarcoma, metastases, nasopharyngeal carcinoma, craniopharyngioma, pituitary adenoma, glomus tumor, meningioma, schwannoma, and epidermoid.

Metastatic Lesions

The most frequent metastatic lesions to the base of the skull are from the prostate, lung, and breast. Prostate metastases are osteoblastic and can simulate meningioma, whereas lung and breast are more commonly lytic. Chloromas (granulocytic sarcoma) are solid tumors of myelogenous cells seen in patients with leukemia. They prefer the paranasal sinuses and the orbit but have been reported in the sphenoid sinus with extension through the clivus. Their intensity characteristics are probably similar to meningioma. Wegener granulomatosis and inflammatory pseudotumor (this lesion can be hypointense on T2WI) can mimic malignant neoplasms of the skull base.

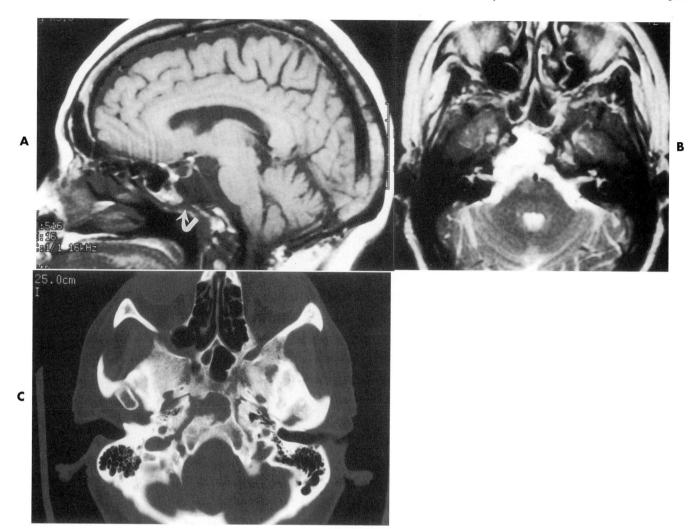

Fig. 11-49 Skull base meningocele. **A,** A CSF intensity lesion *(curved arrow)* erodes the clivus on the T1WI. **B,** Axial T2WI also displays the fluid consistency of the meningocele. **C,** The bone window from the CT study shows erosion of the clivus with smooth margination.

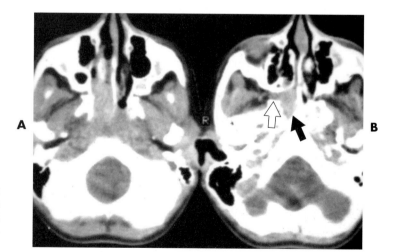

Fig. 11-50 Juvenile angiofibroma. **A,** The CT images demonstrate a mass in the nasopharynx and pterygopalatine fossa. It enhances and expands fossa on the right. Mild skull base erosion *(arrow)* is seen in **B**. Also note the enlargement of the pterygopalatine foramen *(open arrow)*.

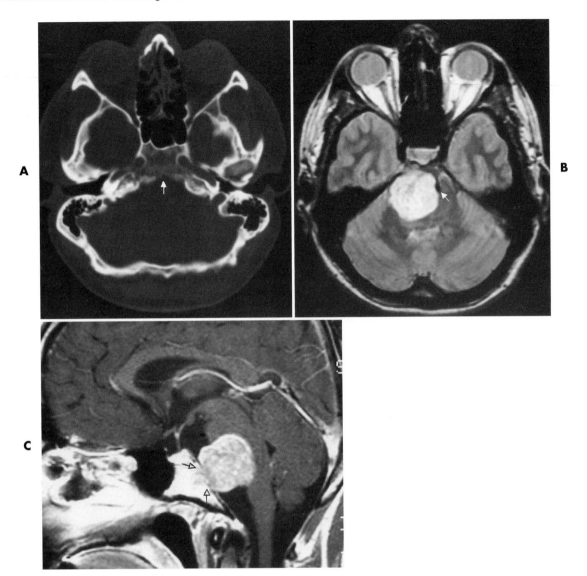

Fig. 11-51   Clivus chordoma. **A,** Axial CT with bone windows reveals slight erosion *(arrow)* in the clivus. This is very significant, suggesting a clivus-based lesion such as chordoma. **B,** Axial PDWI demonstrates a high-intensity mass compressing the pons and deviating the basilar artery *(arrow)*. **C,** Observe attachment to the clivus *(open arrows)* on this enhanced sagittal T1WI.

Other Sphenoid Sinus and Infrasellar Lesions

Miscellaneous sphenoid sinus and infrasellar lesions will be discussed extensively in Chapters 13 and 14. Some lesions of the sphenoid sinus grow superiorly to invade the sella and present as sellar or suprasellar masses. Nasopharyngeal carcinoma, sphenoid metastases, and chordomas arising in the sphenoid sinus can extend to involve the sella in a secondary fashion. Sphenoid sinus mucoceles are expansile lesions that have a variable intensity pattern but have a tendency for high intensity on T1WI. A thin margin of bone is usually present.

Craniopharyngioma can present as an infrasellar mass (see Fig. 11-36). They may calcify in 30% to 50% of cases, show cyst formation, and enhance. Intensity on MR can be variable. The differential includes rhabdomyosarcoma, histiocytic lymphoma, pharyngeal chordoma, squamous cell carcinoma, lymphoepithelioma, adenoid cystic carcinoma, esthesioneuroblastoma, inverted papilloma, juvenile angiofibroma, and metastases.

Jugular Foramen Lesions

Lesions that occur in this location include glomus tumor, neurofibroma or schwannoma, meningioma, and meta-static disease. The diagnosis of glomus tumor is obvious when flow voids are seen in a lesion in the region of the jugular foramen on MR. Unfortunately, many glomus tumors do not have this salt-and-pepper appearance. The glomus tumor, neurofibroma, and metastatic lesion may in certain cases all erode bone in this foramen. CT is again best at demonstrating bony erosion or foraminal enlargement. The glomus tumor can occlude the jugular bulb and grow into the jugular vein. All these lesions enhance, and when no flow voids are in the lesion, differentiation may be difficult. Meningiomas that extend into the jugular foramen usually demonstrate a dural base and an enhancing tail.

> When imaging the skull case,
> You must chase
> A lesion of the face
> All over the place
> Or back to the base,
> To be deemed an ace
> —*With apologies to the late Dr. Theodor Geisel (Dr. Seuss)*

SUGGESTED READINGS

Ahmadi J, North CM, Segall HD, et al: Cavernous sinus invasion by pituitary adenomas, *AJNR* 6:893-898, 1985.

Araki Y, Ashikaga R, Takahashi S, et al: High signal intensity of the infundibular stalk on fluid-attenuated inversion recovery MR, *AJNR* 18(1):89-93, 1997.

Barrow DL, Mizuno J, Tindall GT: Management of prolactinomas associated with very high serum prolactin levels, *J Neurosurg* 68:554-558, 1988.

Benitez WI, Sartor KJ, Angtuaco JCE: Craniopharyngioma presenting as a nasopharyngeal mass: CT and MR findings, *J Comput Assist Tomogr* 12:1068-1072, 1988.

Bonneville JF, Cattin A, Racle A, et al: Dynamic CT of the laterosellar extradural venous spaces, *AJNR* 10:535-542, 1989.

Burton EM, Ball WS, Crone K, et al: Hamartoma of the tuber cinereum: a comparison of MR and CT findings in four cases, *AJNR* 10:497-501, 1989.

Castillo M, Davis PC, Ross WK, et al: Meningioma of the chiasm and optic nerves: CT and MR findings, *J Comput Assist Tomogr* 13:679-681, 1989.

Chung JW, Chang KH, Han MH, et al: Computed tomography of cavernous sinus diseases, *Neuroradiology* 30:319-328, 1988.

Daniels DL, Pech P, Pojunas KW, et al: Trigeminal nerve: anatomic correlation with MR imaging, *Radiology* 159:577-583, 1986.

Daniels DL, Mark LP, Ulmer JL, et al: Osseous anatomy of the pterygopalatine fossa, *AJNR* 19(8):1423-1432, 1998.

Destrieux C, Kakou MK, Velut S, et al: Microanatomy of the hypophyseal fossa boundaries, *J Neurosurg* 88(4):743-752, 1998.

Destrieux C, Velut S, Kakou MK, et al: A new concept in Dorello's canal microanatomy: the petroclival venous confluence, *J Neurosurg* 87(1):67-72, 1997.

Doppman JL, Frank JA, Dwyer AJ, et al: Gadolinium DTPA enhanced MR imaging of ACTH-secreting microadenomas of the pituitary gland, *J Comput Assist Tomogr* 12:728-735, 1988.

Downs DM, Damiano TR, Rubinstein D, et al: Gasserian ganglion: appearance on contrast-enhanced MR, *AJNR* 17(2):237-241, 1996.

Eldevik OP, Blaivas M, Gabrielsen TO, et al: Craniopharyngioma: radiologic and histologic findings and recurrence [see comments], *AJNR* 17(8):1427-1439, 1996.

el-Kalliny M, van Loveren H, Keller JT, et al: Tumors of the lateral wall of the cavernous sinus, *J Neurosurg* 77(4):508-514, 1992.

Elster AD, Chen MYM, Williams DW III, et al: Pituitary gland: MR imaging of physiologic hypertrophy in adolescence, *Radiology* 174:681-685, 1990.

Elster AD, Sanders TG, Vines FS, et al: Size and shape of the pituitary gland during pregnancy and post partum: measurement with MR imaging, *Radiology* 181:531-535, 1991.

Elster AD: Modern imaging of the pituitary, *Radiology* 187:1-14, 1993.

Elster AD, Sanders TG, Vines FS, et al: Size and shape of the pituitary gland during pregnancy and post partum: measurement with MR imaging, *Radiology* 181(2):531-535, 1991.

Faro SH, Koenigsberg RA, Turtz AR, et al. Melanocytoma of the cavernous sinus: CT and MR findings, *AJNR* 17(6):1087-1090, 1996.

Fehlings MG, Tucker WS: Cavernous hemangioma of Meckel's cave: case report, *J Neurosurg* 68:645-647, 1988.

Fujisawa I, Asato R, Kawata M, et al: Hyperintense signal of the posterior pituitary on T1-weighted MR images: an experimental study, *J Comput Assist Tomogr* 13:371-377, 1989.

Fujisawa I, Nishimura K, Asato R, et al: Posterior lobe of the pituitary in diabetes insipidus: MR findings, *J Comput Assist Tomogr* 11:221-225, 1987.

Gammal TE, Brooks BS, Hoffman WH: MR imaging of the ectopic bright signal of posterior pituitary regeneration, *AJNR* 10:323-328, 1989.

Ginsberg LE, De Monte F, Gillenwater AM, et al: Greater superficial petrosal nerve: anatomy and MR findings in perineural tumor spread *AJNR* 17(2):389-393, 1996.

Gudinchet F, Brunelle F, Barth MO, et al: MR imaging of the posterior hypophysis in children, *AJNR* 10:511-514, 1989.

Kaufman B, Tomsak RL, Kaufman BA, et al: Herniation of the suprasellar visual system and third ventricle into empty sellae: morphologic and clinical considerations, *AJNR* 10:65-76, 1989.

Kelly WM, Kucharczyk W, Kucharczyk J, et al: Posterior pituitary ectopia: an MR feature of pituitary dwarfism, *AJNR* 9:453-460, 1988.

Kernaze MG, Sartor K, Winthrop JD, et al: Suprasellar lesions: evaluation with MR imaging, *Radiology* 161:77-82, 1986.

Kleinschmidt-DeMasters BK, Winston KR, Rubinstein D, et al: Ectopic pituitary adenoma of the third ventricle, *J Neurosurg* 72:139-142, 1990.

Kornreich L, Horev G, Lazar L, et al: MR findings in hereditary isolated growth hormone deficiency, *AJNR* 18(9):1743-1747, 1997.

Kornreich L, Horev G, Lazar L, et al: MR findings in growth hormone deficiency: correlation with severity of hypopituitarism, *AJNR* 19(8):1495-1499, 1998.

Kristof RA, Van Roost D, Wolf HK, et al: Intravascular papillary endothelial hyperplasia of the sellar region. Report of three cases and review of the literature, *J Neurosurg* 86(3):558-563, 1997.

Kucharczyk J, Kucharczyk W, Berry I, et al: Histochemical characterization and functional significance of the hyperintense signal on MR images of the posterior pituitary, *AJNR* 9:1079-1083, 1988.

Kucharczyk W, Davis DO, Kelly WM, et al: Pituitary adenomas: high-resolution MR imaging at 1.5T, *Radiology* 161:761-765, 1986.

Kucharczyk W, Peck WW, Kelly WM, et al: Rathke cleft cysts: CT, MR imaging, and pathologic features, *Radiology* 165:491-495, 1987.

Laine FJ, Braun IR, Jensen ME, et al: Perineural tumor extension through the foramen ovale: evaluation with MR imaging, *Radiology* 174:65-71, 1990.

Lewi J, Curtin H, Eelkema E, et al: Benign expansile lesions of the sphenoid sinus: differentiation from normal asymmetry of the lateral recesses, *AJNR* 20(3):461-466, 1999.

Lim TH, Chang KE, Han MC, et al: Pituitary atrophy in Korean (epidemic) hemorrhagic fever: CT correlation with pituitary function and visual field, *AJNR* 7:633-637, 1986.

Linden CN, Martinez CR, Gonzalvo A, et al: Intrinsic third ventricle craniopharyngioma: CT and MR findings, *J Comput Assist Tomogr* 13:362-368, 1989.

McCormick PC, Bello JA, Post KD: Trigeminal schwannoma: surgical series of 14 cases with review of the literature, *J Neurosurg* 69:850-860, 1988.

Meyers SP, Hirsch WL, Jr, et al: Chondrosarcomas of the skull base: MR imaging features, *Radiology* 184(1):103-108, 1992.

Michael AS, Paige ML: MR imaging of intrasellar meningiomas simulating pituitary adenomas, *J Comput Assist Tomogr* 12:944-946, 1988.

Molitch ME, Russell EJ: The pituitary "incidentaloma," *Ann Intern Med* 112:925-931, 1990

Naylor MF, Scheithauer BW, Forbes GS, et al: Rathke cleft cyst: CT, MR, and pathology of 23 cases [published erratum appears in J Comput Assist Tomogr Jan—Feb;20(1):171, 1996], *J Comput Assist Tomogr* 19(6):853-859, 1995.

Okamoto K, Ito J, Furusawa T, et al: Reversible hyperintensity of the anterior pituitary gland on T1-weighted MR images in a patient receiving temporary parenteral nutrition, *AJNR* 19(7):1287-1289, 1998.

Ostrove SG, Quencer RM, Hoffman JC, et al: Hemorrhage within pituitary adenomas: how often associated with pituitary apoplexy syndrome? *AJNR* 10:503-510, 1989.

Peck WW, Dillon WP, Norman D, et al: High-resolution MR imaging of microadenomas at 1.5T: experience with Cushing disease, *AJNR* 9:1085-1091, 1988.

Poussaint TY, Barnes PD, Anthony DC, et al: Hemorrhagic pituitary adenomas of adolescence *AJNR* 17(10):1907-1912, 1996.

Pusey E, Kortman KE, Flannigan BD, et al: MR of craniopharyngiomas: tumor delineation and characterization, *AJNR* 8:439-444, 1987.

Scanarini M, D'Avella D, Rotilio A, et al: Giant-cell granulomatous hypophysitis: a distinct clinicopathological entity, *J Neurosurg* 71:681-686, 1989.

Sparacia G, Banco A, Midiri M, et al MR imaging technique for the diagnosis of pituitary iron overload in patients with transfusion-dependent beta-thalassemia major, *AJNR* 19(10):1905-1907, 1998.

Stuckey SL: Dilated venous plexus of the hypoglossal canal mimicking disease, *AJNR* 20(1):157-158, 1999.

Suzuki M, Takashima T, Kadoya M, et al: Height of normal pituitary gland on MR imaging: age and sex differentiation, *J Comput Assist Tomogr* 14:36-39, 1990.

Tsuha M, Aoki H, Okamura T: Roentgenological investigation of cavernous sinus structure with special reference to paracavernous cranial nerves, *Neuroradiology* 29:462-467, 1987.

Wolpert SM, Osborn M, Anderson M, et al: The bright pituitary gland: a normal MR appearance in infancy, *AJNR* 9:1-3, 1988.

Yeakley JW, Kulkarni MV, McArdle CB, et al: High-resolution MR imaging of juxtasellar meningiomas with CT and angiographic correlation, *AJNR* 9:279-285, 1988.

Yousem DM, Arrington JA, Zinreich SJ, et al: Pituitary adenomas: possible role of bromocriptine in intratumoral hemorrhage, *Radiology* 170:239-243, 1989.

Yousem DM, Atlas SW, Grossman RI, et al: MR imaging of Tolosa-Hunt syndrome, *AJNR* 10:1181-1184, 1989.

CHAPTER 12

Temporal Bone

The temporal bone is the bane of the resident's existence. Just when he or she begins to feel confident in central nervous system (CNS) anatomy, along comes a staff neuroradiologist with an evil grin and a bone-targeted computed tomographic (CT) scan through the temporal bones, eager to stump the resident. Usually this professor has only one more sulcus than there are ossicles, so not to worry.

The detailed bony anatomy of the vestibulocochlear structures of the temporal bone makes CT the primary method of evaluating the erosive and inflammatory lesions of the temporal bone. It is important to appreciate fully the middle ear structures in both an axial and a coronal plane. Although the variety of disease in the temporal bone is actually limited in day-to-day evaluation, it is important to recognize the subtle changes that suggest disease in this region.

We'll start from the outside and work our way inward. Students, fellows, colleagues, lend me your ears!

EXTERNAL AUDITORY CANAL

Normal Anatomy

The external auditory canal (EAC) is derived from the first branchial groove and is an ectodermal structure. First and second branchial arches contribute to the cartilaginous EAC and auricle. Where the ectodermal external auditory canal joins the endoderm of the first branchial pouch is the medial boundary of the EAC, the tympanic membrane. The EAC measures approximately 2.5 cm long and is made of fibrocartilage laterally (0.9 cm) and bone medially (1.6 cm). (Rather than having you study a figure, just look in the mirror or stick your finger in your ear). The posterior border of the glenoid fossa housing the temporomandibular joint serves as part of the anterior wall of the EAC.

Congenital Anomalies

Atresia and hypoplasia Congenital anomalies of the EAC are rather common, more so than middle ear abnormalities. The degree of congenital deformities of the EAC runs the gamut from total atresia to webs, to hypoplasia or stenosis of the EAC, to microtia (a small auricle of the ear) (Fig. 12-1, Box 12-1). Atresias and stenoses may or may not coexist with microtia (see following discussion).

The degree of microtia tends to correlate with the extent of bony stenosis of the external auditory canal. Middle ear malformations also vary with the severity of the auricular anomalies. Pneumatization of the middle ear often follows the degree of microtia—67% of patients with major microtia (absence of normal auricular structures

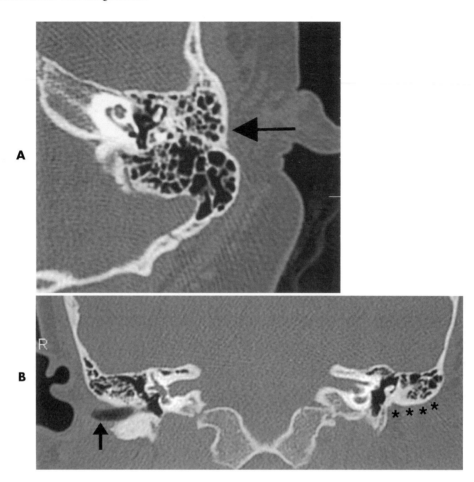

Fig. 12-1 EAC atresia. **A,** Axial CT demonstrates absence of EAC on the left side *(arrow)*. The middle ear osside are deformed. **B,** The finding is confirmed on the coronal image where one can see the normal right EAC *(arrow)*, the absent EAC on the left *(asterisks)*, and the lateralized left middle ear ossides.

and anotia) have reduced pneumatization of the middle ear and mastoid. This is important to note because the surgeon needs to know how much drilling he will have to do and how large a space he will have to work in to reconstruct middle or inner ear structures. In addition, it is important to know whether the inner ear structures are normal. Thirteen per cent of patients with microtia have dysplastic inner ear structures—usually a hypoplastic, lateral, semicircular canal.

In minor microtia (pocket ear, absence of upper helix, absence of tragus, miniear, clefts, and so on), 50% of

the patients have a dysplastic malleus-incus complex whereas with major microtia, 67% are dysplastic and 30% have absent ossicles altogether. The incudostapedial joint is commonly abnormal (>65%) in both minor and major microtia. Abnormalities of the stapes coexist in up to 70% of cases.

Thalidomide embryopathy accounted for a large blip in EAC dysplasias in the early 1960s—rubella infections still account for some these days. Bilateral EAC atresia is seen in 23% to 29% of cases. Microtia coexists in 73% of cases and most of these ears have no definable ear remnants. There is often concomitant abnormality in the temporomandibular joint, with EAC anomalies manifested by flattening or absence of the glenoid fossa. Dysplasia of the mandibular condyle (remember both the EAC and mandibular condyle are formed from first branchial apparatus structures and are associated with the fifth cranial nerve) and defects of the zygomatic arch may be seen. At the extreme, atresia of the EAC may be associated with hypoplasia of the malleus, fusion of the malleus and incus, or other anomalies of middle ear structures (in >50% of cases).

With a stenotic external auditory canal, the slope of the EAC may be more angulated vertically. In addition, keratinous plugs and cholesteatomas may form (see following subsections). Rarely, (11% to 30%) is there an associated anomaly of the inner ear, mainly because inner ear structures are derived from the neuroectoderm as opposed to the branchial system. In patients with EAC atresia, the facial nerve in its horizontal section may have an aberrant course in close proximity to the stapes footplate and may be anteriorly located in its descending portion. Evaluation of the facial nerve position (see Chapter 2), vascular anomalies, middle ear and mastoid air cell pneumatization, ossicular deformities, meningoencephaloceles, sigmoid sinus location, and other features is important for preoperative planning to prevent accidental surgical injury. (Remember the surgeon does not like to be surprised, particularly by "Big Red."). The facial nerve may also be dehiscent in its tympanic course.

Surgery to correct the EAC is fruitless if the inner ear is nonfunctional, eh? Surgery for external ear anomalies is difficult because it often requires grafts of bone and cartilage as well as drilling new canals. Thus, correction just for cosmetic purposes is usually delayed until after adolescence, when growth has slowed down. However, if the ear anomaly leads to learning disabilities it may be treated before schooling. Can't learn well if you can't hear the teacher (Table 12-1).

First branchial cleft cysts   First branchial cleft cysts occur around the ear and/or in the neighboring parotid gland (Fig. 12-2). A fistula from a first branchial cleft anomaly may drain to the EAC at the bone-cartilage interface. Second branchial cleft cysts are 10 times more common than first branchial cleft cysts, but the external ear would be an unusual site for a second cyst to

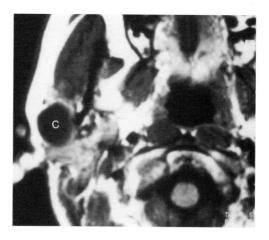

Fig. 12-2   First branchial cleft cyst. Axial T1WI shows a cystic mass *(C)* in the right parotid gland near the external auditory canal. Rarely a first branchial cleft anomaly will communicate with the external ear.

drain. (Check Chapters 14 and 15 for their usual locations.)

Calcifications of the external ear and/or pinna occur in a variety of congenital and acquired lesions. Box 12-2 lists these entities.

Inflammatory Lesions

Malignant otitis externa   The most severe inflammatory condition affecting the EAC is malignant otitis externa, a *Pseudomonas* infection of the EAC seen in elderly diabetic patients (93% of cases). HIV infected patients may also be at risk. Patients present with disgusting-smelling, purulent discharges coming from their ear (capable of clearing out the otologists' waiting room faster than the sound of a dentist's drill!). The infection usually begins at the junction of the cartilaginous and bony portion of the EAC along the fissures of Santorini, which lead to the parapharyngeal space. This process may be incredibly aggressive, extending into the

Table 12-1	Checklist for evaluating for EAC atresia or stenosis

Item	Rationale
Inner ear structures	No sense fixing the outer, middle ear if no sensorineural function
Stapes	Implies inner ear anomaly, means implant
Oval and round window	Access to perilymph, endolymph
Middle ear space	Need place to put, repair ossicles, transmit sound
Facial nerve	Don't want to injure nerve and wake patient up with facial disfigurement for rest of life
Ossicular anatomy	How many need to be replaced? Are there functioning joints?
Carotid artery, jugular vein	Makes for a bloody mess if they are anomalous and in the way

Box 12-2   Calcified External Ear Organs
Acromegaly
Addison disease
Alkaptonuria
Diabetes mellitus
Frostbite
Gout
Hyperparathyroidism
Hypoparathyroidism
Mike Tyson bite
Ochronosis
Pseudogout
Radiation
Relapsing polychondritis

infratemporal fossa, the nasopharynx, the parapharyngeal space, the adjacent bone, the temporomandibular joint, the middle and inner ear structures, and intracranially in the extradural space. Palsies of cranial nerves VI, VII, and IX through XII may reflect extension of the disease at the skull base and into the neural foramina. Venous sinus thrombosis is a complication. The process may mimic an aggressive neoplasm in many respects and often is difficult to control with antibiotics. CT will identify soft tissue in the EAC, bony erosion of the EAC walls, and osteitic changes at the skull base. Magnetic resonance imaging (MR) may demonstrate edema of the external ear, the parapharyngeal fat may be obliterated as the infection extends anteriorly and medially, and the tissue planes around the carotid sheath may be infiltrated (Fig. 12-3). Technetium (Tc) 99m bone scans and gal-

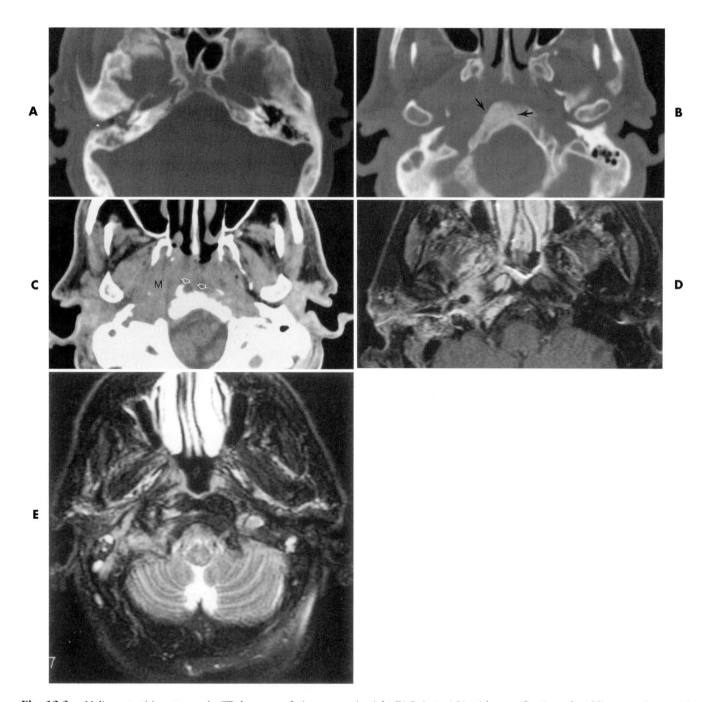

Fig. 12-3   Malignant otitis externa. **A,** CT shows a soft-tissue mass in right EAC *(asterisk)* with opacification of middle ear and mastoid air cells. **B,** Lower section demonstrates bone reaction secondary to osteitis of the clivus *(arrows).* **C,** Obliteration of tissue planes in the nasopharynx and parapharyngeal space by infectious mass *(M). Open arrows* are on the osteomyelitis. **D,** The fat suppressed T1WI MR shows enhancing tissue in the EAC, mastoid, petrous tip, right side of clivus and parapharyngeal space. **E,** High signal on T2WI is present in clivus and longus musculature.

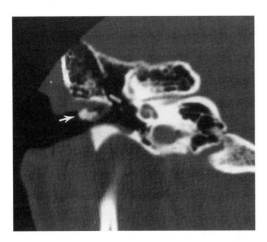

Fig. 12-4   Exostosis of the EAC. Coronal CT reveals a dense EAC exostosis *(arrow).*

lium 67 citrate scans show uptake of radiotracers and may be useful to assess activity of disease.

Keratosis obturans   Keratosis obturans, caused by plugs of keratin in the EAC, is hard to distinguish from a congenital cholesteatoma, which may infiltrate from the middle ear to the EAC. Keratosis obturans, however, is very painful and is usually seen bilaterally in middle-aged adults with histories of bronchiectasis and/or sinusitis. Acquired cholesteatomas are usually unilateral and are seen in older patients. A duller, less severe pain is noted and there is more bone erosion often extending into the middle ear and mastoid bone.

Swimmer and surfer's ear   Swimmer's ear (acute external otitis) is usually due to *Pseudomonas* infection. Rarely, mastoiditis and/or osteomyelitis may complicate swimmer's ear. Patients who swim in cold water are prone to exostoses of the EAC (surfer's ear). Recurrences occur as the swimmers return to the frozen pool or frigid oceans (the polar bear club) (Fig. 12-4). Relapsing chondritis, frostbite, and severe sunburns may affect the auricle of the ear, particularly the upper helix. Remember what your ma said—wear a hat outdoors and use SPF 30 on your ears.

Of course, the most common EAC mass is due to benign wax buildup (cotton swab syndrome). We know one neuroradiologist who had to have an obstetrician paged to the otorhinolaryngology suite to deliver a 3-pound 2-ounce wax ball by forceps delivery from his ear. Mazel Tov!

Benign Neoplasms

Benign tumors of the external ear include hemangiomas (venous vascular malformations), nevi, ceruminomas (adenomas of the ceruminous glands), polyps, and minor salivary gland tumors (included in Box 12-3). All these present as soft-tissue masses that may expand the EAC without destructiveness.

Malignant Lesions

Squamous cell carcinomas   Squamous cell carcinomas of the EAC are the most common neoplastic processes in this location. This is essentially a skin cancer with the associated risk from sun exposure (have you ever seen someone wearing earmuffs at the beach?). The lesion may invade the middle ear and temporal bone. Cartilaginous invasion of the external ear or middle ear extension portends poor prognosis and must be treated aggressively. The 5-year prognosis without middle ear disease is 59% but is 23% if the cancer extends into the middle ear. Deep lesions in the bony canal have the worst prognosis (Fig. 12-5). Pain occurs early because of periosteal spread or extension to the temporomandibular joint, where trismus may also arise. Facial nerve involvement also occurs early in the course. Yousem's law: the probability of anything happening is the inverse ratio to its desirability.

Other skin tumors   Other skin tumors such as basal cell carcinomas or melanomas may also affect the external ear (Fig. 12-6). Lymphatic drainage may be to intraparotid, retropharyngeal, occipital and skull base lymph nodes. Kaposi sarcoma in HIV positive individuals could affect the ear. Carcinoma of the parotid gland commonly invades the temporal bone and EAC, particularly if perineural growth occurs along cranial nerve VII.

Pediatric tumors   In children, rhabdomyosarcomas and lymphomas may present as external ear masses. Spread to the middle ear or along the eustachian tube is not uncommon, and in fact, tumors arising in the na-

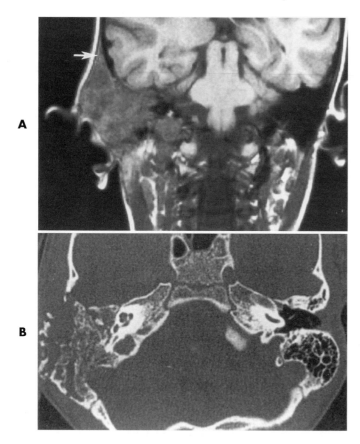

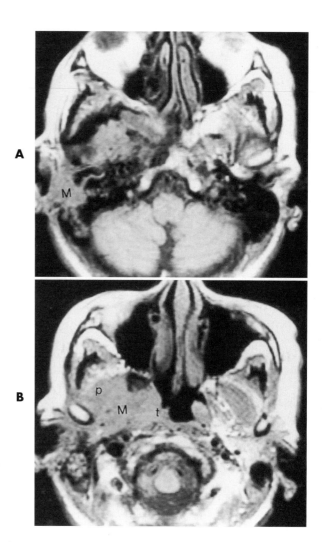

Fig. 12-5 EAC squamous cell cancer. **A,** Coronal T1WI of a patient with an extensive squamous cell carcinoma of the EAC reveals considerable spread into the mastoid air cells and the suprazygomatic portion of the masticator space *(arrow).* **B,** Extensive destruction in the temporal bone by the cancer is seen on CT.

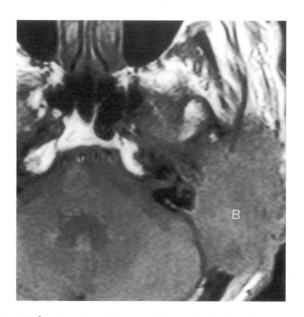

Fig. 12-6 Invasion of temporal bone by basal cell carcinoma *(B)* of the skin. Note the extensive medial extent of this mass, which arose from the skin around the ear in a south Florida sun worshipper. (Case courtesy of Stuart Bobman, another south Florida sun worshipper.)

Fig. 12-7 Retrograde spread of nasopharyngeal cancer. **A,** Patient had pain and discharge emanating from right ear. T1WI shows a soft-tissue mass *(M)* in the right mastoid region that eroded into the EAC. **B,** The ear was the tip of the iceberg. The mass *(M)* arose in the nasopharynx and grew retrograde into the middle ear and EAC via the eustachian tube. Note the parapharyngeal fat and torus tubarius *(t)* obliteration, and invasion of the pterygoid muscle *(p).*

sopharynx can present as ear masses because of retrograde growth along this route. Invasion of the temporal bone is not uncommon (Fig. 12-7).

Metastases Metastases affect the EAC portion of the temporal bone as they would any other osseous structure. Lytic and blastic lesions may occur, depending on the nature of the primary lesion.

THE MIDDLE EAR

Normal Anatomy

The middle ear or tympanic cavity is often divided into a superior attic or epitympanic recess, the mesotympanum at the level of the tympanic membrane, and the hypotympanum lying inferior and medial to the tympanic membrane (Fig. 12-8). Some of the contents of the middle ear cavity and eustachian tube are derived from the first branchial pouch. The first branchial arch forms the bodies of the malleus and incus and the short process of the incus. The second branchial arch forms the superstructure (capitulum and crura) of the stapes and long process of the incus as well as the manubrium of the malleus. The first branchial pouch invaginates into the eustachian tube, mesotympanum, and mastoid air cells.

The tympanic membrane is the lateral border of the middle ear. It has a thin anterosuperior portion known as the pars flaccida and a tougher posteroinferior pars tensa. The tympanic membrane slants down and inward so that the posterosuperior wall is shorter than its anteroinferior wall. The umbo is the attachment of the handle of the malleus to the tympanic membrane. The malleus has a head, which articulates with the body of the incus; a neck, an anterior process that attaches by ligaments to the wall of the mesotympanum and to the tensor tympani muscle; a lateral process; and a manubrium, which connects to the tympanic membrane. The tensor tympani muscle attaches to the upper manubrium and neck of the malleus. The named por-

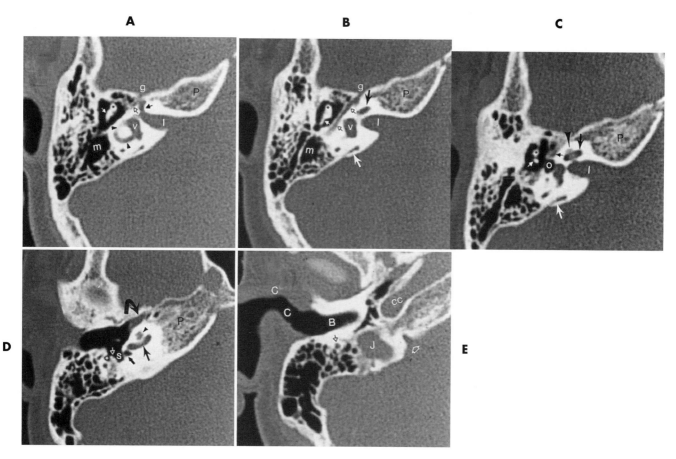

Fig. 12-8 CT of normal anatomy of middle ear, *(A-E)* from superior to inferior region. **A,** Axial view of labyrinthine portion of the facial nerve *(solid black arrow)*, geniculate ganglion of facial nerve *(g)*, proximal portion of the horizontal segment of the facial nerve *(open black arrow)*, head of malleus *(asterisk)*, and short process of incus *(white arrow)*. A joint is barely seen between the incus and malleus (incudomalleal joint), vestibule *(V)* with lateral semicircular canal *(black arrowheads)*, mastoid *(m)*, nonpneumatized petrous apex *(p)*, IAC *(I)*. **B,** Axial view of middle turn of cochlea *(large black arrow)*, geniculate ganglion of facial nerve *(g)*, horizontal segment of the facial nerve *(open black arrows)*, head of malleus *(asterisk)*, short process of incus *(white arrow)*, vestibule *(V)*, mastoid *(m)*, nonpneumatized petrous apex *(p)*, IAC *(I)*, vestibular aqueduct *(large white arrow)*. **C,** Axial view of middle turn of cochlea *(large black arrow)*, apical turn of cochlea *(black arrowhead)*, neck of malleus *(asterisk)*, long process of incus *(small white arrow)*, oval window *(o)*, tensor tympani muscle *(small black arrow)*, nonpneumatized petrous apex *(p)*, IAC *(I)*, vestibular aqueduct *(large white arrow)*. **D,** Axial view of hypotympanum. Basal turn of cochlea *(large black arrow)*, apical turn of cochlea *(black arrowhead)*, nonpneumatized petrous apex *(p)*, round window niche *(small black arrow)*, superior aspect of the eustachian tube and tensor tympani tendon *(curved black arrow)*, sinus tympani *(s)*, pyramidal eminence *(small open white arrow)*, and facial nerve recess *(asterisk)*. **E,** Axial view of region inferior to hypotympanum. Cochlear aqueduct *(open white arrow)*, cartilaginous portion of EAC *(C)*, bony portion of EAC *(B)*, carotid canal *(cc)*, jugular bulb *(J)*, descending portion of facial nerve *(open black arrow)*. Coronal images *(F-J)* from anterior to posterior.

Illustration continued on following page

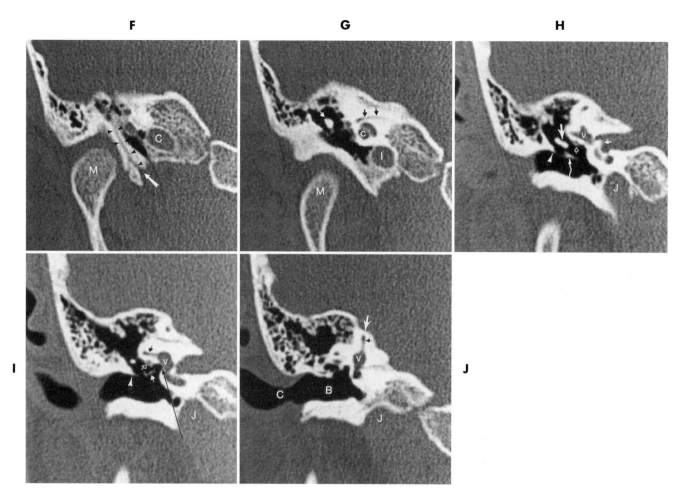

Fig. 12-8   *Continued.* **F,** Coronal view at level of temporomandibular joint. Descending portion of the facial nerve *(black arrowheads),* mandibular condyle *(M),* stylomastoid foramen *(white arrow),* and carotid canal *(C).* **G,** Internal carotid artery *(I),* cochlea *(c),* facial nerve coursing over cochlea *(small black arrows),* head of malleus *(white arrow),* and mandibular condyle *(M).* **H,** Crista falciformis of IAC *(small white arrow),* jugular bulb *(J),* vestibule *(v),* head and neck of malleus *(large white arrow),* tympanic portion of the facial nerve *(open white arrow),* scutum *(arrowhead),* and incus *(squiggly arrow).* **I,** Jugular foramen *(J),* vestibule *(v),* incudostapedial joint *(small white arrow),* tympanic portion of the facial nerve *(open white arrow),* scutum *(arrowhead),* oval window *(long black arrow),* and lateral semicircular canal *(small black arrow).* **J,** Jugular foramen *(J),* arcuate eminence *(white arrow),* superior semicircular canal *(black arrow),* vestibule *(v),* cartilaginous portion of EAC *(C),* and bony portion of EAC *(B).*

tions of the incus are its body, short process, and long process. The short process attaches by ligaments to the posterior tympanic cavity wall, whereas the long process parallels the manubrium posteromedially before bending medially and articulating with the stapes via its lenticular process. The stapes has a head (capitulum), which articulates with the lenticular process of the incus, an anterior crus, a posterior crus, and a footplate.

> To get to learn these little parts
> May put you through some fits and starts
> But those of you with the stoutest hearts
> Are found in the end with the biggest smarts

The footplate of the staples covers the oval (vestibular) window. The stapedius muscle arises from the pyramidal eminence and attaches to the head of the stapes.

This muscle tends to dampen sound by preventing excessive stapedial vibration. This explains the hyperacusis with seventh nerve palsies, as this muscle is innervated by the facial nerve (Fig. 12-9).

The scutum or drum spur is a sharp, bony excrescence seen best on coronal images forming the superomedial margin of the EAC (inferolateral attic wall) from which the tympanic membrane descends. It protrudes from the roof of the epitympanic cavity, the tegmen tympani. The tensor tympani muscle courses parallel to the eustachian tube lateral to the neck of the malleus. The petrosquamous suture connects the lateral tegmen to squamous temporal bone and transmits veins to the intracranial space; this may be a source of spread of infection. The bony ridge over the superior semicircular canal is called the arcuate eminence.

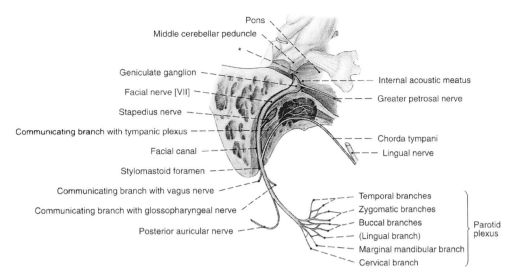

Fig. 12-9   Facial nerve anatomy. Branches from the facial nerve include the greater (superficial) petrosal nerve (for lacrimation), the stapedius nerve (to dampen sound), the tympanic plexus, the chorda tympani (for taste), and infratemporal branches for facial muscles. (From Sobotta Fig 652, p 370.)

The facial nerve courses through the middle ear after entering from the internal auditory canal (IAC) (Box 12-4). The IAC is separated into four quadrants by the transverse crista falciformis and vertically by Bill's bar (not to be confused with the other Bill's Bar at Ninth and Market Street) (Fig. 12-10). Cranial nerve VII is found in the anterosuperior portion of the IAC. The facial nerve has a labyrinthine segment coursing anterosuperiorly and laterally from the IAC to the geniculate ganglion. The geniculate ganglion is superior to the cochlea (see Figs. 12-8 and 12-9). Here it gives off the greater superficial petrosal nerve, which innervates salivation among other things. From the geniculate ganglion, the facial nerve forms its first genu and runs posteroinferolaterally on the undersurface of the lateral semicircular canal and above the oval window niche in its horizontal (or tympanic) segment. The facial nerve then makes its second turn (the second genu) or pyramidal turn to course inferiorly in the mastoid bone in its descending (or intramastoid) segment before exiting at the stylomastoid foramen. Along its course it gives innervation to the stapedius muscle and,

just above the stylomastoid foramen, to the chorda tympani for taste to the anterior two thirds of the tongue. The chorda tympani doubles back on itself running superiorly and reenters the mesotympanum before exiting anteriorly via the petrotympanic fissure to join the lingual nerve.

In the inferoposterior portion of the middle ear cavity, four important structures are visible on axial scans. They are, medially to laterally, the round window niche, the sinus tympani, the pyramidal eminence, and the facial nerve recess (see Fig. 12-8). The sinus tympani and facial nerve recess are indentations in the bone; the eminence is a bony hillock separating the two. The stapedius muscle belly and tendon lie in the pyramidal

---

Box 12-4 Segments of Cranial Nerve VII

Cisternal (cerebellopontine angle cistern)
Intracanalicular
Labyrinthine (fallopian canal) ⎫
Geniculate ganglion (1st genu) ⎪
Horizontal (tympanic)   ⎬ fallopian canal
Intramastoid (2nd genu, descending ⎪
  portion)   ⎭
Intraparotid

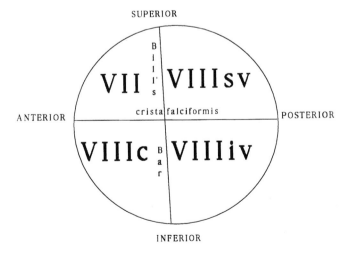

Fig. 12-10   IAC subdivisions. Diagram demonstrating Bill's bar and crista falciformis separating the IAC into four quadrants with cranial nerve VII and cochlear (VIIIc), superior vestibular (VIIIsv), and inferior vestibular (VIIIiv) divisions of cranial nerve VIII.

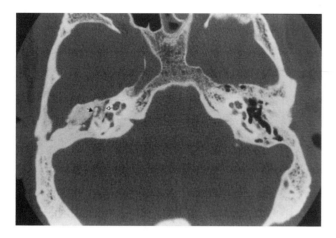

Fig. 12-11 Congenital middle ear deformity. In this patient with EAC atresia, the malleus and incus *(black arrow)* are irregularly shaped, and the middle ear cavity, the long process of the incus, and the stapes are incompletely formed. Tympanic portion of nerve VII *(open arrow)* is normal.

eminence. These recesses are important in that they may become a site for occult inflammatory disease after middle ear surgery. The anatomy here is simple but Yousem's axiom of residents is that no temporal bone anatomy is so simple that it can't be learned incorrectly.

The middle ear cavity connects via the eustachian tube to the nasopharynx at the torus tubarius. This explains the presence of serous otitis media and/or mastoiditis, which are commonly seen with nasopharyngeal carcinoma or adenoidal hypertrophy. The eustachian tube is a conduit for spread of lesions in both directions (e.g., malignant otitis externa from ear to nasopharynx

and squamous cell carcinoma from nasopharynx to mastoid cavity). It is also a conduit of cash from parents to pediatricians as the adenoids obstruct the tube leading to recurrent otitis media (this one's for you, Ilyssa).

Congenital Anomalies

Hypoplasia and fusion The middle ear is also a site of congenital dysplasias that may be associated with EAC stenosis or atresia (Fig. 12-11). Ossicular fusion, hypoplasia, or maldevelopment may occur and may coexist with anomalies of the facial nerve as it runs through the middle ear cavity. Isolated middle ear congenital abnormalities are not as common as those of the EAC or inner ear. When they occur in the absence of external ear anomalies, the distal incus (especially the long process) and the stapes are most commonly affected, followed by the stapes alone and incus alone. These components of the ossicular chain are derived from the second branchial arch (as opposed to the malleus and incus short process from the first arch). Absence, hypoplasia, and fixation to the attic may be seen. Congenital cholesteatomas may also occur with external and middle ear malformations.

Epidermoids To prevent confusion with acquired cholesteatomas use the term epidermoids rather than the older terms congenital cholesteatomas, epidermoidomas, or primary cholesteatomas. Epidermoids may arise in a variety of locations within the temporal bone (Fig. 12-12) from aberrant epithelial rests. The temporal bone is, in fact, the most common skull base site of congenital epidermoids. The classic locations for these lesions

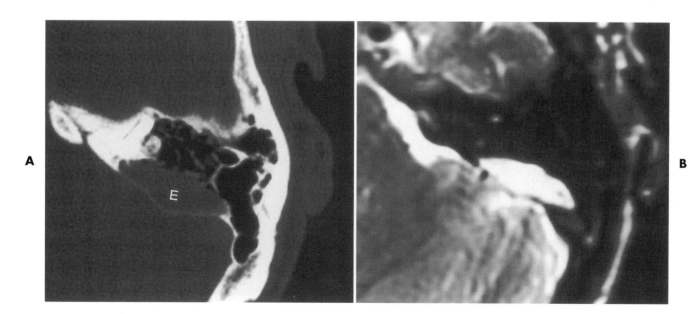

Fig. 12-12 Epidermoid (E) of bone. **A,** A lytic oblong bone lesion is seen along the posterior margin of the top of the petrous bone. **B,** Note how bright the mass is on T2WI. The diagnosis was an intraosseous epidermoid. Contrast this case with that of the enlarged vestibular aqueduct on CT and MR (see Fig. 12-32).

include the petrous apex, along Körner's septum (the petrosquamosal suture) in the mastoid air cells, the Eustachian tube opening, the geniculate ganglion region, and at the middle ear–epitympanum junction. Other common middle ear sites for epidermoids are near the incudostapedial joint and along the sinus tympani and facial nerve recess. Less common locations for epidermoids are in the internal auditory canal, the petrous apex, and the cerebellopontine angle cistern region. These lesions are pearly white to the surgeon's eye (though he also sees the "green" of a potential operation) and are usually hypointense on T1-weighted images (T1WI) and hyperintense on T2-weighted images (T2WI). As in the brain, they are as bright as CSF on T2WI but are more intense than CSF on T1WI. They are bright on FLAIR scanning and brighter than CSF on diffusion weighted scans (DWI). On CT, they appear as noninvasive, low density, erosive, well-circumscribed lesions in the temporal bone with scalloped margins (Fig. 12-13). Although they may be whitish lesions that simulate acquired cholesteatomas, these lesions are not associated with perforation of the tympanic membrane, and the patients have no history of antecedent ear infections or previous surgeries. Presentation often is with deafness, vertigo, or facial nerve palsy. The scutum is usually intact. Epidermoids may be solid or cystic. Epidermoids do not enhance—acquired cholesteatomas may enhance peripherally as any self-respecting inflammatory process should. Treatment for both is surgical excision.

Inflammatory Lesions

Otitis media   Inflammatory disease of the tympanic cavity is common. Opacification of the epitympanic recess with thickening of the tympanic membrane is often seen in patients with otitis media. The most frequent causes of otitis media are *Streptococcus, Moraxella catarrhalis, Haemophilus influenzae,* and *Pneumococcus.* Obstruction of the eustachian tube from nasopharyngeal lymphoid hypertrophy caused by upper respiratory tract infections is responsible for this condition in children. Otitis media generally responds well to antibiotics. Rarely, ossicular erosions, usually a marker for acquired cholesteatoma, can occur in association with otitis media. When they occur, they usually affect the long process of the incus and can lead to conductive hearing defects. The erosions appear on CT as tiny, lytic, punched-out areas in the ossicle. The middle ear is filled with fluid density and intensity on CT and MR in uncomplicated otitis media (Fig. 12-14). Although pneumolabyrinth is more commonly seen in cases of barotrauma or in the postoperative setting, occasionally you may see air in the inner ear structures with infections, presumably from a labyrinthine fistula. Gas-producing organisms may be at fault. (Not you, Bob!)

Ossicular disruptions may be caused by trauma or infection (Fig. 12-15). A gap of greater than 1 mm between the long process of the incus and the head of the stapes is suspected of being disrupted. This finding is equally well displayed on axial or coronal sections. Usually the inflammatory causes are due to erosion of the long process of the incus. Fibrosis may ensue. Because the incus is not well suspended by the anchoring ligaments, the incudostapedial joint is most commonly affected by trauma. Therefore, dislocations and subluxations are common between the incus and stapes. Incudal disarticulation accounts for more than 80% of post-traumatic conductive hearing loss.

Effusions   Middle ear effusions may be present both with infectious and with noninfectious processes. They appear as nonerosive opacification of the middle ear cavity. One may identify an air-fluid level. The process may be due to a pressure phenomenon and can be seen in patients after air travel in poorly pressurized compartments (occasionally seen in the rarefied atmosphere of the first-class cabin).

Mastoiditis   Infection may travel from the middle ear via the aditus ad antrum (the narrow channel connecting the middle ear cavity to the mastoid antrum) to the mastoid air cells. Mastoiditis may occur as a complication of otitis media; coalescence of mastoiditis portends a poor prognosis because it represents bony infection rather than mucositis. β-Hemolytic streptococci and pneumococci are usually the pathogens involved. CT reveals opacification of air cells; bone destruction constitutes a criterion for coalescence. The infection is very bright on T2WI. Occasionally, air-fluid levels within the small mastoid air cells can be seen. Middle ear and/or petrous apex opacification may coexist. Coalescent mastoiditis may also be a complication of cholesteatoma

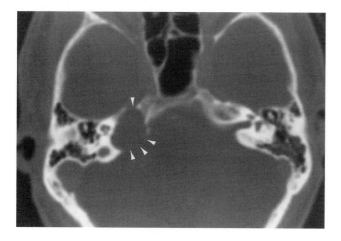

Fig. 12-13   Epidermoid of petrous apex. Axial CT displays a well-defined mass in the petrous apex with a thin bony margin *(arrowheads).* This was a congenital cholesteatoma *(epidermoid).*

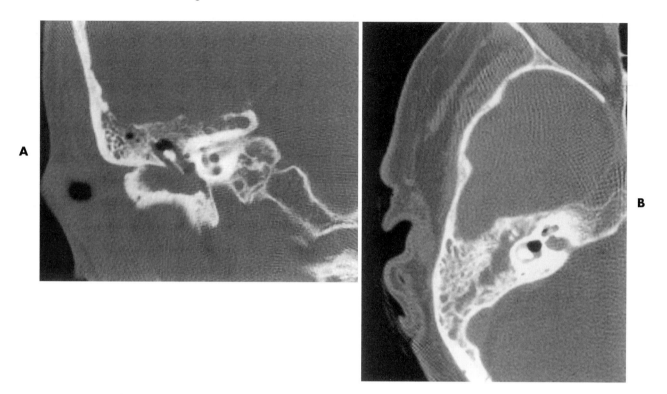

Fig. 12-14   Acute otomastoiditis. **A,** An air fluid level is seen in the epitympanic space with complete opacification of the mesotympanum. The mastoid air cells are also opacified. **B,** Air in the vestibule and in the cochlea (pneumolabyrinth), seen in this patient with otomastoiditis, implies an open connection between the middle ear and the inner ear.

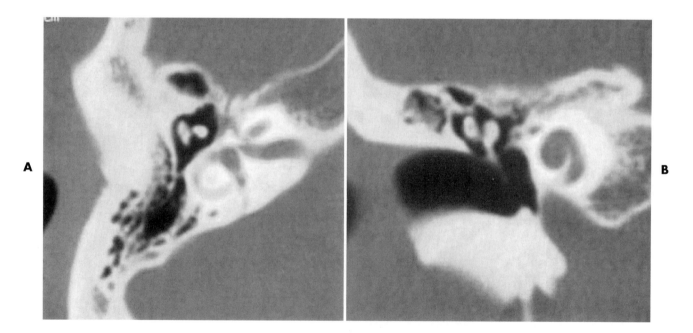

Fig. 12-15   Ossicular dislocation: oops.....splat! **A,** Note that the ice cream (the head of the malleus) seems to be falling off of the ice cream cone (short process of the incus) on this axial scan. This is incudomalleolar dislocation, most often found in the setting of trauma. **B,** The presence of both the incus and the malleus in the same slice on a coronal scan is ABNORMAL! Usually the incus lies posterior to the malleus head.

Illustration continued on following page

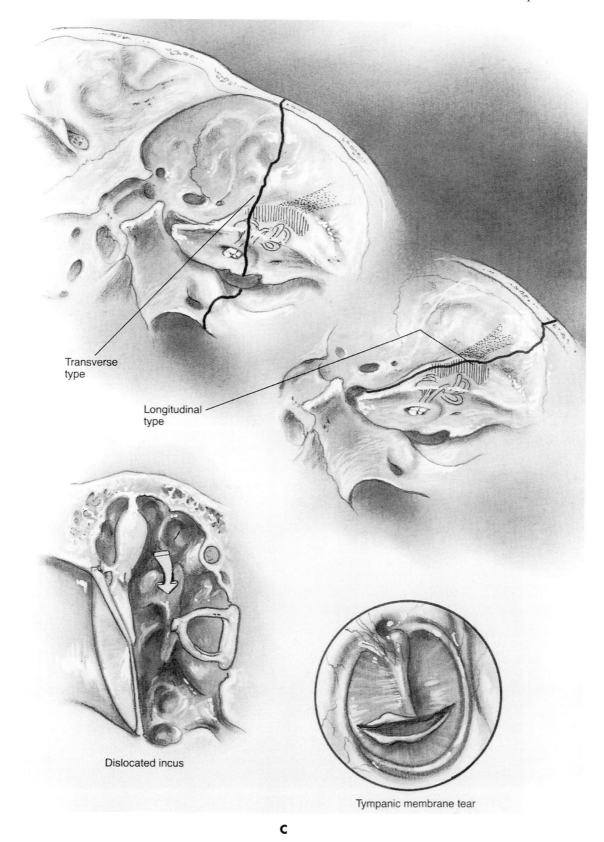

Transverse
type

Longitudinal
type

Dislocated incus

Tympanic membrane tear

C

Fig. 12-15   *Continued.* **C,** Diagrams of fracture lines causing dislocation of incus from stapes. (C from Mathog: Atlas of Craniofacial Trauma. Philadelphia, WB Saunders, 1992.)

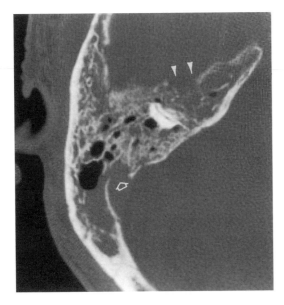

Fig. 12-16 Coalescent mastoiditis. Note the destroyed mastoid air cell septations and the dehiscent area at the transverse sinus anterolateral margin *(open arrow)*. This is a set-up for septic thrombophlebitis. The anterior margin of the petrous bone is also eroded focally *(arrowheads)*.

formation or may develop in and of its own right (Fig. 12-16).

Middle ear effusions and mastoid opacification are a great marker for previous radiation therapy of the brain and/or the head and neck. Alternatively, look for the long-standing nasogastric tube as a predisposing factor.

Sclerosis and poor pneumatization may be seen in patients with chronic mastoiditis.

Complications of acute otomastoiditis include sigmoid sinus thrombosis (see Chapter 4), thrombophlebitis, epidural abscesses, meningitis, subperiosteal abscesses, fistulas, and osteomyelitis. Cerebellar or temporal lobe encephalitis is uncommon. A Bezold's abscess is an inflammatory collection that occurs inferior to the mastoid tip as the infection spreads from the bone to the adjacent soft tissue (Fig. 12-17). It can spread down the plane of the sternocleidomatoid muscle to the lower neck.

Another complication of chronic otitis media ("COM" on the pediatrician's chart) is ossicular fixation. This may cause a conductive hearing loss and may be fibrous (soft tissue around the ossicles) or tympanosclerotic (calcification around ossicles or ossicular ligaments).

Acquired cholesteatomas Long-standing otomastoiditis may result from chronic eustachian tube dysfunction. This may lead to recurrent otitis media and acquired cholesteatomas; these two entities are easier to distinguish in textbooks than in real life, where imaging characteristics may overlap (Table 12-2). Acquired cholesteatomas are erosive collections of keratinous debris from an ingrowth of stratified squamous epithelium through a perforated tympanic membrane. The critical features in identifying a lesion as a cholesteatoma are the presence of bony erosion and/or expansion (Fig. 12-18). This cholesteatoma most often arises from a perforation in the pars flaccida of the tympanic membrane. Once the pars flaccida (Shrapnell's membrane) has been violated,

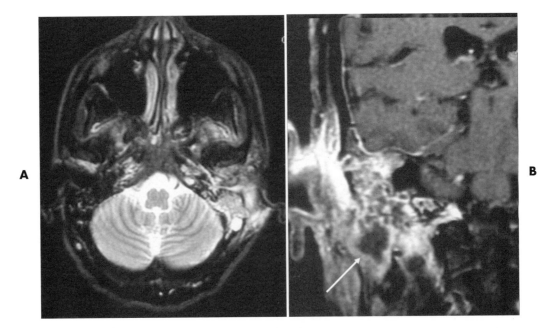

Fig. 12-17 Bezold's abscess. **A,** The T2WI shows the opacified mastoid air cells as well as inflammation extending into the subcutaneous tissue. **B,** The coronal enhanced scan is fantastic: see the ring-enhancing abscess *(arrow)* just below the opacified mastoid tip? Note the meningeal enhancement as well.

Table 12-2   Cholesteatoma versus otitis media

Feature	Cholesteatoma	Otitis media
Middle ear opacified	Yes	Yes
Scutum	Eroded	Normal
Ossicular erosion	Yes	Infrequent
Ossicular displacement	Yes	No
Expansion of aditus ad antrum	Sometimes	No
Lateral semicircular canal fistula	Sometimes	Infrequent
Gadolinium enhancement	Rare	Rare
T2WI signal intensity	Intermediate	Bright
Tympanic membrane retracted	Yes	No
Tegmen tympani erosion	Sometimes	No
Facial nerve canal dehiscence	Sometimes	No

the inflammatory process proceeds into Prussak's space, which is located lateral to the middle ear ossicles in the epitympanic space. One often sees a soft-tissue mass causing erosion of the scutum and medial displacement of the malleus and incus with pars flaccida cholesteatomas. The head of the malleus and body of the incus are the areas most susceptible to erosion by a pars flaccida cholesteatoma; lysis of all the middle ear ossicles is uncommon. From Prussak's space the lesion often spreads through the aditus ad antrum, expanding its waist as the inflammatory process proceeds into the mastoid air cells. On MR, cholesteatomas are hypointense on T1WI and intermediate on T2WI, and do not enhance, as opposed to granulation tissue (postoperative) that does enhance.

Pars tensa cholesteatomas are much less common than pars flaccida cholesteatomas. Although the pars

tensa represents the larger inferior segment of the tympanic membrane, if cholesteatomas arise, they do so from perforation through the posterosuperior most portion of the pars tensa. From this location the sinus tympani, pyramidal eminence, and facial recess may be expanded and/or eroded. Pars tensa cholesteatomas present with a mass in the middle ear, erosion of the long process of the incus or stapes, epitympanic spread, and ossicular displacement. The scutum is usually intact. *Vive la différence avec le pars flaccida!*

Complications of cholesteatomas include fistulization into the semicircular canals (4–25% of cases), with the lateral semicircular canal most commonly affected. This may be identified as a dehiscence in the bony labyrinth with a soft-tissue mass expanding the region of the oval window or lateral margin of the lateral semicircular canal. Alternatively, cholesteatomas may erode the tegmen tympani (the roof of the epitympanic space) and subsequently invade the intracranial compartment (Fig. 12-19). Another area of potential erosion is the lateral or inferior wall of the facial nerve's tympanic portion (Fig. 12-20). If there is dehiscence or skeletization of the facial nerve canal or the sinus tympani, the surgeon must know this preoperatively so that removal of the cholesteatoma is done in a careful fashion so as not to injure the underlying structures. Of course, Yousem's theorem is that if you know something can go wrong and take due precautions against it, something *else* will go wrong, like a stapes gusher.

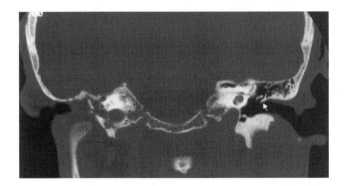

Fig. 12-18   Cholesteatoma. Coronal CT demonstrates destruction of the mastoid air cells with nonvisualization of the scutum on the right side. Compare with normal-appearing scutum on the left side *(white arrow)*. Middle ear ossicles are surrounded by soft tissue and do not have a normal bony appearance, showing some erosive changes along their length. Orientation of the ossicles is also disturbed on the right side.

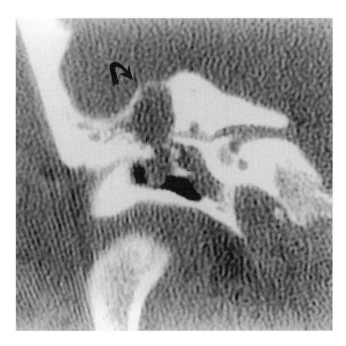

Fig. 12-19   Destruction from a cholesteatoma. The scutum *(arrowhead)* is eroded, the middle ear ossicles fragmented *(tiny arrows)* and the tegmen tympanum skeletonized *(curved arrow)* if not violated.

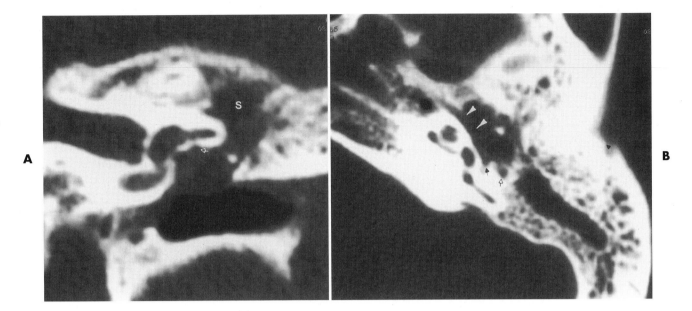

Fig. 12-20   Facial nerve dehiscence from cholesteatoma. **A,** This coronal scan shows absence of the inferior bony canal of the tympanic portion of the facial nerve *(open arrow)*. Some erosion of the scutum is present with opacification of the epitympanic space (s). **B,** The involvement of the lateral wall *(arrowheads)* of the facial (fallopian) canal is seen on the axial scan. Opacification of the sinus tympani *(closed arrow)* and facial nerve recess *(open arrow)* should be reported as they are often hidden from the otoscopist's view.

Surgery for otomastoiditis   Many operations are performed for chronic inflammatory conditions of the middle ear and mastoid air cells. The simple mastoidectomy spares the EAC and ossicular chain but removes the offending mastoid air cells. Another term for the simple mastoidectomy is the canal wall up mastoidectomy and it preserves the posterior wall of the EAC; canal wall down mastoidectomies take this border down. The modified radical mastoidectomy preserves the ossicles but removes the mastoid air cells and EAC. A radical mastoidectomy removes the mastoid air cells and the ossicular chain but preserves the stapes. The incus is the most commonly diseased ossicle; if the stapes can be preserved, a partial prosthesis can be used. The mastoid cavity is usually filled with bone chips, fascia, or fat. In all these surgeries, the facial nerve is preserved at all cost.

Ossiculoplasty or tympanoplasty is a procedure to restore the conductive capability of the ossicular chain usually after damage from cholesteatoma, chronic otitis media, or congenital malformation. There are at least five types of tympanoplasties. In type 1 the procedure spares all the ossicles and the graft rests on the malleus, in type 2 the graft rests on the incus, in type 3 the graft rests on the head of the stapes, in type 4 the graft connects to the footplate of the stapes, and in type 5 the stapes is removed (Fig. 12-21). Type 3 is the most common form of tympanoplasty. A stapedotomy refers to a procedure in which a tiny wire connects the long process of the incus to the stapes footplate with only the superstructure resected. A stapedectomy removes the footplate of the stapes and an implant is placed from the incus

through the oval window into the labyrinth. A variant of the stapedectomy-stapedotomy procedure is one in which the posterior crus of the stapes footplate is preserved—a stupidectomy (just kidding on the name).

Autografts (from the host) for ossicular replacement are hard to sculpt and are rarely used these days. Homografts from cadavers (for the incus) are not commonly used now, because of an unspoken fear of transmitting infectious agents. Synthetic ossicular prostheses (Proplast and Plastipore prostheses) have gained favor. Some ossicular prostheses that an erudite neuroradiologist should be familiar with include the stapes prosthesis, the incus interposition graft (for incudostapedial joint disease), the Applebaum prosthesis (a synthetic prosthesis from long process of incus to capitulum of stapes), the Black oval top synthetic prosthesis (from tympanic membrane to capitulum of stapes or oval window), the Richards synthetic prosthesis (from tympanic membrane to capitulum of stapes or oval window), and the Goldenberg prosthesis (from tympanic membrane to capitulum of stapes or oval window, or stapes to malleus or footplate to malleus) (Fig. 12-22). The latter three ossicular replacement prostheses may be total (TORP) or partial (PORP) depending on whether the stapes superstructure is preserved. They therefore extend from the tympanic membrane to the stapes capitulum (PORP) or footplate (TORP). You may ask who are the TWERPS that developed these TORPS and PORPS, but for the patients who are SOL without these devices, they are STARS. The PORP is the most commonly used synthetic ossicular prosthesis and the prosthesis' hydroxyapatite head at-

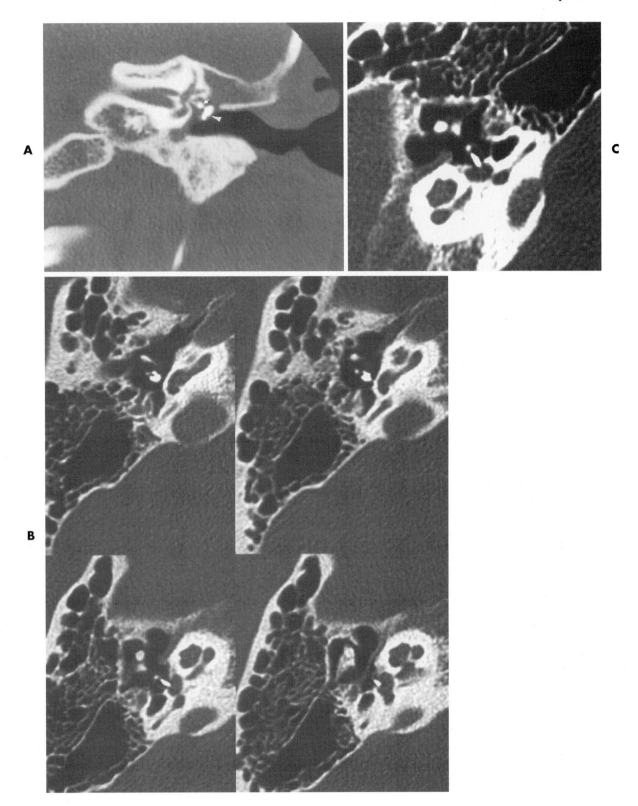

Fig. 12-21   **A,** Incus and stapes prosthesis. In this post-operative case the incus *(arrowhead)* and capitulum of the stapes *(arrow)* have been replaced by a prosthesis. There has been a partial mastoidectomy and the scutum and tympanic membrane cannot be discerned. **B,** This partial ossicular replacement device consists of a component for the incus and a piston for the stapes. It is inserted into the vestibule through the oval window. **C,** The magnified view reveals the stapes footplates with the prosthetic limb extending between the two crura.

Text continued on page 584

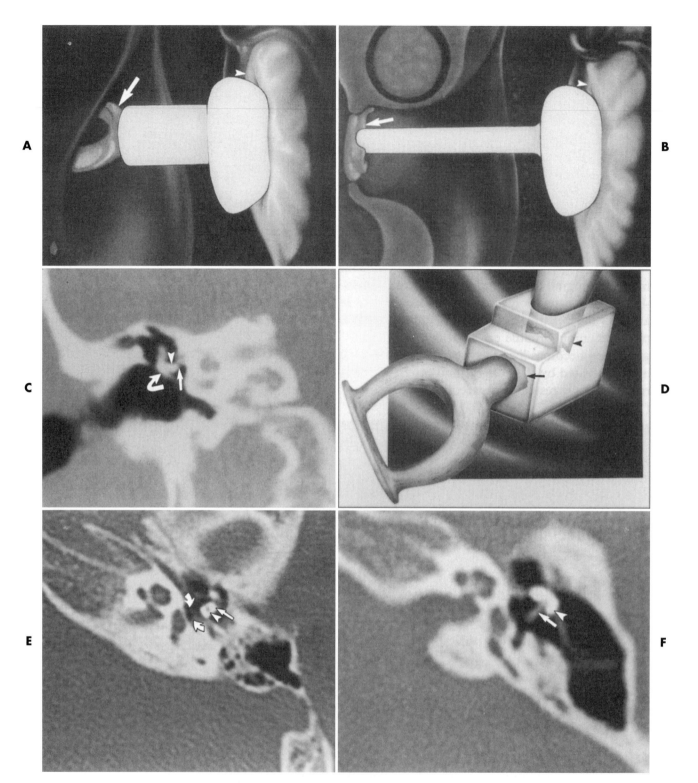

Fig. 12-22 Ossicular replacement prostheses. **A,** PORP extending from the tympanic membrane *(arrowhead)* to the capitulum of the stapes *(arrow).* **B,** TORP extending from the tympanic membrane *(arrowhead)* to the oval window *(arrow).* **C,** Incus interposition graft. Coronal CT scan shows a surgically remodeled incus *(arrowhead)* used as an interposition graft extending from the manubrium of the malleus *(curved arrow)* to the capitulum of the stapes *(straight arrow).* **D,** Applebaum prosthesis, with characteristic L-shaped configuration. A long notch fits over the end of the partially amputated long process of the incus *(arrowhead).* The length of the notch can be varied to accommodate residual long processes of different lengths. The capitulum of the stapes inserts into a hole at the other end of the prosthesis *(arrow).* **E,** Axial CT scan shows an Applebaum prosthesis with the notch *(arrowhead)* medial to the long process of the incus *(straight arrow),* which fits into the notch. The crura of the stapes are also identified *(curved arrows).* **F,** Axial CT scan shows the head *(arrowhead)* and shaft *(arrow)* of a Black PORP. The shaft is made of Plasti-Pore and has significantly lower attenuation than the head. The medial articulation of the prosthesis with the capitulum of the stapes is not seen.

Illustration continued on following page

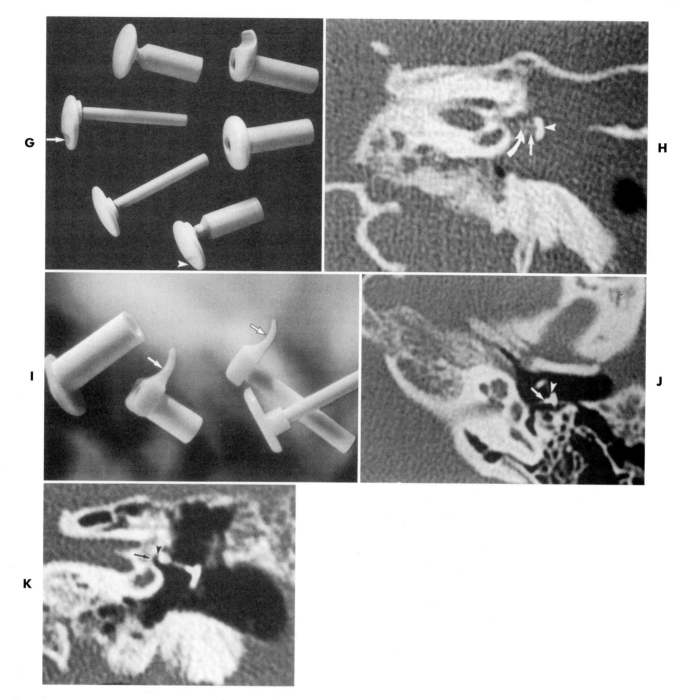

Fig. 12-22 *Continued.* **G,** Various Richards PORPs (short, thick shafts) and TORPs (long, thin shafts). A modified Richards PORP *(arrowhead)* and TORP *(arrow)* with an off-center head and a groove for the malleus are included. **H,** Coronal CT scan shows a Richards PORP, which is encased in granulation tissue but is in normal position with the distal tip in the expected region of the capitulum of the stapes *(curved arrow).* The hollow shaft is centered on a flat hydroxyapatite head *(arrowhead)* and manifests as a linear area of low attenuation *(straight arrow).* **I,** Various Goldenberg PORPs (short, thick shafts) and TORPs (long, thin shafts). The heads of the prostheses are off center relative to the shafts. A prosthesis with a notched head *(arrows)* is used when the malleus is present. The notch fits over the manubrium of the malleus for added stability. **J,** Axial CT scan shows the flat head of a Goldenberg TORP articulating with the tympanic membrane *(arrowhead).* The shaft *(arrow)* is off center relative to the head. The articulation of the medial tip of the shaft with the oval window is not seen. **K,** Coronal CT scan shows the Goldenberg TORP in its entirety. The air gap is seen *(arrowhead),* and a slight superior subluxation of the medial shaft relative to the oval window can be identified *(arrow).* (From Stone JA, Mukherji SK, Jewett BS, et al: CT evaluation of prosthetic ossicular reconstruction procedures: What the otologist needs to know, *Radiographics* 20:593-605, 2000.)

taches to the tympanic membrane and the Plastipore shaft to the capitulum of the stapes.

Failure of ossicular replacement prostheses may be due to recurrent otitis media, recurrent cholesteatoma, reparative granulomas (foreign body reactions), ossicular subluxation or dislocation, adhesions, fracture of the prosthesis, perilymphatic fistula, granulation tissue, recurrence of otospongiotic bone, excessive postoperative bony reaction, or extrusion of the prosthesis. Subluxation of the prosthesis accounts for 50% to 60% of the cases in which there is postoperative hearing loss after ossicular replacement surgery. When PORPS or TORPS are subluxed, it usually occurs at its distal site either with the stapes capitulum or oval window, respectively. In the case of the stapes prosthesis, look for the subluxed prosthesis inferior and posterior to the oval window. The wire between the prosthesis and the incus may also migrate inferiorly. Failed stapedectomy cases may also be caused by persistent perilymphatic fistulae. Evidence for this complication includes air in the labyrinth or persistent fluid in the middle ear. Extrusions of prostheses may occur through holes in the tympanic membrane from surgery or inflammatory perforations. The prosthesis may be found in these cases in the external auditory canal or on the pillow in the morning. Extrusions rarely occur into the vestibule.

Hearing is a complex sense. These procedures were developed to restore native sound transmission: at the extreme, cochlear implants can restore hearing without the ossicles, but the quality of the sound suffers compared with native hearing. Cochlear implants are getting increasingly sophisticated and effective. More on that later!

The postoperative examination of a patient who has undergone temporal bone surgery is fraught with difficulties. How can one tell whether the soft tissue seen in the operative cavity is due to recurrent or residual cholesteatoma, scar tissue, acute inflammation, or non-cholesteatomatous granulation tissue? It is nearly impossible unless the recurrent mass is focal and erosive. If the postoperative soft tissue enhances, it is more likely to be granulation tissue than cholesteatoma. It is best merely to provide landmarks for the surgeon to assess the mass endoscopically or by biopsy. Identifying areas of dehiscence in the base of the skull or near vascular structures (sigmoid sinus, carotid canal, and jugular bulb) may be the most important role of imaging if reoperation is contemplated.

Other inflammatory conditions of the middle ear Wegener's granulomatosis can attack the eustachian tube and from there invade the nasopharynx or skull base. Langerhans cell histiocytosis affects the temporal bones of children as eosinophilic granulomas in isolation or as part of the wider spectrum of disease. Another cause of lysis of the temporal bone is osteoradionecrosis. This has been described most commonly after irradiation for nasopharyngeal carcinoma (Fig. 12-23).

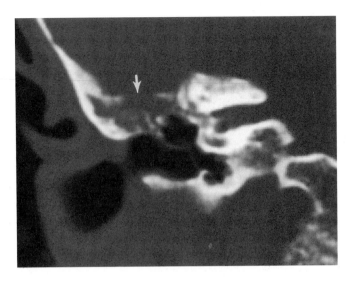

Fig. 12-23 Osteoradionecrosis of the tegmen tympani. Erosion of the tegmen tympani *(arrow)* is seen with sparing of the middle ear cavity. In this case the process was not due to a cholesteatoma but due to osteoradionecrosis in a patient with recurrent nasopharyngeal carcinoma treated with radiotherapy.

Benign Neoplasms

Glomus tympanicum Glomus tympanicum and glomus jugulare tumors are fascinating entities that have interesting anatomic ramifications and pathologic manifestations. They arise from glomus bodies (paraganglioma tissue), which are scattered in the middle ear. Ringing in the ears, unassociated with recent attendance of Rolling Stones concerts (are we "dating" ourselves—we can't get no satisfaction), is a hallmark of these lesions. The glomus tympanicum is a paraganglioma usually identified along the lateral aspect of the cochlea in the middle ear cavity. This tumor is the most common neoplasm of the inferior part of the middle ear, and presents in middle aged women. Its clinical presentation is that of pulsatile tinnitus, a finding that has an extensive differential diagnosis (see Box 12-5). The glomus tym-

---

Box 12-5 Causes of Pulsatile Tinnitus

Aberrant carotid artery, petrous internal carotid artery aneurysms, dissections, persistent stapedial artery
Cholesteatoma, cholesterol granuloma
Dural arteriovenous malformations, cavernous carotid fistulas
Glomus jugulotympanicum (paraganglioma)
Hemangioma
High grade stenosis of internal carotid artery
High jugular bulb, jugular bulb diverticula
Meniere's disease
Meningioma
Pseudotumor cerebri

Box 12-6 Vascular Intratympanic Masses

Aberrant carotid or aneurysm
Arteriovenous malformation
Chronic inflammation (cholesterol granuloma)
Glomus jugulare
Glomus tympanicum
High, dehiscent jugular bulb
Hemangioma
Meningioma
Persistent stapedial artery

panicum, because it produces symptoms relatively early, is usually seen as a small soft-tissue mass bulging behind the tympanic membrane (Box 12-6), which enhances markedly. Its location is variable within the medial aspect of the middle ear. Although classically it presents at the cochlear promontory (Fig. 12-24), it may also reside anterior to the promontory, beneath the cochleariform process and the semicanal of the tensor tympani, inferior to the promontory, in the recess beneath the basal turn of the cochlea or anteroinferiorly. It arises from the glomus bodies (neural crest tissue) along the tympanic branch of cranial nerve IX known as Jacobson's nerve. This nerve runs from the inferior ganglion of cranial nerve IX, through the inferior tympanic canaliculus (between jugular foramen and carotid canal), to the middle ear. Jacobson's nerve forms the tympanic plexus that may cover the cochlear promontory before rejoining as the lesser superficial petrosal nerve. Branches of the tym-

panic plexus may be found near the round window, eustachian tube egress, tensor tympani tendon, and along the inferior tympanic canaliculus. The tumors are classified on the basis of their spread from the cochlear promontory, to the middle ear, the mastoid, and the EAC or carotid canal. The most sensitive study to detect this tumor is a high-resolution, thin-section CT with axial and coronal sections filmed with bone windows and algorithms. As opposed to cholesteatomas and other middle ear masses, the glomus tympanicum does not erode the ossicles but engulfs them. Because a glomus tympanicum is so small, it is usually identified on MR as an enhancing soft-tissue mass of intermediate signal intensity without large vessels (see Fig. 12-24B). The clinical differential diagnosis of these lesions (see Box 12-6) also includes the congenital abnormality of an aberrant internal carotid artery, which deviates posterolaterally near the cochlea. If you want to cause encopresis in a surgeon, send him in to resect what he thinks is a glomus tumor but is really an aberrant carotid artery. There is no right way to do the wrong thing; Yousem's corollary to Murphy's law. Although glomus tympanicum tumors gain blood supply from the inferior tympanic artery branch of the ascending pharyngeal artery, they rarely require preoperative embolization because of their small size.

Tympanic membrane hemangiomas A hemangioma behind the tympanic membrane is another cause of a vascular tympanic mass. It enhances markedly and has nonspecific density and intensity characteristics unless flow voids are seen.

Glomus jugulare Occasionally, a *glomus jugulare* extends from the skull base superiorly into the middle

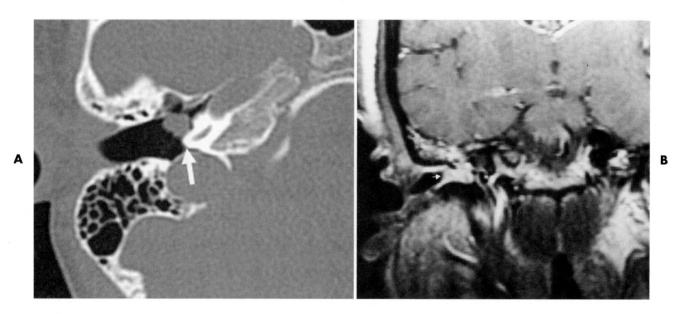

Fig. 12-24 Glomus tympanicum. **A,** If this lesion is white on otoscopy, call it an epidermoid. If it's red, think about an aberrant carotid artery or a glomus tympanicum. If it's green, adjust the color on your set or call it a chloroma. The location, along the cochlear promontory *(arrow)* is perfect for the glomus tympanicum. **B,** Coronal MR reveals an enhancing mass in the middle ear on the right side *(arrow)*. Enhancement above the tumor was due to inflammatory disease in mastoid air cells.

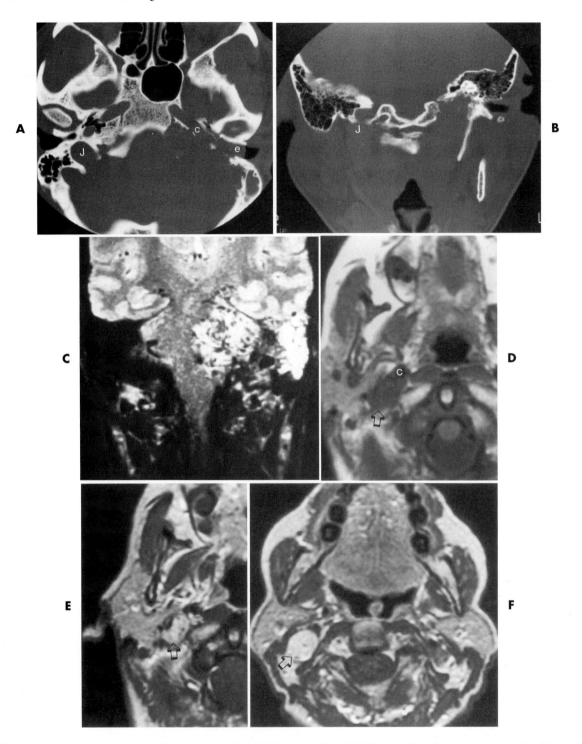

Fig. 12-25   Glomus jugulare. **A,** An erosive process of the left jugular bulb, which has scalloped the posterior wall of the left internal carotid artery *(c)* and has extended into the EAC *(e)* is seen. The contralateral jugular foramen is labelled *J.* **B,** Coronal CT demonstrates erosion and enlargement of the left jugular foramen (normal on right side *J*) with extension of the mass into the labyrinth. **C,** MR of glomus tumor. Coronal T2WI in a patient with a large glomus jugulare illustrates the characteristic flow voids within the mass. This lesion compresses the brain stem on the left side. A lesion of this size may secrete a large amount of adrenergic compounds, the incidence of which in all tumors is approximately 3% to 5%. This has major import if angiography is performed, since a hypertensive crisis may be precipitated in the "secreters." Alpha-adrenergic blocking agents may be required during the arteriogram. **D,** Note the skull base mass *(open arrow)* posterolateral to the carotid artery within the carotid *(c)* space growing in the jugular vein. **E,** It *(open arrow)* shows enhancement but has dots within it (pepper within salt?) **F,** Note also how far inferior this glomus jugulare *(open arrow)* extended (C3—C4 disk level).

ear cavity and may simulate a localized glomus tympanicum (thereby called a glomus jugulotympanicum). Glomus jugulare most commonly arise from the adventitia of the jugular vein in the jugular foramen, though glomus bodies also accompany the auricular branches of the vagus nerve (Arnold's nerve) or the tympanic branch of the glossopharyngeal nerve (Jacobson's nerve). The glomus jugulare has a typical MR appearance on T2WI and enhanced T1WI with what is called a salt-and-pepper look (Fig. 12-25). This is seen as flow voids within the tumor, surrounded by tumor substance. On CT, this mass erodes the jugular foramen of the temporal bone. The mass may grow inferiorly into the jugular vein or may grow from the jugular bulb region into the sigmoid and transverse sinuses. Alternatively, the mass may cause thrombosis of the sinuses or the vein. Mass within the vessel may be distinguished from thrombosis by the presence of enhancement in the former. A hereditary form of paragangliomatosis is associated with multiple glomus tumors including jugulare, vagale, carotid body, and tympanicum. Overall, multiple paragangliomas occur in 15% of patients with a glomus tumor. Rarely, paragangliomas

---

Box 12-7   Jugular Foramen Masses

Chondroid/chondroma lesions
Glomus jugulare
Enlarged jugular bulb (normal variant)
Meningioma
Metastasis
Nasopharyngeal carcinoma
Schwannoma

---

may secrete norepinephrine. This may require α-adrenergic blocking drugs during arteriograms. The arteriographic findings of a hypervascular mass, often supplied by ascending pharyngeal branches, with a persistent stain distinguishes this jugular foramen mass from other differential diagnostic considerations as listed in Box 12-7 and distinguished in Table 12-3.

If the vascularity doesn't show, the diagnosis of glomus must go (with apologies to Johnnie Cochran). Schwan-

Table 12-3   Differential diagnosis of jugular foramen masses

Entity	T2WI intensity	Enhancement	Calcification/ bone erosion	MR technique helpful	Angiographic appearance	CT density
Glomus jugulare	Salt and pepper	Marked, downward dip on dynamic enhancement	Erosion	Dynamic enhancement, MR venogram	Hypervascular with arteriovenous shunting, stain	Hyperdense
Schwannoma	Hyperintense, may have cystic degeneration	Moderate, upward slope on dynamic scanning	No, bone remodeled	Traditional	Hypovascular	Isodense
Metastasis	Hyperintense	Moderate	Erodes bone and infiltrates	Traditional	Most often hypovascular—exceptions include hypervascular metastases such as renal, thyroid	Isodense
Chondroid lesions	Hyperintense with mottling (secondary to calcification)	Moderate	Yes calcified matrix and bone erosion	Gradient echo for calcification	Hypovascular	Areas of high density from matrix
Enlarged jugular bulb	Flow effects	Varies with technique, turbulence	No	MR venogram	Venous phase	Vascular
Nasopharyngeal carcinoma	Hyperintense to intermediate	Moderate	Erodes bone and infiltrates, ? perineural spread	Traditional	Most often hypovascular	Isodense
Meningioma	Isointense to slightly hyperintense	Marked	Osteolysis versus hyperostosis	Traditional	Hypervascular, persistent stain on all tests (Clinton-Lewinsky sign)	Slightly hyperdense

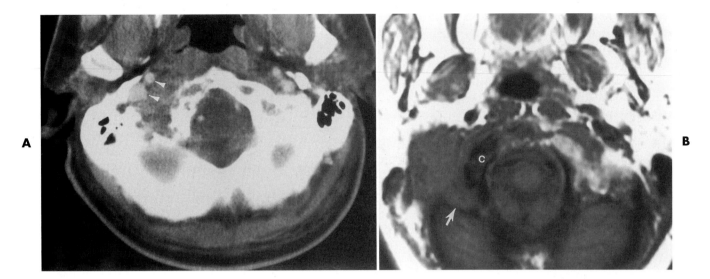

Fig. 12-26 Metastasis in a woman with cervical carcinoma. **A,** CT scan with displaced carotid sheath structures *(arrowheads).* **B,** The occipital condyle *(c)* and region of the stylomastoid foramen *(arrow)* on the right are infiltrated by this mass seen as replaced bright marrow fat by low intensity badness. Involvement of the jugular foramen was seen more superiorly on the T1-weighted scans.

nomas can occur in the jugular foramen because cranial nerves IX through XI run in this region, but are relatively avascular. Metastases (Fig. 12-26), unless from the kidney, thyroid, or choriocarcinoma, are not hypervascular.

Vascular lesions of the temporal bone These lesions mimic glomus tumors and may present similarly on otoscopic examinations a retrotympanic vascular mass. The aberrant internal carotid artery passes through the middle ear cavity and runs anteromedially to the horizontal portion of the cavernous carotid canal (Fig. 12-27). This is easily recognized as a flow void on MR but may be visualized as an enhancing mass of uncertain cause on CT.

The persistent stapedial artery is a rare anomaly (<0.5% of patients) anywhere except in the halls of the Executive West in Louisville (this joke is for American board-fearing radiology residents only) and therefore bears acknowledging. This artery appears transiently in embryologic development as a branch of the hyoid artery (derived itself from the second aortic arch) connecting the external and internal carotid artery. Ultimately, it regresses to form pieces of the caroticotympanic artery. When it persists it may present as a pulsatile middle ear mass. Because it subsumes the role of the middle meningeal artery, its imaging findings include absence of the foramen spinosum, a soft-tissue mass along the horizontal portion of the tympanic facial nerve, and an additional branch leading from the petrous carotid artery. It enters the middle ear to create the obturator foramen of the stapes (between the crura) and leaves the middle ear near the geniculate ganglion (where it can simulate a schwannoma, albeit a bloody one). This anomaly may coexist with an aberrant internal carotid artery

(60%). Associations with trisomy 13, 15, 21, thalidomide exposure, anencephaly (not just in Louisville), and neurofibromatosis have been reported.

Jugular bulb variations are very common and may cause a vascular tympanic mass associated with pulsatile tinnitus. Don't be alarmed by asymmetry in jugular foraminal size; that's the rule, not the exception. Until you see erosion or soft-tissue destruction, don't call it a glomus tumor. Remember also that the jugular foramen has two parts: a pars vasculosa, containing the internal jugular vein and cranial nerves X and XI, and a pars nervosa with cranial nerve IX and continuation of the inferior petrosal sinus. The jugular bulb wall may be dehiscent or nondehiscent; and the jugular vein may rise high into the middle ear cavity. The nondehiscent jugular bulb has preservation of the bony plate of the top of the jugular foramen, whereas the dehiscent jugular bulb shows no bony margin. Aberrantly high jugular bulbs are a common finding, occurring in 7% of the population. The definition of how high above the rim is a high jugular bulb varies between Yao Ming and Shaquille O'Neal but most people use either the inferior rim of the tympanic ring or the inferior margin of the round window as the uppermost limit. High jugular bulbs may extend into the middle ear or into the petrous bone near the endolymphatic sac. Diverticuli of the jugular bulb may enter the middle ear as well.

Dural vascular malformations Another entity that may cause tinnitus is a dural vascular malformation. These commonly affect the transverse sinus and in some cases may be due to previously thrombosed veins or sinuses, resulting in abnormal collateral flow of arteries and veins around the thrombosis. If no soft-tissue mass

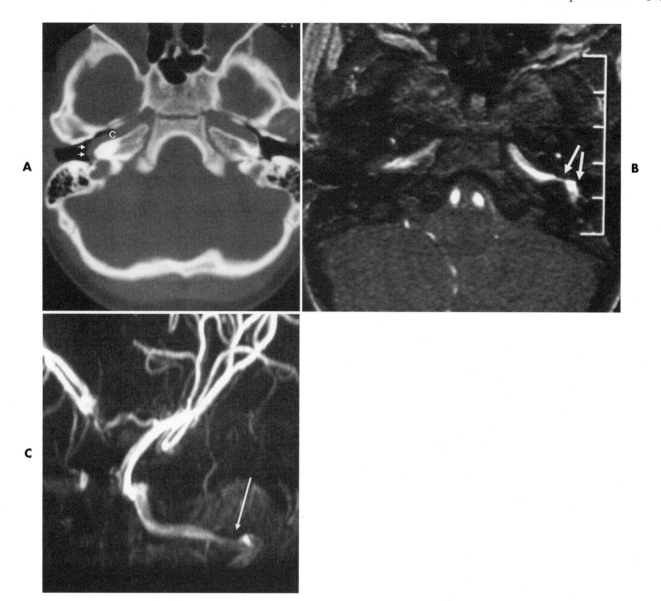

Fig. 12-27   Aberrant right internal carotid artery. **A,** Axial bone targeted CT shows extension of the right petrous carotid *(c)* into the middle ear *(arrows)*. This "mass" may present as a retrotympanic vascular lesion with pulsatile tinnitus. You lose if you recommend biopsy. **B,** Aberrant left internal carotid artery. Raw data from an MRA shows the posterolateral extension of the aberrant carotid *(arrows)* as it enters the middle ear cavity. **C,** The maximum intensity projection clearly shows the aberrant deviation *(arrow)* of the course of the petrous carotid.

in the middle ear or skull base is seen on cross-sectional imaging in patients with objective tinnitus, angiography may be indicated to detect this lesion. At times arteriography is required to distinguish between other lesions that cause pulsatile tinnitus including aneurysms and arteriovenous malformations of the temporal bone, high-flow turbulence associated with stenoses of the internal carotid artery, and high jugular bulbs. Please remember though, the most common neurologic cause of subjective tinnitus is pseudotumor cerebri.

Physicians may separate patients into those with objective pulsatile tinnitus (heard by both physician and patient) and those with subjective tinnitus (heard only by patient). In both cases, the surgeon hears the cash register ring. Objective pulsatile tinnitus is usually evaluated with angiography of the ipsilateral carotid and vertebral arteries initially, with MR or CT to follow. Subjective tinnitus, on the other hand, is best evaluated noninvasively initially with CT or MR. Objective pulsatile tinnitus is usually caused by true vascular malformations, stenoses, or aneurysms. Subjective tinnitus is usually seen in patients with glomus tumors, aberrant internal carotid arteries, and jugular vein abnormalities. Just because the clinician cannot hear the tinnitus does not make the patient a malingerer; in fact, the lesions of subjective tinnitus are often smaller and harder to detect.

Facial schwannomas   Facial schwannomas may arise within the IAC, the labyrinthine portion of the facial nerve, the tympanic portion of the facial nerve, the geniculate ganglion, the mastoid portion of the facial nerve, or within the parotid gland. If you identify expansion of the facial nerve canal, you may make the di-

agnosis of facial schwannomas; however, these lesions often cannot be separated from lesions that occur in neighboring structures such as vestibular schwannomas within the IAC or glomus tumors within the tympanic cavity (Box 12-8). All three of these lesions demonstrate enhancement (Fig. 12-28). If you are fortunate enough to see the flow voids of blood vessels within the glomus tumor, then you may be able to make the differential diagnosis.

Facial hemangiomas   Hemangiomas may also occur in the IAC, around the geniculate ganglion, and at the posterior genu of the facial nerve canal. Bone erosion with a soft-tissue mass is seen by CT and may have a "honeycomb" bony trabecular internal architecture of the ossifying type. These tumors often present with slowly evolving facial paresis and twitching like Kramer on Seinfeld. Hemangiomas of the facial nerve are said to be as common as schwannomas of the facial nerve (This is one of these hard-to-believe facts expounded in the literature, but not matching our collective experience) (Fig. 12-29). Only when the lesions calcify or enhance in a dramatic fashion can facial hemangiomas be distinguished from schwannomas. Without calcification, a glomus tympanicum enters the differential diagnosis. The

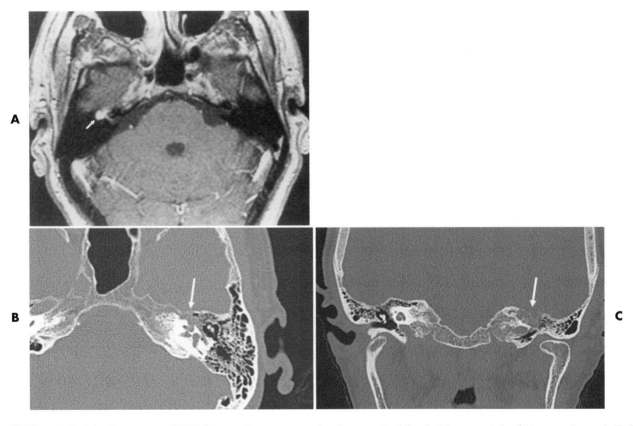

Fig. 12-28   **A,** Facial schwannoma. T1WI shows enhancement and enlargement of the facial nerve at the first genu *(arrow).* **B,** Both the labyrinthine and horizontal segments of the facial nerve on this CT scan are enlarged *(arrow).* As is typical of a schwannoma in this location, the facial nerve function was normal. **C,** The coronal scan shows the erosion of the temporal bone at the geniculate ganglion *(arrow).*

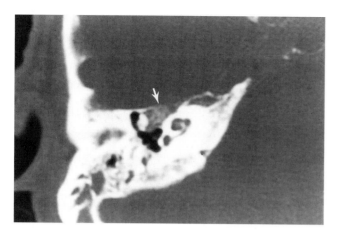

Fig. 12-29 Hemangioma of the facial nerve. Axial CT demonstrates a mass *(arrow)* with spiculated calcification in the region of the geniculate ganglion of the right temporal bone. Internal architecture should suggest the diagnosis of hemangioma.

borders of a hemangioma are indistinct compared with the well-demarcated schwannoma. The distinction is important because a schwannoma is rarely resected without sacrificing the nerve, but a hemangioma can sometimes be separated from the nerve.

One note about the facial nerve: it normally may show some enhancement at the geniculate ganglion and in its horizontal and descending portions. Seventy-six percent of facial nerves enhance in one or more of these portions, and asymmetry may be present in 69% (Fig. 12-30). Enhancement in the IAC, in the labyrinthine portion, and in the parotid gland, on the other hand, is always abnormal. The reason for the normal enhancement is the prolific circumneural arteriovenous plexus around the nerve. The plexus is not present in the IAC or intralabyrinthine and extracranial portions of the nerve. In patients with Bell's palsy, enhancement in the labyrinthine portion of the nerve or at the fundus of the IAC distinguishes the entity from the normal nerve enhancement. This may be because this is the narrowest channel through which the nerve must pass. Hence the swollen, virus-ridden nerve gets inflamed and lights up with contrast on MR. If you see enlargement and enhancement of the tympanic and intramastoid portion in the appropriate setting, you can suggest acute Bell's palsy. Therefore, look side to side when evaluating an MR scan for Bell's.

Please note that most people and managed care case reviewers (are the two mutually exclusive?) believe that

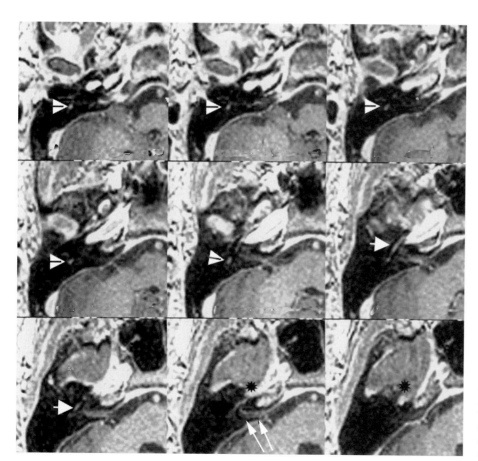

Fig. 12-30 Cranial nerve VII enhancement: There should be no enhancement in the intracanalicular *(thin arrows)* or labyrinthine pregeniculate portions of the facial nerve. However, the geniculate ganglion *(near asterisk)* and the horizontal tympanic *(short closed arrows)* and descending intramastoid portion *(arrowheads)* of the facial nerve will enhance more often than not.

imaging of patients with acute facial nerve palsy should be limited to "atypical Bell's palsy," that is if the symptoms persist longer than 4 weeks, the paralysis is progressive, other cranial nerves are affected, pain is a prominent feature, or hemifacial spasm is present. Justify that scan by citing that 5% of patients with Bell's palsy are ultimately found to have a facial nerve schwannoma. (see Fig. 12-28). If you get it approved, remember that an exception granted becomes a right expected the next time it is requested. You're home free; Ma Belle amie.

Malignant Lesions

Perineural spread Another important source of facial nerve dysfunction is malignant perineural spread. Parotid malignancies, especially adenoid cystic carcinoma or the rare lymphoma, have a propensity for tracking up the facial nerve and presenting with Bell's palsy. Squamous cell carcinomas of the parotid or face also present this way. The lesion is seen as enlargement and enhancement of the nerve itself or secondary enlargement of the stylomastoid foramen.

Other malignancies Malignancies of the middle ear are uncommon. Usually these masses are derived from EAC structures and secondarily invade the middle ear. This is particularly true of squamous cell carcinomas and rhabdomyosarcomas. Primary rhabdomyosarcomas of the middle ear may arise from muscular cells along the eustachian tube opening. Rarely, ectopic salivary gland tissue may be present within the middle ear cavity and neoplasms such as adenocarcinoma or adenoid cystic carcinoma may arise in such ectopic salivary tissue. The most common primary tumors to metastasize to the temporal bone are lung and breast cancer.

INNER EAR

Normal Anatomy

The cochlea and semicircular canals comprise the principal components of the inner ear. The osseous labyrinth (otic capsule) includes the vestibule, semicircular canals, and cochlea. The membranous labyrinth includes the perilymph (within the cochlea's scala vestibuli and tympani) and the endolymph (within the cochlear duct, semicircular canals, and vestibular aqueduct). The cochlea has two and a half (apical [one], middle [one], and basal [one half to three-quarters]) turns. The apical turn amplifies low tones and the basilar turn high tones (seems paradoxical—base, high, apex, low—but that's how She made it).

The vestibule is the common chamber to which the semicircular canals join. There are lateral, superior, and posterior semicircular canals. The superior and posterior semicircular canals share a nonampullated end known as the crus communis. The stapes articulates to the vestibule via the oval window. The vestibule contains the posteriorly located utricle and the round, anterior saccule, the sense organs responsible for balance. The endolymphatic sac (vestibular aqueduct) courses posterolaterally from the vestibule and dilates into a blind-ending sac (see Fig. 12-8 B and C).

The cochlea is filled with perilymph but has an endolymph channel as well. The cochlea has a base and a cupula (or apex), and is divided by a bony central canal known as the modiolus. The round window is located at the basal turn. At the scala vestibuli, perilymph from the vestibule communicates with that of the cochlea. At the end of the scala tympani, the perilymphatic space connects to the round window. The scalae tympani and vestibuli join at the cupula's helicotrema. It takes these scalae to hear the tympani at *La Scala*. The cochlear aqueduct extends from the scala tympani posteromedially to drain perilymph into the subarachnoid space of the posterior fossa. It is seen on sections below the IAC (see Fig. 12-8 E).

Congenital Anomalies

Although most causes of sensorineural deafness are derived from degenerative disorders of the inner ear, several different types of congenital anomalies cause inner ear dysplasias and hearing loss. Underlying causes for these anomalies include thalidomide exposure, congenital rubella or cytomegalovirus infection, and genetic disorders. Each seems to have an eponym associated with it, and rather than tax the brain memorizing these obscure entities, grab a beer, sit back, relax, and learn a few of the prototypical lesions.

Cochlear abnormalities The otic capsule structures develop between the fourth and tenth weeks of gestation. The most common of the congenital cochlear deformities is Mondini's defect, which occurs late in auditory embryologic development, usually at 7 to 8 weeks. The scala separations of the lumen of the cochlea are not developed completely at this point. Essentially, Mondini's defect is incomplete development of the two-and-a-half turns of the cochlea. The basal turn is relatively well formed, but the middle and apical turns may balloon into a cyst. Variations in the number of remaining turns in the cochlea comprise various types of otic dysplasia (Fig. 12-31). In Pendred syndrome, a congenital disease characterized by sensorineural hearing loss and thyroid dysfunction, Mondini malformation is commonly found. Enlargement of the endolymphatic sac in association with a large vestibular aqueduct is present as well in about 20% of Mondini malformations.

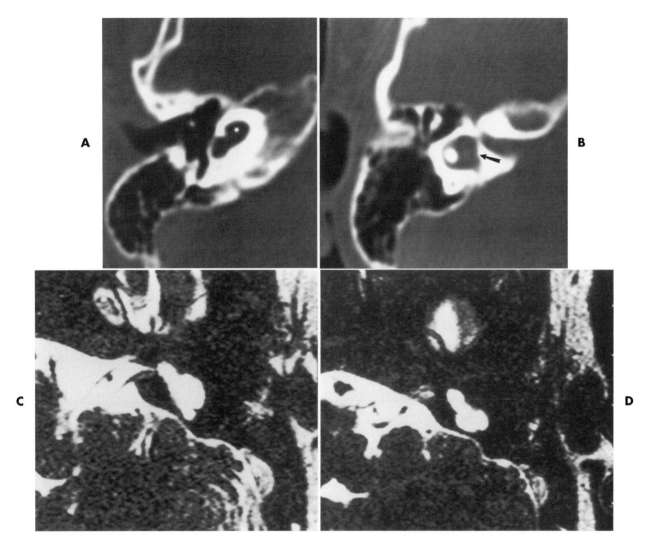

Fig. 12-31   Mondini's deformity. **A,** Observe the absence of well-formed cochlear turns creating a cystic-inner ear structure *(asterisk)* where the cochlea should be located. **B,** Note that the vestibule *(arrow)* is also enlarged in this patient, a not uncommon finding with cochlear abnormalities. **C,** The thin section T2 weighted scan shows absence of the normal turns of the cochlea and a common cavity with the vestibule. **D,** Looks like a Cock's deformity to us....well-hung at that.

In a Cock's deformity (also referred to as Michel's *dysplasia*) there is a common cavity comprising the vestibule and the cochlea. No modiolus of the cochlea is identified. This congenital lesion occurs due to arrest in development at 4 to 5 weeks gestation. Semicircular canals may be normal or affected as well. The differential diagnosis includes complete labyrinthine aplasia where one sees a common cavity but the IAC is absent. After a Mondini deformity, the Cock's deformity is the second most common cochlear malformation.

In cochlear aplasia and hypoplasia, the cochlea fails to develop and you may see no or just one cochlear turn. The patients present with unilateral hearing loss. Perilymph fistulas (communication between the scalae vestibuli and tympani) may coexist. The ipsilateral cochlear nerve may be missing and the IAC small.

Michel's *aplasia* refers to total absence of inner ear structures associated with other skull base deformities (platybasia), abnormal course of the facial nerve and jugular vein anomalies. The stapes does not develop and the oval window is absent. Michel's aplasia is usually due to a defect in the otic placode development at the third week of gestation.

If the cochlear aqueduct is congenitally enlarged, hearing may be impaired. Enlargement is difficult to define with the cochlear aqueduct as it narrows from medially to laterally and may be nearly invisible in its petrous and lateral segments. A medial orifice size of more than 1.5 mm should be considered abnormal and a midportion diameter of more than 1.2 mm is suspicious. An enlarged cochlear aqueduct, because it represents a communication between the scala tympani and the subarachnoid

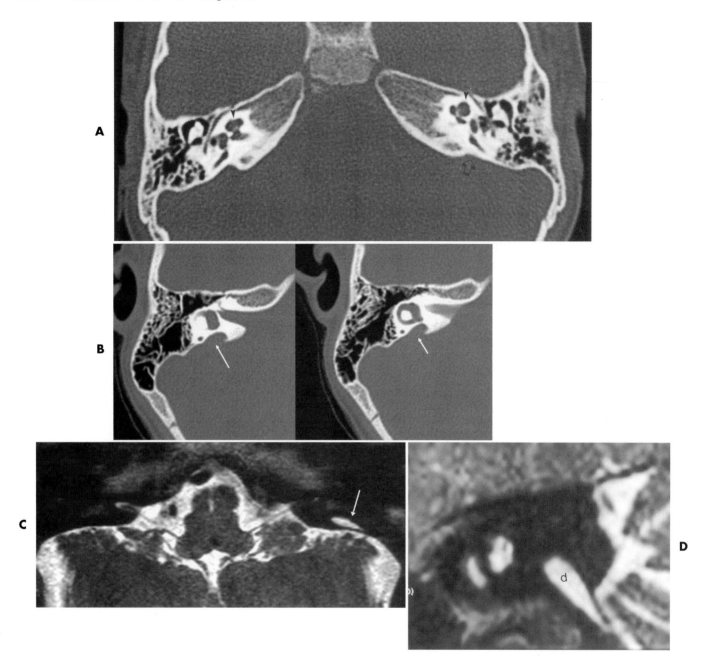

Fig. 12-32   **A,** Bilateral aqueductal enlargement with malformed modiolus. On the *left* the vestibular aqueduct *(open arrow)* is predominantly extra-osseous. **B,** Enlarged aqueduct *(arrow)* on *right.* **C,** Dilated vestibular aqueduct. This high resolution T2 weighted scan demonstrates an enlarged endolymphatic sac *(arrow)* on the left side. It measured 3 mm in diameter. **D,** Sagittal reconstructions demonstrates dramatic dilatation of the proximal portion of the duct *(d).* The patient had left sensorineural hearing loss. (Case courtesy of Stuart Bobman.)

space, has been implicated in children with recurrent meningitis and ear infections. This anomaly has also been associated with the poststapedectomy "gusher," so named because cerebrospinal fluid and perilymphatic fluid intermingle in spurts.

Perilymphatic fistula   A perilymphatic fistula is an abnormal connection between the subarachnoid space and the perilymphatic space of the inner ear. The usual sites of the fistula in children are at the oval and round

windows often with associated stapes superstructure malformations. Spread of middle ear infections to the meninges or of meningitis to the inner or middle ear can occur through perilymphatic fistulae. Labyrinthitis ossificans can result as a sequela of such spread. Congenital sources include enlarged vestibular aqueducts, Mondini malformations, Michel's anomalies, and Cock's deformities. Acquired causes of perilymphatic fistulae include cholesteatomas, chronic otitis media, and trauma.

Semicircular canal abnormalities Maldevelopment of the semicircular canals is another form of otic dysplasia. The lateral semicircular canal is most often affected in the form of hypoplasia because the lateral semicircular canal is the last to form embryologically (superior first, posterior second, lateral last). If the posterior (next most common) or superior (least common) semicircular canal fails to develop, the lateral semicircular canal is also affected. Compensatory enlargement of the vestibule will occur. Hearing loss occurs rather than imbalance. If one sees an isolated semicircular canal deformity without cochlear anomalies it implies that the defect occurred after 8 to 9 weeks of gestation; by that time the cochlea has completely developed.

Apalsia of the semiciricular canals can be seen in CHARGE syndrome.

A recently described entity, superior semicircular canal dehiscence, is characterized clinically by sound and/or pressure induced vertigo. Oscillopsia (the perception that stationary objects are moving) and vertigo evoked by loud noises is Tullio phenomenon, a frequent clinical finding (but is also seen in otosyphilis, Meniere disease, perilymphatic fistulae, and Lyme disease). The presumed etiology is a congenital predisposition superimposed on a traumatic event. This lesion has benefited from the very thin section imaging afforded by multidetector helical CT scanning as the imaging finding, that of a dehiscence of the bone overlying the superior semicircular canal, is pretty subtle unless submillimeter sections are performed. A bilateral finding of dehiscence or thinning, at the least, is not unusual. Surgical exploration of the middle cranial fossa has confirmed the CT findings in selected patients; covering up the gap may lead to symptom relief.

Vestibular aqueductal abnormality Enlargement and flaring of the vestibular aqueduct greater than 1.5 to 2 mm (enlarged vestibular aqueduct syndrome) is the most common cause of congenital sensorineural hearing loss (Fig. 12-32). However, this may also be seen after head trauma—the patient has a predisposition for the condition with a large aqueduct, but increased intracranial pressure associated with the head trauma, leads to the auditory symptoms. The midpoint of the normal duct should have a transverse diameter equal to or under 1.5 mm in size or about the same size as the adjacent semicircular canal if the tick marks on your scale have been erased by the diligent technologist. Enlarged vestibular aqueducts cause high-frequency hearing loss and may be seen in isolation or in association with abnormal cochlea (76%), cystic vestibules (31%), or abnormal semicircular canals (23%). One may see the dilated endolymphatic sac on MR as brighter than CSF on T1WI due to high protein, hyperosmolar fluid. CHARGE syndrome, Pendred syndrome, and congenital CMV infections may predispose to enlarged vestibular aqueducts. Defects in the

modiolus of the cochlea are frequently seen with enlarged endolymphatic sacs. A narrowed vestibular aqueduct less than 0.5 mm in diameter may be seen with Meniere disease. Thus, if you don't see a vestibular aqueduct in a dizzy patient on a high resolution study, think Meniere. Vestibular system anomalies may occur in isolation or concomitant with cochlear abnormalities.

Atresia or stenosis of the IAC is often associated with absent cranial nerves VIII and less commonly VII. Finding a nerve is important in candidates who are considered for cochlear implants. High resolution MRI would be the study of choice. Often the facial nerve will leave the IAC early or aberrantly when cranial nerve VIII is aplastic or hypoplastic. ("I'm getting out while the getting's good," VIII said.)

Achondroplasia Achondroplasia is one source of congenital inner ear anomalies (Box 12-9). Its temporal bone manifestations include (1) poorly developed mastoid air cells, (2) upward tilting ("towering") of the petrous ridges and internal auditory canals from 110 to 129 degrees, (3) rotation of the cochlea and ossicles, (4) changes of chronic otomastoiditis, and (5) narrowing of the skull base and foramen magnum.

Inflammatory Lesions

Labyrinthine ossification After chronic middle or inner ear infections, temporal bone trauma, cholesteatoma, bacterial meningitis, mumps, Cogan's syndrome, or labyrinthectomy, labyrinthine ossificans may develop. Meningitis can cause labyrinthine ossificans through the spread of the infection from the subarachnoid space to the scala tympani by means of the cochlear aqueduct. Fibroblasts in the labyrinth are induced by the inflammatory state to produce fibrosis, and they may differentiate into osteoblasts to form ossific deposits in the cochlea. This is another of the causes of a "dead" (deaf)

Box 12-9 Congenital Syndromes with Inner Ear Anomalies

Achondroplasia
Apert Syndrome
Cock's deformity
Down Syndrome
Fountain syndrome
Michel
Mondini
Neurofibromatosis
Osteogenesis imperfecta
Pendred syndrome
Treacher Collins
Wildervanck syndrome

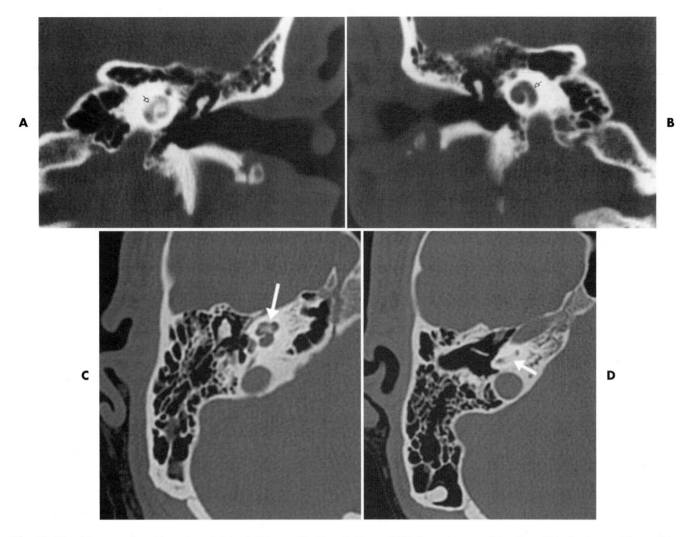

Fig. 12-33   Montage of cochlear stenosis/labyrinthine ossification. **A,** Coronal CT shows increased density within the turns of the cochlea *(open arrow)* caused by prior inflammatory labyrinthitis. **B,** Compare density in **A** with that of the normal contralateral cochlea *(open arrow).* **C,** The middle and apical turns show increased bony obliteration *(arrow).* That's too much for a normal modiolus. **D,** The basal turn *(arrow)* was also involved.

Illustration continued on following page

ear (often with vertigo) that is best evaluated with CT. Bony replacement of the labyrinthine portion of the inner ear with dense sclerosis is identified on CT (Fig. 12-33, Box 12-10). Imaging findings include cochlear stenosis (about 40%), cochlear fibroossific change (perhaps better seen with high resolution T2W MR as the fibrous obliteration may not be evident on CT as in Fig. 12-33G), and cochlear ossification (more than 30%). Obliterative changes in the semicircular canals and vestibule are not uncommon in association with cochlear labyrinthitis ossificans. Osseous obliteration at the round window niche may lead to inadequate cochlear implant insertion—the further into the cochlear turns that a multi-channel electrode can be inserted, the better the quality of hearing.

Cochlear Otospongiosis (Don't call me otosclerosis because I'm usually not sclerotic) Otospongiosis is another cause of sensorineural hearing loss that is usually bilateral (80%) and seen most frequently in young to middle-aged women. Otospongiosis suggests the pathophysiology in which endochondral bone is replaced by spongy bone. In the early phases, one identifies a lytic lucent erosion of the labyrinthine margins of the oval window, the round window niche, and the cochlea. Fenestral otospongiosis or retrocochlear otospongiosis most frequently affects the anterior margin of the oval window (Fig. 12-34). In the cochlear form of otospongiosis, the middle and basal turns of the cochlea are most frequently involved, showing areas of demineralization. A "double ring" (lucent) sign caused by resorption of bone

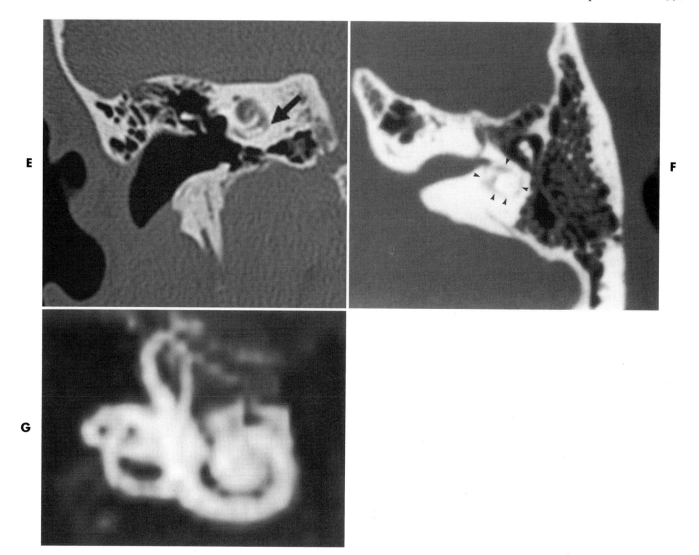

Fig. 12-33 *Continued.* **E,** The coronal CT is definitive. *Arrow* is on basal turn ossification. **F,** Labyrinthitis ossificans. The vestibule and semicircular canal *(arrowheads)* show the same obliterated appearance due to labyrinthitis ossificans. **G,** Example of normal cochlear patency. A 3D reconstruction of the high-resolution MR gradient echo scans shows the complete labyrinthine structures with open turns to the cochlea. Fibrous obliteration would result in a narrowed low intensity area.

Box 12-10   Causes of Labyrinthine Ossification

Cholesteatoma with labyrinthine fistula
Chronic otitis media
Labyrinthectomy
Late or treated otospongiosis
Mumps and measles
Pagets
Post meningitis
Suppurative labyrinthitis
Trauma

---

immediately around the membranous cochlea may be seen as a result of the normal basal turn lucency paralleled by otospongiosis. Rarely, in the late phases of this disease increased bony density caused by recalcification is visualized. If you see demineralization of the cochlea in a child, think osteogenesis imperfecta. The differential diagnosis also includes otosyphilis and rarely fibrous dysplasia (not). Paget disease would be the diagnosis if the entire skull base were involved, but that's rarer then carious hens' teeth.

COCHLEAR IMPLANTS   A cochlear implant may be required in patients with cochlear otosclerosis. This operation consists of inserting an electrode through the round window into the cochlea with the distal end along the cochlea's basal membrane where the auditory nerve

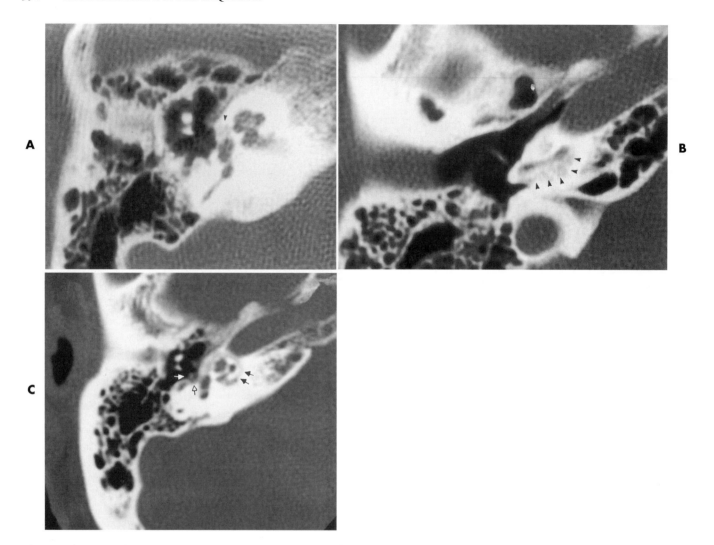

Fig. 12-34 Otospongiosis. **A,** Note the new spongiotic bone growth at the anterior margin of the oval window *(arrowhead)*. This is indicative of fenestral otospongiosis. The cochlea looks fine. **B,** Cochlear otospongiosis. Demineralization of the ultradense labyrinthine bone is seen around the basal turns of the cochlea *(arrowheads)*. **C,** Fenestral and cochlear otosclerosis. This unfortunate individual had evidence of otospongiosis *(black arrows)* manifested as demineralization around the cochlea. The patient also had fenestral otosclerosis seen as increased bone at the oval window *(open black arrows)* with fixation of the footplate of the stapes *(white arrow)*. (C, Courtesy of Joel Swartz, M.D., Philadelphia.)

transmits the sound. Single-channel electrodes are tres passe now, dudes, so go with the much more en vogue multichannel system. Rock n' roll will never sound so good. The multichannel electrodes (e.g., Clarion, Nucleus, or Med-El) must be placed 24 mm deep for optimal function. The more electrodes into the cochlea the better the outcome. Insertion of more than 19 of the 22 electrode arrays of the Nucleus cochlear implant device (Cochlear Corp, East Englewood, Colorado) is considered a good insertion. That means you should count the channels inserted. Preoperative evaluation with CT is sometimes ordered to ensure that the facial nerve is in its normal anatomic position (to prevent injury at surgery) and that cochlear patency is present. If the turns of the cochlea are so thickened that there is obliteration

of the scala tympani, the surgeon may elect to drill out the cochlea's internal walls and lay the implant in the opening to the shallow depth. The results with this type of implant are less favorable than if the cochlea is spared. If the patient has bilateral hearing loss and one cochlear implant is being inserted, the surgeon will place it in the cochlea that is (more) patent. What the surgeon needs to know before implantation is summarized in Box 12-11.

Of children who receive cochlear implants, nearly half have deafness secondary to meningitis. Congenital lesions and viral infections account for most of the rest of the cases. The cochlea of patients with a history of meningitis may be obstructed (labyrinthitis ossificans) and this leads to a higher rate of implant placement failure. One should look for cochlear stenosis (basal turn most commonly affected), cochlear ossification, and round window ossification as predictors for suboptimal placements.

Fenestral otospongiosis Fenestral otospongiosis is more common than cochlear otosclerosis. It typically involves the oval window (80% to 90%) and the round window (30% to 50%) niches. The stapes is essentially glued in position to the oval window, preventing transmission of sound and resulting in conductive hearing loss. The oval window niche is narrowed with fenestral otospongiosis with plaques of bone anteriorly (Fig. 12-34A,C). The density of the fenestral plaques is variable. Although it is usually seen as hyperdense to the normal oval window membrane, it is only rarely (15%) as dense as the otic capsule. The operation of choice for otospongiosis is a small fenestra stapedotomy or total stapedectomy. Stapedial mobilization and stapedioplasty no longer suffice. With a total stapedectomy, a prosthesis must be inserted into the oval window. Metal, Teflon, and wire devices are commonly used. Bilaterality in the ears is seen in up to 85% of patients with fenestral otosclerosis. This is a disease of young adulthood; 70% of cases occur in patients 18 to 30 years old.

Meniere syndrome Imaging findings in Meniere syndrome (endolymphatic hydrops) have eluded neuroradiologists up until this decade. Now various reports suggesting that the absence of visualization of the endolymphatic sac on high-resolution 3D T2-weighted scans is indicative of Meniere disease have surfaced. Some even believe that the stage of the disease can be assessed with this technique, the sac becoming visible once again when the Meniere's is quiescent. Eventually, we will have the resolution to see the dilated scala channels in the cochlea with bulging membranes—it's around

the corner with clinical 3.0 Tesla imaging. Our own experience has found numerous cases of endolymphatic sac enhancement on MRI in patients with Meniere disease.

Paget disease Another of the bone-producing lesions in the inner ear is Paget disease (Box 12-12). Paget disease may cause either sensorineural or conductive hearing loss. In its early phases one identifies a diffuse lytic process involving the bony labyrinth; however, in the late phases increased density is seen. The lytic phase appears to begin medially in the petrous apex and to progress laterally (Fig. 12-35). To distinguish otosclerosis from Paget disease, the adage is that Paget starts peripherally and spreads centrally whereas cochlear otosclerosis begins centrally and spreads outward.

Fibrous dysplasia Fibrous dysplasia may affect the temporal bone, causing increased density in a ground-glass fashion. The mastoid portion is affected most commonly, and the involvement may lead to conductive hearing loss.

Labyrinthitis Enhancement of the labyrinth on MR in patients with sudden hearing loss and vertigo has recently been described as suggestive of labyrinthine infection (Fig. 12-36). Cochlear enhancement or vestibular apparatus enhancement may occur and often correlates with electronystagmogram findings and clinical symptoms. Labyrinthitis may be due to viral, bacterial, luetic, or idiopathic causes. Asymptomatic patients do not show labyrinthine enhancement. Autoimmune labyrinthitis occurs when antibodies to cochlear antigens form; there is often enhancement of the cochlea bilaterally on MR. The differential diagnosis includes the labyrinthine schwannoma. Other causes of labyrinthine enhancement are listed in the Box 12-13.

Petrous apicitis Petrous apicitis is a nondestructive inflammatory condition of the aerated petrous apex (Box 12-14). Pneumatization of the petrous apex is present in only 30% to 35% of people, so petrositis can develop in these (unfortunate) persons, often after what was thought to be successful mastoidectomy surgery for in-

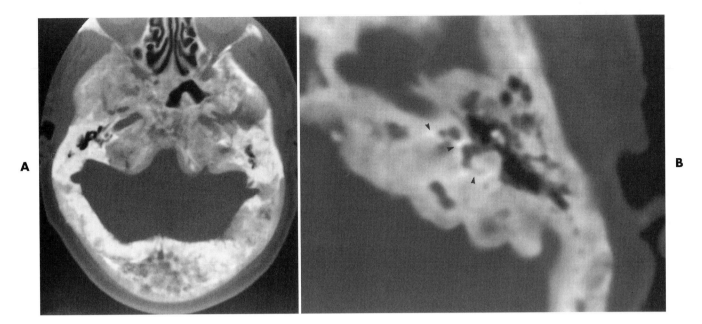

Fig. 12-35 **A,** Paget disease of the temporal bone. Axial CT reveals diffuse increased bone density with thickening throughout the base of the skull. Note the predominance in the petrous apex with relative sparing laterally, especially around the right labyrinth. **B,** Paget disease of the temporal bone. Sparing of the otic capsule around the cochlea and labyrinth *(arrowheads)* is suggestive of Paget disease. The rest of the temporal bone is thickened and dense.

flammatory disease. Associated with this condition is Gradenigo's syndrome, which causes pain in the distribution of cranial nerve V, a VI nerve palsy, and otorrhea. The lesion appears as opacification of the petrous air cells, typically of low signal intensity on T1WI and high intensity on T2WI. If chronic infection persists, the signal intensity of the apicitis may change with the higher protein content and viscosity, causing high signal on T1WI and/or lower signal intensity on T2WI. The dura

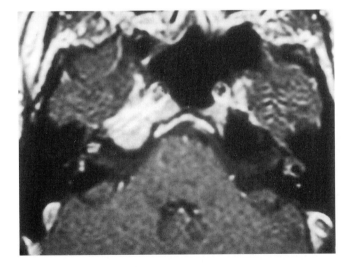

Fig. 12-36 Labyrinthitis. T1WI shows enhancement of the right cochlea and left and right vestibule in this patient with viral labyrinthitis. A cute finding but infrequently seen. Left semicircular canals enhance.

near the gasserian ganglion (Meckel's cave) may enhance on MR. Cranial nerve VI is affected as it passes through Dorello canal, a bony passageway leading from the tip of the temporal bone to the cavernous sinus containing nerve VI and the inferior petrosal sinus (see Chapter 11).

Cholesterol granulomas Cholesterol granulomas are lesions that typically arise in the petrous apex of the temporal bone. The inciting event in the genesis of cholesterol granulomas (also known as chocolate cysts, cholesterol cysts, epidermoids, and blue-domed cysts) seems to be a small blood vessel rupture with recurrent hemorrhage in the petrous apex. This may be caused by negative pressures occurring in the petrous air cells, resulting from chronic obstruction. This elicits a foreign body reaction by the mucosa of the air cells, causing giant cell and fibroblastic proliferation and cholesterol crystal

---

Box 12-13 Causes of Labyrinthine Enhancement

Autoimmune labyrinthitis (antibodies to cochlear antigens)
Cogan syndrome (interstitial keratitis, vestibuloauditory abnormality, vasculitic)
Labyrinthine schwannoma
Labyrinthitis (Viral, bacterial, luetic, etc)
Lyme disease
Postoperative after schwannoma resection
Post-trauma with hemorrhage into labyrinth

Box 12-14   Petrous Apex Masses

Cholesterol granulomas
Chondroid lesions
Chordoma
Cranial nerve V schwannomas
Eosinophilic granuloma (Langerhans' cell histiocytosis)
Epidermoid
Glomus jugulare
Meningioma
Metastases
Mucoceles
Myeloma
Petrous apicitis
Petrous carotid aneurysms

deposition with subsequent recurrent subclinical hemorrhages. The lesion expands as the host response perpetuates itself; nothing is so bad that your body can't help it to get worse. Eventually, the patient develops cranial nerve findings (usually V or VIII). These lesions present as lytic lesions within a pneumatized petrous apex filled with soft-tissue debris on CT. The cholesterol granuloma is lined by fibrous connective tissue as opposed to acquired cholesteatomas, which are encapsulated by stratified squamous epithelium. Cholesterol granulomas and cholesteatomas are commonly confused solely because they share three syllables, but they look nothing alike on MR. A cholesterol granuloma has high signal intensity on all pulse sequences because of the hemorrhagic products and/or the cholesterol debris (Fig. 12-37). Acquired cholesteatomas are not bright on T1WI. The differential diagnosis includes a mucocele of the petrous apex, petrous apicitis, or a hemorrhagic bony metastasis.

A mucocele of the petrous apex can occur and present as an expansile mass similar to a cholesterol granuloma. Depending on the state of hydration of the secretions within a mucocele, the lesion may be bright or dark on all pulse sequences. Enhancement of petrous apicitis and mucoceles is expected to be in a peripheral fashion.

If you're accustomed to using fast spin echo T2W scans on MR beware this pitfall. Both petrous apex fat and

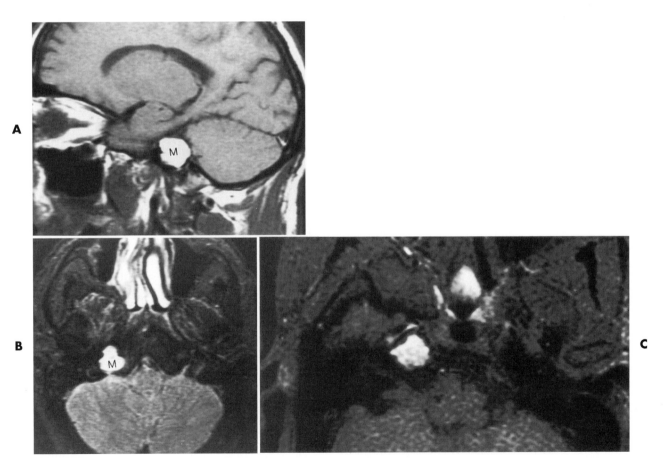

Fig. 12-37   Cholesterol granuloma. **A,** Sagittal T1WI demonstrates a high intensity mass *(M)* in the right petrous apex. **B,** Lesion *(M)* is bright on T2WI as well. This is thought to be secondary to subacute hemorrhagic products caused by recurrent hemorrhage. **C,** A fat suppressed T1WI shows a high signal intensity lesion at the petrous apex near the junction with the clivus. Hemorrhage or protein could account for the intensity.

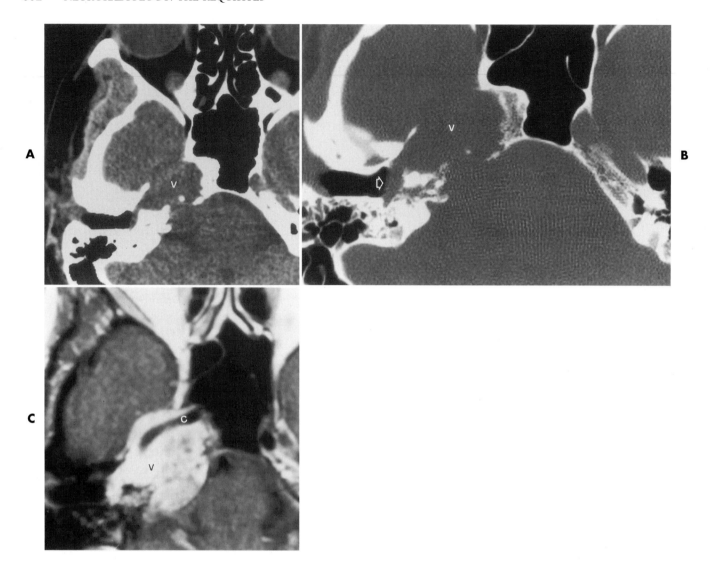

Fig. 12-38 Petrous apex mass *(v)*. **A,** CT scans show erosion of the right petrous apex extending along the carotid artery on the right side. The bone window **(B)** shows the irregular margination to the lesion *(v)* as well as its extension into the middle ear cavity *(arrow)*. Post contrast MR **(C)** shows a rounded enhancing mass displacing and encasing the right internal carotid artery *(C)*. A meningioma, schwannoma, or eccentric chordoma could appear in this fashion, as could a metastasis. Patient refused surgery. Will we ever know?

a cholesterol granuloma will look the same on FSE scans, that is, bright on both T1WI and T2WI. Only by identifying expansion of the bone or by applying fat suppression to the sequence will you be able to get out of this quandary. Performing the antiquated CT may be a last resort to show the lytic bone with cholesterol granulomas.

Other causes of hearing loss The work up of acute hearing loss usually yields an abundance of cases of viral or immune-mediated disease, Meniere disease, vascular disorders, syphilis, neoplasms (vestibular schwannomas), multiple sclerosis, and/or perilymphatic fistulas. Sickle cell disease is associated with intralabyrinthine hemorrhages that may present with sudden hearing loss.

Dural malformations, neoplasms, or other vascular lesions that may cause chronic recurrent hemorrhage may lead to (hemo)siderosis of the CNS. This is an unusual cause of hearing loss in which chronic bleeding leads to hemosiderin deposition on the brain stem and nerves running through the basal cisterns. Cranial nerve VIII is particularly sensitive to the effects of hemosiderin deposition. The characteristic MR appearance, a thin, dark rim around the surface of the brain stem and cerebellum on T2WI, is discussed more completely in Chapter 4.

Benign Neoplasms

Cranial nerve VIII schwannomas The benign masses associated with the inner ear—the glomus tympanicum, facial schwannoma, and IAC schwannomas—have all been described earlier. Intralabyrinthine schwannomas are rare tumors but enhance markedly on MR and can be detected relatively easily. They are usually situated close to the round window niche. They are an unusual cause of hearing loss and, as opposed to the more typical "acoustic" schwannomas, appear to arise from the cochlear (not the vestibular) branch of cranial nerve VIII. Usually the patients are thought to have Meniere disease because of the associated vertigo. The tumors are associated with neurofibromatosis type 2.

Chordomas and chondroid neoplasms Chordomas may occur at the petrous apex from remnants of the notochord that have migrated peripherally from the base of the skull. The tumor calcifies frequently, shows lytic destruction of bone, and has mild enhancement. On T1WI, the lesions are usually isointense (75%) or hypointense (25%), but nearly all are very hyperintense on T2WI. Septations are seen frequently (70%). Chondrosarcomas may appear identical to chordomas and affect the skull base. In this situation, CT may suggest the diagnosis of chondrosarcoma by demonstrating the characteristic whorls of calcification. Signal heterogeneity within chondrosarcomas is seen in 59% of cases but hemorrhage rarely. Enhancement is marked and heterogeneous. Only 6.7% of all chondrosarcomas occur in the head or neck, but as Murphy's law has it, they tend to show up when you're reading cases that day. Chondroblastomas may present as an intraosseous temporal bone mass. They typically have a chondrified matrix, though not always.

Cranial nerve V schwannomas Cranial nerve V schwannomas may also occur along the petrous apex (Fig. 12-38). These lesions begin in an extraosseous location but may erode the medial petrous bone near the trigeminal impression. They enhance (see Chapter 11).

Langerhans cell histiocytosis Eosinophilic granuloma, in the spectrum of Langerhans cell histiocytosis (histiocytosis X, Langerhans granulomatosis), has a propensity for involving the mastoid portion of the temporal bone. This is a disease of childhood and young adulthood that presents as a lytic process in the temporal bone. Hearing difficulties without pain may be the initial complaint. The lesion is dark on T1WI and bright on T2WI, and enhances (Fig. 12-39). It is a cause of lytic temporal bone lesions that spare the middle ear in children and is not uncommon. The differential diagnosis is acute mastoiditis; however, eosinophilic granuloma is usually a nontender lesion in an afebrile, otherwise healthy child.

Other causes of VII nerve enhancement Intracanalicular (IAC) nerve VII enhancement is always abnormal. The differential diagnosis of nerve VII enhancement includes schwannomas, Lyme disease (see Chapter 6), lymphoma, hemangioma, sarcoidosis, Bell's Palsy, viral neuritis, Ramsay-Hunt syndrome (a herpetic infection), Guillain Barre, and perineural tumor spread. Of the two most common lesions, Bell's palsy is thought to account for 80% of facial nerve paralysis, with schwannomas comprising only 5%.

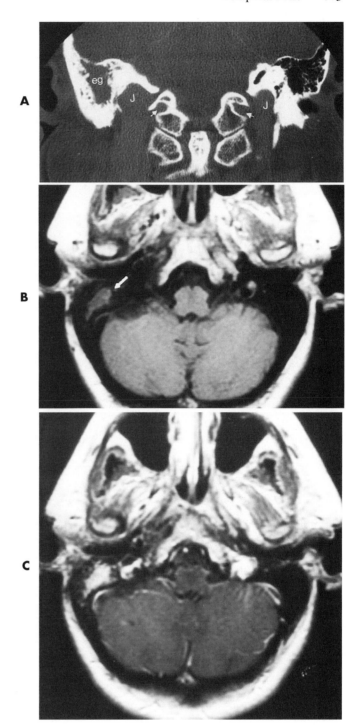

Fig. 12-39 Eosinophilic granuloma. **A,** Coronal CT depicts a destructive process *(eg)* in the right mastoid air cells. Hypoglossal canal is labelled by *arrows. J,* Jugular foramen. We used a special CT that automatically labels the lesions with the proper diagnosis. (It costs approximately $100,000 in present dollars for this educational retrofit.) **B,** Axial T1WI shows isointense lesion *(arrow)* in the same location. **C,** Enhanced T1WI shows enhancement of the lesion. This was an unusual case in that the patient was seen in her forties with eosinophilic granuloma.

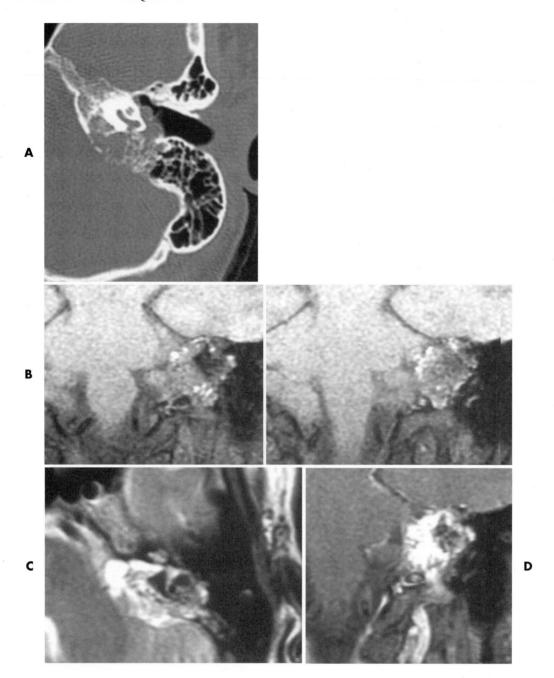

Fig. 12-40 ELST. **A,** This mass arose in the region of the vestibular aqueduct but grew through the temporal bone into the middle ear. **B,** Coronal unenhanced scan reveals that the mass is partially bright on T1WI. **C,** The mass is of mixed intensity on T2WI and extends into the subarachnoid space. **D,** After contrast administration portions of the mass converted from dark to light.

In Bell's palsy, the region of pathology most commonly is located at the narrowest canal that the facial nerve must go through in its course—at the distal intrameatal segment of the IAC. Smooth, linear, abnormally intense contrast enhancement of the distal intrameatal segment, indicating peripheral inflammatory nerve palsy is a common finding indicative of a viral (presumed Bell's) palsy of the facial nerve. This may also be found after facial nerve trauma related to breakdown of the blood/peripheral nerve barrier associated with nerve de-generation and regeneration after traumatic stretching of the greater superficial petrosal nerve. Scar formation along the nerve may also produce thickening and intense enhancement of the affected nerve segments.

Malignant Lesions

There are relatively few primary malignant lesions of the inner ear. Hematogenous metastases may occur in the inner ear, but direct invasion is more common. Rarely,

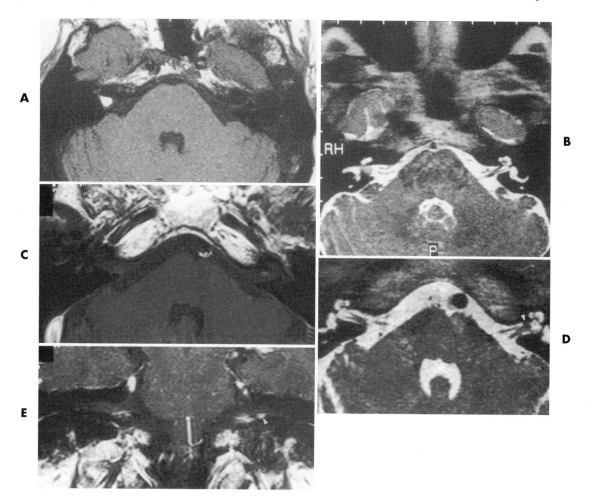

Fig. 12-41   Montage of IAC lesions. **A,** IAC lipomas. Precontrast T1WI shows a bright mass in the right IAC. Could it be a hemorrhagic schwannoma, a melanoma, dropped metastasis, or a lipoma of the IAC? **B,** The T2WI would only be helpful if performed with fat suppression. If the lesion became dark with fat suppression we could say it was a lipoma. The intermediate signal implies this was not a hemorrhagic schwannoma and a melanotic nodule would be most unlikely. **C,** A very subtle lesion in the IAC on the left can be easily missed on this unenhanced T1WI. **D,** The 3D fast spin echo high resolution T2WI shows the mass along the cochlear nerve on the left side *(arrowhead).* **E,** Doubting Thomases? The mass *(arrowhead)* is in the inferior and anterior portion of the IAC on the coronal enhanced scan. That means a cochlear schwannoma is the diagnosis. (Case compliments of [and masterfully imaged by] Stuart Bobman, Naples, Florida.)

neurofibrosarcomas, rhabdomyosarcomas, lymphomas, or malignant hemangiopericytomas may occur in this location. Perineural spread of malignancies along the facial nerve may lead to destructive processes affecting the inner ear. Squamous cell carcinoma is probably the most common malignancy to affect the inner ear. It can arrive there via (1) the EAC, (2) the middle ear, (3) the back of the nasopharynx along the eustachian tube, (4) a cholesteatoma, or (5) the parotid gland.

Endolymphatic Sac Tumors (ELST)   These tumors of the endolymphatic sac were previously called adenomatoid papillary tumors and were initially thought to be thyroid metastases because of the papillary histology. More recently, their site of origin has been reevaluated and it looks now that they need not be of endolymphatic sac origin. Some arise from the top of the jugular bulb, the mucosa of the aerated cells around the jugular bulb,

or the mastoid air cells. The tumors are characterized by aggressive bony destruction and calcified matrix on CT (Fig. 12-40) and bright signal on T1WI, possibly from hemorrhage. Tumors larger than 2 cm may have flow voids owing to branches of the external carotid artery that supply this hypervascular tumor. The orientation of the tumor, parallel to the posterior margin of the petrous temporal bone, simulates the vestibular aqueduct. There is an association with von Hippel-Lindau disease.

A final word about the internal auditory canal (also covered in Chapter 3). Thin section high resolution T2WI MAY in some cases demonstrate small vestibular schwannomas or other intracanalicular lesions without requiring the use of contrast administration (Fig. 12-41). Given all-comers, schwannomas of the IAC far outnumber intralabyrinthine neoplasms as causes of unilateral hearing loss.

Table 12-4 Differentiation of longitudinal and transverse fractures

Feature	Longitudinal	Transverse
Frequency	70%–86%	20%
Site of blow	Temporoparietal region	Frontal, occipital region
EAC involved	Often	Rare
Tympanic membrane perforated	Yes	No
Ossicular disruption	Common, especially incus	Rare
Facial nerve injury site	Geniculate ganglion (10%–20%)	Horizontal portion (40%–50%)
Hearing loss	Conductive (60%)	Sensorineural in lateral type (95%)
Inner ear involved	No	Yes (vertigo)
CSF otorrhea	From tegmen tympani fracture	No
2° cholesteatoma	Possible	Possible

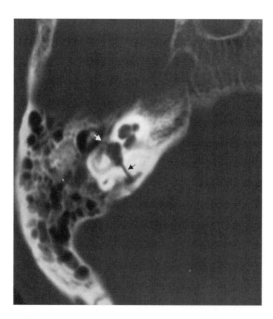

Fig. 12-42 Vertical temporal bone fracture. Vertical fracture *(small black arrow)* through the temporal bone extends across the vestibule *(asterisk)* on the right side perpendicular to the plane of the petrous ridge. One can see that the plane of the fracture would cross the horizontal portion of the facial nerve *(white arrow)*. Fluid in the mastoid air cells is probably hemorrhage from the fracture.

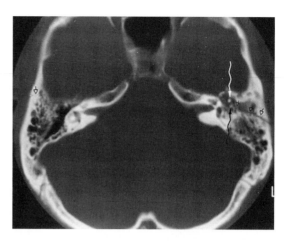

Fig. 12-43 Horizontal fracture of the temporal bone. Axial CT shows bilateral horizontal temporal bone fractures *(open black arrows)*. On the left side, the fracture extends into the middle ear cavity, where incudomalleal separation has occurred. Note the widened space between the neck of the malleus *(squiggly white arrow)* and the incus long process *(squiggly black arrow)*.

TRAUMA

Fractures of the temporal bone are termed vertical (transverse), horizontal (longitudinal), or complex (mixed or oblique) depending on their orientation to the petrous ridge (Table 12-4). Vertical temporal bone fractures traverse in a superoinferior orientation and yield a relatively high rate of injury to the facial nerve. Two types of vertical fractures exist: those that occur laterally through the cochlea or vestibule and those that course medially through the IAC and petrous pyramid. Vertical fractures are only one fifth to one third as common as horizontal fractures, but the facial nerve is injured in up to 40% of the cases. Sensorineural hearing loss is not uncommon, and transection of the cochlear nerve can occur at the IAC apex (Fig. 12-42). A hemotympanum is seen in 50% of vertical fractures.

Horizontal or longitudinal fractures run along the plane of the temporal bone, coursing from the EAC, through the middle ear, toward the sphenoid bone, which also is frequently fractured. This type of fracture is more common (70% to 90%) than the vertical fracture and is often (15% to 20%) associated with ossicular dislocation (Fig. 12-43). The incudostapedial joint, being the weakest of the middle ear articulations, is most commonly affected. This is detected by seeing a fracture of the long process of the incus with separation of more than 1 mm from the stapes head posterolaterally. Incudal dislocations are the source of nearly 80% of the cases of post-traumatic conductive hearing defects attributable to the ossicles. There is also a high rate (>90%) of hemotympanum associated with horizontal temporal bone fractures. Because this may be the only clue to their presence on a scout thick section CT in a traumatized patient, ALWAYS check the middle ear cavity and mastoid for fluid on posterior fossa bone windows. Otorrhea is reported to occur in 50% of cases.

The facial nerve is also traumatized in 10% to 20% of horizontal fractures, usually from local effects at the geniculate ganglion rather than transection. Labyrinthine extension of a longitudinal fracture is rare, because it involves the most resistant portion of the temporal bone. On the other hand, involvement of the EAC and glenoid fossa of the temporomandibular joint is very common.

Now that you have read the classic teaching about temporal bone fractures, here's the bad news. Most temporal bone fractures are actually oblique, and therefore components of each of the two types may coexist. Sorry.

Intracranial complications of temporal bone fractures include meningitis; injuries to the adjacent venous sinuses, causing extraaxial blood collections or thromboses; traumatic meningoencephaloceles; and cerebrospinal fluid leakage.

Dueling rhymes from the authors:

With each passing year
I learn more of the ear
Knowing its trivia
Can make one a diva
At least that's what I hear

A resident stunted by fear
Began to study the ear,
From outer to inner;
He wound up a winner,
But it took him nearly a year.
—D.M.Y.

No more tears, my dears
It may have taken years
But you have finished the ears
Forget the jeers
Of your peers
Go drink some beers
And hear the cheers

A young ENT resident had forgotten
To check the culture that now smelled rotten
She missed the infection
Causing many injection
Had the CT been gotten—no need to swab with cotton
—R.I.G.

SUGGESTED READINGS

Ahlqvist JB, Isberg AM: Validity of computed tomography in imaging thin walls of the temporal bone, *Dento-Maxillo-Facial Radiol* 28:13-19, 1999.

Bemporad JA, Chaloupka JC, Putman CM, et al: Pigmented villonodular synovitis of the temporomandibular joint: diagnostic imaging and endovascular therapeutic embolization of a rare head and neck tumor, *AJNR.* 20:159-162, 1999.

Bigelow DC, Eisen MD, Smith PG, et al: Lipomas of the internal auditory canal and cerebellopontine angle. *Laryngoscope* 108:1459-1469, 1998.

Chakeres DW, Kapila A, LaMasters D: Soft-tissue abnormalities of the EAC: subject review of CT findings, *Radiology* 156:105-109, 1985.

Cobb SR, Shohat M, Mehringer CM, et al: CT of the temporal bone in achondroplasia, *AJNR* 9:1195-1199, 1988.

Curtin HD, Jensen JE, Barnes L Jr, et al: "Ossifying" hemangiomas of the temporal bone: evaluation with CT, *Radiology* 164:831-835, 1987.

Daniels DL, Czervionke LF, Millen SJ, et al: MR imaging of facial nerve enhancement in Bell palsy or after temporal bone surgery, *Radiology* 171:807-809, 1989.

Dietz RR, Davis WL, Harnsberger HR, et al: MR imaging and MR angiography in the evaluation of pulsatile tinnitus [see comments], *AJNR* 15:879-889, 1994.

Fatterpekar GM, Mukherji SK, Alley J, et al: Hypoplasia of the bony canal for the cochlear nerve in patients with congenital sensorineural hearing loss: initial observations, *Radiology* 215:243-246, 2000.

Fayad JN, Linthicum FH, Jr: Temporal bone histopathology case of the month: otosyphilis, *Am J Otol* 20:259-260, 1999.

Fitzgerald DC, Mark AS: Sudden hearing loss: frequency of abnormal findings on contrast-enhanced MR studies, *AJNR* 19:1433-1436, 1998.

Gebarski SS, Telian SA, Niparko JK: Enhancement along the normal facial nerve in the facial canal: MR imaging and anatomic correlation, *Radiology* 183:391-394, 1992.

Goh YH, Chong VF, Low WK: Temporal bone tumours in patients irradiated for nasopharyngeal neoplasm, *J Laryngol Otol* 113:222-228, 1999.

Harnsberger HR, Dart DJ, Parkin JL: Cochlear implant candidates: assessment with CT and MR imaging, *Radiology* 164:53-57, 1987.

Holland BA, Brant-Zawadzki: High-resolution CT of temporal bone trauma, *AJNR* 5:291-295, 1984.

Johnson DW, Hasso AN, Stewart CE: Temporal bone trauma: high resolution CT evaluation, *Radiology* 151:411-415, 1984.

Johnson DW, Voorhees RL, Lufkin RB, et al: Cholesteatomas of the temporal bone: role of computed tomography, *Radiology* 148:733-737, 1983.

Latack JT, Kartush JM, Kemink JL, et al: Epidermoidomas of the cerebellopontine angle and temporal bone: CT and MR aspects, *Radiology* 157:361-366, 1985.

Lo WWM, Solti-Bohman LG, Lambert PR: High-resolution CT in the evaluation of glomus tumors of the temporal bone, *Radiology* 150:737-742, 1984.

Mafee MF, Henrikson GC, Deitch RL, et al: Use of CT in stapedial otosclerosis, *Radiology* 156:709-714, 1985.

Mafee MF, Singleton EL, Valvassori GE, et al: Acute otomastoiditis and its complications: role of CT, *Radiology* 155: 391-397, 1985.

Mafee MF, Valvassori GE, Deitch RL, et al: Use of CT in the evaluation of cochlear otosclerosis, *Radiology* 156:703-708, 1985.

Marsot-Dupuch K, Doyen JE, Grauer WO, de Givry SC: SAPHO syndrome of the temporomandibular joint associated with sudden deafness, *AJNR* 20:902-905, 1999.

Martin N, Sterkers O, Mompoint D, et al: Cholesterol granulomas of the middle ear cavities: MR imaging, *Radiology* 172:521-525, 1989.

Meyers SP, Hirsch WL Jr, Curtin HD, et al: Chondrosarcomas of the skull base: MR imaging features, *Radiology* 184:103-108, 1992.

Michael AS, Mafee MF, Valvassori GE, et al: Dynamic computed tomography of the head and neck: differential diagnostic value, *Radiology* 154:413-419, 1985.

Naidich TP, Mann SS, Som PM: Imaging of the osseous, membranous, and perilymphatic labyrinths, *Neuroimaging Clin North Am* 10:23-34, vii, 2000.

Petrus LV, Lo WW: Spontaneous CSF otorrhea caused by abnormal development of the facial nerve canal, *AJNR* 20:275-277, 1999.

Pisaneschi MJ, Langer B: Congenital cholesteatoma and cholesterol granuloma of the temporal bone: role of magnetic resonance imaging, *Topics in Magnetic Resonance Imaging* 11:87-97, 2000.

Remley KB, Coit WE, Harnsberger HR, et al: Pulsatile tinnitus and the vascular tympanic membrane: CT, MR and angiographic findings, *Radiology* 1974:388-389, 1990.

Rothschild MA, Wackym PA, Silvers AR, Som PM: Isolated primary unilateral stenosis of the internal auditory canal, *Int J Ped Otorhinolaryngol* 50:219-224, 1999.

Sabnis EV, Mafee MF, Chen R, Alperin N: Magnetic resonance imaging of the normal temporal bone, *Topics in Magnetic Resonance Imaging* 11:2-9, 2000.

Sartoretti-Schefer S, Brändle P, Wichmann W, Valavanis A: Intensity of MR contrast enhancement does not correspond to clinical and electroneurographic findings in acute inflammatory facial nerve palsy, *AJNR* 17:1229-1236, 1996.

Sartoretti-Schefer S, Kollias S, Valavanis A: Ramsay Hunt syndrome associated with brain stem enhancement, *AJNR* 20:278-280, 1999.

Sartoretti-Schefer S, Kollias S, Wichmann W, Valavanis A: T2-weighted three-dimensional fast spin-echo MR in inflammatory peripheral facial nerve palsy, *AJNR* 19:491-495, 1998.

Sartoretti-Schefer S, Scherler M, Wichmann W, Valavanis A: Contrast-enhanced MR of the facial nerve in patients with post-traumatic peripheral facial nerve palsy, *AJNR* 18:1115-1125, 1997.

Sartoretti-Schefer S, Wichmann W, Aguzzi A, Valavanis A: MR differentiation of adamantinous and squamous-papillary craniopharyngiomas, *AJNR* 18:77-87, 1997.

Schubiger O, Valavanis A, Stuckmann G, et al: Temporal bone fractures and their complications: examination with high resolution CT, *Neuroradiology* 28:93-99, 1986.

Seemann MD, Seemann O, Bonel H, et al: Evaluation of the middle and inner ear structures: comparison of hybrid rendering, virtual endoscopy and axial 2D source images, *Eur Radiol* 9:1851-1858, 1999.

Seltzer S, Mark AS: Contrast enhancement of the labyrinth on MR scans in patients with sudden hearing loss and vertigo: evidence of labyrinthine disease, *AJNR* 12:13-16, 1991.

Stone JA, Castillo M, Neelon B, Mukherji SK: Evaluation of CSF leaks: high-resolution CT compared with contrast-enhanced CT and radionuclide cisternography, *AJNR* 20:706-712, 1999.

Swartz JD, Faerber EN, Wolfson RJ, et al: Fenestral otosclerosis: significance of preoperative CT evaluation, *Radiology* 151:703-707, 1984.

Swartz JD, Faerber EN: Congenital malformations of the external and middle ear: high-resolution CT findings of surgical import, *AJR* 144:501-506, 1985.

Swartz JD, Mandell DW, Berman SE, et al: Cochlear otosclerosis (otospongiosis): CT analysis with audiometric correlation, *Radiology* 155:147-150, 1985.

Swartz JD, Mandell DW, Faerber EN: Labyrinthine ossification: etiologies and CT findings, *Radiology* 157:395-398, 1985.

Swartz JD: High-resolution CT of the middle ear and mastoid: parts I, II, III, *Radiology* 148:449-464, 1983.

Tekdemir I, Aslan A, Ersoy M, et al: A radiologico-anatomical comparative study of the cochlear aqueduct, *Clin Radiol* 55:288-291, 2000.

Teresi LM, Kolin E, Lufkin RB, et al: MR imaging of the intraparotid facial nerve: normal anatomy and pathology, *AJR* 148:995-1000, 1987.

Torizuka T, Hayakawa K, Satoh Y, et al: Evaluation of high-resolution CT after tympanoplasty, *J Comput Assist Tomogr* 16:779-783, 1992.

Urman SM, Talbot JM: Otic capsule dysplasia: clinical and CT findings, *Radiographics* 10:823-838, 1990.

Yeakley JW: Temporal bone fractures, *Current Problems in Diagnostic Radiology* 28:65-98, 1999.

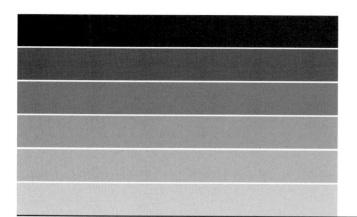

INTRODUCTION TO HEAD AND NECK CHAPTERS

Imaging of the head and neck can be divided into three main regions: sinonasal, mucosal, and extramucosal spaces. Within each of these are subdivisions based on anatomic landmarks, which allow a more organized approach to head and neck imaging. The anatomy of this area is fearsome to most radiologists in training (or out of training). Therefore, the next three chapters emphasize the appropriate parlance of the head and neck specialist.

Although it is important to know the imaging characteristics that may suggest a limited diagnosis in head and neck lesions, the more important role of the radiologist is to provide answers to the specific questions of the otorhinolaryngology clinician that will help in the staging of the lesion and/or treatment of the patient. For this reason, rather than emphasizing the differential diagnosis for a lesion with a given set of density or intensity characteristics, these chapters emphasize the relevant clinical issues associated with a given disease. Because many lesions occur in various locations along the aerodigestive system, we have tended to avoid repeating the *imaging characteristics, imaging characteristics* at each site. The reader will be spared the tedium of *redundancy, redundancy.*

With this approach in mind, this section of the book begins with a border zone between the brain and the head and neck: the sinonasal cavity. Only the cribriform plate separates "Nosage" from "Knowledge."

The concept of reading a chapter on runny noses may not be appealing to you. Take solace in the fact that you don't have to spend your life treating them as do the career rhinologists, who sometimes have their noses in the air, believing they can interpret their own scans. Rather than your taking a snotty approach to imaging, it is important to understand the terminology better than they do. Remember . . . they are only surgeons.

ANATOMY

We will follow the classic approach of reviewing the anatomy of the sinonasal cavity (zzzzz) and then proceed to congenital, inflammatory, and neoplastic categories. There will be some redundancy as we describe classical versus surgical anatomic considerations in some of these categories.

To appreciate the pathogenesis of sinusitis, you must understand the normal anatomic pathways of mucociliary clearance in the paranasal sinuses (Fig. 13-1). The cilia within the maxillary sinus propel the mucous stream in a starlike pattern from the floor of the maxillary sinus toward the *ostium* situated superomedially. In approximately 30% of patients, a second accessory ostium to the maxillary sinus is present inferior to the major opening. From the maxillary sinus ostium, mucus from the maxillary antrum (the maxillary antrum and maxillary sinus are synonymous—but you get head and neck brownie points if you use the former term) gets swept superiorly through the *infundibulum,* which is located lateral to the uncinate process and medial to the inferomedial border of the orbit. The *uncinate process,* a sickle-shaped bony extension of the lateral nasal wall extending anterosuperiorly to posteroinferiorly, is rarely (<2.5% of patients) pneumatized itself. Occasionally, the uncinate process attaches to the lamina papyracea (the medial wall of the orbit). If it does so, the infundibulum does not have a superior opening, thus creating a blind pouch, the recessus terminalis. The *hiatus semilunaris* is a slit-like air-filled space anterior and inferior to the largest

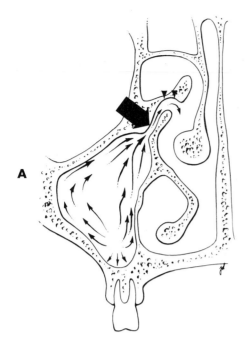

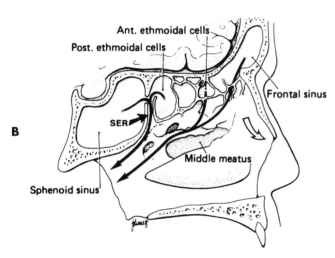

Fig. 13-1   A. Mucociliary clearance passes from the antral floor along the walls of the maxillary sinus toward the main maxillary sinus ostium. It then passes lateral to the uncinate process in the infundibulum *(fat black arrow)* into the hiatus semilunaris *(arrowheads)* and then to the middle meatus. **B,** Note the anterior to posterior flow of mucous from the frontal, ethmoid and sphenoid sinuses. The frontal recess, middle meatus, and sphenoethmoidal recess (SER) are the respective egresses from the sinuses. (Figure modified from Zinreich SJ, Kennedy DW, Rosenbaum AE, Gayler BW, Kumar AJ, Stammberger H. Paranasal sinuses: CT imaging requirements for endoscopic surgery. *Radiology* 1987; 163: 769-775).

ethmoid air cell, the *ethmoidal bulla*, and right above the uncinate process. Mucus is passed through the hiatus semilunaris posteromedially via the *middle meatus,* a channel between the middle turbinate and the uncinate process, into the back of the nasal cavity to the nasopharynx where it is subsequently swallowed. Alternatively, you can "hock a loogie" to get it out.

The ostiomeatal complex (OMC) refers to the maxillary sinus ostium, the infundibulum, the uncinate process, the hiatus semilunaris, the ethmoid bulla, and the middle meatus; the common drainage pathways of the frontal, maxillary, and anterior ethmoid air cells.

The frontal sinuses drain inferomedially via the *frontal recess* (also called the *frontoethmoidal recess)*. The frontal recess connotes the common drainage of the frontal sinus and the anterior ethmoid air cells. The frontal recess is the space between the inferomedial frontal sinus and the anterior part of the middle meatus. The frontal sinus and the anterior ethmoid air cells usually drain directly into the middle meatus via the frontal recess, or less commonly into the superior ethmoidal infundibulum, before passing to the middle meatus.

The most anterior ethmoid air cells located in front of the middle turbinate's cribriform plate attachment are termed *agger nasi cells.* Agger nasi cells lie anterior, lateral, and inferior to the frontal recess. They are present in more than 90% of patients (Fig. 13-2). The roof of the ethmoid sinus is termed the fovea ethmoidalis.

As stated earlier, ethmoidal bulla is the term used for the ethmoid air cell directly above and posterior to the infundibulum and hiatus semilunaris. A very large ethmoidal bulla can obstruct the infundibulum and hiatus semilunaris, and lead to interference with the drainage of the maxillary and anterior ethmoid sinuses. When anterior ethmoid air cells are located inferolateral to the bulla, along the inferior margin of the orbit protruding into the maxillary sinus, they are termed *Haller cells,* maxilloethmoidal cells, or infraorbital cells. They are seen in 10% to 45% of patients. When greatly enlarged, Haller cells may narrow the infundibulum or maxillary sinus ostium (Fig. 13-3).

Between the ethmoidal bulla and the basal lamella (the lateral attachment of the middle turbinate to the lamina

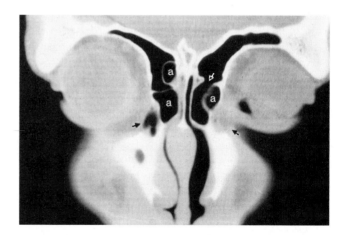

Fig. 13-2   Agger nasi cells. Frontoethmoidal recess *(open arrow)* and agger nasi ethmoid air cells *(a)* are excellently displayed on this coronal CT. Note approximation of lacrimal fossa *(arrows)* to agger nasi cells.

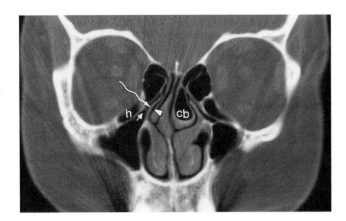

Fig. 13-3   Haller cell. Coronal CT with bone windowing demonstrates a Haller cell *(h)* on the right side seen below the right orbit. This patient also has a concha bullosa *(cb)* on the left side. The maxillary sinus ostium is designated by the *small arrow.* The infundibulum is the air channel extending superomedially from the ostium. The medial wall of the infundibulum is the uncinate process *(squiggly arrow).* The air channel medial to the uncinate process but lateral to the middle turbinate is the middle meatus *(arrowhead)* and, as you can see, extends superiorly toward the nasal vault.

papyracea of the orbit) is the sinus lateralis. The sinus lateralis, comprising the suprabullar and retrobullar recesses, may open into the frontoethmoidal recess or into a space posterior to the bulla, the hiatus semilunaris posterioris.

The posterior ethmoid air cells are located behind the basal (or ground) lamella of the middle turbinate and drain via the superior meatus, the supreme meatus, or other tiny ostia just under the superior turbinate. Ultimately, these ostia drain into the sphenoethmoidal

recess of the nasal cavity (Fig. 13-4), from which the secretions pass to the nasopharynx. In some patients the most posterior ethmoid air cell may pneumatize into the sphenoid bone, superior to the sinus. This is termed an *Onodi cell—related to the Star Wars hero O.B. 1 Konodi.*

The nasal cavity typically has three sets of turbinates: the superior, middle, and inferior turbinates. Occasionally, one may identify a fourth superiormost turbinate, the supreme turbinate. An aerated middle turbinate, which usually communicates with the anterior ethmoid air cells, is termed a *concha bullosa* and is seen in approximately 34% to 53% of patients. Most people believe that, unless huge, the presence of a concha bullosa does not predispose to chronic sinusitis. Significant pneumatization of the inferior or superior turbinates is much less common (<10% of patients).

The nasal septum is the midline structure between the right and left turbinates. The nasal septum is composed of three parts: a cartilaginous anteroinferior portion; a bony posteroinferior portion known as the vomer; and a superoposterior bony portion, the perpendicular plate of the ethmoid bone. The nasal septum is aerated only rarely. Nasal septal deviation, however, is common, and bony spurs often develop at the apex of the deviation. Spurs may cause the sensation of nasal obstruction.

The nasolacrimal duct (see Chapter 10) courses downward from the lacrimal sac bordering the medial canthus, where it is in close association with agger nasi air cells. Inflammation of agger nasi cells may be associated with epiphora because of this close relationship. The duct subsequently runs in the anterior and inferior portion of the lateral nasal wall. Its ending opens below the inferior turbinate at the inferior meatus.

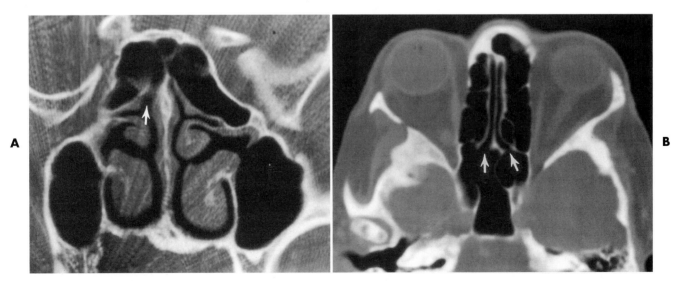

Fig. 13-4   Sphenoethmoidal recess. **A,** The sphenoethmoidal recess leads from the sphenoid and posterior ethmoid sinus into the nasal cavity *(arrow).* **B,** The recesses are oriented both in an anteroposterior plane seen best on this axial scan *(arrows)* and a superior-inferior plane seen best coronally (A).

Paranasal Sinus Development

The frontal sinus is not present at birth but pneumatization evolves from age 1 to 12. Growth over the orbital roof usually occurs from ages 4 to 8. Frontal sinusitis before age 4 is therefore rare. On the other hand, the ethmoid sinuses are present at birth. Rapid expansion of the ethmoid air cells occurs during ages 0 to 4 and again with the adolescent growth spurt from 8 to 12. The ethmoid sinus is usually the source of infection in childhood sinusitis.

The maxillary antrum is also present though small at birth. Its growth continues to age 14, but can be influenced by dental development. Tooth buds will be seen between the maxilla and the aerated sinus and obviously can prohibit an anterior antrostomy in these youngsters.

The sphenoid sinus begins its pneumatization at about age 2 and the growth is slower and more delayed than the other sinuses. The ultimate size of the sphenoid sinus is quite variable. Remember the development of the sinuses by the mnemonic: enraged military fought Saddam (ethmoid, maxillary, frontal, sphenoid).

Note that the OMC is developed at birth and functional endoscopic sinus surgery (FESS) surgery is an option for chronic childhood sufferers of sinusitis. Similarly, the mucosa in the infant is somewhat redundant and easily congested. Therefore, mucosal thickening should not be assumed to be due to sinusitis in a crying child. The clinical evaluation is paramount here. Up to 60% of asymptomatic infants can have complete or near complete opacification of their sinuses.

A metaphysical moment: why did the Omnipotent One design the skull with paranasal sinuses? One answer: the head might be too heavy for the cervical spine if it was rock solid bone. Was it for buoyancy reasons in the primordial soup? We would ask Him directly but do not know His e-mail address.

IMAGING MODALITIES

Sinonasal imaging has progressed methodically as each new generation of imaging modality has encroached on the domain of the former generation. Although plain films once served as the most commonly ordered study to evaluate the sinonasal cavity (in the Eisenhower era), computed tomography (CT) has now supplanted plain films because the endoscopic sinus surgeon has required greater anatomic precision. During the 1970s and 1980s, FESS replaced the more traditional Caldwell-Luc and maxillary antrostomy procedures for treating chronic sinusitis.

The plain film examination, which consists of a Waters (brow up anteroposterior [AP] view), Caldwell (frontal AP view), lateral, and submental vertex view, is as anachronistic in sinonasal imaging as a stethoscope is

for evaluation of coronary artery disease. The drawback of overlapping structures makes the evaluation of the OMC, anterior ethmoid sinus, middle meatus, and sphenoid sinus grossly limited with plain films. Plain films are most often ordered at our hospital in the evaluation of a fever of unknown origin in intensive care unit patients who are unable to be transported for CT, but now these patients may be too sick to be admitted (thanks to your neighborhood HMO). If you need an imaging study to diagnose sinusitis, CT is the way to go. Alternatively, look at the patient's handkerchief, postblow.

FESS is done via an intranasal endoscope rather than with an external approach, so surgeons must know where they are at all times, to prevent complications such as orbital or intracranial entry, particularly when they are operating posteriorly in the sinonasal cavity. CT serves as the road map for this procedure. The goal of FESS is to maintain the normal mucosa of the sinonasal cavity and to preserve the natural pathway of mucociliary clearance. FESS does not attempt to strip the mucosa clean as was sometimes performed in a Caldwell-Luc procedure, so mucociliary motility is preserved. Also, rather than creating an alternate egress of mucus from the maxillary sinus, as in an inferior meatal antrostomy (the Caldwell-Luc procedure), FESS enlarges the natural ostia and passageways of the paranasal sinuses. Whereas in the past maxillary and frontal sinusitis were thought to be the primary processes in patients with chronic sinusitis, it is now believed that these sinuses are secondarily obstructed because of disease in the OMC. The classic theory of FESS is that disease at the ostium and inferior infundibulum obstructs the maxillary sinus, whereas disease in the middle meatus and posterior infundibulum obstructs the frontal and anterior ethmoid air cells. Therefore, surgery is directed toward removing potential obstacles to mucociliary clearance at the OMC. Persistence of chronic sinusitis after nasoantral windows is usually due to anterior ethmoid disease. Therefore amputation of the uncinate process, enlargement of the infundibulum and maxillary sinus ostia, and creation of a common unobstructed channel for the anterior ethmoid air cells are common practices in FESS. Usually FESS also includes complete or partial ethmoidectomies.

The results of 3 decades of FESS have not been wholly satisfying except perhaps to the surgeons ($$$$$). Thus, recurrence rates of sinusitis after FESS remain high, as are the repeat surgery rates ($$$$$$$$$$$$). It may be that the primary abnormality is in fact the inability of the diseased mucosal surface to propel the mucus through the "optimized" ostia even after FESS. We still do not understand this very common malady very well—but do not expect us to blow our nose into a hanky over it.

For the FESS surgeon coronal CT is ideal because it simulates the appearance of the sinonasal cavity from the perspective of the endoscope. At present coronal reconstructions of axial CT data from multi-detector spiral CT scans are nearly as good as direct coronal images and may be able to eliminate some dental amalgam artifact that otherwise is present. To eliminate the effects of reversible sinus congestion, patients undergoing CT for evaluation of chronic sinus disease are best scanned 4 to 6 weeks after medical therapy and not during an acute infection. Some radiology departments also administer nasal spray decongestants or antihistamines to reduce reversible mucosal edema before the patients are placed in the scanner. In our hospital, if we gave the drugs, we'd lose our profit margin. Even with this preparation, surgeons claim that in approximately 10% of cases with "normal CT scans" they find endoscopic evidence of significant sinusitis. This fact is often cited when making that call to the medical director of the MCO to justify payment for the endoscopy.

Magnetic resonance (MR) examination of the sino-nasal cavity can be performed in a standard head coil or, for more precise anatomic resolution, with a surface coil placed over the anterior part of the face. Both T1-weighted images (T1WI) and T2-weighted images (T2WI) are required because of the variability of signal intensity of sinonasal secretions caused by protein concentration. Fat-suppressed enhanced T1WI are employed for the evaluation of complicated sinusitis or for suspected neoplastic disease. Differentiating tumors from infections of the sinonasal cavity may be best achieved with enhanced MR: infected mucosa enhances in a peripheral fashion, whereas tumors usually enhance solidly and centrally (Fig. 13-5).

CONGENITAL DISORDERS

The piriform aperture of the nasal cavity can be narrowed congenitally. A width of less than 11 mm is indicative of congenital nasal piriform aperture stenosis.

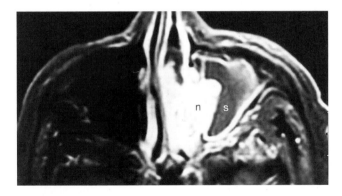

Fig. 13-5 Differentiation of tumor versus inflammation on enhanced scan. Enhanced fat-suppressed T1WI demonstrates solid enhancement within this neoplasm *(n)*. Note that the mucosa of the maxillary sinus enhances peripherally, whereas the sinonasal secretions *(s)* do not enhance. Thus the border of the tumor is well delineated.

Abnormal dentition and a midline bony inferior palatal ridge are confirmatory imaging findings. The most common anomalies that result in infantile airway compromise include posterior choanal stenoses and atresias, bilateral cysts (mucoceles) of the distal lacrimal ducts, and stenosis of the pyriform nasal aperture.

Choanal Atresia

Choanal atresia is usually diagnosed in infancy because neonates are obligate nose breathers as they suck on a bottle or breast (Box 13-1). The child is seen with respiratory distress. Although the diagnosis can be suggested by the inability to pass a nasogastric tube through the nose, imaging is necessary to determine whether the obstruction is membranous (15% of cases) or bony (85%) and whether other congenital CNS or non-CNS anomalies are associated (50%). In addition to the narrowed posterior choana, look for thickening of the vomer (Fig. 13-6). The posterior choanal opening should be over 0.5 cm in width in neonates, 1 cm in adolescents. The vomer should measure less than 0.34 cm in children under 8 years old. Rather than atresia, some patients have mere stenosis of the passageway. Often, unilateral choanal atresia may escape detection into adulthood. Patients may be unaware of the hyposmia often associated with this disorder. Smell is an underrated sense.

A dacryocystocele or piriform aperture stenosis may mimic choanal atresia clinically.

Dermoids, Sinus Tracts, and "Gliomas"

There are several congenital lesions of the sinonasal cavity, including congenital encephaloceles, dermoid cysts, sinus tracts, and nasal gliomas (Table 13-1). These lesions occur as an abnormality in the process of invagination of the neural plate. In embryogenesis, the dura of the brain contacts the dermis at the nasion region as the neural plate

---

Box 13-1   Entities Associated with Choanal Atresia
Achondroplasia
Amniotic band (currently playing in Soho) syndrome
Apert's syndrome
CHARGE syndrome (colobomas, heart disease, atresia of choanae, retarded growth, genital anomalies, ear anomalies)
Crouzon syndrome
Fetal alcohol syndrome
Holoprosencephaly
Thalidomide embryopathy
Treacher Collins syndrome

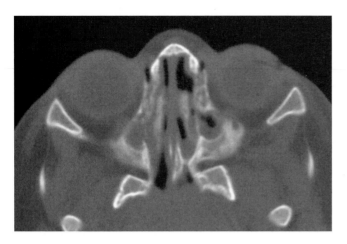

Fig. 13-6 Membranous and bony choanal atresia. On the left side the nasal passageway narrows, the vomer is thicker on that side, and both a bony (posterior) and soft tissue (anterior) plug is seen. No luck passing the tube on the left side.

retracts. Normally, the dermal connection regresses; when it does not, one of these lesions may develop. A cerebrospinal fluid (CSF) connection to the intracranial contents is maintained with meningoencephaloceles (see Chapter 9), whereas the connection is fibrous only with a nasal glioma (Fig. 13-7). Nasal gliomas are NOT neoplasms but congenital anomalies. They are extranasal more commonly than intranasal. (What an oxymoron—nasal gliomas are usually extranasal and are not gliomas—a moronic ox must have coined this term.) Most patients with dermoid sinus tracts have a pit in the middle of the nose. (No, it is not a zit, it is a pit and it can give parents a fit.) Dermoid cysts occur more commonly than tracts; however, tracts may cause more severe symptoms because of their intracranial connection in 25% of cases. Thus meningitis, osteomyelitis, and intracranial abscesses may occur in the setting of dermoid tracts.

Hypoplastic Maxillary Antrum

Congenital hypoplasia of the maxillary sinus occurs in 9% of patients. On plain films, a hypoplastic maxillary antrum (appearing denser) can simulate sinus opacification, but the CT will not fall into this trap.

Bony changes that suggest the diagnosis of a hypoplastic antrum are listed in Box 13-2. Causes of OVER-expansion of paranasal sinuses are listed in Box 13-3. In the differential diagnosis of sinus hypoplasia is the "silent sinus syndrome" or maxillary sinus atelectasis. In this entity, ostial obstruction from chronic sinusitis leads to chronic negative pressure, which leads to hypoventilation, which, over time, reduces the sinus' volume, hence "sinus atelectasis." Patients present with enophthalmos (not sinus symptoms strangely enough) as the orbital floor becomes depressed, the maxillary walls retract centripetally, and the retromaxillary fat fills the space left by the atelectatic sinus. The CT shows the retracted maxillary sinus walls in association with a small volume, opacified sinus (Fig. 13-8).

INFLAMMATORY LESIONS

Sinusitis

From the standpoint of a public health hazard, sinusitis ranks as one of Americans' most common afflictions. It is estimated that more than 31 million people in the United States are affected by sinus inflammatory disease each year and that 16 million visits to primary care physicians annually are for sinusitis and its complications. Adults average two to three colds per year, and 0.5% of viral upper respiratory infections are complicated by sinusitis. Overall, Americans spend more than $150 million per year for over-the-counter cold and sinusitis medicines, $100 million of which is for antihistamine medications. That would buy a lot of CT and MR imaging studies. Mucus means millions.

Most cases of acute sinusitis are related to an antecedent viral upper respiratory tract infection. With mucosal congestion as a result of the viral infection, apposition of mucosal surfaces results in obstruction of the normal flow of mucus, which results in retention of secretions, creating a favorable environment for bacterial

Table 13-1 Congenital nasal lesions			
Lesion	**Imaging findings**	**Clinical examination**	**Treatment**
Nasal glioma	1. Soft tissue mass with characteristics of brain 2. No connection or fibrous connection to brain or CSF	Intranasal or extranasal mass	Excision
Dermoid	1. Fat-containing mass 2. ±Sinus tract 3. Inflammatory changes	1. Nasal dimple 2. Sinus tract	Exploration and excision
Encephalocele	1. Connection to CNS with associated defect in skull bone 2. Brain and/or meninges included 3. Other CNS anomalies	1. Pulsatile mass 2. Dural covering	1. Patch dura 2. Reduce brain tissue

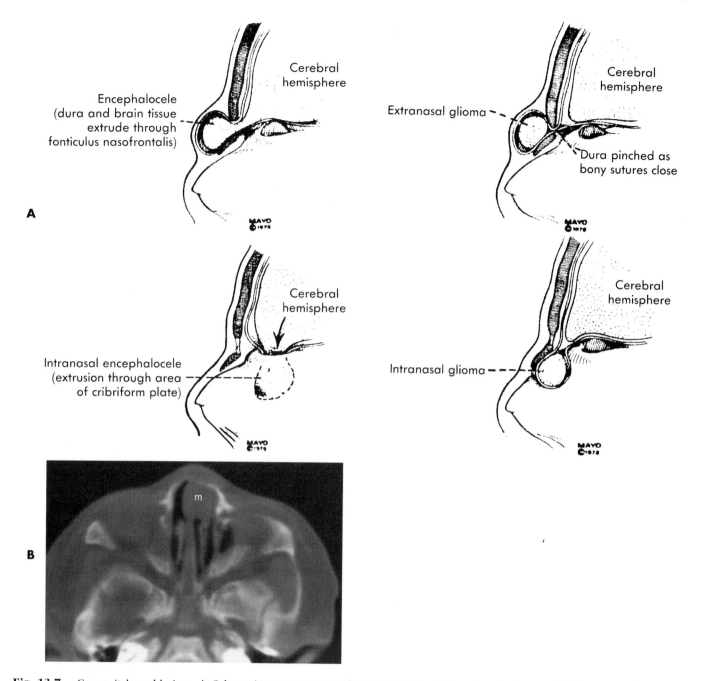

Fig. 13-7   Congenital nasal lesions. **A,** Schematic representation of encephaloceles *(left)* and nasal gliomas *(right)* are provided. (From Gorenstein A et al: *Arch Otolaryngol* 106:536, 1980. Copyright © Mayo Clinic.) **B,** Note the intranasal mass *(m)* in this infant. The left nasal bone is bowed around the mass. In this age group, the differential diagnosis would include a hemangioma, an epidermoid cyst, a polyp, or a nasal glioma. Remember that a nasal glioma is not a neoplasm—think of the lesion as an embryonal rest.

superinfection. The ethmoid sinuses are most commonly involved in sinusitis, possibly because of their position in the "line of fire" as inspired particles collide with and irritate the fragile ethmoid sinus lining. The bacterial pathogens responsible for acute sinusitis include *Streptococcus pneumoniae, Haemophilus influenzae,* β-hemolytic streptococcus, and *Moraxella catarrhalis.* In the chronic phase *Staphylococcus, Streptococcus,* corynebacteria, *Bacteroides,* fusobacteria, and other anaerobes may be responsible. The fungi that may infect the sinuses include *Aspergillus, Mucor, Bipolaris, Drechslera, Curvularia,* and *Candida.*

Anatomic considerations (sorry for the redundancy)   Several issues must be addressed when a patient's CT is evaluated before FESS. Is the uncinate process apposed to the medial orbital wall (an atelectatic infundibulum)? If so, its vigorous removal may result in orbital penetration. Are there areas of dehiscence in the lamina papyracea, or do the orbital contents protrude into the ethmoid sinus (both of which may lead to unintentional orbital entry from the ethmoid sinus)? Defects in the lamina papyracea have been reported in 5% to 10% of autopsy specimens. Because orbital hematomas are the most common orbital complication of FESS, it is important to identify any gaps in the lamina papyracea. CT obviously is the best means for identifying the thin medial bony wall of the orbit.

Are there areas of dehiscence in the cribriform plate and sphenoid sinus walls? Remember that there is an attachment of the middle turbinate to the cribriform plate. If the surgeon tugs too hard, the cribriform will fall and down will come CSF and/or brain through the new foramen in the skull base. The potential for intraorbital, intracranial, carotid, or optic nerve perforation at the time of surgery depends on these anatomic variants, found in 4% to 15% of patients. Three percent of people have optic nerves that are in contact with the posterior ethmoid wall—most course along (90%) or through (6%) the sphenoid sinus. An area of bony dehiscence seen at CT is present in 24% of optic nerves, just waiting for that errant endoscopic rip (Fig. 13-9). There have been limited reports of optic nerve transection during sphenoethmoidectomy from an intranasal approach, and dehis-

cence of the sphenoid wall may be a predisposing factor. An intersinus septum in the sphenoid sinus that attaches to the carotid canal is important to recognize preoperatively and is typically best identified in the axial view (Fig. 13-10). Over-vigorous removal of such an intersinus septum during surgery may result in carotid laceration. Consideration should therefore be given to performing *axial* CT routinely when sphenoid sinus surgery is contemplated.

Appearance on imaging In addition to commenting on the normal anatomic variations in the CT report, the radiologist should identify areas of mucosal thickening and sinus passageway opacification. It has come to be accepted that the *location* of sinusitis is more important in producing a patient's symptoms than the *extent* of the sinusitis. Therefore, a subtle area of opacification in the infundibulum of the OMC may cause more pain and discomfort than nearly complete opacification of the maxillary sinus with a mucous retention cyst and/or polyp.

OMC opacification correlates well with the development of sinusitis (Fig. 13-11). The positive predictive value of infundibular opacification for the presence of

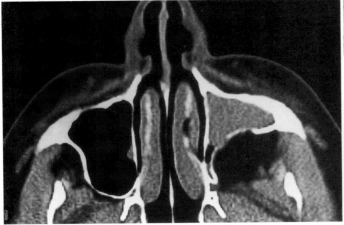
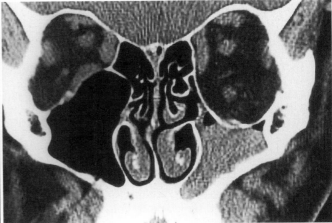

Fig. 13-8   Silent sinus syndrome. **A,** Note the retracted posterior wall of the left maxillary antrum. Fat fills the vacuum. The sinus is nearly completely opacified. **B,** The coronal CT scan demonstrates the depressed orbital floor, the low volume maxillary antrum, and the slightly thickened walls. The sinus has become "atelectactic."

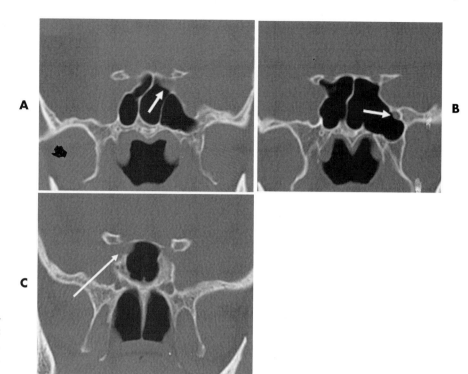

Fig. 13-9   Potential sites of disaster—dehiscent areas in the sinuses. **A,** Along the left optic canal in the sphenoid sinus *(arrow).* **B,** Along the left maxillary nerve *(arrow).* **C,** Along the right optic nerve *(arrow).*

maxillary sinus inflammatory disease is approximately 80%. When the middle meatus is opacified, the maxillary and ethmoid sinuses show inflammatory change in 84% and 82% of patients, respectively. The specificity of middle meatus opacification for maxillary or ethmoid sinus disease is more than 90%. These findings support the contention that obstruction of the narrow drainage pathways leads to subsequent sinus inflammation.

Some head and neck radiologists categorize recurrent

inflammatory sinonasal disease into five patterns: (1) infundibular, (2) ostiomeatal unit, (3) sphenoethmoidal recess, (4) sinonasal polyposis, and (5) sporadic or unclassifiable disease. The infundibular pattern is seen in 26% of patients and refers to isolated obstruction of the inferior infundibulum, just above the maxillary sinus os-

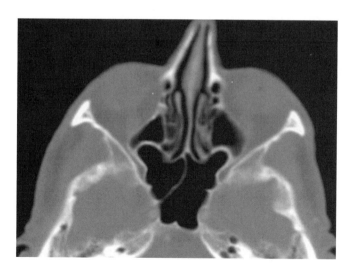

Fig. 13-10   Sphenoid sinus septae. The right septum in the sphenoid sinus attaches to the medial wall of the right internal carotid artery. Over vigorous removal of this septum during sphenoid sinus surgery can cause a laceration in the carotid wall.

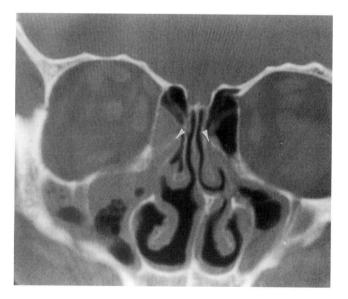

Fig. 13-11   The OMC in sickness. Note that both maxillary sinus ostia and infundibula *(arrowheads)* are opacified in this individual. Associated right ethmoid and bilateral maxillary sinus inflammation is present. Nasal septal deviation to the left does not help matters.

tium. Limited maxillary sinus disease often coexists with this pattern, whereas the ostiomeatal unit pattern, seen in 25% of cases, often has concomitant frontal and ethmoidal disease. The ostiomeatal unit pattern is designated when middle meatus opacification is present. Sphenoethmoidal recess obstruction occurs in 6% of cases and leads to sphenoid or posterior ethmoid sinus inflammation. When the sinonasal polyposis pattern is present, enlargement of the ostia, thinning of adjacent bone, and opacified sinuses are usually seen.

As far as the degree of sinus disease, some use the Lund MacKay Staging system where the frontal, anterior ethmoid, posterior ethmoid, sphenoid, maxillary sinus, and ostiomental complex on each side is assigned a grade. The grades are 0 for clear, 1 for partial opacification, and 2 for complete opacification. Imagine adding that to each dictation!

The presence of air-fluid levels is more typically associated with acute sinusitis than with chronic inflammatory disease. In cases of suspected acute sinusitis air fluid levels and/or complete opacification of a sinus is present in 63% of cases (Fig. 13-12). Of course, acute sinusitis may be superimposed on chronic changes. The findings suggestive of chronic sinusitis include mucosal thickening, bony remodeling, polyposis, mucous retention cysts, and bone thickening secondary to osteitis from adjacent chronic mucosal inflammation (Fig. 13-13).

Hyperdense secretions on CT may be due to four main causes: (1) inspissated secretions, (2) fungal sinusitis, (3) hemorrhage in the sinus, and (4) calcification. The hyperdense sinus may be the only clue to fungal sinusitis and is an important feature to note. However, chronic sinusitis infected with bacteria occasionally is hyper-

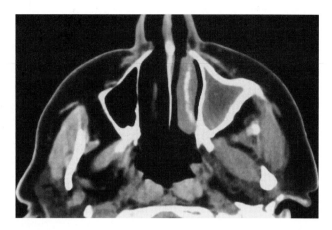

Fig. 13-13   Chronic sinusitis. Marked bony thickening around the opacified left maxillary sinus signifies chronic disease.

dense on CT, particularly in patients who have very long-standing disease or cystic fibrosis. The hyperdense sinus often corresponds to the hypointense sinus on T2WI (Fig. 13-14). Nonetheless, say a fungus is among us if you see dense secretions.

One may also see calcifications in the maxillary antra that may indicate fungal sinusitis, however, once again, the finding may also be present with nonfungal inspissated secretions (though not to the same extent). Here are a few tips: if the intrasinus calcification is central and is fine, punctate like, it is most likely due to fungi. If the calcification is peripheral, curvilinear, and eggshell like, it is probably nonfungal. If you measure the Hounsfield units (HU) you can gain some specificity to the "hyperdense sinus." Those with HUs greater than 2000 have a 93.3% chance of maxillary sinus aspergillosis. The mean CT density of the sinus concretions without aspergillosis is 778 HU. These numbers are like the NASDAQ: great to quote but nonpredictive for your own portfolio of scanners.

The following features of the "calcified" sinus **mass** have been reported. A single discrete hyperdensity is most likely to be an inflammatory mass (aspergilloma, rhinolith), but multiple discrete calcifications could be seen in tumors (enchondromas, inverted papillomas, meningiomas) or inflammatory lesions. If the process is diffusely hyperdense with a well-defined margin, think of a fibroosseous lesion but if it is poorly marginated, consider a high-grade sarcoma (chondrosarcoma, osteosarcoma). Although calcification is not unusual in inverted papillomas it is more likely to be residual bone, not calcifications. On the other hand, esthesioneuroblastomas have intrinsic calcifications.

A rhinolith (stone in the nose) is often due to a foreign body that has become lodged in the nose and has slowly calcified. This may occur in the setting of traumatic or recreational nasal septum injuries (snort, snort).

While you are evaluating coronal CT scans for sinusi-

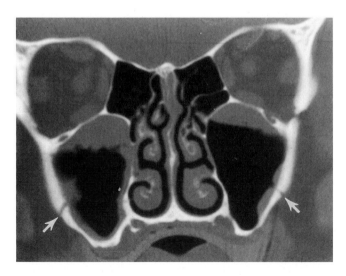

Fig. 13-12   Sinusitis. Coronal supine study shows an air-fluid level in the right maxillary antrum and diffuse mucosal thickening bilaterally in the maxillary sinuses. The lineal radiolucencies in the maxillary sinus laterally represent a normal neural canal *(arrows)*.

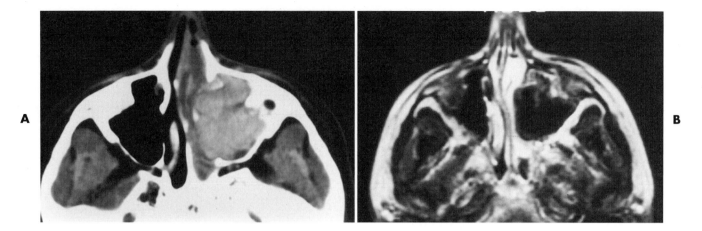

Fig. 13-14   Fungal sinusitis. **A,** Unenhanced CT shows a hyperdense opacified left maxillary antrum. **B,** On T2WI, the secretions were black suggesting inspissation, paramagnetic accumulation, and/or fungal sinusitis. Cultures grew *Drechslera* fungi.

tis, do not forget to look at four other related areas; the teeth, the sella, the nasopharynx, and the temporo-mandibular joints. Pain from odontogenic infections or carious teeth may be mistakenly attributed to sinusitis. Therefore, you will do everyone a favor if you check the maxillary teeth for areas of demineralization or periapi-cal cysts as you check for sinusitis. By the same token, of those patients referred for Denta-scans (a 3D CT of the teeth, mandible, and maxilla) with periodontal dis-ease, 60% had maxillary sinusitis as opposed to those without periodontal disease who had just a 25% rate of maxillary disease. It is very useful to observe the dis-placement of the maxillary sinus wall to distinguish odontogenic cystic lesions, which displace the inferior antral wall superiorly from maxillary sinus lesions like mucoceles that push the bone down.

Malocclusions or temporomandibular joint degenera-tive change may indicate a maxillofacial pain syndrome that may simulate pain from sinusitis. Look for narrow-ing or sclerosis around the joint.

We are also surprised at the high rate of incidental sellar lesions seen on coronal CT that we miss, but are brought to our attention by the FESS surgeons. Naso-pharyngeal carcinomas also savage the unwary neuro-radiologist, but not readers of our book! Look for it. One case found by listening to us is worth a case of *Neuro-radiology: THE REQUISITES*.

Screening sinus CTs are often performed prior to bone marrow transplantation (BMT) in patients with hemato-logic malignancies. Of those showing severe sinusitis on initial screening CT scans, two-thirds experience clinical sinusitis post-BMT. Forty percent of patients with mod-erate sinus abnormalities on pre-BMT CT scans develop clinical sinusitis during their post-BMT course, compared to 23% with normal pre-BMT CT scans. The presence of sinusitis on pre-BMT studies is also associated with a trend toward overall decreased survival. So, do not argue

with the oncologists about whether these studies are warranted—these docs have more important things to do . . . like curing cancer.

Trauma often affects the walls of the paranasal si-nuses. Remember that the floor of the orbit serves as the roof of the maxillary sinus so fractures there cause blood levels in the sinuses. Similarly the medial wall blow out fracture affects the ethmoid sinus and orbital roof frac-tures may affect supraorbital ethmoid cells or the frontal sinus. Direct blows to the forehead may cause inward displacement fractures of the frontal sinuses (Fig. 13-15). Skull base fractures may cross the sphenoid sinus. These air-filled spaces are not necessarily the best buttresses against trauma, being very thin and with nothing but air between them and the directed force.

MR's sensitivity to mucosal thickening accounts for the visualization of the normal *nasal cycle*. There is cycli-cal passive congestion and decongestion of each side of the nasal turbinates, nasal septum, and ethmoid air cell mucosa that rotates from side-to-side over the course of 1 to 8 hours in humans. Thus 1 to 2 mm of ethmoid si-nus mucosal thickening may not be due to inflammatory disease but may reflect the normal intermittent conges-tion of the nasal cycle. Be aware of the nasal cycle so you do not over read increased mucosal signal from the turbinates and ethmoid sinus as disease on MR. Do not fall into this trap. Take a test. Sniff right now and de-termine which side of your nose is dominant. We will check at the end of the chapter to see if your cycle has switched sides. (The authors' long noses are on oppo-site sides at this time, right for Bob and left for Dave. But we are often on opposite sides of the political spectrum, right for Bob and left for Dave. But we both respect Colin Powell.) Even if one uses 5 mm of thickness of the mu-cosa or greater as a determinant of pathology on MR, in-cidental sinus inflammation is present in over 32% of asymptomatic subjects coming to MR scanning.

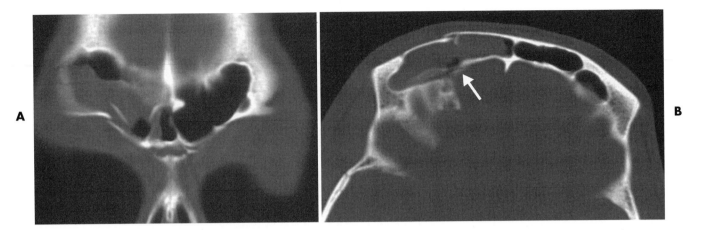

Fig. 13-15   Trauma to the frontal sinus **A,** When a fracture *(arrow)* goes through both walls of the frontal sinus the potential for a CSF leak, meningitis, pseudomeningoceles, and intracranial hemorrhagic complications increases. This is difficult to discern on a coronal scan. **B,** Rely on the axial scans to make this distinction. *Arrow* on posterior wall of frontal sinus.

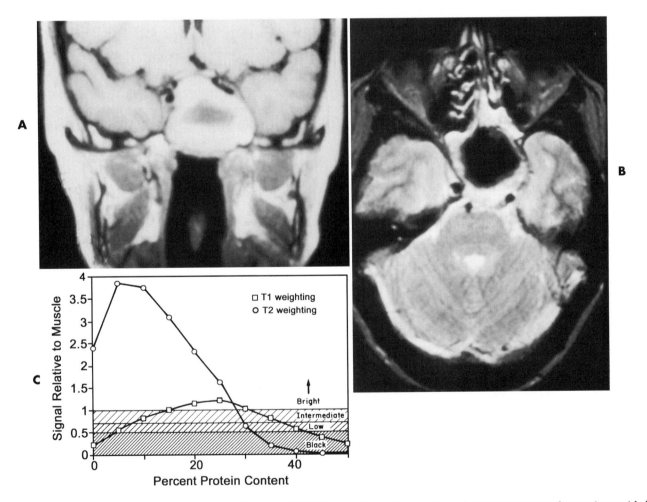

Fig. 13-16   Sinonasal secretions on MR. **A,** On the coronal T1WI, the sphenoid sinus shows hypointense central secretions with hyperintense peripheral contents. **B,** The T2WI also has hypointense central and hyperintense peripheral secretions. This was a mucocele with inspissated obstructed secretions. **C,** The influence of protein content in sinonasal secretions on signal intensity is depicted in this graph. Note that there are regions from low protein content to highest protein content that pass from dark T1-bright T2, bright T1-bright T2, bright T1-dark T2, and dark T1-dark T2 signal intensity. (C reprinted with permission from RSNA publications: Som PM, Dillon WP, Fullerton GD, Zimmerman RA, Rajagopalan B, Marom Z. Chronically obstructed sinonasal secretions: observations on T1 and T2 shortening. *Radiology* 172:515-520, 1989.)

Sinonasal secretions are not always bright on T2WI and dark on T1WI. The change in signal intensity of sinonasal secretions based on protein concentration and mobile water protons has been recently explained. The changes are probably due to the increased cross-linking of glycoproteins in hyperproteinaceous secretions, leading to fewer available free water protons and more bound protons (to glycoproteins). As protein concentration increases, the signal intensity on T1WI of sinus secretions changes from hypointense to hyperintense, to hypointense again. On T2WI, hypoproteinaceous watery secretions are initially bright, but as the protein concentration and viscosity increase, the signal intensity on T2WI decreases. Therefore you can get four confusing intensity patterns for sinus secretions: (1) hypointense on T1WI and hyperintense on T2WI in the most liquid form (total protein concentration <9%), (2) hyperintense on T1WI and hyperintense on T2WI in the mild to moderately proteinaceous form (total protein concentration 20% to 25%), (3) hyperintense on T1WI and hypointense on T2WI in a highly proteinaceous form (total protein concentration 25% to 28%), and (4) hypointense on T1WI and hypointense on T2WI when the secretions are in a nearly solid form (total protein concentration >28%) (Fig. 13-16).

Because air and very hyperproteinaceous secretions appear as a signal void, this is a potential pitfall. You may think the sinus is aerated but it's (s)not. Other potential problems in which hypointensity may be encountered on both T1WI and T2WI include osteomas, odontogenic lesions, osteochondromas, fibrosis, and fungal sinusitis mycetomas. The low signal of fungal sinusitis is thought to result from the paramagnetic effects of either iron or manganese metabolized by the fungi (Box 13-4).

Chronically obstructed sinus secretions may have any combination of signal intensities. Thus, it may be difficult to distinguish inflammation from neoplasm solely based on intensity patterns. For this reason, the presence of peripheral rim enhancement is a reassuring finding that suggests inflammation rather than neoplasm (which enhances

centrally). This point is worth stressing and is sponsored by the contrast agent suppliers in your neighborhood.

Post-FESS scanning Postoperatively, neither CT nor MR is highly accurate in distinguishing fibrosis from inflammation. Both enhance and appear as mucosal thickening. The absence of disease on a postoperative study is reliable, but false-positive studies occur frequently.

Interestingly, although postoperative studies will show open OMCs increasing from 42% to 83% in patients with chronic sinusitis, and from 8% to 45% in patients with polyposis, the overall extent of sinus opacification before and after FESS is more often than not minimally changed (Fig. 13-17). Nonetheless, whether based on physiology or merely cognitive dissonance theory, over 90% of patients say they feel better after FESS.

There is one classification for types of FESS surgeries that is worth putting up your nose through the cribriform plate and into your brain (Table 13-2). If you learn this, the ENT surgeons may provide you with intranasal steroid sprays for life.

CT is the study of choice in the acute setting of orbital complications after FESS, which usually occur within 48 hours after surgery. CT is reliable in diagnosing an orbital hematoma, assessing for optic nerve compression or inadvertent resection, and planning therapy to relieve increased intraorbital pressure. It can be performed in an emergency setting with less image degradation caused by eye motion artifact than MR. Often, however, if vision is deteriorating rapidly, this compli-

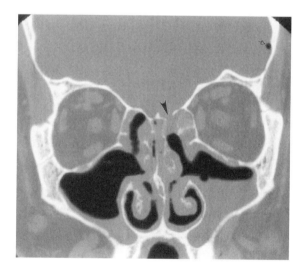

Fig. 13-17 Post-operative study after uncinatectomies and ethmoidectomies. Despite the surgery to open the ostia and ethmoid sinuses, this patient continued to have acute maxillary sinusitis attacks (note the air-fluid levels on the coronal prone study) and chronic mucosal changes in the ethmoid sinuses. Extra credit: Did you catch the dehiscent area in the left fovea ethmoidalis *(arrowhead)*. This may be a manifestation of the disease or the surgery. The dot of intracranial air *(small open arrow)* is the second edge of the film diagnosis. Score 3 if you got that one too.

Box 13-4 Sinonasal Lesions with Signal Voids on MR

Amyloidomas
Chondroid lesions
Fibrosis
Fungus balls
Hemorrhage
Inspissated secretions
Odontogenic masses
Osteomas
Sinoliths
Teeth

Table 13-2	Types of FESS			
Type	Uncinate resected?	Ethmoidectomy		Maxillary sinus surgery
I	Yes	Only agger nasi cells		No
II	Yes	Bulla, anterior ethmoidectomy, frontal sinus opening		No
III	Yes	Bulla ethmoidectomy, frontal sinus opening		Antrostomy
IV	Yes	Anterior and posterior ethmoidectomy		Antrostomy
V	Yes	Anterior and posterior ethmoidectomy PLUS SPHENOIDECTOMY		Antrostomy
S*	Yes	Yes, along with carotid artery, optic nerve, or frontal lobe*		Yes

*Joke—get it? S doesn't stand for simple, but suit, as in legal suit.

cation is treated on the basis of clinical findings. Acute hematomas are usually hyperdense on CT; occasionally, diffuse orbital fat edema may be the most salient finding. Usually, orbital hematomas are due to transection of an ethmoidal artery at FESS. The artery then retracts into the orbit and continues to bleed. The intraorbital pressure rises with the expanding hematoma, leading to compromise of the flow of the retinal artery and ischemia of the optic nerve. Decompression is required rapidly (within hours), or irreversible nerve damage will occur. Canthotomies are emergently performed.

Other complications include trauma to the medial wall of the orbit. While removing the middle turbinate, the lateral attachment to the lamina papyracea (the basal lamella) may be yanked off and injure the medial wall of the orbit (why do you think they call it paper thin as in lamina papyracea?). Contusion to the medial rectus muscle, fat herniation into the sinus, and orbital hematomas may follow in "suit" (if so, sue you later). Orbital emphysema may be seen.

CSF leaks due to trauma to the cribriform plate and damage from over vigorous removal of the superior attachment of the middle turbinate at the fovea ethmoidalis are other potential FESS complications. This may lead to postoperative meningitis, epidural abscess, or pneumocephalus. Fortunately, the FESS surgeons are getting good at patching their own dural holes with mucosal free grafts or septal flaps. (Cover ups?)

Osteoplastic frontal sinus grafts are often placed during frontal sinus obliterative procedures when FESS has been unsuccessful in opening the frontal recess. Postoperatively, patients may develop pain that may be secondary to neuromas, mucoceles, or recurrent sinusitis if the sinus is not plugged completely. Most surgeons use fat to obliterate the sinus. MRI with fat suppression can evaluate the frontal sinus after obliteration with adipose tissue to look for mucoceles and to differentiate viable adipose tissue from fat necrosis in the form of oil cysts.

The amount of fat intensity in the sinus obliteration decreases over time as fibrosis occurs. Concomitant intensity changes occur.

Uncommon Inflammatory Conditions of the Sinuses

Rhinoscleroma refers to the granulomatous, mass-like infection caused by *Klebsiella rhinoscleromatis,* a gram-negative aerobic coccobacillus. This disease is endemic to Africa, Central and South America, South Central and Eastern Europe, the Middle East, and China. This is a disease of young (often impoverished) adults where sinonasal inflammation is seen extending bilaterally in the anterior and posterior nares. The hard and soft palate may be affected as well. The signal intensity on both T1WI and T2WI is bright often simulating a fungal infection or a melanoma. There may be heterogeneous low intensity foci within the nasal masses. The masses may obstruct the OMCs and lead to secondary obstructive sinusitis. The lesion ultimately leads to sclerosis and chronic nasal occlusion.

Granulomatous Diseases

Sarcoidosis may affect the sinonasal cavity and is one of the sources of nasal septal perforation (along with cocaine abuse, syphilis, leprosy, and Wegener's granulomatosis) (Fig. 13-18). The entities of lethal midline granuloma, Stewart syndrome, midline granuloma syndrome, polymorphic reticulosis, lymphomatoid granulomatosis, and pseudolymphoma have recently been reclassified into cases of Wegener's granulomatosis and/or non-Hodgkin T-cell lymphoma. The generic term of "midline destructive lesions of the sinonasal tract" has also been applied to these entities (Box 13-5). Both Wegener's granulomatosis and non-Hodgkin T-cell lymphoma may present with nasal septal perforations and soft-tissue

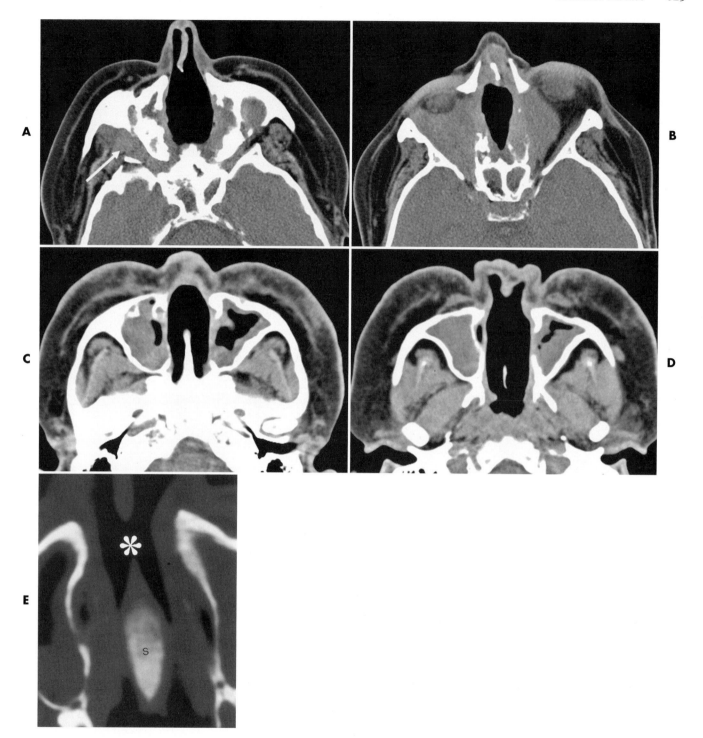

Fig. 13-18   Septal perforations. **A,** This patient had Wegener's granulomatosis. The nasal septum is gone and the patient had infiltration of the orbits and the soft tissue around the right maxillary antra *(arrow)* **B. C** and **D,** Similar findings with less soft tissue destruction are seen in this case of sarcoidosis. Steroid use accounted for the prominence of the facial fat. **E,** Another case of sarcoidosis with nasal septal perforation *(snowflake)* and ground glassy, thickened vomer (S).

masses in the sinonasal cavity. Wegener's granulomatosis shows noncaseating multinucleated giant cell granulomas and necrotizing vasculitis histopathologically. Disease onset is usually in the 40s with 90% of individuals having upper or lower respiratory involvement. CNS

Wegener's granulomatosis occurs in up to 5% of cases, usually manifesting with cranial neuropathies. Meningeal inflammation, vasculitis, or direct spread from parameningeal sources are the etiologies of CNS Wegener's granulomatosis. Hypophysitis may also occur. Reports of meningeal spread of Wegener's granulomatosis and/or cavernous sinus involvement have been published (and even read by your humble [not!] authors).

Non-Hodgkin T-cell lymphoma shows monoclonal lymphocytes with positive CD45 and CD45RO markers, without CD20 positivity. Bony erosion may be seen, particularly involving the medial wall of the maxillary antrum or the hard palate.

Foreign body granuloma, polyarteritis nodosa, lupus, and hypersensitivity angiitis may also present with destructive sinonasal masses. Pseudotumor, an idiopathic inflammatory disease characterized by fibroblasts, histiocytes, and inflammatory cells can simulate an aggressive sinus process.

Meningitis Secondary to Sinusitis

Although MR has a limited role in the evaluation of uncomplicated sinusitis, it has great potential for evaluating intracranial and intraorbital complications, including meningitis, thrombophlebitis, subdural empyemas, intracranial abscesses, and perineural or perivascular spread of infection. For detection of meningitis, contrast is required to identify abnormal meningeal enhancement (Fig. 13-19). Coronal scans are particularly good for identifying meningitis adjacent to frontal or ethmoidal sinusitis. Subdural and epidural collections associated with infection are discussed in Chapter 6.

Orbital complications of sinusitis may include preseptal and postseptal cellulitis, subperiosteal abscesses (the most common intraorbital complication in pediatric patients), and phlegmons. These entities are described fully in Chapter 10 assuming Bob does his job.

Thrombophlebitis

Thrombophlebitis is an important complication to recognize as a consequence of sinusitis. Although thrombosed veins and venous sinuses may occur as a result of adjacent sinusitis it is more commonly seen with mastoiditis. Sigmoid sinus venous thrombosis and venous infarction may complicate mastoiditis and petrous apicitis. In the paranasal sinuses, the most common venous channel involved is the cavernous sinus, and thrombosis is usually associated with sphenoid sinus inflammation.

Fungal Sinusitis

The advantages of MR are of particular value in a patient who has an aggressive fulminant fungal sinus infection such as mucormycosis or aspergillosis (see Chapter 6). These fungal infections in their fulminant or invasive form have a propensity for invasion of the or-

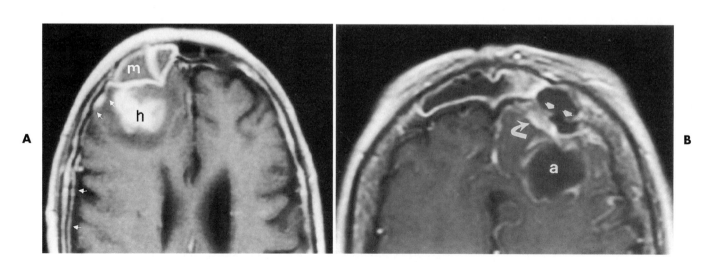

Fig. 13-19 Meningitis associated with sinusitis. **A,** The dura is enhancing *(arrows)* on this enhanced T1WI in a patient with a frontal mucocele *(m)*. Note that there is rim mucosal enhancement in the sinus. The intraparenchymal hemorrhage *(h)* was presumed to be due to venous infarction. **B,** In this case of a mucocele gone bad, the extension through the inner table of the frontal sinus *(arrows)* led to a thick rind of meningeal inflammation *(curved arrow)* and an intraparenchymal abscess *(a)*.

bit, the cavernous sinus, and the neurovascular structures. Numerous case reports have described MR's ability to identify spread of mycotic infections from the turbinates to the sinuses, orbit, and intracranial cavity. Fungi may cause vascular insults such as thrombosis or cerebral infarcts. Mucormycosis in particular appears to spread intracranially along the vessels. This fungus grows in the internal elastic membrane of blood vessels; its hyphae may penetrate the lumen of the vessel to occlude it. Prompt detection of this complication can lead to life- or orbit-saving therapy.

Periantral soft-tissue infiltration either anterior or posterior to the maxillary sinus, should suggest the possibility of invasive fungal sinusitis in the appropriate clinical setting. Early detection may save the patient from a significant face-ectomy so scout the walls of the antrum for fatty infiltration and save a "shana punim" (pretty face).

With regard to fungal sinus infections, one must understand that there are different levels of aggressiveness to mycotic infections. Sinonasal mycotic infection is similar in this regard to pulmonary fungal disease. Extramucosal fungal infection may be manifested as *polypoid lesions* (i.e., allergic aspergillosis caused by saprophytic growth on retained secretions in patients with atopy) or as *fungus balls*. These are benign conditions usually caused by *Aspergillus*. They are often dense on CT as well but are much more benign-looking and localized than allergic fungal sinusitis (AFS). Fungus balls are usually rounded masses, perhaps with a lamellated appearance. They have high signal on T1WI and low on T2WI (Fig. 13-20).

Allergic fungal sinusitis (AFS), a nonvirulent form of the disease is characterized on CT by increased attenuation within the sinuses. Bilateral involvement is frequently present. Complete opacification with expansion, erosion or remodeling and thinning of the sinuses are signature features of AFS. The signal intensity on T2WI is usually low.

Steroid therapy and local excision are sufficient treatment for extramucosal fungal infections like AFS or fungus balls. *Infiltrating fungal sinusitis* occurs in an immunocompetent host but is not as aggressive as the *fulminant infection* seen in the immunocompromised person. The fulminant disease is the lethal form of infection and may be caused by *Mucor* or *Aspergillus*. Wide, local excision and intravenously administered antifungal drugs are required for extirpation of the invasive mycotic infections. Orbital exenteration, hyperbaric oxygen treatment, and radical surgical therapy often are necessary for fulminant cases, and even then the prognosis is grim. Invasive fungal sinusitis is often hyperdense on CT and hypointense on MR.

Cystic Fibrosis

Cystic fibrosis (mucoviscidosis) is a common autosomal recessive disease characterized by viscous secretions and hence chronic sinusitis (>90%) and polyposis (46%). Mucociliary clearance is inhibited by the thick grundgy secretions. Sinonasal development in this childhood disease is often retarded by the chronic infections. The mucosa is often polypoid in its appearance and mucocele formation is not infrequent. The triad of frontal sinus hypoplasia, medial bulging of the lateral nasal wall (indicative of polyposis), and ethmoid opacification in a child is highly suggestive of cystic fibrosis. Add in some high density of the secretions and polyps on the turbinates and you are home free. Hypoplasia of the

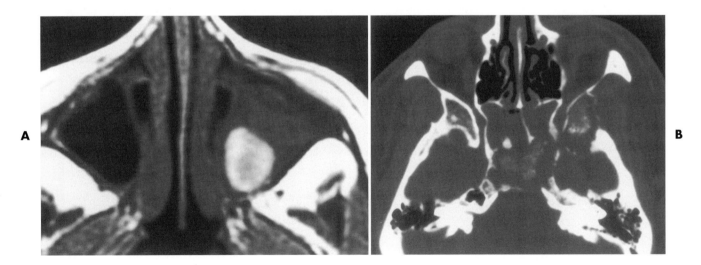

Fig. 13-20 Two forms of aspergillus. **A,** The hyperintense focus in the opacified left maxillary antrum may have been an inspissated mucous retention cyst but they are usually of water intensity. Au contraire, this proved to be an aspergilloma. **B,** Destruction of the sphenoid wing, septations of the sphenoid sinus, clivus, and petrous tips occurred in this diabetic patient who developed invasive sinonasal aspergillosis. Image used bone window settings.

sphenoid sinus is present also to such a degree that if you do see pneumatization of the basisphenoid, you should question the diagnosis of cystic fibrosis.

Mucocele

Another complication of sinusitis is a mucocele. Although CT best demonstrates the bony distortion and thinning associated with mucocele formation and the remodeling of the osseous structures suggesting chronicity, MR can detect its interface with intracranial or intraorbital structures. When infected, the term used is *mucopyocele*. The density of the secretion on CT is usually high indicative of chronicity and inspissation. The signal intensity of mucoceles may vary considerably because of protein content. Mucoceles are most common in the frontal (65%) and ethmoid (25%) sinuses, with maxillary (10%) and sphenoid sinus mucoceles the least common (Fig. 13-21). A peripheral rim enhancement pattern is seen on MR. This pattern is useful for distinguishing mucoceles and obstructed secretions from neoplasms such as inverted papillomas or malignancies, which may also remodel bone but show solid enhancement. Tumors, fibro-osseous bone lesions, trauma, postoperative scarring, and hematomas can cause mucoceles.

Postoperative Encephaloceles and CSF Leaks

Encephaloceles are better distinguished from sinonasal inflammation by MR than by CT (Fig. 13-22). Encephaloceles may occur from congenital defects (see Chapter 9) or may arise in the postoperative setting when the cribriform plate has been violated. In the postoperative encephalocele, rhinorrhea is the presentation that elicits the imaging study, but this may occur as late as 18 months after surgery. Is the rhinorrhea due to a dural tear or a postethmoidectomy encephalocele? Dural tears occur most commonly on a patient's right side because most surgeons are right handed, making the right sinonasal cavity more difficult to surgerize. Persistent postoperative leaks caused by dural tears are probably best assessed with a combination of studies. Nuclear medicine studies in which indium–diethylene triamine pentaacetic acid (DTPA) is injected intrathecally are highly accurate for detecting leaks when active flow is present, even at a slow rate. Pledgets are placed in the nose; counts are recorded; and right and left sides, and superior and inferior quadrants, are compared. However, the anatomic definition afforded with CT with or without intrathecal contrast instillation is more useful to the clinician and is gradually replacing nuclear medicine studies. These scans are best performed with the patient in the prone position. If active CSF leakage is rapid, the CT may show the contrast dye in the adjacent sinus or at the site of intracranial bony defect (Fig. 13-23). Perform these studies with both soft tissue and bone windows for optimal detection and localization of the leak.

If there is the possibility of brain herniating through the dehiscent area, MR is valuable. It may also distinguish postoperative scar tissue, recurrent polyps, or inflammation from meninges, CSF, and brain. Some people have

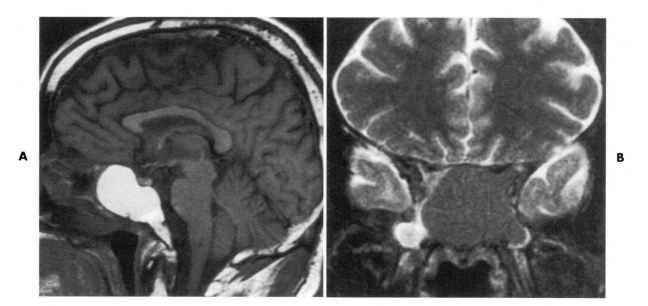

Fig. 13-21 Mucocele. **A,** T1WI reveals a very bright sphenoid sinus. **B,** The T2WI shows low signal. This likely represents a stage of hyperproteinaceous secretions that exceeds 35% protein content according to Som's study (see Fig. 13-16C). The atypical feature of this mucocele which could be debated is the absence of sinus expansion—could this just be dense secretions or a melanoma as opposed to a mucocele? Cut once, but measure twice.

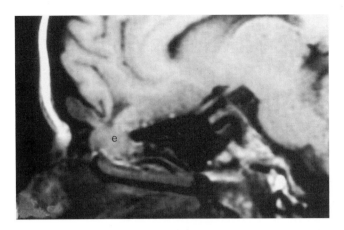

Fig. 13-22   Postoperative encephalocele. Parasagittal T1WI demonstrates herniation of brain *(e)* in a postoperative defect through the cribriform plate after functional endoscopic sinus surgery. Dysfunction was noted after the functional surgery. Biopsy of the mass did not help.

advocated using a heavily T2-weighted MR study, "MR cisternography," to detect the site of CSF leaks, but the authors of this text, being minimalists of cerebrum, are skeptical of the role of MR in this scenario. Nonetheless, this is gaining popularity with the otherwise MR-wary rhinologists and rhinoradiologists and rhinoceroseses. We are more supportive of the notion that an unenhanced 1-mm coronal section CT may be able to answer most questions related to rhinorrhea. Although it may be like shooting ourselves in the wallet, we believe that in

many ways direct endoscopic visualization of intrathecally instilled fluorescein actively leaking from the cribriform plate is the most reliable test in a skilled endoscopist's hands. (Often the ENT surgeons instill an agent for nuclear medicine cisternography at the same time.) A CT scan before or after this test will often solve the CSF leak riddle; where's the leak?

Polyposis

One of the manifestations of allergic sinusitis is sinonasal polyposis. Polyps may also occur in the absence of allergies and are due to nonneoplastic hyperplasia of inflamed mucous membranes.

From an imaging standpoint, this entity is somewhat problematic because the lesion, although benign, may demonstrate aggressive bony distortion. On CT, the findings suggestive of polyposis include enlargement of sinus ostia, rounded masses within the nasal cavity, expanded sinuses or portions of the nasal cavity, thinning of bony trabeculae, and, less commonly, erosive bone changes at the anterior aspect of the skull base (Fig. 13-24). Most cases of sinonasal polyposis show bilateral changes and nasal involvement (>80%). Truncation of the bony middle turbinate, where the bulbous part of bony middle turbinate is missing is found in over half of cases with this disease.

Because the aggressive skull base erosion might suggest a malignancy, it would be useful if specific findings on MR or CT distinguished polyposis from cancer. Unfortunately, this is not always possible. Although the signal intensity of most sinonasal polyps on T2WI is bright, this overlaps with some of the neoplasms seen in the paranasal sinuses, including sarcomas, adenoid cystic car-

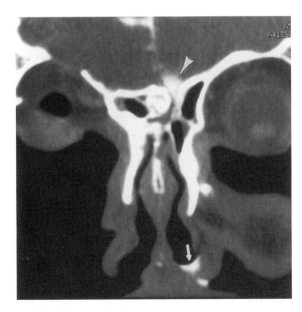

Fig. 13-23   CSF leak. The gap in the cribriform plate on the left side and the intrathecal contrast seeping through the defect *(arrow)* are demonstrated on this case of traumatic CSF leak. Check out the contrast in the left nostril *(arrow)*—it doesn't get any better than that.

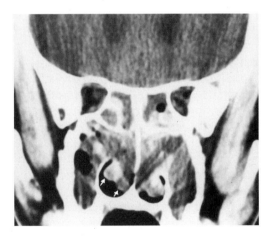

Fig. 13-24   Polyps. This patient has extensive polyps in the nasal cavity bilaterally, opacifying the airway. The coronal view shows the polypoid excrescences *(arrows)* from the inferior turbinates to best advantage. Expansion of ostia is another hallmark of polypoid disease.

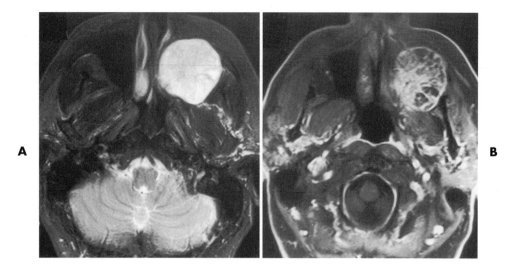

Fig. 13-25   Fool me once, shame on you. Fool me twice shame on me. **A,** A hyperintense mass in the left maxillary antrum is identified on T2WI. Would you bet on a pleomorphic adenoma or a mucocele or something else? **B,** The enhancement is predominantly solid. Therefore, it's not a mucocele. Pleomorphic adenoma? Nope . . . adenoid cystic carcinoma.

cinomas (Fig. 13-25), and other, less common, minor salivary gland neoplasms. Polyps usually enhance peripherally because they represent hypertrophied mucosa, but, occasionally, when the mucosa folds repetitively on itself, they may enhance solidly like neoplasms.

Antrochoanal (Killian) polyps arise in the maxillary sinus but may protrude into the nasal cavity or the nasopharyngeal airway. The polyp usually extends through the accessory ostium of the sinus and projects posteriorly through the posterior choana to the nasopharynx. A CT classification of the three stages of antrochoanal polyp natural history has been proposed. If the polyp does make it to the nasopharynx it is staged as stage I (early development). If the polyp extends to the nasopharynx and the accessory ostium of the maxillary sinus is fully occluded it is graded as stage II (fully mature) (Fig. 13-26). If the polyp extends to the nasopharynx and the accessory ostium is only partially occluded by the neck of the polyp it is called Stage III (regressive stage). Antrochoanal polyps are smooth hypodense masses that often remodel bone and enlarge the maxillary sinus accessory ostium on CT, features indicative of slow sustained growth. On MR they are very bright on T2WI and have a variable amount of usually peripheral enhancement. Choanal polyps are seen in children and young adults with a strong male preponderance.

Sphenochoanal polyps track from . . . well, you can guess. They can usually be found between the nasal septum and the middle turbinate and track through the sphenoethmoidal recess.

Polyps occur in 1.3% of the general population and 16.2% of patients with chronic sinusitis.

They are commonly associated with aspirin intolerance, nickel exposure (4%), cystic fibrosis (10% to 20%), asthma

(30%), allergic rhinitis (25%), and Kartagener's syndrome (Box 13-6). The latter refers to the immotile cilia syndrome in which patients have recurrent sinusitis, situs inversus, bronchiectasis, and infertility. Kartagener's syndrome is an autosomal recessive disorder with variable penetrance.

Steroids may retard the growth or decrease the size of sinonasal polyps through an effect on insulin-like growth factor 1. Depending upon the severity of the patient's symptoms, intranasal or oral steroid treatment may be prescribed for sinonasal polyposis. Unfortu-

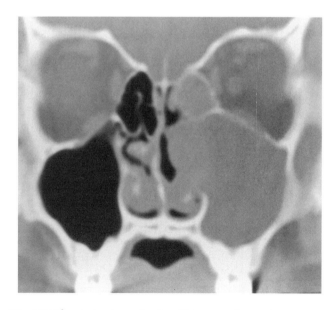

Fig. 13-26   Antrochoanal polyp. This coronal scan shows a mass spilling over from the maxillary antrum into the nasal cavity. The accessory ostium is occluded and expanded; therefore the antrochoanal polyp would be considered Stage II.

Box 13-6   Congenital Causes of Sinonasal Polyps

Aspirin intolerance
Cystic fibrosis
Immotile cilia syndrome
Kartegener syndrome
Peutz-Jeghers syndrome

nately, like rejected HMO claims, the disease often keeps coming back. The patient is then faced with a choice of pulsed intermittent steroid therapy or surgery. For cystic fibrosis children, this often means recurrent surgery.

Retention Cysts

Mucous retention cysts develop as a result of obstruction of small seromucinous glands, usually in the maxillary sinus. In most cases, it is impossible to distinguish a polyp from a retention cyst. The distinction is of little clinical relevance. If the endoscopist is told that a patient has a mucous retention cyst, he or she will pay particular attention to that OMC for possible intermittent obstruction. The cyst itself is not addressed unless obstructive in size. Retention cysts are smooth domed homogeneous lesions usually found in the maxillary sinus and often in the dependent portion. They are bright on T2WI. Any site that has minor salivary gland tissue could have a mucous retention cyst.

BENIGN NEOPLASMS

The stereotypic benign neoplasm expands and remodels the bone as a result of its slow, nonaggressive growth. This is contrasted with malignancies that destroy bone and invade in an ill-defined, poorly marginated manner. Four types of skull base erosion have been described in relation to sinonasal masses. These are (1) resorption of the central skull base, (2) enlargement of the foramina of the central skull base, (3) thinning of the central skull base, and (4) displacement of the bone. The first two are more common with malignant lesions and the last two with benign tumors.

Some malignancies, however, may show bony bowing, and some benign tumors aggressively destroy bone. Don't bet the farm on this one—instead, be a stockbroker and cultivate a hedge!

Osteomas

Of the benign neoplasms to affect the sinonasal cavity, osteomas, enchondromas, papillomas, schwannomas,

and juvenile angiofibromas are the most commonly seen. Osteomas are usually identified in the frontal sinus and may infrequently be a source for recurrent headache and/or recurrent sinusitis (Fig. 13-27). Occasionally, the osteoma (or osteochondroma) results in mucocele formation and/or pneumocephalus as the posterior wall of the frontal sinus is breached (Fig. 13-28). The classic history associated with a frontal sinus osteoma narrowing the sinus opening is a patient who has severe sinus pain

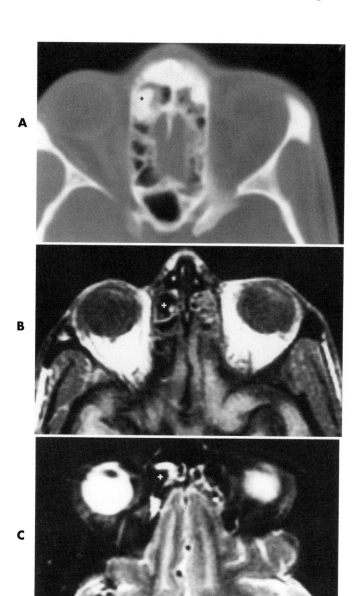

Fig. 13-27   Osteoma. **A,** An osteoma *(asterisk)* in a right anterior ethmoid air cell is seen well on CT. **B,** Tl WI fails to demonstrate the lesion (+), although mucosal thickening is present elsewhere. Remember MR is insensitive to cortical bone and calcification. **C,** The T2WI again highlights the inflammation around the osteoma (+), but the lesion is black, simulating aeration. Now you know why CT remains preeminent in the sinuses.

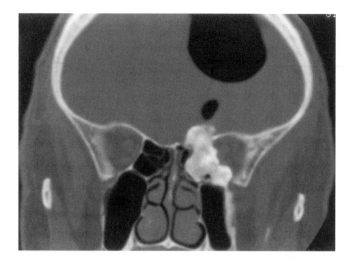

Fig. 13-28   Osteochondroma and pneumocephalus. Classically osteomas are said to be the tumors that can cause pneumocephalus. This osteochondroma must have misread the book—from its ethmoid sinus origin, it perforated the anterior cranial fossa and led to a communication with the brain—hence pneumocephalus.

associated with takeoffs from airplane flights (unrelated to the six free drinks in the first-class cabin of the last remaining American Airline). Osteomas are benign masses that often are completely invisible on MR because of the presence of dense compact bone making up the mass. On the other hand, they are easily identified on CT as markedly hyperdense bony masses protruding in the sinus. Remember that a patient with colonic polyps

and osteomas may have Gardner syndrome. This is an autosomal dominant syndrome associated with malignant transformation of the polyps in 100% of cases if left untreated. Another syndrome associated with osteomas is Ollier disease.

Papillomas

Papillomas come in many different varieties, the most common of which (around 75%) is the inverted papilloma. This benign neoplasm is remarkable for the coincidence of squamous cell carcinoma in approximately 15% of cases. Inverted papillomas may show a rather aggressive bone destruction pattern and have been known to cross the cribriform plate into the anterior cranial fossa. The lesion typically arises from the lateral nasal wall or maxillary sinus, and it accounts for approximately 4% of all tumors of the nasal cavity. Staging classification has been proposed to include: Stage I—limited to the nasal cavity alone; Stage II—limited to the ethmoid sinuses and medial and superior portions of the maxillary sinuses; Stage III—extension to the lateral or inferior aspects of the maxillary sinuses or extension into the frontal or sphenoid sinuses; and Stage IV—spread outside the nose and sinuses (Fig. 13-29). CT may demonstrate a nonspecific enhancing mass along the lateral nasal wall. The diagnosis is not evident except when, as in approximately 20% of cases, it contains stippled calcium. On MR the lesion is typically isodense to muscle on T1WI and is isointense to hypointense on T2WI. Most of the other benign polypoid masses are bright and ho-

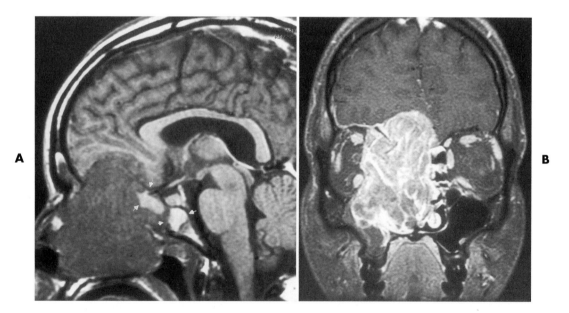

Fig. 13-29   Intracranial growth of inverted papilloma. **A,** A large tumor eroding through the anterior cranial fossa and extending inferiorly to the level of the hard palate is seen on this sagittal T1WI. Inspissated hyperintense secretions *(arrows)* in the frontal, ethmoid, and sphenoid sinuses were present. **B,** The enhancement pattern suggests an inverted papilloma with the striations. Note also the right orbital invasion in addition to the intracranial spread (stage IV disease).

mogeneous in intensity on T2WI. The lesion enhances in a solid fashion and in roughly 50% of cases is heterogeneous in both its signal intensity and enhancement. There seems to be a crenated/convoluted cerebriform appearance to this enhancement that is typical of this entity. If you see this pattern and correctly make this diagnosis, we'll call you "cerebriform" also. The inverted papilloma can erode the skull base in a manner similar to aggressive cancers; because its signal intensity characteristics overlap those of malignancies, there is no way to preoperatively predict the diagnosis. The lesion is particularly problematic to the surgeons who treat it as if it were a malignant neoplasm by an aggressive surgical approach. Unfortunately, the recurrence rates are around 22% to 40% despite aggressive operations. Recurrences may be distinguished from postoperative thickening by dynamic enhanced MR; recurrent inverted papillomas have earlier and greater enhancement than granulation tissue.

Enchondromas

Enchondromas are rare neoplasms of the sinonasal cavity. On CT, they often have "popcorn" calcification, different from the "stippled" calcification of inverted papillomas. The nasal septum is one of the favored sites of enchondromas.

Meningiomas

One percent of meningiomas occur outside the CNS, presumably from embryologic arachnoid rests. The most common sites for these "extradural" meningiomas are the sinonasal cavity. The upper nasal cavity, the ethmoid sinuses, and the frontal sinuses are the most common sinonasal sites. As with all meningiomas they are usually slightly hyperdense masses on CT, intermediate in intensity on MR pulse sequences, and will avidly enhance. A dural attachment may be present or absent, best seen on postcontrast MR studies.

MALIGNANT NEOPLASMS

CT and MR probably play complementary roles in the evaluation of sinonasal malignancies because of CT's superiority in defining bony margins and MR's superior soft-tissue resolution, multiplanar capability, and ability to define intracranial, meningeal, or intraorbital spread. One of the advantages of MR is its ability to distinguish sinus neoplasm from postobstructive secretions. Skull base invasion is another area where MR has gained ascendancy. MR provides more information than CT with regard to demonstrating dural invasion, cavernous sinus infiltration, tumor and muscle differentiation in the in-

---

Box 13-7   T System of Staging Maxillary Sinus Cancer

T1   Tumor limited to maxillary sinus mucosa with no erosion or destruction of bone
T2   Tumor causing bone erosion or destruction including extension into the hard palate and/or middle nasal meatus, except extension to posterior wall of maxillary sinus and pterygoid plates
T3   Tumor invades any of the following: bone of the posterior wall of maxillary sinus, subcutaneous tissues, floor or medial wall of orbit, pterygoid fossa, ethmoid sinuses
T4a Tumor invades anterior orbital contents, skin of cheek, pterygoid plates, infratemporal fossa, cribriform plate, sphenoid or frontal sinuses
T4b Tumor invades any of the following: orbital apex, dura, brain, middle cranial fossa, cranial nerves other than maxillary division of trigeminal nerve (V_2), nasopharynx, or clivus

From Greene FL, Page DL, Fleming ID, et al (eds): *AJCC Cancer Staging Manual,* ed 6. New York, Springer-Verlag, 2002, p. 61. Used with permission.

---

fratemporal fossa and masticator space, optic nerve identification amid adjacent tumor, and fat-suppressed enhancing tumor separation from the internal carotid artery and cavernous sinus. The T system of staging sinus cancers is summarized in Boxes 13-7, 13-8. Bear with us, faithful consumer and perspicacious reader, the next section is a long one but has lots of fun facts.

Box 13-8   T System of Staging Ethmoid Sinus Cancer

T1   Tumor restricted to any one subsite, with or without bony invasion
T2   Tumor invading two subsites in a single region or extending to involve an adjacent region within the nasoethmoidal complex, with or without bony invasion
T3   Tumor extends to invade the medial wall or floor of the orbit, maxillary sinus, palate, or cribriform plate
T4a Tumor invades any of the following: anterior orbital contents, skin of nose or cheek, minimal extension to anterior cranial fossa, pterygoid plates, sphenoid or frontal sinuses
T4b Tumor invades any of the following: orbital apex, dura, brain, middle cranial fossa, cranial nerves other than (V_2), nasopharynx, or clivus

From Greene FL, Page DL, Fleming ID, et al (eds): *AJCC Cancer Staging Manual,* ed 6. New York, Springer-Verlag, 2002, p. 61. Used with permission.

Squamous Cell Carcinoma

Squamous cell carcinoma (relatively hypointense on T2WI) should be distinguished from most inflammation (hyperintense on T2WI). Inflammation and neoplasm can be distinguished in 95% of cases on the basis of T2WI and enhancement (Fig. 13-30). Even when the sinus secretions become increasingly inspissated and the signal intensity on T2WI decreases, the neoplasm can be distinguished from the obstructed secretions by its typical heterogeneity as opposed to the smooth homogeneous appearance of sinus secretions. This is also true in the case of mucoceles, which may occur after or in association with sinus neoplasms. However, do not count on this trend all the time—low intensity on T2WI is an inconstant finding in sinonasal malignancies. The signal intensities of nonsquamous cell tumors (especially minor salivary gland tumors, sarcomas, and lymphoma), can show some overlap with inflammation.

Squamous cell carcinomas of the sinonasal cavity enhance in a solid fashion as opposed to a peripheral rim of enhancement in sinus secretions and/or mucoceles. Unfortunately, lymphomas, undifferentiated carcinomas, inverted papillomas, and some sarcomas may have identical signal intensity and enhancement characteristics as squamous cell carcinoma. Therefore, among sinonasal tumors, specific histologic diagnoses are elusive. The knee-jerk reaction by we jerks is to call everything a squamous cell carcinoma and accept being wrong in 25% of cases (still a passing grade). The hallmark of imaging malignancies of the sinonasal cavity is bony destruction, seen in approximately 80% of scans of sinonasal squamous cell carcinomas at initial presentation. Maxillary sinus carcinomas are confined to the maxillary antrum in only 25% of cases at presentation.

Contrast is particularly useful for demonstrating epidural or meningeal invasion of neoplasms. Often, enhanced coronal scans with fat-suppression techniques are necessary to identify enhancement amid the abundant skull base fat. In one series, 75% of patients with intracranial extension of sinonasal malignancies had additional information about tumor extent demonstrated with postcontrast MR studies. It should be noted that meningeal enhancement need not necessarily imply neoplastic invasion; just as in cases of meningioma, the dura may enhance because of reactive fibrovascular changes alone. Discontinuous dural enhancement without intervening hypointense epidural margination favors neoplastic invasion. Nodular enhancement and enhancing tissue over 5 mm thick imply neoplasm over reactive changes.

Squamous cell carcinomas account for 80% of the malignancies affecting the paranasal sinuses and 80% occur in the maxillary antrum. Seventy-five percent of patients affected are more than 50 years old and there is a male preponderance. Occupational exposures to nickel and chrome pigment and the use of Bantu snuff and cigarettes have been implicated as risk factors. The staging of maxillary sinus cancers used to be based on Ohngren's line from the medial canthus of the eye to the angle of the mandible separating the anteroinferior infrastructure from the superoposterior suprastructure. The superoposterior tumors did worse. The new staging is based more on the site of spread from the maxillary antrum (see Box 13-7).

When you encounter a sinonasal mass that is eroding intracranially, you should consider carcinoma, olfactory neuroblastoma, sarcoma, lymphoma, metastasis, sinonasal polyp, and inverted papilloma. Twelve percent of polyps and mucoceles eventually erode the skull base. Bone remodeling in this location is a rarity; a permeative pattern is the norm for all lesions. Necrosis, hemorrhage, or calcification in carcinomas, olfactory neuroblastomas, or sarcomas may cause signal heterogeneity. Malignancies have a broad, flat base of skull erosion; benign conditions have a rounded, polypoid intracranial excrescence.

Sinonasal Undifferentiated Carcinoma (SNUC)

SNUCs are very aggressive malignancies associated with a very poor prognosis. These most commonly occur in the ethmoid sinus and show early bone destruction. Involvement of the adjacent structures of the nose, skin, orbit, and calvarium is common even at presentation. Their imaging appearance is similar to that of a squamous cell carcinoma gone wild, often with necrosis (Fig. 13-31). They enhance heterogeneously. Histopathologi-

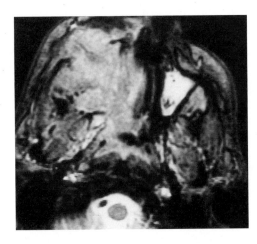

Fig. 13-30 Differentiation on T2WI of cancer and secretions. This right maxillary sinus squamous cell carcinoma is easily distinguished in intensity from the nonviscous secretions in the left maxillary antrum. This differentiation is not foolproof (thank heavens for fools), particularly with minor salivary gland tumors and sarcomas. Thus the need for MR contrast agents (see Fig. 13-5).

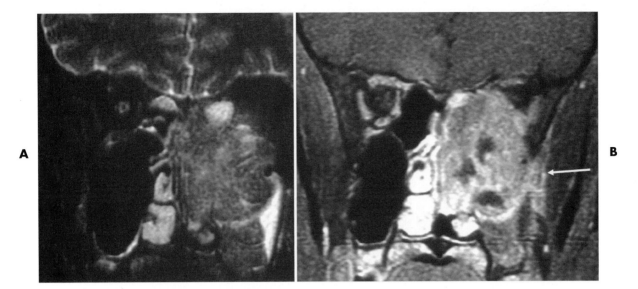

Fig. 13-31   SNUC (sinonasal undifferentiated carcinoma). **A,** When you see a sinonasal mass which is low intensity on a T2WI, you'd better worry about a malignancy like squamous cell carcinoma or SNUC. **B,** SNUCs are usually large and the enhance. Necrosis is an ominous sign as is the spread into the left infratemporal fossa *(arrow)*. Bad luck, you're a dead duck if you have a SNUC.

cally one sees a high mitotic rate, tumor necrosis, and prominent vascularity. Just as these are poor prognostic signs if you have an astrocytoma, they imply a similar fate with a SNUC.

Minor Salivary Gland Cancers

Minor salivary gland tumors and melanoma are the next most common malignancies to affect the sinonasal cavity after squamous cell carcinoma. The minor salivary gland tumors represent a wide variety of histologic types including adenoid cystic carcinoma, mucoepidermoid carcinoma, adenocarcinoma, and undifferentiated carcinoma. Of these tumors, adenoid cystic carcinoma is the most common variety. Its signal intensity may be high or low on T2WI (Fig. 13-32), possibly related to the degree of tubular or cribriform histologic pattern as well as to cystic spaces, necrosis, and tumor cell density. Tissue specificity is not readily achievable with MR or CT except perhaps in some melanomas.

Contrast is of particular use with adenoid cystic carcinomas, which have a propensity (60%) for perineural spread. With sinonasal cavity malignancies, one should always attempt to trace the branches of cranial nerve V via the pterygopalatine fossa, foramen rotundum, foramen ovale, and orbital fissures to identify perineural neoplastic spread. Retrace your steps. Check the hard palate for spread down the greater and lesser palatine foramina.

Adenocarcinomas of the paranasal sinuses have a predilection for the ethmoid sinuses and appear more commonly in woodworkers. This tumor also tends to have low signal intensity on T2WI but may have high signal intensity in a small percentage of cases.

Melanoma

Melanoma is a tumor that is usually identified in the nasal cavity (two to three times more common than in the paranasal sinuses) and is sometimes associated with melanosis, in which there is diffuse deposition of melanin along the mucosal surface of the sinonasal cavity (Fig. 13-33). Therefore, multiplicity of lesions may suggest melanoma as a diagnosis. The nasal septum is the most common site of malignant melanoma, followed by the turbinates. Neither CT nor MR is particularly helpful in identifying the field "cancerization" of melanoma. When melanoma contains melanin, there is paramagnetism, which causes T1 and T2 shortening, accounting for high signal intensity on T1WI and low signal intensity on T2WI. However, an amelanotic melanoma may have low intensity on T1WI and bright signal intensity on T2WI. The presence of hemorrhage associated with the melanoma, a common occurrence because of the coincidence of epistaxis, may further obfuscate the signal intensity pattern. Melanoma is another tumor that has a propensity for neurotropic spread. It also readily metastasizes via hematogenous routes.

Olfactory Neuroblastoma

A calcified malignancy high in the nasal cavity or ethmoid vault is usually an olfactory neuroblastoma (esthesioneuroblastoma) (Fig. 13-34). This tumor arises from olfactory epithelium in the nasal vault from cells derived from the neural crest. Olfactory neuroblastomas have a bimodal peak seen both in males 11 to 20 year olds and

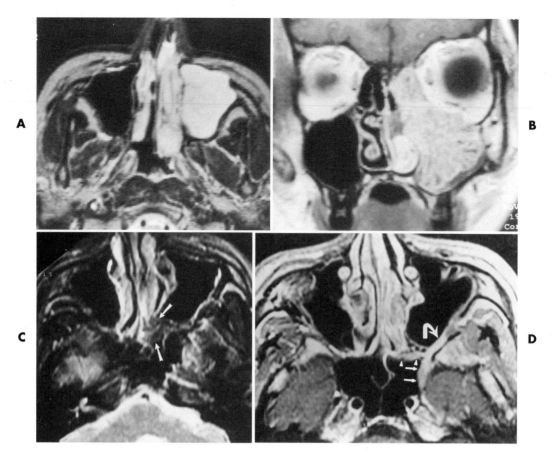

Fig. 13-32   The tricky case. Although the T2W scan shows a hyperintense left maxillary sinus **(A),** the enhanced scan **(B),** by virtue of demonstrating a solid homogeneous pattern of enhancement, implies a neoplasm. This was an adenoid cystic carcinoma. Although it would be extremely rare for a squamous cell carcinoma to be so bright on a T2WI, other minor salivary gland cancers including low grade mucoepidermoid carcinomas and adenocarcinomas could look this way. Another case of adenoid cystic carcinoma. **C,** Axial T2WI demonstrates a low intensity mass in the posterior left nasal cavity *(arrows).* This mass invaded the pterygopalatine fossa on the left side. **D,** Axial enhanced T1WI demonstrates enhancing tumor traveling along the foramen rotundum on the left side *(arrows)* and extending through the pter-ygopalatine fossa *(arrowheads)* and pterygomaxillary fissure *(curved arrow).* This is perineural spread of adenoid cystic carcinoma.

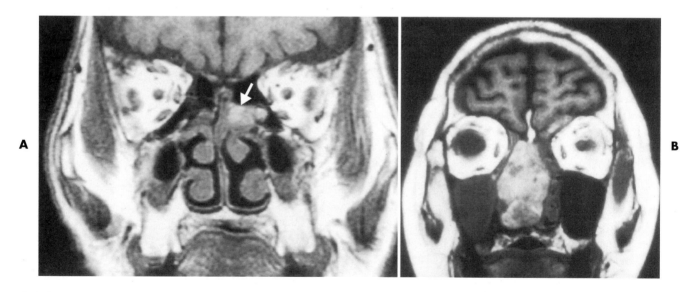

Fig. 13-33   Sinonasal melanoma. **A,** Bright on T1WI, this nasal cavity melanoma *(arrow)* was very well localized. Sinonasal melanomas span the gamut from tiny discolored mucosal lesions identified incidentally for epistaxis to much larger and more aggressive invasive masses **(B).** Remember that they need not be bright on T1WI—that's merely a reflection of quantity of melanin. This one had a lot.

636

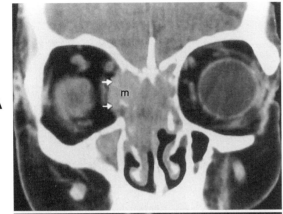

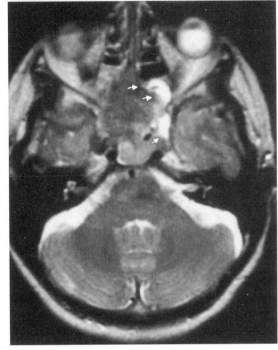

Fig. 13-34   Olfactory neuroblastoma. **A,** A superior nasal cavity mass *(m)* has eroded through the lamina papyracea into the right orbit *(arrows).* **B,** On T2WI the mass is low intensity probably due to its hypercellularity. Note trapped bright secretions on the left side *(arrows).*

in middle-aged adults (sixth decade of life). Patients present with a history of nasal obstruction, epistaxis, or decrease in olfactory function. As with squamous cell carcinoma, olfactory neuroblastomas typically have low signal intensity on T2WI. Intracranial cysts associated with this tumor have been described and are virtually pathognomonic for this malignancy. Esthesioneuroblastomas have a particular propensity for crossing the cribriform plate to enter the intracranial space. In fact, the staging classification of olfactory neuroblastomas is based on extension into the intracranial compartment (stage C) or into the paranasal sinuses or orbit (stage B). When intracranial extension is identified, a craniofacial approach with a

neurosurgical-otorhinolaryngologic team is required. In this type of surgery the frontal lobe is retracted to gain optimal exposure to the cribriform plate so that the tumor can be removed en bloc. A fascia lata or galeal pericranial graft is placed between the brain and resected dura, and is sutured closed. This is followed by skin grafting under the dural surface. Craniofacial resections have decreased the recurrence rates from upper nasal vault–cribriform plate tumors such as adenocarcinomas, olfactory neuroblastomas, squamous cell carcinomas, and sarcomas.

Olfactory neuroblastomas can have lymphatic and hematogenous metastases. Recurrence rates are over 50%.

Sarcomas

Sarcomas of the sinonasal cavities are very rare, with chondrosarcoma the most common. Again, the histologic diagnosis is probably better suggested by CT based on characteristic whorls of calcification. It arises most commonly along the nasal septum (in the cartilaginous portion). Their aggressiveness is variable.

Rhabdomyosarcomas are not uncommon in the sinonasal cavity, although one sees them in the orbit, pharynx, and temporal bone more commonly. They are usually of the embryonal cell type and often have a benign appearance to the manner in which they erode bone—some expand the bone rather than destroy it. Most are homogeneous in CT density, T1 and T2 signal intensity, and contrast enhancement. Intratumoral hemorrhage is not a rarity.

Lymphoma

Non-Hodgkin lymphoma occurs in the paranasal sinuses and may have variable signal intensity as well. It is characterized by homogeneous signal intensity without necrosis and is associated with cervical lymphadenopathy. Nasal lymphoma often presents with nasal obstruction (80%), nasal discharge (64%) and epistaxis (60%). Septal perforations occur. Most (75%) are of T-cell lineage as opposed to nasopharyngeal carcinoma, which is more commonly of B-cell clonality (69%). Five-year survival rates for T-cell nasal lymphomas are less than 40%. Advanced age and bulky disease are associated with reduced survival. T-cell lymphomas occur mostly in the nasal cavity and ethmoid sinus. Of the B-cell lymphomas of the sinonasal cavity (25%) most arise in the maxillary sinus. Five-year survival rates of B cells lymphomas are better than T cell lymphomas.

Nasal natural killer cell lymphomas in posttransplant patients have recently been reported. This appears in the overall spectrum of posttransplant lymphoproliferative diseases (PTLD) but is one of the more aggressive varieties. Nasal T-cell/natural killer cell lymphoma presents with obliteration of the nasal passages and maxillary sinuses, erosion of the maxillary alveolus or hard palate, and/or invasion of the orbits and nasopharynx in over half the cases. Necrosis and erosion of the nasal septum is typical of this entity. It's a killer.

Neuroendocrine Tumors

Neuroendocrine tumors of the sinonasal cavity can be divided into those referred to as typical carcinoid (well differentiated), atypical carcinoid (moderately differentiated), and small cell neuroendocrine (poorly differentiated) carcinomas. Small cell varieties are most common. Paranasal sinus neuroendocrine carcinomas expand and destroy sinus walls. They show intermediate T2WI signal intensity and enhance.

Metastases

Metastatic disease to the paranasal sinuses is extremely rare. Of the primary causes of metastases to the sinuses, renal cell carcinoma is the most common. This is a very vascular tumor that also has a propensity for hemorrhage. Depending on the stage of hemorrhage, the renal cell carcinoma metastasis may have variable density and signal intensity. A quick aside about renal cell carcinoma: it is the most common tumor to metastasize to the nasal cavity, larynx, and skin. After lung and breast carcinoma, renal cell carcinoma is the most common tumor to metastasize to the head and neck in general. Approximately 15% of patients with hypernephroma have metastases to the head and neck, and the most common site is the thyroid gland.

Myeloma may affect the walls of the paranasal sinuses as can plasmacytomas. These are lytic lesions that can have soft-tissue masses associated with them (Fig. 13-35).

One should also note that there is a high rate of sinonasal involvement by nasopharyngeal carcinoma. In a Hong Kong series of 150 cases of nasopharyngeal carcinoma, extrapharyngeal spread occurred at rates of 63% for the skull base, 56% for the parapharynx, 53% for the nasal cavity, 17% for oropharynx spread, 27% for the sphenoid sinus, 14% for the ethmoid sinus, 5% for the orbit, and 5% for the maxillary antrum. Spread to the maxillary sinus and the orbit were among the worse prognostic indicators.

LYMPH NODE DRAINAGE OF NEOPLASMS

The lymph node drainage of sinonasal neoplasms is poorly understood. The drainage of sphenoid and posterior ethmoid sinus malignancies is to retropharyngeal lymph nodes and from there to the high jugular chain. Maxillary sinus cancers drain to the submandibular

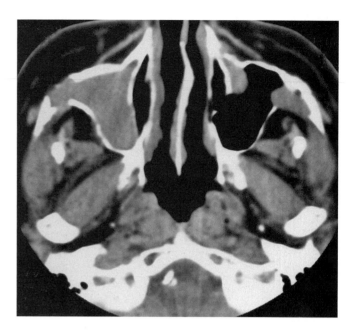

Fig. 13-35 Multiple myeloma. See the numerous punched out lytic lesions of the sinus walls in this patient with myeloma.

lymph node chains. At presentation, only 9% to 14% of sinonasal cancers have spread to the lymph nodes; this figure has justified routine radiation therapy after surgery for lesions in this area. Limited supraomohyoid neck dissections (see Chapter 14) may be performed as well.

OPERABILITY OF SINONASAL TUMORS

What makes a sinonasal tumor inoperable, and what should you be particularly cognizant of when reviewing these cases? See Boxes 13-7 and 13-8 for stage 4b disease! There are five general criteria for nonresectability: (1) distant metastases, (2) optic chiasm invasion, (3) extensive cerebral involvement, (4) bilateral carotid infiltration, and (5) very poor general health. In some university settings (uh oh!) cavernous sinus and/or chiasm invasion no longer constitute contraindications for surgery.

Quickly, sniff through your nose. Has your nasal cycle switched from 20 pages ago? (Bob is still to the right of center . . . as always!)

SUGGESTED READINGS

Anon JB, Klimek L, Mosges R, Zinreich SJ: Computer-assisted endoscopic sinus surgery. An international review, *Otolaryngol Clin North Am* 30:389-401,1997.

Babbel R, Harnsberger HR, Nelson B, et al: Optimization of techniques in screening CT of the sinuses, *AJR* 157:1093-1098, 1991.

Babbel RW, Harnsberger HR, Sonkens J, et al: Recurring patterns of inflammatory sinonasal disease demonstrated on screening sinus CT, *AJNR* 13:903-912, 1992.

Baredes S, Cho HT, Som ML: Total maxillectomy. In Blitzer A, Lawson W, Friedman WH, eds: *Surgery of the paranasal sinuses,* Philadelphia, 1985, WB Saunders.

Barkovich AJ, Vandermarch P, Edwards MSB, et al: Congenital nasal masses: CT and MR imaging features in 16 cases, *AJNR* 12:105-116, 1991.

Barnes L, Verbin RS, Gnepp DR: Diseases of the nose, paranasal sinuses and nasopharynx. In Barnes L, ed: *Surgical pathology of the head and neck,* vol 1, New York, 1985, Marcel Dekker.

Baroody FM, Hughes CA, McDowell P, et al: Eosinophilia in chronic childhood sinusitis, *Arch Otolaryngol—Head and Neck Surg* 121:1396-1402, 1995.

Batsakis JG: *Tumors of the head and neck: clinical and pathological considerations,* ed 2, Baltimore, 1979, Williams & Wilkins.

Bingham B, Shankar L, Hawke M: Pitfalls in computed tomography of the paranasal sinuses, *J Otolaryngol* 20:414-418, 1991.

Bolger WE, Butzin CA, Parsons DS. Paranasal sinus bony anatomic variations and mucosal abnormalities: CT analysis for endoscopic sinus surgery, *Laryngoscope* 1:56-64, 1991.

Buus DR, Tse DT, Farris BK: Ophthalmic complications of sinus surgery, *Ophthalmology* 97:612-619, 1990.

Clary RA, Cunningham MK, Eavey RD: Orbital complications of acute sinusitis: comparison of computed tomography scan and surgical findings, *Ann Otol Rhinol Laryngol* 101:598-600, 1992.

Conner BL, Roach ES, Laster W, et al: Magnetic resonance imaging of the paranasal sinuses: frequency and type of abnormalities, *Ann Allergy* 62:457-460, 1989.

Cooke LD, Hadley DM: MRI of the paranasal sinuses: incidental abnormalities and their relationship to symptoms, *J Laryngol Otol* 105:278-281, 1991.

Digree KB, Maxner CE, Crawford S, et al: Significance of CT and MR findings in sphenoid sinus disease, *AJNR* 10:603-606, 1989.

Dillon WP, Som PM, Fullerton GD: Hypointense MR signal in chronically inspissated sinonasal secretions, *Radiology* 174: 73-78, 1990.

Dolgin SR, Zaveri VD, Casiano RR, et al: Different options for treatment of inverting papilloma of the nose and paranasal sinuses: a report of 41 cases, *Laryngoscope* 102:231-236, 1992.

Driben JS, Bolger WE, Robles HA, et al: The reliability of computerized tomographic detection of the Onodi (Sphenoethmoid) cell, *Am J Rhinol* 12:105-111, 1998.

Drutman J, Babbel RW, Harnsberger HR, et al: Sinonasal polyposis, *Semin Ultrasound CT MR* 12:561-574, 1991.

Duvoisin B, Landry M, Chapuis L, et al: Low-dose CT and inflammatory disease of the paranasal sinuses, *Neuroradiology* 33:403-406, 1991.

El Gammal T, Brooks BS: MR cisternography: initial experience in 41 cases, *AJNR* 15:1647-1656, 1994.

El Gammal T, Sobol W, Wadlington VR, et al: Cerebrospinal fluid fistula: detection with MR cisternography, *AJNR* 19:627-631, 1998.

Evans FO, Sydnor JB, Moore WEC, et al: Sinusitis of the maxillary antrum, *N Engl J Med* 290:135-140, 1974.

Friedman RA, Harris JP: Sinusitis, *Annu Rev Med* 42:471-489, 1991.

Fuji K, Chambers SM, Rhoton AL Jr: Neurovascular relationships of the sphenoid sinus, *J Neurosurg* 50:31-39, 1979.

Furuta Y, Shinohara T, Sano K: Molecular pathologic study of human papillomavirus infection in inverted papilloma and squamous cell carcinoma of the nasal cavities and paranasal sinuses, *Laryngoscope* 101:79-85, 1991.

Graamans K, Slootweg PJ: Orbital exenteration in surgery of malignant neoplasms of the paranasal sinuses: the value of preoperative computed tomography, *Arch Otolaryngol Head Neck Surg* 115:977-980, 1989.

Harnsberger HR, Babbel RW, Davis WL: The major obstructive inflammatory patterns of the sinonasal region seen on screening sinus computed tomography, *Semin Ultrasound CT MR* 12:541-560, 1991.

Havas TE, Motbey JA, Gullane PJ: Prevalence of incidental abnormalities on computed tomographic scans of the paranasal sinuses, *Arch Otolaryngol Head Neck Surg* 114:856-859, 1988.

Hong SC, Leopold DA, Oliverio PJ, et al: Relation between CT scan findings and human sense of smell, *Otolaryngol—Head and Neck Surg* 118:183-186, 1998.

Hudgins PA, Browning DG, Gallups J, et al: Endoscopic paranasal sinus surgery: radiographic evaluation of severe complications, *AJNR* 13:1161-1167, 1992.

Hyams DJ: Papillomas of the nasal cavity and paranasal sinuses, *Ann Otol Rhinol Laryngol* 80:192-206, 1971.

Katsantonis GP, Friedman WH, Sivore MC: The role of computed tomography in revision sinus surgery, *Laryngoscope* 100:811-816, 1990.

Kennedy DW, Zinreich SJ, Kumar AJ, et al: Physiologic mucosal changes within the nose and ethmoid sinus: imaging of the nasal cycle by MRI, *Laryngoscope* 98:928-933, 1988.

Kennedy DW, Zinreich SJ, Rosenbaum AE, et al: Functional endoscopic sinus surgery: theory and diagnostic evaluation, *Arch Otolaryngol* 111:576-582, 1985.

Kennedy DW, Zinreich SJ: Functional endoscopic approach to inflammatory sinus disease: current perspectives and technique modifications, *Am J Rhinol* 2:89-96, 1988.

King AD, Lam WW, Leung SF, et al: MRI of local disease in nasopharyngeal carcinoma: tumour extent vs tumour stage, *Br J Radiol* 72:734-741, 1999.

Kuhn JP: Imaging of the paranasal sinuses: current status, *J Allergy Clin Immunol* 77:6-9, 1986.

Lanzieri CF, Shah M, Krauss D, et al: Use of gadolinium-enhanced MR imaging for differentiating mucoceles from neoplasms in the paranasal sinuses, *Radiology* 178:425-428, 1991.

Lawson W, Le Benger J, Som P, et al: Inverted papilloma: an analysis of 87 cases, *Laryngoscope* 99:1117-1124, 1989.

Lenglinger FX, Krennmair G, Muller-Schelken H, Artmann W: Radiodense concretions in maxillary sinus aspergillosis: pathogenesis and the role of CT densitometry, *Eur Radiol* 6:375-379, 1996.

Leopold D, Zinreich SJ, Simon BA, et al: Xenon-enhanced computed tomography quantifies normal maxillary sinus ventilation. *Otolaryngol—Head and Neck Surg* 122:422-424, 2000.

Li C, Yousem DM, Hayden RE, et al: Olfactory neuroblastoma: MR evaluation, *AJNR* 14:1167-1172, 1993.

Lloyd GA, Barker PB: Subtraction magnetic resonance for tumors of the skull base and sinuses: a new imaging technique, *J Laryngol Otol* 105:628-631, 1991.

Lloyd GA, Lund VJ, Phelps PD, et al: MRI in the evaluation of nose and paranasal sinus diseases, *Br J Radiol* 60:957-968, 1987.

Lloyd GA: CT of the paranasal sinuses: study of a control series in relation to endoscopic sinus surgery, *J Laryngol Otol* 104:477-481, 1990.

Loevner LA, Yousem DM, Lanza DC, et al: MR evaluation of frontal sinus osteoplastic flaps with autogenous fat grafts. *AJNR* 16:1721-1726, 1995.

Lund VJ, Harrison DF: Craniofacial resection for tumors of the nasal cavity and paranasal sinuses, *Am J Surg* 156:187-190, 1988.

Lyons BM, Donald PJ: Radical surgery for nasal cavity and paranasal sinus tumors, *Otolaryngol Clin North Am* 24:1499-1521, 1991.

Malen I, Lindahl L, Andeasson L, et al: Chronic maxillary sinusitis: definition, diagnosis, and relations to dental infections and nasal polyposis, *Acta Otolaryngol* 101:320-327, 1986.

Mantoni M, Larsen P, Hansen H, et al: Coronal CT of the paranasal sinuses before and after functional endoscopic sinus surgery, *Eur Radiol* 6:920-924, 1996.

Moseley IF: The plain radiograph in ophthalmology: a wasteful and potentially dangerous anachronism, *J R Soc Med* 84:76-80, 1991.

Moser FG, Panush D, Rubin JS, et al: Incidental paranasal sinus abnormalities on MRI of the brain, *Clin Radiol* 43:252-254, 1991.

Mosesson RE, Som PM: The radiographic evaluation of sinonasal tumors: an overview, *Otolaryngol Clin North Am* 28:1097-1115, 1995.

Mukherji SK, Figueroa RE, Ginsberg LE, et al: Allergic fungal sinusitis: CT findings, *Radiology* 207:417-422, 1998.

Myers EN, Fernau JL, Johnson JT, et al: Management of inverted papilloma, *Laryngoscope* 100:481-490, 1990.

Paller AS, Pensler JM, Tomita T: Nasal midline masses in infants and children: dermoids, encephaloceles, and gliomas, *Arch Dermatol* 127:362-366, 1991.

Rak KM, Newell JD 2d, Yakes WF, et al: Paranasal sinuses on MR images of the brain: significance of mucosal thickening, *AJR* 156:381-384, 1991.

Razek AA, Elasfour AA: MR appearance of rhinoscleroma, *AJNR* 20:575-578, 1999.

Shapiro MD, Som PM: MRI of the paranasal sinuses and nasal cavity, *Radiol Clin North Am* 27:447-475, 1989.

Sisson GA Sr, Toriumi DM, Atiyah RA: Paranasal sinus malignancy; a comprehensive update, *Laryngoscope* 99:143-150, 1989.

Som PM, Dillon WP, Curtin HD, et al: Hypointense paranasal sinus foci: differential diagnosis with MR imaging and relation to CT findings, *Radiology* 176:777-781, 1990.

Som PM, Dillon WP, Fullerton GD, et al: Chronically obstructed sinonasal secretions: observations on T1 and T2 shortening, *Radiology* 172:515-520, 1989.

Som PM, Dillon WP, Sze G, et al: Benign and malignant sinonasal lesions with intracranial extension: differentiation with MR imaging, *Radiology* 172:763-766, 1989.

Som PM, Lawson W, Lidov MW: Simulated aggressive skull base erosion in response to benign sinonasal disease, *Radiology* 180:755-759, 1991.

Som PM, Lidov M: The significance of sinonasal radiodensities: ossification, calcification, or residual bone? *AJNR* 15:917-22, 1994.

Som PM, Shapiro MD, Biller HF, et al: Sinonasal tumors and inflammatory tissues: differentiation with MR imaging, *Radiology* 167:803-808, 1988.

Stammberger H, Posawetz W: Functional endoscopic sinus surgery: concept, indications and results of the Messerklinger technique, *Eur Arch Otorhinolaryngol* 247:63-76, 1990.

Terk MR, Underwood DJ, Zee CS, et al: MR imaging in rhinocerebral and intracranial mucormycosis with CT and pathologic correlation, *Magn Reson Imaging* 10:81-87, 1992.

Van Tassel P, Lee Y-Y, Jing B-S, et al: Mucoceles of the paranasal sinuses: MR imaging with CT correlation, *AJR* 153:407-412, 1989.

Van Tassel P, Lee YY: Gd-DTPA enhanced MR for detecting intracranial extension of sinonasal malignancies, *J Comput Assist Tomogr* 15:387-392, 1991.

Yoon JH, Na DG, Byun HS, et al: Calcification in chronic maxillary sinusitis: comparison of CT findings with histopathologic results, *AJNR* 20:571-574, 1999.

Yousem DM, Fellows DW, Kennedy DW, et al: Inverted papilloma: MR evaluation, *Radiology* 185:501-506, 1992.

Yousem DM, Kennedy DW, Rosenberg S: Ostiomeatal complex risk factors for sinusitis: CT evaluation, *J Otorhinolaryngol* 20:419-424, 1991.

Yousem, DM, Galetta SL, Gusnard DA, et al: MR findings in rhinocerebral mucormycosis, *J Comput Assist Tomogr* 13:878-882, 1989.

Yousem DM, Li C, Montone KT, et al: Primary malignant melanoma of the sinonasal cavity: MR imaging evaluation, *Radiographics* 16:1101-1110, 1996.

Zinreich J: Imaging of inflammatory sinus disease, *Otolaryngol Clin North Am* 26:535-547, 1993.

Zinreich SJ, Kennedy DW, Kumar AJ, et al: MR imaging of normal nasal cycle: comparison with sinus pathology, *J Comput Assist Tomogr* 12:1014-1019, 1988.

Zinreich SJ, Kennedy DW, Malat J, et al: Fungal sinusitis: diagnosis with CT and MR imaging, *Radiology* 169:439-444, 1988.

Zinreich SJ, Kennedy DW, Rosenbaum AE, et al: Paranasal sinuses: CT imaging requirements for endoscopic surgery, *Radiology* 163:769-775, 1987.

Zinreich SJ: Functional anatomy and computed tomography imaging of the paranasal sinuses, *Am J Med Sci* 316:2-12, 1998.

Zinreich SJ: Imaging of chronic sinusitis in adults: X-ray, computed tomography, and magnetic resonance imaging, *J Allergy Clin Immunol* 90:445-451, 1992.

Zinreich SJ: Imaging of the nasal cavity and paranasal sinuses, *Current Opinion in Radiology* 4:112-116, 1992.

Zinreich SJ: Paranasal sinus imaging, *Otolaryngol—Head & Neck Surg* 103:863-868; discussion 868-869, 1990.

Mucosal Disease of the Head and Neck

The approach to this chapter on mucosal disease is divided along anatomic lines starting from top (nasopharynx) to bottom (subglottic larynx).

When you are dealing with diseases of the mucosa, the pathology is rather monotonous. If you predict squamous cell carcinoma for the histologic findings of any mucosal lesion in the head and neck, you'll probably be correct in nearly 90% of cases. (You should only have such good odds on your next internet stock pick.) Also, because the routine inflammatory lesions of the upper aerodigestive system are easily diagnosed clinically with a tongue depressor or otoscope without the need for imaging studies, more than 80% of the radiology studies of the head and neck for mucosal disease consist of staging scans of biopsy-confirmed squamous cell carcinoma. Although it may seem that this makes the role of the head and neck imager rather dull (matching his intellect) as you will see, the anatomic considerations of cancer's spread will keep your interest—we hope.

An old adage allows that adding alliteration to already authoritative authors augments educational allure. Can you find 10 examples in this chapter?

NASOPHARYNX

Anatomy

The nasopharynx is broadly defined as that area of the mucosal surface that encompasses the superior, lateral, and posterior walls of the aerodigestive tract, above the soft and hard palate. Below the nasopharynx lies the oral cavity anteriorly and the oropharynx posteriorly. The nasopharynx is lined by stratified squamous and ciliated columnar epithelium and includes the mucosa overlying the eustachian tube orifice, the cartilaginous portion of the eustachian tube (torus tubarius), and the posterolateral pharyngeal recesses known as the fossa of Rosenmüller (Fig. 14-1). The mucosa of the nasopharynx is

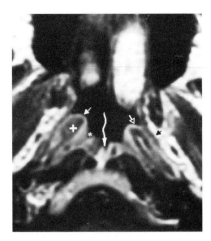

Fig. 14-1 Normal nasopharyngeal anatomy. The torus tubarius *(white arrow)*, eustachian tube orifice *(open white arrow)*, and fossa of Rosenmüller (*) are labelled. The tensor veli palatini *(black arrow)*, and levator veli palatini (+) are seen. A midline pit *(squiggly arrow)* may be due to early Tornwaldt cyst formation.

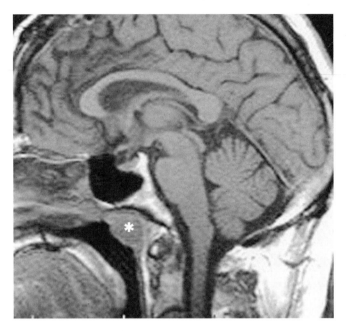

Fig. 14-2 Adenoidal hypertrophy. The width of the nasopharyngeal adenoid tissue *(asterisk)* is enlarged in HIV patients and is one of the findings to check for on sagittal T1WI of the brain. Diminished marrow signal intensity, posterior triangle nodes, and parotid cysts may be other signs of early HIV.

separated from the deep retropharyngeal space by the pharyngobasilar fascia. The pharyngobasilar fascia forms a rather stiff barrier to the spread of mucosal diseases but it has openings within it through the sinus of Morgagni to emit the eustachian tubes (on a good day) or nasopharyngeal carcinoma (on a bad day). The buccopharyngeal fascia is deep to the pharyngobasilar fascia and serves as another of the fascial barriers from nasopharynx to retro- and parapharyngeal spaces.

On either side of the eustachian tube orifice lie, anterolaterally, the tensor veli palatini (innervated by cranial nerve V-3) and posteromedially the levator veli palatini muscle (innervated by cranial nerve IX), deep to the mucosa (see Fig. 14-1). These muscles elevate and tense the soft palate into which they insert, preventing nasal regurgitation during swallowing (an embarrassing occurrence). Between these muscles is a slip of fat (typically obliterated in early nasopharyngeal carcinomas) and posterolateral to these muscles lies the fat-filled parapharyngeal space. Fixate on fat—a fine friend for finding faryngeal foulness.

The nasopharynx also houses the adenoidal lymphoid tissue. The amount of adenoidal tissue present depends on the age of the patient, because it atrophies by the fourth decade of life. Nonetheless, in a young adult the normal adenoidal tissue may simulate a lymphoma or an exophytic squamous cell carcinoma. In normal controls (age range 24 to 55 years, mean 34.5 years), the maximal dimension of the nasopharyngeal lymphoid tissue on sagittal MR scans is only 3.36 mm (SD 2.48). In HIV age matched subjects, the mean adenoidal width is 6.76 mm (SD 5.82) (Fig. 14-2). Be hesitant to call a malignancy in the high nasopharyngeal vault where the adenoids live until you see deep invasion, infiltration of the parapharyngeal fat, or obscuration of the planes between the

tensor and levator veli palatini muscles. Adenoidal tissue is usually slightly hyperintense on T1-weighted images (T1WI) and hyperintense on T2-weighted images (T2WI) and enhances. These characteristics would be unusual for a squamous cell carcinoma but could occur in a lymphoma. The adenoids, the palatine (also known as faucial) tonsils, and the lingual tonsils make up *Waldeyer's ring* of lymphoid tissue (Fig. 14-3). All of these may show lymphoid hyperplasia in cases of HIV infection and mononucleosis or because of exposure to chronic irritants (cigarette smoke, alcohol, chewing tobacco, and mothers-in-law).

Minor salivary gland tissue is present throughout the aerodigestive system and is relatively abundant in the nasopharynx, oropharynx, and oral cavity. The hard and soft palate has the highest concentration of minor salivary glands (and consequently the highest rates of minor salivary gland neoplasms).

Congenital Lesions

The most common congenital lesion of the nasopharynx is the Tornwaldt's cyst (Fig. 14-4). This results from apposition of the mucosal surfaces of the nasopharynx in the midline as the notochord ascends through the clivus to create the neural plate. A Tornwaldt's cyst usually is hypodense on computed tomography (CT). The intensity on MR varies with the protein content but is usually bright on T1WI and T2WI. The cyst is usually well defined and characteristically occurs in the midline,

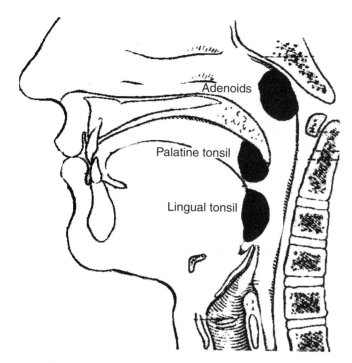

Fig. 14-3   Waldeyer's ring. While the adenoids and lingual tonsils are basically midline structures, the palative tonsils are found bilaterally framed by the pharyngeal faucial arches. These arches are created by the palatoglossus (anteriorly) and palatopharyngeus (posteriorly) muscles.

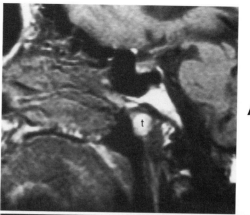

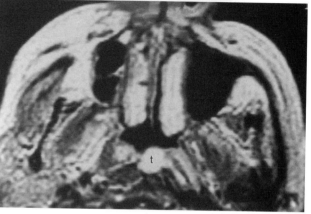

Fig. 14-4   Tornwaldt's cyst. **A,** Sagittal T1WI demonstrates a hyperintense mass *(t)* high in the nasopharynx. **B,** On T2WI the mass is seen to be just para-midline *(t)* and most likely represents Tornwaldt's cyst. High signal intensity is due to elevated protein content within the cyst.

although it may be seen off midline in a small percentage of cases. The cysts become infected on rare occasions and may be a source of persistent halitosis. (This halitosis, caused by microbsis anaerobsis, is ferosis.)

Transsphenoidal encephaloceles may present as a nasopharyngeal mass. Usually the endoscopist is able to identify dura, dural blood vessels, or pulsating brain tissue. This entity is seen most commonly in Southeast Asians (see Fig. 9-19). Encephaloceles often include unexpected items of intracranial origin (did you catch this one?). Teratomas tend to transgress transsphenoidally too and transmit totitensity tissue.

The craniopharyngeal canal is the route by which the anterior pituitary gland ascends from the pharynx to the pituitary fossa. Nasopharyngeal craniopharyngiomas are very uncommon but represent neoplasms related to the craniopharyngeal duct that ascends from the pharynx to the suprasellar region. They are mentioned here in the congenital section for confusion purposes and also in Chapter 11 sella and central skull base for redundancy sake.

Inflammatory Lesions (Box 14-1)

The nasopharynx may be a site of spread of malignant otitis externa (MOE), a *Pseudomonas aeruginosa* infection that extends widely from the external auditory canal (EAC). The infection usually passes from the fis-

sures of Santorini at the cartilaginous EAC, along the skull base, and into the soft tissues of the parapharyngeal space. Otitis externa often causes reaction in adjacent osseous organs. It may also spread to the nasopharynx via the eustachian tube (Fig. 14-5). Patients with MOE are characteristically elderly with poorly controlled diabetes. Fortunately, the demographics of the lesion, together with the finding of *Pseudomonas* on bacterial cul-

---

Box 14-1   Inflammatory Lesions of the Nasopharynx

1. Adenoidal hypertrophy (HIV)
2. Infected Tornwaldt's cyst
3. Infectious mononucleosis
4. MOE
5. Mucous retention cyst
6. Pharyngitis
7. Retropharyngeal abscess/adenitis
8. Tonsillitis affecting adenoids

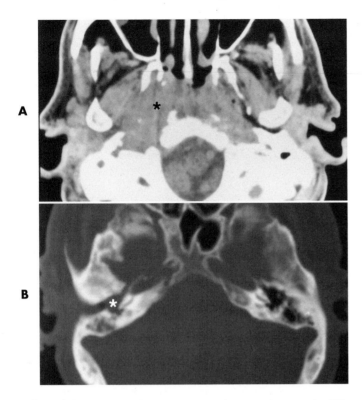

Fig. 14-5   MOE with extension to the nasopharynx. **A,** CT through the nasopharynx demonstrates a soft-tissue mass affecting the right side of the nasopharynx *(asterisk)* with obliteration of the parapharyngeal fat planes on the right side. **B,** Bone-targeted CT demonstrates involvement in the right ear *(asterisk)*.

ture, directs the clinician to the correct diagnosis. This generally presents as a submucosal mass. Stranding or obliteration of the adjacent fat, erosion of the ear canal, and opacification of the EAC, middle ear, and/or mastoid air cells may suggest this diagnosis. Unfortunately, tumors that block the eustachian tube also cause a serous otitis media and mastoiditis, and the distinction between nasopharyngeal cancer, carcinoma of the EAC, and MOE may enter a differential diagnosis (Table 14-1). When the EAC involvement with MOE is minimal, but the parapharyngeal component is large, you may confuse a nasopharyngeal process for MOE and vice versa. Tell the clinicians to take what you say with a grain of salt if the history is classic for MOE. Osteomyelitis of the skull base, seen as hyperostosis or lysis on CT, may coexist with MOE. Curly and Larry may also coexist with MOE. Treatment of MOE is with aggressive antibiotics and a punch in the stomach nyuk, nyuk.

Submucosal cysts that occur in the nasopharynx as sequela of previous infections are most often seen around the fossa of Rosenmüller. These cysts usually have low signal intensity on T1WI and high signal intensity on T2WI. Occasionally, one identifies a true abscess in the nasopharynx, although this is uncommon. Retropharyngeal extension of such an infection is a complication to be excluded on imaging studies. Pharyngitis and retropharyngitis can lead to Grisel syndrome; torticollis with rotatory subluxation of C1 on C2 secondary to an adjacent inflammatory mass. More often, one sees retropharyngeal lymphadenitis due to pharyngitis, tonsillitis.

As mentioned previously, lymphoid hyperplasia as a response to inflammation in adjacent regions, may affect the adenoidal tissue. When this is seen, check for pharyngitis or tonsillitis in children, mononucleosis in hormonally active teenagers, HIV infection in adults, and cigarette butts in the ashtrays of your waiting room in "risky" adults.

As one will read shortly, calcifications in the lymphoid tissue of Waldeyer's ring, including the adenoids, are not uncommon. They simply symbolize sequelae of successful sanatory of such sickness.

Benign Neoplasms

The classic benign nasopharyngeal tumor is the juvenile nasopharyngeal angiofibroma (JNA) (also see Chapter 11). This is a tumor that is characterized by its high vascularity and its propensity for bleeding. The typical

Table 14-1   Distinction between MOE from malignancies of nasopharynx or ear

Feature	MOE	Ear malignancy	Nasopharynx malignancy
Nasopharyngeal mass	Common	Rare	Yes
Submucosal spread	Yes	Rare	Yes
Skull base involvement	Yes	Yes	Yes
Patient demographics	Elderly diabetic patient/ immunosuppressed	Elderly sun-worshipper/golfer	Young Asian or elderly patient with positive Epstein-Barr virus antibodies
Opacification of middle ear	Yes	Possible	Yes
Opacification of EAC	Yes	Yes	Rare
Cranial nerves involved	Yes	Yes	Yes
Response to antibiotics	Yes	No	No

Box 14-2   Staging of JNA

IA   Tumor limited to posterior nares or nasopharyngeal vault
IB   Extension into one or more paranasal sinuses
IIA Minimal lateral extension through sphenopalatine foramen into medial pterygomaxillary fossa
IIB Full occupation of pterygomaxillary fossa, displacing posterior wall of antrum forward; superior extension eroding orbital bones
IIC Extension through pterygomaxillary fossa into cheek and temporal fossa
III Intracranial extension

patient is a male adolescent who has recurrent epistaxis, unassociated with nose-picking. This lesion is incredibly uncommon in females so don't bet the Y-chromosome on this diagnosis if he is a she. The lesion has been said to arise from the nasopharynx, the sphenopalatine foramen (a medial egress from the pterygopalatine fossa), the pterygopalatine fossa itself, the vidian canal, and/or the nasal cavity. The tumor, although benign, often has aggressive growth with spread via the pterygopalatine fossa into the infratemporal fossa and the intracranial compartment. A grading system for the juvenile angiofibroma has been derived that forces the "A" student to learn some of the skull base foramina (Box 14-2). Remember that the sphenopalatine foramen leads to the nasal cavity, the vidian canal to the foramen lacerum, carotid canal, and skull base and the pterygomaxillary fissure to the infratemporal fossa. Extension into adjacent structures is exceedingly common (Table 14-2).

On CT the tumor is isodense to muscle before contrast administration but demonstrates marked enhancement. By the time it is diagnosed the tumor usually spans the nasal cavity, the nasopharynx, and the pterygopalatine fossa with bowing of the posterior wall of the maxillary antrum anteriorly and widening of the pterygomaxillary fissure. JNA used to be a classic plain film (base view) diagnosis and occasionally may still be seen on residents' boards. Be careful if you have an old geezer for an examiner.

Table 14-2   Spread of juvenile angiofibromas

Site of spread	%
Pterygopalatine fossa	89
Infratemporal fossa	85
Sphenoid sinus	61
Maxillary sinus	43
Intracranial	20

On MR the salient feature of the angiofibroma is the abundance of flow voids from its high vascularity. The tumor has a characteristic "salt (tissue) and pepper (flow voids)" appearance, which is also described with glomus tumors (Fig. 14-6). The salt and pepper may be "served" both on T2WI and contrast-enhanced T1WI. (Radiologists seem to like those salt-and-pepper analogies.) When the tumor is small this finding may be absent. The extent of the tumor should be mapped relatively easily on postcontrast fat-suppressed MR. One should pay particular attention to the skull base foramina and the numerous exits from the pterygopalatine fossa (Fig. 14-7).

On angiography these tumors are highly vascular, and are usually supplied by branches of the ascending pharyngeal artery and the internal maxillary artery. Often bilateral supply as a result of rich pharyngeal anastomoses is present. Recruitment from internal carotid artery tributaries including petrous and cavernous carotid branches may occur, with extension of the tumor through the base of the skull. Embolization of the tumor may be useful preoperatively to reduce blood loss.

Recurrence rates are as high as 60% because the tumor tends to infiltrate the pterygoid bone, base of skull, and sphenoid bone. It can reactivate from there. Tumor recurrences can be treated with primary radiation therapy.

Other than an occasional benign minor salivary gland tumor, such as the pleomorphic adenoma (Fig. 14-8), often benign neoplasms of the nasopharynx are not seen.

Posttransplant lymphoproliferative disease (PTLD) can affect the adenoids and tonsils and is usually seen after solid organ transplantations (lung is most common). The onset of this process may range from months to years after the transplant. The aggressiveness of the entity also ranges widely from benign lymphoid hypertrophy to myeloma, to monoclonal lymphomas, to polyclonal lymphomas. The same virus that brought you mono, brings you PTLD—EBV leading to B cell proliferation at your service. Surprisingly, PTLD can present as a necrotic mass in the nasopharynx (Fig. 14-9).

Malignant Neoplasms

TNM staging   The TNM staging system is used to classify head and neck cancers. T refers to primary Tumor extent, N to regional lymph Nodes, and M for distant Metastases. On the basis of the TNM stage of a tumor, treatment regimens are planned, prognoses are predicted, and treatment efficacy is assessed. The TNM staging of squamous cell carcinoma is used throughout the aerodigestive system.

Nasopharyngeal Carcinoma   For the purposes of TNM staging the nasopharynx used to be divided into four "subsites": (1) posterior wall, (2) superior wall, (3) lateral wall (fossa of Rosenmüller), and (4) anterior inferior wall (including the superior soft palate). How-

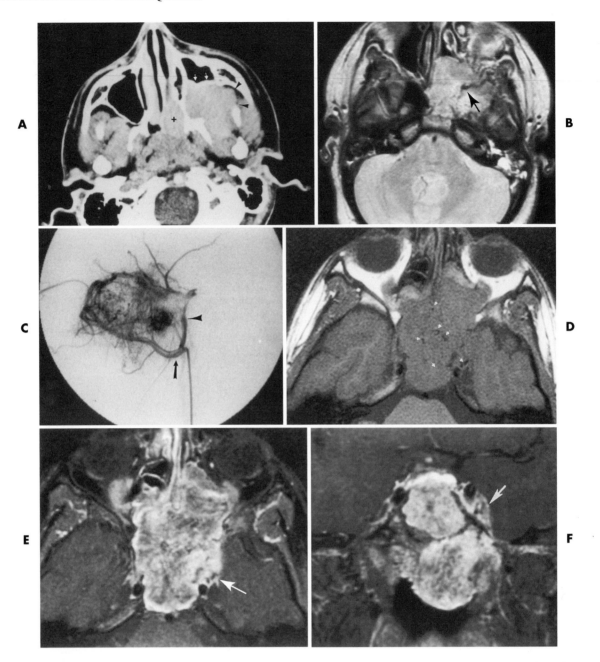

Fig. 14-6   Juvenile angiofibroma. **A,** Note the mass displacing the maxillary sinus' posterior wall *(arrows)* anteriorly and growing into the nasal cavity (+) and infratemporal fossa *(arrowheads).* **B,** A large vessel *(arrow)* coursing through the tumor is seen on PDWI. Middle ear and mastoid fluid is present, probably secondary to eustachian tube obstruction. **C,** Extensive blood supply from internal maxillary *(arrow)* and enlarged middle meningeal *(arrowhead)* branches are seen on this selective subtraction arteriogram. **D,** Precontrast T1WI shows a mass that has a few tiny flow voids *(arrows)* within it. The mass has invaded the left orbit, sphenoid sinus and ethmoid sinus, and the left cavernous sinus also is suspect. **E,** The enhancing tumor clearly invades the left cavernous sinus to Meckel's cave *(arrow)* **(F).** The coronal scan **(F)** shows the polypoid nasopharyngeal component and skull base invasion. Given the cavernous sinus invasion, call it Grade III JNA.

ever the latest American Joint Commission on Cancer staging guide has eliminated the subsite designations and now considers T1 nasopharyngeal cancer to be confined to the nasopharynx. Tumor spread to the soft tissues of the oropharynx or nasal fossa is graded T2. For T2b or not 2b, the parapharyngeal fat is the question. If there is no parapharyngeal spread into that lovely little fat we mentioned previously, call it T2a; if the fat is infiltrated it would be T2b. T3 designates invasion into bony structures and/or paranasal sinuses whereas intracranial, infratemporal fossa, hypopharyngeal, orbital, or cranial nerve involvement merits a T4 lesion. The World Heath

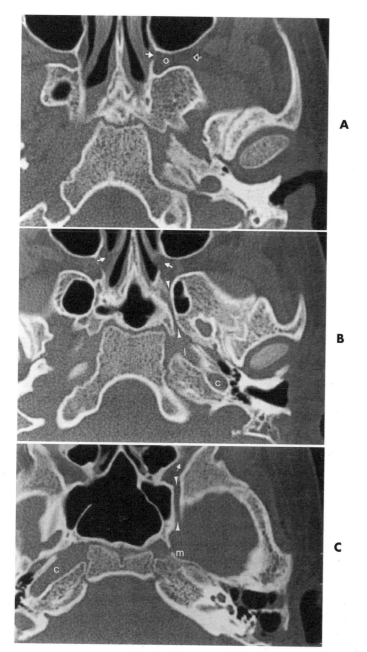

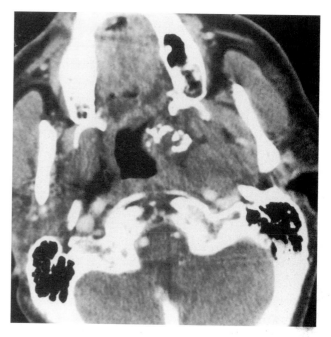

Fig. 14-8 Unusual appearance in an unusual location of a common lesion. This is a calcified pleomorphic adenoma of the nasopharynx. Although one might consider a chondroid lesion of the Eustachian tube or a calcified node, the location is not ideal for those lesions. If you place this lesion in the parapharyngeal space (see Chapter 15), a minor salivary gland pleomorphic adenoma becomes the best diagnosis.

Fig. 14-7 Anatomy of the pterygopalatine fossa. **A,** The openings from the pterygopalatine fossa *(o)* into the nasal cavity via the sphenopalatine foramen *(arrow)* and into the infratemporal fossa via the pterygomaxillary fissure *(open arrow)* are labeled. **B,** *Arrowheads* denote the vidian canal, another egress from the pterygopalatine fossa. Foramen lacerum (l) will become the floor of the internal carotid artery in its horizontal course. Arrows = sphenopalatine foramina. **C,** New *arrowheads* in more superior section outline the foramen rotundum while small *arrow* shows the inferior orbital fissure. These are the upper terminations of the pterygopalatine fossa. V-2 will pass thorugh rotundum to get to Meckel's cave (M). C = horizontal petrous carotid artery—lacerum would be just below.

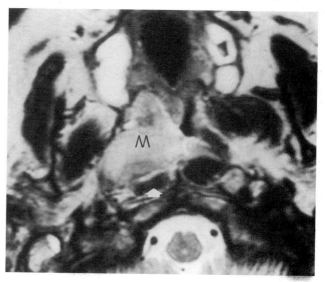

Fig. 14-9 PTLD of the nasopharynx. This mass *(M)*, which extended from the nasopharynx into the pharyngeal tissues in a patient who had undergone lung transplant, was a case of PTLD. The lesion infiltrates the retropharyngeal space and compresses the longus musculature *(arrow)*. Another common finding in transplant patients is sinusitis.

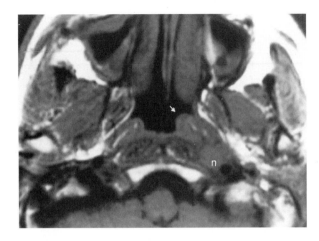

Fig. 14-10 Nasopharyngeal carcinoma with a retropharyngeal lymph node. T1WI demonstrates enlargement of the torus tubarius *(white arrow)* on the left side resulting from a nasopharyngeal carcinoma in this 20-year-old Southeast Asian man. Retropharyngeal lymph node *(n)* is identified medial to the carotid artery on the left side.

Organization (Who is WHO?) classifies nasopharyngeal carcinomas into three types; Type 1 squamous cell carcinoma, Type 2 nonkeratinizing carcinoma (with or without lymphoid stroma), and Type 3 undifferentiated carcinoma (with or without lymphoid stroma). Of these types, types 2 and 3 are the most common varieties of carcinoma and all types of nasopharyngeal carcinomas account for 80% of nasopharyngeal malignancies, followed by lymphoma, minor salivary gland tumors, and rhabdomyosarcoma. Nasopharyngeal carcinoma is notorious for demonstrating minimal mucosal disease while having a large submucosal component, which is best evaluated by cross-sectional imaging techniques. In fact, often the lesion may be completely inapparent to the endoscopist because of the frequent apposition of mucosal surfaces around the fossa of Rosenmüller, which hides the primary tumor (Fig. 14-10). In this case fat is your friend—its loss suggests bad news neoplasms. Patients may have symptoms referable to the middle ear as a result of the eustachian tube obstruction, which often occurs early in the disease. Whenever new serous otitis media occurs in an adult, think nasopharyngeal carcinoma and be sure that you scrutinize this area.

The most common site for nasopharyngeal carcinoma is the lateral pharyngeal wall around the fossa of Rosenmüller. Nasopharyngeal carcinoma is also notorious for its spread beyond the mucosal surface of the head and neck, into the parapharyngeal space (65% to 84% of cases), the retropharyngeal space (40%), the masticator space (15%), the carotid space (23%), and the perivertebral space (15%) (see Chapter 15). The sphenoid sinus (27%), nasal cavity (22%), and ethmoid sinus (18%) are also frequently invaded. Situated as it is near the base of the skull, nasopharyngeal carcinoma also is notorious for

direct and/or perineural spread through the various skull base foramina to the intracranial space (31% to 48%). To detect this superior migration of the neoplasm, coronal scanning is very helpful. Axial scans should identify nasal cavity or oropharyngeal spread that would make the lesion grade T2.

A bimodal distribution appears in the incidence of nasopharyngeal carcinoma. A younger age group (15 to 25 years old) is seen with undifferentiated nasopharyngeal carcinoma in Southeast Asia, particularly in the Chinese population where it accounts for 18% of all cancers. Chinese Americans have a seven fold increased risk of nasopharygeal carcinoma over non-Chinese counterparts. The Westerners who get nasopharyngeal carcinoma are usually older, from 40 to 60 years old, who have more squamous and nonkeratinizing carcinomas. Exposure to the Epstein-Barr virus (EBV) has been suggested to lead to an increased incidence of carcinoma of the nasopharynx, particularly in the nonkeratinizing and undifferentiated varieties. Late membrane protein (LMP) 1, LMP2, and EBNA1 proteins are coded by the EBV genome incorporated into the nasopharyngeal carcinoma cells and are now the target of systemic immunotherapies directed at this tumor. In addition, some investigators say that acquired immunodeficiency syndrome (AIDS) may predispose to nasopharyngeal carcinoma. In these instances the patient is younger than those in the second peak of nasopharyngeal carcinoma, the late-middle-aged adult. The latter patients often carry risk factors of cigarette smoking and alcohol abuse, although the association with nasopharyngeal carcinoma is less strong than elsewhere in the aerodigestive system.

On CT, nasopharyngeal cancers demonstrate density similar to that of muscle. Because of the low differentiation between muscle and the tumor, subtle nasopharyngeal carcinomas may be difficult to diagnose. Infiltration of the parapharyngeal space is the most reliable (and a very frequent) sign of nasopharyngeal carcinoma. Thus, it is critical to assess the fat around the fossa of Rosenmüller for any evidence of infiltration, particularly the loss of planes between the levator and tensor veli palatini muscles. Looking just at the mucosal surface is fraught with difficulty because of the frequent asymmetry in the aeration of the fossa of Rosenmüller. For every early nasopharyngeal carcinoma diagnosed because of tiny mucosal asymmetries, there are probably three cases in which only mucosal apposition or secretions are seen at endoscopy. This is a classic "overcall" region. For this reason one must emphasize analysis of the parapharyngeal and intermuscular fat. Have we beaten this point home enough to all you non–head-and-neck dilettantes.

Another important finding described on CT is widening of the preoccipital soft tissue in the midline by more than 1.5 to 2.0 cm. This may signify extensive submucosal disease and may necessitate taking deep biopsy specimens of the nasopharynx even in the face of normal endoscopy. Be wary of this finding, however. Without invasion of fat planes and adjacent muscles, you may be fooled into calling prolific adenoidal tissue cancer.

Invasion intracranially or along the cranial nerves is difficult to diagnose early with CT. One must identify enlargement of the nerves, enlargement of skull base foramina, or infiltration of the bone. Scans with contrast and bone windows may help identify the skull base disease on CT. By the time the skull base foramina have enlarged, however, the tumors are probably far advanced. In addition, the evaluation of the base of the skull and/or meninges is problematic with CT because of difficulties associated with beam-hardening artifact. For this reason and because of its superior soft-tissue resolution, MR is the recommended study for evaluation of nasopharyngeal carcinoma. The involvement of cranial nerve V from the pterygopalatine fossa up to the cavernous sinus and/or cranial nerve VII via the stylomastoid foramen are much better seen with unenhanced T1W scans and/or

fat suppressed enhanced T1W scans. Skull base involvement through the sinus of Morgagni along the eustachian tube or to the foramen lacerum is also well demonstrated on unenhanced T1WI.

On T1WI, the carcinoma in the nasopharynx may be isointense to the muscles. One should be able to identify readily the levator (posteromedial) and tensor (anterolateral) veli palatini muscles around the torus tubarius. Expect to see bright signal for that over-emphasized fatty strip between these muscles, in the parapharyngeal space and in the retropharyngeal space located posterior to the pharyngobasilar fascia and anterior to the longus colli-capitis muscles. Retropharygeal spread occurs in 45% of nasopharyngeal carcinomas (Fig. 14-11).

On T2WI, carcinoma of the nasopharynx is often of low to intermediate signal intensity but is always brighter than the dark signal of muscle. However, some tumors may be very bright on T2WI, making differentiation with mucosal edema very difficult. To make matters worse, the normal nasopharyngeal mucosa, the adenoidal tissue, and carcinomas all enhance. In the performance of post-contrast MR of the nasopharynx, fat saturation should be used to better evaluate the invasion of skull base foramina and fat.

Treatment of nasopharyngeal carcinoma is nonsurgical. Early stage disease (Box 14-3) is treated with radiation therapy alone with 3 year survival rates in the 90% range. More recently intensity modulated radiotherapy (IMRT) has been used to great effect in treating nasopharyngeal carcinoma. This technique employs variable intensity beams through static multileaf collimators that shape the radiation field. Tumor tissue can, in this way, get doses up to 70 to 80 gray while vital intracranial and spinal structures are spared from the harmful rays. Sequential tomography with multiple arcs and multiple fields of radiation beams may also be employed for

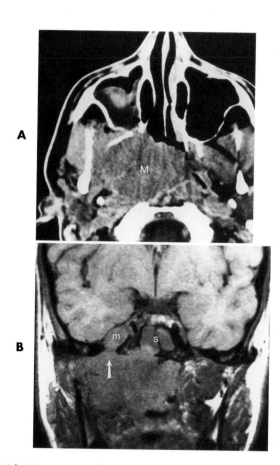

Fig. 14-11 Extensive nasopharyngeal carcinoma with intracranial invasion. **A,** Axial CT shows a large right-sided nasopharyngeal mass *(M)* measuring more than 4 cm in diameter. **B,** Coronal MR demonstrates infiltration into the sphenoid sinus *(s)* as well as extension through the foramen ovale *(arrow)* by the tumor. Meckel's cave *(m)* is enlarged and invaded, and the inferolateral aspect of the cavernous sinus appears to be bulging.

Box 14-3   Staging of Nasopharyngeal Carcinoma

Nasopharynx

T1 Tumor confined to the nasopharynx
T2 Tumor extends to soft tissues
    T2a Tumor extends to the oropharynx and/or nasal cavity without parapharyngeal extension*
    T2b Any tumor with parapharyngeal extension*
T3 Tumor involves bony structures and/or paranasal sinuses
T4 Tumor with intracranial extension and/or involvement or cranial nerves, infratemporal fossa, hypopharynx or orbit, or masticator space

From Greene FL, Page DL, Fleming ID, et al (eds): *AJCC Cancer Staging Manual;* ed 6. New York, Springer-Verlag, 2002, p 35. Used with permission.

T4 disease. These techniques, with chemotherapy, have rendered nasopharyngeal carcinoma an eminently curable disease at a local level—unfortunately for the patient, the tumor has a relatively high propensity for hematogenous spread.

Recent studies have suggested that tumor volume may be a better predictor of radiation/chemotherapy response than T staging, at least for high-grade nasopharyngeal carcinomas. (But do not forget that T-staging just yet, mon ami). The cumulative survival for T3 and T4 patients with less than 30 cc of tumor (>80%) is better than that for patients with 30 to 60 cc of tumor (45%), and for those with more than 60 cc of tumor (<10%) at 5 year follow-up. Presumably, hypoxia and radioresistance occur in large tumor volume cancers, making cure less likely.

With concomitant chemotherapy added (*cis* platinum and flourouracil) to stage II disease the survival rates get bumped up by about 5% to 10% over radiotherapy alone into the 85% to 90% range. Stage III and IV nasopharyngeal carcinomas are treated with chemotherapy and concomitant radiotherapy. Undifferentiated (Type 3) cancers seem to respond the best. However, do not expect the images of the nasopharynx to normalize. Au contraire you may expect to see residual asymmetry and mucosal apposition forever more (quoth the Baltimore Raven).

Bulky disease, small recurrences after radiotherapy, and persistent nodal disease may occasionally be managed surgically. These tumors have traditionally not been part of the bailiwick of the surgeon. However, a few centers are starting to operate primarily on patients with localized nasopharyngeal cancers. It is important to recognize that the major role of the radiologist in the evaluation of a nasopharyngeal tumor is not in predicting histology but in identifying and mapping the tumor for therapeutic planning. The cowboy role—shooting off diagnoses from the hip and possibly hitting yourself in the foot—is not a wise one to play here. Rather, evaluate the anatomy and morphology of the lesion and leave histology and the shooting to the pathologist and the NRA (Nasopharyngeal Radiotherapy Association). Be a detecter and cartographer, not a radiographer—identify and map the lesion.

First echelon nodal spread from nasopharyngeal carcinoma is to retropharyngeal and high jugular (level II) lymph nodes. Nodal spread is assumed with nasopharyngeal carcinoma since it occurs at a rate of about 80%. Disease in the nodes and the size of the nodes show less correlation with nasopharyngeal carcinoma (NPCA) than other head and neck carcinomas. Even a tiny NPCA spreads to the nodes early—that's probably why the T staging of NPCA is not based on size criteria the way oral cavity and other pharyngeal cancers are.

Lymphoma Squamous cell carcinoma does not have a monopoly on bad news in the nasopharynx. Because of the abundant lymphoid tissue associated with the adenoids of the nasopharynx, lymphoma also occurs here. It is usually in the form of non-Hodgkin lymphoma and affects young adults. Its appearance is identical to that of carcinoma except that necrosis is uncommon in lymphoma. Otherwise density and intensity characteristics overlap. Remember that B-cell lymphomas are part of the spectrum of PTLD to affect the adenoidal region and can cause a necrotic mass. Nodes are present in 80% of patients with "extranodal" lymphoma. Lymphoma in the nasopharynx has the opportunity to spread to the skull base and cranial nerve foramina.

Hodgkin disease rarely affects Waldeyer's ring and afflicts adults of younger age than non-Hodgkin lymphoma.

Minor salivary gland tumors The extensive minor salivary gland tissue in the nasopharynx accounts for neoplasms such as adenoid cystic carcinoma (the most common minor salivary gland malignancy), mucoepidermoid carcinoma, acinic cell carcinoma, adenocarcinoma, pleomorphic low grade adenocarcinoma, and undifferentiated carcinoma. Adenoid cystic carcinomas may be particularly difficult to treat because of their tendency to spread perineurally (seen in 60% of individuals). The skull base foramina are easy targets for nasopharyngeal adenoid cystic carcinomas, and from there the tumor marches up the nerves to the intracranial compartment. Atten-shun! The perineural predilection portends a poor prognosis, potentially paralyzes, and produces paresthesias.

Rhabdomyosarcoma In children the predominant tumor of the nasopharynx is rhabdomyosarcoma, an eminently treatable tumor with chemotherapy (Fig. 14-12). Intracranial extension is common with rhabdomyosarcomas, and rhinorrhea may be a presenting symptom. Rhabdomyosarcoma rapidly races retropharyngeally reaping the wrath of rancorous radiotherapists. The sur-

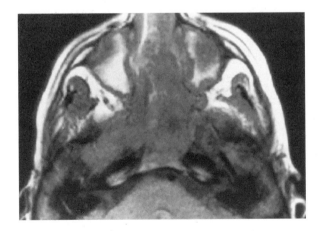

Fig. 14-12 Rhabdomyosarcoma of the nasopharynx. Axial T1WI demonstrates a large mass that obliterates the nasopharyngeal airway and grows into the nasal cavity. Infiltration into the skull base and parapharyngeal tissues is noted, as is obstruction of the paranasal sinuses.

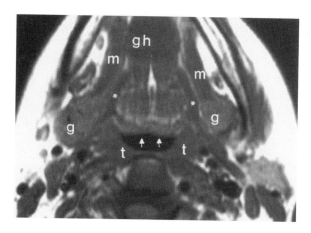

Fig. 14-13 Normal anatomy of the oropharynx. On this axial T1WI one can identify the base of the tongue with lingual tonsil tissue *(small arrows)* and the palatine tonsils *(t)*. Also identifiable on this scan are the submandibular glands *(g)*, the sublingual space extending from the submandibular glands anteriorly, and the midline fatty lingual septum with genioglossus muscles on either side. Muscles on either side of the sublingual space are the mylohyoid muscles *(m)* laterally and the hyoglossus *(asterisk)* medially. Geniohyoid muscle *(gh)* makes up the bulk of the tissue anteriorly in the tongue usually below genioglossus.

vival rate with combined chemotherapy and radiation is more than 50% at 5 years.

Plasmacytomas Plasmacytomas can occur in the nasopharynx, palatine tonsils, and base of tongue. They are usually oval in shape and have similar intensity to muscle on T1WI and are only slightly hyperintense on T2WI. They enhance notably, often with a heterogeneous center.

It is nearly impossible to distinguish among the major histologic types of tumor that involve the nasopharynx. Age is probably the best discriminator, although lymphomas and nasopharyngeal carcinomas do show some overlap. If you identify necrosis within the tumor, suggest the diagnosis of carcinoma or PTLD. Necrosis would be seen as an area of high signal intensity on T2WI amid the tumor, generally centrally, or as an area of

nonenhancement centrally. On the other hand, lymphoma frequently has a homogeneous bland appearance even when the tumor is large. Its signal intensity may be variable but usually is indistinguishable from that of nonnecrotic carcinoma. Lymphoma often grows in a more exophytic pattern, with less deep infiltration than carcinoma. Minor salivary gland tumors have a variable pattern of signal intensity on MR. Occasionally, one may identify a very bright minor salivary gland tumor on T2WI, which usually represents either adenoid cystic carcinoma or low-grade mucoepidermoid carcinoma. Perineural spread will suggest the former. Finally, of the tumors of the nasopharynx that may be hemorrhagic, rhabdomyosarcoma is the most common. Rhabdomyosarcomas are usually seen in patients less than 10 years old.

OROPHARYNX

Anatomy

The oropharynx includes the posterior third of the tongue (also known as the tongue base); the vallecula; the palatine tonsils and tonsillar fossa; the posterior and superior pharyngeal walls from the level of the soft palate down to the pharyngoepiglottic folds; the uvula; and the soft palate (Fig. 14-13). The circumvallate papillae of the tongue separate the oral tongue (a part of the oral cavity) anteriorly from the oropharynx posteriorly. The hard palate is part of the oral cavity, but the soft palate is part of the oropharynx. The floor of the mouth, the undersurface of the tongue, and the buccal mucosa are all parts of the oral cavity, not the oropharynx.

Besides the palatine tonsils, the oropharynx also contains the lingual tonsillar tissue seen at the base of the tongue. Just as in the nasopharynx, where the adenoidal tissue may mimic a lymphoma, the lingual tonsillar tissue may also simulate an exophytic lymphoma (Fig. 14-14).

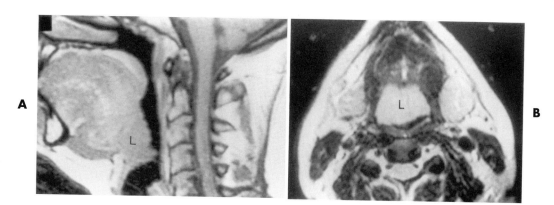

Fig. 14-14 Lingual tonsillar hypertrophy. **A,** Tech student posing as a normal subject for anatomy shows marked lingual tonsillar enlargement *(L)*. **B,** The tissue is bright on T2WI. Note small right submandibular nodes. Does this deserve a biopsy? (See Figure 14-23).

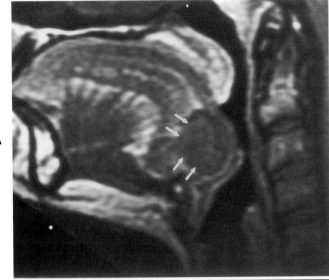

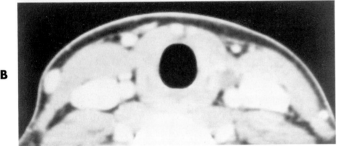

Fig. 14-15 Lingual thyroid. **A,** Sagittal T2WI shows a mass at the base of the tongue *(arrows)* that is low in signal intensity. This would be unusual for lingual tonsillar hypertrophy. **B,** The CT scan of the same patient reveals absence of normal thyroid tissue in its native position. (Remember that it is harder to identify something that should be there but isn't there than something that should not be there.) (Case courtesy of Suresh Mukherji, University of Michigan Medical Center.)

Although the oropharynx is lined by squamous epithelium, the presence of the lymphoid tissue of the tonsils and minor salivary gland tissue accounts for the diversity of tumors in this region.

Congenital Lesions

Thyroid tissue may be seen embedded in the posterior tongue because of arrested descent from the foramen cecum, which is located at the junction of the two sides of the circumvallate papillae along the anterior edge of the base of the tongue. This thyroid tissue is typically in the midline, hyperdense on CT because of its natural iodine content, and enhancing. After identifying the lingual thyroid tissue, the radiologist must next image the neck for any additional thyroid gland residua (Fig. 14-15). In 80% of cases the lingual thyroid tissue is the only functioning thyroid tissue in the body. Although treatment is excisional due to a risk of airway compro-

mise in adolescence, the surgeon may elect to leave a little length of lingering lingual thyroid in place if this is the case. Incomplete descent of the thyroid gland to its normal location in the lower part of the neck is an uncommon congenital anomaly. Thyroglossal duct cysts may also occur in the tongue base or floor of mouth. They are much more common entities than lingual thyroid glands but are usually infrahyoidal. This entity is covered in the thyroid gland section of Chapter 15.

Congenital cysts (unilocular) and lymphangiomas (usually multilocular) may occur in the tongue but usually in its oral portion. Venous vascular malformations, with or without evidence of phleboliths, frequent the tongue as well. Previously, these were called hemangiomas, but this term is now relegated to those lesions that tend to regress in adolescence or in response to steroids.

Diffuse macroglossia may be present in patients with hypothyroidism, amyloidosis, Down syndrome, glycogen storage diseases, mucopolysaccharidoses, and neurofibromatosis among other conditions (see Box 14-4). Macroglossia makes meals of meat moot—merely a miserable malnutritive manipulation.

Narrowings of the oropharynx can cause obstructive sleep apnea (OSP) and the Pickwickian syndrome (Who you calling "fat boy"?). Pickwickian syndrome refers to morbid obesity, hypoventilation, and polycythemia. ZZZZZZZZZZZZZZZ

Ooops we nodded off there for a second. The narrowing of the airway may be due to obesity, redundancy of mucosal and muscular tissue, hypertrophy of lymphoid tissue, or on a congenital basis (hence discussed herein). In general cross-sectional diameters of the oropharynx are reduced in patients with OSP at the soft palate, base of tongue, or uvula levels. The normal cross-sectional airway measurement should be about 100 mm². Patients with OSP often have values at or below a minimum width of 50 mm². Airways are smaller in diameter

---

Box 14-4 Macroglossia

Acromegaly
Amyloidosis
Beckwith-Weidemann Syndrome
Down Syndrome
Familial macroglosia
Glycogen storage diseases
Hemangioma
Hypothyroidism
Infants of diabetic mothers
Lingual thyroid tissue
Lymphoma
Mucopolysaccharidoses

during hypnotic relaxation (sleep simulation) than during the awake state in these patients and may correspond with oxygen desaturation episodes. Treatment options for OSP are varied and include behavioral modification such as weight reduction (did Sarah Ferguson use to snore?—only Prince Andrew knows), sleep hygiene, intraoral appliances that advance the mandible, positional training, and continuous positive airway pressure (CPAP) applied via a nasal mask. Uvulopalatopharyngoplasty or other surgical interventions are reserved for those who fail conservative therapy and who experience significant deoxygenation/hypoxia in their sleep.

Inflammatory Lesions

Pharyngitis and abscess Benign inflammatory disease occurs frequently in the oropharynx, mostly manifesting as tonsillitis and pharyngitis. Because this is an easily made clinical diagnosis in the proper setting, no imaging of these conditions is typically required. Nonetheless, occasionally one may find a peritonsillar abscess in a patient who does not respond to antibiotics for tonsillitis. The typical microorganisms that cause a tonsillar abscess include *Streptococcus pneumoniae, Streptococcus viridans,* and occasionally gram-negative anaerobes. Often one is dealing with multiple bugs at once (call Terminix). After recurrent tonsillitis one may see tiny tonsillar concretions (calcifications). These are of no import and do not implicate granulomatous infections. Abscesses have low-density centers and a peripheral rim of enhancement on CT. Adjacent inflammation of the fat is due to neighboring cellulitis and fasciitis. On MR, inflammatory lesions are very bright on T2WI because of the marked amount of edema and swelling associated with lesions such as abscesses.

A peritonsillar location is the most common site of abscess in children, followed by the retropharyngeal region. Remember that most of these actually represent necrotizing adenitis as opposed to direct spread into parapharyngeal spaces.

Fistula If a fistula in the tonsil is identified, consider a branchial cleft anomaly as a possible cause. Typically, the second branchial cleft fistulas drain to the tonsil and may or may not be associated with a cystic lesion in the soft tissues of the neck near the angle of the mandible. Alternatively, actinomycosis is an unusual cause of peritonsillar fistulas.

After infections it is common to see retention cysts within the palatine tonsils or calcifications . . . or tonsilloliths.

Benign Neoplasms

Pleomorphic adenoma Minor salivary gland tumors occur within the oropharynx, especially along the soft

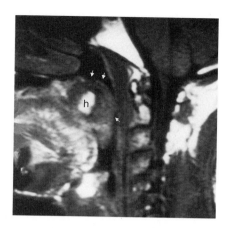

Fig. 14-16 Pleomorphic adenoma. Sagittal T1WI depicts a mass *(arrows)* in the soft palate in this patient. Bright signal centrally *(h)* represents a hematoma from a heavy-handed resident who performed a biopsy of the lesion before scanning. At least that way we got pathologic proof that this was a pleomorphic adenoma.

palate. In this location benign tumors approximate malignant minor salivary gland tumors in nearly equal abundance. The most common benign tumor of the soft palate minor salivary glands is the pleomorphic adenoma (Fig. 14-16). Pleomorphic adenomas are usually very bright on T2WI. They enhance.

Hemangioma Hemangiomas (venous vascular malformations and such) are the most frequent pediatric benign oropharyngeal lesion. These tumors are characterized by their avid enhancement. Look for phleboliths.

Schwannomas of the hypoglossal or lingual nerve present as well defined masses that are intermediate in signal intensity on T2WI and show enhancement. Seeing cysts synchronously in schwannomas seems standard stock.

Amyloidosis may affect the tongue base and tonsils as a cause of macroglossia or may affect other portions of the airway or lymph nodes (Fig. 14-17).

Malignant Neoplasms

Squamous cell carcinoma As opposed to the nasopharynx, which is classified by spread, staging of the oropharynx for squamous cell carcinoma is based largely (tee hee) on size criteria (Box 14-5) (big is bad!). With the T4 lesion, tumor invades adjacent structures such as the bone (mandible or maxilla), the soft tissues of the neck, pterygoid muscles, larynx, or the deep muscles of the tongue. The staging criteria necessitate measuring all lesions of the oropharynx to assist the surgeon in the proper therapy for a given oropharyngeal squamous cell carcinoma. Rulers rule. In addition, it is critical to assess for invasion into the mandible or maxilla or the soft tissues of the neck (Fig. 14-18). Invasion of the deep muscles and soft tissues of the neck may be equally well vi-

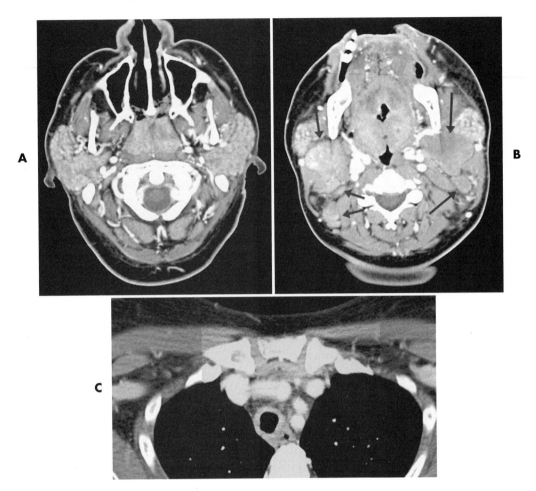

Fig. 14-17   Diffuse amyloidosis. This patient had amyloidosis that affected the nasopharynx **(A)**, tonsils **(B)**, larynx, trachea **(C)**, and the lymph nodes (seen in **B**, *arrows*) of the neck. Unusual, yes, first edition, no.

sualized with MR and CT; however, the increased soft tissue resolution on MR with T1WI, T2WI, and enhanced fat-suppressed imaging makes MR the preferable examination. On CT there is less conspicuity between tumors and muscle because both have similar densities.

Box 14-5   T-Staging of the Oropharynx

T1   Tumors 2 cm or less in greatest dimension
T2   Tumor more than 2 cm but not more than 4 cm in greatest dimension
T3   Tumor more than 4 cm in greatest dimension
T4a Tumor invades invades the larynx, deep/extrinsic muscle of tongue, medial pterygoid, hard palate, or mandible
T4b Tumor invades lateral pterygoid muscle, pterygoid plates, lateral nasopharynx, or skull base or encases carotid artery

From Greene FL, Page DL, Fleming ID, et al (eds): *AJCC Cancer Staging Manual;* ed 6. New York, Springer-Verlag, 2002, p 35. Used with permission.

Other issues that must be addressed with respect to oropharyngeal carcinomas are listed below:

Pre-epiglottic fat invasion   From the base of the tongue a tumor may extend into the vallecula, the air space anterior to the epiglottis but posterior to the tongue base. Once the vallecula is infiltrated, the critical space to be evaluated by the radiologist is the pre-epiglottic fat. When the pre-epiglottic fat space is infiltrated with tumor, it is surgically impossible to remove the fat while maintaining the integrity of the epiglottis' petiole (inferior stem). A tumor of the base of the tongue that does not involve the pre-epiglottic fat can be resected without requiring a portion of the supraglottic larynx to be included in the operative specimen. On the other hand, if the pre-epiglottic fat is invaded, the patient will often require an epiglottectomy, partial supraglottic laryngectomy or, at worse, a total laryngectomy. The combination of base of tongue surgery with laryngeal surgery often leads to a poor quality of life in which both swallowing and speaking are compromised. (Basically you can't complain about the quality of the food on an airplane for example.) The pre-epiglottic fat is best

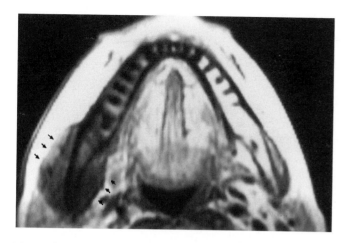

Fig. 14-18 Squamous cell carcinoma invasion into the mandible. This T1WI shows a large mass *(arrows)* that has invaded through the right mandible at the mandibular angle. Bone marrow of the right mandible has been replaced by the infiltrating tumor. Lesion arose in the right tonsil (not shown).

assessed with sagittal T1 weighted scans and axial T1 weighted scans in which soft-tissue signal intensity within the fat suggests cancerous involvement. Occasionally, adjacent inflammation or peritumoral edema or partial volume effects might simulate pre-epiglottic fat invasion. Massive pre-epiglottic fat disease also often makes radiation therapy undesirable because of the bulk of the tumor, thereby limiting curability. Pre-epiglottic invasion also predisposes one to lymph node spread so there is a worse prognosis associated with this feature.

Mandibular invasion Although periosteal invasion is nearly impossible to identify by any current imaging technique, cortical invasion is equally well seen on CT and MR with T1WI showing loss of the hypintense cortex, fat-suppressed T2WI showing high signal infiltration, and postcontrast fat suppressed T1WI showing enhancement of the cortical defect. Infiltration of the bone marrow of the mandible or the maxilla is better appreciated with MR, appearing as low signal on T1WI infiltrating the high intensity fatty marrow. Scans will identify tumor adjacent to the mandible, cortical erosions, infiltration of marrow fat, and/or tumor on both sides of the mandible. Particularly when a lesion arises on the alveolar surface of the mandible, single plane imaging may be insufficient to determine mandibular invasion. For this reason, when the issue of mandibular involvement is raised, axial and coronal images are recommended either with CT or with MR. Depending on the extent of involvement, the oral cavity/oropharyngeal cancer adjacent to the mandible is treated differently. If tumor abuts the mandible but is not fixed to the periosteum or mandible, the periosteum is resected as the margin. For tumor fixed to or superficially invading the periosteum and/or cortex, inner cortex resection (corticectomy) can

be performed for margin control. Marginal resection can be performed for superficial alveolar (oral cavity) cancers. Once the cortex has been violated or marrow has been infiltrated, a more extended mandibular resection is required for cure as primary radiation incurs the risk of osteoradionecrosis at doses high enough to sterilize the bone disease. In most cases, microvascular osteomusculocutaneous free flaps are used to replace the bone and to achieve a cosmetic result in which facial deformity is not evident.

Flaps are usually separated into several categories: Site (local, regional, or distant), tissue (cutaneous, fasciocutaneous, musculocutaneous, or osteomusculocutaneous), and blood supply (random, axial, pedicled, or free). Modern techniques of inserting osteo-integrated implants into bone grafts (often distant osteomusculocutaneous free flaps of the fibula) afford the patient an opportunity to have a dental surface capable of chewing those delicious airplane granola bars and pretzels. After radiation therapy and/or in individuals who have carious teeth, marrow changes may occur that might simulate tumoral infiltration but may actually represent radiation fibrosis, osteoradionecrosis (Fig. 14-19), osteomyelitis, or periodontal disease.

Prevertebral muscle invasion If a cancer is fixed to the prevertebral musculature (longus capitus-longus colli complex) the patient is deemed unresectable. Although the imaging findings of high signal intensity on T2 weighted scans in the muscles, contrast enhancement of the muscle, or nodular infiltration of the muscles would suggest neoplastic infiltration, in fact these findings have not been very reliable. The surgical evaluation at the time of panendoscopy or open exploration remains the gold standard, despite the fact that in rare instances a plane can be found between tumor and the prevertebral musculature. Because the prevertebral musculature is so close to the spinal canal and spinal cord, there are some issues with regard to curative radiotherapy in individuals who have infiltration in this location. At the very least the radiologist should suggest the possibility of violation of the prevertebral musculature when the aforementioned findings are present and/or there is obliteration of the retropharyngeal fat stripe by cancer. At that point the surgeon must take over and evaluate for fixation at panendoscopy (shake that tumor, baby) or at surgery (trying to create a plane in the retropharyngeal space between tumor and longus muscles). Sending surgeons searching for spurious squamous cells in this space squanders seconds and subsidizes civil suits.

Pterygopalatine fossa invasion Extension to the pterygopalatine fossa or to other avenues of the fifth cranial nerve raises the possibility of perineural spread of the cancer to the skull base. "Losing the tumor at the skull base" because of spread along the cranial nerves happens infrequently with squamous cell carcinoma

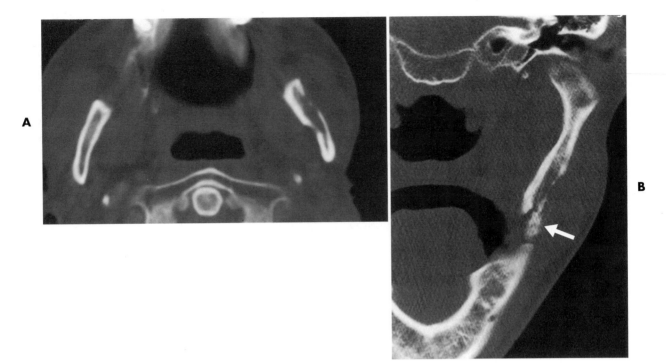

Fig. 14-19 Osteoradionecrosis. The absence of a corresponding mass despite the fracture, cortical thinning, and marrow replacement seen on the axial (**A**) and coronal (**B**) scan might suggest the diagnosis of osteoradionecrosis. Note also the dense piece of bone (sequestrum) on the coronal scan *(arrow)* that may provide a clue here.

when the radiologist cautions the surgeon about this possibility—on the other hand this is typical for adenoid cystic carcinoma where remote perineural spread is almost the norm. Once again, MR appears to have some advantages in evaluating the nerves over CT, showing abnormal enlargement and enhancement of the nerve. Foraminal enlargement and bony infiltration is a reliable finding on CT, but is pretty uncommonly seen. If one sees infiltration of the fat of the pterygopalatine fossa, atrophy of the muscles innervated by the trigeminal nerve, or abnormal enhancement in Meckel's cave on CT, perineural invasion is implied (see Chapter 11) . Perineural spread of tumor may be antegrade or retrograde and may show "skip lesions" radiographically.

Pterygomandibular raphe invasion The pterygomandibular raphe stretches from the medial pterygoid muscle's insertion on the medial pterygoid plate to the mylohyoid ridge of the mandible. It serves as the origin or insertion of the buccinator muscle and the pharyngeal constrictor muscles. The pterygomandibular raphe is one of the boundaries between the oral cavity and the oropharynx as it effectively divides the anterior tonsillar pillar and the retromolar trigone (Fig. 14-20). The retromolar trigone, a portion of the oral cavity, is the area behind the maxillary teeth but in front of the coronoid process and ascending ramus of the mandible. Tumor can spread along this plane superiorly to the temporalis muscle, medially into the pterygomandibular space

where the lingual and inferior alveolar nerves run, or inferiorly into the floor of the mouth. If tumors spread anteriorly from the medial pterygoid plate they enter the pterygopalatine fossa.

Bilateral or deep invasion of the tongue base Tongue base lesions also have characteristic problems inherent to their location. Because the neurovascular bundle, including the hypoglossal nerve, the lingual nerve, and the lingual artery, enters from the base of tongue, infiltration of these structures makes surgical excision, while preserving function, more difficult. These same neurovascular structures then course along the styloglossus-hyoglossus complex and the floor of the mouth to supply the anterior aspect of the tongue. If the base of the tongue is infiltrated bilaterally, there is a relatively limited chance that a patient will be able to have functioning tongue available after surgical removal of the tumor. The surgical guideline to abide by is that you need 25% of the base of the tongue and one hypoglossal nerve and one lingual artery to have a functioning tongue that can do more than hang out there like a dog's (Little Bow Wow).

The tongue is one of the most critical organs of the aerodigestive system, being instrumental in both swallowing and phonation. Without a tongue or a viable reconstruction, the patient is left with a permanent feeding tube and, in many cases, a tracheostomy as the airway becomes unprotected. Part of the emphasis in head and

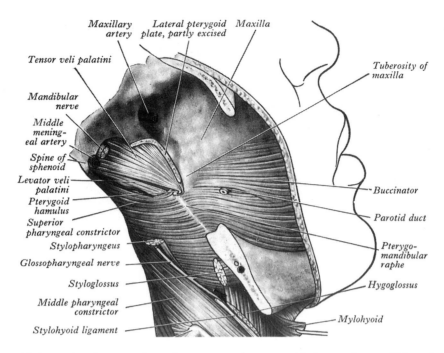

Fig. 14-20   Pterygomandibular raphe; the muscular raphe connects the pterygoid plate to the mandible and represents both a barrier to spread of tumor as well as a route of growth. (From Williams PL, Warwick R: Gray's Anatomy, ed 36, Philadelphia, Saunders, 1980, p 532. Used with permission.)

neck surgery is the creation of sophisticated flaps that can be constructed to allow swallowing (like a seal) without bolus formation. For this reason it is important for the radiologist to identify spread of tumor across the fatty lingual septum that defines the midline of the tongue. If unilateral disease only is present, tongue function will often be sufficient for near normal lifestyle. Patients who undergo hemiglossectomies can form a bolus and can speak reasonably intelligibly if not a little garbled. Nowhere else in the head and neck is bilaterality of disease more important with respect to patient quality of life. Once the base of the tongue has been resected, neurovascular grafting can not be achieved to preserve function in the anterior aspect of the tongue. If the midline of the base of the tongue has been violated to any significant degree by cancer, the possibility of having a complete resection with adequate margins while maintaining a functioning tongue is remote. If a small mobile portion of the base of the tongue is preserved, functional recovery with flap reconstruction is much improved. In some institutions total glossectomies are never performed, leaving radiotherapy and chemotherapy with or without brachytherapy implants the only options for cancer cure. With large pectoralis, rectus abdominus free flaps, or bulky microvascular flaps, one can usually get the patient swallowing again after total glossectomy so that lifelong feeding by gastrostomy tubes is not required. The risk of aspiration into the larynx is also reduced when bulky flaps are used.

Some programs follow the adage that a total glossectomy means a laryngectomy. Although this is certainly true in patients who have already had radiation, have supraglottic spread of oropharyngeal tumors, have huge disease, or are respiratorily compromised (defined as unable to walk two flights of stairs chased by an HMO regulator without getting winded), in the advanced cancer centers this need not be the case in all comers. The pectoralis or bulky free flap allows the patient to swallow with a head tilt and the supraglottis protects the airway. The patient is taught to cough after swallowing to prevent the petite pois passing by the petiole and to protect the laryngeal passageway.

The tongue undergoes predictable changes after it has been denervated (usually as a result of primary tumor resections, neck nodal surgery, anterior horn cell disease [ALS], and occasionally from primary neoplasms of the hypoglossal nerve). In the first few months one will see high signal on T2WI in the ipsilateral hemitongue and a relatively normal T1WI. After about 5 months fatty infiltration of the tongue, manifesting as high signal on T1WI (and low density on CT), and volume loss ipsilaterally may be seen. The same pattern is seen with denervated muscles of mastication.

The most common locations for a primary squamous cell carcinoma of the oropharynx are the anterior portion of the tonsil (Fig. 14-21) and the tongue base. Tonsillar carcinomas have a propensity for invasion into the tongue musculature beyond the circumvallate papillae,

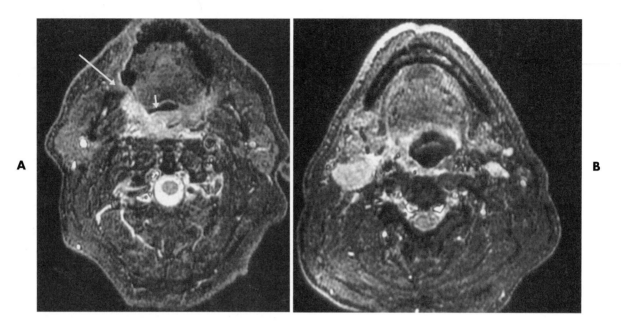

Fig. 14-21   Tonsil carcinoma. **A,** Tonsillar squamous cell carcinomas often invade anterolaterally to enter the retromolar trigone *(long arrow),* medially to enter the soft palate *(short arrow),* and anteriorly to invade the tongue base (not seen here). **B,** Nodal disease is well-depicted on fat-suppressed T2WI and is very common with carcinomas of the tonsil. In fact, bilateral adenopathy should be assumed until proven otherwise.

thereby spreading across the anatomic boundary between the oropharynx and oral cavity. Tonsillar carcinomas also may spread laterally and superiorly to invade the retromolar trigone (Fig. 14-22). Once the retromolar

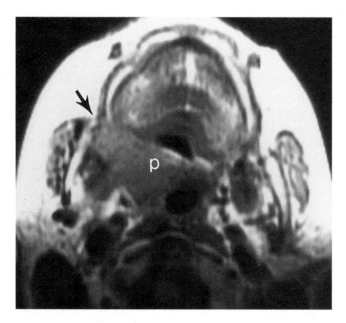

Fig. 14-22   Tonsillar carcinoma extending into the retromolar trigone. T1WI demonstrates anterolateral extension of a tonsillar carcinoma into the region posterior to the maxilla and anterior to the mandible *(arrow).* This mass also extends into the soft palate *(p).*

trigone has been invaded, tumors may ascend the pterygomandibular raphe to the medial pterygoid plate or via the pterygopalatine fossa along the fifth cranial nerve.

Nonetheless, tonsillar carcinomas are also the most common source of occult primary tumors that present as cervical adenopathy alone (the dreaded "carcinoma of unknown primary"). These microscopic cancers may be deep within the crypts of the lymphoid tissue and may be invisible to both endoscopy and imaging. Other sites for carcinomas of unknown primary that should be assiduously studied include the nasopharynx, piriform sinus, base of tongue, and chest.

The appearance of oropharyngeal squamous cell carcinoma is similar to that elsewhere in the aerodigestive system on both CT and MR. It should be noted, however, that the base of tongue drains to bilateral lymphatic systems, and therefore one must critically assess both sides of the neck for associated lymphadenopathy. Primary drainage is to upper jugular and submandibular lymph node chains. Cystic nodes are possible with a tonsillar carcinoma primary.

The prognosis for oral cavity and oropharyngeal carcinoma for all-comers is about 50% for 5 year survival. Obviously, the smaller the tumor the better the prognosis. Surgery, radiation therapy, and chemotherapy all play roles in treatment with the latter generally reserved for more advanced, widespread, or unresectable disease. Markers for a worse prognosis include expression of mutated tumor suppressor gene p53, enhancement of oncogene cyclin D1, and high levels of vascular endothelial

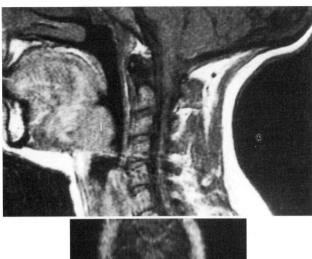

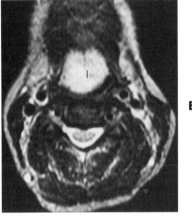

Fig. 14-23 Oropharyngeal lymphoma. **A,** Sagittal T1WI reveals a round exophytic mass in the base of the tongue *(l)* secondary to lymphoma. **B,** On T2WI the signal intensity of the lesion *(l)* is markedly hyperintense, which would be highly unusual for squamous cell carcinoma. (Compare with Figure 14-14.)

growth factor. The latter works to increase radioresistance and increase hematogenous metastases and leads to lower survival and disease-free rates.

Lymphoma Because of the presence of faucial and lingual tonsillar tissue along the tongue base, the incidence of lymphomatous involvement of the oropharynx is significant. Once again these lesions may appear as exophytic masses and must be distinguished from tonsillar lymphoid hypertrophy. Both lymphoma and lymphoid hyperplasia may be relatively high in signal intensity on T2WI and may show enhancement, thereby making their differentiation very difficult (Fig. 14-23). The presence of associated lymphadenopathy may not even be helpful. Biopsy may be necessary. This quandary is an issue in AIDS patients with suspected lymphoma.

Don't forget PTLD of the palatine tonsils also (see previous discussion under nasopharyngeal lesions).

Minor salivary gland tumors Nearly half of minor salivary gland tumors of the oropharynx are pleomorphic adenomas with the other half being malignant. Minor salivary gland malignancies of the oropharynx are

usually due to adenoid cystic carcinoma. The most common site of occurrence is the soft palate.

Sarcomas Rhabdomyosarcomas may also occur within the tongue. Rhabdos run rampant in rug rats requiring radiation for remissions. Also in the sarcomatous category, hemangiopericytomas and synovial sarcomas may occur in the oropharynx.

ORAL CAVITY

Anatomy

The oral cavity includes lips, the anterior two thirds of the tongue, the buccal mucosa, the gingiva, the hard palate, the retromolar trigone, and the floor of the mouth. The pterygomandibular raphe at the underlying retromolar trigone serves as one junction point for the oral cavity and oropharynx. The circumvalate papillae of the tongue and the hard palate-soft palate junction function as other boundary zones.

For the radiologist the phrase "the floor of the mouth" should be equated with the mylohyoid musculature (which constitutes the inferior sling of the mouth) and the sublingual space, between the mylohyoid muscle and the hyoglossus muscle (Fig. 14-24). To repeat, the lingual nerve from the trigeminal nerve and the hypoglossal nerve run together from the floor of the mouth into the tongue base and sublingual space and are important to identify intraoperatively to maintain tongue function. The radiologist must identify whether tumor is in the sublingual space, to alert the surgeon regarding the potential for the sacrifice of these nerves. The chorda tympani from the facial nerve supplies taste to the anterior two thirds of the tongue and its branches join that of the

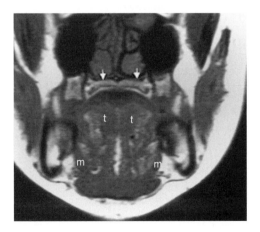

Fig. 14-24 Normal anatomy of the oral cavity. The hard palate *(small arrows)*, the anterior two thirds of the tongue *(t)*, and the gingival surfaces of the mandible constitute portions of the oral cavity. The oral cavity also includes the floor of the mouth, seen as the mylohyoid *(m)* muscular sling inferolaterally.

lingual nerve. The glossopharyngeal nerve supplies taste to the posterior third of the tongue. The patients (and surgeons) would like to have the nerves for taste preserved. Gustatory pleasures (chocolate-lovers unite!) are important for quality of life.

Congenital Lesions

Besides thyroid migrational anomalies and simple cysts, the congenital lesions of the oral cavity are mainly due to dermoid cysts (a term generically used to include epidermoid, dermoid, and teratoid cysts) and cystic hygromas (lymphangiomas). The dermoids contain fat or fluid and are usually in the floor of the mouth. Epidermoid cysts usually occur in the sublingual space and have fluid density and signal intensity (Fig. 14-25). The lesion may have geometric designs within the cyst. The lymphangiomas are generally more infiltrative than dermoids and are characterized by large cystic spaces, which may have high protein content or hemorrhage within them. Therefore, their signal intensity on MR may be mixed on all pulse sequences. Both these lesions may be bright on T1WI, but the fatty lesion is hypodense on CT and has lower signal intensity on T2WI.

Cherubism Cherubism can occur in patients with familial fibrous dysplasia of the mandible, neurofibromatosis, Noonan syndrome (male Turner's syndrome), and Ramon syndrome (cherubism, gingival fibromatosis, epilepsy, and mental retardation). The ground glass appearance and "bubbliness" are typical of this bilateral bony lesion.

Inflammatory Lesions

Odontogenic lesions Numerous odontogenic abnormalities may be found within the oral cavity, the most common of which is the lytic lesion known as the radicular (periapical) cyst (Table 14-3). This is a lucent lesion of either the mandible or the maxilla, and is associated with an infected tooth. These lesions rarely come to the medical radiologist; usually the dentist on bite-wing films diagnoses them. The second most common odontogenic cystic lesion is the dentigerous cyst. This cyst is associated with an unerupted tooth and is usually seen in the mandible, particularly around the molar region. Both the radicular cyst and the dentigerous cyst are usually unilocular, as opposed to the keratocyst and the ameloblastoma, which are benign but aggressive multilocular cystic lesions most commonly affecting the mandible (Fig. 14-26). Keratocysts are associated with the *basal cell nevus (Gorlin's) syndrome,* in which patients have proliferative falcian calcification, multiple basal cell carcinomas of the skin, scoliosis, ribbon-shaped ribs, CNS tumors, and keratocysts of the mandible.

Of the congenital cysts in the maxilla, the nasopalatine cyst (incisive canal cyst) is the most common. This cyst usually arises in the midline incisive canal and slowly expands the maxilla and hard palate. Usually the cyst is painless and the teeth are unaffected. Therefore, it is not considered an odontogenic cyst.

Sclerotic dental lesions also span the spectrum of inflammatory, benign neoplastic, and malignant lesions (Table 14-4).

SAPHO (synovitis, acne, palmoplantar pustulosis, hyperostosis, and osteitis) syndrome is associated with diffuse sclerosing osteomyelitis of the mandible. Superficial stigmata (skin scars) of SAPHO syndrome subject sufferers to shameless scorn. The inflammation can spread from the TMJ to the skull base to the cochlea, leading to deafness.

Ranula The final inflammatory lesion of the oral cavity is the ranula (mucus escape cyst). This is a cystic lesion that is due to obstruction of the sublingual gland duct or minor salivary gland of the floor of the mouth, which causes a backup of secretions. The obstruction may be due to previous infection, trauma, or calculi. Depending on whether the ranula protrudes through the mylohyoid musculature, the lesion may be termed sim-

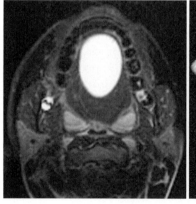
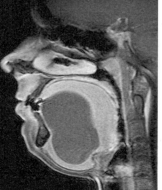

Fig. 14-25 (Epi) Dermoid cyst of tongue. **A,** Axial T2WI is dominated by the very bright midline mass in the oral tongue. It is too anterior to be a thyroglossal duct cyst and not lateral or inferior enough to be a ranula. **B,** The sagittal post-contrast T1WI confirms the cystic nature of the mass by virtue of the absence of enhancement.

Table 14-3   Benign lytic dental lesions

Lesion	Imaging appearance	Typical clinical findings
Ameloblastoma	Multiloculated (60% of cases) lytic lesion often associated with dentigerous cysts; hyperostotic margins; cortex eroded or penetrated	85% in mandibular molar area with expanded jaw; painless, male predominance
Brown tumor	Lytic lesion with erosion of lamina dura; ill-defined borders	Hyperparathyroidism
Central odontogenic fibroma	Multilocular lesion with sclerotic borders	Expanded mandible
Cherubism	Bilateral, symmetric multilocular lucencies (soap bubble) in posterior mandible; expanded cortex without perforation; simulates fibrous dysplasia	Painless; bilateral enlargement of lower part of face; angelic appearance; autosomal dominant inheritance; regression after adolescence
Dentigerous (follicular) cyst	Lytic, lucent, expansile lesion adjacent to unerupted tooth; spares cortex; sclerotic margins	Unerupted asymptomatic 3rd molar or canine tooth
Giant cell granuloma	Well-defined multilocular lucency with sclerotic margins involving mandible	Asymptomatic in children and young adults
Globulomaxillary cyst	Lucent lesion between lateral incisor and canine in maxilla	Asymptomatic
Incisive canal cyst (nasopalatine duct cyst)	Lucent lesion in midline hard palate with hyperostotic borders at canal	Swollen anterior hard palate; asymptomatic
Keratocyst (primordial cyst)	Unilocular or multilocular expansile lucent lesion; erodes cortex but does not perforate it	Recurrent posterior mandibular lesion with thin walls; associated with basal cell nevus syndrome
Radicular (periapical) cyst	Lytic; lucent at apex of erupted tooth; loss of lamina dura; hyperostotic borders	Carious, tender nonvital tooth

ple (above the mylohyoid) or plunging (through the muscle). Do not poo-poo this minutia as it makes a difference to the surgeon—the simple ranula is approached via an intraoral resection, whereas the plunging ranula

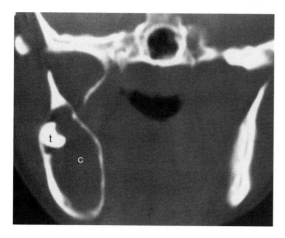

Fig. 14-26   Dentigerous cyst. Coronal bone targeted CT demonstrates a large unilocular cystic mass *(c)* in the mandible with an associated unerupted tooth *(t)*. This is virtually pathognomonic for a dentigerous cyst.

requires a submandibular or transcervical or combined intraoral and cervical resection. The ranula's wall usually enhances. The ranula may have a pointed edge along its anterior extent in the sublingual space at the site of obstruction (Fig. 14-27). Rupture of a ranula can cause an encapsulated mucus-containing infection in the deep tissue of the neck.

Benign Tumors

Osteomas   Benign lesions of the oral cavity are common and include bony lesions such as osteomas and tori palatini, which are benign bony outgrowths from the hard palate that present as ossified masses. Tori mandibuli occur—where else—along the inner cortex of the mandible.

Hemangiomas   Within the tongue, hemangiomas may occur. The hemangiomas are generally well defined in the tongue and demonstrate marked enhancement.

In the buccal/cheek region one may find a disgusting benign tumor of the hair follicles, the pilomatrixoma. They are usually found in the subcutaneous tissue of adolescent girls and contain calcification. They are well-circumscribed and noninvasive.

Table 14-4 Sclerotic dental lesions

Lesion	Imaging appearance	Typical clinical findings
Adenomatoid odontogenic tumor	Calcified well-defined lesions with thick capsule; associated with impacted tooth; involves crown of tooth	Teenagers with impacted maxillary front teeth; painless; female predominance
Cementoblastoma	Circular radiodensity attached to a mandibular tooth with pencil-thin border; surrounded by lucency; radial spicules	Expanded mandible with vital tooth; occurs 1st–3rd decades of life
Chondrosarcoma	Moth-eaten appearance with chondroid whorls; may be lucent or dense	Maxillary swelling; painful in adults
Ewing's sarcoma	Onion-skinning; destructive lesion; poorly defined	5–25 yr of age with painful mandibular mass, fever, rapid growth, loose teeth
Fibrous dysplasia	Ground-glass appearance, homogeneous in later stages	Focal painless mass; slow growth; posterior maxilla
Garré's sclerosing osteomyelitis	Predominantly sclerotic bony lestion; hot on scintigrams; often with periosteal reaction and apical lucency	Bony-hard cortical swelling of mandible; carious molars; nonvital teeth
Lymphoma	"Moth-eaten," sclerotic bone	Often systemic symptoms
Metastases	Dense permeative lesions	Lung, breast, prostate, colon, kidney, thyroid primary tumors; loose teeth; often painful
Odontoma	Compound: Miniature teeth (enamel) within maxilla with peripheral lucent zone Complex: Irregular opaque mass in mandibular molar region	Young patient with mass between canines or in mandible; painless; young adults or children
Osteoma	Dense benign excresence; well-defined	Associated with Gardner's syndrome with colonic polyps, supernumerary teeth, cysts; seen as a torus on palate; painless, slow-growing
Osteosarcoma	Sclerotic or lytic; poorly defined with opaque spicules with sunray appearance; resorbs roots	Maxillary or mandibular mass; rapid growth; painful; loose teeth
Paget's disease	Dense thickened bone with risk of osteosarcoma; cotton-wool appearance in maxilla; loss of lamina dura	Elderly patient with dentures no longer fitting commonly in maxilla
Pindborg's tumor	Multiple small calcifications within lytic lesion associated with impacted teeth	Mass in mandibular molar

Ameloblastoma The ameloblastoma is a benign neoplasm of the oral cavity that is hard to remove completely and has a high rate of recurrence (Fig. 14-28). These characteristics may also be seen with keratocysts, myxomas, and aneurysmal bone cysts. Ameloblastoma is the second most common odontogenic tumor and arises in the mandible in 81% of cases. The molar region is affected in 70% of cases. The lesion is painless unless superinfected and has scalloped margins, multiloculation, and expanded cortical surfaces. Solid and cystic components are seen on MR with frequent mural nodules. Enhancement is marked in the periphery, not in the cysts. High intensity on T1WI sometimes occurs and may be due to hemorrhage or cholesterol crystal accumulation.

Other dental tumors Other benign dental tumors are beyond the scope of this textbook and most neuroradiologists, but are summarized in the previously cited Tables 14-3 and 14-4. Suffice it to say that dental radiology is a specialty worthy of respect by the nondental ra-

diologic community. Dental disease is daunting due to dumbfounding and redundant distributions and depictions of different dense and destructive diagnoses. All the lesions look the same to us.

Malignant Neoplasms

Squamous cell carcinoma The risk factors for oral cavity squamous cell carcinoma include smoking, alcohol abuse, and chewing tobacco. Chewing betel nuts has also been associated with an increased risk of squamous cell carcinoma. Surprisingly the lower lip is the second most common site of squamous cell carcinoma in the head and neck after the skin. Radiologists are not aware of this fact, because lip lesions usually are not imaged. Lower lip cancers are many times more common than upper lip tumors due to the sun exposure, gravitational effects and to the reluctance of most Moms to apply SPF #30 to their kids' lips. PABA tastes pretty bad.

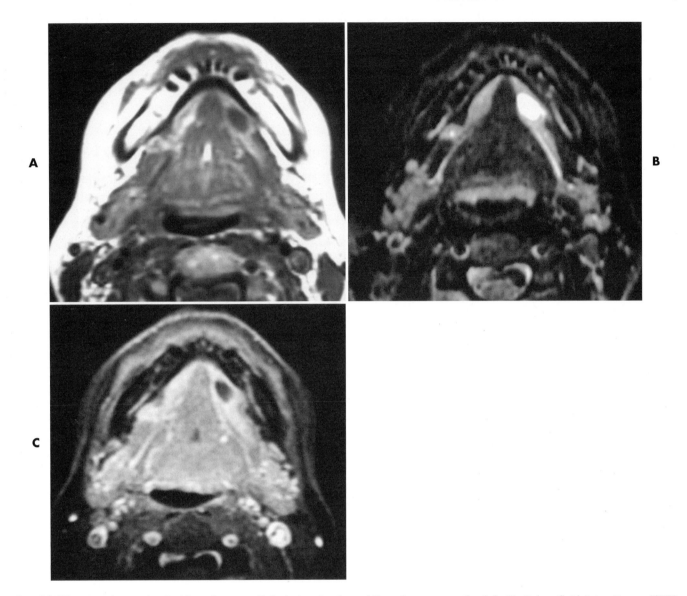

Fig. 14-27   Simple ranula. **A,** Note the cute little lesion in the sublingual space on the left. **B,** It has fluid intensity on T2WI. **C,** Only peripheral enhancement is seen. This is a quintessential simple ranula, probably from a sublingual duct obstruction.

The presentation of patients with oral cavity cancer may be delayed because people often assume that the lesions in the mouth are due to trauma from biting or chewing rather than from a neoplastic proliferation. Denial also plays a large role. Therefore it is not uncommon for a patient to have the minor complaint of "ill-fitting dentures" or a nonhealing ulcer of the oral cavity, only to find that the lesion is an aggressive, deeply infiltrative squamous cell carcinoma.

The T staging of oral cavity cancer is very similar to that of the oropharynx and is divided by size criteria from T1 to T3 (Box 14-6). A stage T4 tumor shows infiltration to bone or soft tissue. The combined metachronous (lesions that *will* develop) and synchronous (two lesions at the same time) rate with squamous cell carcinoma of the

oral cavity is 40%, and therefore these patients are followed up closely for the rest of their lives with panendoscopy for the possibility of the second tumor. In addition, because of the uniform presentation of the carcinogens to the oral cavity, there is the possibility of "field cancerization," in which multiple sites of carcinoma in situ, severe dysplasia, and invasive carcinoma may be present within the oral cavity at presentation.

The critical questions that the radiologist must address with oral cavity cancer are as follows: (1) Is there mandibular or maxillary invasion? (Fig. 14-29) (2) Is there extension into the retromolar trigone and pterygomandibular raphe? (3) Is there extension into the oropharynx? (4) Is there spread into laryngeal soft tissues, necessitating a laryngectomy? (5) Is there extension across the mid-

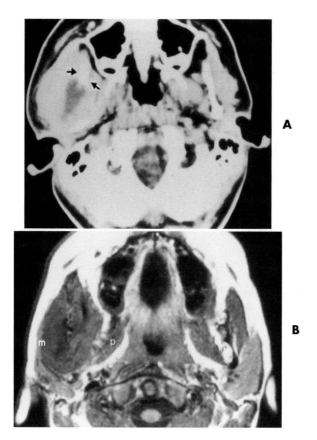

Fig 14-28   Ameloblastoma. **A,** A mass with central necrosis, centered on the coronoid process *(arrows)* of the mandible, can be seen on this unenhanced CT. **B,** The T1WI shows the tissue planes around the mass and the infiltration of the masseter *(m)* and preservation of the pterygoid *(p)* muscles to better advantage.

line of the tongue requiring total glossectomy versus a radiation-chemotherapy cocktail? (6) Is there perineural spread of the tumor? Life without a tongue is for the birds. People do not appreciate how critical their tongue is to all types of functions and pleasures. If they did, they would never stick their tongue out and subject it to the elements. Mick Jagger, Michael Jordan, and Linda Lovelace, beware!

The maxilla is more commonly involved with oral cavity and specifically retromolar trigone cancers than with oropharyngeal cancers. Rarely, a soft palate cancer may affect the maxilla and tonsillar cancers may spread to the retromolar trigone and from there infiltrate the maxilla. Partial maxillectomies are relatively well tolerated by patients as long as appropriately tailored obturators are constructed, which separate the nasal cavity from the oral cavity and oropharynx. Otherwise, regurgitation of food products into the nasal cavity and/or phonation difficulties such as velopharyngeal insufficiency may arise from this common cavity. After the maxilla the tumor may grow into the maxillary sinus or the pterygopalatine fossa (vide infra).

From Greene FL, Page DL, Fleming ID, et al (eds): *AJCC Cancer Staging Manual;* ed 6. New York, Springer-Verlag, 2002, p 24–25. Used with permission.

Although bilaterality is important with all tongue lesions, it is the base of the tongue that is the critical component to the swallowing mechanism. Therefore you can be reasonably functional after oral tongue resections as long as you have most of your posterior tongue still wig-

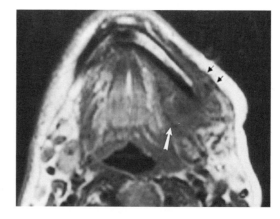

Fig. 14-29   Oral cavity cancer. Axial T1WI depicts a soft tissue mass along the floor of the mouth *(arrow)* that has a component *(small black arrows)* superficial to the mandible. Note that the marrow signal is preserved although the lesion sweeps around its posterolateral edge. Corticectomy could cure confined cortical carcinoma.

gling around after the surgeon's knife filets you. Phonatory issues also are different between oral tongue and oropharyngeal tongue resections. The tip and anterior portion of the tongue are more important with creating certain consonant sounds such as Ts, Ds, Gs, Js, and Zs. With total glossectomies you take out not only the tongue, but a lot more consonants and vowel sounds.

Nodal disease is less frequent with superficial oral cavity primary cancers than oropharyngeal ones. The exact numbers from different series vary widely, but roughly 30% of patients with oral cavity cancers have nodes at presentation whereas the percentage for oropharyngeal cancers runs approximately 65%. Nodal spread impacts significantly on patient outcome (reducing 5 year survival by 50%), emphasizing the importance of identifying pathologic nodes in all patients with cancer. Drainage of the anterior two thirds of the tongue goes to the submandibular lymph nodes and from there to the high internal jugular chain. Because reactive lymph nodes in the submandibular region may grow to more than 1 cm in size, submandibular nodes are not suggested to be neoplastic until they are more than 1.5 cm in diameter.

With oral cavity cancers, the issues of depth of skin invasion, pterygomandibular raphe invasion, maxilla invasion, and pterygopalatine fossa invasion (the latter secondary to retromolar trigone cancer) remain important. If the disease is limited or superficial, transoral resection with reconstruction by skin grafting, local flaps, or healing by secondary intention can be used. More extensive skin grafting may be required with oral cavity cancers that invade superficially than the oropharyngeal cancers, which tend to occur in the deeper tissues of the head and neck.

Because of the low soft tissue discrimination with CT, MR is the study of choice to evaluate the extent of tongue cancers. Too often, tongue cancers are isodense to the normal intrinsic muscles of the tongue, which leads to underdiagnosis on CT. In addition, dental amalgam creates such tremendous artifact on CT that unless one is able to tilt the gantry at multiple complementary angles to avoid metallic artifact, the tongue and gingival surfaces of the gums are not well seen. On MR, however, the dental amalgam creates a much more localized artifact, which does not obscure the anatomy to the same extent as CT.

The two pulse sequences that are of the greatest use with MR of the tongue are (1) the T2WI, because tumors are brighter than the very dark intrinsic musculature of the tongue, and (2) the fat-suppressed enhanced scans, which often demonstrate marked enhancement in tongue cancers. Mandibular marrow invasion can be diagnosed by soft-tissue infiltration across the dark cortical margin of the mandible into the bright signal intensity fat on T1WI. On CT this diagnosis requires demonstration of direct bony erosion.

Floor of mouth cancers may cause obstruction of the submandibular duct. This causes an enlarged, edematous, painful, submandibular gland that may simulate inflammation caused by calculous disease and lead to delayed diagnosis. For the evaluation of a painful salivary gland, unenhanced CT is recommended to exclude calculi.

One must also be cognizant of the role of the nasopalatine nerves, greater and lesser palatine canals, inferior alveolar canal, and pterygopalatine fossa as avenues for the possible spread of cancers along nerves. Ultimately, the foramen rotundum and foramen ovale should be assessed with imaging to insure that intracranial extension of tumor along the cranial nerves has not occurred.

Other oral cavity malignancies Although squamous cell carcinomas constitute more than 90% of the malignancies of the tongue, there is a small incidence of rhabdomyosarcomas, minor salivary gland malignancies, and lymphomas in this location. Gingival lymphomas infiltrate the bone causing subtle erosions. Surprisingly, many of these lymphomas are unassociated with lymph nodes.

Osteosarcomas of the craniofacial region account for less than 10% of all osteosarcomas. When they occur, they favor the mandible (50%) and the maxilla (25%). Most are lytic in appearance—the mandibular ones may be blastic. Some occur in sites of Paget disease or radiation portals. Familial retinoblastomatosis may predispose to osteosarcomas by virtue of the chromosome 13 oncogene. These osteosarcomas often occur in the portals of the retinoblastoma.

HYPOPHARYNX

Anatomy

The hypopharynx is a nebulously defined space that includes three major subsites: the pyriform sinus, the postcricoid region (pharyngoesophageal junction), and the posterior pharyngeal wall above the inferior border of the cricoid cartilage (Fig. 14-30). The top of the hypopharynx is at the epiglottic level, and its inferior border is the pharyngoesophageal junction. The mucosa over the posterior surface of the cricoarytenoid joints is part of the hypopharynx. The anteromedial wall of the pyriform sinus is the aryepiglottic fold, a structure of the supraglottic larynx.

The pyriform sinus is best evaluated with the patient undergoing Valsalva's maneuver because this distends the airway down to its inferiormost portion, the pyriform apex. This maneuver is best employed during barium studies or ultrafast CT scans (spiral CT). Performing Valsalva's maneuver for 6 minutes (for an MR scan) is nearly impossible unless you've been coached in the

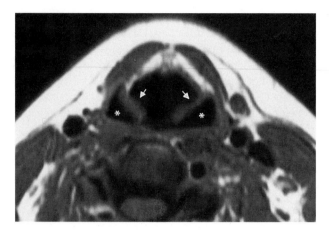

Fig. 14-30 Anatomy of the hypopharynx. Axial T1WI demonstrates the air-filled pyriform sinuses *(asterisks)*, which are delineated anteromedially by the aryepiglottic folds *(small arrows)*. Other subsites of the pharynx in this location include the posterior and lateral pharyngeal walls.

Lamaze method or have sufficient reading material and sphincter tone—try it yourself if you are a nonbeliever. The apposition of mucosal surfaces in the pyriform sinus often makes lesion localization difficult. You may not be able to distinguish extension to the adjacent aryepiglottic fold, the lateral pyriform sinus mucosa, or the posteromedial mucosa without maneuvers to increase distention.

Minor salivary gland tissue is present in the hypopharynx amid the squamous mucosa lining the space.

Congenital Lesions

The pyriform sinus is a drainage site for third branchial cleft cysts, and the pyriform sinus apex may be a site of sinus tracts leading from fourth branchial cleft cysts (see Table 15-2, Fig. 15-63). The third branchial cleft sinus tract passes between the common carotid artery and vagus nerve to the anterior border of the inferior sternocleidomastoid muscle. The fourth branchial cleft sinus tract passes around the great vessels and the aortic arch on the left side. This lesion is so rare (as with the otic artery, absent from this text), that some people say it does not exist. Nonetheless, the fourth branchial cleft sinus tract lives on in this chapter.

Inflammatory Lesions

Besides superinfected branchial cleft anomalies and postinflammatory submucosal cysts, no specific inflammatory lesions are unique to the hypopharynx. Pharyngoceles may occur in patients with chronic increased intrapharyngeal pressure such as in horn blowers (Dizzy Gillespie), shofar blowers (Hymie Gillespie), glass blowers (John Gillespie), and shaft blowers (Monica Gillespie). These are usually air filled but occasionally may become obstructed and fill with fluid. No study has shown that politicians, who also blow a lot of hot air, have increased rates of pharyngoceles.

Zenker's diverticulae occur near the cricopharyngeus muscle and protrude posteriorly. They are best demonstrated by gastrointestinal radiologists and barium. They increase in frequency and size with age and develop at Killian's dehiscence, an area of weakness between the cricopharyngeus and the inferior pharyngeal constrictor muscles. The patient may complain of dysphagia, bad breath, aspiration pneumonia, or regurgitation of undigested food. A Killian-Jamieson lateral pharyngoesophageal divertculum protrudes laterally and is typically smaller than a Zenker's diverticulum. It can occur at any age and is less likely to cause symptoms than a Zenker or a chancre.

Pyriform sinus fistulae are usually associated with fourth branchial apparatus abnormalities. They may pass to the thyroid gland causing acute suppurative thyroiditis or open to the skin. The vast majority of these fistulae are left sided. Recurrence rates are about 40%. Most occur in children.

Benign Tumors

No benign tumors are specific to the hypopharynx. Minor salivary gland pleomorphic adenomas and/or schwannomas are infrequently seen here.

Malignant Tumors

The staging of hypopharyngeal cancer depends on the number of subsites that are invaded, the size of the lesion, as well as the presence or absence of fixation of the hemilarynx (Box 14-7). Once again, whip out that measuring stick because you must make distinctions between tumors—less than 2 cm, 2 to 4 cm, and over 4 cm in size. Size matters!

If the tumor invades adjacent structures such as the thyroid or cricoid cartilage, or extends out into the soft tissues of the neck, the lesion is considered a T4 cancer. The anatomy of the hypopharynx gets somewhat confusing because the anteromedial margin of the pyriform sinus is the lateral aspect of the aryepiglottic fold, which is considered a portion of the supraglottic larynx. The anterolateral wall of the pyriform sinus is the posterior wall of the paraglottic space more inferiorly. Because tumors in the pyriform sinus often obliterate the space between the lateral/pharyngeal mucosa of the aryepiglottic fold and the mucosa of the pyriform sinus, it is often difficult to determine whether a tumor is supraglottic (arising from the aryepiglottic fold), or hypopharyngeal (arising along the lateral aspect of the pyriform sinus). Endoscopists have a much better appreciation of this distinction because they are able to slide the endoscope

Box 14-7 T Staging of the Hypopharynx

Hypopharynx

T1 Tumor limited to one subsite of hypopharynx and 2 cm or less in greatest dimension

T2 Tumor invades more than one subsite of hypopharynx or an adjacent site, or measures more than 2 cm but not more than 4 cm in greatest diameter without fixation of hemilarynx

T3 Tumor more than 4 cm in greatest dimension or with fixation of hemilarynx

T4a Tumor invades thyroid/cricoid cartilage, hyoid bone, thyroid gland, esophagus, or central compartment soft tissue*

T4b Tumor invades prevertebral fascia, encases carotid artery, or involves mediastinal structures

Subsites: Postcricoid region, pyriform sinus, aryepiglottic fold (pharyngeal wall), posterior pharyngeal wall (to cricoarytenoid joint)

Note: Central compartment soft tissue includes prelaryngeal strap muscles and subcutaneous fat.

From Greene FL, Page DL, Fleming ID, et al (eds): *AJCC Cancer Staging Manual;* ed 6. New York, Springer-Verlag, 2002, p 35. Used with permission.

medial to the tumor if it is a lateral pyriform sinus cancer or lateral to the tumor if the lesion is arising from the aryepiglottic fold. However, endoscopy is limited in the evaluation of very large tumors that obscure the pyriform sinus apex; this may be an area where either cross sectional imaging with reconstructions or barium studies may be of particular use.

Most hypopharyngeal cancers (60%) arise in the pyriform sinus with the remainder evenly split between postcricoid and posterior pharyngeal locations. The pyriform sinus cancers do not behave well—they metastasize early, invade aggressively into the soft tissue of the neck, and present late (because this area is clinically silent) (Fig. 14-31). There seems to be a particular affinity for pyriform sinus cancers to spread through the thyrohyoid membrane or cricothyroid membrane into the neck where they may encircle the carotid arteries. This is not good, as some deem cancerous carotid encasement a criterion for cancelling curative cutouts.

As in laryngeal carcinoma, one of the major issues regarding hypopharyngeal tumors is the invasion of cartilage. The superior aspect of the thyroid cartilage is particularly vulnerable to hypopharyngeal cancer. At this time most radiologists believe that MR is superior to CT in the evaluation of early laryngeal cartilage invasion (but hedge during the boards in case your examiner bucks the majority trend—see discussion that follows). MR may be able to detect the more subtle cartilaginous invasion

before through-and-through disease is present. For this indication enhanced fat-suppressed MR appears to be a particularly valuable pulse sequence. In the later stages infiltration of the strap muscles superficial to the cartilage is seen equally well on MR and CT.

Watch for prevertebral muscle invasion with posterior pharyngeal wall hypopharyngeal carcinomas. Findings include bright signal intensity on T2WI and enhancement of the longus musculature. Watch for Plummer-Vinson syndrome references (glossitis, anemia, cervical esophagus or hypopharyngeal webs) in patients with postcricoid carcinomas.

Pyriform sinus cancers also have a high rate of metastasis to the adjacent lymphatics and lymphadenopathy in some cases is reported to occur in 75% of patients at presentation. Jugular lymph nodes in levels II, III, and IV are the primary drainage sites. Necrosis in these nodes seems more common with a hypopharyngeal primary tumor.

The other malignancies seen in the hypopharynx include synovial sarcomas, lymphomas, and minor salivary gland tumors. A well-defined yet heterogeneous mass with septations, hemorrhage, cysts, calcification, or multilocularity should raise suspicion of a synovial sarcoma. These lesions DO NOT arise from synovial structures. This is a misnomer. Saying "synovial sarcoma" should not suggest a synovial source, simply cell shape.

Because histology is really not an issue, the critical questions the radiologist must answer are (1) Is there cartilaginous invasion? (2) Is there extension into deep tissues of the neck? (3) Is lymphadenopathy present?

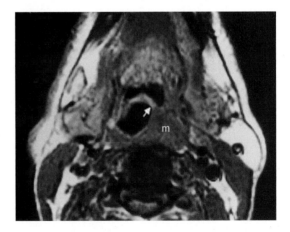

Fig. 14-31 High hypopharyngeal lesion. This mass *(m)* is located at the top of the pyriform sinus and invades the lateral pharyngeal wall below the level of the epiglottis *(arrow)*. Because the lesion is apposed to the lateral aspect of the epiglottis, it is difficult to determine whether this is a supraglottic lesion of the aryepiglottic fold or a lesion in the high pyriform sinus. Fortunately, the endoscopist can determine the lesion's origin because if the scope passes medially, it suggests a pyriform sinus origin; if the scope passes laterally, it suggests aryepiglottic fold origin.

(4) Is there evidence of infiltration into the posterior paraspinal musculature? (5) Is there extension into the larynx or paraglottic space? So many questions and, too often, so few correct answers. But now you will know better.

Most patients require a resection of supraglottic structures and pharyngectomy for pyriform sinus cancers. Occasionally, when the paraglottic space is infiltrated, a total laryngectomy and pharyngectomy is necessary.

LARYNX

Anatomy

The larynx is broadly separated into the supraglottis, the glottis, and the subglottis (Fig. 14-32). Each of these areas is dealt with individually by the head and neck oncologic surgeon, although lesions often cross these boundaries of the larynx (transglottic cancers). The supraglottis includes the false vocal cords, the arytenoids, the epiglottis, and the aryepiglottic folds. The glottis includes the true vocal cords, the anterior and posterior commissures, and the vocal ligament extending from the arytenoid cartilage. The laryngeal ventricle is said to separate the supraglottis and glottis, but is itself a part of the supraglottis. The subglottis begins 1 centimeter below the ventricle and extends to the first tracheal ring.

The larynx is anchored on a framework composed of the hyoid bone, the epiglottis, the thyroid cartilage, the cricoid cartilage, and the arytenoids, each of which has an integral function. Of these, the complete ring of the cricoid cartilage is the only indispensable strut for preservation of airway patency. The major role of the epiglottis is to protect the airway during swallowing. From the inferior portion of the arytenoid cartilage the vocal ligament stretches to the thyroid cartilage anteriorly and supports the vocal cord. The lower cricoarytenoid joint is the marker for the level of the true vocal cord (Fig. 14-33).

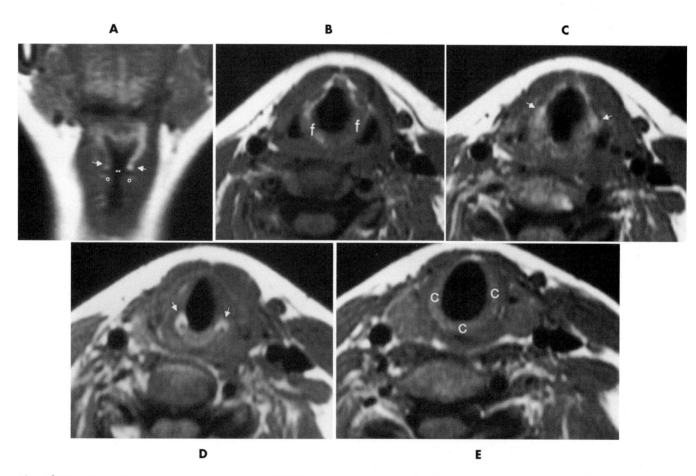

Fig. 14-32 Normal laryngeal anatomy. **A,** Coronal T1WI shows the laryngeal ventricle (••), which separates the false cord above from the true cord below. Note that at the false cord level the paraglottic tissue is high intensity from fat *(arrows)*, whereas below the ventricle the soft tissue is muscular *(o)* from the thyroarytenoid muscle, which makes up the bulk of the true cord. One centimeter below the ventricle is the margin of the subglottic region. **B,** Axial T1WI demonstrates the supraglottic structures including the aryepiglottic fold *(f)* extending posteroinferiorly toward the arytenoid region. **C,** At the false cord level one again can identify the fat *(arrows)* in the paraglottic space. **D,** At the true cord level the paraglottic tissue is made up of the thyroarytenoid musculature. The landmark for the true cord level is the cricoarytenoid joint *(arrows)*. **E,** Subglottic region is marked by the full cricoid *(c)* ring.

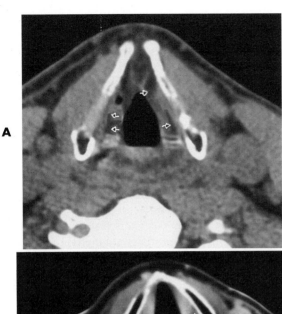

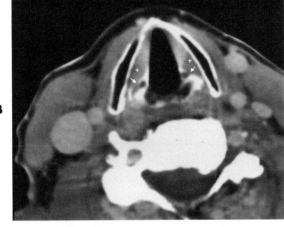

Fig. 14-33 False cord and true cord levels. **A,** The false cord is characterized by low density fat *(arrows)* in the paraglottic space. **B,** The true cord is located at the lower cricoarytenoid joint *(arrows).* The thyroarytenoid muscle *(+)* makes up the "paraglottic" tissue and this muscle attaches to the vocal process of the arytenoid.

On the lateral side of the laryngeal mucosal surface is the paraglottic space, which contains fat, lymphatics, and small muscles. At the false cord level the paraglottic space contains fat, whereas at the true cord level it contains the thyroarytenoid muscle, another important landmark to define laryngeal levels. Thus, you can tell if you are at a supraglottic level by seeing fat deep to the mucosa—at the glottic level it is muscle that is seen submucosally. The thyroarytenoid muscle makes up the bulk of the true vocal cord and parallels the vocal ligament. The cricoarytenoid muscle moves the arytenoids to narrow or open the glottic airway for speech. The true vocal cords meet in the midline at the anterior commissure. This junction should be no more than 1 to 2 mm of thickness. The posterior commissure refers to the mucosa between the two vocal processes on the anterior surface of the arytenoid cartilage.

The vagus nerve innervates the larynx through two branches: the recurrent laryngeal nerve and the superior laryngeal nerve. The only muscle supplied by the latter is the cricothyroid muscle, and its paralysis causes only minor changes in the voice. The course of the vagus and recurrent laryngeal nerve is important to understand in patients with vocal cord paralysis. The nerve descends from the medulla through the jugular foramen into the carotid sheath. The vagus follows the carotid sheath inferiorly with the recurrent laryngeal nerve looping under the aortic arch on the left and the subclavian artery on the right, before ascending in the tracheoesophageal groove. The branches of the recurrent laryngeal nerve perforate the cricothyroid membrane to supply the intrinsic musculature of the larynx.

The larynx is lined by squamous epithelium. Minor salivary glands are present predominantly in its supraglottic portion. The lymphatics of the supraglottis are abundant, whereas in the glottis they are sparse. The amount of lymphatics in the subglottis is intermediate between the two.

Congenital Lesions

Webs can occur in the larynx, usually at the true cord level. When subglottic narrowing is seen in an infant, the differential diagnosis is usually between a hemangioma and idiopathic subglottic stenosis. Both these conditions are benign, and the infant may outgrow the lesions if supportive care is provided. These are plain film diagnoses with findings of airway narrowing.

Tracheolaryngomalacia is another neonatal entity that can cause airway narrowing and that is usually outgrown with time. The children have inspiratory stridor because the floppy laryngeal cartilages collapse under the effects of negative inspiratory pressure. The collapse of the airway with inspiration can be demonstrated at fluoroscopy.

Inflammatory Lesions

Laryngitis Almost all of us have experienced the inconvenience (and serendipitous benefits) of laryngitis. This condition is usually associated with a viral upper respiratory tract infection and is benign and self-limited. Chronic laryngitis may actually be due to laryngeal nodules, a nonneoplastic reaction to chronic voice abuse—a clear contraindication to incessant nagging or politicking. (Attention, all presidential hopefuls reading this book!) This is also an occupational hazard for professional singers, though it does not seem to stop the hip-hop rappers.

Submucosal cysts The most common benign mass in the larynx is a submucosal cyst. This is thought to be due to obstruction of small minor salivary or mucous glands and occurs most commonly in the supraglottis. Rarely, these lesions may grow large enough to cause airway compromise. Anterior to the epiglottis, one may find the low density, nonenhancing vallecular cyst. It may simulate a thyroglossal duct cyst but is usually off midline.

Laryngocele The laryngocele is an outpouching of the laryngeal ventricle caused by obstruction of the ventricular saccule. The saccule is a superolateral extension of the ventricle into the paraglottic space. A laryngocele may be filled with either air or fluid (so-called saccular cyst) and is seen frequently in people playing wind instruments, who have chronic increased intraglottic pressure—basically hard blowers or blow-hards. The laryngocele is characterized as being internal, mixed, or external in its location. The internal laryngocele remains confined by the thyrohyoid membrane, whereas the external laryngocele protrudes through the thyrohyoid membrane. By definition the lesion arises within the laryngeal ventricle so that an isolated external laryngocele is almost unheard of; most lesions are in fact mixed laryngoceles, which have both a component internal and external to the membrane. Occasionally the laryngocele becomes infected and it is then termed a pyolaryngocele.

Occasionally, a laryngocele may arise because of inflammatory or neoplastic processes (Fig. 14-34). To exclude a carcinoma at the saccule, endoscopy to evaluate the ventricle is recommended in patients with laryngoceles. Imaging studies should allow careful scrutiny of lesions in this region which may be blind to endoscopy because of the overhanging shelf of the false cord.

Subglottic stenosis Subglottic stenosis may occur from previous intubation and/or as a result of previous inflammatory disease in this region of the larynx. In this case the narrowing of the subglottic portion of the larynx is generally symmetric. Granulation tissue or tracheomalacia may contribute to the airway narrowing after prolonged intubation.

Supraglottitis We use the term supraglottitis because most cases of "epiglottitis" will affect the aryepiglottic folds and even the superior aspects of the arytenoids. In some cases the soft palate and prevertebral swelling may be the predominant factor in creating upper respiratory symptoms. Epiglottitis is a life-threatening illness that generally is seen in 2- to 4-year-old children. This is a bacterial infection of the epiglottis that is usually caused by *Haemophilus influenzae*. The epiglottis is markedly thickened (thumb-shaped), and dilatation of the airway above the epiglottis is present. Manipulation of the epiglottis in the acute setting may cause diffuse laryngeal edema, producing acute respiratory compromise. Fifty percent of infants with this disorder ultimately require intubation. Epiglottitis is generally a clinical diagnosis with imaging limited to a confirmatory upright lateral plain film (Fig. 14-35). The patients often have increased stridor when they are placed supine, and therefore cross-sectional imaging is not recommended—unless you have a gutsy radiologist. Furthermore, you want to keep the patient in a location close to where an emergency tracheostomy can be performed, which is usually not in an outpatient imaging center.

Streptococcus may predominate as an organism in adult supraglottitis. The infection is milder in adults and is less likely to cause acute respiratory arrest or obstruction. Adult supraglottitis is a more indolent infection than pediatric epiglottitis because adults can tolerate more supraglottic and prevertebral swelling than children. In adults, the ratio of the width of the epiglottis to the anteroposterior width of C-4 should not exceed 0.33 (sensitivity, 96%; specificity, 100%), the prevertebral soft tissue to C-4 should not exceed 0.5 (sensitivity, 37%; specificity, 100%) and the hypopharyngeal airway to the width of C-4 should be less than

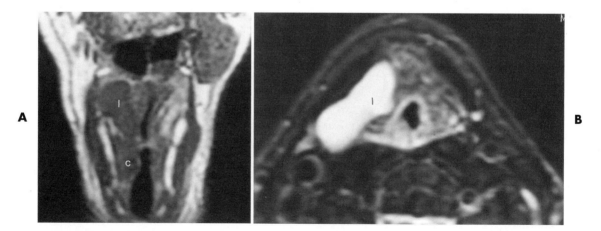

Fig. 14-34 Laryngocele associated with laryngeal carcinoma. **A,** This patient had a transglottic squamous cell carcinoma (*c*) that obstructed the saccule of the laryngeal ventricle on the right side. Internal laryngocele (*l*) developed in the paraglottic soft tissue. **B,** T2WI demonstrates the fluid-filled laryngocele (*l*), also known as a saccular cyst, in the paraglottic tissues. This should not be confused with squamous cell carcinoma, which would not be as bright on the T2WI.

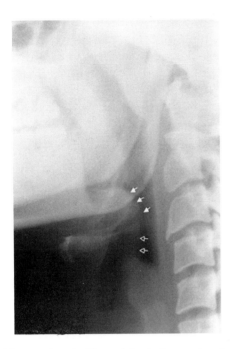

Fig. 14-35 Epiglottitis. The epiglottis *(arrows)* and aryepiglottic folds *(open arrows)* are markedly thickened in this patient with epiglottitis. The case is unusual in that it occurred in an adult (note the degenerative change in the cervical spine). Make this diagnosis on an upright lateral plain film, one of the last indications for plain radiography in neuroradiology.

1.5 (sensitivity, 44%; specificity, 87%) or epiglottitis should be suspected. Look for aryepiglottic folds enlargement and arytenoid swelling.

Croup Epiglottitis must be distinguished from croup. Croup is a viral infection that occurs in children younger than those affected by epiglottitis. Parainfluenza 1 or 2 and influenza A are the most common pathogens. Croup is characterized by edema of the glottis and subglottis such that the normal contours of the laryngeal ventricle and true cords are obliterated, and a smooth steeple-shaped laryngeal airway is produced. Croup is a much less morbid disease than epiglottitis and should be distinguishable on the basis of plain films (Table 14-5).

Wooof, wooof—sounds like the classic barking cough of croup.

Laryngotracheal papillomatosis Laryngotracheal papillomatosis refers to a viral infection that is seen most commonly in children and is probably due to transmission of the human papilloma (DNA) virus types 6 and 11 at the time of passage through the birth canal. The true cords are the most common laryngeal site. This disease is currently treated with laser surgery and steroids, but the papillomas commonly recur. When the branches of the trachea and bronchi are affected, postobstructive pneumonias and respiratory compromise may occur.

Granulomatous inflammatory conditions, including tuberculosis (TB), sarcoidosis, giant cell reparative granulomas, Wegener's granulomatosis, Langerhans histiocytosis, and candidiasis may affect the larynx. Of these, TB has a propensity for invading the cartilage. Relapsing polychondritis can affect the cricoarytentoid joints.

Crush injuries Crush injuries of the adult larynx usually involve fractures of the thyroid cartilage and/or cricoarytenoid joint dislocation. The classic scenario is an impact of the larynx against the steering wheel of a car. A mucosal tear may occur as an isolated finding or in combination with the cartilaginous fracture. Pneumomediastinum or subcutaneous air or air leakage into the paraglottic spaces may be present. The primary danger to the patient is loss of airway patency, particularly if swelling occurs or the cricoid cartilage is affected. Late sequelae include infection and chondritis as an exposed cartilaginous surface is a neat culture medium for bacteria. Crushed cartilages from car crashes can create crepitus, chondritis, and chondromalacia culminating in chili con carne for cricoids.

Benign Tumors

Papilloma The laryngeal papilloma is a true neoplasm (as opposed to a polyp) and, although benign, has a small association with squamous cell carcinoma. It appears as a small focal lesion on the vocal cord.

Hemangioma In childhood some lesions are to be considered in the subglottic region. These include the

Table 14-5 Differentiation of croup from epiglottitis		
Feature	Croup	Epiglottitis
Organism	Parainfluenza virus	*Haemophilus influenza* (children); streptococcus (adults)
Radiographic findings	Steeple-shaped subglottis	Thickened epiglottis, arytenoids, and aryepiglottic folds
Region of larynx	Glottic/subglottic	Supraglottic
Fever	No	Yes
Age at onset (yr)	<2	>2
Dysphagia	No	Yes

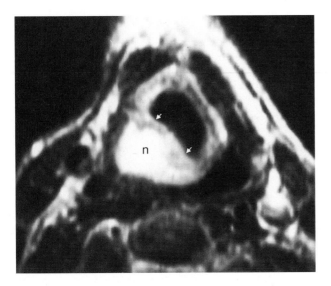

Fig. 14-36 Neurofibroma of the aryepiglottic fold. Axial T2WI portrays a submucosal mass arising from the left aryepiglottic fold. Note that the mucosa *(arrows)* appears to be normal and lower in intensity than the submucosal neurofibroma *(n).*

subglottic hemangioma and congenital subglottic stenosis. The subglottic capillary hemangioma is a benign neoplasm that generally occurs in 1- to 2-year-olds. Fifty percent of patients with subglottic hemangiomas have cutaneous hemangiomas as well. This is a benign tumor that often responds to steroid therapy, benign neglect (because it regresses with age) and/or laser therapy. In general, excisional treatment is not required except in those cases where extensive laryngeal narrowing is produced by the mass. On plain films the subglottic hemangioma causes an asymmetric narrowing of the airway of the subglottis. CT and MR reveal a smooth, enhancing mass that is asymmetric in the subglottis and that compromises the airway. In adults hemangiomas are usually supraglottic lesions.

Neurogenic tumors Another uncommon benign neoplasm that may be seen in children or adults and that usually affects the supraglottis is the schwannoma or the neurofibroma. The aryepiglottic fold and arytenoid region are most commonly involved, presumably because of superior laryngeal nerve involvement by the tumor (Fig. 14-36). These neoplasms appear as exophytic or submucosal masses that enhance.

Other rare benign tumors of the larynx include granular cell tumors, leiomyomas, and rhabdomyomas. Most extracardiac rhabdomyomas arise from pharyngeal constrictor muscles, the floor of the mouth, and the tongue base not the larynx. Paragangliomas and lipomas infrequently frequent the larynx.

Amyloidoma An amyloidoma of the larynx has a characteristic appearance on MR. The lesion is very hypointense on T1WI and T2WI and usually does not show enhancement. After the larynx (61% of cases), focal amyloidosis of the head and neck most commonly affects the

tongue and oropharynx (23%) (see Fig. 14-17), the trachea (9%), the orbit (4%), and the nasopharynx (3%). Rarely, amyloidosis may calcify. Chondromas of the larynx, on the other hand, have a signature appearance on CT, with whorls of calcification, usually centered on the cricoid cartilage.

Malignant Tumors

As opposed to a discussion of congenital, inflammatory, and benign masses in the larynx, an analysis of malignancies requires separation by anatomic subsites because of the different issues relevant to each site. Most of the dissertation that follows relates to the issues involved with treatment of squamous cell carcinoma, because minor salivary gland malignancies, lymphomas, sarcomas, and chondrosarcomas are so rare in the larynx.

Supraglottic squamous cell carcinoma Staging of supraglottic carcinoma is based on subsites of the supraglottis, cord mobility, and deep invasion (Box 14-8).

Because laryngeal conservation therapy is a hot area in head and neck surgery, the indications for supraglottic laryngectomy as opposed to total laryngectomy must be reviewed. In a supraglottic laryngectomy the epiglottis, false vocal cords, aryepiglottic folds, and preepiglottic fat are totally removed. If tumor extends to or below the laryngeal ventricle, a horizontal supraglottic laryngectomy, in which the surgical cut is through the plane

---

Box 14-8 T Staging of Supraglottic Cancer

T1 Tumor limited to one subsite of supraglottis with normal vocal cord mobility

T2 Tumor invades mucosa of more than one adjacent subsite of supraglottis or glottis, or region outside the supraglottis (e.g., mucosa of base of tongue, vallecula, medial wall of pyriform sinus) without fixation of the larynx

T3 Tumor limited to larynx with vocal cord fixation and/or invades any of the following: postcricoid area, pre-epiglottic tissues, paraglottic space, and/or minor thyroid cartilage erosion (e.g., inner cortex)

T4a Tumor invades through the thyroid cartilage and/or invades tissues beyond the larynx (e.g., trachea, soft tissues of neck including deep extrinsic muscle of the tongue, strap muscles, thyroid, or esophagus)

T4b Tumor invades prevertebral space, encases carotid artery, or invades mediastinal structures

Subsites: False cords, arytenoids, suprahyoid epiglottis, infrahyoid epiglottis, aryepiglottic folds

From Greene FL, Page DL, Fleming ID, et al (eds): *AJCC Cancer Staging Manual;* ed 6. New York, Springer-Verlag, 2002, p 48. Used with permission.

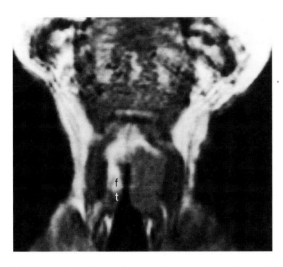

Fig. 14-37 Transglottic laryngeal carcinoma. Coronal T1WI shows a large mass in the left larynx. Lesion infiltrates the region of the false cord *(f)* and true cord *(t)* on the left side, and compresses the airway.

of the ventricle removing all laryngeal structures above but preserving thyroid cartilage cannot be performed (Fig. 14-37). Therefore, the presence of tumor at the upper margin of the true vocal cord is a critical branch in the surgical decision-making tree. In addition, if there is cartilaginous, postcricoid, or anterior commissure invasion, a supraglottic laryngectomy is not possible. The incidence of thyroid cartilage invasion is much higher than that of hyoid bone, arytenoid cartilage, or cricoid cartilage invasion, but thyroid cartilage extension usually occurs when the tumor is transglottic. Other contraindications to supraglottic laryngectomy (be it supracricoid or horizontal) include involvement of both arytenoid cartilages, arytenoid fixation (which implies cricoid cartilage invasion to the "blades"), or extensive bilateral involvement of the base of tongue and/or pre-epiglottic fat (Fig. 14-38).

It is important to understand that a supraglottic cancer may have extensive submucosal glottic and subglot-

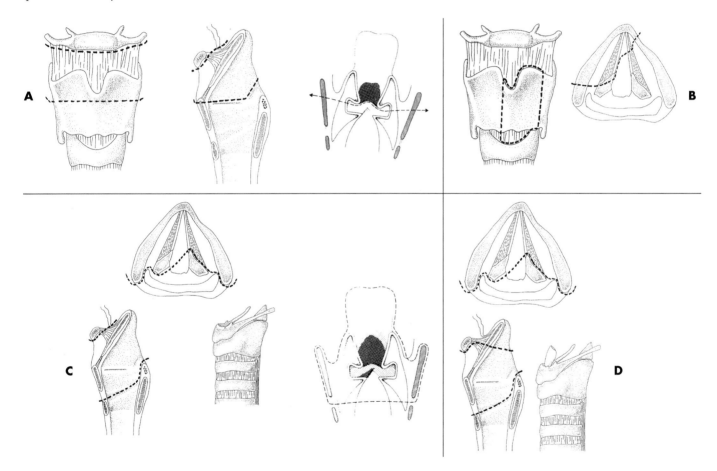

Fig. 14-38   A, The horizontal supraglottic laryngectomy removes the epiglottis and the upper margin of the thyroid cartilage. The plane of section crosses just above the laryngeal ventricle. The true vocal cords are preserved and the voice is good. **B,** The vertical hemilaryngectomy (VHL) removes a significant portion of the thyroid cartilage unilaterally and may extend anteriorly across the midline. If the VHL does not cross the midline, it may be called a frontolateral VHL; if it captures portions of the contralateral vocal cord, with or without the arytenoids, it may be termed an anterolateral VHL. The epiglottis is spared. **C,** The supracricoid laryngectomy with cricohyoidopexy removes all of the thyroid cartilage and epiglottis. One of the arytenoids is usually removed ipsilateral to the tumor. **D,** If a portion of the epiglottis is spared, the reconstruction is called a cricohyoidoepiglottopexy. The hyoid bone is spared with all voice conservation procedures. (From Maroldi R, Battaglis G, Nicolai P, et al: The appearance of the larynx after conservative and radical surgery for carcinomas, *Eur Radiol* 7:418-431, 1997.)

tic invasion, but look totally normal by endoscopy. The route of spread is submucosally into the paraglottic space, where the normal fat is readily permeable for the invasion of tumor. Epiglottic carcinoma likes to spread to the preepiglottic fat and from there can spread inferiorly to affect the petiole and anterior commissure of the glottis. Paraglottic spread is the mode du jour for aryepiglottic fold and false cord tumors. Invasion to the postcricoid region is usually limited to those affecting the posterior commissure or interarytenoid region. Because of these modes of deep spread, cancers can grow extensively invisible to endoscopy and masquerade as a relatively limited neoplasm. Coronal MR may be very helpful in deciding therapy by defining the extent of the tumor, because the tumor is well outlined by paraglottic fat at the false cord and ventricle levels. In contrast, the soft tissue lateral in the paraglottic space at the true cord level is the thyroarytenoid muscle and is readily separable from the fat above. The true cord is below the laryngeal ventricle.

Of all the laryngeal cancers, supraglottic and transglottic squamous cell carcinomas have the highest frequency of nodal metastases at presentation. This is because of the abundant lymphatics associated with the supraglottis as opposed to the relatively sparse lymphatics of the glottis.

As noted previously, the distinction between supraglottic and hypopharyngeal lesions gets blurred when the tumor extends from the aryepiglottic fold to the pyriform sinus and/or the posterior pharyngeal wall. Often it is difficult to determine the site of origin of a cancer that has spread in this fashion, but in either case an extended resection (partial laryngectomy), taking the pyriform sinus, may be required (Table 14-6).

The debate on whether CT or MR is the better method for evaluating the larynx for cartilaginous invasion has not been settled. The irregular ossification-calcification of the thyroid cartilage is particularly troublesome, and you will note that the T4 staging for supraglottic and glottic laryngeal carcinoma refers to thyroid cartilage invasion. Thus, the elastic cartilage of the epiglottis and the hyaline cartilage of the arytenoids are not considered in TNM staging, although they often are invaded with cancer. Cancer is said to preferentially invade ossified cartilage, infiltrating the bone marrow with ease compared with nonossified cartilage.

On CT, the absolute findings diagnostic of thyroid cartilage invasion are through-and-through erosion with extension of the mass into the strap muscles. Sclerosis of the cartilage may be a harbinger of cartilaginous invasion; in a recent study only 50% of patients with this finding had invasion, with the remainder showing only perichondrial involvement (Fig. 14-39). A cautionary note however. Areas of arytenoid sclerosis occur in 16% of normal subjects especially in the body of the arytenoid and more commonly in women. Other CT findings in-

clude lysis or destruction of cartilage or obliteration of the marrow space of ossified cartilage. Unfortunately CT tends to be relatively insensitive to cartilage invasion.

On MR, involvement of the strap muscles is a sure sign of thyroid cartilage invasion, but enhancement of tissue in the fat suppressed walls of the cartilage and brightening of intracartilaginous tissue on fat suppressed fast spin echo T2WI suggest early invasion (Fig. 14-40). Using these criteria, one finds that MR is very sensitive (85%) to cartilage invasion. Unfortunately, this is at a cost of decreased specificity as we now know that there is a ton of peritumoral inflammation around that can simulate neoplasm and can brighten signal on T2WI and cause enhancement. The patient and clinician end up in the radiologic nightmare—order a CT and you may underestimate disease, get caught with residual tumor, and have a worse prognosis, but save a voice box. Choose MR and you may remove a "clean" larynx, render the patient "speechless", but have a better chance of tumor free margins. AAAAAAAAAHHHH.! What a choice. Flip a coin.

Glottic squamous cell carcinoma (Fig. 14-41) The staging of squamous cell carcinoma of the glottis is also based on cord mobility and fixation as well as extension into adjacent soft tissue and/or cartilage (Box 14-9).

Because patients with squamous cell carcinoma of the glottis are seen early because of voice changes, the prog-

	Table 14-6 Supraglottic surgical procedures	
Lesion	**Minimal supraglottic procedure**
Small suprahyoid epiglottic lesion	Laser epiglottectomy
Infrahyoid epiglottic lesion (into preepiglottic fat)	Supraglottic laryngectomy
Unilateral arytenoid involvement	Extended supraglottic laryngectomy, taking arytenoid or supracricoid laryngectomy
Tongue base involvement (limited)	Extended supraglottic laryngectomy, taking unilateral tongue base
Aryepiglottic fold involvement	Extended supraglottic laryngectomy, taking unilateral pyriform sinus
True cord involvement or close to true cords	Supracricoid laryngectomy with cricohyoidopexy
Pyriform sinus involvement unilateral	Supracricoid hemilaryngopharyngectomy
Extension deep into subglottis, T4 lesions, or extensive pyriform sinus involvement	Total laryngectomy

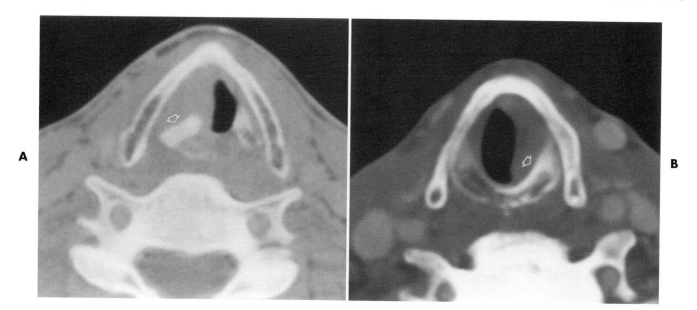

Fig. 14-39 Cartilage sclerosis. **A,** This glottic carcinoma has led to arytenoid sclerosis *(arrow)* on the right side. Although that is pretty obvious, the density change in the anterior half of the thyroid cartilage may be entirely normal. **B,** Do you buy the left cricoid sclerosis *(arrow)* in this patient with left vocal cord carcinoma?

nosis associated with this lesion is better than that elsewhere in the larynx. The cancer is usually detected at an earlier stage. If you're hoarse for very long, you usually see a doctor. See an ENT doc—she is more likely to pick up the cancer. Let the health care economist see the generalist who may treat his cancer as an inflammatory condition for 9 months (but at half the cost at least—dead people are cheaper to treat).

Just as the principal issue in treatment of supraglottic laryngeal carcinoma is its superior-inferior extension, the critical features in analyzing primary glottic carcinoma are its transverse and anterior-posterior dimensions. One

of the potential surgical treatments for primary glottic carcinoma is the vertical hemilaryngectomy (unilateral removal of the cord and supraglottic structures, sparing the contralateral side). This surgery leaves the patient with a working voice and is the preferred modality of treatment in the appropriate patient population. However, consideration of this therapy is contingent on the tumor not extending contralaterally beyond the anterior third of the opposite vocal cord (Table 14-7). Posterior extension into the arytenoid cartilages or the cricoid cartilage is also a contraindication to the vertical hemilaryngectomy. If the tumor extends superiorly or inferi-

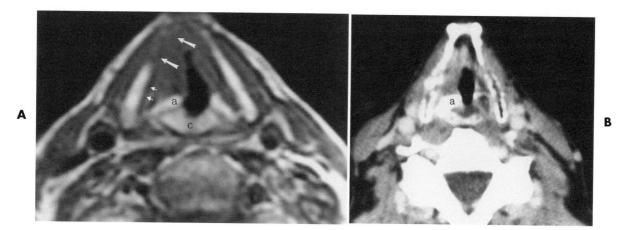

Fig. 14-40 Cartilaginous invasion by laryngeal carcinoma. **A,** Axial T1WI reveals invasion of the anterior aspect of the right thyroid cartilage *(large arrows)* by a glottic cancer. Note that the high signal intensity of the cartilaginous marrow and the low signal intensity of the edge of ossified cartilage *(small arrows)* are preserved. True cord level is well demonstrated at the crico*(c)*-arytenoid *(a)* joint. **B,** Axial CT scan demonstrates sclerosis of the arytenoid *(a)* cartilage on the right side of another patient with glottic carcinoma. Presence of sclerosis suggests perichondral invasion, which may be a harbinger of true cartilaginous invasion.

Illustration continued on following page

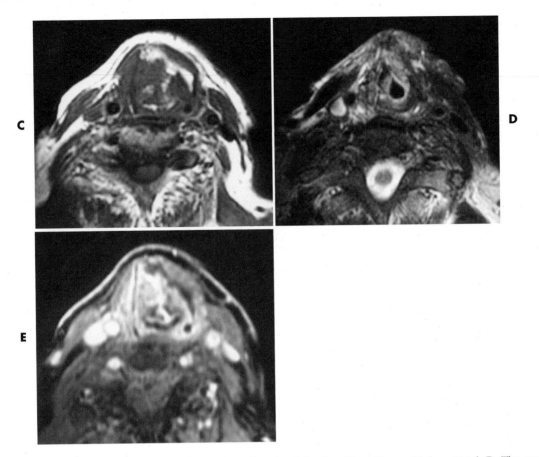

Fig. 14-40 *Continued.* **C,** T1WI shows replacement of the right side of the thyroid cartilage with low signal. **D,** The cartilage appears expanded and brighter than the contralateral side on the T2WI with fat suppression. **E,** With contrast, the cartilage shows pathologic enhancement with involvement of the strap muscles.

orly into the supraglottic or subglottic region, the possibility of a vertical hemilaryngectomy is lowered.

Glottic carcinomas may spread from the anterior commissure, via the neurovascular perforations through the thyrohyoid membrane to the soft tissues of the neck, to the paraglottic space, or to the subglottic compartment. This is difficult to visualize at office endoscopy and sometimes the presence of subglottic disease is initially

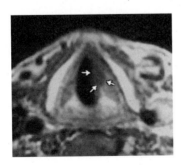

Fig. 14-41 T1 glottic carcinoma. Axial T1WI delineates a small focal mass *(arrows)* in the left true vocal cord. Mass did not impair cord mobility and was localized to the left side, thereby classifying it as a T1a lesion.

Box 14-9 T Staging of Glottic Cancer

T1   Tumor limited to the vocal cord(s) (may involve anterior or posterior commissure) with normal mobility

T1a Tumor limited to one vocal cord

T1b Tumor involves both vocal cords

T2   Tumor extends to supraglottis and/or subglottis, and/or with impaired vocal cord mobility

T3   Tumor limited to the larynx with vocal cord fixation and/or invades paraglottic space, and or minor thyroid cartilage erosion (e.g., inner cortex)

T4a Tumor invades through the thyroid cartilage and/or invades tissue beyond the larynx (e.g., trachea, soft tissues of neck including deep extrinsic muscle of the tongue, strap muscles, thyroid, or esophagus)

T4b Tumor invades prevertebral space, encases carotid artery, or invades mediastinal structures

Subsites: True cords including anterior commissure, posterior commissure

From Greene FL, Page DL, Fleming ID, et al (eds): *AJCC Cancer Staging Manual;* ed 6. New York, Springer-Verlag, 2002, p 48. Used with permission.

Table 14-7 Glottic surgical procedures

Lesion	Minimal glottic procedure
Very small midcord lesion	Excisional biopsy
Moderate-sized midcord lesion	Laser cordectomy
Large midcord lesion	Open cordectomy with false cord imbrication
Whole unilateral cord T1a	Vertical hemilaryngectomy
Bilateral cord T1b	Supracricoid laryngectomy with cricohyoidoepiglottopexy
T3, unilateral subglottic extension, pyriform sinus involvement	Near-total laryngectomy
T4	Total laryngectomy

Re: T2, T3 and selected T4 (eg, involving but not through thyroid cartilage) glottic cancer can be resected with SCL with CHEP or CHP.

borne out by imaging studies showing thickening in this location.

Supracricoid laryngectomies remove the supraglottic structures and the entire thyroid cartilage. This surgery requires at least one freely mobile arytenoid with no interarytenoid tumor and a clean cricoid cartilage for providing this option to the patient. Pharyngeal involvement and subglottic spread also are contraindications in most settings. Effectively, what happens is that the arytenoid apposes to the tongue base to allow speech and sphincteric function. This requires a "pexy" procedure in which the cricoid is suspended from the hyoid bone.

As with all laryngeal carcinomas, the presence of cartilaginous invasion or extension into the adjacent soft tissues is very important. As stated previously, the risk of lymphatic invasion is much lower with glottic carcinoma. Only when the tumor extends to the supraglottis or subglottis is expectant treatment of the lymph nodes required.

T1 and T2 glottic carcinomas may be treated with radiation therapy alone in some instances. The cure rates for T1 glottic carcinoma with either surgery or radiation are approximately 90%. However, the quality of the voice is generally better after focal localized radiation therapy. The radiation therapy usually does not include the lymph node chains because of the sparse lymphatics involved.

Chondroradionecrosis One of the most catastrophic of iatrogenic mishaps to affect the larynx is chondroradionecrosis. This may occur in some unusual individuals after standard doses of radiotherapy for laryngeal neoplasms, but is, thankfully, rare to see. The hallmarks of chondroradionecrosis are soft-tissue swelling of the larynx, sloughing of the arytenoid cartilage with subluxation, fragmentation, sclerosis, and collapse of the thyroid cartilage, and/or the presence of gas bubbles around the cartilage (Fig. 14-42). Super infection often occurs. Invariably, this entity requires a total laryngectomy, which often was the surgical extreme that the therapists were hoping to avoid by going with radiation therapy for the cancer.

Chondroid tumors The malignancies other than squamous cell carcinoma that affect the vocal cords include the chondroid tumors. The cricoid cartilage is associated with chondromas and chondrosarcomas. These lesions are identified on CT by their "popcorn-like" whorls of calcification caused by the chondroid matrix of the tumor. Distinguishing a benign from a malignant chondroid tumor is sometimes difficult; in the larynx the chondrosarcomas are usually low-grade and slow growers. They are often treated with piecemeal resection. Chondrosarcomas account for less than 1% of laryngeal malignancies, are seen in the 40 to 60 age range and predilect males by 5 to 10 to 1. Over 70% arise in the cricoid cartilage.

A neoplasm that has characteristics of both squamous cell carcinoma and sarcoma is known as the spindle cell sarcoma or carcinosarcoma. This lesion is rarely seen

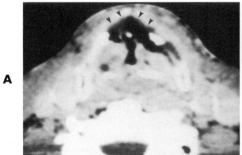 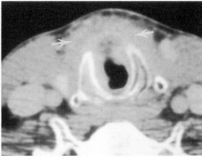

A   **B**

Fig. 14-42 Chondronecrosis of the larynx. **A,** Loss of the anterior portions of the thyroid cartilage bilaterally is coupled with extralaryngeal air in the pre- and paraglottic soft tissues *(arrowheads)*. Fragmentation is typical. Note the absence of fat planes characteristic of the irradiated neck. **B,** At the cricoid level the necrotic tissue *(arrows)* is seen projecting anteriorly into the strap muscles. (A, compliments of Hugh Curtin, M.D., Boston MA).

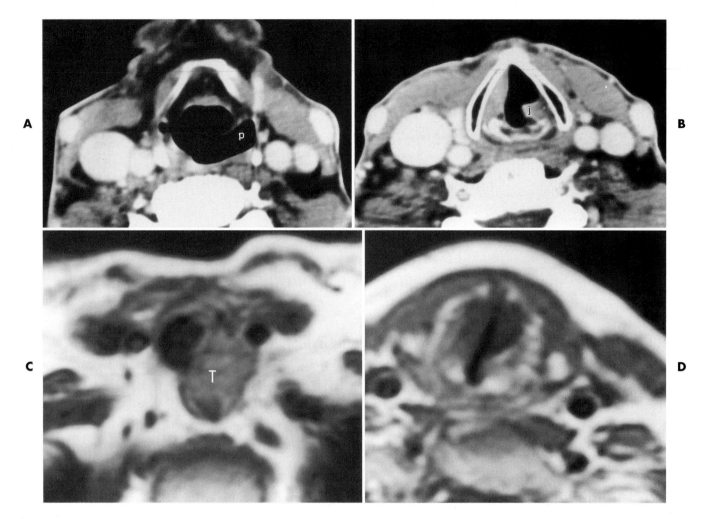

Fig. 14-43   Montage of vocal cord paralysis. Case 1. Left-sided vocal cord paralysis. **A,** Axial CT through the supraglottic larynx demonstrates dilatation of the left pyriform sinus *(p).* Aryepiglottic fold on the left side is more medially oriented than that on the right. **B,** Note the cord atrophy suggesting chronic vocal cord paralysis on the left side. In addition, there is medial orientation of the cricoarytenoid joint *(j)* and the remaining vocal cord tissue. The source of this patient's vocal cord paralysis was not evident because the resident forgot to scan inferiorly to the aortic arch, where the nerve circles before doubling back in the tracheoesophageal groove. That same resident has become a very successful imaging center entrepreneur. Case 2. **C,** The culprit: Residual thyroid carcinoma *(T)* in the left tracheoesophageal groove, picking off the left recurrent laryngeal nerve. **D,** The effect: Arytenoid rotation, reduced size of the left posterior cricoarytenoid muscle, and cord atrophy.

Illustration continued on following page

elsewhere in the aerodigestive tract besides the larynx. Its prognosis is similar to that of squamous cell carcinoma in the larynx, and therefore the histologic distinction does not generally alter therapy or prognostic consideration. Radiation therapy in carcinosarcoma produces similar control rates to irradiated patients with similar volume disease with the more typical squamous cell carcinoma.

Vocal cord paralysis   In the investigation of vocal cord paralysis, you should follow the course of the vagus and recurrent laryngeal nerve on the scans and include the skull base and the superior mediastinum. Remember the anatomy from a couple pages back? Or do you not have the vagus node-tion of what we are talk-

ing about? The recurrent laryngeal nerve loops around the subclavian artery on the right side and the aortic arch on the left. Separate causes of vagal neuropathy into those lesions above the hyoid bone and those below. Metastases to the jugular foramen, glomus tumors, schwannomas, nasopharyngeal carcinomas, and chordomas account for the majority of skull base causes of vocal cord paralysis (Fig. 14-43). Because slips of the vagus also supply the pharynx at the suprahyoid level, some swallowing and gag reflex dysfunction should be associated with lesions of the high vagus. If you find pharyngeal muscle atrophy or a deviated uvula on your imaging studies, insist the etiology is an upper vagus nerve lesion—remember that the gag is sensory IX and motor

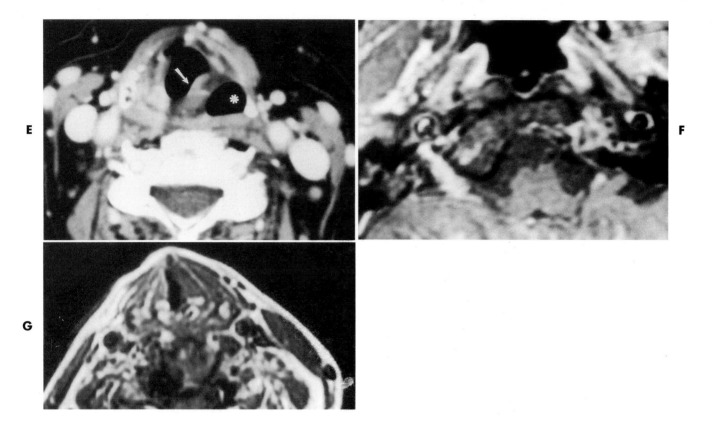

Fig. 14-43   *Continued.* **E,** Other findings on CT: left piriform sinus dilatation as the left aryepiglottic fold slides medially. Case 3. **F,** Second culprit: Lymphoma in jugular foramen affecting vagus nerve. **G,** Atrophic fatty replaced right true vocal cord implies long-standing disease.

X and can be politically motivated. Cranial nerves IX, XI, and XII travel with the vagus in its uppermost segment; therefore lesions affecting the vagus superiorly usually (95%) affect one or all of these cranial nerves as well.

Below the hyoid bone, an isolated vocal cord paralysis may be seen without pharyngeal effects. The common lesions causing lower vagus abnormalities are related to lesions in and around the carotid sheath including squamous cell carcinoma, thyroid masses, glomus vagale tumors, schwannomas, posttraumatic dissections and pseudoaneurysms, intraoperative injury, and lymphadenopathy. In the mediastinum lymphoma, bronchogenic carcinoma, lymphadenopathy, patent ductus arteriosus, mitral stenosis (due to the associated pulmonary artery dilatation), aneurysms, and arterial dissections may cause recurrent laryngeal nerve paralysis. Situated in the tracheoesophageal groove as it ascends to the larynx after exiting the mediastinum, the nerve is susceptible to lesions in the thyroid gland (cancer, goiter, and trauma), the parathyroid tissue (adenoma and carcinoma), and esophagus (Zenker's diverticulum, perforation).

Several imaging findings suggest the presence of vocal cord paralysis: (1) atrophy of the cord (thyroarytenoid muscle), (2) dilatation of the laryngeal ventricle, (3) medial orientation of the vocal cord, (4) dilatation of the ipsilateral pyriform sinus and vallecula, (5) medial orientation and angulation of the aryepiglottic fold, and (6) anteromedial deviation of the arytenoid cartilage (see Fig. 14-43). Recently, a new finding has been brought to our attention, that of posterior cricoarytenoid (PCA) muscle atrophy as this is one of the intrinsic muscles of the larynx innervated by the recurrent laryngeal nerve. Atrophy of the PCA muscle is found in over half of patients with vocal cord paralysis but less than 5% of radiologists can identify this muscle (Fig. 14-44). Curious.

Subglottic squamous cell carcinoma   Subglottic squamous cell carcinomas constitute less than 5% of all laryngeal carcinomas. These lesions are very difficult to identify at indirect or fiberoptic endoscopy because visualization of the undersurface of the vocal cord or the proximal trachea may be obscured by the shadow of apposed true cords. The best views are obtained under supported direct laryngoscopy in the operating room.

The staging of subglottic laryngeal carcinoma is similar to that in the glottis and supraglottis and deals principally with cord mobility, cartilaginous destruction, or extension to the soft tissues of the neck (Box 14-10). The prognosis for subglottic lesions is generally poor because by the time the diagnosis is made, the lesion is generally fairly extensive. It may infiltrate the trachea,

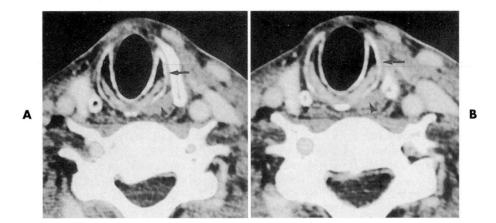

Fig. 14-44   Right vocal cord paralysis. **A** and **B,** Two consecutive axial CT scans in a patient with a right-sided glomus vagale show atrophy of the right PCA muscle and right cricothyroid muscle relative to the normal left side (*arrowhead* indicates normal left PCA muscle; *arrow,* normal left cricothyroid muscle). (From Romo LV, Curtin HD: Atrophy of the posterior cricoarytenoid muscle as an indicator of recurrent laryngeal nerve palsy. *AJNR* 20:467-471, 1999.)

esophagus, and even the thyroid gland. Remember to look at the paratracheal, esophageal, anterior visceral (Delphian-level VI), and upper mediastinal nodal chains when you find a subglottic cancer. The mucosa of the subglottis is pencil thin. Any nodularity or thickening must be suspected of being cancerous on any imaging modality (Fig. 14-45).

The major issue when examining a patient for subglottic carcinoma is whether there is paraglottic, glottic and/or supraglottic extension at the time of diagnosis. Because surgical resection of subglottic carcinomas nearly always requires cricoid cartilage resection, total laryngectomy is usually performed. Take it from the noted head and neck surgeon, Johnnie Cochran: "If over 1.0 cm of subglottic extension is in doubt, the larynx must come out."

Below the inferior surface of the cricoid cartilage the tumors are referred to as tracheal lesions rather than sub-

glottic laryngeal lesions. Tracheal carcinomas are much less common than laryngeal carcinomas and enter the realm of pulmonary radiology. We will stop here.

To detect recurrences of squamous cell carcinoma nuclear medicine studies and a prayer may be useful. Pray that the clinicians actually get the baseline CT or MR study you recommend at 8 weeks after all therapies (Fig. 14-46). Since that is not likely, rely on PET and thallium-201 SPECT scans for differentiating recurrent squamous cell carcinoma from posttreatment changes if the CT findings are not clear cut. As expected, growing tumors are hot. The limitations of these studies are predominantly attributable to lower resolution and the nuclear medicine doctors not understanding the anatomy of

---

Box 14-10   T Staging of Subglottic Cancer

T1	Tumor limited to the subglottis
T2	Tumor extends vocal cord(s) with normal or impaired mobility
T3	Tumor limited to larynx with vocal cord fixation
T4a	Tumor invades cricoid or thyroid cartilage and/or invades tissues beyond the larynx (e.g., trachea, soft tissues of neck including deep extrinsic muscles of the tongue, strap muscles, thyroid, or esophagus)
T4b	Tumor invades prevertebral space, encases carotid artery, or invades mediastinal structures

From Greene FL, Page DL, Fleming ID, et al (eds): *AJCC Cancer Staging Manual;* ed 6. New York, Springer-Verlag, 2002, p 48. Used with permission.

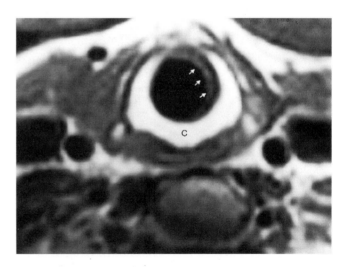

Fig. 14-45   Subglottic carcinoma. Axial T1WI demonstrates thickening of the mucosa (*arrows*) along the left subglottic region. At this level one should not see any thickness to the mucosa of the subglottic larynx. Note the high signal of the cricoid cartilage (*c*).

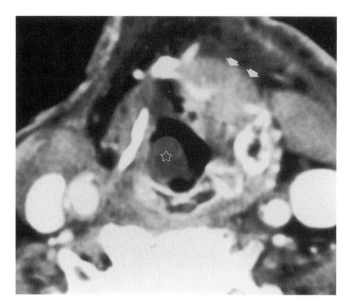

Fig. 14-46 Recurrent carcinoma after radiation. Note the soft tissue mass *(arrows)* along the left thyroid cartilage in this patient with recurrent squamous cell carcinoma. An unusual mucous retention cyst *(star)* protrudes into the lumen of the larynx.

this region and not being able to speaky dee Eenglishp langage. Combined PET-CT scanners are ideal for detecting primary tumor or nodal recurrences. PET-CT studies may also predict response to therapy. Be careful of scans within 6 weeks of treatment; false positive studies abound.

LYMPH NODES

Although the lymph nodes are not a part of the mucosa of the head and neck, it seems more relevant to discuss the nodes in the chapter dealing with squamous cell carcinoma. The most common cause of nodal disease in an adult is a squamous cell carcinoma metastasis from a mucosal primary tumor.

Anatomy

The nomenclature of the lymph nodes of the neck has undergone a recent change, which is supported by various societies of head and neck surgeons. (Because we support the notion that the customer is always right similar to Arthur Anderson and ENRON, we will learn this new classification of nodes.) This nomenclature identifies the lymph nodes by a grading system from I to VII (Fig. 14-47). Little labor in learning levels of lymph nodes leads to learned lymphatic luminaries. Level I lymph nodes include the submental and submandibular lymph node chains. Level II lymph nodes include the internal jugular lymph node chain above the hyoid bone. These

nodes include the jugulodigastric node, a node that sits along the posterior belly of the digastric muscle at the upper pharyngeal level. Level III lymph nodes involve the jugular chain between the hyoid and cricoid cartilage, and level IV lymph nodes involve the jugular chain below the cricoid cartilage. Level V is designated as all the lymph nodes of the posterior triangle of the neck (deep and posterior to the sternocleidomastoid muscle and above the clavicle). Level VI lymph nodes are those which previously were identified in the anterior jugular and visceral chain in front of the thyroid gland. Finally, level VII nodes are in the superior mediastinum region. Although some now split level I nodes into Ia (submental) and Ib (submandibular nodes) and classify level V nodes into Va (above cricoid) versus Vb (below cricoid to clavicle), this has yet to be universally accepted and only adds letters to a number system that already taxes the radiologist's capabilities. Add a IIa, IIIa, and IVa to

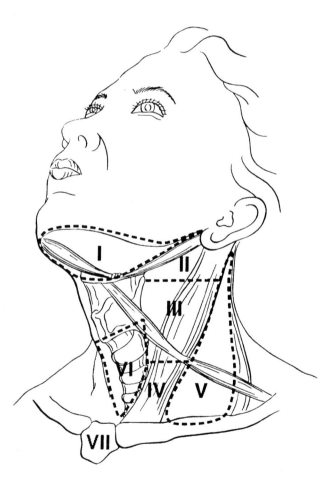

Fig. 14-47 Nomenclature of lymphadenopathy. The seven nodal regions are displayed in this diagram. The true delineation between levels II and III is the carotid bifurcation, but it has been accepted to use the hyoid as that landmark. Similarly, the boundary between III and IV is the omohyoid muscle, but radiologists use the cricoid cartilage on axial scans as the landmark. (From Greene FL, Page DL, Fleming ID, et al (eds): AJCC Cancer Staging Manual, 6th ed, New York, Springer, 2002, p 19.)

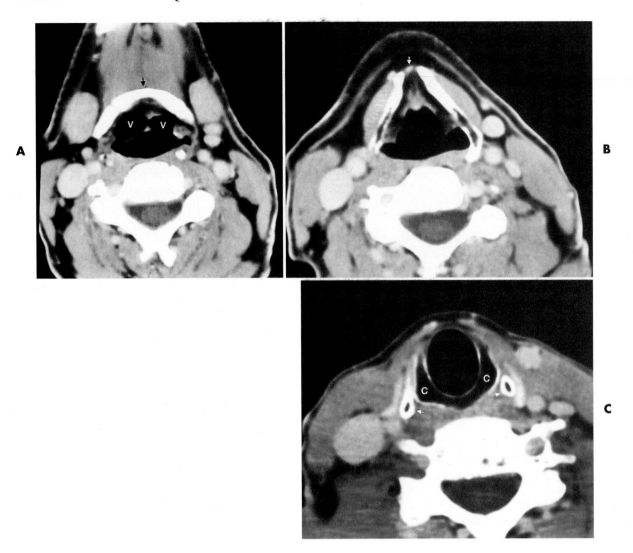

Fig. 14-48 Hyoid, thyroid, and cricoid levels. **A,** Often the hyoid bone is completely ossified *(arrow)*. It is characterized by a smooth arching curvature and is usually located at the level of the carotid bifurcation, vallecula *(v)*, or epiglottic tip. **B,** The thyroid cartilage usually is more angulated, less curved than the hyoid, and, at the upper levels, will have a midline notch *(arrow)*. The aryepiglottic folds, false and true cords will identify this level. **C,** The cricoid cartilage is the only one with a complete posterior ring (signet-shaped, smaller in front). The true cords and subglottic region are seen at the level of the cricoid ring. The inferior cornua of the thyroid cartilage *(arrows)* are seen in this section.

account for nodes around the jugular whereas IIb, IIIb, and IVb are posterior to the jugular vein and whoa, you have reached the saturation point. This classification assumes that you know how to distinguish the hyoid bone from the thyroid cartilage and the cricoid cartilage (complete ring), because most nodes are found in levels II to IV (Fig. 14-48).

"**To be a node, or not to be a node: that is the question**" How did William Shakespeare, LMD, FMG, differentiate a lymph node from a vessel or a slip of muscle? On rapid-bolus enhanced CT, nodes are distinguished from vessels by their lack of bright enhancement. A vessel is seen to track down or up the neck and usually bifurcates. Nodes, although they may be oblong, do not

appear tubular as does a vessel. To distinguish a node from muscle on CT is sometimes difficult unless you know the muscular anatomy well. Usually, the only area of confusion is distinguishing a jugulodigastric node from the posterior belly of the digastric. The latter courses anteromedially and ultimately travels along the undersurface of the mylohyoid muscle as the anterior belly of the digastric muscle. On MR, vessels demonstrate flow voids whereas nodes are soft tissue. Vessels often have phase ghosting artifacts caused by flow, whereas nodes are stationary. On T2WI muscles are very hypointense whereas the nodes are bright especially on fat-suppressed fast spin echo imaging. On T1WI nodes are isointense with muscle. Again, knowing the muscular anatomy will help you,

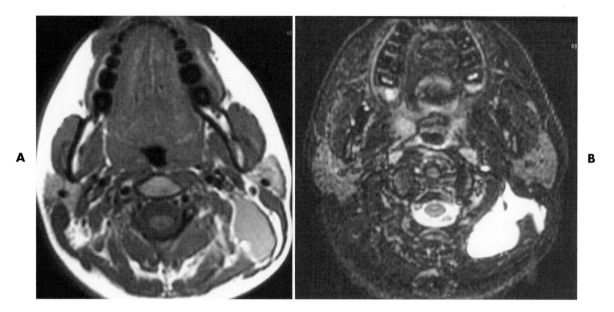

Fig. 14-49   Cystic hygroma. Riddle me this, Batman: What is bright on a T1WI **(A)**, intensely bright on a T2WI **(B)**, nonenhancing, multiloculated, and located in the posterior triangle of the neck in a child? Two points for a cystic hygroma, Robin!

until you cheat and look at the T2WI for brightness (designating a node). If they are large and bright, the surgeon's knife will bite.

Congenital Lesions

Cystic hygroma   Congenital lymphatic lesions of the head and neck (in decreasing size) include cystic hygromas, cavernous lymphangiomas, and capillary lymphangiomas. Most cystic hygromas are apparent at birth (50% to 60%) and are seen most commonly in the neck (75%) and axilla (20%) (Fig. 14-49). Cystic hygromas may transilluminate. Occasionally, they may be diagnosed in utero because of polyhydramnios. They are usually hypodense and multiloculated on CT and have variable intensity on T1WI and T2WI because of their proteinaceous-chylous-hemorrhagic content. The mass may present acutely as a result of spontaneous or posttraumatic intralesional hemorrhage. The cystic hygroma is not invasive, being compressible and distorted by arteries. The cause of these lesions is thought to be obstruction of the primitive lymphatic channels that are derived from the venous system early in gestation. An association with Turner syndrome, Noonan syndrome, and fetal alcohol syndrome is well-described.

Inflammatory Lesions

Adenitis   Children seem to have a predilection for dramatic adenitis. Posterior triangle reactive adenopathy often accompanies the ubiquitous middle ear infections of young childhood. Pharyngitis can lead to complica-

tions of retropharyngitis, now recognized as an inflammatory process usually mediated by retropharyngeal adenitis, not direct spread (Fig. 14-50). Nonetheless, it can be a fulminant infection that can require surgical intervention.

Tuberculous adenitis   The classic cause of an inflammatory cervical adenitis is tuberculous adenitis (scrofula), usually seen in Southeast Asians. The patients have painless posterior neck masses with or without systemic symptoms. The source of the infection is usually contaminated milk associated with *Mycobacterium bovis,* causing a subclinical pharyngitis. In the United States *Mycobacterium tuberculosis* is the most common cause. Atypical mycobacteria (*Mycobacterium scrofulaceum* especially) may also cause tuberculous adenitis. Concomitant pulmonary tuberculosis is relatively uncommon. The disease manifests as bilateral low density necrotic lymph nodes, often in the level 5 posterior triangle distribution (Fig. 14-51). The nodes often have ring-like thick enhancement and appear multiloculated. Adjacent fat planes are obscured or edematous. The nodes often calcify after treatment (Box 14-11). The differential diagnosis of calcified nodes should include tuberculosis, other granulomatous diseases (fungi, sarcoidosis, and Thorotrast granulomas) treated lymphoma, anthrosilicosis, and metastatic thyroid carcinoma, adenocarcinoma, or squamous carcinoma.

Castleman disease   Castleman disease (angiofollicular hyperplasia) is a nodal disease that can be seen in the chest (70% of cases) and the head and neck (10%). Usually the patient is asymptomatic and less than 30 years old. The unique feature of these nodes is their avid en-

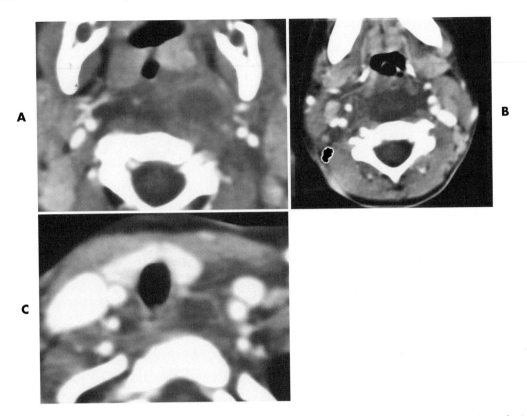

Fig. 14-50 Retropharyngeal adenitis. **A,** A retropharyngeal low density collection likely represents necrotizing adenitis from the antecedent pharyngitis. Note the low density in the retropharyngeal space away from the node that may be due to either edema or phlegmon. **B,** Spread inferiorly from the nasopharyngeal level can occur due to the potential space afforded by the retropharyngeal fat and "danger space." (Ah! but that is better left for a discussion in Chapter 15, Virginia) **C,** Spreading all the way down to the tracheal level is possible—and beyond.

hancement because of hypervascular stroma (Fig. 14-52). The nodes are nonnecrotic. There may be a stellate area of nonenhancement in the center of the enhancing nodes.

Mononucleosis Mononucleosis, caused by Epstein-Barr virus infection, is another inflammatory source of multiple enlarged nonnecrotic lymph nodes. The differential diagnosis includes AIDS and sarcoidosis. In AIDS and mononucleosis the lymphoid tissue of Waldeyer's ring (adenoids, palatine tonsils, and lingual tonsils) may be hypertrophied and bilateral nodes are the rule (Fig. 14-53). If intraparotid lymphoepithelial cysts are present, human immunodeficiency virus infection is more likely. If the parotid glands are enlarged and infiltrated diffusely, sarcoidosis may be suggested but a chest radiograph with bihilar adenopathy may be the best clue. Otherwise the differential diagnosis may rely on serology or the appropriate (kissing) history.

Cat scratch fever Another "zebra" that can cause bilateral lymph nodes, including intraparotid nodes, is cat scratch fever. There often is edema surrounding the nodes. The etiologic agent in this infection has recently been characterized as a gram negative intracellular bacterium (*Bartonella henselae*). If you quiz the clinician about a cat scratch history and actually come up with the

diagnosis, you'll be a star in his or her eyes forever. It is a self-limited disease that may manifest regional lymphadenopathy, fever, and malaise, but can progress to encephalopathy and neuropathy after a cat scratch or flea bite. Parinaud oculoglandular syndrome, characterized by unilateral conjunctivitis with polypoid granuloma of the palpebral conjunctiva, and preauricular, parotid, and periparotid lymphadenopathy can be caused by *Bartonella* infections. The diagnosis is confirmed by positive serologic tests or positive PCR assays to the bacterium.

Sinus histiocytosis Sinus histiocytosis may cause massive nodes. These may develop egg-shell calcification after interferon therapy.

Kikuchi disease Kikuchi disease, histiocytic necrotizing lymphadenitis, predominantly affects young adults of Asian ethnicity. The etiology is unclear, but is probably viral, and the patients present with adenopathy, fever, and leukopenia. It is associated with large necrotic and nonnecrotic, enhancing and nonenhancing adenopathy. The CT appearance of Kikuchi disease can simulate lymphoma and other nodal diseases that have necrosis, such as metastasis and tuberculosis. Ki Kareful not to Miss Kikuchi!

Kimura disease Kimura disease is another import from the Far East. It is a chronic inflammatory process

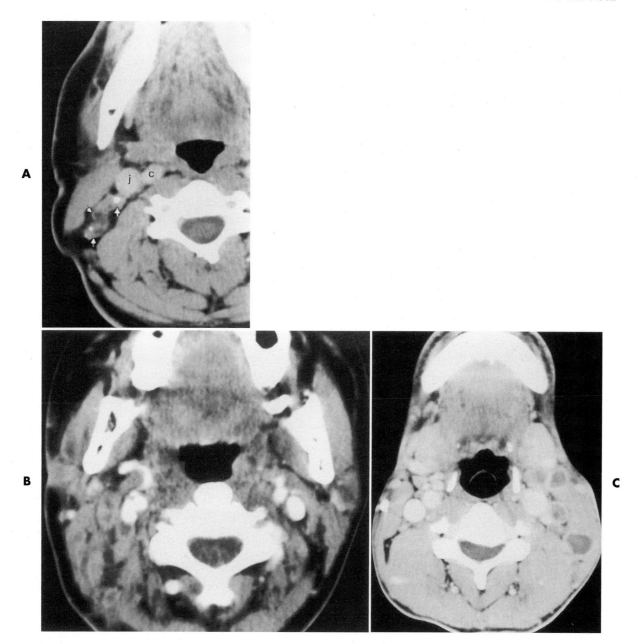

Fig. 14-51   Gallery of tuberculous adenitis. **A,** Scrofula. Axial enhanced CT demonstrates calcified lymph nodes *(arrows)* in the posterior triangle (level V) of the neck in this patient with a history of tuberculous adenitis. Note that the lymph nodes are well differentiated from jugular *(j)* and carotid *(c)* vessels seen anteriorly and medially. **B,** The necrotic nodes in the right neck with soft tissue stranding and irregular margination begs the diagnosis of TB adenitis especially in a young person. **C,** Enhanced CT shows rim enhancing nodes in the left neck infiltrated with "red snappers."

Box 14-11   Causes of Calcified Lymph Nodes

1. Tuberculous adenitis
2. Radiated lymphoma nodes
3. Thyroid metastases
4. Mucinous adenocarcinoma metastases
5. Rarely inactive (burnt-out) inflammatory nodes
6. Granulomatous (nontuberculosis) infections
7. Thorotrast

---

with associated diffuse hypervascular adenopathy in the cervical chains favoring the submental and submandibular regions, eosinophilia, and a predilection for Asian men aged 10 to 30. The salivary glands may be swollen and tender. The nodes are round, solid, hypoechoic, and homogeneous. They have hilar hypervascularity on power doppler scans (hey, since this is an Asian import, the sonographic features are what is best known about the disease).

Posttransplant lymphoproliferative disorder Posttransplant lymphoproliferative disorder (PTLD) is one of

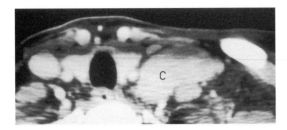

Fig. 14-52   Castleman disease. The nodal mass on this enhanced CT scan is of the same density as the thyroid gland. Such enhancing node *(c)* is suggestive of angiofollicular hyperplasia (Castleman disease), thyroid carcinoma, Kaposi sarcoma, some lymphomas, and Kimura disease.

these cross-over diseases between a reactive node, a benign neoplasm, and a malignant neoplasm. Basically, you can find enlarged nodes in the abdomen, chest, and neck (in descending order of frequency) in patients after whole organ transplants (heart, liver, kidney, or bone marrow). The inciting event appears to be an infection by Epstein Barr virus, leading to a proliferation of B cells. If the T cells are deficient, as in transplant patients or HIV infections, this B-cell mass production gets revved up. Although this may result in a polyclonal lymphoproliferation, if unabated, a monoclonal dominant spike may appear. In some of these patients, lymphoma develops; in others the adenopathy resolves with manipulation of medications to produce a reduction in the degree of immunosuppression. Chemotherapy may be required in some. In addition to enlarged lymph nodes,

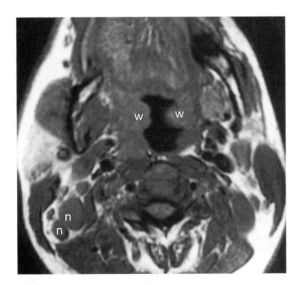

Fig. 14-53   Large lymph nodes with Waldeyer's ring lymphoid hyperplasia. Note the enlarged lymph nodes *(n)* in the neck and the enlargement of Waldeyer's ring tissue in the palatine tonsils *(w)*. Differential diagnosis includes AIDS, mononucleosis, lymphoma, sarcoidosis, or pharyngeal carcinoma with malignant lymphadenopathy.

adenoidal, lingual, and palatine tonsillar hypertrophy may be present with PTLD.

Benign Neoplasms

No benign neoplasms typically cause lymphadenopathy (short section, yea!).

Malignant Neoplasms

Squamous cell carcinoma   The staging of lymph nodes and distant metastases in the TNM classification is noted in Boxes 14-12, 14-13, 14-14.

The critical numbers to remember are less than or equal to 3 cm for N1 nodes, 3 to 6 cm for N2 lymph nodes, and greater than 6 cm for the N3 classification. Nodal infiltration from carcinoma of the nasopharynx is present in 80% of patients and is bilateral in 50%. The first echelon of drainage is to lateral retropharyngeal nodes. From there, the high jugular (level II, jugulodigastric) and posterior triangle (level V) chains are next to be infiltrated. The nodal staging for the nasopharynx is "special"; N0 no nodes, N1 unilateral supraclavicular node 6 cm or less, N2 bilateral supraclavicular nodes 6 cm or less, and N3 nodes greater than 6 cm or into the supraclavicular region. Issues other than pure size criteria include the presence (or absence) of central nodal necrosis, which suggests tumor no matter what the size.

Box 14-12   N (Nodal) Staging Criteria for Oral Cavity, Oropharynx, Hypopharynx, Paranasal Sinuses, and Larynx

NX: Regional lymph nodes cannot be assessed
N0:   No regional lymph node metastasis
N1:   Metastasis in single ipsilateral lymph node, ≤3 cm in greatest dimension
N2:   Metastasis in single ipsilateral lymph node, >3 cm but ≤6 cm in greatest dimension, or multiple ipsilateral lymph nodes, none >6 cm in greatest dimension, or bilateral or contralateral lymph nodes, none >6 cm in greatest dimension
N2a: Metastasis in single ipsilateral lymph node >3 cm but ≤6 cm in greatest dimension
N2b: Metastasis in multiple ipsilateral lymph nodes, none >6 cm in greatest dimension
N2c: Metastasis in bilateral or contralateral lymph nodes, none >6 cm in greatest dimension
N3:   Metastasis in lymph node >6 cm in greatest dimension

From Greene FL, Page DL, Fleming ID, et al (eds): *AJCC Cancer Staging Manual;* ed 6. New York, Springer-Verlag, 2002, p 36. Used with permission.

When the lymph nodes are being evaluated, it is important to analyze whether extracapsular extension (spread outside the confines of the lymph node to the adjacent soft tissue) is present because it reduces the 5-year prognosis by 50% and often leads to local treatment failure (Box 14-15). The incidence of extracapsular spread of tumor correlates with the nodal size. Histopathologically, 23% of nodes less than 1 cm, 53% of nodes 2 to 3 cm, and 74% of nodes greater than 3 cm in transverse diameter have extracapsular extension (Fig. 14-54). Measure those nodes!

The clinical evaluation of the lymph nodes relies on the gift of palpation. The numbers argue that even in the best of hands, over 20% of patients with N0 necks clinically have occult nodal metastases. Our mission is to improve on that number. Most patients with T2 cancers undergo a neck disection even if they are N0. Of the positive specimens from neck disections of N0 patients (around

30% of cases), 25% reveal metastases less than 3 mm in size. Can we honestly expect to find these lesions?

There has been considerable debate about the appropriate size criteria to identify lymph nodes as enlarged and therefore infiltrated with neoplasm. Again and again size does matter in the head and neck. Masters of the mucosa must measure masses. But, for a change, smaller is better. The debate centers on millimeters, some favoring 10 mm, some 12 mm, and some 15 mm as the maximum normal transverse diameter of a reactive node. Most would agree that at greater than 15 mm the node should be considered neoplastic until proved otherwise. Retropharyngeal nodes should not exceed 8 mm in diameter. More leeway is given to the highest jugular node (jugulodigastric node) and submandibular nodes, but read on, faithful student, and you will see that despite these guidelines, radiology ain't cutting the mustard in predicting neoplastic infiltration of nodes.

A recent dog of an RDOG (Radiology Diagnostic Oncology Group) study looked at how well we in imaging do at predicting neoplastic invasion in nodes. The answer is that we are abysmal. In this large multi-institutional study of thousands of nodes they found that using

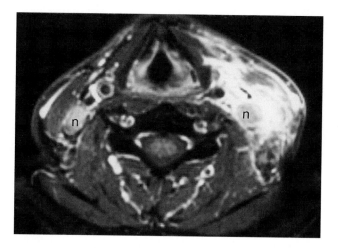

Fig. 14-54   Extranodal spread of tumor. Fat-suppressed, enhanced T1WI readily depicts the spread of neoplasm from the lymph node *(n)* into the soft tissues of the neck. The presence of extracapsular spread portends a worse prognosis and problems obtaining "clean margins" at surgery.

Table 14-8   Lymph node size and pathology

Size	CT sensitivity	CT specificity	MR sensitivity	MR specificity
5mm	98%	13%	92%	20%
8mm	95%	22%	87%	31%
10mm	88%	39%	81%	48%
12mm	74%	67%	66%	72%
15mm	56%	84%	51%	86%

(From Curtin HD, Ishwaran H, Mancuso AA, Dalley RW, et al: Comparison of CT and MR imaging in staging of neck metastases, *Radiology*, 207:123–130, 1998)

the 10 mm cut off, CT was only 39% specific and 88% sensitive for detecting disease and MR did not fare much better (48% and 81% respectively). With use of a 10-mm size or central necrosis to indicate a positive node, CT had an NPV of 84% and a PPV of 50%, and MR imaging had an NPV of 79% and a PPV of 52% (Table 14-8).

RDOG found that one had to use a 5 mm cut-off to achieve a 10% error rate of a negative study (1 − the negative predictive value), but that left a false positive rate of 56%. Why are we even doing these studies then? Good question! In many cases, whether we say there are nodes or not, the surgeons go ahead and treat the necks. They want to pick up the 20% to 30% of cases with microscopic disease. They know that some primary tumors, such as oropharyngeal, hypopharyngeal, and supraglottic cancers have such a high rate of nodal involvement (in the 60% range) that they are simply going to treat regardless of what they feel, you see, and Aunt Minnie wants. Furthermore, they tend to take out the nodes because it affords them better access to the primary tumor with that fatty nodal stuff removed. It is in the way! Get it out! They realize that the incidence of malignant cervical lymphadenopathy with squamous cell carcinoma varies with the primary tumor from site to site (Table 14-9).

The sonographers, led by our European and Asian counterparts are strong advocates for the use of ultrasound (US) in the evaluation of lymph nodes. Power doppler US will show round nodes with no hilar flow and peripheral parenchymal nodal flow in most metastatic nodes. Hilar vessels with branching suggest lymphadenitis whereas peripheral vessels suggest metastases. If you combine a short axis diameter of 5 to 7 mm with absence of hilar blood flow the sensitivity can rise to near 90% and specificity to around 95%. If that isn't good enough you can use ultrasound to provide guidance for fine needle aspiration of nodes for cytologic evaluation. This technique is very accurate (with a specificity approaching 99%) but requires the patience and expertise that many Americans do not possess.

So what is the big deal about nodes? Remember Dave and Bob's 50% rule of lymph nodes. Having a lymph node with your primary tumor cuts your 5 year prognosis by 50%, having bilateral nodes cuts it another 50%, having extracapsular spread of tumor cuts it another 50%, having fixation to vital structures (carotids, vertebral arteries, paraspinal muscles, transverse processes, brachial plexi) cuts it another 50%, and 50% of our school age children have lymph nodes palpable 50% of the time.

Lymph node morphology   The shape of the lymph node may also be a secondary indication of whether it is involved by tumor. More rounded lymph nodes have a greater chance of being neoplastic than those which have a kidney bean shape. Most authors agree that a lymph node that has central necrosis no matter what its size should be considered malignant until proved other-

Table 14-9   Primary sites of squamous cell carcinoma versus presence of lymphadenopathy

Primary site	Nodes at presentation (% of cases)	Bilateral nodes (% of cases)	Nodes after therapy (% of cases)	Nodal drainage levels
Nasopharynx	72–85	25–33	15–20	2–5
Oropharynx	66–76	20–25	15–20	2, 3, 5
Hypopharynx	59–65	9–13	15–20	2–5
Supraglottic larynx	55–80	21	10–20	2–4
Oral cavity	3–36	8–12	8–28	1–3
Sinonasal	10–17	<5	16	1–3
Glottis	3–7	<5	<5	2–4

wise, unless the patient has active tuberculosis or has been treated with radiation in the past for lymphoma. A lymph node with fat centrally is benign and may signify previous inflammation and/or radiation.

Another important issue to consider when you are dealing with internal jugular chain lymph nodes is the presence or absence of carotid invasion by lymphadenopathy. Presently, no ideal radiographic study can predict whether the carotid artery is invaded by tumor when there is contiguous lymphadenopathy. It has generally been accepted that if less than 270 degrees of the circumference of the carotid artery is encircled by squamous cell carcinoma, the likelihood of carotid wall invasion is small. This suggests that the surgeon may be able to "scrape" the tumor off the carotid artery. However, when the tumor encircles the carotid artery greater than 270 degrees, the carotid wall is nearly always invaded and the carotid artery may need to be sacrificed. The surgeon may spend a great deal of time palpating the lymph nodes to assess clinically whether they are fixed to the carotid artery; however, imaging, particularly MR, may be more useful than the clinical examination. At least we radiologists would like to believe that. Carotid angiography may not be as useful because the lumen of the artery may be entirely normal whereas its adventitia and media may be infiltrated with cancer. On the other hand, the arteriogram is invaluable in determining whether the patient can tolerate carotid sacrifice at the time of surgery via reversible balloon occlusion testing. By the time the carotid is encased, the long-term prognosis is abysmal and even sterling surgeons with sharpened scalpels shan't stunt the Stygian survival.

Extension of lymph nodes into the posterior musculature of the neck, paraspinal soft tissue and/or the base of the skull also makes surgical resection much more difficult if not impossible. The presence of these findings suggests that the tumor may be extensive beyond visible dimensions and may require heroic surgery for a small chance of cure.

Some lymph nodes that are located deep in the head and neck are not clinically palpable. Retropharyngeal lymph nodes, which commonly accompany nasopharyngeal carcinoma, are impossible to detect clinically (Fig. 14-55). Sometimes, deep parapharyngeal lymph nodes and/or lymph nodes in the jugular digastric chain (level 2) may not be readily palpable. For this reason it is generally accepted that 15% to 30% of all malignant lymph nodes escape clinical detection. The role of the radiologist is to identify these lymph nodes and the very small lymph nodes that demonstrate central nodal necrosis that may be dismissed by the clinician (and unsophistocated radiologist) as insignificant.

Most head and neck radiologists agree that CT is the easiest method for identifying the lymph nodes in the neck, provided that a large bolus of contrast has been

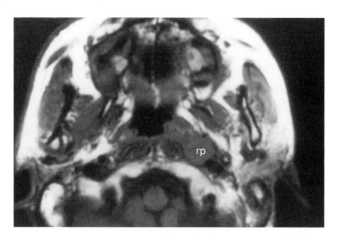

Fig. 14-55   Retropharyngeal lymph node. Axial T1WI demonstrates an enlarged retropharyngeal lymph node *(rp)* on the left side. Note that this lymph node would be impossible to palpate clinically, highlighting the benefit of preoperative imaging of patients with squamous cell carcinoma. If this figure looks somewhat familiar, you are right. This is the same patient with nasopharyngeal carcinoma seen way back in Fig. 14-10. (Mail in your coupon for a discount.)

delivered to the blood vessels to distinguish them from lymph nodes. In addition, there is some evidence that central nodal necrosis may be more readily identified by CT than by MR.

In general, clinicians use relatively rigid clinical staging criteria to determine whether the lymph nodes are to be removed. In many instances to remove the possibility of microscopic disease, the surgeon operates on a clinically N0 neck. The alternative treatment option is to treat these patients with postoperative radiation therapy to eliminate microscopic lymph node disease. Often, however, the clinicians hold radiation therapy in abeyance because of the 15% likelihood of a metachronous primary squamous cell carcinoma in a patient with head and neck cancer. Radiation may be held in reserve to treat the secondary primary tumor. This may be a rationale for a surgical approach to disease in a younger patient. In some cases radiation is used before surgery to reduce the overall bulk of the disease so that the surgical removal is easier. Nonetheless, no study has shown that cure rates with surgery after radiation therapy are significantly better than those with radiation therapy after surgery.

Occasionally, a patient has malignant lymphadenopathy without a clinically apparent primary tumor. The most common head and neck sites for an occult primary neoplasm invisible to endoscopy are the nasopharynx, the tonsil, the pyriform sinus apex, and the tongue base. Therefore, in those patients who have unknown primary tumors, these areas should demand greater attention by the radiologist. The workup should include either CT or MR as well as a barium swallow and upper gastrointestinal examination. In patients who have cervical adenopathy with an unknown primary tumor by clinical and endoscopic examination, imaging will identify the primary tumor in 25% of cases. In many instances the primary tumor is never discovered. Occasionally, the patient who has lymphadenopathy in the lower part of the neck may have an esophageal, tracheal, bronchial, or pulmonary primary tumor.

The results of using FDG PET to identify the primary sites of cancers when malignant adenopathy is present without a clinical or radiographic source for it have been mixed. PET potentially predicts primaries proactively in pretty high percentages; 25-50% of otherwise occult primary cancers are discovered with PET (interpreted by a head and neck radiologist, however rather than an unclear medicine imager). However, performing bilateral tonsillectomies with the neck node dissection probably reveals an equal number of primary tumors.

Thyroid carcinoma Lymphadenopathy from thyroid carcinoma is unique in many senses. In 50% of cases the nodal disease is the presenting sign of the cancer and in 25% of cases the thyroid cancer may be occult to palpation and imaging (we just made up these numbers—pretty good, eh?). Thyroid papillary carcinoma lymph nodes may be (1) cystic, (2) calcified, (3) highly vascular, (4) highly enhancing, (5) colloid containing and therefore, (6) bright on T1WI, (7) tiny, (8) retropharyngeal, (9) hemorrhagic, and (10) worthy of their own separate paragraph. The nodes may be treatable with iodine therapy. Remember also that papillary carcinoma, though known for its regional lymphatic spread may also produce a miliary pattern in the lungs and so make sure you flip to the lung windows once you hit the apices on your CT scans. For once, do not just think like a neuroradiologist.

Lymphoma The most common noninflammatory cause for a unilateral neck mass in a patient between 20 and 40 years old is lymphoma. Non-Hodgkin lymphoma (NHL) (75% of lymphomas) is more common in the head and neck than Hodgkin lymphoma (25%), and usually Waldeyer's ring is also involved with NHL. Fifty percent of patients with Waldeyer's ring NHL have nodes at presentation. When one has isolated nodal disease in the neck or mediastinal involvement, the odds shift more in favor of Hodgkin disease (HD). A history of mononucleosis is present in many patients with HD and may play a role in the etiology. Classically HD proceeds in an organized fashion through the lymphatic chains, from one echelon to the next. NHL is more likely to jump around and have pulmonary, osseous, and noncontiguous nodal involvement. The head and neck is the second most common site of NHL after the gastrointestinal tract (although franchises of the NHL may be found throughout the United States and Canada).

Either gallium scanning or thallium scanning may be used to identify lymph nodes with Hodgkin disease.

POSTTREATMENT IMAGING

Do not just shrug your shoulders and murmur something about your inability to distinguish normal postoperative or postradiotherapeutic changes from recurrent disease when these cases come across your screen. You can contribute some information about the possibility of recurrence, particularly if you have a baseline posttreatment study when edema has resolved (after approximately 8 weeks). Ninety percent of head and neck cancer recurrences take place within the first 12 months and 96% within 2 years. For this reason patients are not considered cured of their tumor until 5 years have passed and no evidence of tumor is identified. Recurrences are usually split evenly between those at the primary site, those in the nodes, and those at both the primary site and the nodes. Therefore, the survey for residual or recurrent disease should be performed frequently within the first 2 years, usually at 6-month intervals, and must cover the primary site and the cervical lymph nodes. Growth of tissue after the 8-week posttreatment scan should make one worry about recurrence. Focal exophytic (into the extramucosal deep soft tissue) or endophytic (into the aerodigestive airway) soft-tissue bulges should be histologically examined for recurrence. Morphology is the key here. MR intensity, CT density, and enhancement features are useless, particularly after radiotherapy. Growth with time is the only sure-fire sign to hang your hat on for recurrence! Unfortunately, we rarely have a baseline scan to work with after therapy despite entreaties (and donuts) sent to our clinical colleagues.

Before you are able to identify recurrences, you must be familiar with the terminology of operations on the neck. Neck dissections are performed to remove suspected adenopathy. The nodes may have been identified by palpation or imaging preoperatively, or sometimes the nodes are removed in an N0 neck because of a high rate of microscopic disease with that particular primary site (e.g., supraglottic larynx, base of tongue, and tonsil). If the sternocleidomastoid muscle, the spinal accessory nerve (XI), the submandibular gland, and the jugular vein are removed with level I to V nodal chains, the procedure is called a radical neck dissection. The side of the neck is flattened, and minimal tissue is left besides skin, arteries, and the anterior viscera. A modified neck dissection usually spares either the spinal accessory nerve (allowing a functional trapezius muscle), the sternocleidomastoid muscle, and/or the internal jugular vein. A supraomohyoid neck dissection removes level I to III nodes above the cricoid cartilage and usually spares the sternocleidomastoid muscle, internal jugular vein, and spinal accessory nerve. This dissection is commonly performed for N0 primary tumors high in the aerodigestive system, with a low to intermediate rate of occult metastases. An anterior neck dissection may be performed for thyroid cancer to remove anterior visceral chain nodes (level VI). Bilateral neck dissections may also be performed. It is important to remember that once the normal pathway of lymphatic drainage from a primary site has been removed surgically, nodal metastases may subsequently occur in unusual locations for that particularly primary tumor. After both nodal chains have been removed, watch out for dermal lymphatic drainage of tumor cells because the nodes are no longer available to sequester the neoplasm. This is identifiable as subcutaneous stranding and thickening on CT or MR. Unfortunately this may be indistinguishable from the edema associated with acute radiation treatment.

A word about head and neck cancer radiation: it is vitally important for the patient to receive the radiotherapy for the cancer with as little interruption as possible, so do not overcall lumps that may delay therapy. A recent study has shown that with treatments less than 55 days apart, 56 to 65 days apart, and more than 66 days apart, the 5-year survival rates were 56%, 46%, and 15%, respectively in patients undergoing sequential chemotherapy and radiation therapy. Treatment interruptions during definitive radiation therapy are a no-no. Try to soft call anything in this time range.

Most radiologists have a hard time understanding flaps and grafts beyond shaking down your local equipment vendors. For this reason we reiterate some of the terminology of these surgical procedures. Surgical reconstruction of defects in the head and neck after operation requires the interposition of flaps and grafts. Surgeons have a whole host of skin (cutaneous), muscle (myo-), bone (osteo-), and fat (lipo-) plugs that they are capable of inserting these days. These are usually defined with the prefixes provided, so that an osteomyocutaneous flap is one that contains bone, muscle, and skin.

The site from which the flap is taken precedes the description of what is taken. A "free" flap is not one for which there has been no charge (far from it!). It really is one that is "far from it," at a distant site and wholly separated from the original surgical defect. So a fibular free flap may be used to reconstruct the mandible, or a radial forearm free (cutaneous) flap frequently fixes florid flaws in the floor of the mouth. Free flaps require anastomoses of blood vessels (and sometimes nerves) from the donor site to the surgical bed with microvascularization techniques.

A local or regional flap requires rotation or "pedicling" a piece of adjacent tissue into a surgical gap without disrupting the original blood supply of the flap. Thus a local muscular (myocutaneous) temporalis flap may be rotated down to fill the gap of an infratemporal fossa resection, or a pedicled pectoralis major flap may re-

construct a large base of tongue or floor of mouth defect. Often on imaging the most striking feature of these flaps is the dominance of the fat in the graft. Granted, some of the appearance varies with patient habitus, nationality, whether Oprah is staying on her diet, and the type of graft used (in Americans the rectus abdominis graft usually has more fat than a radial forearm flap), but the muscle of the graft often atrophies to a greater extent than the fat. A graft that has been irradiated often has a denser appearance on CT and MR than one that has not been irradiated and may appear as a sheet of fibrous-like tissue without good tissue planes.

FUTURE CANCER RISK

A general adage among head and neck clinicians is that tumors recur at surgical margins along the periphery of the tumor, whereas they recur centrally within the tumor bed when radiation therapy is the primary modality of treatment. Recurrent squamous cell carcinoma may be very difficult to identify when small and this has been another area where FDG PET has shown value. Nonetheless, for the rest of their lives patients with head and neck cancers generally are surveyed for the possibility of a secondary malignancy. If a surgeon has a few of these patients as long-term survivors, he can keep his office schedule filled for years. As stated previously, the incidence of synchronous or metachronous oral cavity cancers in a patient who has had a previous cancer is approximately 40%. In patients who have head and neck cancers outside the oral cavity, the metachronous rate is still 15%.

Another fascinating fact: 19% of patients with head and neck carcinoma who undergo thoracic CT have one or more primary or metastatic neoplasms discovered. Synchronous primary lung cancers are twice as common as metastatic lesions to the lungs. Of the second lesions, less than one third were discovered on chest radiographs. The primary sites of the head and neck cancers that had second lesions were fairly evenly distributed between larynx, pharynx, and oral cavity and most had stage IV lymphadenopathy. Most series of patients with head and neck cancers report a second lung primary incidence of 0.8% to 6% and lung metastases incidence of 5% to 7%. Bottom line: Recommend a chest CT in patients with head and neck squamous cell carcinomas to pick up additional lesions so that the head and neck surgery will not be for naught.

Do not be too morose after reading this chapter with its emphasis on cancer and head and neck surgery. By chewing tobacco, smoking and excessive drinking, humans abuse their mucosa and the mucosa strikes back in a vicious way: squamous cell carcinoma. Although beauty may be only skin (mucosa) deep, cancer may go clear down to the bone. So be good to your mucosa. Kick the habit!

> Those who smoke
> On cancer may choke
> Surgeons must wage
> A war on T-stage
> To save the poor bloke.

For a quick pick-me-up, read the next chapter (extramucosal diseases). There are a lot more benign tumors and interesting infections there.

Our authors' outstanding alliterations are over, allowing uninterrupted ease in education.

SUGGESTED READINGS

Ahuja A, Ying M, Mok JSW et al: Gray scale and power doppler sonography in cases of Kimura Disease, *AJNR* 22: 513-517, 2001.

Anzai Y, Blackwell KE, Hirschowitz SL, et al: Initial clinical experience with dextran-coated superparamagnetic iron oxide for detection of lymph node metastases in patients with head and neck cancer [see comments], *Radiology* 192:709-715, 1994.

Anzai Y, Brunberg JA, Lufkin RB: Imaging of nodal metastases in the head and neck, *J Mag Res Imaging* 7:774-783, 1997.

Anzai Y, McLachlan S, Morris M, et al: Dextran-coated superparamagnetic iron oxide, an MR contrast agent for assessing lymph nodes in the head and neck, *Am J Neuroradiol* 15:87-94, 1994.

Anzai Y, McLachlan S, Morris M, et al: Dextran-coated superparamagnetic iron oxide, an MR contrast agent for assessing lymph nodes in the head and neck, *AJNR* 15:87-94, 1994.

Aspestrand F, Kolbenstvedt A, Boysen M: Carcinoma of the hypopharynx: CT staging, *J Comput Assist Tomogr* 14:72-76, 1990.

Atlas SW, Braffman BH, LoBrutto R, et al: Human malignant melanomas with varying degrees of melanin content in nude mice: MR imaging, histopathology, and electron paramagnetic resonance, *J Comput Assist Tomogr* 14:547-554, 1990.

Avrahami E, Englender M, Chen E, et al: CT of submandibular gland sialolithiasis, *Neuroradiology* 38:287-290, 1996.

Avrahami E, Englender M: Relation between CT axial cross-sectional area of the oropharynx and obstructive sleep apnea syndrome in adults, *AJNR* 16:135-140, 1995.

Avrahami E, Katz R: An association between imaging and acute posttraumatic ear bleeding with trismus, *Oral Surg Oral Med Oral Pathol Oral Radiol Endodontics* 85:244-247, 1998.

Avrahami E, Solomonovich A, Englender M: Axial CT measurements of the cross-sectional area of the oropharynx in adults with obstructive sleep apnea syndrome, *AJNR* 17:1107-1111, 1996.

Ballantyne AJ, McCarten AB, Ibanez ML: The extension of cancer of the head and neck through peripheral nerves, *Am J Surg* 106:651-667, 1963.

Bansberg SF, Harner SG, Forbes G. Relationship of the optic nerve to the paranasal sinuses as shown by CT, *Otolaryngol Head Neck Surg* 96:331-335, 1987.

Barakos JA, Dillon WP, Chew WM: Orbit, skull base, and pharynx: contrast-enhanced fat-suppression MR imaging, *Radiology* 179:191-198, 1991.

Batsakis JG: *Tumors of the head and neck: clinical and pathological considerations,* ed 2, Baltimore, 1979, Williams & Wilkins.

Biller HF, Ogura JF, Pratt LL: Hemilaryngectomy for T2 glottic, *Arch Otolaryngol* 93:238-243, 1971.

Bonadona G, Santoro A, Viviani S, et al: Treatment strategies for Hodgkin's disease, *Semin Hematol* 25:51-57, 1988.

Brasnu D, Laccourreye H, Dulmet E, et al: Mobility of the vocal cord and arytenoid in squamous cell carcinoma of the larynx and hypopharynx: an anatomical and clinical comparative study, *Ann Otolaryngol Chiru Cervicofac* 105:435-441, 1988.

Braun IF: MR of the nasopharynx, *Radiol Clin North Am* 27:315-330, 1989.

Carvalho P, Baldwin D, Carter R, et al: Accuracy of CT in detecting squamous carcinoma metastases in cervical lymph nodes, *Clin Radiol* 44:79-81, 1991.

Castelijns JA, Doornbos JN, Verbeeten B: MR imaging of the normal larynx, *J Comput Assist Tomogr* 9:919-925, 1985.

Castelijns JA, Gerritsen GJ, Kaiser MC, et al: Invasion of laryngeal cartilage by cancer: comparison of CT and MR imaging, *Radiology* 166:199-206, 1987.

Castelijns JA, Golding RP, van Schaik C, et al: MR findings of cartilage invasion by laryngeal cancer: value in predicting outcome of radiation therapy, *Radiology* 174:669-674, 1990.

Cocke EW, Wange CC: Cancer of the larynx: selecting optimal treatment, *CA* 26:194-200, 1976.

Curtin HD, Williams R, Johnson J: CT of perineural tumor extension: pterygopalatine fossa, *AJNR* 5:731-737, 1984.

Curtin HD: Imaging of the larynx: current concepts, *Radiology* 173:1-11, 1989.

Curtin HD, Ishwaran H, Mancuso AA, Dalley RW, Caudry DJ, McNeil BJ. Comparison of CT and MR imaging in staging of neck metastases. Radiology 1998;207:123-30.

Daniels, DL, Rauschning W, Lovas J, et al: Pterygopalatine fossa: computed tomographic studies, *Radiology* 149:511-516, 1983.

De Pena CA, Van Tassel P, Lee Y-Y: Lymphoma of the head and neck, *Radiol Clin North Am* 28:723-743, 1990.

DeVita VT Jr, Hubberd SM, Longo DL: Treatment of Hodgkin's disease, *Monogr Natl Cancer Inst* 10:19-28, 1990.

DiSantis DJ, Balfe DM, Hayden R, et al: The neck after vertical hemilaryngectomy: computed tomographic study, *Radiology* 151:683-687, 1984.

Dodd GD, Dolan PA, Ballantyne AJ, et al: The dissemination of tumors of the head and neck via the cranial nerves, *Radiol Clin North Am* 8:445-461, 1970.

Fayos JV: Carcinoma of the pharynx, *Radiology* 138:675-681, 1981.

Ferlito A, Som PM, Rinaldo A, Mondin V. Classification and terminology of neck dissections. *Orl; Journal of Oto-Rhino-Laryngology and Its Related Specialties* 62:212-216, 2000.

Fleming ID, Cooper JS, Henson DE et al. (editors) AJCC Cancer Staging Manual, ed 5. Philadelphia 1997. Lippincott-Raven

Foster JA, Wulc AE, Yousem DM, et al: *Computed tomography in lacrimal outflow obstruction,* Meeting of ESOPRS, Seville, Spain, 1992 (abstract).

Friedman M, Shelton V, Mafee MM, et al: Metastatic neck disease: evaluation by CT, *Arch Laryngol* 110:443-447, 1984.

Ghossein NA, Bataini JP, Ennuyer A, et al: Local control and site of failure in radically irradiated supraglottic cancer, *Radiology* 12:187-192, 1974.

Glasier CM, Mallory GB Jr, Steele RW: Significance of opacification of the maxillary and ethmoid sinuses in infants, *J Pediatr* 114:45-50, 1989.

Goaz PW, White SC: *Oral radiology: principles and interpretation,* ed 2, St Louis, 1987, CV Mosby.

Goepfert H, Dichtel WJ, Medina JE, et al: Perineural invasion in squamous cell skin carcinoma of the head and neck, *Am J Surg* 148:542-547, 1984.

Gussack GS, Hudgins PA: Imaging modalities in recurrent head and neck tumors, *Laryngoscope* 101:119-124, 1991.

Harnsberger HR, Mancuso AA, Muraki AS, et al: The upper aerodigestive tract and neck: CT evaluation of recurrent tumors, *Radiology* 149:503-509, 1983.

Harvey RT, Ibrahim H, Yousem DM, Weinstein GS. Radiologic findings in a carcinoma-associated laryngocele. *Annals of Otology, Rhinology & Laryngology* 1996;105:405-408

Hennig J, Friedburg H: Clinical applications and methodological developments of the RARE technique, *Magn Reson Imaging* 6:391-395, 1988.

Hennig J, Nauerth A, Friedburg H: RARE imaging: a fast imaging method for clinical MR, *Magn Reson Med* 3:823-833, 1986.

Hoe J: CT of nasopharyngeal carcinoma: significance of widening of the preoccipital soft tissue on axial scans, *AJR* 153:867-872, 1989.

Hunink MG, de Slegte RG, Gerritsen GJ, et al: CT and MR assessment of tumors of the nose and paranasal sinuses, the nasopharynx and the parapharyngeal space using ROC methodology, *Neuroradiology* 32:220-225, 1990.

Jacobs CJM, Harnsberger HR, Lufkin RB, et al: Vagal neuropathology: evaluation with CT and MR imaging, *Radiology* 164:97-102, 1987.

Johnson JT: A surgeon looks at cervical lymph nodes, *Radiology* 175:607-610, 1990.

Jones KM, Mulkern RV, Schwartz RB, et al: Fast spin-echo MR imaging of the brain and spine: current concepts, *AJR* 158:1313-1320, 1992.

Kassel EE, Keller MA, Kucharczyk W: MR of the floor of the mouth, tongue and orohypopharynx, *Radiol Clin North Am* 27:331-351, 1989.

Kikinis R, Wolfensberger M, Boesch C, et al: MR imaging at 2.35 T, *Radiology* 171:165-170, 1989.

Kraus DH, Lanzieri CF, Wanamaker JR, et al: Complementary use of computed tomography and magnetic resonance imaging in assessing skull base lesions, *Laryngoscope* 102:623-629, 1992.

Laine FJ, Braun IF, Jensen ME, et al: Perineural tumor extension through the foramen ovale: evaluation with MR imaging, *Radiology* 174:65-71, 1990.

Lewis M, Perl A, Som PM, Urken ML, Brandwein MS. Osteogenic sarcoma of the jaw. A clinicopathologic review of 12 patients. *Archives of Otolaryngology—Head and Neck Surgery* 1997;123:169-174

Loevner LA, Ott IL, Yousem DM, et al. Neoplastic fixation to the prevertebral compartment by squamous cell carcinoma of the head and neck. *AJR American Journal of Roentgenology* 1998;170:1389-1394

Loevner LA, Yousem DM, Montone KT, Weber R, Chalian AA, Weinstein GS. Can radiologists accurately predict preepiglottic space invasion with MR imaging? *AJR. American Journal of Roentgenology* 1997;169:1681-1687

Loevner LA, Yousem DM, Montone KT, Weber R, Chalian AA, Weinstein GS. Can radiologists accurately predict preepiglottic space invasion with MR imaging? *American Journal of Roentgenology* 1997;169:1681-1688

Lufkin RB, Hanafee WN, Wortham D, et al: Larynx and hypopharynx: MR imaging with surface coils, *Radiology* 158:747-754, 1986.

Lufkin RB, Hanafee WN: Application of surface coils to MR anatomy of the larynx, *AJR* 145:483-489, 1985.

Lufkin RB, Hanafee WN: Magnetic resonance imaging of the head and neck, *Invest Radiol* 23:162-169, 1988.

Lufkin RB, Wortham DG, Dietrich RB, et al: Tongue and oropharynx: findings on MR imaging, *Radiology* 161:69-76, 1986.

Mancuso AA, Hanafee WN: Elusive head and neck carcinomas beneath intact mucosa, *Laryngoscope* 93:133-139, 1983.

Mandell DL, Brandwein MS, Woo P, Som PM, Biller HF, Urken ML. Upper aerodigestive tract liposarcoma: report on four cases and literature review. *Laryngoscope* 1999;109:1245-1252

Mehra YN, Mann SB, Dubey SP, et al: Computed tomography for determining pathways of extension and a staging and treatment system for juvenile angiofibromas, *Ear Nose Throat J* 68:576-589, 1989.

Melki PS, Mulkern RV, Panych LP, et al: Comparing the FAISE method with conventional dual-echo sequences, *J Magn Reson Imaging* 1:319-332, 1991.

Miller EM, Norman D: The role of computed tomography in the evaluation of neck masses, *Radiology* 133:145-149, 1979.

Mishell JF, Schlif JA, Mafee MF: Chondrosarcoma of the larynx: diagnosis with magnetic resonance imaging and computed tomography, *Arch Otolaryngol Head Neck Surg* 116:1338-1341, 1990.

Mittl RL Jr, Yousem DM, Turner RS: Frequency of unexplained meningeal enhancement in the brain following lumbar puncture, presented at Radiological Society of North America, 1992, Chicago, Dec 2, 1992.

Morgan K, MacLennan KA, Narula A, et al: Non-Hodgkin's lymphoma of the larynx (stage IE), *Cancer* 64:1123-1127, 1989.

Nusbaum AO, Som PM, Rothschild MA, Shugar JM. Recurrence of a deep neck infection: a clinical indication of an underlying congenital lesion. *Archives of Otolaryngology—Head and Neck Surgery* 1999;125:1379-1382

Oloffson J, Sokjer H: Radiology and laryngoscopy for the diagnosis of laryngeal cancer, *Acta Radiol* 4:449-476, 1977.

Paling MR, Black WC, Levine PA, et al: Tumor invasion of the anterior skull base: a comparison of MR and CT studies, *J Comput Assist Tomogr* 11:824-830, 1987.

Pandolfo I, Gaeta M, Blandino A, et al: MR imaging of perineural metastasis along the vidian nerve, *J Comput Assist Tomogr* 13:498-500, 1989.

Parker GD, Harnsberger HR: Clinical-radiologic issues in perineural tumor spread of malignant diseases of the extracranial head and neck, *Radiographics* 11:383-399, 1991.

Reede DL, Bergeron RT: Cervical tuberculous adenitis: CT manifestations, *Radiology* 154:701-704, 1985.

Reid MH: Laryngeal carcinoma: high-resolution computed tomography and thick anatomic sections, *Radiology* 151:689-696, 1984.

Robbins KT, Medina JE, Wolfe GT, et al: Standardizing neck dissection terminology, *Arch Otolaryngol Head Neck Surg* 117:601-605, 1991.

Rothrock SG, Pignatiello GA, Ronald MH: Radiologic diagnosis of epiglottis: objective criteria for all ages, *Ann Emerg Med* 19:978-982, 1990.

Sack MJ, Weber RS, Weinstein GS, Chalian AA, Nisenbaum HL, Yousem DM. Image-guided fine-needle aspiration of the head and neck: five years' experience. *Archives of Otolaryngology—Head & Neck Surgery* 1998;124:1155-1161

Sack MJ, Weber RS, Weinstein GS, Chalian AA, Nissenbaum HL, Yousem DM. Image-guided fine needle aspiration of the head and neck. *Archives of Otolaryngology-Head and Neck Surgery* 1999;(in press):

Segal R: MR imaging of head and neck adenoid cystic carcinomas: a study of twenty-seven cases with clinical pathological correlation, *Radiology* 184:95-101, 1992.

Sham JST, Cheung YK, Choy D, et al: Nasopharyngeal carcinoma: CT evaluation of patterns of tumor spread, *AJNR* 12: 265-270, 1991.

Silverman PM, Bossen EH, Fisher SR, et al: Carcinoma of the larynx and hypopharynx: computed tomographic-histopathologic correlations, *Radiology* 151:697-702, 1984.

Solbiati L, Rizzatto G, Bellotti E, et al: High-resolution sonography of cervical lymph nodes in head and neck cancer criteria for differentiation of reactive versus malignant nodes, *Radiology* 169(P):113, 1988 (abstract).

Som PM, Bergeron RT: *Head and neck imaging,* ed 2, St Louis, 1991, Mosby-Year Book.

Som PM, Curtin HD, Mancuso AA. An imaging-based classification for the cervical nodes designed as an adjunct to recent clinically based nodal classifications [see comments]. *Archives of Otolaryngology—Head and Neck Surgery* 1999;125:388-396

Som PM, Curtin HD, Mancuso AA. Imaging-based nodal classification for evaluation of neck metastatic adenopathy. *Ajr. American Journal of Roentgenology* 2000;174:837-844

Som PM, Curtin HD, Mancuso AA. The new imaging-based classification for describing the location of lymph nodes in the neck with particular regard to cervical lymph nodes in relation to cancer of the larynx. *Orl; Journal of Oto-Rhino-Laryngology and Its Related Specialties* 2000;62:186-198

Som PM, Norton KI, Shugar JMA, et al: Metastatic hypernephroma to the head and neck, *AJNR* 8:1103-1106, 1987.

Som PM, Shapiro MD: MR of the head and neck, *Radiol Clin North Am* 27:331-393, 1989.

Som PM: Imaging the postoperative neck, *Radiology* 187:593-603, 1993.

Som PM: Lymph nodes of the neck, *Radiology* 165:593-600, 1987.

Stevens MH, Harnsberger HR, Mancuso AA: Computed tomography of cervical lymph nodes: staging and management of head and neck cancer, *Arch Otolaryngol* 11:735-739, 1985.

Sutton RT, Reading CC, Charboneau JW, et al: US-guided biopsy of neck masses in postoperative management of patients with thyroid cancer, *Radiology* 168:769-772, 1988.

Teatini G, Simonetti G, Salvolini U, et al: Computed tomography of the ethmoid labyrinth and adjacent structures, *Ann Otol Rhinol Laryngol* 96:239-250, 1987.

Teresi LM, Lufkin RB, Vinuela F, et al: MR imaging of the nasopharynx and floor of the middle cranial fossa. Part II. Malignant tumors, *Radiology* 164:817-821, 1987.

Unger JM: The oral cavity and tongue: magnetic resonance imaging, *Radiology* 155:151-153, 1985.

Van den Brekel MWM, Castelijns JA, Croll GA, et al: Magnetic resonance imaging vs. palpation of cervical lymph node metastasis, *Arch Otolaryngol Head Neck Surg* 117:666-673, 1991.

Van den Brekel MWM, Castelijns JA, Stel HV: Detection and characterization of metastatic cervical adenopathy by MR imaging: comparison of different MR techniques, *J Comput Assist Tomagr* 14:581-589, 1990.

Vassallo P, Wernecke K, Roos N, et al: Differentiation of benign from malignant superficial lymphadenopathy: the role of high-resolution US, *Radiology* 183:215-220, 1992.

Vermund H, Gollin FF: Role of radiotherapy in the treatment of cancer of the tongue, Cancer 32:333-345,1973.

Vogl T, Bruning R, Grevers G, et al: MR imaging of the oropharynx and tongue: comparison of plain and Gd-DTPA studies, *J Comput Assist Tomogr* 12:427-431, 1988.

Vogl T, Dressel S, Bilaniuk LT, et al: Tumors of the nasopharynx and adjacent areas: MR imaging with Gd-DTPA, *AJR* 154:585-592, 1990.

Wallace C, Ramsay AD, Quiney RE: Non-Hodgkin's extranodal lymphoma: a clinico-pathological study of 24 cases involving head and neck sites, *J Laryngol Otol* 102:914-922, 1988.

Weinstein GS, Laccourreye O, Brasnu D, Yousem DM. The role of computed tomography and magnetic resonance imaging in planning for conservation laryngeal surgery. *Neuroimaging Clinics of North America* 1996;6:497-504

West MS, Russell EJ, Breit R, et al: Calvarial and skull base metastases: comparison of nonenhanced and Gd-DTPA-enhanced MR images, *Radiology* 174:89, 1990.

Woodruff WW, Yeates AE, McLendon RE: Perineural tumor extension to the cavernous sinuses from superficial facial carcinoma: CT manifestations, *Radiology* 161:395-399, 1986.

Yousem DM, Chalian AA. Oral cavity and pharynx. *Radiologic Clinics of North America* 1998;36:967-981, vii

Yousem DM, Geckle RJ, Bilker WB, McKeown DA, Doty RL. Posttraumatic olfactory dysfunction: MR and clinical evaluation. *Ajnr: American Journal of Neuroradiology* 1996;17:1171-1179

Yousem DM, Hatabu H, Hurst RW, et al. Carotid artery invasion by head and neck masses: prediction with MR imaging. *Radiology* 1995;195:715-720

Yousem DM, Hurst RW. MR of cervical lymph nodes: comparison of fast spin-echo and conventional spin-echo T2W scans. *Clinical Radiology* 1994;49:670-675

Yousem DM, Lexa FJ, Bilaniuk LT, et al: Rhabdomyosarcomas in the head and neck: MR imaging evaluation, *Radiology* 177:683-686, 1990.

Yousem DM, Loevner LA, Tobey JD, Geckle RJ, Bilker WB, Chalian AA. Adenoidal width and HIV factors. *AJNR American Journal of Neuroradiology* 1997;18:1721-1725

Yousem DM, Montone KT, Sheppard LM, Rao VM, Weinstein GS, Hayden RE. Head and neck neoplasms: magnetization transfer analysis. *Radiology* 1994;192:703-707

Yousem DM, Montone KT. Head and neck lesions. Radiologic-pathologic correlations. *Radiologic Clinics of North America* 1998;36:983-1014, vii

Yousem DM, Schnall MD, Dougherty L, Weinstein GS, Hayden RE. Magnetization transfer imaging of the head and neck: normative data. *Ajnr: American Journal of Neuroradiology* 1994;15:1117-1121

Extramucosal Diseases of the Head and Neck

As opposed to the mucosal diseases of the head and neck, in which the differential diagnosis usually revolves around well, moderately, or poorly differentiated squamous cell carcinoma 90% of the time, the extramucosal space allows the radiologist to exercise his or her finely honed skills in forming a differential diagnosis. Rumination, differentiation, and pontification may follow—and not just in this chapter. As opposed to the mucosal surface, the anatomy of the extramucosal space does not lend itself to a stepwise superior-to-inferior progression, and therefore the organization of this chapter is a little more haphazard.

The reader should understand that more comprehensive dry texts dealing with head and neck imaging are readily available for reference (at a much more expensive price). This chapter will be bargain basement head and neck radiology but, at the same time, give you 95% of what you need to interpret cases well—which is probably better than 95% of the radiologists practicing now and at a 95% discount compared to those multi-authored texts that no one ever reads anyway.

In the suprahyoid and infrahyoid neck, layers of the deep cervical fascia serve to encapsulate regions of the anatomy that lend themselves to specific analysis. Although these layers of fascia are rarely visualized, they do represent a subtle barrier that restricts the free movement of pathology from one area of the neck to the other. Although it is true that some entities easily cross the deep cervical fascia and other lesions are multispatial in their distribution, this framework is quite useful as a learning tool for studying the head and neck.

We shall begin the discussion of the extramucosal lesions of the head and neck with the salivary glands, to get the juices flowing (pun intended). In the context of spatial anatomy, the major salivary glands are encapsulated in the parotid space and the submandibular space.

SALIVARY GLANDS

Anatomy

The three major salivary glands are the parotid gland, the submandibular gland, and the sublingual gland. The parotid gland is located superficially under the skin around the ear and extends over the ascending ramus of the mandible. The parotid space includes the gland, branches of the external carotid artery and retromandibular vein, cranial nerve VII, the investing layers of deep cervical fascia, and a few branches of the auriculotemporal rami of the third division of cranial nerve V. Although the external carotid artery branches and the retromandibular vein are readily identifiable on scans of the normal parotid gland, the branches of the facial nerve may be detected only when one performs fine imaging cuts through the anatomy. The parotid gland's consistency changes with age. As you get older, your gland gets more fatty (just like the rest of your body). The size and the consistency of the gland also depend on body habitus: in someone who gives the gland a good workout and grows corpulent, the gland tends to be bigger and fattier.

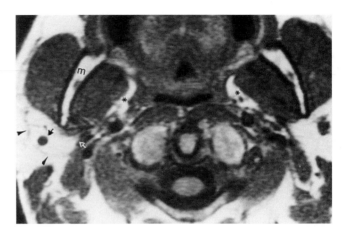

Fig. 15-1 Normal parotid anatomy. Retromandibular vein *(arrow)*, facial nerve *(arrowheads)*, deep portion of the parotid gland *(open arrow)*, mandible *(m)*, and parapharyngeal fat *(asterisk)* can be identified on this T1WI through the right parotid gland.

A portion of the parotid gland extends deep to the plane of the facial nerve (identified radiographically by the stylomandibular tunnel from the styloid process to the ascending ramus of the mandible) and is termed the *deep lobe* of the parotid. The *superficial lobe* extends from just under the skin and usually has an accessory tongue of tissue that passes over the masseter muscle. These lobes do not exist; it is an arbitrary distinction dividing the gland into anatomic sections based on the facial nerve. The importance of differentiating the deep and superficial portions of the parotid stems from the different surgical approaches to tumors in each section and the relationship to the facial nerve (Fig. 15-1). If a lesion is in the superficial portion of the parotid gland, it is usually approached from an external periauricular incision, the facial nerve is dissected deep to the mass to ensure its safety, and the lesion is plucked (excised) from the gland superficial to the nerve. If a mass in the deep portion of the parotid is well defined and noninfiltrative, it is also approached from the same incision and the facial nerve is dissected and then lifted up to

Lesion location (space)	Displacement of parapharyngeal fat	Displacement of styloid musculature	Displacement of longus musculature
Parotid deep portion	Anteromedial	Posterior	Posterior
Masticator	Posteromedial	Posterior	Posterior
Carotid	Anterior	Anterior	Posterior
Mucosal	Posterolateral	Posterior	Posterior
Retropharyngeal	Anterolateral	Anterior	Posterior
Perivertebral	Rarely displaced	Anterior	Anterior
Parapharyngeal	Self	Posterior	Posterior

Table 15-1   How to place a lesion

shell out the deep lobe mass. However, if the lesion is infiltrating through the deep portion and may encase the nerve, the approach is as above, but may be combined with a parapharyngeal space approach via a neck incision below the ear. Unfortunately, with infiltrating deep lobe lesions the facial nerve must often be surgically sacrificed (if it has not already been sacrificed by the tumor itself).

Deep parotid space lesions displace the parapharyngeal fat anteromedially and maintain a fat plane between the lesion and the mucosal surface of the pharynx. The parapharyngeal fat is a good marker for telling what space a lesion is in (Table 15-1).

The parotid duct is termed Stensen's duct, and it passes over the masseter muscle before curving medially to insert in the cheek at the second maxillary molar. Because the parotid gland is late in its encapsulation, lymphoid tissue lies within it. For that reason the parotid gland alone of the salivary glands has the potential for lymphadenitis, metastases to intraglandular lymph nodes, lymphoma, and autoimmune lymphocytic disorders.

The submandibular space (Box 15-1) encompasses the tissue below the mucosa of the floor of the mouth yet above the fascia connecting the mandible to the hyoid bone. As such it contains the sublingual compartment with the mylohyoid muscle, sublingual gland, portions of the submandibular gland, the associated ducts, and the corresponding neurovascular structures. Below the sublingual space is the submaxillary space with the main portion of the submandibular gland, the level Ia and Ib lymph nodes (see previous chapter or reread if you've forgotten already).

The submandibular gland is located in the floor of the mouth, deep to the angle of the mandible (Fig. 15-2). The submandibular gland secretes seromucinous saliva as opposed to the parotid gland, which secretes serous saliva. In addition, the pH of the saliva produced by the submandibular gland is more alkaline and the fluid is more viscous. The duct of the submandibular gland is called Wharton's duct, and it drains on either side of the

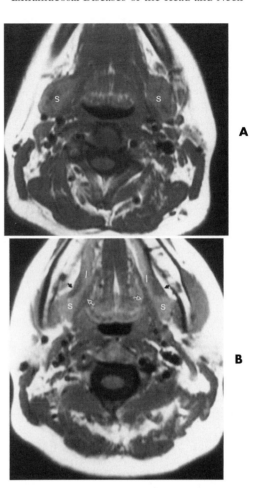

Fig. 15-2   Normal submandibular-sublingual anatomy. **A,** Submandibular glands *(s)* can be seen on this T1WI anterior to the carotid sheath vessels. Note that there normally is some heterogeneity to the gland because of its hilum and ductal system. **B,** Superior portion of the submandibular gland *(s)* can be seen on this section, which also nicely demonstrates the sublingual gland tissue *(l).* Note that the sublingual space is bounded by the mylohyoid musculature *(closed arrows)* laterally and the styloglossus-hyoglossus complex *(open arrows)* medially.

Box 15-1   Submandibular Space Compartments and Contents

Submandibular space
  Sublingual space
    Mylohyoid muscle
    Portions of submandibular gland
    Sublingual gland
    Wharton's duct
  Submaxillary space
    Level I lymph nodes
    Submandibular gland main portion

---

frenulum of the floor of the mouth. The duct has a tighter orifice but is wider than Stensen's duct and is more easily traumatized in the mouth. The duct of the submandibular gland courses anteriorly and superiorly before reaching its orifice.

The sublingual gland is located in the sublingual space between the mylohyoid muscle and the genioglossus muscle in the floor of the mouth. The size of the sublingual gland ranges from being inapparent on imaging studies to a readily identifiable structure in the floor of the mouth. The sublingual gland has many draining ducts (known as ducts of Rivinus) into the floor of the mouth. If a dominant sublingual duct opens to Wharton's duct, it is called the duct of Bartholin. The saliva produced by the sublingual gland is also seromucinous. It is the smallest of the major salivary glands and has the fewest lesions associated with it. But it does get in the path of floor of the mouth squamous cell carcinoma.

Minor salivary glands are found scattered throughout the aerodigestive system but abound in the oral cavity (especially the palate). Minor salivary glands can also be found in the oropharynx, nasopharynx, sinonasal cavity, the parapharyngeal space, the larynx, the trachea, the lungs, and even into the middle ear and eustachian tube. These glands secrete mucinous saliva. Minor salivary glands do not have readily identifiable ducts; however, they are the source of the many retention cysts that are seen as benign lesions in the aerodigestive system.

Now that the hors d'oeuvres have been served and your appetite has been whetted, you are ready to start the meal.

Congenital Disorders

Branchial cleft cyst First branchial cleft cysts (BCCs) classically occur in the parotid gland or around the external auditory canal (Box 15-2). Several classifications of first BCCs have been developed including Arnot type I (intraparotid cyst) and Arnot type II (cyst in the anterior neck that may drain with a tract through the deep portion of the parotid gland to get to the external auditory canal) (Figs. 15-3, 15-4). Work type I first BCCs are anterior and inferior to the pinna and may communicate with the EAC. Work type II BCCs occur at the angle of the mandible (where we typically see second BCCs) and extend to the junction of the bony and cartilaginous EAC. They may drain into the external auditory canal and are of CSF density and intensity unless otherwise infected or traumatized. Because second BCCs are so much more common, they probably outnumber first BCCs in the periparotid location (Table 15-2). Who really cares whether it is a first or a second BCC? Be happy if you come up with that diagnosis. Although these lesions usually have fluid density and intensity characteristics, if infected or traumatized, their appearance may be more confusing (see Fig. 15-3). Adjacent inflammation may be present, and the whole complex may sim-

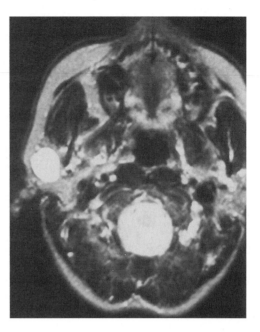

Fig. 15-3   First BCC. This intraparotid cyst with a sharply defined wall is very bright on T2WI. There is no way of knowing whether this is an inflammatory cyst, a posttraumatic sialocele, or a BCC.

ulate an infiltrative process. Fistulization to the bone-cartilage junction of the external ear may occur with first branchial cleft anomalies.

Simple cyst Simple congenital cysts, unassociated with the branchial apparatus, also occur in the salivary glands. Solitary lymphoepithelial cysts are found only in the parotid gland because of its encapsulation of lymphoid tissue; more often they are seen multiply in patients positive for human immunodeficiency virus (HIV) (see later discussion).

Venous vascular malformations Venous vascular malformations (formerly called hemangiomas) may occur in the submandibular space as well as in other spaces of the head and neck. On CT they may show calcification, but invariably one identifies a lobulated, heterogenously enhancing mass. Areas of enhancement that are as extensive as that of the neighboring jugular vein are not unusual. If you perform a fine needle aspiration (FNA) of this lesion you will be faced with the bane of the aspirator's existence—recurrent samples of "nothing but blood." Do not bother. Interestingly enough, there is a 20% coincidence rate of developmental venous anomalies (venous angiomas) of the brain in those subjects with head and neck venous malformations.

Inflammatory Lesions

Calculous disease Calculous disease (in the non-mathematical sense) is the most common benign condition to affect the salivary glands by a factor of the ($\pi \times$

Box 15-2   Cystic Masses in the Parotid Gland

Abscesses, infected collections
Branchial cleft cysts (BCCs)
Lymphoepithelial cysts
Pleomorphic adenomas and Warthin's tumors
Pseudocysts
Sialectasis
Sialoceles
Simple cysts

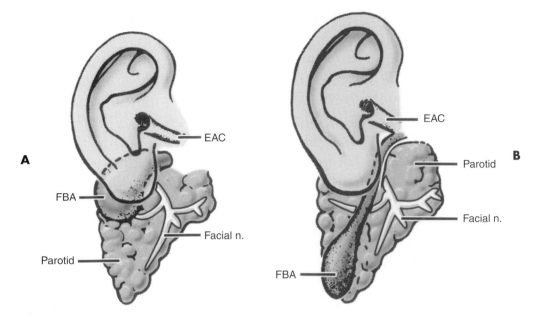

Fig. 15-4   First BCC's Arnot types. **A,** Type I first branchial cleft anomaly (FBA). The cyst is located in the parotid gland. There is no communication with the external auditory canal (EAC). **B,** Type II first branchial cleft anomaly (FBA). The proximal portion of the anomaly communicates with the EAC. The cyst tract typically extends inferiorly within the deep lobe of the parotid gland. The main portion of the cyst is usually located inferior to the parotid gland. Consequently, these masses may present as submandibular masses. (From Mukherji SK, Fatterpekar G, Castillo M, et al: Imaging of congenital anomalies of the branchial apparatus. *Neuroimaging Clin North Am* 10:76-77, 2000.)

!3)[4]. Because the submandibular gland secretes a more mucinous, viscous, alkaline saliva and the wider duct must drain in an uphill direction with greater possibility of stasis, calculi occur most commonly in the submandibular duct (Fig. 15-5). In fact, submandibular gland calculi outnumber those in the parotid gland by a "calculation" of four to one. Sublingual gland calculi and minor salivary gland calculi are extremely uncommon. Although most of the calculi associated with the salivary glands are radiopaque, a small percentage of calculi

(20%) may not be so radiodense as to be visible on plain films.

Patients who have calculous disease usually have painful glands, exacerbated by chewing foods that precipitate salivation. If the clinician suspects calculous disease, the usual workup includes plain films to evaluate for large radiopaque calculi. If no calculi are identified by plain films, or if the patient has a fever associated with a painful salivary gland and an abscess is suspected, computed tomography (CT) should be done because it

Table 15-2	Branchial cleft anomalies			
Features	**BCC type 1**	**BCC type 2**	**BCC type 3**	**BCC type 4**
% of all BCCs	7	90	2	1
Location	1. Inferopostero-medial to pinna 2. Angle of mandible to EAC 3. Periparotid	1. Anterior to mid-SCM, deep to ICA 2. Angle of mandible 3. At CCA bifurcation 4. Parapharyngeal	1. Anterior to lower SCM, superficial	1. Low, anterior to SCM 2. Left side in >90% 3. Follows recurrent laryngeal nerve
Sinus drainage	Ear, skin	Tonsillar fossa, skin	Pyriform sinus	Pyriform apex
Etiology	Persistent cleft	Failure of arch to proliferate, persistent cervical sinus	Persistent cervical sinus	Persistent cervical sinus

BCC, Branchial cleft cyst; *CCA,* common carotid artery; *EAC,* external auditory canal; *ICA,* internal carotid artery; *SCM,* sternocleidomastoid muscle.

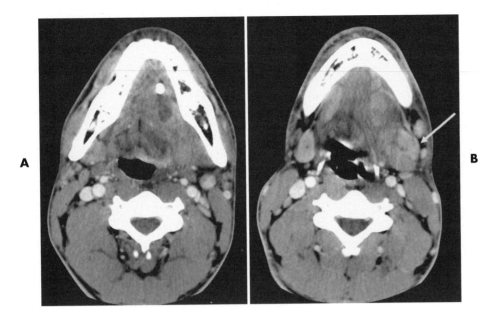

Fig. 15-5 Submandibular sialadenitis. **A,** A large stone with a dilated Wharton's duct is seen in the left sublingual space. **B,** Note the swollen gland *(arrow)* with the effaced sublingual space fat planes.

is more sensitive for the detection of calcification and inflammatory masses (Fig. 15-6). Remember that magnetic resonance imaging (MR) is less sensitive to calcified or noncalcified tiny calculi; larger calculi can be seen as low intensity areas on T2 weighted scans but flow voids may simulate calculi. In the instance of a calculus that is not radiopaque on CT, one might be forced to perform conventional sialography (cannulation of the salivary duct with injection of contrast). MR sialography is a new technique that neuroradiologists have stolen from the MR cholangiopancreatography protocol of the body MR guys. One can use either a single shot fast spin echo heavily T2-weighted sequence that highlights the ducts alone or perform a high resolution 3D fast spin echo T2 weighted sequence that can be prescribed through the gland and duct. Sialography is useful in demonstrating strictures of the ducts after passage of a calculus and intraluminal filling defects from nonopaque stones. Do not confuse an air bubble on conventional sialography with a calculus; one moves with positioning, the other does not. Guess which. Ductal strictures may predispose to recurrent calculous disease. However, the use of sialography for diagnosing calculi has dramatically decreased as CT is so effective here.

Most of the sialograms that are performed at our institution are for chronic sialadenitis from autoimmune causes. These studies are done because patients are seen with hard glands, worrisome for masses, but cross sectional imaging shows no lesion. The sialogram suggests the diagnosis of autoimmune chronic sialadenitis if there are pruned, truncated main ducts with punctate/globular collections peripherally in the glandular parenchyma.

Treatment of sialolithiasis (a catchy seven-syllable word for salivary gland stones) generally consists of administering solutions to increase salivation with the hope of passing the calculi naturally. Transoral resection of sialoliths and sialodochoplasty can be performed for isolated distal duct (close to ampulla) sialoliths. Imaging may help define the location of isolated nonpalpable or multiple sialoliths. For proximal or glandular sialoliths the surgeon may decide to treat the patient with resection of the gland. This is often the preferred treatment with recurrent bouts of sialolithiasis with sialadenitis. A cervical (submandibular) approach may be taken with sialoliths that extend beyond the mylohyoid (in the proximal duct).

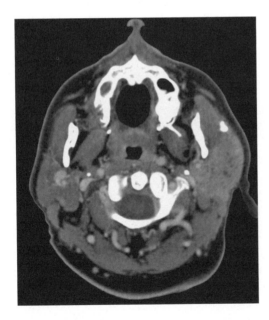

Fig. 15-6 Parotid sialolithiasis. That is a big stone in a small Stenson's duct. Note how much larger the inflamed left parotid gland is when compared to the right.

With a classic clinical history suggesting stones, treatment may proceed without antecedent imaging.

Sialosis   Sialosis is a painless enlargement of the parotid glands that has been associated with numerous causes, including (1) diabetes, (2) alcoholism, (3) hypothyroidism, (4) medications including phenothiazines and some diuretics, (5) obesity, (6) starvation, and (7) idiopathic causes. This usually is a bilateral and symmetric process that may resolve when the underlying cause has been removed. It should be noted, however, that the normal range of parotid gland size and consistency is varied and often it is difficult to state definitively that the glands are larger than normal. On imaging studies the glands with sialosis generally have a CT density and signal intensity on T2-weighted images (T2WI) slightly greater than that of normal fatty parotid glands. The glands in sialosis usually are not as bright on T2WI as glands that are infected. You may see distortion of the facial contour by the enlarged glandular tissue.

Sialadenitis   Sialadenitis refers to glandular inflammation, whereas sialectasis refers to dilatation of ductal spaces. Sialadenitis is often associated with sialectasis, or dilatation of the ductal system. The most common cause of these conditions is calculous disease. Microabscesses within the parotid tissue may be seen in a person who has sialectasis and/or sialadenitis. They are identified on CT as areas of low density with peripheral rim enhancement and on MR as areas of very bright signal intensity on T2WI of the salivary glands. Microabscesses often are multiple and may be a source of painful parotid glands with fever. Abscesses may develop around the mandible, sublingual gland, or submandibular gland in association with dental infections (Fig. 15-7).

A wide variety of inflammatory conditions may affect the salivary glands. Although mumps may be the most common infection to affect the salivary glands (specifically the parotid glands), it is virtually never imaged; the diagnosis is a clinical one. On the other hand, inflammatory conditions that enlarge the parotid glands in the adult may be evaluated to rule out masses. Other viral etiologies include HIV, coxsackie, and influenza viruses. Bacterial infections are uncommon and are usually due to *Streptococcus, Haemophilus,* and *Staphylococcus* species.

Other etiologies of acute parotitis include granulomatous (tuberculosis, candida, cat scratch fever) and idiopathic causes (postpartum parotitis). Poor dental hygiene may contribute to the development of infections affecting the submandibular, sublingual, and parotid glands. The minor salivary glands rarely show inflammatory change other than mucous retention cysts from local obstruction. Vallecular minor salivary gland cysts can get huge.

Sialodochitis   Sialodochitis refers to inflammation of the main salivary ductal system. A number of autoim-

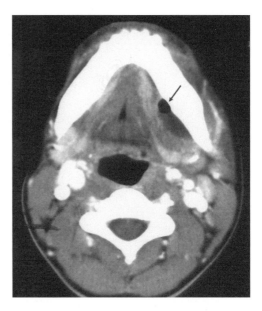

Fig. 15-7   Abscess. An abscess in the sublingual space is usually a result of carious teeth or treatment for such. A pocket of air and fluid is marked by the *arrow.*

mune conditions may cause sialadenitis and sialodochitis. When the process is limited to the salivary glands without other associated findings, the disease is termed Mikulicz's disease, or in the most recent classification Sjögren type 1 disease (poor Dr. Mikulicz is getting squeezed out). This is an autoimmune disorder that causes chronic sialadenitis and sialodochitis and leads to fibrous salivary gland tissue (primarily of the minor glands) with resultant dry mouth. This disorder usually affects middle-aged women. When the disease is associated with a collagen-vascular disease (most commonly rheumatoid arthritis more so than systemic lupus erythematosus) and involvement of the lacrimal glands, the disorder is classified as Sjögren syndrome (Sjögren type 2). Sjögren syndrome is an autoimmune disorder that causes dry eyes, dry mouth, and arthritis. Patients with Sjögren syndrome have tenfold increased risk of lymphoma, which may have its first manifestations in the parotid glands. The lymphoma is usually of the non-Hodgkin variety and may affect any other area of the head and neck as well (Fig. 15-8). Often these patients are scanned to survey for the possibility of lymphoma.

Sjögren syndrome is characterized on conventional or MR sialography by punctate, globular, cavitary, or destructive appearance of the ducts of the parotid glands. Tiny pools of contrast may be seen in the gland. With increasing severity of disease there is greater and greater replacement of glandular tissue with fat. Thus, some have suggested that the severity of fat deposition correlates well with the impairment of salivary flow in Sjögren patients. Sjögren syndrome is also associated with the presence of lymphoepithelial cysts and nodules akin

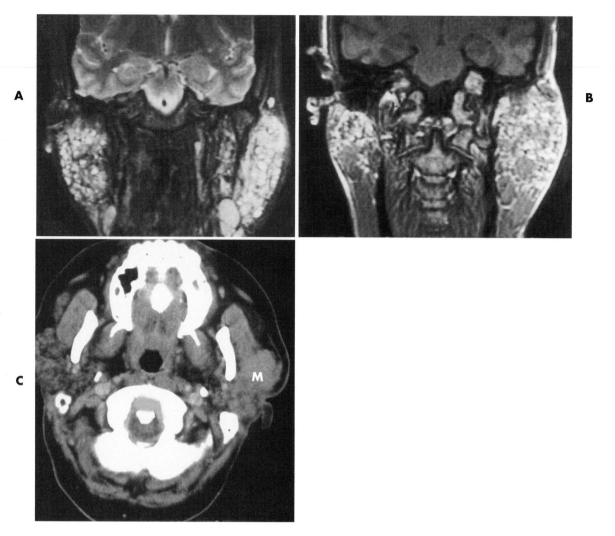

Fig. 15-8   Sjögren syndrome. **A,** The coronal T2WI reveals many tiny benign lymphoepithelal lesions (BLELs) as well as nodes inferiorly and bilaterally. **B,** Dominant masses are seen on the T1WI, but which do you biopsy? FNA revealed lymphoid aggregates. **C,** Lymphoma of the parotid gland and Sjögren's syndrome in another case. The axial CT scan shows a mass *(m)* in the left parotid gland diffusely infiltrating its superficial and deep portion. The right gland is not normal, assuming an acinar pattern of glandular density and fatty replacement.

to those seen in patients with HIV associated parotid lesions (see following discussion).

The cross-sectional imaging appearance of parotid glands in patients who have Sjögren disease may range from normal to a dried up, scarred down, atrophic gland, to one with lots of large and/or tiny cysts and nodules within it, to one with a dominant mass within it. This looks very much like AIDS-related parotid disease (see below).

The glands with autoimmune sialadenitis generally are denser than normal (Fig. 15-9). Some authors have described a "salt and pepper" appearance (there is that same old food analogy) to the gland on both T1WI and T2WI in 46% of patients with Sjögren syndrome, presumably reflecting fibrosis and lymphocytic infiltration intermixed with sialectasis. Biopsy should be performed on any dominant mass, to rule out lymphoma.

Lymphoepithelial lesions   Since the ascent of acquired immunodeficiency syndrome (AIDS) in the young population, lymphoepithelial lesions of the parotid gland have become much more common. These may include purely cystic lesions or solid lesions of lymphoid aggregates (Fig. 15-10). Therefore in a younger patient with multiple lesions in the parotid gland you should consider lymphoepithelial lesions as opposed to multiple Warthin's tumors. The differential diagnosis also includes multiple intraparotid lymph nodes and/or lymphoma. The lymphoepithelial lesions of the parotid have been associated with HIV seropositivity, and the presence of these abnormalities may predate the infection that classifies the patient as having AIDS. Associated findings with the HIV-related parotid disease include diffuse generalized lymphadenopathy in the neck and prominence of adenoidal

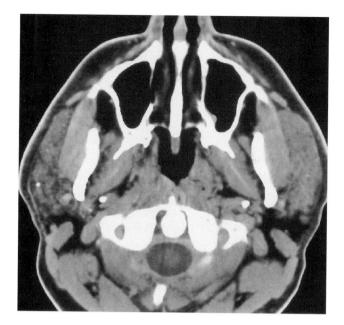

Fig. 15-9   Autoimmune sialadenitis. Axial unenhanced CT shows bilateral enlargement and increased density to the parotid glands. This patient had Mikulicz disease with superimposed small calculi. Calculate the number of punctate high-density areas in the parotid glands from the calculi.

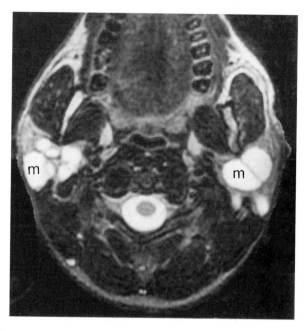

Fig. 15-10   Lymphoepithelial lesions associated with HIV. Parotid glands have multiple high intensity masses *(m)* on this fat-suppressed fast spin echo T2WI, typical of lymphoepithelial cysts in this HIV-positive man.

and tonsillar tissue. Bone marrow signal intensity on T1WI may be lower than normal. When the lympho-epithelial lesion is cystic, it has low density on CT and signal intensity characteristics of cerebrospinal fluid on T1WI and T2WI. However, the lymphoepithelial solid nodules may have a more variable density and signal intensity on cross-sectional imaging.

Som and colleagues have coined the term "acquired immunodeficiency syndrome-related parotid cysts" (ARPCs) to describe the cysts associated with human immunovirus infection and note that they are hard to distinguish from Sjögren-related benign lymphoepithelial lesions (BLELs). In patients who are HIV positive but do not have AIDS, one can see similar cysts or lymphoid nodules in the parotid glands. As these lesions often are not cystic but may be solid, the use of the term ARPCs seems inaccurate to us. Perhaps the term HIV established random parotid entities (HERPES) would be a better term.

Sialocele   A sialocele refers to a collection of saliva that communicates with the parent duct in a manner similar to that of a pharyngocele or a laryngocele filled with fluid (Fig. 15-11). The most common cause of sialoceles is penetrating trauma, although blunt trauma may also cause disruption of the duct and leakage of salivary contents into the parenchyma and outside the gland. This most commonly occurs in the parotid gland, either from a punch to the side of the face or from a stab wound. The entity is distinguished from a pseudocyst because it communicates with the parent duct and is not lined by fibrous tissue.

Ranula   Another entity, more fully described in Chapter 14 in the discussion of oral cavity lesions, is the ranula. This is a postinflammatory cystic lesion that results from obstruction of either the sublingual or submandibular duct and that produces a cystic mass either

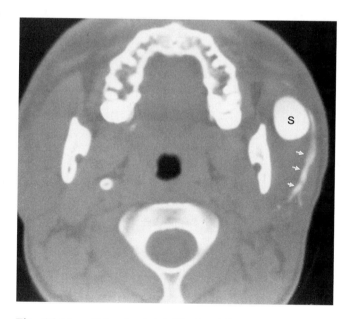

Fig. 15-11   Sialocele. Axial CT after left parotid sialography demonstrates opacification of a sialocele *(s)*. One can see the normal parotid duct *(arrows)* coursing to and communicating with the sialocele on the left side. This patient had been punched in the left side of the face.

confined by the mylohyoid muscle (simple ranula, epithelial lined) or extending to the submandibular region (a plunging ranula, not epithelial lined) (see Fig. 14-27). A ranula has also been termed a "mucous escape cyst," a mucous retention cyst, and a mucocele of the sublingual gland or neighboring minor salivary glandular tissue. The simple ranula is usually addressed transorally, but may be treated with resection or, in some cases, marsupialization. The lingual and hypoglossal nerves must be carefully identified during the operation. A plunging ranula may be excised through a transcervical submandibular incision with a neck dissection. This allows complete resection of the cyst and will help spare the lingual and hypoglossal nerve. Alternatively, the surgeon may excise the sublingual gland transorally and pack the cyst or place a drain in it. By treating the gland, some believe the plunging cyst will resolve on its own.

Retention cysts Retention cysts are very common benign "masses" that result from inflammation and obstruction of minor salivary gland ducts and therefore may be seen throughout the aerodigestive system's mucosal surface.

Miscellaneous inflammatory disorders Sarcoidosis may also affect the parotid gland, usually manifesting as bilaterally enlarged glands with multifocal nodules. Gallium uptake on nuclear medicine scans may be striking.

A mucus plug in the duct may also cause a painful swollen gland (Kussmaul's disease). One pseudomass associated with calcifications in the gland is termed the "Kuttner tumor," a focal masslike firmness of the submandibular gland due to chronic sialadenitis from sialolithiasis.

Benign Neoplasms

There is an adage in head and neck imaging that the larger the salivary gland in the adult, the lower the incidence of malignant tumors associated with it. Thus, the rate of malignancy increases from 20% to 25% in the parotid gland to 40% to 50% in the submandibular gland and 50% to 81% in the sublingual glands and minor salivary glands. In children, 90% to 95% of salivary tumors occur in the parotid and 5% occur in the submandibular and sublingual glands. Sixty-five percent of salivary gland neoplasms in children are benign. In contradistinction to adults the larger the gland of origin in children the more likely the tumor will be malignant.

Although CT and MR dominate the evaluation of the major salivary glands for neoplasms, do not count sonography out completely, particularly if you live on the wrong side of the Atlantic. It has been reported that 95% of space-occupying lesions of the major salivary glands can be completely delineated by sonography. All salivary gland neoplasms are hypoechoic to normal glandular tissue. Ultrasound (US) correctly assesses whether a lesion is benign or malignant in 90% on the basis of definition of the margins of the tumor, but 28% of malignant lesions may be misinterpreted as being benign. Sonography differentiates extraglandular from intraglandular lesions with an accuracy of 98% (all mistakes were periparotid lymph nodes). The authors hope that this last paragraph will help the overseas sales of our book despite France's arguments with our foreign policy—now back to CT and MR.

Pleomorphic adenoma Nearly 80% of benign parotid neoplasms are pleomorphic adenomas (Box 15-3). Pleomorphic adenomas, also known as benign mixed tumors (BMT), occur most commonly in middle aged women. Monomorphic adenomas and myoepitheliomas are the other common benign tumors and may arise in both parotid and submandibular glands. Most pleomorphic adenomas are well-defined lesions that commonly appear solid and round. Pleomorphic adenomas are well identified on both CT and MR against the fatty background of the normal adult's parotid gland (Fig. 15-12). On CT, the lesions have density similar to that of muscle and demonstrate mild to moderate enhancement. With a delay, one may see an increase in the degree and homogeneity of enhancement in parotid pleomorphic adenomas. On MR, the lesions are best identified on T1WI amid the bright signal of the parotid fat; however, they are usually seen on T2WI as very bright lesions (add that to your 80% rule—80% of bright lesions in the parotid are pleomorphic adenomas). Additional MR findings include a complete capsule (often low intensity on T2WI) and a lobulated contour. Pleomorphic adenomas inconstantly have cystic degeneration or calcification within them. Because the incidence of calcification is so much lower in other types of parotid tumors, the presence of calcification nonetheless suggests pleomorphic adenoma.

A small percentage of pleomorphic adenomas degenerate into carcinomas. It is not known whether a carcinoma is present within the pleomorphic adenoma from its outset or whether this is a manifestation of malignant

---

Box 15-3   Eighty Percent Rule of the Parotid Gland
1. 80% of tumors are benign
2. 80% of benign parotid gland tumors are pleomorphic adenomas
3. 80% of salivary gland pleomorphic adenomas occur in parotid gland
4. 80% of parotid pleomorphic adenomas occur in superficial lobe
5. 80% of untreated pleomorphic adenomas remain benign; 20% ultimately undergo malignant change
6. 80% of what people read is not retained after 2 weeks

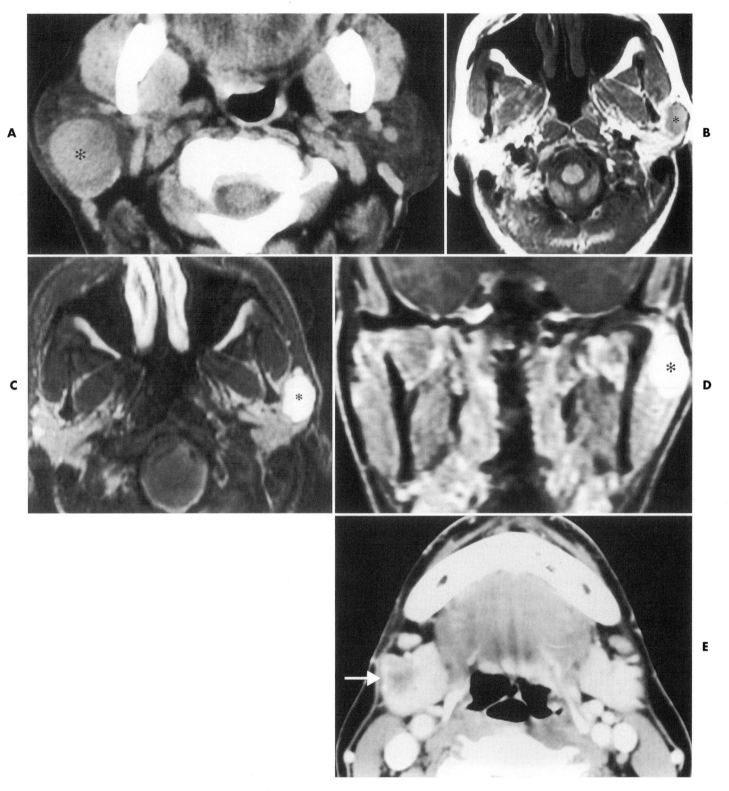

Fig. 15-12   Pleomorphic adenoma. **A,** The well-defined mass (*) in the superficial portion of the right parotid gland turned out to be a pleomorphic adenoma, following the 80% rules of the parotid gland (see text). **B,** A different patient had a mass (*) identified incidentally on this T1WI in the left parotid gland. **C,** The brilliant bright signal on the T2WI, in the face of a T1WI that does NOT look like a cyst, suggests a pleomorphic adenoma (*)—80% of the time. **D,** Avid enhancement (*) on postcontrast T1WI is characteristic as well. **E,** Monomorphic adenoma of the right submandibular gland *(arrow),* low in density, well defined, easily removed.

transformation, but most pathologists favor the latter theory. In any case it is because of this carcinomatous association that pleomorphic adenomas are removed in their entirety with a cuff of normal salivary tissue in most instances. Pleomorphic adenomas are the most common tumor of the parotid gland in both its superficial and deep portions. In fact, pleomorphic adenomas are the most common benign tumor of the submandibular, sublingual, and minor salivary glands. If you guess pleomorphic adenoma, you will have a better batting average than Ted Williams. They are multicentric in 0.5% but as they account for 80% of benign tumors and benign tumors are 80% of all tumors, this means that approximately 3% of multiple parotid neoplasms are pleomorphic adenomas.

Monomorphic adenomas (myoepitheliomas, oncocytic adenomas, canalicular adenomas) look very much like pleomorphic adenomas but are more commonly seen in submandibular glands. They are well-defined and enhance.

Warthin's tumor Warthin's tumors are also known as cystadenoma lymphomatosum. Guess what? They can be cystic or lymphoma-like in their appearance. These tumors are nearly exclusive to the parotid gland and are the most common multiple and bilateral tumors in the parotid (Box 15-4). As opposed to pleomorphic adenomas, which are generally seen in middle-aged women, Warthin's tumors are most commonly seen in elderly men. Warthin's tumors may have a tumoral cyst and favor the parotid's tail (dirty old tumor!). These lesions are entirely benign and show no evidence of malignant transformation. Therefore if an FNA identifies a lesion as a Warthin's tumor, surgeons may conservatively watch the tumor rather than remove it, although that may break their heart. On MR, the lesions are well seen on T1WI opposite the high signal intensity of the parotid gland (Fig. 15-13). However, the signal intensity on T2WI is often heterogeneous and variable and may overlap that of the bright signal of pleomorphic adenomas or the darker intensity of malignancies of the parotid gland (see fol-

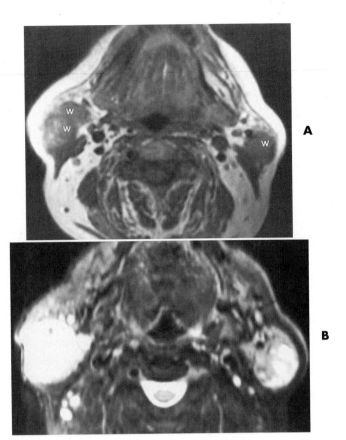

Fig. 15-13 Warthin's tumor. **A,** Axial T1WI demonstrates bilateral Warthin's tumor *(w)*. Note heterogeneity to the signal intensity in the posterior tumor on the right side, which is typical of Warthin's tumors. **B,** In a different patient the T2WI shows bilateral masses with heterogeneity most marked on the left side.

lowing section). Warthin's tumors, like oncocytomas, have increased uptake on technetium 99m pertechnetate nuclear medicine scans. Therefore, if an FNA is equivocal or nondiagnostic, recommend a nuclear medicine technetium scan to make the diagnosis of Warthin's tumors.

Oncocytoma The oncocytoma is a relatively rare benign tumor almost exclusively seen in the parotid gland. It contains oncocytes with abundant pink cytoplasm. These lesions have an MR appearance similar to that of pleomorphic adenomas, being generally bright on T2WI. However, because they are sufficiently rare, the signal intensity characteristics of these tumors have not been well delineated. The tumors may also take up technetium on nuclear medicine scans.

Hemangioma Hemangiomas are the most common salivary gland tumor seen in children, girls more than boys. The lesion enhances brightly and is very hyperintense on a T2WI. Cutaneous hemangiomas may coexist. Congenital capillary hemangiomas represent 90% of parotid gland tumors in neonates. They will undergo spontaneous resolution by adolescence in most cases.

Box 15-4 Multiple Masses in the Parotid Gland

Acinic cell carcinomas
Lymph nodes
Lymphoepithelial lesions
Lymphoma
Metastases
Pleomorphic adenomas
Sarcoidosis
Sjögren's syndrome
Warthin's tumors

Lymphangiomas are the second most common benign lesion to effect pediatric parotid gland. The third most common benign tumor of the pediatric parotid gland is the pleomorphic adenoma.

Venous vascular malformations also occur in salivary glands. They enhance and may have associated phleboliths.

Other benign tumors Lipomas, schwannomas, and neurofibromas may also be seen in association with the salivary glands, most commonly the parotid. Lipomas have fat density and present in children. The neurogenic tumors generally follow cranial nerves V (submandibular, sublingual, and parotid glands) or VII (parotid glands). Be careful to trace these tumors along the expected course of the nerves, even to their foramina.

Malignant Neoplasms

Patients with parotid malignancies usually have a palpable, discrete, painless mass (98% of cases). Other presentations include facial nerve dysfunction (24%) and cervical adenopathy (6%). Facial nerve paralysis associated with a parotid mass usually means a malignancy is present. Of the malignancies to cause a facial nerve paralysis, adenoid cystic carcinoma and undifferentiated carcinoma predominate, with an incidence of 17% to 26%. The mean delay in reporting the mass to a physician is 3 months. The staging of malignant salivary gland lesions is outlined in Box 15-5.

The differentiation of deep or superficial parotid malignancies is critical from the standpoint of the extent of dissection needed to separate the nerve from the tumor or to gain access to the tumor, the attendant risk to the facial nerve, and in the case of tumors extending into the parapharyngeal space, the need for a cervical approach with or without mandibulotomy. Demonstration or suspicion of direct invasion of the nerve at the stylomastoid foramen (or above) prods the surgeon to plan for transmastoid identification of the facial nerve to control disease and prevent tumor spillage. The superficial parotidectomy thereby becomes skull base surgery with its attendant risks (to the other cranial nerves, venous sinuses, carotid artery, and temporomandibular joint function) and morbidity. If the skull base is invaded, the cartilaginous auditory canal may have to be addressed and possibly resected. A radical mastoidectomy is contemplated and even the ascending ramus of the mandible may be removed. MR does well in demonstrating the perineural, vascular, and dural invasion that may be present with parotid malignancies.

Mucoepidermoid carcinoma While the most common malignant lesion of the parotid gland is mucoepidermoid carcinoma, in the submandibular, sublingual, and minor salivary glands it is adenoid cystic carcinoma. Mucoepidermoid carcinomas, like squamous cell carci-

Box 15-5 Classification of Salivary Gland Malignancies

PRIMARY TUMOR (T)

TX: Tumor that cannot be assessed
T0: No evidence of primary tumor
T1: Tumor ≤2 cm in diameter without extraparenchymal extension
T2: Tumor >2 cm but ≤4 cm in diameter without extraparenchymal extension
T3: Tumor >4 cm and/or tumor having extraparenchymal extension*
T4a: Tumor invades the skin, mandible, ear canal, and/or facial nerve
T4b: Tumor invades skull base and/or pterygoid plates and/or encases carotid artery

*Note: Extraparenchymal extension is clinical or macroscopic evidence of invasion of soft tissues. Microscopic evidence alone does not constitute extraparenchymal extension for classification purposes.

NODAL INVOLVEMENT (N)

NX: Regional lymph nodes cannot be assessed
N0: No regional lymph node metastasis
N1: Metastasis in single ipsilateral lymph node, <3 cm in greatest dimension
N2: Metastasis in single ipsilateral lymph node, <3 cm but ≤6 cm in greatest dimension, or multiple ipsilateral lymph nodes, none >6 cm in greatest dimension, or bilateral or contralateral lymph nodes, none >6 cm in greatest dimension
  N2a: Metastasis in single ipsilateral lymph node >3 cm but ≤6 cm in greatest dimension
  N2b: Metastasis in multiple ipsilateral lymph nodes, none >6 cm in greatest dimension
  N2c: Metastasis in bilateral or contralateral lymph nodes, none >6 cm in greatest dimension
N3: Metastasis in lymph node >6 cm in greatest dimension

DISTANT METASTASIS (M)

MX: Presence of distant metastasis cannot be assessed
M0: No distant metastasis
M1: Distant metastasis

From Greene FL, Balch CM, Fleming ID, et al (eds): *AJCC Cancer Staging Manual*, ed 6. New York, Springer-Verlag, 2002, p 70. Used with permission.

noma, can be graded from low to high, and the prognosis varies with the grade. Mucoepidermoid carcinomas account for 30% of all salivary gland malignancies, and 60% of them occur in the parotid gland (Fig. 15-14). Mucoepidermoid carcinoma is the most common pediatric salivary gland malignancy. Thirty-five percent of salivary gland neoplasms in children are malignant and of these, 60% are mucoepidermoid carcinomas. Primary salivary

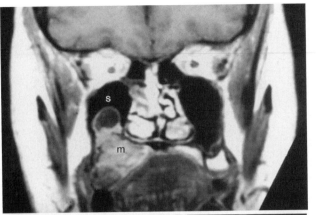

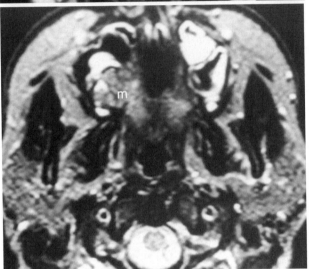

A

B

Fig. 15-14 Mucoepidermoid carcinoma. **A,** Coronal enhanced T1WI delineates a mass *(m)* emanating from the hard palate minor salivary gland tissue, which protrudes into the maxillary sinus *(s)*. Mass has moderate enhancement. **B,** On the T2WI, note that the mass *(m)* has intermediate signal intensity. Higher signal intensity anteriorly is caused by inflammatory change associated with the lesion.

gland lymphoma does occur in the parotid gland as can leukemic infiltration in children.

In the parotid gland, a lesion's morphology may be misleading as far as predicting benignity versus malignancy. Some pleomorphic adenomas have tentacles with an irregular margin. By the same token, some mucoepidermoid carcinomas are well defined by a pseudocapsule and do not appear to be invasive. Therefore, you cannot rely on shape to distinguish cancer from benign tumors. We favor shapely masses that make you salivate—like Hershey kisses (the G-rated version of this book).

Unfortunately, density and intensity provide paltry clues to a lesion's identity. On CT, most tumors of the parotid gland have a density equal to muscle—no help there. Low-grade mucoepidermoid carcinomas may have high signal intensity, and high-grade, poorly differenti-

ated mucoepidermoid carcinomas are usually low in intensity on T2WI. Therefore, a low-grade mucoepidermoid carcinoma may have intensity characteristics that are identical to those of a pleomorphic adenoma, and a Warthin's tumor may simulate a high-grade mucoepidermoid carcinoma. Thus, a lesion's T1 or T2 signal intensity, margination, and internal architecture cannot necessarily predict benignity or malignancy (high or low grade). Gridlock! For this reason, *chère radiologiste,* refrain from predicting histology when dealing with parotid masses; just define the lesion for the surgeon so that adequate removal, with attention to the facial nerve, can be achieved or offer to do an FNA for diagnosis.

Adenoid cystic carcinoma Adenoid cystic carcinoma, the second most common primary malignancy of the parotid gland and the most common tumor of the submandibular, sublingual, and minor salivary glands, is notorious for its propensity for perineural spread (50% to 60%) and persistence despite "complete surgical removal." They are like dust mites; you can not get rid of them, they keep multiplying, and you learn to live with them for a small price. Similar to the mucoepidermoid carcinoma, variable intensity occurs with the T2WI, which allows a weak guess at histology—but, again, do not bet the farm or even a cow pie (Fig. 15-15). Noncystic masses in the parotid gland have muscular CT density, low intensity on T1WI, and mild to moderate enhancement. An adenoid cystic carcinoma of the parotid gland may spread via the ramifications of cranial nerve VII retrograde into the temporal bone or may spread via the auriculotemporal branches of cranial nerve V to the

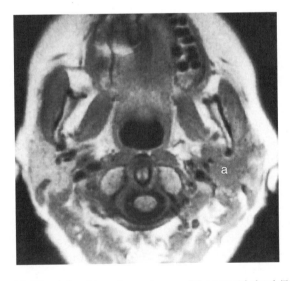

Fig. 15-15 Adenoid cystic carcinoma of the parotid gland. T1WI of the left parotid shows infiltrative mass *(a)* extending into both superficial and deep portions of the gland. Note how well the mass is identified by the replacement of the normal high intensity parotid tissue. Better watch cranial nerve VII on this lesion. Mind your facials!

Meckel's cave region through the foramen ovale. Again, adenoid cystic carcinomas may be very well defined within the parotid gland, and the diagnosis of a malignancy may not be suspected before biopsy. In the other salivary glands adenoid cystic carcinoma generally demonstrates perineural extension along the branches of the second and third divisions of cranial nerve V. This cancer is a relentless, slow-growing tumor whose prognosis is generally measured in terms of decades rather than 5-year survival rate because of its prolonged course.

Squamous cell carcinoma   Squamous cell carcinoma may be seen within the parotid gland. Sometimes it is difficult to tell whether the squamous cell carcinoma is present secondarily because of invasion of lymph nodes from a primary site outside the parotid or is intrinsic to the parotid gland (Fig. 15-16). How it gets there is mysterious; it is presumably caused by metaplasia of the ductal columnar epithelium into squamous cells. This same difficulty lies with lymphoma of the parotid—is it a primary parotid tumor or secondary spread? When multifocal in the parotid, it is generally accepted that the squamous cell carcinoma is probably within lymph nodes in the parotid gland. A search for a primary tumor is undertaken. The overlying skin and ear are the primary sites that drain to the parotid gland; however, the parotid lymph nodes may be involved with diffuse lesions such as lymphoma. Squamous cell carcinoma does not generally occur in submandibular, sublingual, or minor salivary glands as a primary site, although it certainly spreads from adjacent mucosal surfaces or lymph nodes. As mentioned in Chapter 14, obstruction of submandibular or sublingual gland ducts may be a presenting symptom of floor of mouth cancers.

Squamous cell carcinomas are virtually always hypointense on T2WI unless necrosis coexists.

Adenocarcinoma   Adenocarcinomas may also arise within the parotid gland, sublingual gland, submandibular gland, or minor salivary glands (Fig. 15-17). This lesion generally has a worse prognosis than that of mucoepidermoid carcinoma and adenoid cystic carcinoma (Box 15-6). This tumor is derived from the glandular tissue itself as opposed to ductal tissue. Signal intensity is variable, depending on mucinous, cystic, or solid contributions. Some adenocarcinomas occur from malignant degeneration of pleomorphic adenomas.

The polymorphous low-grade adenocarcinoma of the salivary gland (PLAC) is a low-grade neoplasm that predominantly occurs in the minor salivary glands of the oral cavity (mucosa of the soft and hard palates, in the buccal mucosa, and in the upper lip) but can be seen in the parotid gland. It has a much more benign prognosis and course than the traditional butt-kicking adenocarcinoma.

Acinic cell carcinoma   Acinic cell carcinoma is the most common primary multifocal malignancy to affect the parotid gland. Its prognosis is intermediate be-

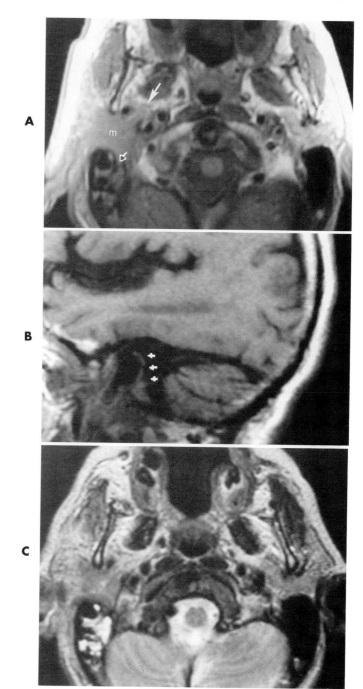

Fig. 15-16   Squamous cell carcinoma of the parotid gland. **A,** Axial T1WI demonstrates an ill-defined mass *(m)* in the right parotid gland invading the deep portion *(arrow)* and extending posteriorly to the stylomastoid foramen *(open arrow)*. **B,** There is perineural spread up the intramastoid cranial nerve VII *(below the arrows)* on this sagittal T1WI. **C,** As is typical of squamous cell carcinoma in the parotid gland, the lesion has low intensity on T2WI.

tween that of mucoepidermoid carcinoma and adenocarcinoma of the parotid gland. This tumor is seen exclusively in the parotid gland, and the incidence of bilateral acinic cell carcinomas is approximately 3%. No

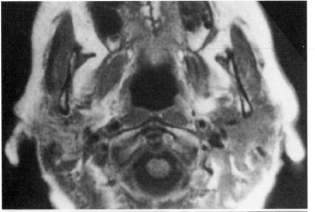

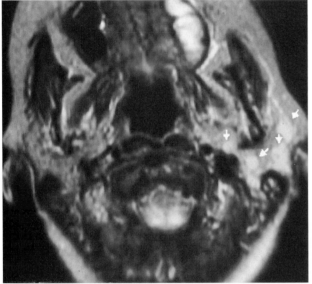

Fig. 15-17 Adenocarcinoma of the parotid gland. **A,** This T1WI shows the left parotid mass to look similar to that of the adenoid cystic carcinoma seen in Fig. 15-15. T1WI is not useful in predicting histologic identity. **B,** On T2WI the lesion is heterogeneous with what appears to be cystic portions *(arrows)*. Adenocarcinoma may have variable signal intensity on T2WI depending on the content of cystic, mucinous, or hypercellular sections.

specific imaging features other than its multifocality suggest this diagnosis.

Undifferentiated carcinoma Undifferentiated carcinoma is also seen as a salivary gland tumor. This lesion has a very poor prognosis but fortunately is rarely seen (<10% of cases).

Carcinoma ex pleomorphic adenoma As mentioned previously, if left alone to grow, a pleomorphic adenoma will degenerate into or coexist with a carcinoma in a significant (10% to 25%) percentage of cases. Cut it out! Usually the histologic subtype is an adenocarcinoma, and the lesion may be seen with rapid growth or even distant metastases (lung, bone, and nodes). An entity known as benign metastasizing pleomorphic adenoma, in which lesions may be present distant to the

Box 15-6 Five-Year Prognosis of Parotid Malignancies (Percentage of Parotid Malignancies)

GOOD

Acinic cell carcinoma (12%)
Adenoid cystic carcinoma (6%–15%)
Low-grade mucoepidermoid carcinoma (25%)

POOR

High-grade mucoepidermoid carcinoma (20%)
Adenocarcinoma (8%)
Squamous cell carcinoma (1%–7%)
Carcinoma ex pleomorphic adenoma (9%)
Undifferentiated carcinoma (9%)

parotid gland but with the same histology, has been reported. How this can be called a benign tumor is baffling; however, the term should be familiar to radiologists. It is similar to the entity of benign metastasizing meningiomas or leiomyomas of the uterus.

The incidence of nodal metastases in untreated parotid cancers is low except in T3 or T4 lesions. Although mucoepidermoid carcinoma and squamous cell carcinoma metastasize to nodes in 37% to 44% of cases, the other histologic types are only associated with lymphadenopathy in 5% to 21%, with adenoid cystic carcinoma being the lowest.

MASTICATOR SPACE

Anatomy

The masticator space is defined by layers of the deep cervical fascia and encompasses the muscles of mastication (the medial and lateral pterygoid, masseter, and temporalis muscles) as well as the condyle and ascending ramus of the mandible, branches of the external carotid artery and third division of cranial nerve V, and venous branches from the jugular system (Fig. 15-18). Of the muscles of mastication, the small lateral pterygoid has a primary function of opening the mouth, whereas the bulky medial pterygoid, masseter, and temporalis muscles serve to keep the mouth closed. Given that the Lord has given us three huge muscles to keep our yappers shut and only one small one to open our mouth, you can see why we feel politicians and lawyers are defying the rightful laws of nature and should have their lateral pterygoids removed.

How do you identify a lesion as being within the masticator space? When a masticator space lesion is present, the parapharyngeal fat is displaced posteromedially and

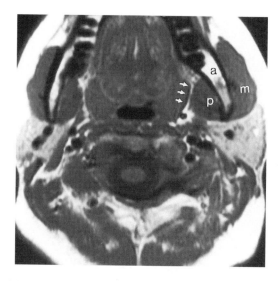

Fig. 15-18   Normal masticator space. Masseter muscle *(m)*, pterygoid muscle *(p)*, and angle of the mandible *(a)* are well visualized on this T1WI. Note that a masticator space lesion would displace parapharyngeal fat *(arrows)* medially and predominantly posteriorly.

may be infiltrated along its anterolateral aspect (see Table 15-1). Even if the lesion does not arise within the muscles, bone, or cranial nerve V, you will be able to identify a masticator space lesion by this characteristic displacement of the parapharyngeal fat. Have faith.

Congenital Disorders

Once again, branchial cleft cysts are one of the congenital lesions that occur in or around the masticator space and may be seen in its deep (along the pterygoids) or superficial (over the masseter) compartments.

Lymphangiomas (loculated, infiltrative, multicystic, nonenhancing lesions with high signal on T1WI and T2WI) and hemangiomas (venous vascular malformations that enhance, are solid, and are dark on T1WI and bright on T2WI) may also infiltrate the masticator space (Fig. 15-19). Both of these lesions are usually evident at birth.

Accessory parotid gland lobes may simulate a masticator space lesion, presenting as a palpable mass over the masseter. Low density on CT and relatively high intensity compared to muscle on T1WI should suggest the diagnosis and obviate the need for biopsy. This is really a pseudomass of the masticator space—it is outside of the investing deep cervical fascia.

Diseases that may infiltrate the muscles of mastication are listed in Box 15-7.

Inflammatory Lesions

Odontogenic lesions   Most of the inflammatory lesions of the masticator space relate to infections of odon-togenic origin. Therefore, abscesses around the teeth, osteomyelitis of the mandible, and cellulitis associated with carious teeth are the prime offenders in this category (Fig. 15-20). Occasionally, cellulitis and myositis of the masticator space develop as a result of penetrating injuries, superficial facial infections, or adjacent parotitis. Most inflammatory lesions of the masticator space can be readily identified on CT or MR. On CT, look for thickening of the adjacent muscle, infiltration of the nearby fat, subcutaneous tissue, or skin with a strand pattern to it. If an abscess has developed, it will appear in a fashion similar to abscesses elsewhere, with a low-density center and a peripheral enhancing rim. On MR, inflammatory lesions, because of their high water content from edema, are very bright on T2WI. There are some exceptions to this rule, namely actinomycosis (because of sulfur granule deposition) and fungal infections (because of paramagnetic iron and manganese accumulation).

Bruxism and atrophy   Bruxism may develop in patients who constantly gnash their teeth. This is a fancy word for (usually) bilateral enlargement of the muscles of mastication. It occurs most commonly idiopathically but may develop as a result of malocclusion, excessive chewing, or clenching the teeth (as occurs when radiologists are called to the witness stand). Rarely, this may be a unilateral phenomenon. Alternatively, one may see atrophy of the muscles of mastication when one has a cranial nerve V abnormality (Fig. 15-21). This may be caused by lesions in the peripheral branches of the third division of cranial nerve V or by loss of central input to the motor portion of the trigeminal nerve from lesions in the frontal cortex. Perioperative injury may cause denervation atrophy as can trauma. With denervation atrophy one may see enhancement after gadolinium administration and/or high signal intensity on T2W scans in the muscles of mastication. Neurogenic tumors may also induce these imaging characteristics.

Fibrous dysplasia   Fibrous dysplasia causes enlargement of the mandible with expansion of the outer cortex of the bone, generally without erosion through the bone. This may affect the entire portion of the mandible and is more commonly seen there than in the maxilla. McCune-Albright syndrome refers to precocious puberty, café-au-lait spots, and polyostotic fibrous dysplasia, (which may affect the mandible unilaterally) in girls. When a patient has bilateral bubbly bone lesions with a ground-glass appearance, consider either fibrous dysplasia or cherubism, which is a related disorder. Both of these disorders tend to expand during adolescence, are possibly related to hormonal influences, and either regress or stabilize in young adulthood.

The skull and facial bones are involved in 10% to 25% of cases of monostotic fibrous dysplasia and in 50% of polyostotic fibrous dysplasia. The mandible, maxilla, and calvarium are frequently involved.

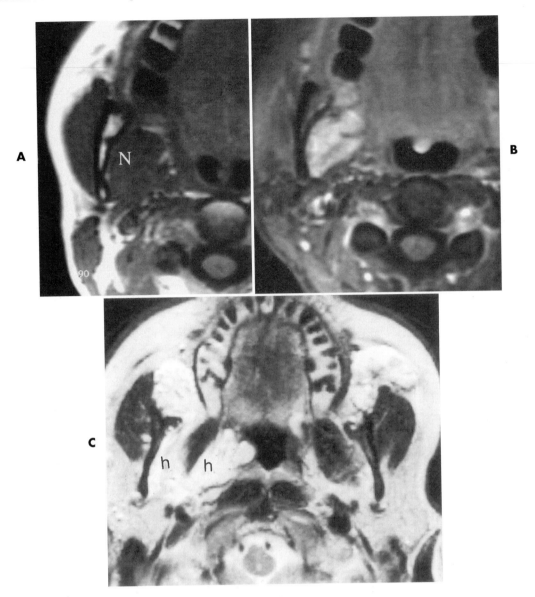

Fig. 15-19 Venous vascular malformation of masticator space. Note how this mass *(N)* that is isointense to muscle in **A,** enhances so dramatically in **B.** This is typical of soft tissue "hemangiomas." **C,** Different case, and same diagnosis: T2WI shows infiltrating venous vascular malformations *(h).*

Most of the lesions of the mandible are odontogenic in origin. As explained earlier in the discussion of the oral cavity (Tables 14-3 and 14-4), radicular cysts from carious teeth and dentigerous cysts associated with unerupted teeth are the most common causes of cystic lesions of the mandible.

Temporomandibular joint syndrome The temporomandibular joint (TMJ) falls under the rubric of the masticator space. The TMJ may be the source of chronic facial or head pain. TMJ (or chronic maxillofacial pain) syndrome is seen in women nine times more frequently than men, is often precipitated by a traumatic event, and is very poorly understood. Presently, most imaging is per-

Box 15-7   Infiltrative Lesions of the Muscles of Mastication

Beckwith Weidemann syndrome (craniofacial dysmorphism, macroglossia, omphalocele, gigantism, visceromegaly, abdominal neoplasms)
Bruxism
Glycogen storage disease
Hypothyroidism
Lipodystrophy
Neurofibromatosis
Proteus syndrome

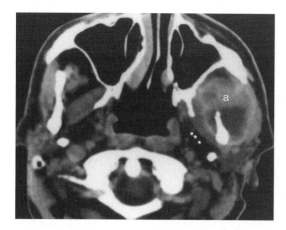

Fig. 15-20 Abscess in masticator space. Axial CT shows an abscess *(a)* centered on the left mandible. Note that the parapharyngeal fat *(asterisks)* is displaced posteromedially by this masticator space infection. This is what happens when dentists do not wash their instruments of torture properly.

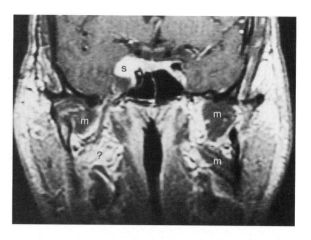

Fig. 15-21 Atrophy of muscles of mastication. This enhanced T1WI demonstrates the differential size of the right masticator musculature from that of the left masticator musculature *(m)*. This finding should prompt a search for nerve V lesions. Voilà! One can find a trigeminal schwannoma *(s)* in the cavernous sinus on the right side. It is amazing how sometimes these things work out so nicely in textbooks. ? = small right lateral pterygoid.

formed with MR where the meniscus, condyle, glenoid fossa, and surrounding soft tissues may be evaluated. Rarely, arthrography may be performed through injection of the joint under fluoroscopy. The meniscus has an anterior triangular band and a larger posterior band, which are joined in the middle by an intermediate zone (Fig. 15-22). The posterior band is attached to the posterior joint by the retrodiskal tissue, or bilaminar zone. The meniscus should be centered over the condylar head in open- and closed-mouth positions with the posterior margin of the posterior band between the 11 and 12 o'clock point of the condyle in the closed-mouth position. The joint itself has an anterosuperior compartment and an inferior compartment, which usually do not communicate. The lateral pterygoid muscle opens the jaw and inserts on the anterior portion of the meniscus. The medial pterygoid, temporalis, and masseter muscles close the jaw.

Anterior meniscal dislocations are the most common type in patients with TMJ complaints. In this setting the meniscus' posterior band is dislocated anteriorly from directly over the condyle. This displacement is more than 10 degrees anterior to the 12 o'clock position, more like the 9–10 o'clock position. It may be far in front of the condyle in the closed-mouth position on sagittal T1WI (Fig. 15-23). The dislocation may reduce on opening (often with a clicking sound—the "opening click") and may redislocate on closing (a closing click). The timing of the opening click may correlate with the degree of anterior dislocation of the meniscus. Alternatively, the meniscus may remain anteriorly dislocated even on opening. The location of the disk in front of the condyle may restrict the joint's motion (a closed-lock situation).

A medial or lateral component to the anterior dislo-

cation (rotational dislocation) is not uncommon (Fig. 15-24). Isolated medial and lateral (termed "sideways") dislocations are relatively rare; however, with a transverse component the possibility of nonsurgical reduction of the dislocation is decreased (from 46% to 9%). For this reason a coronal MR should be performed. Posterior dislocations are extremely rare.

A stuck disk is one that does not move in open or closed-mouth positions. It may or may not be anteriorly displaced but it is usually fibrosed in and immobile. This may be associated with pain and disability.

Because approximately 35% of subjects without TMJ symptoms have anterior dislocations, many researchers believe that internal derangement, as defined by meniscal displacement, is not the only source of pain. Nonetheless, 78% of patients with TMJ symptoms have disk displacements. The degree of disk displacement is greater in symptomatic than asymptomatic individuals and recapture of the displaced disk is less frequent in patients than volunteers (where it is the norm). Bilateral involvement is twice as common in patients than volunteers. A recent study of whiplash victims and age and gender matched controls found that although 53% of the subjects in the car accident had meniscal displacement, as did 45% of the control group. Effusions were found in 8% of controls and 6% of whiplashed patients. Clearly, the baseline incidence of this disease is very high. The size of TMJ effusions correlates well with pain scales. A T2WI in the sagittal plane demonstrates joint fluid if it is present in substantial amounts (see Fig. 15-24C and E). Other authors have focused on the retrodiskal tissues and believe that inflammation (again bright on T2WI)

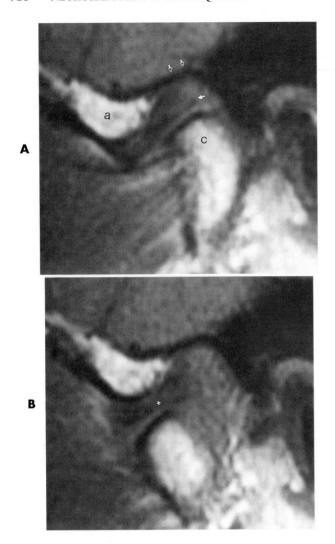

Fig. 15-22   Normal TMJ anatomy. **A,** The meniscus in the closed mouth view has its posterior edge *(arrow)* between 11 and 12 o'clock in relationship to the condylar head *(c)*. The cortex of the glenoid fossa *(open arrows)* and the articular eminence *(a)* make up the superior landmarks of the TMJ. Note the meniscus has an anterior and posterior triangular band. **B,** In the open mouth view, the condyle translates forward to a position under the eminence. The meniscus maintains its "bow-tie" configuration with its intermediate zone (+) centered over the condyle.

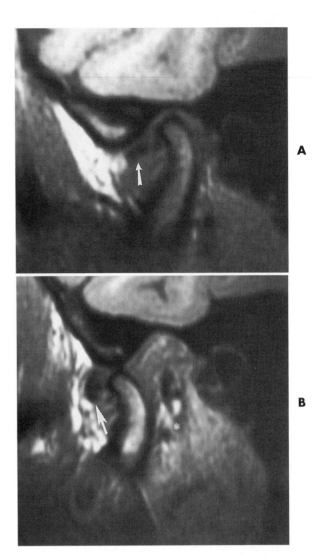

Fig. 15-23   Anterior dislocation of the meniscus. **A,** Meniscus *(arrow)* is far anterior and inferior on the closed mouth view. There is decreased distance between the condyle and glenoid fossa. The next issue is whether the meniscus returns to a normal appearance on the open mouth view (relocates or recaptures) or remains anteriorly dislocated. **B,** Bad news. This meniscus *(arrow)* remains anteriorly located and misshapen on the open mouth view. Note good range of motion (sometimes mobility is restricted by the meniscus—"closed locked position"), but you can imagine the friction between the condyle and eminence in this patient. Ouch.

there may irritate nerve fibers, accounting for the pain. Still others believe that a fixed immobile meniscus may be the causative factor. Looking for movement of the meniscus in relation to the condyle is important in comparing open- and closed-mouth views. The fact that the cause of the patients' symptoms has not been well characterized has not stopped the government from the "*t*hrow *m*oney at *j*unk" syndrome (TMJ research).

MR is not able to detect disk perforations other than showing secondary findings of joint effusion and meniscal displacements. Arthrography or arthroscopy is the only means of demonstrating perforations. Perforations usually occur at the junction of the bilaminar zone with

the posterior band. They occur more frequently with a transverse component to meniscal dislocations.

Initial treatment for TMJ syndrome is splinting, analgesics, behavior modification, and muscle relaxants. If the patient fails to respond to this noninvasive therapy and has meniscal abnormalities, plication of the meniscus into a more normal location or meniscal removal with or without prosthesis may be attempted. Adhesions may be lysed if present under arthroscopy. Suffice it to say that some patients have persistent meniscal dislocations after surgery but get pain relief, whereas others re-

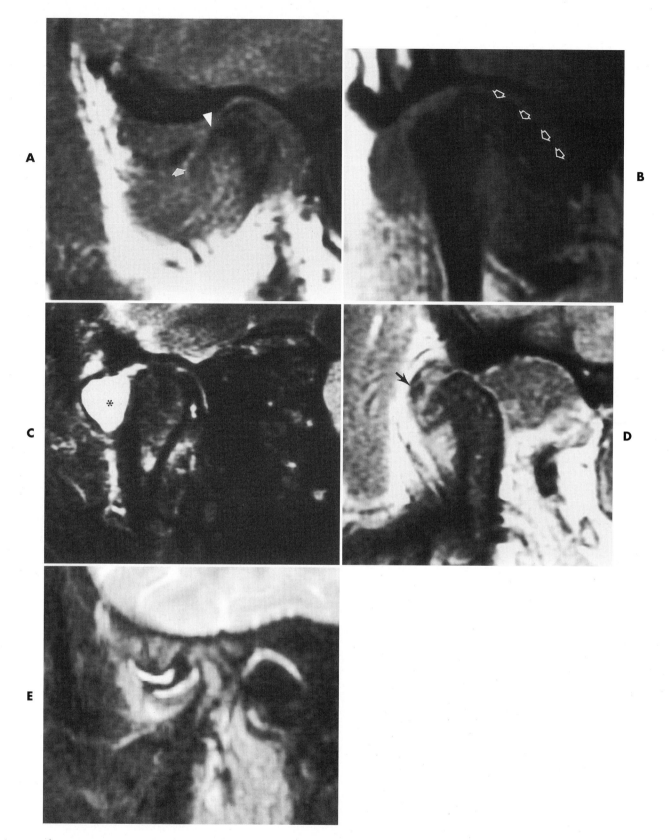

Fig. 15-24 Anteromedial dislocation of the disc. **A,** The low meniscus *(arrow)* is displaced far anteriorly on the sagittal closed mouth T1WI and there are degenerative changes to the condylar head including "bird-beaking" *(arrowhead)* and sclerosis. **B,** The meniscus *(open arrows)* is displaced medially off the top of the condyle on the coronal T1WI. The dark condylar signal should raise the spectre of avascular necrosis. **C,** A large effusion (*) is present on the T2WI. **D,** The meniscus *(arrow)* becomes bunched up anteriorly and does not recapture on the open mouth sagittal view. **E,** TMJ effusion. The different anterior compartments of the temporomandibular joint can be identified on this T2WI, separated by the anteriorly displaced meniscus. The fluid produces bright signal.

main in discomfort. Still others may have complications related to the surgery including foreign body reactions, granular cell reactions, or avascular necrosis of the condylar head (which may occur without surgery) that worsen symptoms. The Teflon Proplast TMJ prosthesis has been associated with numerous postoperative complications such as described above.

In the long term, degenerative changes in the joint may develop and include narrowing, osteophytic bird-beaking of the condyle, eburnation, ankylosis, and, as noted previously, chronic avascular necrosis. The latter may be identified as low signal intensity on all pulse sequences in the condylar head. Sclerosis is seen on CT (Fig. 15-25). Finally we have imaging findings to account for patients' symptoms.

Rheumatoid arthritis may also affect the TMJ. Usually erosions of the condyle are seen with a soft-tissue component (see Fig. 15-25B). Effusions and meniscal perforations also complicate the rheumatoid joint. Other arthritides include septic arthritis, gout, and pseudogout of the TMJ.

The TMJ may be affected by such lesions as pigmented villonodular synovitis (characterized by hemosiderin or other blood products seen as dark signal on T2* MR), synovial chondromatosis (Fig. 15-26), and tumoral calcinosis.

Benign Neoplasms

In 1982, a new classification of hemangiomas and vascular malformations was proposed by Mulliken and Glowacki and has since been adopted. In this new design, infantile hemangiomas have been relegated to those benign neoplasms of endothelial cells that may or may

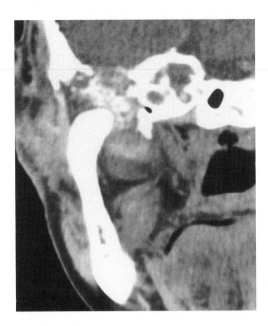

Fig. 15-26 Calcified lesion of TMJ. This temporomandibular joint lesion shows a calcified matrix and destruction of the temporal bone making up the glenoid fossa. The differential diagnosis would include synovial chondromatosis, a chondrosarcoma, a chondroblastoma, calcium pyrophosphate dihydrate deposition disease, tumoral calcinosis, and Brown tumor, in decreasing order of likelihood.

not be present at birth, have a rapid proliferative phase shortly after birth, and often involute during early childhood with 50% completely resolved by 5 years of age and 72% by 7 years old. Such hemangiomas occur more frequently in Caucasians and girls. They may be in the skin, subcutaneous tissues, or deep spaces of the head

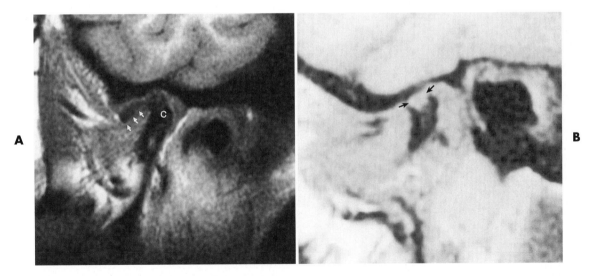

Fig. 15-25 Avascular necrosis of the TMJ. **A,** Sagittal T1WI shows decreased intensity in the mandibular condyle *(c)* in this patient with chronic TMJ syndrome. Note that the meniscus *(arrows)* is anteriorly dislocated in this closed mouth view. This patient had avascular necrosis of the condyle, confirmed by wedge resection. **B,** Erosive synovitis of the TMJ. Note the erosion *(arrows)* of the condylar head on the sagittal T1WI in this patient with rheumatoid arthritis.

and neck. If the lesions fail to involute on their own, they may be prodded to do so with steroids, alpha interferon, or chemotherapy. The masses are low signal on T1WI, bright on T2WI, and enhance. As they involute fibrofatty infiltration occurs and they enhance less.

Kasabach-Merritt syndrome refers to a syndrome in which infantile hemangiomas are associated with consumptive coagulopathy, high output congestive heart failure, and respiratory distress with or without splenomegaly.

Vascular malformations are the other "hemangiomas" that have been re-classified. They may be primarily venous, lymphatic, or combination lesions when they are low-flow ones. They are comprised of dysplastic vessels, are present at birth, grow during fast growth phase of the child, and persist. The majority of these lesions are venous and therefore are seen as slow flow vascular channels on MR. They too are dark on T1WI, bright on T2WI, and enhance. These lesions may show calcifications on CT. Mafucci syndrome may include venous malformations and enchondromatosis. Klippel-Trenaunay-Weber syndrome hasmixed capillary-venous-lymphatic malformations with hemihypertrophy. Sclerosis may be the treatment of choice, even using ethanol under general anesthesia.

The more lymphatic the lesion the more cystic it may appear but the cystic components usually have brighter signal than CSF on T1W and fluid-attenuated inversion recovery (FLAIR) scans.

Purely lymphatic malformations, that is, the cystic hygroma family of lesions, are increased in patients with Turner syndrome, Noonan syndrome, Down syndrome, and trisomy 13. High flow vascular malformations contain an arterial component and may contain a nidus or a fistula. They are the least frequent of the childhood vascular malformations but may be seen with Osler-Weber-Rendu syndrome.

The infantile hemangioma is the most common pediatric, benign neoplasm of the masticator space. This generally begins in the superficial tissues but may extend deeply into the muscles and adjacent fat of the masticator space. Hemangiomas enhance dramatically on CT and MR and have very high signal intensity on T2WI. Generally, because most are capillary hemangiomas, you do not see the large vascular structures with flow voids that you see with lesions such as glomus tumors or venous vascular malformations of the head and neck. Angiofibromas may also arise in the muscles of mastication though their more common head and neck site is at the sphenopalatine foramen associated with the nasopharynx (Fig. 15-27).

Ameloblastoma A relatively common benign bony tumor of the mandible is the ameloblastoma. It is labeled benign because it does not metastasize, but it is highly aggressive locally and may have malignant growth pat-

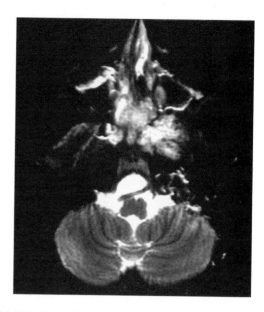

Fig. 15-27 Juvenile nasopharyngeal angiofibroma (JNA). The T2WI shows the mass in the nasopharynx and masticator space on the left. It grows through the pterygopalatine fossa.

terns. Ameloblastomas present as solitary masses of the mandible. They are usually multiloculated and have septations within the lesion. There may be an extraosseous component to this lesion as it expands beyond bony confines. The lesion is seen as a lytic process within the mandible on CT with fine septations running within it. On MR, it is high intensity on T2WI and may have enhancing septa within it (see Fig. 14-28).

Neurogenic tumors Other benign neoplasms of the masticator space include schwannomas and neurofibromas. Because the masticator space is permeated by

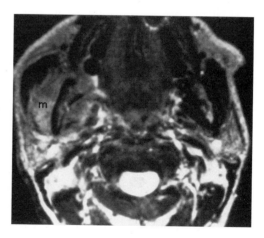

Fig. 15-28 Ewing sarcoma of the mandible. Note the large soft tissue mass (*m*) centered on the mandible on the right side of this T2WI. Again, the parapharyngeal fat is displaced posteromedially. Ewing sarcoma, because it is a small cell tumor with a high nuclear/cytoplasmic ratio, may be low to intermediate in signal intensity on T2WI.

branches of cranial nerve V, this may be a site of neural tumor development. Isolated schwannomas are the most common neurogenic tumor of the masticator space. Plexiform neurofibromas may be extensive and may be a cause of a diffuse masticator space mass. A small percentage of patients with neurofibromatosis may have malignant neurogenic tumors, which may affect the masticator space. Usually, the inferior alveolar canal is eroded by malignant neurofibromas, and the tumor may ascend into and through the skull base (foramen ovale) via the third division of cranial nerve V.

Schwannomas may rarely undergo fatty degeneration that may cause them to simulate lipomas (which favor the buccal region).

Malignant Neoplasms

Osteosarcoma and Ewing sarcoma Most of the malignancies of the masticator space relate to tumors of the mandible. Therefore, osteosarcoma and Ewing sarcoma should be mentioned early in the discussion of malignancies of the masticator space (Fig. 15-28). Both of these lesions may demonstrate periosteal reaction and either a dense hyperostotic destructive mass or a lytic process in the mandible. Ewing sarcomas occur in a younger age group than osteosarcomas, which affect patients in their third and fourth decades of life. Rarely, ameloblastomas may demonstrate malignant potential as well. When an ameloblastoma metastasizes, it usually goes to the lung.

Squamous cell carcinoma Squamous cell carcinoma of the mucosa is the most common malignancy outside the masticator space to invade this region. Typically, the squamous cell cancers arise in the region of the oral cavity (especially the retromolar trigone), oropharynx, or nasopharynx, where extension to the pterygoid musculature is not uncommon. Alternatively, oral cavity tumors may spread into the mandible (Fig. 15-29). Buccal cancers may invade the masseter muscle. Only the temporalis muscle is relatively spared from squamous cell carcinoma spread.

Metastasis Metastases to the bones of the masticator space are not uncommon and typically arise from kidney, breast, or lung cancer. Thyroid cancer may also be a source of metastatic involvement of the mandible. The most common metastasis to the mandible is an adenocarcinoma from the breast, and mandibular involvement occurs five times more commonly than maxillary involvement. Metastases to the mandible are more common than primary mandibular bony tumors. In children, neuroblastomas may go to the bones or soft tissue of the masticator space (Fig. 15-30).

Soft tissue sarcoma In addition to malignant lesions of the bone and spread from adjacent mucosal surfaces, some soft-tissue sarcomas affect the masticator space. Rhabdomyosarcomas are the most common of these tu-

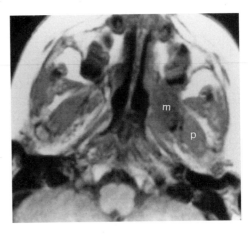

Fig. 15-29 Squamous cell carcinoma extending into the masticator space. This hard palate squamous cell carcinoma *(m)* grew through the retromolar trigone into the pterygoid musculature *(p)*, thereby invading the masticator space. From this region, the lesion may invade the pterygopalatine fossa.

mors and are generally seen in children. Rhabdomyosarcomas have a propensity for intratumoral hemorrhage and are generally bright on T2WI (Fig. 15-31). Fibrosarcomas and osteosarcomas have also been reported in the head and neck, often in association with retinoblastoma. This association may be related to the oncogene found with bilateral retinoblastomas. Osteosarcomas may have bony matrix; fibrosarcomas may be dark on T2WI. Malignant neurofibrosarcomas may also affect the masticator space.

Lymphoma Lymphoma in the facial nodes may present as a superficial masticator space lesion, but lym-

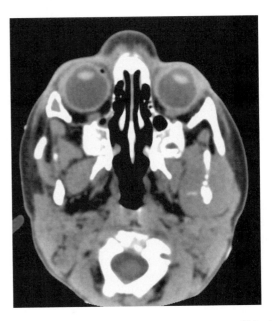

Fig. 15-30 Metastasis from neuroblastoma to mandible. There is a soft tissue mass centered about the left mandible on this scan. Note that this is a child. Diagnosis: neuroblastoma.

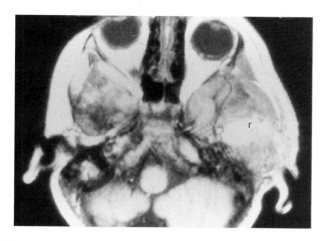

Fig. 15-31 Rhabdomyosarcoma. Axial T1WI shows a rhabdomyosarcoma with intratumoral hemorrhage invading the masticator space and the infratemporal fossa. The incidence of hemorrhage within a rhabdomyosarcoma *(r)* is approximately 30%.

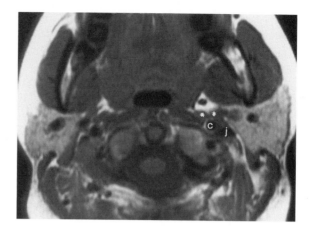

Fig. 15-32 Normal parapharyngeal space. Axial T1WI shows the high signal intensity of the prestyloid parapharyngeal space fat. Separating the prestyloid and poststyloid parapharyngeal space is the styloid musculature *(asterisks)*. Directly behind the styloid musculature one can identify the carotid artery *(c)* and jugular vein *(j)* within the carotid space. On CT, the styloid process may be the best anatomic landmark to separate the two spaces.

phoma may also permeate the mandible and/or infiltrate the muscles of mastication. This is most commonly seen in non-Hodgkin lymphoma.

You got your juices flowing with salivary lesions. You have chewed on a few masticator processes. Now you will be served the foie gras, a fatty infiltrated region, the parapharyngeal space. As you read this next section, pour yourself a glass of Sauterne with the additional income you will make from the knowledge you have already gained. Wash down the foie gras.

PARAPHARYNGEAL SPACE

Anatomy

The parapharyngeal space is classically separated into a prestyloid compartment and a poststyloid compartment (Fig. 15-32). The poststyloid parapharyngeal space contains the carotid sheath and has been called the carotid space by many authors. When cognoscenti refer to the parapharyngeal space, however, they are generally referring to the prestyloid portion. The fascia of the stylopharyngus, styloglossus, and tensor veli palatini muscle separates prestyloid and poststyloid spaces, but one can also use the styloid process for this boundary. Only fat, lymphatics, and very small branches of the internal maxillary artery, ascending pharyngeal artery, and mandibular (V-3) nerve are within the parapharyngeal space. Occasionally, you may find ectopic minor salivary gland tissue; however, the space is dominated by its fat.

Fat is a readily mobile substance (as the middle-aged abdomen can attest) and therefore is readily displaced and infiltrated by adjacent disease. By observing the direction

of displacement of this fat, you can identify a lesion as arising from one of the deep spaces of the head and neck (see Table 15-1). Bet you never thought fat could be so useful. Just do not let it metastasize to your head.

Congenital Disorders

Other than a rare second branchial cleft cyst (see Table 15-2) and lymphangioma, congenital lesions of the parapharyngeal space are rare (Box 15-8). The tract of the sec-

---

Box 15-8   Differential Diagnosis of Prestyloid Parapharyngeal Space Lesions

1. Branchial Cleft Cysts
2. Castleman's disease
3. Cystic hygroma
4. Fibromatosis
5. Inflammatory pseudotumor
6. Lymph nodes
7. Minor salivary gland tumors—Pleomorphic adenoma rules
8. Neurogenic tumors
9. Paragangliomas
10. Parapharyngeal space abscess
11. Parotid deep lobe tumors
12. Solitary fibrous tumor
13. Spread of adjacent tumors such as nasopharyngeal and oropharyngeal carcinoma, chordoma, and synovial sarcoma

ond branchial cleft extends to the oropharyngeal tonsillar fossa and thus a second branchial cleft cyst may rarely arise here. Mechanical compression of adjacent cranial nerves IX to XII can cause symptoms. Cystic schwannomas would be in the differential diagnosis but concurrent solid tissue in schwannomas, not branchial cysts, should steer you to the Louisville slugger diagnosis.

Inflammatory Lesions

Intrinsic inflammatory disease of the parapharyngeal space is also rare. Infections may spread secondarily from (1) mucosal infections such as tonsillitis or pharyngitis, (2) masticator space lesions such as odontogenic abscesses, and (3) parotid infections. Adenitis related to any of these primary infections may coexist.

Benign Neoplasms

Primary lesions arising within the prestyloid parapharyngeal space are extremely uncommon. Because only fat, ectopic minor salivary gland tissue, and lymph nodes are present in this region, the most common intrinsic lesions of the prestyloid parapharyngeal space are enlarged lymph nodes, either inflammatory or neoplastic. Occasionally, minor salivary gland tumors occur with the pleomorphic adenoma being the most common (Fig. 15-33). As elsewhere these tumors are very bright on T2WI and have a well-defined, lobulated margin. Lipomas also may arise primarily in the parapharyngeal space. A tumor in the parapharyngeal space must be completely surrounded by fat on all sides to call it primary to that region; if you lose a fat plane, the lesion may be creeping in from another space of the neck.

Of intrinsic tumors that infiltrate the prestyloid parapharyngeal space, major and minor salivary gland tumors are most common (40% to 50%), followed by neurogenic tumors (17% to 25%) and glomus tumors (10% to 15%). Parotid masses in the deep lobe, mostly pleomorphic adenomas (80% to 90%), are the most common benign neoplasm to invade the parapharyngeal space secondarily. Malignant parotid tumors rarely arise in this location. The distinguishing feature between a deep lobe of the parotid mass and a primary parapharyngeal space minor salivary gland tumor is the location of the parapharyngeal fat. If the parapharyngeal fat is displaced anteromedially, suggest the diagnosis of a deep lobe parotid mass. If the parapharyngeal fat is seen between the le-

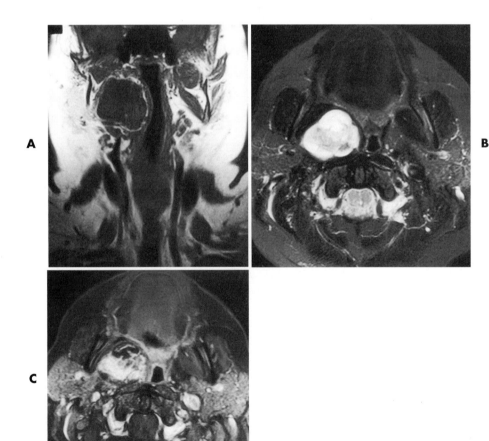

Fig. 15-33 Parapharyngeal space pleomorphic adenoma. **A,** If you transplanted this mass to the parotid gland this would be a "no-brainer" pleomorphic adenoma. After all, it is bright on T2W **(B)** and enhances **(C).** The parapharyngeal space location should not dissuade you. Pleomorphic adenomas arise from minor salivary gland tissue there. (Case courtesy of Stuart Bobman, M.D., Naples Florida.)

sion and the deep lobe of the parotid, then the lesion is either mucosal in origin or arose within the ectopic tissue of the prestyloid parapharyngeal space.

Malignant Neoplasms

Secondary invasion of the parapharyngeal space occurs often, usually spreading from a mucosal space abnormality. Of the various sites of the mucosal space, the nasopharynx and tonsils represent the most frequent sources of secondary invasion of the parapharyngeal space (Fig. 15-34). Nasopharyngeal squamous cell carcinoma has been described to invade the parapharyngeal space in 65% of cases at the time of diagnosis. Because this tumor has a propensity for submucosal growth as opposed to exophytic growth, the infiltration of the parapharyngeal fat may be the only indicator of a nasopharyngeal primary cancer. From the tonsil, lateral growth leads to the parapharyngeal fat. A tumor deep within the crypts of the tonsil

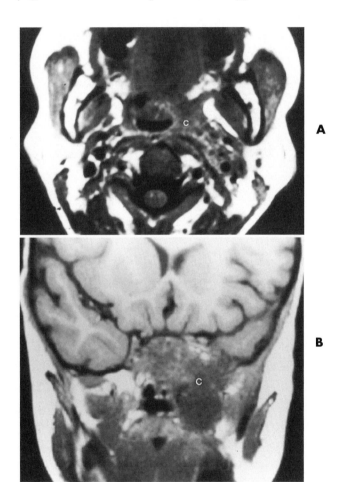

Fig. 15-34   Malignant spread of cancer into parapharyngeal space. **A,** Axial T1WI demonstrates a tonsillar carcinoma *(c)* growing laterally into the parapharyngeal space. Fat is being displaced laterally. **B,** In another patient, a coronal T1WI shows growth of a nasopharyngeal cancer *(c)* into the parapharyngeal fat. Note the preservation of the fat on the contralateral side.

may escape the endoscopist's attention and the radiologist may be the only one who can identify the primary tumor, on the basis of its infiltration of the parapharyngeal fat.

Synovial sarcomas can arise in the parapharyngeal space. These masses are not derived from the synovium and are unrelated to joints. Good name, eh? Trust the pathologists to confuse the poor radiologists, but we return the favor with our 25-gauge fine needle aspirations. They are distinguished by their propensity for fluid levels, encystment, intratumoral hemorrhage, calcification, and multiloculation. They may be well defined and have excellent prognoses . . . for sarcomas!

Only malignant lymphadenopathy and minor salivary gland neoplasms qualify as intrinsic malignancies of the parapharyngeal space. Minor salivary gland malignancies are far outnumbered by mucosal tumors that invade the area secondarily.

Plasmacytomas can occur in the parapharyngeal space, either de novo or via growth from the pharynx. These tumors occur four times more frequently in men than women. Eighty percent of extramedullary plasmacytomas occur in the head and neck (nose > sinus > nasopharynx > tonsil). They may fill the parapharyngeal space with tumor that is similar in intensity to muscle on T1WI and intermediate in intensity on T2WI. They enhance more uniformly in the periphery than in the center.

If you are still awake after your foie gras and Sauterne, you will find out next what the pâté may do to your carotid space.

CAROTID SPACE

Anatomy

The carotid space (poststyloid parapharyngeal space) deserves to be treated as a separate entity because of the numerous tumors associated with the carotid sheath and because this space is partially encapsulated by deep cervical fascia. The fascia around the carotid sheath is complex in that it may be incomplete in parts or absent in some people, and is uniformly intact only below the bifurcation. The normal contents of the carotid space include the carotid artery, internal jugular vein, vagus nerve (X), sympathetic nervous plexus, branches of the ansa cervicalis/hypoglossi (C1–3 roots), and cranial nerves IX, XI, and XII. Lymph nodes abound around and within the carotid sheath. The carotid space courses down the entire length of the neck and begins at the skull base. Superiorly, the carotid space is separated from the prestyloid parapharyngeal space by the styloid musculature, seen as small slips of the styloglossus and stylopharyngeus muscles just anterior to the carotid sheath but posterior to the parapharyngeal fat (Fig. 15-32).

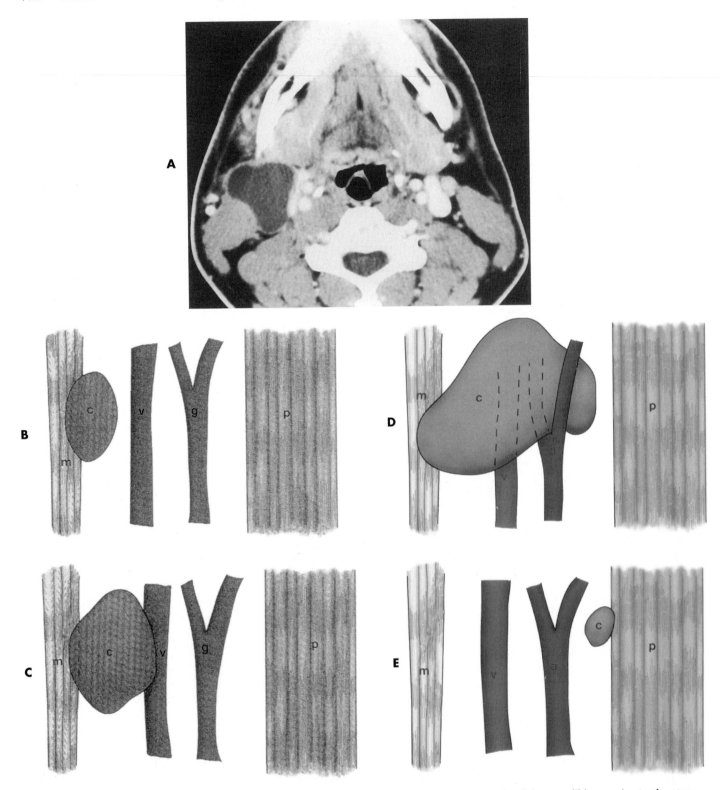

Fig. 15-35 Branchial cleft cyst. **A,** Bailey Type 2. What will you call a cystic mass at the angle of the mandible anterior to the stern-ocleidomastoid muscle, which approaches the carotid sheath and has a thin rim? A second branchial cleft cyst, if you are smart! **B,** Type I second branchial cleft cyst anomaly. The cyst lies superficial to the anterior border of the sternocleidomastoid muscle beneath the cervical fascia. m = sternocleidomastoid; v = internal jugular vein; a = common carotid artery; c = cyst; p = pharynx. **C,** Type II second branchial cleft cyst anomaly. The cyst abuts the carotid sheath and is varyingly adherent to the internal jugular vein. **D,** Type III second branchial cleft cyst anomaly. The cyst passes characteristically medially between the internal and external carotid arteries and extends toward the lateral wall of the pharynx. **E,** Type IV second branchial cleft cyst anomaly. This is a columnar-lined cyst located deep to the carotid vessels abutting the pharynx. (B-E from Mukherji SK, Fatterpekar G, Castillo M, et al: Imaging of congenital anomalies of the branchial apparatus. *Neuroimaging Clin North Am* 10:86-87, 2000.)

Congenital Disorders

Branchial cleft cyst and lymphangioma Second BCCs may be intimately associated with the carotid bifurcation. These cysts probably arise because of incomplete closure of the cervical sinus of His (not hers). If they connect to the external skin or the pharyngeal mucosa they are called branchial cleft sinus tracts. If they connect from pharynx to skin they are considered fistulae (see Table 15-2). They may occur anywhere along the path from the palatine tonsil to the supraclavicular region but are most commonly found near the angle of the mandible along the carotid sheath. The Bailey type II cyst is most classic, posterior to the submandibular gland and along the sternocleidomastoid muscle, in close association with the carotid bifurcation (Fig. 15-35). Bailey type I is located anterior to the surface of the sternocleidomastoid muscle, deep to the platysma. Bailey type III may extend between the internal and external carotid artery and may send a tail to the mucosal space. Bailey type IV is actually in the pharyngeal mucosa or submucosa and is deep to the carotid arteries.

In a similar fashion lymphangiomas may infiltrate the contents of the carotid space. These lesions are seen in children and/or neonates and may have variable signal intensity on MR because of their protein content and/or propensity for hemorrhage. Lymphangiomas develop as a result of sequestration of lymphatic sacs. They may be combined with vascular malformations in a lymphangiohemangioma. Septations are present in most lymphangiomas, and the signal intensity on T1WI may simulate muscle (75%) or fat (25%). Heterogeneity within the lesion is present in more than 80% of cases. Most (75%) occur in the posterior triangle of the neck, with the axilla the next most common site.

Inflammatory Lesions

Cervical adenitis Inflammation that involves the carotid space usually comes from adjacent adenitis or extension from mucosal space infections. The source of pericarotid cervical adenitis may be mucosal, odontogenic, or perimucosal abscesses; tuberculous adenitis; or suppurative adenopathy associated with any pharyngitis. Diffuse adenopathy in the neck should make you think of AIDS-related illnesses, mononucleosis, sarcoidosis, sinus histiocytosis, and lymphoma (see Chapter 14).

Vascular inflammatory lesions Primary carotid space inflammatory processes include thrombophlebitis of the internal jugular vein. The latter is associated with peritonsillar inflammation and the entity known as Ludwig's angina. Iatrogenic causes secondary to venous line placement or surgery may also account for some cases of thrombophlebitis. Often, one will see a halo of edema around the thrombosed vein and with fat suppressed MR, enhancement of the vessel wall and the peri-venous soft tissue. Typical scenario: a patient with leukemia with an internal jugular line left in just a tad too long.

Pseudoaneurysms of the carotid artery may present as a neck mass. Somber is the surgeon who rushes to perform a biopsy of this "lesion" before consulting the radiologist. The cause of a pseudoaneurysm may be parapharyngeal space abscesses, syphilis, fibromuscular dysplasia, carotid dissection (Fig. 15-36), Ehlers-Danlos syndrome, trauma, surgery, neoplastic "blow-out," or idiopathic causes. Accelerated atherosclerosis may appear as thickening around the carotid bifurcation, and occasionally you may see intramural hemorrhage into an ulcerated carotid plaque. This may be the result of all that foie gras.

Unfortunately, as a neuroradiologist, one of the dreaded calls in the middle of the night is from the Trauma Service for "gun-shot wound to the neck" arteriogram. As you wiggle and jiggle and try to get out of this study you should know a few clues that may help predict whether a carotid sheath vessel has been damaged. Prevertebral soft-tissue swelling, bullet fragments, and metal foreign bodies adjacent to major vessels are useful but nonspecific radiographic signs. More importantly, one must rely on the clinical assessment of an expanding hematoma, entry and exit wounds, and neurologic deficits to guide the angiographic study.

Carotidynia is a syndrome associated with tenderness, swelling, or increased pulsations over the carotid artery with pain in the ipsilateral neck. This is a self-limited syndrome usually lasting less than 2 weeks. Although very few imaging studies have explored this entity, a recent report has noted enhancing soft tissue around the distal common carotid artery and bifurcation region. The tissue, measuring less than 8 mm in thickness and covering 1.5 to 3.5 cm in length resolves with nonsteroidal anti-inflammatory medication. Differential diagnosis includes giant cell arteritis, dissection, fibromuscular dysplasia, Takayasu arteritis, and wall hematoma.

Benign Neoplasms

Schwannoma The majority of carotid space masses are benign. Of these, two classic lesions are the vagus schwannoma and the glomus tumor. Situated posterior to the carotid artery, vagus nerve lesions tend to displace the carotid artery and parapharyngeal fat in an anterior direction. Schwannomas of the vagus nerve are usually well-defined, rounded structures hypodense to muscle on CT and enhance moderately. The lesions are circumscribed on T1WI because of the high signal intensity fat around the carotid sheath and around the parapharyngeal space. Whereas on an enhanced CT the border between the schwannoma and carotid artery or

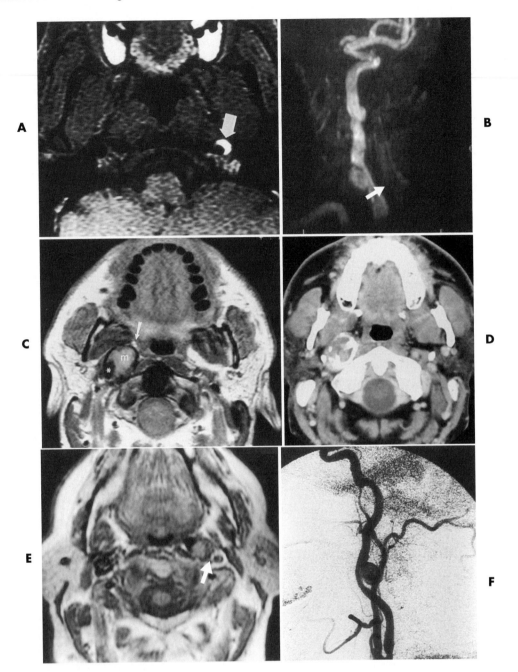

Fig. 15-36. Carotid dissection. **A,** Fat suppressed T1WIs are the best studies to show the subacute clot in the wall of a dissected carotid *(arrow)* or vertebral artery. This stands out as bright as a DWI and stroke—which may be the next study to perform. **B,** Pseudoaneurysm. A left cervical carotid artery pseudoaneurysm *(arrow)* can be identified on the MRA of the neck in this patient who suffered a penetrating wound to the neck. **C,** Pseudoaneurysm of the right internal carotid artery. Axial PDWI shows a right carotid space mass *(m)* that has variable signal intensity. Note the peripheral rim of signal void and the posterolateral area of dark signal *(asterisk).* Is that due to flow void, calcification, or hematoma? Only the surgeon will know for sure if you are unfortunate enough to recommend biopsy. Note also that the parapharyngeal fat *(arrow)* is displaced anteromedially by this carotid space lesion. **D,** Axial CT shows that the majority of the mass is calcified in its rim. We debated whether there was enhancement, suggesting flow on this CT, but it was left to the arteriogram to make the final decision. No guts, no glory. Beware the pericarotid nodule. **E,** No this is not a node *(arrow).* This is a clot in a partially thrombosed carotid pseudoaneurysm. **F,** See, we told you so!

jugular vein may be indistinguishable, on MR it is possible to identify the flow voids of the carotid artery and jugular vein as opposed to the enhancing solid tumor (Fig. 15-37). On T2WI the signal intensity of schwanno-

mas is variable, depending on its content of Antoni A and Antoni B tissue. Occasionally, schwannomas may be cystic and demonstrate characteristic density and intensity features for cyst fluid. Schwannomas also may

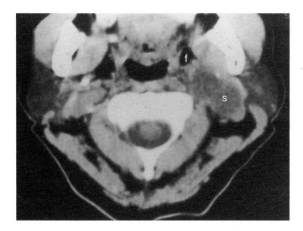

Fig. 15-37 Schwannoma in carotid space. Axial CT shows a low-density schwannoma *(s)*. Again, note that a carotid space lesion displaces prestyloid parapharyngeal fat *(f)* anteriorly.

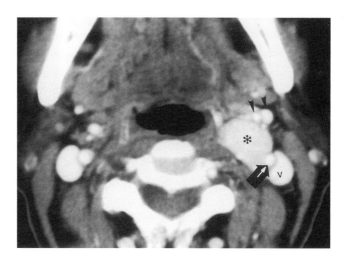

Fig. 15-38 Carotid body tumor. Internal carotid *(superimposed arrows)* and external carotid branches *(arrowheads)* are splayed apart by the carotid body tumor *(asterisk)* on the enhanced CT. The jugular vein *(v)* is posteriorly located.

hemorrhage within themselves. Remember that these schwannomas in the high neck may arise from either cranial nerves IX, X, XI, XII, the sympathetic plexus, or cervical spine nerve roots.

Glomus tumor Carotid body tumors (paragangliomas) usually arise at the carotid bulb. Therefore, they tend to splay the internal and external carotid arteries away from each other. These tumors are highly vascular and demonstrate dramatic enhancement (Fig. 15-38). If sequential CT or MR images during contrast infusion are performed, you can readily distinguish the schwannoma from the carotid body tumor (Table 15-3). The glomus tumor dynamic contrast curve shows rapid uptake of contrast, an early dip (MR), a high peak contrast, and rapid washout, whereas the schwannoma has a slower wash-in and a lower peak. The other lesions with the glomus-type dynamic curve include hemangiomas, aneurysms, arteriovenous malformations, and angiofibromas. Meningiomas have a rapid uptake phase and a high peak but have persistent contrast accumulation with a prolonged washout. You can perform a dynamic scan by repetitive imaging at the same level while giv-

ing a large (30 to 40 mL) bolus of contrast injected for 5 seconds. It only takes about 1 to 2 minutes of scan time.

On unenhanced MR you may identify numerous flow voids within a carotid body tumor; however, quite frequently these tumors do not demonstrate the characteristic salt-and-pepper appearance (again!) of vessels that is seen with glomus tumors elsewhere (Fig. 15-39). Nonetheless, a lesion arising at the carotid bifurcation that demonstrates marked enhancement should be considered to be a glomus tumor until proved otherwise. Conversely, tumors that do not avidly enhance are NOT glomus tumors. Angiography demonstrates the high vascularity of the glomus tumor (despite the absence of flow voids on MR) as opposed to the schwannoma, as well as its characteristic persistent staining and early arteriovenous shunting. Remember to check for the metanephrine secretion (seen in 3% to 5% of paragangliomas) before performing the angiogram, or else you

Table 15-3 Differentiation of carotid space glomus tumors from schwannomas

Feature	Schwannoma	Glomus tumor
Carotid displacement	Pushes anteriorly	Splays internal and external carotid arteries apart and displaces them anteriorly
Contrast uptake	Slow uptake	Rapid uptake dynamically, early dip
Flow voids on MR	No	Yes
Vascularity on angiography	Variable	Hypervascular
Density on unenhanced CT	Usually hypodense	Usually isodense
Morphology	May have cysts	Speckled

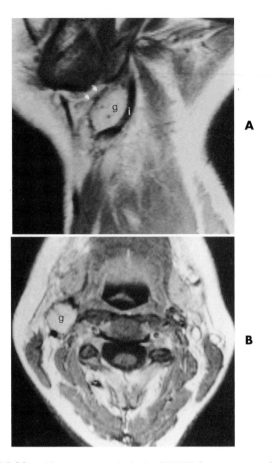

Fig. 15-39 Glomus tumor. **A,** Sagittal PDWI demonstrates a high intensity carotid body paraganglioma situated between the internal carotid artery *(i)* and external carotid artery *(arrows)* just above the bifurcation. **B,** On the enhanced T1WI the lesion *(g)* is dramatically enhancing and can be seen splaying the carotid vessels above the bifurcation.

may find the blood pressure monitor (and neurointerventionalist) going through the roof.

Glomus jugulare tumors also may grow thru the skull base to involve the carotid space. In most cases, when they do so, they infiltrate the lumen of the jugular vein. Erosion of the jugular spine is the sina qua non at the skull base.

Glomus vagale (glomus intravagale tumor or vagal paraganglioma) tumors may also present in the poststyloid parapharyngeal space and may displace the carotid artery anteriorly as opposed to splaying it at the bifurcation. The tumor is derived from the nodose ganglion, one of the vagal ganglia in the upper neck, which lies within the carotid sheath. The most common level of involvement in the neck is near the angle of the mandible and above the hyoid bone. Cranial nerves IX to XII may be affected or the patient may present with a Horner syndrome. Glomus vagale tumors are relatively uncommon, being overshadowed by the carotid body tumors. These two tumors can sometimes be differentiated on

the basis of the displacement of the external carotid artery (ECA) as glomus vagales displace the ECAs anteriorly with the ICA (and the jugular vein posteriorly), whereas carotid body tumors will push the ECA posterolaterally away from the ICA. The distinction between a vagus schwannoma and the glomus vagale tumor has to be made on the basis of flow voids and/or characteristic vascular flow curves on dynamic imaging, as opposed to the displacement of the carotid blood vessels.

Treatment of glomus vagale tumors almost always results in sacrifice of the vagus nerve and subsequent vocal cord paralysis. Look for the medialized ipsilateral true vocal cord (thyroplasty) after such surgery. Implants, silastic or otherwise, may be seen in the cord.

A small percentage of patients have a familial incidence of glomus tumors where the multiplicity rate may be as high as 30%. These patients also may demonstrate bilateral involvement, which is said to occur in 5% to 15% of patients with carotid body tumors.

Indium 111 octreotide scintigraphy enables distinction of glomus tumors from schwannomas and other masses of the carotid space as uptake occurs in the former but not the latter. False positive cases can be seen in other neuroendocrine-like lesions such as medullary thyroid carcinomas, thyroid adenomas, Merkel cell tumors, and carcinoid lesions. However, for the detection of multicentric paragangliomas (greater than 1.5 cm—it is a nuclear medicine study after all) in patients with familial paragangliomatosis this is a useful nukes exam (score one for the guys glowing in the dark outside of North Korea).

Malignant Neoplasms

Lymphadenopathy Lymphadenopathy from squamous cell carcinomas ranks as the third most common carotid space lesion after schwannomas and glomus tumors (Fig. 15-40). The lymph nodes are part of the internal jugular chain (levels II, III, and IV) and may be associated with either inflammatory or neoplastic processes involving the mucosal space. Lymph nodes may be present anterior, posterior, medial, and lateral to the carotid sheath and therefore may displace the blood vessels in any possible direction. Lymphomas may also involve the carotid sheath nodes.

Often, one is called on to determine whether the carotid artery wall is invaded by spread from mucosal primaries or malignant lymphadenopathy. This conundrum has already been discussed in Chapter 14 under Lymphadenopathy. Although no absolute criteria have been developed to determine carotid wall invasion, involvement of greater than 270 degrees of its circumference by neoplasm strongly suggests the wall is infiltrated with tumor, particularly if you are dealing with squamous cell carcinoma (Fig. 15-41).

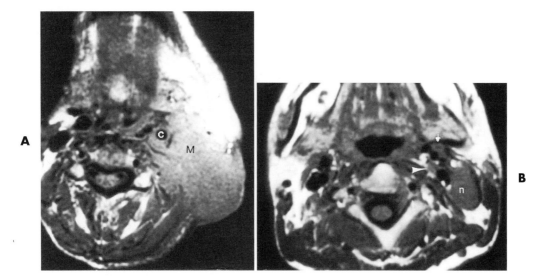

Fig. 15-40   Carotid space lymph nodes. **A,** Note circumferential encasement of the carotid artery *(c)* by this huge nodal mass *(M)*. The jugular vein is obliterated and the carotid space infiltrated. **B,** Nodes can be seen posterior *(n)*, anterior *(arrow)*, and medial *(arrowhead)* to the carotid sheath structures.

Mucosal disease spread   The carotid artery and space may also be invaded from extension of mucosal cancers rather than lymphadenopathy. When a tumor surrounds the carotid sheath contents by over 270 degrees, carotid invasion is implied. Intraluminal tumor is another not-so-subtle sign. Carotid blow-out in encased vessels figures into the therapeutic planning of the mucosal space squamous cell carcinoma. Radiation oncologists are generally reluctant (no guts, no glory) to radiate

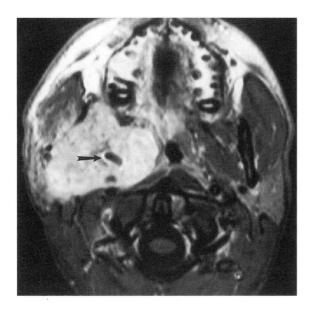

Fig. 15-41   Encased carotid artery *(arrow)*. When the carotid artery is encircled by tumor, you can bet that the surgeons will call the mass unresectable. If the tumor envelops less than 270 degrees of the vessel's circumference it may be saved.

the bed of a tumor where the carotid artery may rupture. The incidence of rupture during radiotherapy is relatively small but is many times greater if the patient has already undergone surgery in the neck. Rarely, the radiologist may occlude the diseased carotid artery before an attempt at complete surgical resection or radiotherapy.

RETROPHARYNGEAL SPACE

The retropharyngeal space may be likened to the intermezzo between the pharynx and the perivertebral space. Eat on.

Anatomy

The retropharyngeal space is a potential space defined by the deep cervical fascia. It is located deep to the pharyngeal mucosa and anterior to the longus colli and capitis muscles. The normal contents of the retropharyngeal space are fat and lymph nodes above the hyoid bone and fat alone below the hyoid bone. The retropharyngeal space extends from the base of the skull to the upper thoracic spinal level and is a site for spread from pharyngeal or esophageal lesions. The "danger space" is a term used to refer to a potential space associated with the retropharyngeal space arising from splitting of layers of the deep cervical fascia's deep layer into the alar fascia, ventral to the perivertebral space. Whereas the middle layer of the deep cervical fascia fuses with the deep layer at T-6, the split in the deep layer may track to the level of the diaphragm. Some people have studied the danger space and the deep layers of the cervical fascia ad nauseum, all because they have seen two or three lesions there in their storied careers. Do not succumb to this minutia, stick with the biggies: low back pain, headaches, sinusitis, Alzheimer disease, and stroke. Even MS is overstated, Bob.

Characteristically, the parapharyngeal fat is displaced in an anterolateral fashion by retropharyngeal space lesions. However, one must introduce a separate structure, the muscular longus colli and capitus complex, for the differentiation of a retropharyngeal mass from a prevertebral mass. A retropharyngeal mass remains anterior to the longus musculature, whereas a perivertebral space mass displaces the muscle anteriorly.

Congenital Disorders

Retropharyngeal carotid artery Of the benign congenital lesions to affect the retropharyngeal space, the medially deviated internal carotid artery is a potentially dangerous normal variant. When the carotid artery is located in the retropharyngeal space, it may simulate a deep submucosal mass to the endoscopist looking from within. He or she may be tempted to perform a deep biopsy to identify the source of the bulge in the pharyngeal mucosa. This may lead to a catastrophic pulsatile complication. Malpractice lawyers will appear like vultures circling carrion.

Inflammatory Lesions

Retropharyngeal abscesses, suppurative adenitis, and cellulitis are usually sequelae of pharyngitis (adenoidal or tonsillar infections) or sinusitis (in children). Initially, the infection spreads to a retropharyngeal lymph node (Fig. 15-42). From there a diffuse cellulitis of the retropharyngeal space and/or lymphedema may occur as the capsule of the node is violated. Most people believe that what we radiologists called retropharyngeal abscesses in yesteryear (the

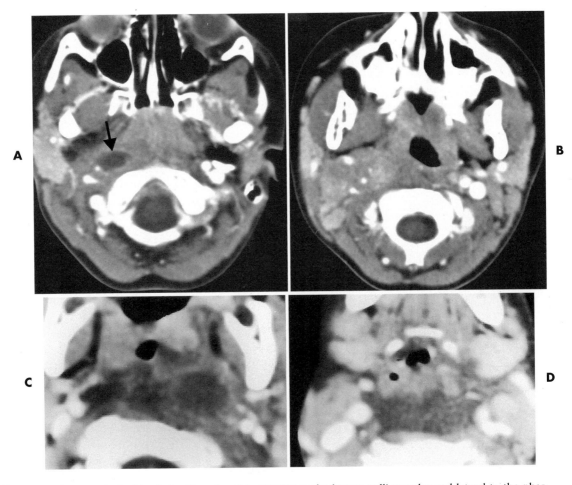

Fig. 15-42 Retropharyngeal adenitis. **A,** Positioned as it is anterior to the longus colli muscles and lateral to the pharynx, this most likely represents a necrotic suppurative right retropharyngeal node *(arrow)*. Adenoidal hypertrophy and/or inflammation are present as well. **B,** Lower down one can see the narrowed right carotid artery and the inflammation of the carotid space. Thrombophlebitis of the jugular veins or arteritis of the carotid may ensue. Jugular nodes are enlarged. **C,** This peritonsillar abscess resulted in edema in the retropharyngeal space (just anterior to the longus musculature). **D,** This extended to the hyoid level.

20th century) actually represented suppurative adenitis and not a separate inflammatory collection (see Fig. 14-50 in the Mucosal Space chapter). By the same token it is important to understand that the retropharyngeal fat may become quite edematous with adjacent inflammatory masses. Therefore, one should not jump to the conclusion that low density in this space represents an abscess. Until the collection is loculated or has a ring enhancement picture, hold off on sending in the clowns to drain the collection or it may be you who is shown to be the joker. Infected fluid density that is ill-defined may be a phlegmon.

Internal carotid artery thickening, spasm, and even thrombosis may accompany a retropharyngitis and/or lymphadenitis in children. Neurologic findings may be absent or subtle despite the carotid changes.

Mononucleosis may also cause lymphadenopathy in the retropharyngeal space and elsewhere in the head and neck.

Benign Neoplasms

Lipomas, fibromyxomas, and hemangiomas may occur in the retropharyngeal space. To make these calls, look for fat in the lipomas (Fig. 15-43), an oval shaped mass for fibromyxoma, or highly enhancing tissue for a hemangioma.

Malignant Neoplasms

Lymphadenopathy Just as in the prestyloid parapharyngeal space, malignant lesions primarily emanating from the retropharyngeal space are very uncommon. The most common is lymphadenopathy associated with nasopharyngeal or oropharyngeal abnormalities. In the nor-

mal child one may identify retropharyngeal lymph nodes associated with infections; however, lymph nodes greater than or equal to 1 cm in the adult are pathologic in almost all cases (see Fig. 14-54). Lymph node spread from nasopharyngeal squamous cell carcinoma is the most common malignant lesion of the retropharyngeal space. This is the first echelon of spread of nasopharyngeal cancer before the high jugular lymph node chain. Lymph node enlargement in the retropharyngeal space may also be caused by lymphoma. The parotid gland may also drain to retropharyngeal nodes.

Other sources of lymphadenopathy in the retropharyngeal space include papillary carcinoma of the thyroid gland and malignant melanoma. For this reason an examination of the thyroid gland for the possibility of malignancy must extend to the skull base to include retropharyngeal lymph nodes.

Contiguous spread from mucosal disease Contiguous spread from nasopharyngeal carcinoma may also lead to invasion of the retropharyngeal space and displacement of the longus colli muscles posteriorly. Retropharyngeal space infiltration is present in 40% of patients with nasopharyngeal carcinoma at the time of diagnosis (Fig. 15-44; see also Fig 14-9, a case of PTLD into the retropharyngeal space). If the posterior deep cervical fascia of the retropharyngeal space and the longus colli musculature are involved with cancer, the likelihood of surgical cure is markedly diminished.

Rhabdomyosarcoma Rhabdomyosarcomas also occur in the retropharyngeal space. Rhabdomyosarcomas usually invade the retropharyngeal space from their primary site in the nasopharynx. Of the various types of

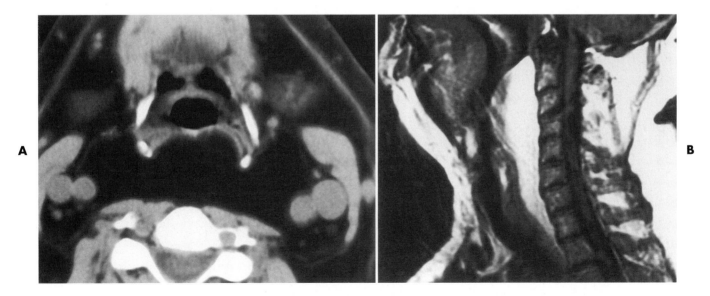

A   **B**

Fig. 15-43   Lipoma of the retropharyngeal space. **A,** The CT shows a mass anterior to the longus muscles, which has fat density. It is posterior to the pharyngeal musculature and resides in the retropharyngeal space. **B,** Sagittal T1WI shows the high intensity fat that narrows the airway at the tongue base level. The patient was having sleep apnea and was cured not with CPAP, but with liposuction.

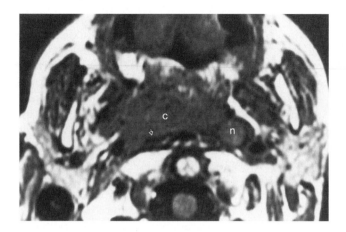

Fig. 15-44   Nasopharyngeal carcinoma with retropharyngeal infiltration. Axial T1WI shows infiltration of the retropharyngeal space by nasopharyngeal carcinoma *(c)*. Again, the longus colli muscles *(open white arrow)* are seen to be flattened against the vertebral body. Lateral retropharyngeal lymph node *(n)* is also seen on the left side.

rhabdomyosarcomas, the embryonal histologic type is the most common to affect the head and neck.

Leukemic infiltration   Although non-Hodgkin lymphomas are a more frequent source for lymphatic infiltration of the retropharyngeal space, acute leukemia may diffusely infiltrate this region.

PERIVERTEBRAL SPACE

Anatomy

To clump the remaining portions of the neck into one catchall category, you will note the use of the phrase *the perivertebral space.* In this way lesions in front of (prevertebral) and within, behind, and on the side of the spine (posterolateral neck) can be captured in this section (Fig. 15-45). It is an arbitrary distinction, but lesions here are diverse enough that they defy organization. Play through.

The perivertebral space includes the longus colli-capitus muscle complex, the paraspinal musculature, the vertebral body, the posterior triangles of the neck, the neurovascular structures within the spinal canal, and the brachial plexus (see following discussion). Perivertebral space lesions displace the longus colli musculature anteriorly and when large enough displace the parapharyngeal fat anterolaterally. The deep cervical fascia of the perivertebral space encircles the paraspinal and prevertebral muscles, the vertebral bodies, the nerves, and vessels, and it divides the space into two compartments by attaching to the transverse processes.

Congenital Disorders

The classic congenital mass in the perivertebral space is the cystic hygroma located in the posterior triangle of the neck. This lesion has been discussed in the previous chapter and will also be addressed with respect to the brachial plexus.

Inflammatory Lesions

The most common benign condition of the perivertebral space is spondylosis of the vertebral bodies. When a vertebral body osteophyte is large enough, it may simulate a submucosal pharyngeal or retropharyngeal mass and produce dysphagia. Large anterior osteophytes are

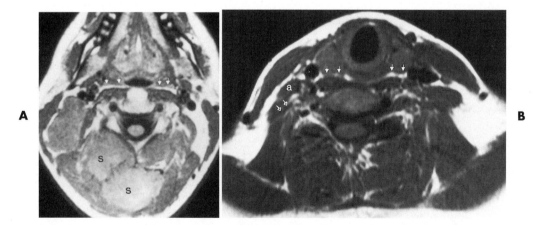

Fig. 15-45   Normal retropharyngeal space-perivertebral space anatomy. **A,** Axial T1WI in the suprahyoid region demonstrates fat *(arrows)* in the retropharyngeal space anterior to the longus colli muscles. Ignore the incidental soft tissue sarcoma *(s)* invading the perivertebral space of the neck. **B,** Once again in the infrahyoid region the retropharyngeal fat *(arrows)* can be identified. Additionally, one can identify the anterior scalene muscle *(a)*, which is the marker for the brachial plexus. The brachial plexus nerves run posterior to the anterior scalene muscle but anterior to the middle scalene muscle and may be faintly seen on the right side *(open arrows)*.

not uncommon in elderly patients, even without a history of cervical spine trauma. In cases of diffuse idiopathic skeletal hyperostosis and/or ossification of the posterior longitudinal ligament, there may be large anterior osteophytes that coexist.

Infections of the perivertebral space center on diskitis and osteomyelitis. These are unusual in patients with normal immune responses except in those patients in whom surgery on the cervical spine has been performed or in intravenous drug abusers (Fig. 15-46). The radiographic findings of diskitis and osteomyelitis are discussed fully in Chapter 17.

Rotatory subluxation of the atlanto-axial joint may coexist with retropharyngitis in the entity known as Grisel syndrome.

Esophageal perforation may lead to mediastinitis and infection of the perivertebral space.

Acute calcific prevertebral tendinitis has findings of calcifications within the tendons of the longus colli muscles and therefore represents a perivertebral process. However, there may be retropharyngeal effusions associated with this entity.

Nodular fasciitis occurs in the neck. It may present as a lateral neck mass and be misdiagnosed clinically as a lymph node. It may enhance brightly but is usually intermediate in intensity on T2WI. Most people feel this represents a low-grade soft-tissue tumor, not an inflammatory process.

Necrotizing fasciitis was in "fasciion" a few years back. Imaging findings consist of (1) diffuse thickening and infiltration of the skin and subcutaneous tissue (cellulitis); (2) diffuse enhancement and/or thickening of the super-ficial and deep cervical fasciae (fasciitis); (3) enhancement and thickening of the platysma, sternocleidomastoid muscle, or strap muscles (myositis); and (4) fluid collections in multiple neck compartments. This disease could result in sloughing of tissue, gas containing abscesses, and pulmonary manifestations of adult respiratory distress syndrome, mediastinitis, and pneumonia.

Aggressive fibromatosis (desmoid tumor) may also infiltrate the muscles of the perivertebral space/posterior triangle. Although there are reports that this lesion is always dark on T1W and T2W scans and is isodense to muscle on CT, other studies have shown isointensity on T1WI and hyperintensity on T2WI relative to adjacent normal muscle. Enhancement is variable. This lesion may be a precursor to or in the family of malignant fibrous histiocytoma.

Fibrosing inflammatory pseudotumor can affect the perivertebral space and spread to the skull base. As expected from its appearance in the orbit, the lesion shows characteristic MR findings of bone destruction and hypointensity on T2WI. Enhancement on MR images is weak.

Benign Neoplasms

The benign neoplasms of the perivertebral space are relatively uncommon. They include lipomas, schwannomas from the cervical nerve branches, hemangiomas of the musculature, and benign bony tumors. By sheer numbers hemangiomas dominate the benign bone neoplasm category, but as they are most often confined to the vertebral bodies and rarely affect the head and neck surgeon, they will not be addressed here.

Benign bony tumors will be addressed in the spine chapters but we will mention chordoma in this section as the prototypical perivertebral benign bony lesion.

Lipomas can occur anywhere in the head and neck, but have a predilection for the lateral subcutaneous tissues, the supraclavicular fossa, and the posterior perivertebral space. The differential diagnosis will include liposarcomas, which may or may not have nonfatty soft tissue associated with them. Another bizarroma is Madelung disease, an entity with massive lipomatosis of the posterior neck. Excess fat can be seen predominantly in the posterior part of the neck, under the trapezius and sternomastoid muscles, in the supraclavicular fossa, between the paraspinal muscles, and in the anterior part of the neck (suprahyoid and infrahyoid). The patients may present with respiratory symptoms secondary to tracheal compression, neuropathies, weakness, macrocytic anemia, and venous stasis.

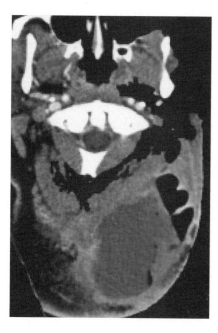

Fig. 15-46   Abscess. A large air-containing collection in the posterior perivertebral space is seen in this frequent flyer to the Hopkins ER. Drug abuse and neglect contributed to the appearance. Retropharyngeal edema.

Chordoma   Of the histologically benign bony neoplasms, chordomas preferentially affect the cervical perivertebral space. The characteristic cell type is the physaliferous cell. Chordomas though histologically benign should be considered malignant tumors because they tend to invade aggressively into the skull base and metastasize in 7% to 20% of cases. Patients usually have cranial nerve symptoms (nerve VI most commonly; then nerves III, V, VII, and VIII) as the tumor invades the cavernous sinus or skull base. Chordomas often affect the clivus, the C1–C2 region, or the sacrococcygeal portion of the vertebral column. The tumor is destructive and lytic and is often associated with calcifications. It displaces the longus colli musculature anteriorly and may cross the boundaries of the C1–C2 region. The signal intensity of these lesions often is bright on T2WI (Fig. 15-47). The tumor demonstrates minimal enhancement. The differential diagnosis includes chondrosarcoma.

These tumors are also discussed in Chapter 17.

Malignant Neoplasms

Metastasis   Malignancies of the perivertebral space center on the vertebral bodies. Metastases from blood-borne sources are the most common lesions in the vertebral body, often from breast, lung, or kidney primary tumors. Primary vertebral body malignancies include osteosarcomas and Ewing sarcomas in addition to plasmacytomas. Multiple myeloma may affect the cervical spine as well. Invasion by Pancoast tumors extending from the lung apex may also present as a perivertebral or supra-

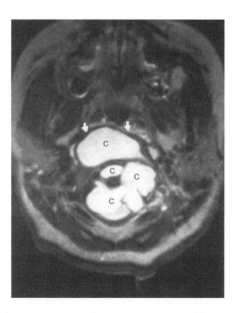

Fig. 15-47   Chordoma of the perivertebral space. This T2WI demonstrates a high intensity C1 chordoma *(c),* which stretches the longus colli muscles *(arrows)* anteriorly, typical of a perivertebral mass.

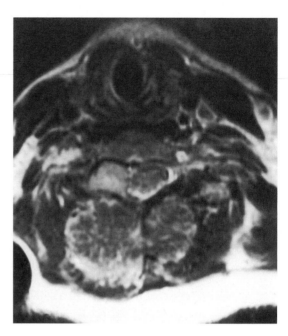

Fig. 15-48   Hemangiopericytoma. The mass that infiltrated the paraspinal musculature and swung around to enter the neural foramen was not of neurogenic origin. The differential diagnosis would include a lymphoma and soft tissue sarcoma.

clavicular mass and may cause a brachial plexopathy (see following discussion).

Soft-tissue malignant masses in the perivertebral musculature include lymphoma, rhabdomyosarcoma, malignant fibrous histiocytoma, and neurofibrosarcoma. Less commonly found soft-tissue neoplasms include hemangiopericytomas (Fig. 15-48) and synovial sarcomas.

Lymphadenopathy   Lymphadenopathy is perhaps the most common perivertebral space lesion to affect the region. The primary site of abnormality may be above or below the head and neck. Lymphoma may also account for nodes in the posterior triangle (level 5) of the neck or may present as a supraclavicular mass. Classically Hodgkin disease manifests as a posterolateral neck mass. A case of a calcified lymph node from pediatric neuroblastoma can be seen in Fig. 15-49.

BRACHIAL PLEXUS

The brachial plexus is considered a part of the perivertebral space. The brachial plexus is derived from the C5–T1 cervical nerve roots, which pass inferolaterally to the axilla for supply to the upper extremity. The mnemonic for remembering the anatomy here is "rad techs drink cold beer" The Roots merge into Trunks (upper, middle, and lower) at the scalene muscular Triangle. The Trunks divide into Divisions (anterior and posterior) which then form Cords (lateral, posterior, and middle) at the Clavicle. The cords form the

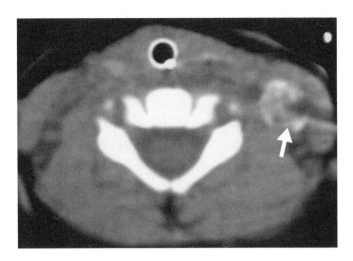

Fig. 15-49   Calcified node. This one stumped us—a neonate with a palpable and calcified nodule in the left side of the neck *(arrow)*. Consider it to be paraspinal and you may get the correct diagnosis: metastatic neuroblastoma.

Branches again in an unnecessarily complicated manner. Usually His designs are simpler. Suffice it to say the brachial plexus runs between the anterior and middle scalene muscles and then with the subclavian artery to the level of the clavicles. At that point the plexus runs with the axillary artery, posterior to the larger axillary vein.

Congenital Lesions

Lymphatic malformations and venous malformations are the most common congenital lesions to affect the brachial plexus. The posterior neck is the most common site for cystic hygromas, followed by the axilla. In both of these locations the brachial plexus may be affected. Consider whether the patient has a "webbed neck" to suggest a radiographic diagnosis of Turner syndrome on the neck CT study. Lymphangiomas infiltrate and encase the brachial plexus and adjacent vessels but usually they do not enhance, unlike venous vascular malformations. Multiloculation, fluid-fluid levels, bright fluid on T1WI are all ancillary findings highly suggestive of lymphatic malformations.

Two types of perinatal injuries may affect the brachial plexus: an Erb palsy and a Klumpke palsy. Both of these may occur as a result of shoulder dystocia at the time of delivery. In the former, the avulsion of nerve roots occurs at the C5–C6 level and the intrinsic muscles of the hand are unaffected, though the shoulder is weak (Fig. 15-50). In the latter, the C7, C8, and even T1 roots are torn and therefore the hand muscles are affected. The patient may have a coincident Horner syndrome secondary to involvement of the sympathetic nervous system structures and/or stellate ganglion opposite the C7–T1 level.

Traumatic injuries in the adults are usually from "braking a fall by a motocross racer" injuries (i.e., Harley Davidson syndrome). Avulsions of nerve roots ensue.

Cervical ribs also can cause a brachial plexopathy (Fig. 15-51). The incomplete cervical ribs often have a band leading from them to the clavicle that traps the plexus and therefore are more often symptomatic than the complete cervical ribs. Either way a thoracic outlet syndrome may be produced. Women are affected more than men. They are unilateral in the majority of cases.

Inflammatory Lesions

Brachial plexitis (neuralgic amyotrophy) most commonly is viral in origin. However, this may also occur as a complication of radiotherapy, especially after treatment of supraclavicular adenopathy and/or breast cancer axillary nodes. Radiation brachial plexitis is characterized by its symmetry, high signal on fat-suppressed T2WI, and variable enhancement.

Nodular fasciitis is a nonspecific sclerosing inflammatory condition that can lead to loss of planes around the brachial plexus. It is often low in intensity on T2WI.

Benign Neoplasms

Lipomas and neurogenic neoplasms predominate in this category. Both are late to produce symptoms and are easily characterized by density (lipoma = fat) or shape (fusiform = schwannoma).

Malignant Neoplasms

Primary malignancies that affect the C5–T1 nerves include malignant fibrous histiocytoma and other lesions akin to fibrosarcoma (Figure 15-52), liposarcomas, and, in children, rhabdomyosarcomas and neurofibrosarcomas (in the NF-1 population). Soft-tissue lymphomas may also infiltrate here.

Secondary invasion may be caused by contiguous involvement or lymphadenopathy. Direct invasion by Pancoast tumors or chest wall sarcomas may lead to a brachial plexopathy. Often there is an associated Horner syndrome.

The most common sources of lymphadenopathy producing a brachial plexopathy are primary tumors and lymphomas of the breast, lung, esophagus, head, and neck. Usually an infiltrative nodal mass erases the planes between the brachial plexus and the scalene muscles (Fig. 15-53). Sometimes the plexopathy only appears after radiotherapy, but the radiation oncologists will claim it was there from the outset, just overlooked.

Now that you have digested the spaces of the head and neck, it is time to stimulate the head and neck hormones with a discussion of the thyroid and parathyroid glands.

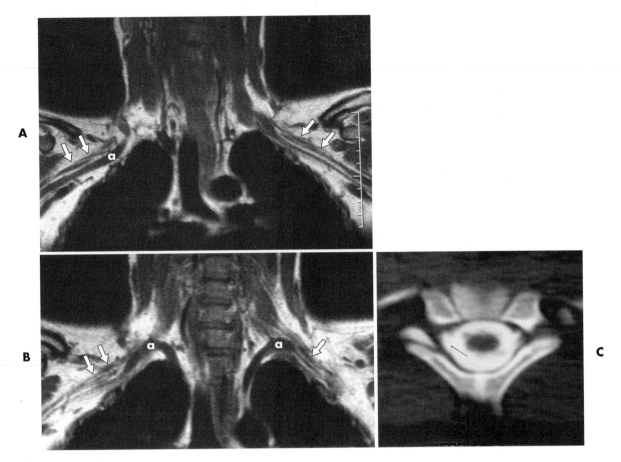

Fig. 15-50 Brachial plexus anatomy. **A,** Note the relationship of the brachial plexus *(arrows)* to the subclavian artery *(a)* on these coronal scans (i.e., posterior and superior for the most part). **B,** A more posterior section shows plexus with artery anterior. **C,** Avulsed nerve root (Better seen on the film). One can just make out the anterior and posterior nerve rootlets on the left, but on the right an empty sac is seen. The beginnings of a pseudomeningocele can be identified *(arrow).*

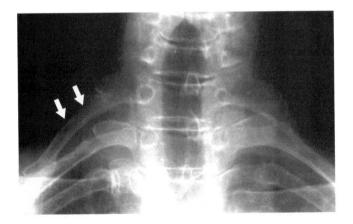

Fig. 15-51 Cervical rib. There is a complete cervical rib on the right *(arrows)* and an incomplete one on the left. The patient had a left brachial plexopathy. At surgery, a fibrous band across the left brachial plexus from the cervical rib stump to the manubrium was present.

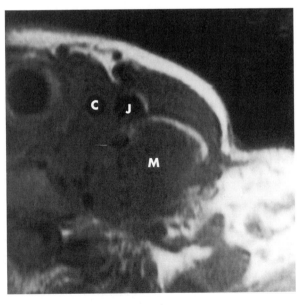

Fig. 15-52 Desmoid tumor of brachial plexus. This infiltrative mass *(m)* involved the anterior scalene muscle (no longer discernible) and was associated with a brachial plexopathy. The carotid *(C)* and jugular vein *(v)* are being displaced anteriorly.

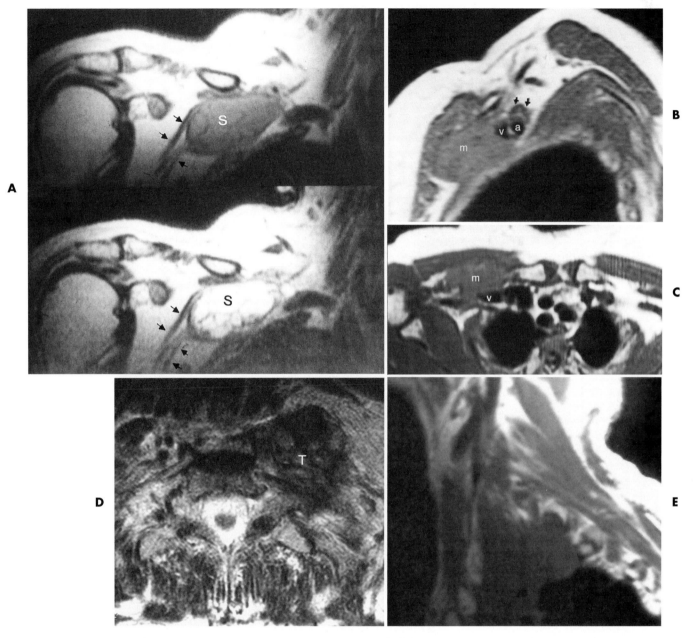

Fig. 15-53   Brachial plexopathy pathology. **A,** A malignant schwannoma *(s)* on unenhanced *(above)* and enhanced *(below)* coronal T1WI can be seen intertwined with the brachial plexus nerve roots *(arrows)*. **B,** A different patient with adenopathy from a lung cancer has a mass *(m)* anterior to the axillary artery *(a)* and vein *(v)* on the sagittal T1WI. The brachial plexus *(arrows)* is predominantly posterosuperior to the mass, intimately associated with the axillary artery. **C,** On axial T1WI, the mass *(m)* is located anterior to the subclavian vein *(v)*, infiltrating the plexus in the supraclavicular fossa on the right. **D,** Brachial plexus infiltration. The space between the anterior scalene muscle and the middle scalene muscle has been infiltrated by this Pancoast tumor *(T)* which grew through the lung apex into the lower neck. **E,** On sagittal scanning the lesion is seen to emanate from the upper lobe of the lung.

THYROID GLAND

Anatomy

A plethora of lesions, both benign and malignant, affect the thyroid gland. Head and neck radiologists and pulmonary radiologists have laid claim to the thyroid gland as within their turf. If most thyroid gland abnormalities would stay in the neck (unlike goiters, retrosternal thyroids, and ectopic thyroidal tissue), head and neck radiologists would have more clout in claiming the gland as their own.

The thyroid gland has two lobes connected by a midline isthmus. The gland is located at the C5-T1 level and is encapsulated in fascia that is attached to the trachea, accounting for its movement with swallowing. A pyramidal lobe is variably present and projects upward from the isthmus. The gland is supplied by superior thyroidal arteries from the external carotid and inferior thyroidal arteries from the thyrocervical trunk off the subclavian artery.

Congenital Disorders

Agenesis and ectopic thyroid tissue One third of congenital thyroid lesions are due to total agenesis. The remainder are due to ectopic thyroid tissue. Of the ectopic locations, 50% are in the base of the tongue (lingual thyroid) and 50% between the tongue and the normal location of the gland. Congenital intrathyroidal cysts are uncommon. They are usually due to degenerated adenomas or cysts within multinodular goiters.

The work-up of the lingual thyroid gland requires an iodine based nuclear medicine study to search for other thyroid tissue. In 80% of the cases the lingual thyroid gland is the ONLY source of thyroid hormone in the individual. This will influence therapy timing as thyroid hormone is important for healthy growth as a child. Imagine removing what you believe is a hemangioma of the tongue (because it enhances and you did not perform an unenhanced scan to see that it was bright [from iodine] beforehand) in a child. Pathology comes back 10 days later as lingual thyroid tissue. In the meantime the patient is in myxedema coma because you never thought to replace the thyroid hormone because you never suspected the diagnosis. Now the patient is on thyroid hormone for life from childhood. In many cases the surgeon will leave the lingual thyroid tissue in through adolescence (unless it is obstructing the airway) and beyond if this is the only thyroid tissue in the body. It is that time you wish for struma ovarii or struma cardia (other ectopic sites). Leaving the lingual thyroid tissue in does have its drawbacks. The incidence of papillary carcinoma runs as high as 3% to 5%—about what you find at autopsy studies of cervical thyroid tissue.

Thyroglossal duct cyst Thyroglossal duct cysts (TGDC) represent the most common nonodontogenic cysts in the head and neck. They account for 70% of con-

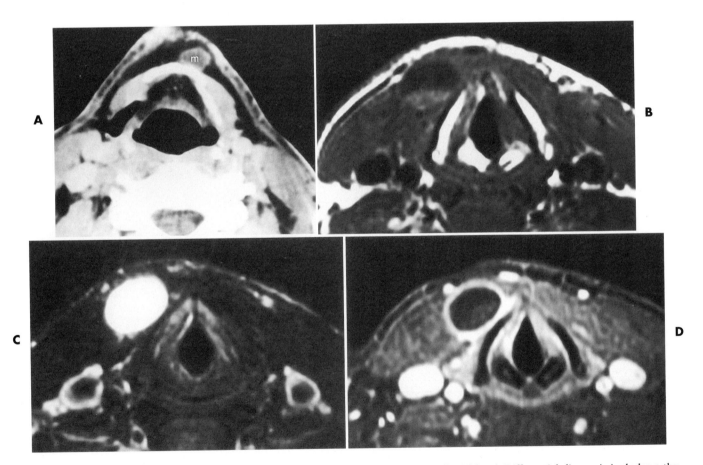

Fig. 15-54   Thyroglossal duct cyst. **A,** Axial CT demonstrates a cystic mass *(m)* at the hyoid level. Differential diagnosis includes a thyroglossal duct cyst, a necrotic lymph node (unusual in this location), a dermoid (wrong density), or a thymic cyst (too high). **B,** Despite what appears to be a fluid-fluid level which may distract you from the correct diagnosis, this lesion, embedded in the strap muscles, is a thyroglossal duct cyst until proven otherwise. **C,** TGDCs are classically very bright on T2WI and enhance only on the periphery if at all **(D).**

genital neck masses. TGDC are due to a remnant of the duct along the pathway of descent of the thyroid gland and may occur anywhere from the foramen cecum of the tongue to the natural location of the thyroid gland. TGDCs are most often infrahyoid (65%) but can occur at the hyoid level (15%) or in the suprahyoid soft tissue (20%). A cystic lesion embedded in the strap muscles (thyrohyoid, geniothyroid, and so on) is a TGDC with little question about it. For this you can stick your neck and TGDC out. Unlike ectopic thyroid tissue located between the tongue and lower neck, TGDCs do not typically contain functioning thyroidal tissue though microscopic rests are present in some cases. Three fourths of TGDCs are in the midline. For math aficionados this means that 25% are off midline (Fig. 15-54). Cysts look like cysts, but sometimes they may have high protein. That leads to bright signal on T1WI. Rim enhancement is not uncommon.

On ultrasound the appearance is more variable. The cysts may be anechoic (28%), homogeneously hypoechoic with internal debris (18%), solid appearing (28%), and heterogeneous (28%). The majority show posterior back wall enhancement (88%) and only half show a classic typical thin wall.

Carcinoma in a TGDC is rare, arising in approximately 1% of cases. When it occurs, its histologic appearance is usually papillary, although squamous and follicular varieties have also been reported. As one might expect, medullary carcinoma does not occur in TGDCs as these tumors arise from the parafollicular cells, not thyroid derivatives. Thyroglossal duct carcinoma can be suspected when mural nodules, calcifications, or combinations thereof are present in the cyst.

The Sistrunk procedure, in which the tract of the thyroglossal duct, the midline tongue base, and the midportion of the hyoid cartilage are resected, is the definitive procedure for treating TGDC.

If you see fat or a solid nodule associated with a cyst in the thyroid gland, consider the diagnosis of teratoma.

Autoimmune and Inflammatory Lesions

Goiter   A goiter is a diffuse enlargement of the thyroid gland often found in association with iodide deficiency. Goiters may have areas of cystic degeneration, hemorrhage, colloid formation, or nodularity within them and therefore are difficult to analyze on the basis of nuclear medicine, ultrasound, CT, or MR characteristics (Fig. 15-55). Goiters are usually evaluated by nuclear medicine studies in which a lesion is classified into three main categories: hot (hyperaccumulation of radiotracer), warm (increased uptake with suppression of background thyroidal tissue), or cold (nonfunctioning, low uptake). Warm and hot nodules, because they represent hormonally active tissue, usually have a benign cause. Cold

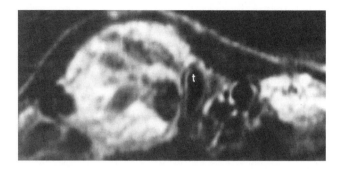

Fig. 15-55   Thyroid goiter. Axial T2WI demonstrates a multinodular mass compressing the trachea *(t)* to the left side. Note the inhomogeneity of the signal. As one might expect, there may be photopenic areas within this mass on a nuclear medicine study.

nodules are more worrisome for malignancy. A cold nodule in a goiter is malignant in less than 15% of cases, so unless a mass in a goiter is growing, biopsy is usually not performed. Nonetheless, many thyroid nodules, discovered clinically or serendipitously while scanning for other sites, get aspirated. Once the cytologists see macrophages, colloid, and papillary cells they call it multinodular goiter (Fig. 15-56). The surgeon may still operate if cosmesis, airway, or esophageal compromise dictate. Often a trial of hormone suppression is offered beforehand—to limited benefit.

Suppurative thyroiditis   Suppurative thyroiditis may occur because of bacterial infection or as a complication of branchial cleft fistulas from the piriform sinus that inflame the adjacent thyroid gland. These are

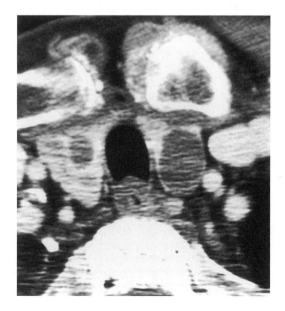

Fig. 15-56   Thyroid cysts. Enhanced CT shows a well defined left thyroid lobe cyst and several right thyroid lobe cysts and/or low-density nodules. With this diffuse bilateral pattern we would suggest a multinodular, multicystic goiter and not be concerned.

usually due to third or fourth branchial cleft abnormalities and may have a cutaneous opening at the clavicular level. The ratio of left to right congenital pyriform sinus fistulae is 4 to 1.

Subacute thyroiditis   Inflammatory conditions of the thyroid gland include subacute, Hashimoto, radiation-induced, Riedel, and acute lymphocytic thyroiditis. Subacute (de Quervain) thyroiditis is due to an as yet unidentified virus. Like most thyroid disorders, de Quervain thyroiditis is more common in women. Patients are febrile, and the thyroid gland becomes swollen and tender. The disease is self-limited, and most patients are euthyroid after the acute bout, with a small percentage becoming hypothyroid.

Hashimoto thyroiditis   As opposed to subacute thyroiditis, the other inflammatory disorders are not associated with fever or a tender thyroid gland. In Hashimoto thyroiditis the gland is infiltrated with lymphocytes and plasma cells, and the disease is thought to be due to autoantibodies to thyroid cell proteins, especially thyroglobulins. Antimicrosomal antibodies are elevated. Although initially the patient may be euthyroid, eventually hypothy-roidism sets in because of replacement of functioning tissue with lymphocytes and fibrosis. Goitrous enlargement of the gland is commonly seen in Hashimoto thyroiditis. An increased rate of thyroid lymphomas has been reported in women who have this disease. Other autoimmune disorders such as Sjögren syndrome, pernicious anemia, lupus erythematosus, rheumatoid arthritis, and diabetes occur with increased frequency in patients with Hashimoto thyroiditis. Increased, but still exceptionally low.

Riedel thyroiditis and radiation-induced thyroiditis   Riedel thyroiditis and radiation-induced thyroiditis both lead to fibrosis of the gland in the long run and are chronic in their courses. The thyroid gland may feel firm and woody in both these disorders. Hypothyroidism occurs in up to 50% of patients. Riedel thyroiditis may be associated with retroperitoneal fibrosis, orbital pseudotumor, mediastinal fibrosis, and sclerosing cholangitis. The term multifocal fibrosclerosis has been coined for this entity. On imaging Riedel thyroiditis is homogeneously hypoechoic on ultrasound (US), hypodense on CT, and hypointense on all sequences with MR. Enhancement is variable.

Graves disease   Graves disease is synonymous with diffuse toxic goiter and is a common cause of hyperthyroidism. The disease has an ophthalmopathy associated with proptosis, lid retraction, fatty infiltration, and extraocular muscle enlargement. The orbital manifestations of this syndrome have been explained in Chapter 10. Graves is an autoimmune disease associated with increased levels of long-acting thyroid stimulator (LATS), antibodies to thyroid stimulating hormone (TSH) receptors that circulate in 80% to 90% of persons with Graves disease. The gland is enlarged and is hot diffusely.

Diffuse nontoxic goiters and multinodular goiters usually develop as a response to increased TSH levels and are seen in euthyroid patients. The gland is enlarged, with nodularity.

Colloid cyst   A colloid cyst is another common lesion of the thyroid gland. This may have high density on CT and most characteristically has high intensity on T1WI. Colloid and hemorrhage may be difficult to distinguish on the basis of CT and MR. This lesion may cause a cold spot on a technetium or iodine nuclear medicine scintigram.

Benign Neoplasms

Adenoma   The most common benign tumors of the thyroid gland are adenomas. More than 70% of solitary neoplasms in the thyroid glands are benign adenomas, either follicular or papillary. The lesion may be inhomogeneous, but the margins by and large are well circumscribed on CT or MR. Thyroid adenomas may be associated with calcifications; however, the same is true of thyroid carcinomas.

If you were to perform thyroid US as a screen in middle-aged women, you would find that more than one third have nodules in their thyroid glands. On autopsy specimens 50% of thyroid glands have nodules. Fortunately, the vast majority of these are benign degenerated nodules: 4.2% of nodular glands have malignancies. The percentages shift toward malignancies when the patient has a history of radiation exposure especially after two or three decades.

More highly differentiated adenomas may concentrate radiotracers and appear as hot or warm nodules on thyroid scintigrams. Because they are often autonomously secreting (independent of TSH stimulation), they suppress the remaining normal thyroid tissue. If necrosis or intralesional hemorrhage develops, the nodule will become cold.

Malignant Neoplasms

Only 4% to 7% of histologically examined thyroid nodules are positive for cancer, but a solitary nodule in a male patient or a child has a higher rate of being neoplastic. Papillary, follicular, and mixed papillary-follicular carcinomas account for 80% of thyroid malignancies. Medullary carcinoma (10% of thyroid malignancies), undifferentiated or anaplastic carcinoma (3%), and Hürthle cell (2%) are less common cancers of the thyroid gland. All these lesions may have well-circumscribed or poorly circumscribed margins and do not have a characteristic CT or MR appearance to distinguish them from adenomas.

As in some adenomas, the lesions demonstrate a photopenic area on technetium or iodine scans. Nonetheless, only 20% of cold nodules are cancerous (the remainder are adenomas, colloid cysts, focal thyroiditis, or other benign cysts). Thyroid carcinomas may be cystic, hemorrhagic, calcified, or hyperproteinaceous. They may spread diffusely to the lymphatics and/or hematogenously and therefore be seen with cervical lymphadenopathy or with distant metastases (Box 15-9). They may infiltrate the trachea and esophagus seen as circumferential involvement, endoluminal spread, enhancement of the wall or focal nodularities.

If a complete pseudocapsule (an even-thickness band of low intensity around the mass) is present on MR, this usually signifies cystic degeneration of an adenoma. If the capsule is irregular in thickness (yet continuous) or discontinuous with nodular penetrating excrescences,

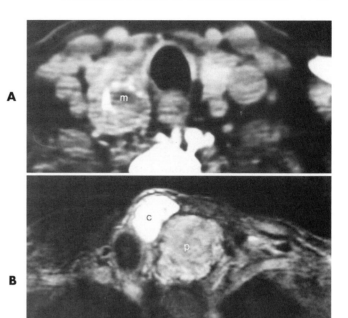

Fig. 15-57   Thyroid carcinoma's multiple faces. **A,** Axial CT demonstrates a mass *(m)* with peripheral calcification in the posterior portion of the right thyroid gland. Do not be fooled by the presence of calcification. It need not suggest benignity in the thyroid gland. This was follicular carcinoma. **B,** This patient had papillary carcinoma *(p)*, which was associated with a large cyst *(c)*. Hemorrhage, calcification, cyst formation, and lymphatic and hematogenous metastases may all be characteristic of thyroid cancer.

Box 15-9   TNM Classification of Thyroid Malignancies

PRIMARY TUMOR (T)

TX: Primary tumor cannot be assessed

T0: No evidence of primary tumor

T1: Tumor 2 cm or less, limited to thyroid

T2: Tumor >2 cm but ≤4 cm, limited to thyroid

T3: Tumor >4 cm limited to thyroid or any tumor with minimal extrathyroid extension

T4a: Tumor of any size beyond capsule to subcutaneous tissues, larynx, trachea, esophagus, or recurrent laryngeal nerve

T4b: Tumor invades prevertebral fascia or encases carotid artery or mediastinal vessels

(All anaplastic carcinomas are considered T4 tumors)

Note: All categories may be subdivided: (a) solitary tumor, (b) multifocal tumor (the largest determines the classification).

REGIONAL LYMPH NODES (N)

NX: Regional lymph nodes cannot be assessed

N0: No regional lymph node metastasis

N1: Regional lymph node metastasis

   N1a: Metastasis to level VI nodes

   N1b: Metastasis in bilateral, midline, or contralateral cervical or mediastinal lymph node(s)

DISTANT METASTASIS (M)

MX: Presence of distant metastasis cannot be assessed

M0: No distant metastasis

M1: Distant metastasis

From Greene FL, Page DL, Fleming ID, et al (eds): *AJCC Cancer Staging Manual,* ed 6. New York, Springer-Verlag, 2002, p 78. Used with permission.

---

carcinoma is more likely (Fig. 15-57). Discontinuous pseudocapsules without areas of penetration are commonly seen in adenomatous goiters. Hemorrhagic degeneration is more common in adenomas and goiters but may also be present in cancer.

Papillary carcinoma   Papillary carcinomas are the most common malignancies of the thyroid gland, accounting for half of thyroid cancers. In a patient less than 40 years old papillary adenocarcinomas outnumber all other cancers of the thyroid by a 5 to 1 margin. Women are more commonly affected than men, and cervical lymphadenopathy is the most common presentation (50% of cases). Lymphatic rather than hematogenous spread is the rule. The prognosis with papillary carcinoma is the best of the thyroid malignancies. A propensity for cystic appearing nodes has been demonstrated. The nodes may also be calcified, colloid containing, highly vascular, and tiny. The nodes may be bright on T1WI or have calcification evident on CT.

Despite its relatively favorable prognosis there are several features that portend decreased survival in some cases of papillary carcinoma. Large tumors, esophageal invasion (said to occur in 20% to 30%), tracheal invasion (seen in a similar percentage), lymphadenopathy, and carotid encasement are unfavorable characteristics. Imaging findings indicative of tracheal invasion include abnormal T2WI signal in the wall, circumferential involvement of more than 180 degrees, intraluminal masses, and displacement over 2.5 cm from the midline. Esophageal invasion by tumors is suggested if the wall has abnormal MR signal, the wall enhances, there is tumor encasement greater than 270 degrees, or if there is intraluminal tumor.

Univariate analysis has shown that increased age, male gender, large size, ill-defined margin, carotid invasion, esophageal invasion, lymph node metastases, and extrathyroidal extension are predictors of poor prognosis with papillary carcinoma. Tumor size, nodal metastases, and esophageal invasion were independent variables of poor prognosis.

Follicular carcinoma Follicular carcinomas tend to spread hematogenously. The prognosis is much worse than that for papillary carcinoma. The imaging appearances of this thyroid carcinomas is identical to papillary carcinoma.

Medullary carcinoma Medullary carcinoma is a rare neoplasm of the thyroid gland, accounting for only 7% to 10% of thyroid malignancies. Ten percent are associated with the multiple endocrine neoplasia (MEN) II syndrome, and some cases are familial without other endocrine lesions (Table 15-4). MEN IIa and IIb signify

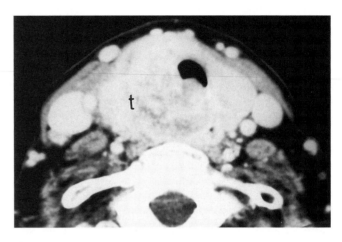

Fig. 15-58 Dominant mass in the thyroid gland. The large size of this right thyroid mass *(t)*, the degree of tracheal displacement, the effacement of the wall of the esophagus, and the heterogeneous density in a gland otherwise homogeneous on the left side in an elderly chap makes one write a run-on sentence and also suspicious of the correct diagnosis of anaplastic carcinoma.

syndromes with increased rates of pheochromocytoma and parathyroid hyperplasia. MEN IIb may be associated with marfanoid facies and mucocutaneous neuromas. Medullary carcinoma is derived from parafollicular cells that secrete calcitonin; elevated serum calcitonin levels may be a marker for the disease. Stippled calcification may be the clue to making this diagnosis.

Anaplastic carcinoma Anaplastic carcinomas are

Table 15-4 MEN syndromes

Feature	MEN I	MEN II or IIa	MEN III or IIb
Eponym	Wermer syndrome	Sipple's syndrome	Mucosal neuroma syndrome, Froboese syndrome
Parathyroid abnormality	Hyperparathyroidism (90% of cases) more commonly caused by hyperplasia than by adenoma	Parathyroid hyperplasia in 20%–50%	Very rare
Thyroid lesion	Goiter, adenomas, thyroiditis are rare	Medullary thyroid carcinoma (100%)	Medullary thyroid carcinoma (100%)
Pituitary lesions	Adenomas (20%–65%)	No	No
Pheochromocytoma	No	Yes (>50%, bilateral)	Yes (50%)
Other manifestations	1. Pancreatic islet cell adenomas (insulinoma or gastrinoma) in 30%–80% 2. Adrenal cortex adenomas or carcinomas (30%–40%) 3. Rarely glucagonomas, VIP-omas, carcinoid tumors 4. Zollinger-Ellison syndrome	1. Pheochromocytoma 2. Scoliosis	1. Mucocutaneous neuromas (100%) 2. Marfanoid facies 3. Café-au-lait spots 4. Intestinal ganglioneuromatosis (100%)
Chromosomal linkage	Autosomal dominant, chromosome 11	Autosomal dominant, chromosome 10	Autosomal dominant, chromosome 10

VIP, Vasoactive intestinal polypeptide.

highly aggressive, large bulky lesions that occur in an older population than papillary carcinomas (Fig. 15-58). The tumors do not take up iodine usually, but may be thallium or gallium avid. At the time of diagnosis there is usually infiltration of adjacent trachea, esophagus, or extrathyroidal tissues and the prognosis is grim, very grim. Spread to the trachea is the rule with these lesions as the larger the tumor, the higher the rate of invasion. Twenty-nine percent of patients with thyroid carcinoma have tracheal invasion, but the rate is over 80% for anaplastic carcinoma. Intraluminal mass and greater than or equal to 180 degrees of circumferential tracheal involvement has 100% positive predictive value. Three MR findings, soft tissue through cartilage, intraluminal mass, or circumferential involvement of over 180 degrees suggest the presence of tracheal invasion by thyroid carcinomas.

Non-Hodgkin lymphoma Non-Hodgkin lymphoma may also occur in the thyroid gland and is usually manifested by solitary nodules (44% to 86% of cases), multiple nodules (13%), or diffuse enlargement (7% to 11%). Bilateral disease has been reported in up to 53%. Tumor often invades outside the thyroid gland into the carotid sheath. The lymphoma may be primary to the thyroid gland or may result from systemic dissemination. Women are affected more than men, and this disease is seen with greatest frequency in elderly adults. Hashimoto thyroiditis may be a predisposing risk factor. Between 20% and 52% of patients are hypothyroid. On US the lesions are hypoechoic (pseudocystic), whereas on CT lymphoma is hypodense to normal thyroid tissue.

Metastasis Renal cell carcinoma ranks third after lung and breast carcinoma in its propensity to metastasize to the thyroid gland.

PARATHYROID GLANDS

Anatomy

The parathyroid glands are usually located in a perithyroidal location (duh?). Ninety percent of patients have four glands, but there may be two to six parathyroid glands, usually situated along the upper and lower poles of the thyroid gland. Rarely, parathyroid glands are located in the upper mediastinum, within the thyroid gland, in the tracheoesophageal groove, or at the thoracic inlet. The parathyroid glands are derivatives of the third and fourth pharyngeal pouches.

Congenital Disorders

Most parathyroid cysts are due to degeneration of adenomas. Rarely, a congenital parathyroid cyst may be seen, usually within the lowermost glands.

The MEN syndromes are associated with parathyroid adenomas or hyperplasias (see Table 15-4). MEN I can manifest with parathyroid hyperplasia or adenoma and one may define anterior pituitary, islet cell pancreatic, thymic, adrenal, foregut, and bronchial neoplasms as well. Remember P³AT (pituitary, parathyroid, pancreas and adrenal and thyroid). Collagenomas and facial angiofibromas may also coexist. The gene for MEN I has been localized to the eleventh chromosome. This gene must be deleted or inactivated because it expresses a protein, menin, which is a tumor-suppressor protein. Most patients with MEN I have hyperparathyroidism and this is the most common presenting symptom.

Inflammatory Lesions

No infections typically affect parathyroid tissue. Hallelujah!

Benign Neoplasms

When a patient is seen with hypercalcemia, a search for a parathyroid adenoma and/or parathyroid gland hyperplasia may lead to imaging. Although some surgeons operate on the parathyroid glands without preoperative imaging, feeling confident that they can identify the glands in the surgical field and can separate a normal gland from one that is hyperplastic or adenomatous, others employ imaging techniques to identify a parathyroid adenoma preoperatively. The surgical success rate for removal of a hypersecreting gland is 95% without any imaging at all at initial exploration, but is only 60% on repeat cervical exploration after initial failed surgery.

In a patient whose hypercalcemia persists after initial surgery for resection of the parathyroid glands, imaging may be helpful because the reoperation success rate drops to as low as 62% without imaging. In these cases aberrant or ectopic parathyroid tissue may be present. Fool me once, shame on you; fool me twice, shame on me. Get some imaging! The most common location for an ectopic parathyroid gland is the anterior mediastinum, and MR is superior to ultrasound because it is able to look below and deep to the sternum.

A running debate about whether CT (Fig. 15-59), US (Fig. 15-60), nuclear medicine (Fig. 15-61), or MR (Fig. 15-62) is the best study for identifying parathyroid adenomas continues. However, we believe that technetium sestamibi (99m technetium 2-methoxy-isobutyl-isonitrile [MIBI]) is the best study to perform when searching for a parathyroid adenoma. The study has accuracies between 90% to 95% for adenomas with equally high specificity. Unfortunately, for parathyroid hyperplasia the sensitivity is only 60%, but that is still better than the

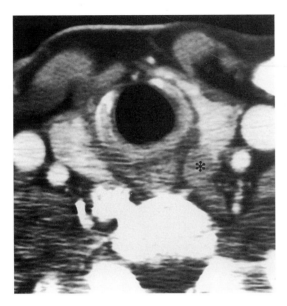

Fig. 15-59 Parathyroid adenoma on CT. The mass posterior to the left lobe of the thyroid gland is a parathyroid adenoma (*). They are usually slightly lower in density than muscle. Heterogeneity to the thyroid gland is the norm.

competitive procedures. In the past, nuclear medicine studies required a subtraction of a technetium Tc 99m or I-123 scan of the thyroid gland from a thallium 201 scan, which identifies the parathyroid adenomas. The sensitivity of these scintigrams was approximately 65% in untreated necks. Now, sestamibi has bumped these sensitivities into the mid 90% range with single agent use. Ten to 25 mCi of MIBI is given with images obtained in the first minutes after injection and again at 2 hours

after injection of the radiotracer. If needed, Tc pertechnetate can be administered to localize the thyroid gland and even subtract the pertechnetate activity in the thyroid from the MIBI activity in the parathyroids and thyroid. Add single photon emission CT (SPECT) scanning and you get another 1% to 2% bump up, in sensitivity, but an additional couple hundred bucks from your HMO and HCFA agent. CT sensitivity is reported as approximately 75%, US as around 60%, and MR as 75%. The specificities of US, nuclear medicine, and CT are greater than 95%, whereas MR has a specificity of about 90%.

In the postoperative patient with hyperparathyroidism, MR has a sensitivity of 74%: 72% in the neck, and 86% in the mediastinum. US (36% to 57%) (see Fig. 15-59) and CT (46% to 55%) do not do nearly as well in the previously operated neck.

For patients who were unsuccessfully treated surgically and have persistent hypercalcemia, technetium sestamibi is a valuable tool. Results from a recent study found that sestamibi scintigraphy achieved an 85% sensitivity and 89% positive predictive value and was equivalent to MR scanning in overall accuracy at a significantly reduced cost. Combining the 2 studies can yield accuracy rates in the mid 90% range for recurrent/residual disease. Ectopic adenomas in the thymus, parapharyngeal region, chest, thyroid gland, and lower neck are better detected than those in the tracheoesophageal groove, a blind spot for MR and MIBI imaging. For hyperplastic, nonadenomatous glands MR (82%) and MIBI (90%) fare pretty well but with hypercellular glands the success rates of MR (77%) and MIBI (64%) drop significantly.

On MR parathyroid adenomas are typically very bright on T2WI and can usually be readily distinguished

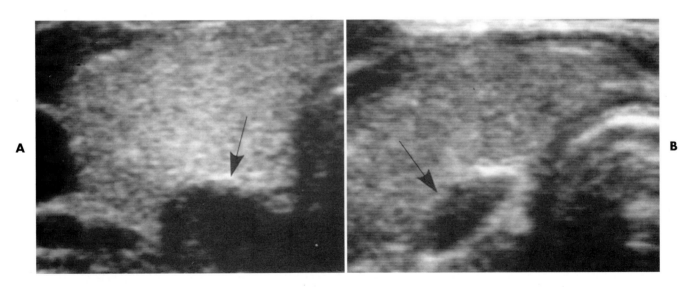

Fig. 15-60 Sonogram of parathyroid adenoma. **A,** The *arrow* marks a parathyroid adenoma posterior to the thyroid gland on this longitudinal scan. **B,** On a transaxial sonogram a different sonolucent adenoma *(arrow)* may be discerned.

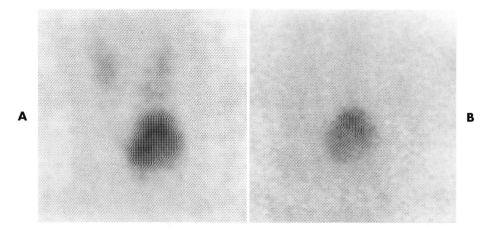

Fig. 15-61   Parathyroid adenoma studies by technetium-sestamibi. **A,** While the initial 15-minute study shows both the normal thyroid gland (faintly seen) and the large adenoma, the 2-hour follow-up study **(B)** shows only the adenoma. Normal thyroid uptake has washed out.

from normal glands (see Fig. 15-61B). In 30% of cases the MR findings may be atypical—high intensity on T1WI or intermediate on T2WI. These atypical cases have been correlated histopathologically with cellular degeneration, intratumoral hemorrhage, fibrosis, and hemosiderin deposition. Parathyroid adenomas enhance brightly.

A problem arises when bright signal is encountered on the MR. The same appearance may be due to a lymph node, parathyroid adenoma, or even an intrathyroid nodule. Remember, the goal of the study is to direct the surgeon to the *possible* location of the parathyroid adenoma. Another potential pitfall is the intrathyroidal parathyroid adenoma. This may simulate a thyroid nodule or cyst and be misdiagnosed.

On US parathyroid adenomas are usually oval sonolucent masses.

Malignant Neoplasms

Rarely one may identify a parathyroid carcinoma. The distinction is based on spread to lymph nodes and rapid growth. Carcinomas account for 1% of cases of hyperparathyroidism.

CYSTIC MASSES IN THE NECK

Throughout this and the preceding chapters you have read about numerous cystic masses that can appear in

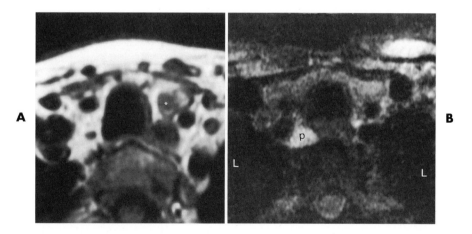

Fig. 15-62   Parathyroid adenoma on MR. **A,** See the paratracheal mass (*) on the left side. It is below the thyroid gland and was hot on sestamibi. **B,** Parathyroid adenoma. Parathyroid adenomas are best seen on axial T2WI and appear as very bright lesions. Although this image of a parathyroid adenoma *(p)* has low signal to noise, we included it to show that even with lesions in the superior mediastinum (lung apices [L] and with miserable quality you can visualize the abnormality. This is the advantage of MR over ultrasound and nuclear medicine.

the head and neck. This section organizes these entities for you before you hit the final summary chapter. These lesions usually present as nontender, palpable masses without associated lymphadenopathy. Rarely, they may declare themselves from superimposed infection. The specifics about each "cyst" are summarized in Table 15-5. To understand one of the most common of these cysts, the BCC, one must have an understanding of normal branchial arch derivatives (see Tables 15-2, 15-6, and 15-7).

Table 15-5 Cystic masses in the neck

Cyst	Clinical presentation	Imaging appearance
Abscess	Fever, pain, systemic reaction	1. Thick-walled mass 2. Infiltration, edema of subcutaneous fat 3. Rim enhancement
BCC	Painless mass in 10- to 40-yr-old patients; occasionally infected	1. Mass anterior to SCM, at CCA bifurcation 2. Thin walled unless infected 3. Unilocular
Cystic hygroma	Painless mass in neonate	1. Mass posterior to SCM 2. High intensity to T1WI (25%) because of blood, protein, fat 3. Multiloculated 4. Insinuates 5. Posterior triangle or submandibular
Cystic, necrotic node	Associated thyroid cancer or squamous cell carcinoma	1. Necrotic node with thick rim 2. Possible extracapsular extension
Dermoid	Midline cyst in tongue, oral cavity in young adult, dorsum of tongue	1. Fat often seen 2. Thin wall
Epidermoid	Off-midline cyst in mouth	1. Cystic (no fat) 2. Unilocular; may be in sublingual space
Laryngocele/ pharyngocele	Often asymptomatic	1. Air- or fluid-containing sac emanating from saccule of laryngeal ventricle or pharynx 2. Thin walled
Lipoma	Soft, compressible mass in posterior triangle in middle-aged patient with rapid weight gain	1. Fat density/intensity on CT, MR
Parathyroid cyst	Painless cyst below thyroid gland, rarely hyperparathyroid as result of PTH secretion, adult	1. Cyst with or without nodule 2. 95% below thyroid gland 3. Thin-walled
Parotid cysts	Painless masses, sometimes seen in HIV-positive patients	1. Usually cyst intensity, density in the parotid 2. Multiple 3. Associated with lymph nodes, Waldeyer's ring hyperplasia
Ranula	Cystic mass in floor of mouth located in sublingual space; may protrude into submandibular region, often superinfected	1. If not infected, thin-walled mass, homogeneous unilocular in sublingual space, possibly protruding through mylohyoid (plunging ranula) 2. Tail pointed to obstructed sublingual or submandibular duct 3. If infected, thick walled
Thyroglossal duct cyst	Midline painless mass in adult	1. Unilocular cyst embedded in strap muscles 2. Suprahyoid, 20%; hyoid, 15%; infrahyoid, 65% 3. May have high protein 4. 75% midline
Thyroid cysts	Enlarged lobe of thyroid with palpable mass and/or goiter	1. Colloid cysts are dense on CT, hyperintense on T1WI 2. Follicular cysts may have high or low intensity on T1WI 3. Often have hemorrhage
Thymic cyst	Midline cyst low in neck in child, ectopic thymus may be on left side	1. Anterior mediastinum or low neck cyst 2. Multiloculated

BCC, Branchial cleft cyst; CCA, common carotid artery; PTH, parathyroid hormone; SCM, sternocleidomastoid muscle.

Table 15-6   Arch derivatives and anomalies

Arch	Arch artery derivative (mesoderm)	Arch nerve derivative	Arch cartilage derivative	Arch anomalies
1	Degenerates	V-3	Mandible; malleus; most of incus; tensor tympani; masticator, tensor veli palatini, anterior digastric muscles; middle ear cavity; tonsils	1. Treacher Collins syndrome; abnormal external ear, hypoplastic mandible 2. Pierre Robin syndrome: hypoplastic mandible, cleft palate, low ears, eye defects
2	Degenerates	VII	Manubrium of malleus; long process of incus; stapes; styloid process; parts of hyoid stapedius, facial, posterior digastric muscles; inferior facial canal; tonsils; parathyroid; tonsillar fossa	Persistent stapedial artery
3	Carotid arteries	IX	Part of hyoid, stylopharyngeus muscles; parathyroid; thymus; pyriform sinus	DiGeorge's syndrome: absent thymus and 3rd parathyroid gland
4	Left = Aorta; Right = Proximal subclavian	X (superior laryngeal)	Thyroid cartilage; cuneiform cartilage, inferior pharyngeal constrictor, cricopharyngeus muscles; inferior pyriform sinus	R = Aberrant subclavian artery
5	This arch is MIA			
6	Pulmonary arteries	X (recurrent laryngeal)	Cricoid, arytenoids, trachea, intrinsic muscles of the larynx	

The main differential features of these lesions are their age at onset, location, and cystic contents. The pediatric lesions include the cystic hygroma (60% evident at birth and 90% by 3 years) and the thymic cyst. In young adulthood you will see BCCs, thyroglossal duct cysts, dermoids, and ranulas. Older patients have thyroid and parathyroid cysts, lipomas, or cystic/necrotic lymph nodes.

The head and neck is the third most common site for dermoids after the gonads and superior mediastinum. In the head and neck region, the orbit, oral cavity, and nasal cavity account for most. A classic location of a dermoid is along the anterior floor of the mouth where they may simulate a ranula or lymphatic vascular malformation. One may see internal cobblestone architecture on MR that suggests the final diagnosis of a dermoid.

Thyroglossal duct cysts classically present in the midline and are associated with the infrahyoid strap muscles: the second BCC is anterior to the sternocleidomastoid muscle at the carotid bifurcation level (see Fig. 15-35); the thymic cyst is low in the midline of the neck; the cystic hygroma is in the posterior triangle of the neck; and the thyroid, parotid, and parathyroid cysts are in their native tissue. Lower down in the neck one may find third and fourth branchial apparatus lesions/cysts (Fig. 15-63).

The presence of fat identifies lipomas and dermoids. High protein or hemorrhage may be seen in thyroid, parathyroid, lymphatic, and epidermoid cysts as well as in a cystic hygroma (Fig. 15-64). Most parotid cysts and noninfected BCCs have density and intensity that simulates CSF. If a thyroglossal duct cyst has high CT density,

Table 15-7   Branchial apparatus derivatives: cleft and pouch

Branchial apparatus	Cleft/Groove (Ectoderm) Derivative	Pouch (Endoderm) Derivative	Nerve associated
1	External auditory canal	Eustachian tube, mastoid air cells	V-3
2	Cervical sinus of His	Palatine tonsil, tonsillar fossa	VII
3	Cervical sinus of His	Thymus, inferior parathyroid gland	IX
4	Cervical sinus of His	Ultimobranchial body, superior parathyroid	X

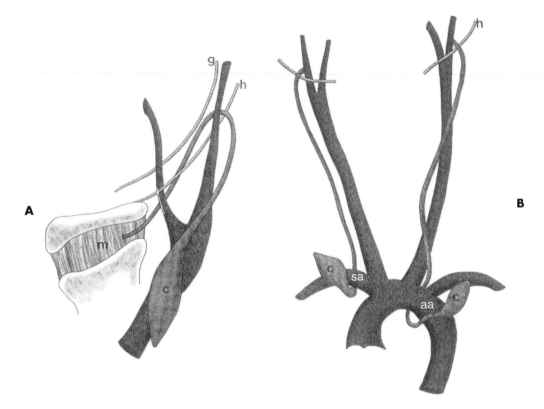

Fig. 15-63 Branchial cleft cysts. **A,** Third branchial cleft cyst anomaly. The epithelium-lined cyst is located posterior to the sternocleidomastoid muscle. The cyst tract typically ascends posterior to the internal carotid artery. It then courses medially to pass over the hypoglossal nerve (*h*) and below the glossopharyngeal nerve (*g*). It then pierces the posterolateral thyrohyoid membrane to communicate with the pyriform sinus. **B,** Fourth branchial cleft cyst anomaly. The nonkeratinized stratified squamous epithelium-lined cysts are located anterior to the aortic arch on the left and the subclavian artery on the right, respectively. The sinus tract is seen to hook inferiorly around the adjacent vascular structures (like the recurrent laryngeal nerve) and ascends to the level of the hypoglossal nerve posterior to the common and internal carotid arteries. It then loops over the hypoglossal nerve to pass deep to the internal carotid artery. C = cyst; aa = aortic arch; sa = subclavian artery; h = hypoglossal nerve. (From Mukherji SK, Fatterpekar G, Castillo M, et al: Imaging of congenital anomalies of the branchial apparatus, *Neuroimaging Clin North Am* 10:89, 92, 2000.)

it usually means that it has previously been infected. This reasoning also applies to other primary congenital cysts. Thick-walled lesions are usually abscesses or necrotic lymph nodes.

You have consumed the offerings we have laid out for you, and hopefully you are attempting to digest all this fabulous food for thought. We hope its transit time through your brain is slower than it would be through your intestines.

SUGGESTED READINGS

Ahuja AT, Chan ES, Allen PW, et al: Carcinoma showing thymiclike differentiation (CASTLE tumor), *AJNR* 19:1225-1228, 1998.

Ahuja AT, Ho SS, Leung SF, et al: Metastatic adenopathy from nasopharyngeal carcinoma: successful response to radiation therapy assessed by color duplex sonography, *AJNR* 20:151-156, 1999.

Ahuja AT, King AD, Chan ES, et al: Madelung disease: distribution of cervical fat and preoperative findings at sonography, MR, and CT, *AJNR* 9:707-710, 1998.

Ahuja AT, King AD, Kew J, et al: Head and neck lipomas: sonographic appearance, *AJNR* 19:505-508, 1998.

Ahuja AT, King AD, King W, Metreweli C: Thyroglossal duct cysts: sonographic appearances in adults, *AJNR* 20:579-582, 1999.

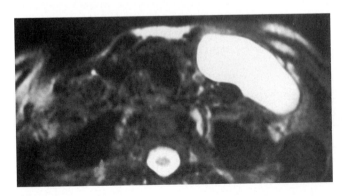

Fig. 15-64. Lower neck cyst. The differential diagnosis of this cystic mass on T2WI in the lower neck would include a third or fourth branchial cleft cyst, a cystic hygroma/lymphangioma, a thymic cyst, a thyroid cyst, or a jugular lymphatic cyst/lymphocele. (Last one is IT.)

Armington WG, Harnsberger HR, Osborn AG, et al: Radiographic evaluation of brachial plexopathy, *AJNR* 8:361-367, 1987.

Auffermann W, Clark OH, Thurnher S, et al: Recurrent thyroid carcinoma: characteristics on MR images, *Radiology* 168:753-757, 1988.

Auffermann W, Guis M, Tavares NJ, et al: MR signal intensity of parathyroid adenomas: correlation with histology, *AJR* 153:873-876, 1989.

Batsakis JG: *Tumors of the head and neck: clinical and pathological considerations,* ed 2, Baltimore, 1979, Williams & Wilkins.

Berry MP, Jenkin RDT: Parameningeal rhabdomyosarcomas in the young, *Cancer* 48:281-288, 1981.

Brander A, Viikinkoski P, Nickels J, et al: Thyroid gland: US screening in middle-aged women with no previous thyroid disease, *Radiology* 173:507-510, 1989.

Casillas J, Sais GJ, Greve JL, et al: Imaging of intra- and extra-abdominal desmoid tumors, *Radiographics* 11:959-968, 1991.

Casselman JW, Mancuso AA: Major salivary gland masses: comparison of MR imaging and CT, *Radiology* 165:183-189, 1987.

Chong J, Som PM, Silvers AR, Dalton JF: Extranodal non-Hodgkin lymphoma involving the muscles of mastication [see comments], *AJNR* 19:1849-1851, 1998.

Chong VF, Fan YF: Radiology of the jugular foramen, *Clin Radiol* 53:405-416, 1998.

Chong VF, Fan YF: Radiology of the parapharyngeal space, *Australasian Radiol* 42:278-283, 1998.

Coit WE, Harnsberger HR, Osborn AG, et al: Ranulas and their mimics: CT evaluation, *Radiology* 163:211-216, 1987.

Cross RR, Shapiro MD, Som PM: MR of the parapharyngeal space, *Radiol Clin North Am* 27:353-378, 1989.

Curtin H: Separation of the masticator space from the parapharyngeal space, *Radiology* 163:195-204, 1987.

Curtin HD, Williams R, Johnson J: CT of perineural tumor extension: pterygopalatine fossa, *AJNR* 5:731-737, 1984.

Davis WL, Harnsberger HR, Smoker WRK, et al: Retropharyngeal space: evaluation of normal anatomy and diseases with CT and MR imaging, *Radiology* 174:59-64, 1990.

Freling NJM, Molenaar WM, Vermey A, et al: Malignant parotid tumors: clinical use of MR imaging and histologic correlation, *Radiology* 185:691-696, 1992.

Gean-Marton AD, Kirsch CFE, Vezina LG, et al: Focal amyloidosis of the head and neck: evaluation with CT and MR imaging, *Radiology* 181:521-526, 1991.

Gotway MB, Reddy GP, Webb WR et al. Comparison between MR imaging and 99m-Tc MIBI scintigraphy in the evaluation of recurrent or persistent hyperparathyroidism. *Radiology* 218:783-790, 2001.

Hardin CW, Harnsberger HR, Osborn AG, et al: Infection and tumor of the masticator space: CT evaluation, *Radiology* 157:413-417, 1985.

Harnsberger HR, Dillon WP: Major motor atrophic patterns in the face and neck: CT evaluation, *Radiology* 155:665-670, 1985.

Harnsberger HR, Mancuso AA, Muraki AS, et al: Brachial cleft anomalies and their mimics: computed tomographic evaluation, *Radiology* 152:739-748, 1984.

Higgins CB, Auffermann W: MR imaging of thyroid and parathyroid glands: a review of current status, *AJR* 151:1095-1106, 1988.

Holiday RA, Cohen WA, Schinella RA, et al: Benign lymphoepithelial parotid cysts and hyperplastic cervical adenopathy in AIDS-risk patients: a new CT appearance, *Radiology* 168:439-441, 1988.

Kane WJ, McCaffrey TV, Olsen KD, et al: Primary parotid malignancies: a clinical and pathologic review, *Arch Otolaryngol Head Neck Surg* 117:307-315, 1991.

Karpati RL, Loevner LA, Cunning DM, et al: Synchronous schwannomas of the hypoglossal nerve and cervical sympathetic chain, *AJR* 171:1505-1507, 1998.

Lanzieri CF, Shah M, Krauss D, et al: Use of contrast-enhanced MR imaging for differentiating mucoceles from neoplasms in the paranasal sinuses, *Radiology* 178:425-428, 1991.

Lee KJ: Embryology of clefts and pouches. In Lee KJ, ed: *Essential otolaryngology,* New York, 1987, Medical Examination Publishing.

Lo WWM, Shelton C, Waluch V, et al: Intratemporal vascular tumors: detection with CT and MR imaging, *Radiology* 171:445-448, 1989.

Mancuso AA, Dillon WP: The neck, *Radiol Clin North Am* 27:407-434, 1989.

Mandelblatt SM, Braun IF, Davis PC, et al: Parotid masses: MR imaging, *Radiology* 164:411-414, 1987.

Mees K, Vogl T, Kellerman O: MR of salivary glands, *Laryngol Rhinol Otol* 67:355-361, 1988.

Mikulis DJ, Chisin R, Wismer GL, et al: Phase-contrast imaging of the parotid region, *AJNR* 10:157-164, 1989.

Naidich TP, Osborn RE, Bauer BS, et al: Embryology and congenital lesions of the midface. In Som PM, Bergeron RT, eds: *Head and neck imaging,* St Louis, 1991, Mosby-Year Book.

Noma S, Kanaoka M, Minami S, et al: Thyroid masses: MR imaging and pathologic correlation, *Radiology* 168:759-765, 1988.

Olsen WL, Jeffrey RB Jr, Sooy CD, et al: Lesions of the head and neck in patients with AIDS: CT and MR findings, *AJNR* 9:693-698, 1988.

Oot RF, Melville GE, New PFJ, et al: The role of MR and CT in evaluating clival chordomas and chondrosarcomas, *AJR* 151:567-575, 1988.

Peck WW, Higgins CB, Fisher MR: Hyperparathyroidism: comparison of MR imaging with radionuclide scanning, *Radiology* 163:415-420, 1987.

Reede DL, Bergeron RT, Som PM: CT of thyroglossal duct cysts, *Radiology* 157:121-125, 1985.

Robinson JD, Crawford SC, Teresi LM, et al: Extracranial lesions of the head and neck: preliminary experience with Gd-DTPA enhanced MR imaging, *Radiology* 172:165-170, 1989.

Russell EJ, Levy JM, Breit R, et al: Osteocartilaginous tumors in the parapharyngeal space arising from bone exostoses, *AJNR* 11:993-997, 1990.

Serpell JW, Campbell PR, Young AE: Preoperative localization of parathyroid tumours does not reduce operating time, *Br J Surg* 78:589-590, 1991.

Siegel MJ, Glazer HS, St Amour TE, et al: Lymphangiomas in children: MR imaging, *Radiology* 170:467-470, 1989.

Sigal R, Monnet O, de Baere T, et al: Adenoid cystic carcinoma of the head and neck: evaluation with MR imaging and clinical-pathologic correlation in 27 patients, *Radiology* 184:95-102, 1992.

Silver AJ, Mawad ME, Hilal SK, et al: Computed tomography of the carotid space and related cervical spaces, *Radiology* 150:723-728, 1984.

Som PM, Biller HF: High-grade malignancies of the parotid gland: identification with MR imaging, *Radiology* 173:823-826, 1989.

Som PM, Braun IF, Shapiro MD, et al: Tumors of the parapharyngeal space and upper neck: MR imaging characteristics, *Radiology* 164:823-829, 1987.

Som PM, Sacher M, Lanzieri CF, et al: Parenchymal cysts of the lower neck, *Radiology* 157:399-406, 1985.

Som PM, Sacher M, Stollman AL, et al: Common tumors of the parapharyngeal space: refined imaging diagnosis, *Radiology* 169:81-86, 1988.

Som PM, Scherl MP, Rao VM, et al: Rare presentations of ordinary lipomas of the head and neck: a review, *AJNR* 7:657-664, 1986.

Som PM, Shapiro MD: MR of the head and neck, *Radiol Clin North Am* 27:1-479, 1989.

Stevens SK, Chang J-M, Clark OH, et al: Detection of abnormal parathyroid glands in postoperative patients with recurrent hyperparathyroidism: sensitivity of MR imaging, *AJR* 160:607-612, 1993.

Swartz JD, Rothman MI, Marlowe FI, et al: MR imaging of parotid mass lesions: attempts at histopathologic differentiation, *J Comput Assist Tomogr* 13:789-796, 1989.

Tabor EK, Curtin HD: MR of the salivary glands, *Radiol Clin North Am* 27:379-392, 1989.

Takashima S, Ikezoe J, Morimoto S, et al: Primary thyroid lymphoma: evaluation with CT, *Radiology* 168:765-768, 1988.

Tefft M, Fernandez C, Donaldson M, et al: Incidence of meningeal involvement by rhabdomyosarcoma of the head and neck in children, *Cancer* 42:253-258, 1978.

Teresi LM, Lufkin RB, Vinuela F, et al: MR imaging of the nasopharynx and floor of the middle cranial fossa. Part II. Malignant tumors, *Radiology* 164:817-821, 1987.

Teresi LM, Lufkin RB, Warthan DG, et al: Parotid masses: MR imaging, *Radiology* 163:405-409, 1987.

Tien RD, Chu PK, Hesselink JR, et al: Intra- and paraorbital lesions: value of fat-suppression MR imaging with paramagnetic contrast enhancement, *AJNR* 12:245-253, 1991.

Tien RD, Hesselink JR, Chu PK, et al: Improved detection and delineation of head and neck lesions with fat suppression spin-echo MR imaging, *AJNR* 12:19-24, 1991.

Van Tassel P, Lee YY: Gd-DTPA-enhanced MR for detecting intracranial extension of sinonasal malignancies, *J Comput Assist Tomogr* 15:387-392, 1991.

Vogl TJ, Dresel SHJ, Spath M, et al: Parotid gland: plain and contrast-enhanced MR imaging, *Radiology* 177:667-674, 1990.

Wake M, Phelps PD: View from within: *Radiology* in focus. Adenoid cystic carcinoma: a comparison between CT, MR and Gd MR imaging techniques, *J Laryngol Otol* 104:662-664, 1990.

Whiteman ML, Serafini AN, Telischi FF, et al: 111In octreotide scintigraphy in the evaluation of head and neck lesions, *AJNR* 18:1073-1080, 1997.

Yousem DM, Huang T, Loevner LA, Langlotz CP: Clinical and economic impact of incidental thyroid lesions found with CT and MR, *AJNR* 18:1423-1428, 1997.

Yousem DM, Lexa FJ, Bilaniuk LT, et al: Rhabdomyosarcomas in the head and neck: MR imaging evaluation, *Radiology* 177:683-686, 1990.

Yousem DM, Sack MJ, Scanlan KA: Biopsy of parapharyngeal space lesions, *Radiology* 193:619-622, 1994.

Yousem DM, Sack MJ, Weinstein GS, Hayden RE: Computed tomography- guided aspirations of parapharyngeal and skull base masses, *Skull Base Surgery* 5:131-136, 1995.

Yousem DM, Scheff AM: Thyroid and parathyroid gland pathology. Role of imaging, *Otolaryngolc Clin North Am* 28:621-649, 1995.

Yousem DM: Parathyroid and thyroid imaging, *Neuroimaging Clin North Am* 6:435-459, 1996.

CHAPTER 16

Anatomy and Degenerative Diseases of the Spine

SPINAL PARLANCE

This chapter begins with a brief review of the anatomy of the spine. Imaging techniques are then discussed, followed by the normal imaging appearance of the spine on magnetic resonance imaging (MR) and computed tomography (CT). We then consider degenerative diseases of the spine. These common diseases may manifest as localized back pain, radiculopathy (pain radiating in a spinal root distribution), or myelopathy (signs of spasticity, increased tone, and increased reflexes). The radiologic differential diagnosis of spine lesions is based on localizing the lesion to a particular space. This has fortunately become less of an issue in the MR era than in the days of the giants, when the savants would meditate over myelographic minutiae and the word Chad was just a male name.

A brief word concerning terminology. Understanding the terminology used in localizing spinal lesions is critical in framing your differential diagnosis as well as presenting yourself as a knowledgeable radiologist. So a little repetition would not hurt. The anatomic algorithm historically used by radiologists was predicated on myelographic interpretation as to whether lesions were extradural, intradural extramedullary, or intramedullary. Intramedullary lesions are indigenous to the spinal cord, tend to expand it, and narrow the subarachnoid space. They include spinal cord tumors such as astrocytoma, ependymoma, and spinal cord metastases, as well as nonneoplastic lesions such as syringohydromyelia, infections, and inflammation such as transverse myelitis, acute disseminated encephalomyelitis, or human immunodeficiency virus (HIV) infection. Intradural extramedullary lesions are lesions outside the spinal cord but within the thecal sac. These include meningioma, neurofibroma, or vascular mass lesions such as angiomatous malformations or varices. Those, which are intradural but extramedullary (outside the cord), expand the subarachnoid space on the ipsilateral side (producing a meniscus) and shove the cord over to the contralateral side. Obviously, intradural lesions below the termination of the spinal cord are extramedullary.

Extradural lesions occur outside the dural tube and may originate from the disk (herniated disk), disk space (epidural infection), or the vertebral bodies (osteophytes, primary bone and metastatic tumors). Lesions that compress or are intrinsic to the cord produce myelopathy, whereas those, which compress and irritate the roots, cause radiculopathy.

Although spinal anatomy lacks the sex appeal of other anatomic sites, it does have certain features that are intriguing and may even keep your attention.

The bony spine is divided by region into the cervical spine containing seven vertebrae (the first two of which are rather unique and are discussed further), the thoracic spine, consisting of 12 vertebral bodies; and the lumbar spine, with five vertebral bodies. The distal spine consists of the sacrum and coccyx. The spine encases the spinal cord, which normally terminates at a variable level from approximately T12 to L2.

The orthopod ordered an MR of the spine
The history, as usual, was worth less than a dime
  With multilevel protrusions
  An impression of confusion
The lawyers bellowed—another failed-back, divine!

ANATOMY

Spinal Nerves

The spinal cord contains eight cervical, 12 thoracic, five lumbar, five sacral, and one coccygeal paired spinal nerves. These nerves are rather easily identified on CT with intrathecal contrast or MR. It is important to appreciate that C1, which is a sensory nerve, exits above the C1-2 interspace so that the C2 nerve exits between C1 and C2, and so on. Therefore, the C8 nerve root ex-

its between C7 and T1. In the thoracic region, T1 exits between T1 and T2, and T12 exits between T12 and L1. In the lumbar spine the L1 root exits between L1 and L2 and so forth, so that the L5 root exits between L5 and S1. However, a funny thing happened on the way to creation. The bodies in the lumbar region became much longer. The nerve roots in this region leave the thecal sac right under the pedicle (Fig. 16-1), well above the interspace. Paracentral disk herniations in the lumbar region characteristically strike the root in the thecal sac that will exit below the interspace. This is because the disk space is inferior to the same numbered exiting root at that level. Thus, an L4-5 disk herniation most often compresses the L5 root because the L4 root is already in the foramen. Very lateral herniated disks may compress the upper root; that is, an L4-5 lateral herniation can compress the L4 root. Larger disks can compress many roots in the thecal sac. Furthermore, disk fragments may migrate superiorly and compress the root exiting at the appropriate interspace, that is, an L4-5 free fragment can compress the L4 root or a combination of both the L4 and L5 nerve roots.

An anatomic variation is the conjoined nerve root, which occurs in less than 5% of patients, with L5-S1 being the most common disk space. This normal variation consists usually of two nerve roots traveling in the same dural pouch and exiting through the same or through different foramina. The problem is really the radiologist's. She or he should not mistake the conjoined root on myelography for an epidural defect with obliteration of the thecal sac below the conjoined root. The most significant mistake occurs on CT of the lumbar region without intrathecal contrast. Here conjoined roots can appear

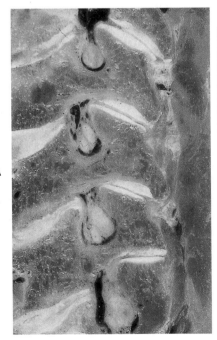

A

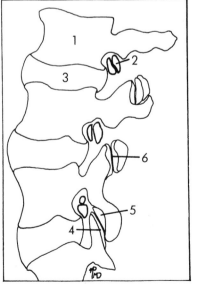

B

Fig. 16-1 Nerve roots in cervical neural foramina. **A,** Cervical roots. **B,** Lumbar roots (*2*) travel in the upper half of the foramen. *1,* Vertebral body; *3,* disk; *4,* superior articular facet; *5,* inferior articular facet; *6,* facet joint. (From Firooznia H, Golimbu C, Rafii M, et al: *MR and CT of the musculoskeletal system,* St Louis, Mosby-Year Book, 1992.)

as disk herniations. The key is that the density of the conjoined root/CSF complex is similar to the thecal sac and not that of disk. Furthermore, conjoined roots have a characteristic position (like the ears of Mickey Mouse) as opposed to disk. Conjoined roots have been reported occasionally to enlarge the neural foramen. Today with MR, this normal variant is not usually a problem.

In the cervical region, the disks generally compress the roots at the foramen at the same level. THUS, a C5–6 disk compresses the C6 root. In the cervical region, the roots are in the lower portion of the foramen whereas in the lumbar region they are in the upper aspect of the neural foramen. In the thoracic region, disk herniations may cause myelopathic changes; however, they can also produce thoracic radiculopathy. Lesions at the given thoracic spine body level might also produce sensory symptoms one to two segments below the compression. This is because the cord ends at approximately T12 to L2 so that cord lesions result in neurologic deficits that are localized below their vertebral body anatomic location.

Each spinal nerve is divided into a dorsal or sensory root and a ventral or motor root. The dorsal root ganglion is a distal dilatation of the dorsal root just proximal to its joining with the ventral root to form the spinal nerve (Fig. 16-2).

Vertebrae

The generic vertebra is composed of the cylindric vertebral body, which contains cancellous bone with marrow and fat, covered by a thin layer of compact bone, and the vertebral arch or posterior elements, covered by a thick layer of compact bone (cortex), including the pedicles, laminae, superior and inferior facets, transverse processes, and spinous process (Fig. 16-3). The vertebral configuration is modified in the different regions of the spine. The cervical vertebrae have their neural foramina between the transverse processes. The superior and in-

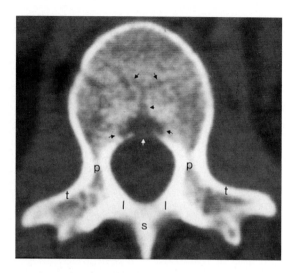

Fig. 16-3   Vertebral anatomy. This CT of a lumbar vertebral serves as a model for a generalized vertebra. Pedicle *(p)*, lamina *(l)*, transverse process *(t)*, basivertebral venous plexus *(arrows)*, and spinous process *(s)* are labeled.

ferior articular facets are fused in the cervical region to form the articular pillar (Fig. 16-4). The lower five cervical vertebrae have five joints connecting them. They are the intervertebral disk, two facet (zygapophyseal) joints, and two uncovertebral joints. The uncovertebral joints (neurocentral joints, joints of Luschka) originate from the lateral posterior portion of the vertebral body, articulate with the contiguous vertebral body, and in-

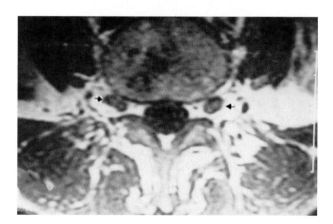

Fig. 16-2   Dorsal root ganglia. Axial T1WI demonstrates normal appearance of the dorsal root ganglia *(arrows)*.

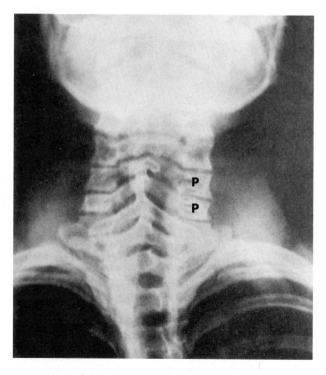

Fig. 16-4   Articular pillor view. (P) is pillor.

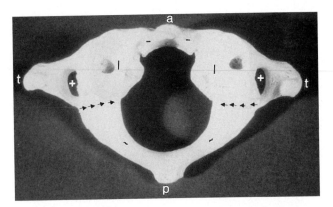

Fig. 16-5 Atlas. Axial view of atlas from above. The following structures are identified: anterior tubercle *(a)*, posterior tubercle *(p)*, foramen transversarium *(+)*, transverse process *(t)*, anterior arch *(−)*, posterior arch *(,)*, sulcus for vertebral arteries *(arrows)*. The holes in the lateral mass *(l)* were placed by Ilyssa Yousem who was playing with her father's tool chest.

sinuate themselves between the disk and the nerve root canal. The vertebral artery enters the foramen transversarium (in the cervical transverse process, naturally) at approximately C6 and travels superiorly.

The first cervical vertebra (atlas) has no body but rather just an anterior arch connected to two lateral masses and a posterior arch (Fig. 16-5). On the upper surface of the posterior arch is a groove over which the vertebral artery courses after it leaves the foramen transversarium of C1. The vertebral arteries pass through the posterior atlantooccipital membrane and course anteriorly superiorly upward through the foramen magnum. As it pierces the dura the vertebral artery may be slightly narrowed, and this caliber change can serve as a marker for the beginning of the intradural segment of the vertebral artery. The first spinal nerve exits here as well.

The second cervical vertebra, the axis, is unique, with

a superior extension from its body termed the dens (odontoid process) (Fig. 16-6). The dens represents the lost vertebral body of the atlas and is usually found fractured by residents on their first call. The articulation between the atlas and axis is composed of multiple synovial joints: one medial between the dens and the anterior arch, one on each side between the inferior articular facet of the lateral mass of the atlas and the superior facet of the axis, and multiple ones between the dens and the atlantoaxial ligaments (transverse, cruciate, and alar). Rheumatoid arthritis has a propensity for the atlantoaxial joint with pannus formation, leading to bone erosions and subluxations.

The thoracic vertebrae have an articulation on the transverse process for the rib and no foramen transversarium, whereas the lumbar vertebrae have neither a foramen transversarium nor a facet for the rib articulation. The lumbar vertebral articulations are composed of the lumbar disk and two facet joints posteriorly. The lateral recess of the lumbar spine is in the anterolateral portion of the spinal canal, with boundaries consisting of the posterior margin of the vertebral body and disk anteriorly, the medial margin of the pedicle laterally, and

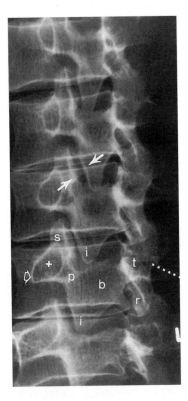

Fig. 16-7 Right posterior oblique film of scottie dog. Right facet joint is seen *(arrows)*. At the disk space below, components of the scottie dog are identified: eye = right pedicle *(+)*, neck = right pars interarticularis *(p)*, ear = right superior articular facet *(s)*, front leg = right inferior articular facet *(i)*, nose = right transverse process *(open arrow)*, tail = left superior articular facet *(t)*, rear leg = left inferior articular facet *(r)*—oops! Scottie had an accident *(. . . .)* !

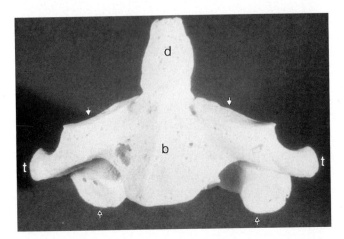

Fig. 16-6 Axis. Anterior view demonstrates dens *(d)*, body *(b)*, superior articular facets *(arrows)*, inferior articular facets *(open arrows)*, and transverse processes *(t)*.

the superior articular facet, the medial insertion of the ligamentum flavum, the lamina, and the pars interarticularis posteriorly (Fig. 16-7).

Intervertebral Disks

The diskovertebral complex is composed of three components: the cartilaginous end-plate, annulus fibrosis, and nucleus pulposus. The end-plate consists of a flat bony disk with an elevated rim (attached ring apophysis), which produces a central depression in the endplate occupied by hyaline cartilage.

The annulus fibrosus surrounds the nucleus pulposus (the remnant of the notochord). The nucleus is eccentrically located near the posterior surface of the disk. The lamellae of the annulus are fewer in number, thinner, and more closely packed posteriorly than anteriorly. This anatomic arrangement may account for the propensity for posterior herniation. The external fibers of the annulus are connected to the bone of the vertebral bodies by Sharpey's fibers, which usually cannot be distinguished by imaging. Annular fibers also merge with both anterior and posterior longitudinal ligaments. Important ligaments of the vertebral column are (1) the anterior longitudinal ligament, running along the anterior aspect of the vertebral bodies; (2) the posterior longitudinal ligament, running along the posterior aspect of the verte-

bral bodies anterior to the thecal sac; (3) the ligamentum flavum, connecting the laminae and extending from the midline laterally to the facets; and (4) the interspinous ligament, joining the superior portion of the spinous process below to the inferior portion of the spinous process above and meeting the ligamentum flavum in the midline (Fig. 16-8). There are also small ligaments in the neural foramen, which may play a role in foraminal stenosis.

Spinal Cord

The spinal cord extends from the medulla oblongata, at the level of the upper border of the atlas, to T12 to L2, where it terminates in the conus medullaris. At the apex of the conus, continuous with the pia mater (i.e., "the tender mother"), is the filum terminale, which descends initially in the thecal sac and then becomes covered with adherent dura as it leaves the thecal sac to insert in the coccyx. The cauda equina emanates from the conus medullaris and contains the nerve roots of the lumbar and sacral nerves. The spinal cord has two enlargements in its course, one in the cervical region from approximately C4 to approximately T1 (cervical enlargement) and the other in the lower thoracic region from approximately T9 to T12 (lumbar enlargement). Do not mistake these normal expansions for a pathologic

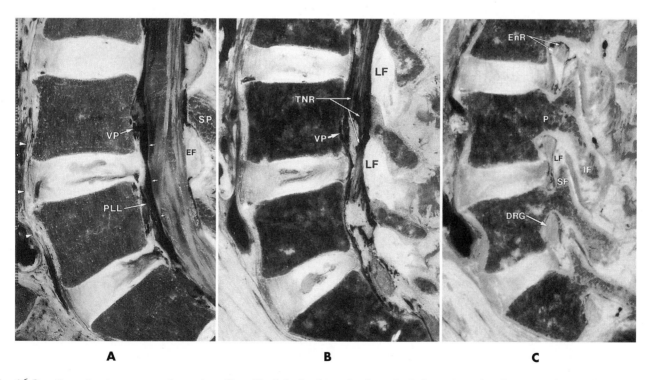

A   **B**   **C**

Fig. 16-8   Cryomicrotome anatomic sections (**A** to **C**) of the lumbar spine in sagittal plane. *Arrowheads,* anterior longitudinal ligament; DRG, dorsal root ganglion; EF, epidural fat; EnR, existing nerve root; IF, inferior facet; LF, ligamentum flavum; P, pedicle; PLL, posterior longitudinal ligament; *small arrows,* dura mater; SF, superior facet; SP, spinous process; TNR, traversing nerve root; VP, venous plexus.

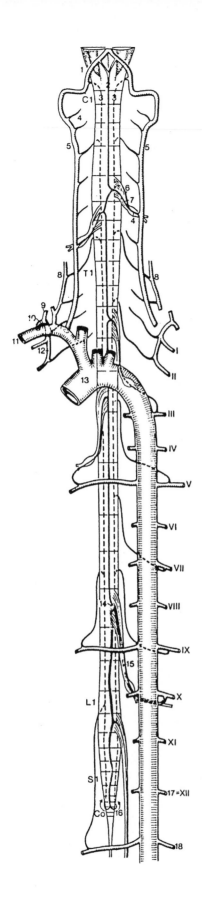

A

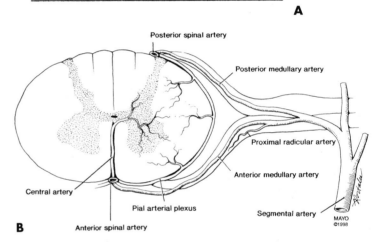

Posterior spinal artery

Posterior medullary artery

Proximal radicular artery

Anterior medullary artery

Segmental artery

Central artery

Pial arterial plexus

Anterior spinal artery

MAYO ©1998

B

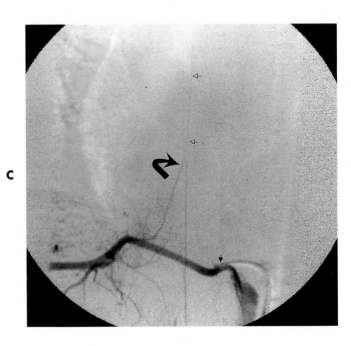

C

process; otherwise you will need a return ticket to your board examination. These enlargements correspond to the locations in the cord that supply the spinal nerves for the upper and lower extremities.

Blood Supply to the Spinal Cord

The blood supply to the spinal cord depends on the particular location (Fig. 16-9). In the cervical region the anterior spinal artery is formed by branches that originate from the vertebral arteries just before joining the basilar artery. The anterior spinal artery supplies the anterior aspect of the spinal cord. In addition, paired posterior spinal arteries originate from the vertebral arteries and supply the dorsal portion of the cord. These two arterial systems do not usually have significant anastomoses between them. The anterior spinal artery supplies the anterior two thirds to four fifths of the cord; including the anterior column of the central gray matter, the corticospinal, spinothalamic, and other tracts. The paired posterior spinal arteries supply the posterior columns and the posterior horn of the central gray matter. The anterior spinal artery is in the midline whereas the posterior spinal arteries lie off the midline (see Fig. 16-9B). The anterior and posterior spinal arteries rarely originate at the same level. The caliber of the anterior spinal artery at a particular spinal level is proportional to the metabolic demands of the spinal gray matter.

At the C3-4, C5-6, and C7-T1 levels, radicular feeders from the vertebral, ascending cervical (anterior to the transverse process), and deep cervical (posterior to the transverse process) arteries anastomose with the spinal arteries. The radicular feeders enter the thecal sac through the intervertebral foramina and divide into the anterior and posterior branches coursing with the nerve roots. Because they follow the nerve root, the spinal arteries have a sharper angle in the lumbar region than in the cervical region. However, not all spinal nerves have radicular arteries. The cervical and upper two thoracic levels comprise one vascular territory. The midthoracic region T3-7 is supplied by intercostal branches from the aorta, branches of the supreme intercostal arteries from the subclavians, and lumbar arteries. This region may have a tenuous blood supply. The lower thoracolumbar region to the filum terminale is supplied by the artery of Adamkiewicz. It is commonly located on the left side between T9 to L2 (85% of the time) and T5 to T8 (15% of the time). It enters the spinal canal with the nerve roots and makes a characteristic hairpin loop, giving off a small superior branch from the apex of the turn and a large descending branch, which supplies the anterior spinal cord and anastomoses with the posterior spinal arteries in the region of the conus medullaris.

Uncommonly, an artery named the artery of Lazorthes arises from the common or internal iliac arteries and accompanies one of the sacral roots of the cauda equina to supply the conus medullaris. The venous blood supply is comparable to the arterial blood supply with a variable amount of anterior and posterior spinal veins running with the spinal arteries.

RADIOLOGIC WORKUP

Imaging Fundamentals and Techniques

Although imaging techniques vary, important concepts in the spine should be appreciated. These generalizations hold true for the vast majority of situations encountered, regardless of the type of equipment available. Presently, MR is the technique of choice in most situations. However, CT, myelography, and myelography supplemented by CT (myelo-CT) all have roles in particular situations and with particular surgeons. The customer is always right, there are many ways to skin a cat, variety is the spice of life—remember the radiologist does not have to take care of the patient, so "Just Do It."

MR technique Dollar for dollar, MR is the best single method for imaging the spine. Complete MR examination requires an excellent sagittal image. Take care to scan from neural foramen to neural foramen with thin sections, with the minimum interslice gap that your particular instrument permits. This sagittal image should be a T1-weighted image (T1WI). Assess the foramina for bony constriction and the normal fat and nerves. Osteophytic narrowing can be identified on good sagittal images. In the lumbar region, the foramina have a vertical orientation. The nerve root is in the superior portion of the foramen under the pedicle. Fat packs the foramen, particularly in the lumbar region. Lesions obliterating the fat are easily detected on T1WI (Fig. 16-10). These include lateral disk herniations, neurofibromas, soft tissue from inflammatory changes, postoperative scar, and spondylolisthesis.

In the cervical region, thin-section axial images are also necessary. A thin section volumetric acquisition through the cervical spine enables sections of 1.5 mm or less with contrast such that the cerebrospinal fluid (CSF) is high signal and osteophytes are low signal

Fig. 16-9 Arterial anatomy of the spine. **A,** Schematic representation. (From Nieuwenhuys R, Voogd J, van Huijen C: *The human central nervous system: A synopsis and atlas,* rev ed 3, Berlin, Springer-Verlag, 1988.) **B,** Arterial blood supply at a single segment. Both the anterior and posterior are illustrated. This is not the typical arrangement. It is unusual for both anterior and posterior medullary arteries to enter at the same segment in any region of the cord. (From Krauss WE: Vascular anatomy of the spinal cord. Neurosurg Clin North Am 1999; 10:10.) **C,** Spinal arteriogram. Injection into an intercostal artery (*arrow* is on catheter tip) reveals filling of artery of Adamkiewicz with its characteristic hairpin turn (*curved arrow*). Anterior spinal artery is filling (*open arrows*).

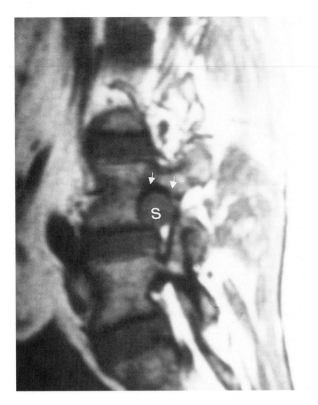

Fig. 16-10   Mass in foramen. Sagittal T1WI of the lumbar spine shows a schwannoma *(s)* filling the neural foramen. Note that the bone is remodeled with scalloping of the pedicle above *(arrows)*.

intensity (Fig. 16-11). Osteophytic compression of the roots or impingement on the spinal canal is obvious. On this T2W sequence it is best to have the disk brighter than bone but darker than CSF; however, usually there is plenty of conspicuity between disk and CSF. If you are uncomfortable that disk and CSF conspicuity are less than adequate, other sequences (use of a larger flip angle 30 degrees gradient echo images or proton density weighted images) increases contrast between the high signal disk and low signal CSF.

Gradient echo MR may tend to exaggerate bony lesions (foraminal or central bony stenosis) of the spine, and what appear as high grade or complete blocks on MR may not be as severe on myelography, CT myelography, or T1WI. Fast spin echo (FSE) T2WI is the routine technique used for imaging the CSF, spinal cord, and nerve roots. One advantage for FSE imaging derives from its relative insensitivity to susceptibility effects compared with gradient and conventional spin echo techniques. Thus, spinal osteophytes are not as exaggerated on sagittal images as with the other techniques and there is better visualization of the extent of thecal sac compression, cord compression, and intrinsic cord pathology.

Another benefit of the FSE technique is edge enhancement. This provides excellent delineation of nerve roots and spinal cord. Intrinsic cord lesions can be exquisitely defined on sagittal FSE images. Short tau inver-

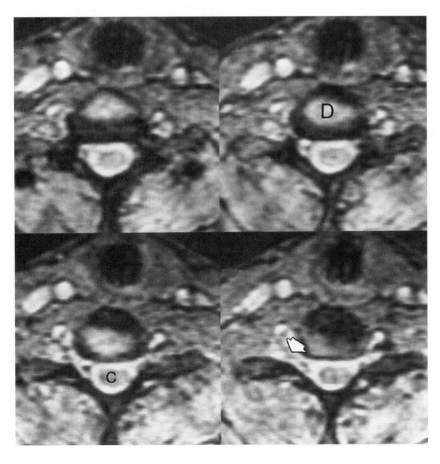

Fig. 16-11   Axial three-dimensional Fourier transform gradient echo image of the spine. This scan was obtained with a 5-degree flip angle. Observe that the disk *(D)* and cord *(c)* are lower in intensity than the surrounding high intensity of CSF. Nerve in the neural foramen in the lower right image is identified *(arrow)* and outlined by bright CSF.

sion recovery images (STIR) are excellent for detection of ligamentous injury.

Although not presently employed, diffusion-weighted imaging of the spinal cord will probably be perfected before the next edition. It will have a role in the diagnosis of ischemic, inflammatory, traumatic, and demyelinating lesions of the spinal cord as well as studying the normal maturation of the cord in pediatric patients. Potentially, its greatest role may be in the evaluation of myelopathy from spondylosis. Before it is ready for prime time, it must deal with adequate signal-to-noise, physiologic motion, spatial resolution, and susceptibility effects. Nevertheless, we predict that its role will be similar to that in the brain when the geeks torque it up.

Although MR is the best technique for demonstrating spinal cord compression, it cannot definitively judge whether a particular lesion will produce a complete block on myelography. This may be less of an issue with new imaging techniques, because treatment protocols are directed more toward lesions as opposed to the consequences of the lesions (the myelographic block). Indeed, the "block" has gone the way of the typewriter—only used by the old curmudgeon.

Enhancement is necessary in the postoperative back to distinguish between scar and disk, in infectious and inflammatory conditions of the spine to assess the full extent of disease, and in the evaluation of the spinal cord to rule out tumor. Although enhancement is in many cases useful in metastatic disease to the vertebral bodies, it is not always necessary. Many times, replacement of the fatty marrow by tumor is obvious on unenhanced images. However, care must be taken not to proceed with a contrast examination of the spine, before performing a nonenhanced scan. In such circumstances diffuse metastases to the spine enhance and appear as "normal fatty marrow" on T1WI (see Fig. 17-27). This is less of an issue if you employ fat suppression on your post-gadolinium images.

For lumbar degenerative disease, thicker axial sections (3 to 5 mm) are adequate. It is important in the lumbar region to scan in the axial plane from pedicle to pedicle rather than just through the disk space, otherwise migrated free fragments of disk material behind the vertebral body may be undetected. For disk herniations, scans should generally be performed parallel to each disk space. This necessitates angulation of the imaging plane in the lower lumbar spine. Another approach is to decrease the axial section thickness to 3 mm or less and to minimize the gap between slices. This enables axial imaging without angulation and does not exaggerate (by volume averaging) normal disks to appear as though they are herniated. This also offers an evaluation for lumbar spinal stenosis. Fast spin echo axial and sagittal images in the lumbar spine are also useful in unambiguously defining the subarachnoid space. This has been a problem in certain situations because most of the imaging protocols in the lumbar region are generally T1-weighted so that both disk and CSF are hypointense, and conspicuity, particularly on axial images, can be difficult.

Myelography "What presently is the role for myelography?" the Grasshopper asks. It is presently reserved to answer those questions that cannot be answered or addressed by MR or CT. Although not performed as often as it once was, myelography, almost always combined with CT (myelo-CT), is still a sensitive and useful technique for disk herniation and, more importantly, osteophytic impingement on cervical roots. Myelo-CT is excellent in patients with cervical radiculopathy for visualizing small spurs compressing nerve roots or in cases of cord compression (Fig. 16-12). Other roles include detecting subarachnoid spread of tumor, small tumor implants on nerve roots, and arachnoiditis. The advantage of the myelo-CT is the exquisite bone detail superimposed upon the subarachnoid contrast. In the opinion of the authors, myelo-CT is more precise than MR at evaluating the effect of uncovertebral joint disease on nerve roots. However, if you are the patient do you want a spinal tap, with the possibility, although remote, of infection or other complications? Some patients report that the postmyelogram headache is worse than the backache before or after surgery. That is an advantage of MR, not to mention it is the method of choice for visualizing the spinal cord and soft tissues.

Patients in whom MR is contraindicated, such as persons with metallic implants or cardiac pacemakers, or those who cannot tolerate MR, can be easily examined by myelo-CT. This is an issue for metallic hardware for spine stabilization such as pedicle screws and anterior metallic plates (Fig. 16-13). Other potential uses are in cases where ambiguity in the diagnosis exists, such as for demonstrating small tumor nodules on nerve roots

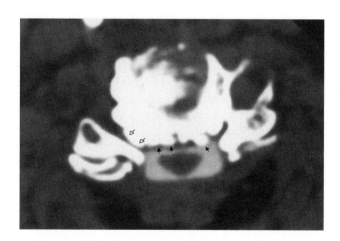

Fig. 16-12   Osteophytic spur. CT myelography faithfully demonstrates osteophytic spurs both centrally *(closed arrows)* and laterally *(open arrows)*. Note that the patient already had a laminectomy. CT myelogram is a reliable method for detecting osteophytic impingement.

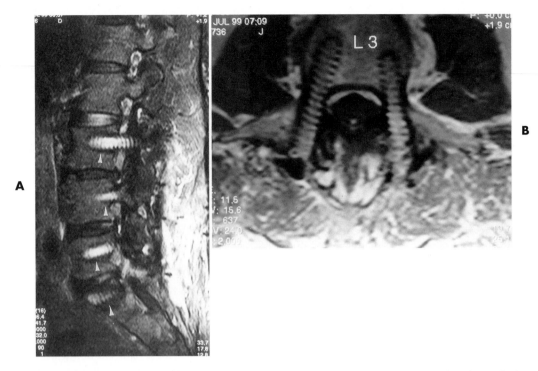

Fig. 16-13 MR of pedicle screws. **A,** What? How can the MR show the pedicle screws so well. You thought we had said they obscure anatomy on MR images. The high signal on the T2WI likely represents the screw tracks *(arrowheads)* from screws that have been removed. (Either that or we have a screw loose ourselves or we've been screwed by the history). **B,** Axial post contrast T1WI shows the correct anatomic placement of the screws in the pedicles but not extending beyond the vertebral body anterior margin.

or for visualizing dilated veins in patients with spinal arteriovenous malformations. MR is excellent at depicting compression of the cord and, although it cannot detect a spinal cord block with respect to intrathecal contrast, there is no down side to patients having a block deteriorating after spinal tap.

When you perform a myelogram be very careful that the contrast agent is instilled in the appropriate compartment. Subdural injections of contrast are not uncommon, and myelograms performed with contrast in the subdural compartment can be misleading (Fig. 16-14). After contrast is instilled into the lumbar region, it is critical to visualize the individual nerve roots of the cauda equina. If these are not demonstrated, you are probably dealing with either a subdural injection or severe arachnoiditis. Another clue to a subdural injection is in the lateral projection, where subdural contrast may collect in the posterior aspect of the thecal sac as opposed to its normal ventral position. In the thoracic region, the cord and its surrounding space should be apparent. Failure to separate cord density from surrounding contrast material again suggests subdural injection. The subdural space in the spine is continuous with that of the brain. On CT, you may see contrast along the clivus, because of subdural injections.

Epidural space extravasations are less common. Irregular streaky collections of contrast can be observed

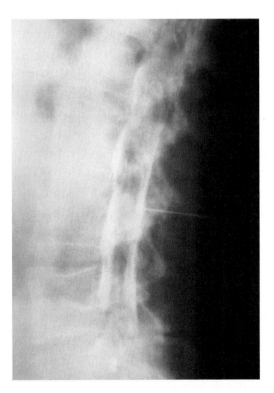

Fig. 16-14 Subdural injection. A lateral myelographic film reveals filling of subdural space. Note that the nerve roots are not clearly seen. There is contrast anterior and posterior to the thecal sac in a characteristic pattern indicating a subdural injection.

throughout the lumbar region, sometimes following nerve roots well beyond the vertebral column, and occasionally in the epidural venous plexus.

Disk herniation on myelography is diagnosed by effacement of the root pouch. Compression of the opacified thecal sac by the disk may also be visualized (Fig. 16-15). It is important to evaluate the myelogram in the anteroposterior (AP), oblique, and lateral planes. A double density can be seen on the lateral radiograph in the paramedian herniated disk. The thecal sac at L5–S1 is convex at its lateral margin as it tapers to the sacrum. Concavity in this region should suggest disk herniation even if the roots do not appear to be effaced. You should appreciate that myelography can be normal in cases of lateral disks and may be insensitive at the L5–S1 level when the cul-de-sac ends at or above this interspace. Needle defects and epidural varices can produce defects on myelography similar to disk herniations.

On AP myelographic films with an extradural lesion, the spinal cord may appear to be enlarged (Fig. 16-16). It is most important to view lesions involving the cord in two planes! Many mistakes have been made by just gunning from the hip because of the AP film, and some clinicians have been shot between the legs by acting on this single image. This is much less of a problem presently because myelography is usually performed in combination with CT.

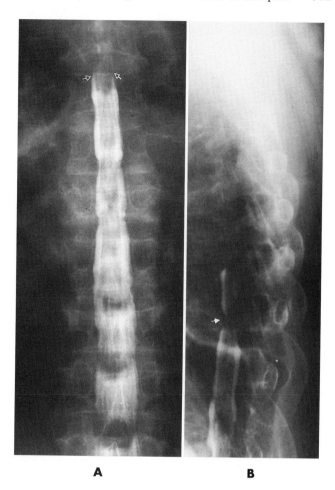

A   **B**

Fig. 16-16 Spinal block producing the appearance of an intramedullary process on AP myelogram. **A,** AP myelographic projection reveals a high-grade block to the flow of contrast in the thoracic region *(arrows)*. The cord appears expanded with narrowing of the lateral contrast margins simulating an intramedullary process. **B,** Lateral projection demonstrates that this is an extradural tumor mass *(arrow)* compressing the cord.

Computed tomography   Just a short word concerning CT. Myelo-CT unambiguously reveals extradural bony lesions compressing the subarachnoid space, roots, and spinal cord. CT without intrathecal contrast is adequate for the lumbar region, where natural contrast exists between epidural fat, disk, and bone (Fig. 16-17). However, there is usually little contrast between the spinal cord and the subarachnoid space in the cervical and thoracic regions, so that intradural processes are suboptimally imaged without intrathecal contrast.

The postmyelogram lumbar CT is best performed, if tolerated, with the patient in the prone position. This enables the contrast to pool in the anterior thecal sac and along the root pouches, making it most sensitive to root effacement by disk or bone. However, the supine position is more easily tolerated and in most cases is acceptable, especially after the patient has turned on the table to mix CSF and contrast. Thin sections, from pedi-

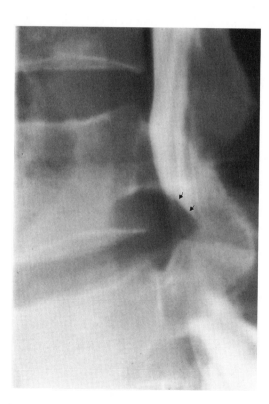

Fig. 16-15 Lateral myelogram of a large herniated disk. Thecal sac and nerve roots are abruptly cut off *(arrows)* by this large herniated disk.

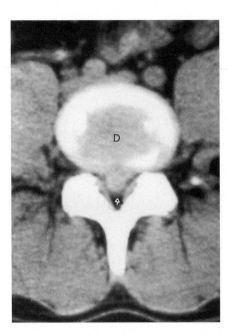

Fig. 16-17 Herniated disk on unenhanced CT. Huge central herniated disk is squashing the thecal sac *(open white arrow)*. Herniated disk and the parent disk *(D)* have the same density.

cle to pedicle, are recommended. This is really a precise unambiguous technique for evaluating radiculopathy. It is just too bad that you have to stick a needle into the subarachnoid space and inject a contrast agent to make it work.

In the cervical and thoracic regions, localization of the abnormality is important (that is usually the purpose of the myelogram). It is unrealistic to think that you can do thin sections through the entire spine despite what your back surgeons think—pin them down to a level. Imaging is ideally performed with bone and soft-tissue windows to optimize for disk and bone.

Intravenous contrast CT of the cervical spine This technique had been advocated years ago (BMR—before MR) to evaluate cervical degenerative disease. Remember the cervical spine contains a large venous plexus around the nerve roots. Following contrast, disk herniation and osteophytes can be seen impinging upon and distorting the enhancing venous plexus. The method has been recently rediscovered and used with spiral CT. The ability to perform 1-mm slices and to reformat the image in multiple planes is potentially of great value. The downside of the technique is the use of intravenous contrast and radiation. Presently, the technique has not been fully evaluated in the marketplace to determine its ultimate role.

Diskography This is a most controversial topic. The procedure calls for injection of contrast material within the nucleus itself. After injection, plain radiographs are made and additional CT images can be performed. There are several observations to be made that include whether the contrast is confined by the annulus, streaks into the annulus, or leaks into the epidural space. Here you may be able to diagnose an unsuspected annular tear. Equally important is the reproduction of patient symptoms from the injection of contrast material. Thus, the injector must have enough experience to perform the technique in a reproducible manner and hopefully the injectee will have a rather standardized response. Yes, we agree it sounds more like art than science and more subjective than most studies we perform. That is why most of these studies are not performed by neuroradiologists but rather by orthopods and physiatrists. Do these procedures add anything? For one thing, they are useful in cases of considerable pain and no definitive imaging findings. Potentially, you can find the level that is producing the symptoms. A second possible useful application is in cases with multiple disk herniations and no definitive notion of which level is the symptomatic culprit. We do not want to belabor this but as neuroradiologists we have found cases of diskograms performed where the keen observational skill of our radiology technologist picked up lateral disk herniations that were missed by the visually impaired orthopod.

Low tech: plain spine films Plain spine films are still performed and are useful particularly when looking for small fractures in cases of trauma and to check alignment of the vertebral bodies, the position of bone grafts, pedicle screws, cages, plates, and abnormal motion of vertebrae during flexion and extension. Every view contains potential aids in demonstrating disease, but we will briefly focus on a few specific regions and important information to be gained. In the standard AP view of the cervical spine, the uncovertebral joints and their relationship to the neural foramina are best demonstrated (Fig. 16-18). There is reasonably good correlation between uncovertebral spurs and myelographic impingement associated with radiculopathy. Alignment of the spinous processes should be assessed for rotational injury to the spine. Subluxations caused by trauma can be detected by noting differences in distance between the spinous process tips of C5-6 and C6-7 and are important because the lateral radiograph may not visualize C6-7. Unilateral facet dislocations produce rotation of the spinous processes in the transverse plane.

The lateral cervical spine radiograph provides an excellent view of the odontoid process and the anterior arch of C1. The distance between the anterior aspect of the odontoid and the posterior surface of the anterior arch of C1 should not be greater than 3 mm in an adult and 5 mm in a child. Alignment of the spine and the disk spaces is easily evaluated with the lateral view. The minimal sagittal diameter of the cervical spinal canal between C3 to T1 is 13 mm corrected for magnification. Pay attention to the distance between the back of the articular facets and the spinolaminar line on a nonrotated

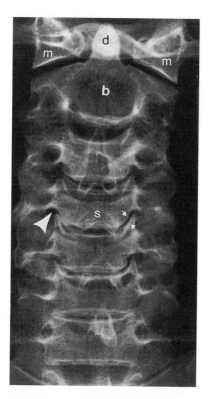

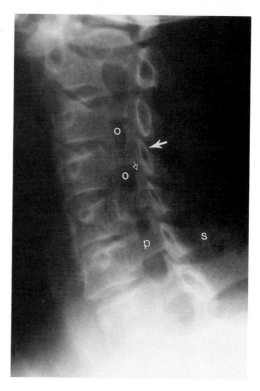

Fig. 16-18   AP view of cervical spine. Lateral masses of C-1 *(m)*, dens *(d)*, body of C-2 *(b)*, bifid spinous process *(s)* C-4, uncovertebral joint *(arrows)*, and a neural foramen *(arrowhead)* are identified.

Fig. 16-19   Oblique radiograph of the cervical spine. Right posterior oblique demonstrates the left neural foramina *(o)*, the pedicle *(p)*, the superior articular facet *(open arrow)*, the lamina *(arrow)*, and the spinous process *(s)*.

cervical spine lateral. If there is little or no distance between the posterior margins of the spinal facets of the cervical vertebra and the spinolaminar line, think spinal stenosis! With the lateral view, you receive at no extra charge the prevertebral soft tissues and the sella turcica. Occasionally, you will note unexpected findings including an enlarged sella or prevertebral mass. A "swimmer's" view is used to study C7–T1 if it cannot be visualized on the lateral, and consists of a lateral view with the tube-side arm depressed and the film-side arm elevated. Ossification of the posterior longitudinal ligament and diffuse idiopathic skeletal hyperostosis (DISH) are identified on the lateral radiograph.

The right and left cervical oblique radiographs are obtained to view the neural foramina, the uncovertebral joints, and the facets (Fig. 16-19). Remember in the cervical region the foramina are directed anterior and lateral; therefore in the right posterior oblique projection with the film behind the neck the left foramina are being visualized. Of course, the opposite is true for the left posterior oblique film.

Thoracic AP films visualize the pedicles and vertebral bodies. Carefully, determine whether there is pedicle erosion, a sign of metastatic disease, or whether the interpediculate distance is abnormal. This indicates an intraspinal lesion, or a possible congenital spinal problem.

The lateral thoracic radiograph provides information on thoracic alignment, abnormal calcifications in a disk or in a meningioma, and the state of the vertebral body and its associated disk spaces.

Information obtained from the lumbar spine AP and lateral films is similar to that of the thoracic spine; however, the oblique radiographs produce the well-known "scottie dog," which provides an excellent view of the pars interarticularis. Fractures of the "neck" of the dog indicate spondylolysis (Fig. 16-20). Spondylolysis is associated with spondylolisthesis (anterior slippage of a vertebral body), both of which are readily detectable on plain films and are discussed later in this chapter. In the right posterior oblique view the right superior articular facet is the ear, the right pedicle is the eye, the right transverse process is the nose, the right inferior articular facet is the front leg, the right lamina is the body, the left superior articular facet is the tail, and the left inferior articular facet is the hind leg (see Fig. 16-7).

NORMAL MR APPEARANCE OF THE SPINE

Enough with the anachronistic imaging—let us rock with the music of WMRI. The beauty of MR is its ability to provide multiplanar images of both the bone and soft

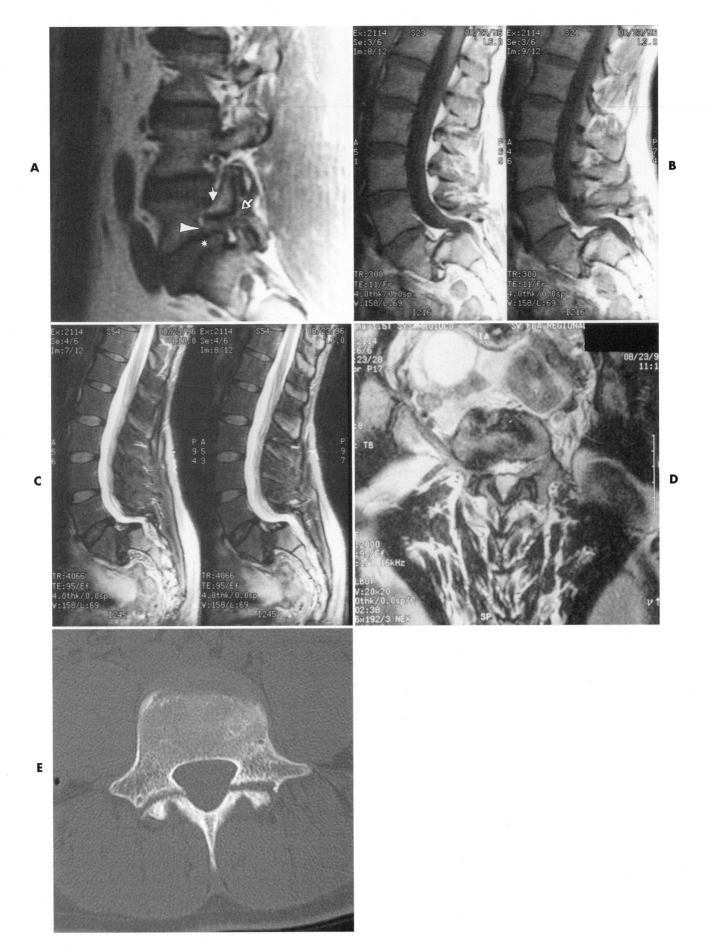

Fig. 16-20   Spondylolysis and spondylolisthesis. **A,** Saggital T1WI beautifully illustrates spondylolisthesis of L-5 on S-1. Note the elongation of the pedicle *(arrow)* and the pars interarticularis defect *(open arrow).* The disk *(asterisk)* is compressing the nerve root in the compromised neurla foramen *(arrowhead).* Normally the foramen has a keyhole appearance on the sagittal image, with an abundance of fat, whereas in spondylolisthesis the orientation of the neural foramen goes from vertical to horizontal and little foraminal fat can be seen. **B,** Sagittal T1WI shows grade 3 spondylolisthesis with endplate degenerative changes at L5-S1. **C,** The effect on the thecal sac is better illustrated on the sagittal T2WI. **D,** Axial T1WI through the defect. **E,** In another patient, a pars defect is well depicted on the axial CT. The horizontal orientation of the defect indicates that this is unlikely to be a facet joint (a first year professor mistake).

tissues of the spine. In the adult, the normal vertebral marrow generally has intermediate to high signal intensity on T1WI and low signal intensity on conventional T2WI with bone marrow hypointense to the disk and CSF hyperintense (Fig. 16-21). This appearance is variable, depending on the exact pulse sequence and the age of the patient. On T2WI fast spin echo images, the normal vertebral marrow is high intensity making lesion detection in the vertebral body more challenging. Fat saturation is important when vertebral body lesions are suspected and FSE techniques are being employed. However, the saturation may not be uniform particularly when large field-of-views are employed.

In children, the marrow is lower in intensity than in adults because of the low fat content of hematopoietic marrow. In young adults, a small region of high intensity on T1WI is observed at the entry of the basivertebral veins. With aging, the hematopoietic (red) marrow is gradually converted to fatty (yellow) marrow. In older patients, this process can result in focal regions of high intensity on T1WI (focal fatty replacement) with a heterogeneous appearance. In children, the normal marrow may enhance; however, in adults normal marrow does not enhance significantly. In patients with anemia, fatty marrow is replaced by hematopoietic marrow with decreased and heterogeneous signal intensity on T1WI.

The epidural plexus of veins has a variable appearance on MR, depending on the particular pulse sequence used. The plexus enhances. Occasionally, this plexus may be prominent and masquerade as a disk. In this situation enhancement is useful. A prominent venous plexus may also be visualized above or below a herniated disk or in spinal stenosis.

DEGENERATIVE DISEASES

Unlike great wines, the spinal column does not improve with age—it degenerates. It is important to separate the process of disk degeneration from disk herniation. The pathophysiology of the degenerative process consists of loss of water in the nucleus pulposus and decreased tissue resiliency (intervertebral chondrosis) with decrease in the height of the disk space. This is manifested on MR by decreased signal intensity on T2WI. Early MR abnormalities representing disk degeneration include infolding of the anterior annulus and a hypointense central dot within the disk on T2WI. Disk degeneration is noticeable by the age of 20 years.

Initially, the nucleus pulposus is soft and gelatinous; however, with aging it is replaced by fibrocartilage and the distinction between nucleus and annulus fibrosus becomes less well defined. The cartilaginous end-plate becomes fissured and more hyalinized. The annulus, which is initially attached to the anterior and posterior longitudinal ligaments, loses its lamellar configuration and develops fissures. The cracks have negative pressure so that gas, primarily nitrogen, comes out of solution and deposits in the intervertebral disk, close to the subchon-

Fig. 16-21   Normal spine MR. **A,** T1WI shows the vertebral bodies to be of higher intensity than the disks. CSF is low intensity. The spinal cord is higher in intensity than the CSF. The basivertebral plexus *(closed arrow)* and the epidural fat *(open arrow)* are identified. **B,** Conventional T2WI reveals the vertebral bodies to be lower in intensity compared with the disks. The CSF is high intensity and the spinal cord is low intensity. The basivertebral plexus is high intensity.

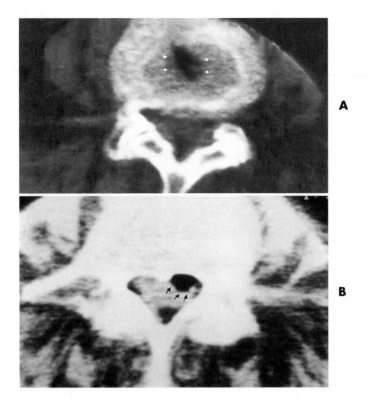

A

B

Fig. 16-22   Vacuum phenomenon. **A,** Very low-density gas *(arrows)* can be seen within the disk. **B,** In this case the gas *(arrows)* is the only evidence of the herniation, which is displacing the thecal sac to the right.

dral bone plate or in other locations. This is termed the vacuum phenomenon (Fig. 16-22). These degenerative changes permit disk material to bulge and subsequently to herniate. Remember that disk herniation may occur in the absence of significant disk degeneration.

Disk calcification commonly occurs in the elderly, and is part of the normal aging process. It is also associated with other conditions (Box 16-1). Increased intensity on T1WI of the disk can be seen uncommonly with mild calcification associated with degeneration. As calcification increases the intensity on T1WI decreases.

Disk Herniation

Degenerative processes may be accompanied by disk herniation. In such an instance, the nuclear material squeezes itself through the annular fissures. The radiologic descriptions that are associated with various imaging findings of disk rupture are imprecise and confusing. A simple approach to this problem is proffered by the authors. You ask, "Why do we do this?" The answer is that (1) we are simple folk; (2) we prefer intracranial zebras to degenerative joint disease (DJD); (3) the more complex the discussion, the greater the lawyers' fees; (4) the interauthor variability is great; (5) this is "The Requisites Series" (we

> **Box 16-1   Diseases Associated with Disk Calcification**
>
> Acromegaly
> Amyloidosis
> Anklyosing spondylitis
> Calcium Pyrophosphate Deposition Disease (CPDD)
> Chondrocalcinosis
> Diabetes Mellitus
> DISH
> Gout
> Hemochromatosis
> Homocysinuria
> Hyperparathyroidism
> Hypothyroidism
> Ochronosis
> Osteoarthritis
> Poliomyelitis
> Sequelae of disk infection

think) and not the *Encyclopaedia Britannica.* Having said that please keep in mind that low back pain alone costs the USA more than 14 billion dollars in compensation and treatments—so it turns out to be vital to your style of life.

When to image? HMOs believe you should wait 4 to 6 weeks. The radicular symptoms and motor signs tend to improve over time and they can save big bucks. However, how does the HMO executive behave? He or she wants to be imaged immediately to know the true diagnosis (believing the only diagnosis is cancer) and how large it is. The authors agree with the HMO executive. Waiting 4 to 6 weeks while you suffer is not tolerable, and HMO executives do not feel your pain. Threaten them by letters and calls to Congress. If you actually have weakness and muscle loss go see the take-no-insurance surgeon.

Here are some definitions that have been advocated to more precisely define degenerative lesions in the lumbar spine. An annular tear (annular fissure) is a separation between anular fibers, avulsion of fibers from their vertebral body insertions, or breaks through fibers that extend in a particular direction (see following discussion) (Fig. 16-23). Such lesions may or may not be secondary to trauma.

Herniation is a localized displacement of disk material (nucleus, cartilage, fragmented apophyseal bone, annulus, or any combination of the constituents of the disk) beyond the limits of the intervertebral disk space. The disk space is defined cranially and caudally by the vertebral body end-plates and peripherally by the outer edges vertebral ring apophyses, exclusive of osteophytic formations. "Localized" is defined as less than 50% (180 degrees) of the periphery of the disk whereas "generalized" is greater than 50%. In the axial plane "focal" is de-

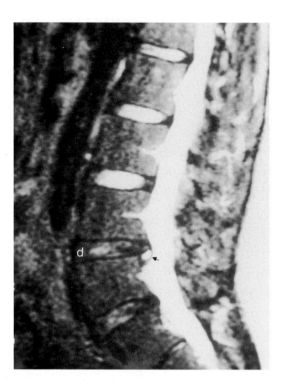

Fig. 16-23   High signal intensity (small arrow) at the margin of this disk (d) likely represents an annular tear. Recent studies have noted that the annular tears enhance and can remain hyperintense on T2WI for years after their occurrence. Hence, high intensity and enhancement of annular tears do not connote acuity.

fined as less than 25% of the disk circumference, "broad based" between 25% to 50% of the disk circumference, and the presence of disk between 50% to 100% beyond the edges of the apophyses is termed "bulging."

Herniations may be described as protrusions or extrusions. Protrusions occur if the greatest distance, in any direction, between the edges of the disk material beyond the disk space is less than the distance between the edges of the base (cross-sectional area of disk material at the outer margin of the disk space), when measured in every plane. Extrusion is defined when any one distance between the edges of the material beyond the disk space is greater than the distance between the edges of the base, or when no continuity exists between the disk material beyond the disk space and that within the disk space. If the displaced disk material is not in continuity with the parent disk it is considered to be a sequestered disk. If the herniated disk is displaced from the extrusion (regardless of whether it is sequestered or not) it is thought to be migrated disk. If the disk herniation is covered by the outer anulus it is considered contained and uncontained if it is through the outer anulus beyond the confines of the annulus (Fig. 16-24). Further description includes the location of the herniation and the extent, if any, that a particular structure (nerve root, thecal sac, spinal cord) is compressed by the herniation. The hard question is whether small focal bulges should be termed small disk herniations, focal disk protrusions (a term used for disk material confined by residual an-

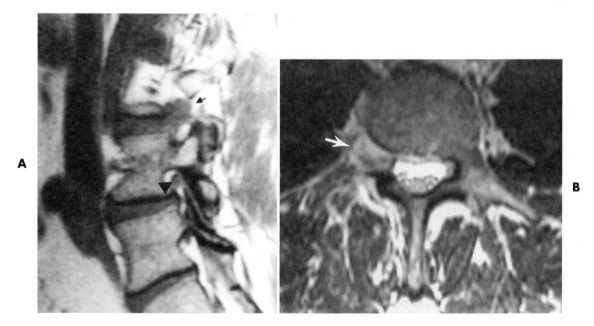

Fig. 16-24   Herniated lateral disk at L3-4. **A,** Sagittal T1WI of this large lateral herniated disk *(arrow)* shows the neural foramen fat replaced by disk, and the nerve root cannot be seen. Nerve root below is identified *(arrowhead)*. **B,** Large lateral disk herniation *(arrow)* is present. This affects the L3 root, as opposed to most herniations at this level, which affect the L4 root.

Illustration continued on following page

C

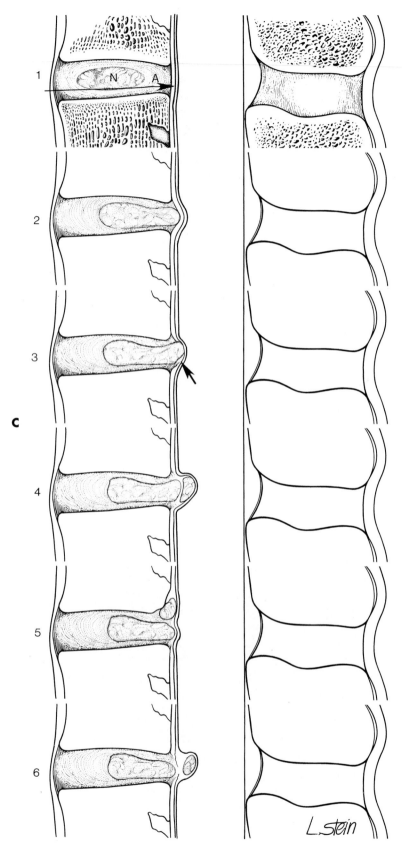

L. stein

Fig. 16-24 *Continued.* **C,** Diagram of lateral spine demonstrating spectrum of disk lesions. *1.* Normal configuration of nucleus pulposus *(N),* intact annulus fibrosis *(A),* posterior longitudinal ligament, and dura. *2.* Bulging disk with intact annulus fibrosus. *3.* Subligamentous herniated disk with rupture of the annulus fibrosus *(arrow). 4.* Herniated disk with a free fragment. *5.* Herniated disk with a free fragment that has migrated superiorly. *6.* Herniated disk that has ruptured through the posterior longitudinal ligament and is against the thecal sac. In extremely rare instances the disk can continue to head east and become intradural. This is so rare that it may be seen only in the operating room when the surgeon inadvertently traverses the dura (oops!).

nulus), or focal disk bulges. The authors' opinion is that these are all small herniations, and it makes more sense to term them small focal disk herniations than to be more cryptic so that the referring physician must ask what the difference is between a protrusion or focal bulge and a herniation. Thus, focal extensions of disk beyond its normal anatomic margin should be deemed herniations. Period. Diffuse extension of a disk beyond the vertebral bodies is termed a bulging disk. There is no focality. This is a "natural" part of the degenerative process.

Extruded disk occurs when the nucleus perforates the annulus but remains in contact with the parent disk. Some authors attempt to localize disk herniations further into those that penetrate the annulus but not the posterior longitudinal ligament. These have been designated to be subligamentous herniations. Remember, the posterior longitudinal ligament merges with the outer annular fibers identified on T2WI as a discrete low intensity curvilinear structure at the posterior margin of the disk. MR criteria suggesting subligamentous herniation includes: (1) continuous low signal line posterior to the herniation; (2) herniation of less than 50% of the spinal canal; and (3) absence of disk fragment. The diagnostic accuracy for differentiating subligamentous from supraligamentous lumbar disk herniations (not contained by the posterior longitudinal ligament) is not impressive (<62% accurate) even if you combine all of the criteria. Probably it is not worth the perseveration in most cases (Fig. 16-25).

In the lumbar region, a sagittal midline septum connects the posterior longitudinal ligament to the vertebral body (see Fig. 16-25C). Thus, subligamentous disk herniations are usually constrained by this membrane and are generally lateral (see Fig. 16-25F). When disk material perforates the annulus fibrosis and is not in continuity with the parent disk, it is termed a free fragment (or sequestered disk), which can migrate to any location. The free fragment can lodge above or below the disk space with equal frequency (see Fig. 16-25E). In extremely rare instances, disks have been reported to transgress the dura and lie intradurally (see Fig. 16-25H and I). This description has also been used as an asset preserver in operative reports by disk jockeys after the dura has been inadvertently breached during surgery.

The diagnosis of disk herniation presently can be made by MR or CT. On MR, you note the presence of disk material focally compressing the thecal sac or nerve roots. This can be demonstrated in the axial or sagittal planes and, if detected, should be confirmed in the other plane. A useful generalization is that all disk material from the same disk should have similar intensity or density, that is, herniated disk material should have similar intensity (or density on CT) to the parent disk. On MR, this is not always the case. Disk fragments may have different intensities depending on their state of hydration and the par-

ticular pulse sequence used. Degenerated disks on MR generally have lower intensity on T2WI than normal disks, and disks containing gas (vacuum disks) have very low intensity on all pulse sequences. Remember that degenerated disks may or may not herniate, but with a few exceptions, herniated disks have degenerated. These exceptions include young persons with acute herniations from such strenuous activities as football, weight-lifting, writing books, and playing tiddlywinks.

Lisse syndrome   This is dedicated to the wife of one of the authors. She presented with acute excruciating medial scapular pain at about the level of T3-4. The pain was so severe the patient could not stand and she rapidly also developed aschtupia without agraphia. MR of the shoulder and cervical spine were initially read as not compatible with the pain level. An astute neurologist noted atrophy of the first dorsal interosseous muscle and weakness in apposition of the thumb and little finger and said it was a C8 root problem, go find it! Thin section CT demonstrated absence of fat in the C8 neural foramen. Thin section MR showed a totally foraminal disk herniation, which was confirmed at surgery (Fig. 16-26). Take home points include: (1) that foraminal disks are difficult, at times, to detect, so that you should look carefully at the contents of the neural foramen at every level; (2) C8 radicalopathy can present as only back pain without arm pain; (3) a good neurologic examination is critical in evaluation of acute disk disease; (4) if the symptoms do not fit, make sure you do not quit; (5) C7-T1 is a blind spot for most MR studies, and (6) aschtupia is a treatable disease. If not detected, C8 disks lead to atrophy of intrinsic hand function and disability. Unfortunately, Lisse reherniated 10 months later with the same symptoms. Again the diagnosis was difficult in spite of knowing where the disk was, however, a postgadolinium image found the fragment and repeat surgery was successful (see Fig. 16-26D). The moral of the second herniation was that despite excellent imaging and surgery TA TA happens.

Annular tears   There are three types of annular tears: concentric, radial and transverse with the latter two being identifiable on MR. Transverse tears are peripheral disrupting Sharpey's fibers. Radial tears start from the nucleus and course through the annulus. On MR, globular or linear high intensity can be observed on T2WI within the posterior annulus (see Fig. 16-23). Anterior radial annular tears are rare but can be associated with back pain. This can be associated with pain or segmental instability. Acute and sometimes chronic annular tears can enhance and T2 hyperintensity may persist for years.

Muscle spasm   Paravertebral muscle spasm is associated with disk herniation. This can be seen as scoliosis with the concavity on the side of the spasm. Patients

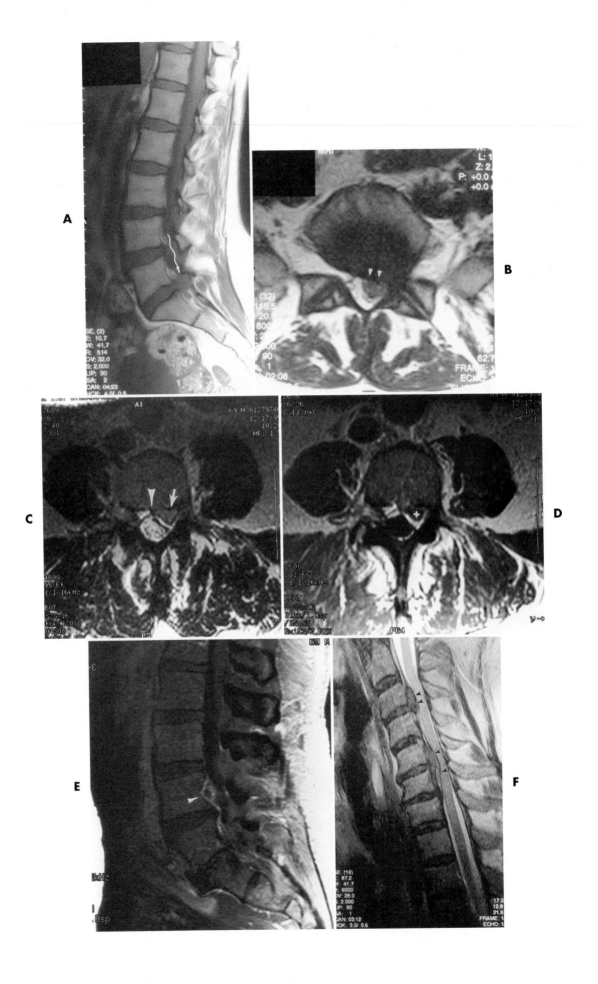

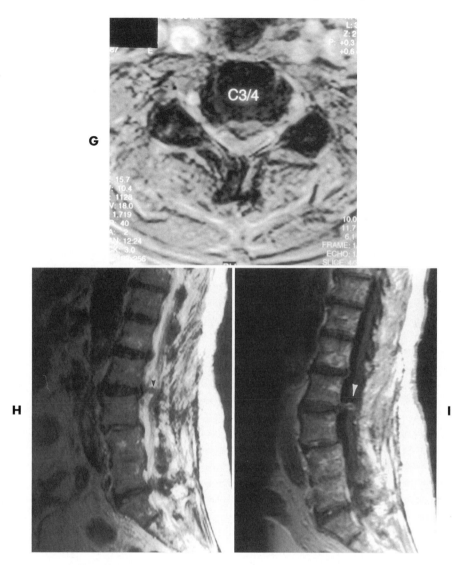

Fig. 16-25   Montage of disk herniations. **A,** Sagittal T1WI reveals a huge L5-S1 herniated disk *(squiggly arrow)* obliterating the epidural fat and the thecal sac. **B,** The disk *(arrowheads)* is low in intensity on T2WI. **C,** A midline septum *(arrowhead)* confines this free disk fragment *(arrow)* seen on this T2WI. **D,** The postcontrast axial T1WI shows minimally enhancing granulation tissue around the non-enhancing disk *(+).* **E,** The absence of communication of the herniated disk *(arrowhead)* with the parent disk is borne out on this sagittal postcontrast T1WI. People use the term "sequestered disk," "sequestration" or "free fragment" for this entity. **F,** Sagittal T2WI shows multiple subligamentous cervical herniated disks (extrusions since the longitudinal extension dimension exceeds the attachment to the parent disk). The posterior longitudinal ligament is outlined by *arrowheads* and has been displaced posteriorly by the mass of the disks. **G,** The 3DFT gradient echo scans highlights the contrast between the gray disk and the dark bone. **H,** An intradural disk fragment *(arrowhead)* is outlined by CSF on this T2WI. **I,** Granulation tissue around the disk enhances and again highlights the intradural location of the free fragment on this sagittal postcontrast T1WI.

with low back and leg pain have been observed to show paraspinal muscle atrophy. This is most obvious in the multifidus muscle, the largest and most medial of the lumbar paraspinal muscles. These muscles originate from the spinous process and spread laterally as they course inferiorly to insert in the iliac crest and sacrum. They are innervated by the medial branch of the dorsal ramus. They are best assessed on axial images. The muscle loss may be caused by pain or lesions affecting the dorsal ra-

mus nerve. The same case can be made for the psoas muscle and is indicative of L2-3 disk.

Time course   Disks can improve over time and spontaneous reduction of herniations, particularly those larger than 6 mm, are reported 6 to 12 months after the initial event. This is associated with clinical improvement (if you have a high pain threshold and no significant neurologic deficit to tolerate the wait). Exactly how this occurs is unknown but investigators have hypothesized

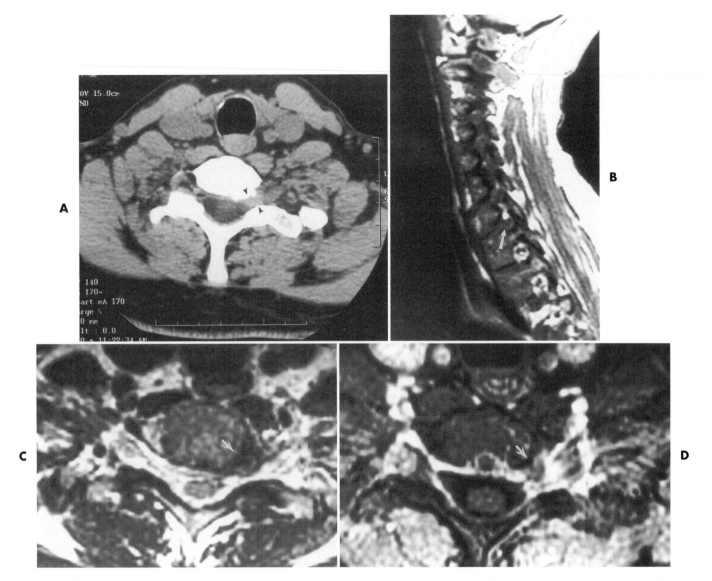

Fig. 16-26 CT and MR of C7-T1 herniated disk (Lisse syndrome). **A,** Cervical CT scan shows loss of the left C7-T1 fat in the left neural foramen *(arrowheads).* Osteophytic ridging and a herniated disk account for the pathology. **B,** The disk is occupying the lower portion of the foramen as seen on the sagittal T1WI *(arrow).* Remember that the nerve roots in the cervical spine usually exit in the lower aspect of the foramen—the opposite of what is taught with respect to the lumbar foramina. **C,** The axial T2WI shows the lateral disk *(arrow)* abutting on the exiting C8 nerve rootlet. **D,** A postoperative study 9 months after operation to remove the herniated disk and after new onset of recurrent symptoms shows a nonenhancing new fragment at the same location. Bad luck, but thanks for the contribution to the book, honey.

about dehydration with disk shrinkage, fragmentation, and phagocytosis as possible factors in the reduction of disk herniation. With the onset of herniation, there is an associated inflammatory process. Neovascularity occurs at the periphery of the herniated disk and the combination of inflammation and neovascularity may contribute to resorption of the disk material. Acute epidural enhancement around a free fragment has been reported with acute disk herniation to occur in 73% of cases. The enhancement proceeds inward over time. Peridiskal enhancement has been associated with a good clinical out-

come. The inflammatory component has also been suggested for the reason why epidural steroids have been used successfully for the nonsurgical treatment of herniated disks. A torn anulus can heal with vascularized granulation tissue and thus can demonstrate different patterns of enhancement too with intradiskal linear enhancement corresponding to concentric tears and an intradiskal nodular pattern representing a radial or transverse tear.

Interpretative skills Just how good are we with respect to our interpretation? A study of the interobserver and intraobserver variability in the lumbar spine using two different nomenclatures (normal, bulge, herniation vs normal, bulge, protrusion, extrusion) reported interobserver variability of 80% and intraobserver variability of 86%. Disagreement arose in calls between normal disk and bulge and bulge versus herniation or protrusion. The reader should also be aware that surgical observations are not the "gold standard" either. This is because of the variety of terms used by the blades to describe their surgical findings, some of which may be confounded by the fact that no surgeon likes to operate on a normal disk. Without excellent surgical/radiologic correlates it is easy to understand why we have such variability in our radiologic analysis. One additional thought—disk herniation can be seen in asymptomatic patients. Just how often? This varies with respect to the reports, techniques, and the location. Suffice to say that about a third of asymptomatic patients will have significant abnormalities in their lumbar spine and probably a great fraction in the cervical region. This is a medical-legal alert—radiologic findings in the absence of clinical correlation is worth about as much as the veracity of the statement pleading "I never had sex with that women." With respect to interpretation of MR spine images—the radiologist may have the last word but certainly not the final say.

Schmorl's Node

Herniation of disk material through the end-plate is termed Schmorl's node (recently termed intravertebral herniation), which usually has discrete margins and intensity similar to disk material, and reveals rim enhancement. Schmorl's nodes can be identified in asymptomatic patients and have been associated with infection, trauma, malignancy, osteopenia, and intervertebral osteochondrosis (Fig. 16-27). On MR, they appear as extension of disk into the vertebral body surrounded by a rim of low intensity on T2WI representing reactive sclerosis. Occasionally, Schmorl's node may be associated with bone marrow edema, which can be confused with infection or metastatic lesion. Chronic Schmorl's nodes may be associated with fatty end-plate changes.

If the disk herniates into the anterior ring apophysis, it is termed a limbus vertebra (seen in children and associated with back pain).

Scheuermann disease This degenerative disease is noted in children with the onset at puberty and a male predominance. It consists of vertebral wedging resulting in lower thoracic kyphosis. It requires the involvement of three contiguous vertebra with wedging of more than 5 degrees. Schmorl's nodes are common. The etiology is thought to be stress related through either congenitally or traumatically weakened portions of the cartilaginous end-plates.

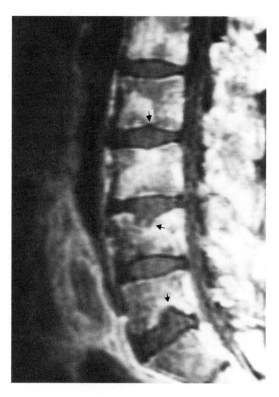

Fig. 16-27 Schmorl's nodes. Sagittal T1WI demonstrates multiple intrabody disk herniations (Schmorl's nodes) *(arrows)* in this patient who incidentally has AML.

Thoracic Disk Herniation

Herniated thoracic disks have a reported incidence of 0.2% to 0.5%. They have an insidious onset with back pain, radicular paresthesias, and myelopathy. MR is the first imaging choice for demonstrating the herniated disk compressing the subarachnoid space and possibly the cord (Fig. 16-28). Occasional problems may arise in specifically diagnosing calcified herniated thoracic disks because of MR's inability to detect calcification. CT myelography is useful for confirmation of the MR findings in this situation. Thoracic disk herniations are associated with straight or curvilinear lines in the posterior vertebral body, which can be visualized on CT or MR and which probably display the path of the end-plate herniation. On CT, disk material is of slightly higher density than the thecal sac containing CSF. Appreciation of this can aid in making stellar calls and winning your '61 Petrus.

Osteophyte Formation

The combination of loss of disk height and disk shrinkage is associated with abnormal motion, particularly in the cervical region. Loss of height (but not of stature) and tissue shrinkage are what we have to look forward to with advancing age. Abnormal stress caused by the

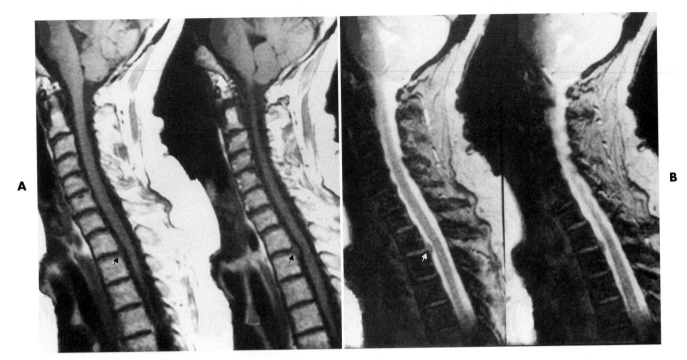

Fig. 16-28 Thoracic disk herniation. **A,** Sagittal T1WI identifies a thoracic disk at T1–2 level *(arrow)*. **B,** T2WI of the disk *(arrow)* is nicely outlined by high intensity CSF.

loss of disk height produces osteophyte formation and posterior displacement of the vertebral body. Because of the abnormal stress, subluxation of the facet joints may occur. Spur formation in the cervical region takes place at the uncovertebral joints. Osteophyte formation at the uncovertebral joints produces compression of the nerve root and clinical signs of cervical radiculopathy. Large osteophytes (sometimes referred to as bars) may also form at the posterior edge of adjacent vertebral bodies, with narrowing of the subarachnoid space and spinal cord compression, producing myelopathy (Fig. 16-29).

A diagnostic dilemma (on MR) is the differentiation between disk and bony osteophyte, the so-called hard disk. It is difficult at times to separate osteophytic compression, ossification of the posterior longitudinal ligament, and a calcified hard disk (Fig. 16-30). All may produce compression of the thecal sac or roots. Calcified disk and osteophyte appear identical, whereas soft disks appear as a different intensity compared with bone on most pulse sequences. Most of the time there is a soft-tissue component to the hard disk. On sagittal T1WI, osteophyte and disk can usually be distinguished. In fact, this may be of little significance if the disease is treated surgically, but CT-myelo can resolve the issue if necessary.

Spondylosis Deformans

The end-plate osteophytes associated with significant degenerative disease in the spine (spondylosis deformans) and uncinate spurs result from traction stress at the osseous site of attachment of the annulus (Sharpey's fibers). Indeed, the end-plate is probably the most vulnerable region of the lumbar vertebral body as it bears the axial load (and we do mean load in the average healthy burger chewing beer guzzling American male). This leads to mechanical fatigue fractures and concave depression of the vertebral end-plate. Characteristically, spondylosis deformans is associated with anterolateral disk protrusion. The nucleus pulposus in this case has normal turgor so that its displacement leads to traction on the Sharpey's fibers of the annulus with the development of osteophytes several millimeters from the diskovertebral junction. These osteophytes extend first in a horizontal and then in a vertical direction. Other findings include preservation of disk height, peripheral vacuum phenomenon, absence of subchondral vertebral eburnation, and a cup-shaped defect in the vertebral rim. Osteophyte formation also occurs at the facet joints; however, this is less significant in the cervical region than in the lumbar region.

With increased degeneration at the articular surfaces, loss of vertebral height is usually manifested by loss of the normal cervical lordosis. This occurs because the posterior joints are already in apposition from degenerative changes and the disk itself has a larger space than the posterior joints. Further loss of disk height results in kyphosis of the cervical spine. In the lumbar region, osteophytic compression occurs primarily in the lateral recess and at the neural foramen. Hypertrophy of the superior articular facets in the lumbar region is most important because it lies anterior to the inferior articu-

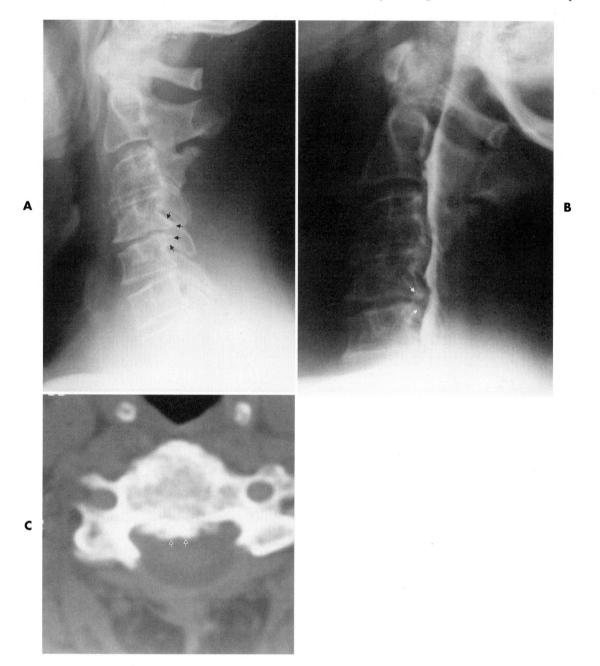

Fig. 16-29   Osteophytic spur. This patient received the full treatment with plain films, CT, myelogram, myelographic CT, and MR. He was studied in the era before cost effective medicine. **A,** Plain lateral film reveals large osteophyte *(arrows)* extending posteriorly. The spinous processes are missing indicating a previous laminectomy. **B,** Myelogram demonstrates compression of the thecal sac by this large osteophyte. **C,** CT of cervical spine in the same patient shows the same large osteophyte *(arrows).*

lar facet and closer to the nerve in the lateral recess and neural foramen (Fig. 16-31).

Recently, some experts have endeavored to refine the definition of spondylosis deformans to only include a degenerative process of the annulus fibrosus, characterized by anterior and lateral marginal osteophytes arising from the vertebral body apophyses with either normal or slightly decreased vertebral height. This is in contrast to the term intervertebral osteochondrosis involving the vertebral body end-plates, the nucleus pulposus, and annulus fibro-

sis. This is associated with disk space narrowing, vacuum phenomenon, and vertebral body reactive changes.

End-plate Changes

In degenerative disease the signal intensity of the end-plate vertebral marrow can be variable on conventional spin echo images with decreased intensity on T1WI and increased intensity on PDWI and T2WI (type I changes), evolving at times to increased intensity on T1WI and

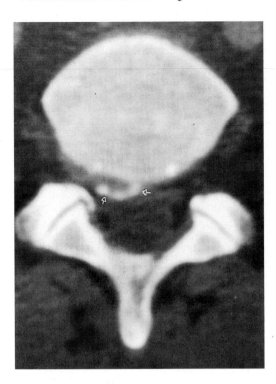

Fig. 16-30 CT of a calcified disk *(arrows)* in the lumbar region. Surgeon may feel a "hard disk" at operation.

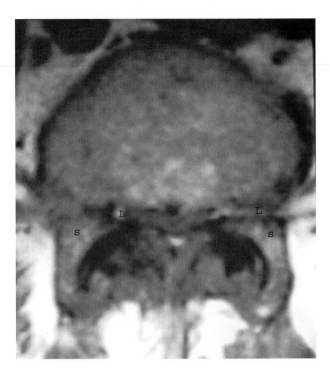

Fig. 16-31 Foraminal stenosis axial T1WI MR. Observe the hypertrophy of the superior articular facets (S) and the compression of the lateral recess (L). (Courtesy of E. Knopp, M.D.) See also Figure 16-38.

isointense to slightly high signal on PDWI and T2WI (type II changes) (Fig. 16-32). These have been associated with histopathologic findings representing fibrous tissue or bone marrow edema associated with acute or subacute inflammatory change (type I) and yellow marrow (type II). Hypointensity on T1WI and T2WI has also been noted and represents bony sclerosis (type III). These should not be mistaken for pathologic disease by unknowing residents (type 0) representing neuroanemia.

Vacuum Phenomenon

Another aspect of degenerative disease (which bears repeating) is the vacuum phenomenon, with gas (nitrogen) in the disk space or facet joints. Gas from the vacuum disk that is in the spinal canal implies disk herniation (see Fig. 16-22B). On CT and MR, air is easily appreciated as linear low density and intensity.

Juxtaarticular Cyst

Juxtaarticular cysts are associated with DJD occurring in a characteristic location, budding from the facet joint and producing a rounded posterolateral extradural mass but they may occur in the posterior paraspinal tissue. The vast majority of these lesions are synovial cysts, although some may actually have a connective tissue capsule (ganglion cyst). They occur in the lumbar region, L4-5 more commonly than L5-S1, although they have

rarely been reported in other regions of the spine. Hemorrhage in these lesions, precipitating acute neurologic symptoms, has been reported. The diagnosis is made by the characteristic location and association with degenerative disease, including disk space narrowing, eburnation, and hypertrophic changes. CT can detect calcification in the cyst wall and gas in the cyst. On MR, the intensity pattern is variable on the basis of the contents of the cyst (Fig. 16-33). These lesions can display enhancement if associated with an inflammatory process. The lesions can present with pain, usually radicular, and neurologic deficits. The major differential diagnosis is extruded posterior disk. There is an association with spondylolisthesis and abnormal movement of the facet joint.

Ossification of the Posterior Longitudinal Ligament

Ossification of the posterior longitudinal ligament (OPLL) is an inflammatory degenerative condition usually associated with degenerative disease of the cervical spine. It was originally described in the Japanese (2% prevalence) but may be seen in any patient population. OPLL affects men and women in the fifth to seventh decades of life. It can produce compression of the spinal cord with myelopathic symptoms. The diagnosis can be tricky on MR because of its insensitivity to calcium. Thin

Text continued on page 780

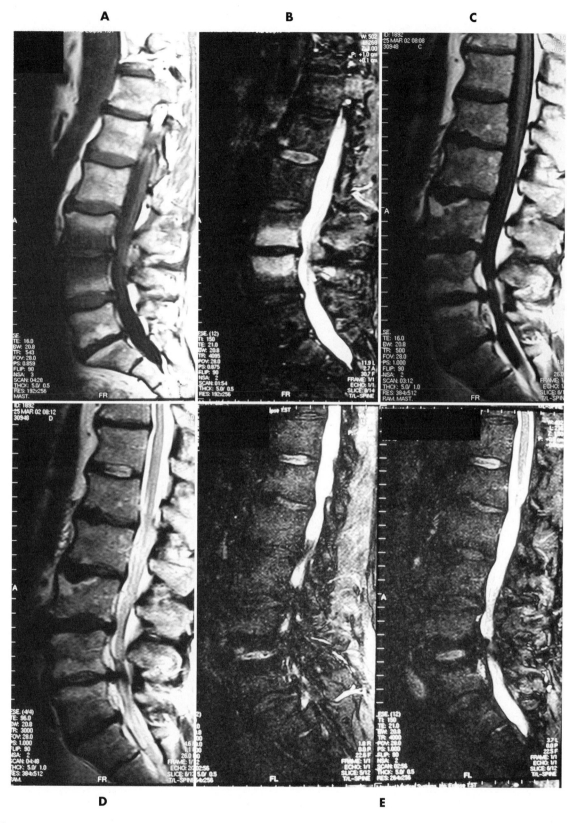

Fig. 16-32   Endplate changes. (Courtesy of D. Panasci, M.D.) **A,** Type 1 change on T1WI. Note the hypointensity in the endplate vertebral marrow. **B,** Type 1 change on T2WI (STIR). There is now high intensity in the end-plate marrow. **C,** Type 2 changes on T1WI. Observe hyperintensity in the end-plates. **D,** Type 2 changes on T2WI. There is slightly increase intensity on this T2WI. **E,** Type 3 change on T2WI. There is marked hypointensity of the L4–L5 endplate on this T2WI. The disk between the endplates is hyperintense.

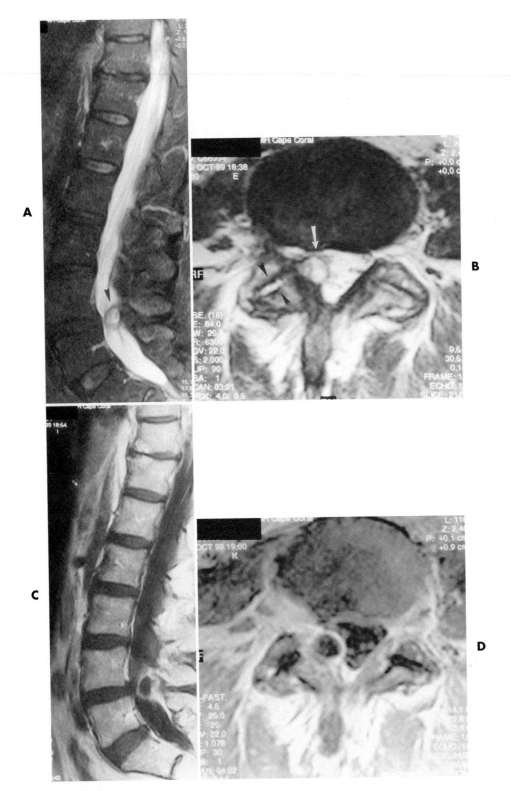

Fig. 16-33   Montage of synovial/juxtaarticular cysts; a great mimicker. **A,** Sagittal T2WI shows a synovial cyst *(arrowhead)* that has a dark intensity rim and hyperintense center. **B,** The origin from the facet joint *(arrowheads)* and the effect on the right-sided nerve roots *(arrow)* is demonstrated on the T2W axial scan. **C** and **D,** After contrast, the wall of the cyst enhances. Note that cyst contents in this case are dark.

Illustration continued on following page

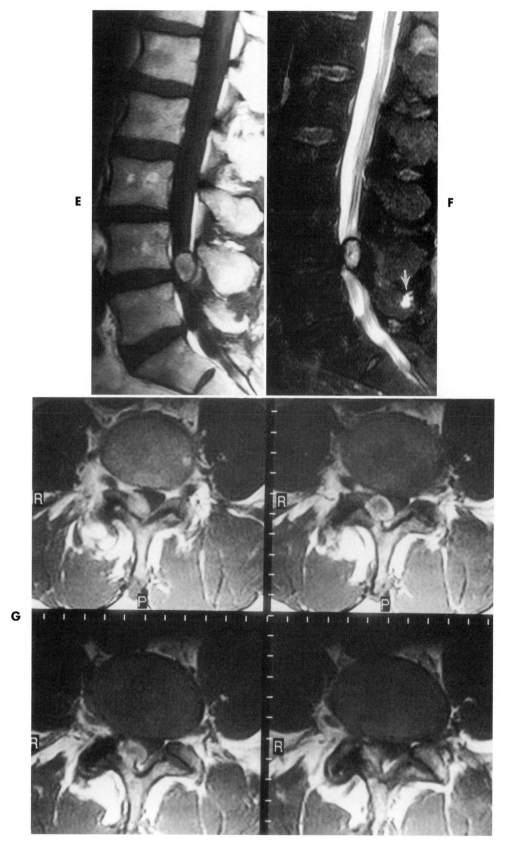

Fig. 16-33 *Continued.* **E,** Contrast the former case with this case where the cyst is high intensity on the sagittal T1WI, likely from inflammatory proteins and/or hemorrhage. **F,** Either hemosiderin or calcification can account for the very low signal intensity of the wall of the cyst on this sagittal T2WI. Note a second juxta-articular cyst projecting posteriorly *(arrow)* at the L5-S1 level. **G,** The corresponding axial T1Wis show compression of the thecal sac. The cyst may elicit radicular symptoms.

Illustration continued on following page

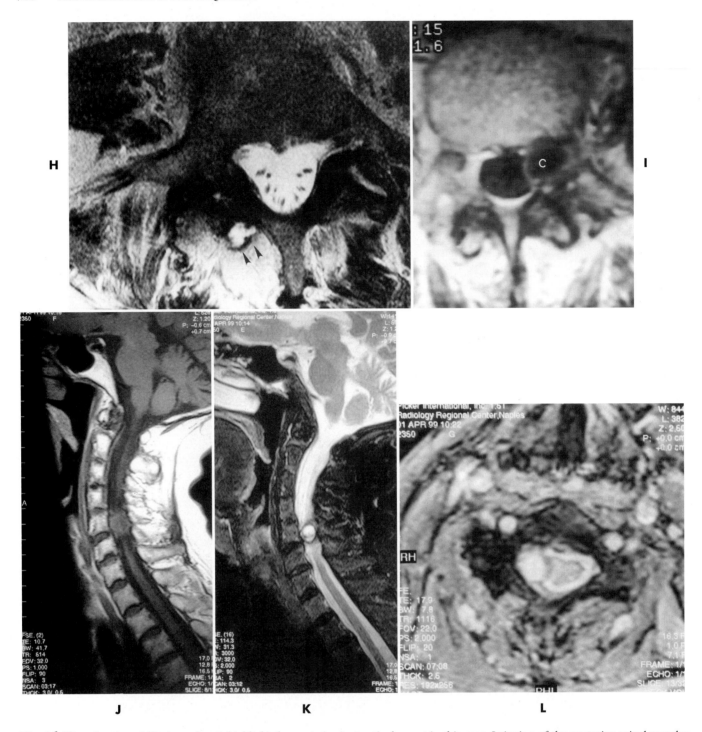

Fig. 16-33 *Continued.* **H,** *Arrowheads* highlight the posterior juxtaarticular cyst in this case. Irritation of the posterior spinal muscles and localized or radiating pain may be produced by the inflammation associated with this cyst. **I,** Is this a herniated disk fragment or a cyst? The "C" gives the diagnosis away. Note that these cysts may present anteriorly and can displace the thecal sac posteriorly like a disk. **J,** This sagittal T1WI of the cervical region appears to show an intrathecal mass. **K,** Au contraire, the "mass" has the typical appearance of a synovial cyst (see figure **F**). **L,** The axial T2WI shows the right-sided synovial cyst. The patient presented with myelopathic symptoms.

ossifications on sagittal MR are difficult to detect, even for a spine hot shot. Detection of this lesion at times is dependent on identification of compression of the cord. On T1WI, CSF and calcium have almost the same intensity. Axial T2WI aid in confirming extraaxial compres-

sion; however, OPLL may be superficially confused with osteophytic compression. The differential diagnosis is important here. OPLL may have fat from marrow in the ossification and is often associated with ligamentum flavum calcification. Remember that OPLL occurs along the full course of the posterior longitudinal ligament whereas osteophytes are present only at the disk space. Calcified herniated disks usually do not occur at multiple levels. A calcified meningioma is usually round, intradural, and unlikely to extend longitudinally, as does OPLL. OPLL makes a strong case for CT and plain films to establish the diagnosis, because less than 50% of cases can be diagnosed by sagittal MR (or so it has been reported) (Fig. 16-34). OPLL occurs in 50% of patients with DISH (see following discussion).

Diffuse Idiopathic Skeletal Hyperostosis

Diffuse idiopathic skeletal hyperostosis (DISH; Forrestier disease) is characterized by ossification along the anterior and to a lesser extent, lateral aspect of the spine (Fig. 16-35). In addition, hyperostosis at the sites of tendon and ligament attachment to bone, ligamentous ossification, and paraarticular osteophytes in both the axial and appendicular skeleton are present. Osseous bridging of at least four contiguous vertebral bodies is one criterion for diagnosis of this condition. The spine has a bumpy contour anteriorly, with the greatest amount of bone being deposited at the level of the intervertebral disks. Hypertrophy and ossification can be identified about the spinous process. Posterior osteophytes are infrequent and small, although ossification of the posterior longitudinal ligament has been observed. DISH differs from spondylosis deformans in that calcification/ossification is present in the anterior longitudinal ligament with an associated prolifera-

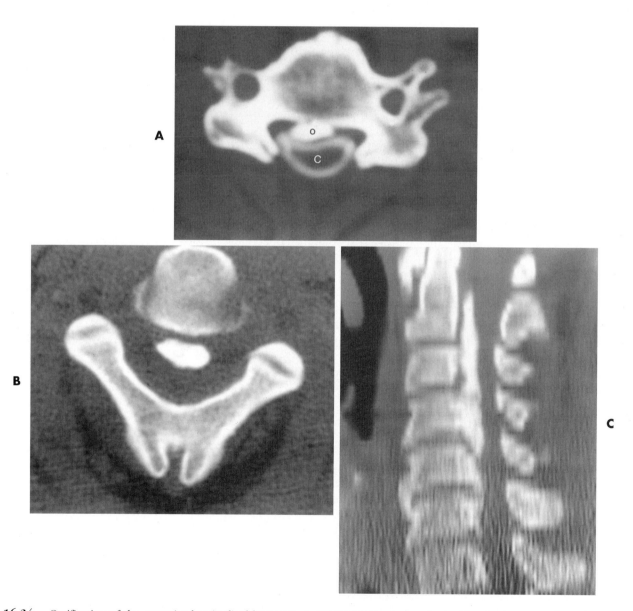

Fig. 16-34   Ossification of the posterior longitudinal ligament. **A,** CT myelogram in a patient with a laminectomy shows contrast outlining the cord *(C),* which is still compressed by the OPLL *(o),* despite surgery. Note that the lesion is not at the disk space. **B** and **C** are CT scans demonstrating the ossification in the posterior longitudinal ligament.

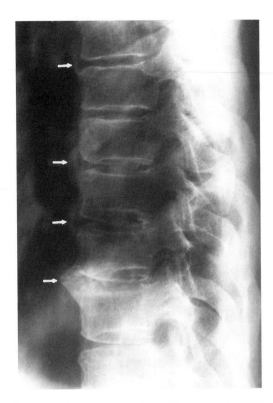

Fig. 16-35 Diffuse idiopathic skeletal hyperostosis (DISH). Note the appearance of osseous bridging *(arrows)* at multiple disk levels throughout the thoracic spine. This is characteristic of DISH.

tive enthesopathy at the site of attachment of the anterior longitudinal ligament to the anterior vertebral body surface. The disk space is preserved (height and intensity) in DISH. The facet joints are not involved. The differential diagnosis of DISH includes ankylosing spondylitis, which is not as florid as DISH and is associated with sacroiliitis (usually the first manifestation of the disease). You can observe erosion of the superior and inferior vertebral margins, producing squaring and bridging of the vertebral bodies (bamboo spine) in ankylosing spondylitis. The facet joints are involved in ankylosing spondylitis and not DISH, and the former is also associated with HLA-B27 and osteoporosis.

Spondylolysis and Spondylolisthesis

In the lumbar region, the articular processes have an oblique orientation. The plane of the joint between the superior and inferior articular facets is from medial to lateral, from the anterior to posterior aspect of the joint. The term *spondylolisthesis* is defined as slippage of one vertebra onto another whereas *spondylolysis* is a fracture through the pars interarticularis, which may or may not be associated with vertebral slippage (see Fig. 16-20). Pars defects can be easily seen on plain spine films, and CT. Spondylolysis is the commonest pathology to affect the pars with a prevalence of 3% to 10%. SPECT imaging is useful for detection of symptomatic pars defects. T1WI can detect a

break in the cortical margin of the pars. Another MR observation is a break in the marrow signal between the superior and inferior articular facets. Spondylolysis may be best detected on sagittal MR with 3mm slices particularly on T1WI. Unfortunately, in a significant portion of cases (about 25%) the pars may not be adequately visualized. Spondylolysis without spondylolisthesis is a cause of chronic low back pain particularly in children and young adults. In fact, in this cohort of patients, if there is any question, plain films are strongly recommended to unequivocally answer the question of a pars defect.

There are many different causes of spondylolisthesis, and a classification based on the anatomy of the articular processes and the pars interarticularis is useful. You can divide lesions producing vertebral slippage into (1) congenital spondylolisthesis, which is associated with dysplastic articular processes, abnormal orientation of articular processes, or conditions such as kyphosis, all of which may produce slippage of vertebrae (widens the spinal canal at the level of the spondylolisthesis), and (2) acquired spondylolisthesis including (a) pars interarticularis lesions produced by stress fractures with persistent defects of the pars or healing of the fracture resulting in elongation of the isthmus, (b) the effects of degenerative facet disease associated with joint instability, most often occurring at L4–5, with a higher incidence in diabetics and associated with compression of the cauda equina against S1 (narrows spinal canal), (c) postsurgical lesions, which may be seen in the cervical or lumbar regions, resulting from altered stress on the joints after cervical fusions or surgery for spinal stenosis, (d) acute trauma with pedicle fractures (widens the spinal canal), and (e) pathologic conditions such as osteoporosis, metastasis, infection, osteopetrosis, or arthrogryposis. Spina bifida of L5 and particularly of S1 is associated with congenital and isthmic spondylolisthesis.

In evaluating spondylolisthesis on MR the sagittal image is probably the most useful in identifying compression of a particular root. Significant findings in this condition include altered shape of the neural foramen with the long axis from vertical to horizontal configuration, loss of the foraminal fat, nerve root compression from reactive changes in the posterior longitudinal ligament, fibrocartilaginous tissue at and surrounding the site of the pars defect, and sharp angulation of the nerve root (pediculate kinking) caused by slippage. Disk herniation at the level of spondylolisthesis is unusual, but disk herniation at the level above the spondylolisthesis is more common. Axial images tend to exaggerate the disk in a region of spondylolisthesis because the posterior margin of the slipped vertebral body appears far anterior to the posterior margin of the disk (pseudoherniation). A grading system is used on the basis of the position of the posterior margin of the subluxed vertebral body compared with the posterior margin of the inferior vertebral body.

When the superior body is subluxed up to one fourth of a vertebral body width on the lateral film it is termed grade 1 spondylolisthesis; half a vertebral body, grade 2; three fourths, grade 3; and a whole width is grade 4. Spondyloptosis refers to a vertebral body plopping over the lower vertebral body (ptosis—grade 5).

Congenital posterior element variations Congenital anomalies of the posterior elements occur and can, at times, confuse even the Professor. Facets can be catawampus ($20 word) at the same level. In this situation, the facets are sagittally (or axially) oriented. This is a particular issue when the facet on one side is medial at its posterior tip than its anterior tip and is termed facet tropism. When present one side slips more than the other and there is vertebral rotation. The subluxation is more severe on the side of the more sagittally oriented facet. Facet tropism may be mild and asymptomatic but can produce symptoms. A facet may also be congenitally absent or hypoplastic. This results in hyperplasia of the contralateral facet with accelerated degenerative changes and stress fractures in the facet.

Ankylosing spondylitis (AS)

AS is a common rheumatologic disorder with an incidence of 1.4% with young men affected more than women (at least 4:1) with HLAB27 positive in 97% of cases. The sacroiliac joints and lumbar spine are the most commonly affected locations but with time, the entire spine can become involved. Plasma cells and lymphocytes infiltrate the soft tissues of the subligamentous bone and diskovertebral junction in this disease. Vascularization and ossification in the ligamentous attachments (enthesopathy) affecting Sharpey's fibers result in classic syndesmophyte formation (bamboo spine). Erosion at the vertebral endplates in combination with ligamentous insertion ossification is the cause of squaring of the anterior vertebral concavity. The anterosuperior and anteroinferior aspects of the vertebral bodies ("shiny corner" on plain films) and sacroiliac joints are subject to reactive changes with bony sclerosis. On MR, there is low intensity in the vertebral body on T1WI and high intensity on T2WI with enhancement. Calcification in the disk in a variety of patterns commonly occurs by a process of enchondral ossification, and can appear as areas of decreased or increased intensity on T1WI (Fig. 16-36). There are a number of conditions associated with AS enumerated in Box 16-2.

Spinal fractures (either traumatic or pseudoarthrosis), progressive spinal deformity, subluxation (atlanto-occipital/atlantoaxial) and rotatory instability, and spinal stenosis are common. Spinal pseudoarthrosis with associated instability is the most significant biomechanical

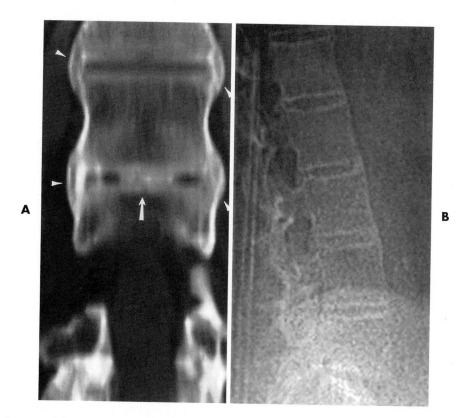

Fig. 16-36   Ankylosing spondylitis. **A,** Coronal reconstruction of axial CT data reveals findings characteristic of ankylosing spondylitis including syndesmophytes *(arrowheads)* and calcification of the disk *(arrow).* **B,** The scout view (a poor man's plain film) showed the "squaring off" of the vertebral bodies and the bridging syndesmophytes anteriorly.

complication of this disease. It is the result of mobile nonunion usually after occult stress fracture. There is reactive sclerosis in the vertebral bodies adjacent to a widened area of destruction across the fractured ankylosed disk. Dural ectasia can also be noted in AS (see Fig. 16-41).

Spinal Stenosis

Many conditions result in compression of lumbar nerve roots and produce symptoms including radicular or nonradicular pain, claudication-like symptoms (which can be misdiagnosed as vascular disease), numbness, and tingling. The syndrome is usually divided anatomically into central stenosis and lateral stenosis, and both may coexist in a single patient. There are many reports on normal measurements and on problems with such measurements. The authors are not obsessive-compulsive measurers. Rather, we believe that a good template in the occipital gray matter to what is normal is the best approach. Nevertheless, some measurements are provided as a guide. The lumbar canal increases in midsagittal diameter, proceeding from superior to inferior; however, the minimal bony sagittal diameter of the lumbar central canal is approximately 11.51242 mm (we are not compulsive). The smallest sagittal measurement occurs between the posterior boundary of the vertebral body and the anterosuperior margin of the spinous process. Interpediculate measurements of less than 16 mm at L4-5 or less than 20 mm at L5–S1 and canal cross-sectional areas of less than 1.45 cm² are considered abnormal. The *interpediculate* distance increases from T12 to L5. Minimal interpediculate distances occur at the midpedicle. For the radiologic etymologic entomologist, the *interpedicular* distance is the distance between two lice.

It should be pointed out that the bony sagittal diameter may not be a sensitive indicator of stenosis because it does not take into account soft tissues such as ligamentum flavum, disk, fat, and facet osteophytes. The normal ligamentum flavum is 2 to 4 mm thick. It is considered to be hypertrophied if it is greater than 5 mm thick. Ossification of the cephalic attachment of the ligamentum flavum is occasionally noted and may be a normal anatomic variant. It has also been described in calcium pyrophosphate dihydrate deposition disease, where it has been associated with spinal stenosis. Images of central stenosis are usually vivid, revealing degenerated disks, hypertrophied ligamentum flavum, loss of epidural fat at the pedicle and lamina level, and facet hypertrophy (Fig. 16-37). Posterior epidural fat can compress the thecal sac when there is narrowing by ligamentum flavum, lamina, and/or facets. In the lower lumbar region the stenotic canal takes on a T shape or what has been termed a trefoil shape, which results from a combination of a narrow canal and facet hypertrophy. This condition is usually the result of degenerative processes superimposed on a bony canal that is borderline normal or slightly small, and is seen in adults in their fifth to sixth decades of life. Short pedicles predispose to spinal stenosis.

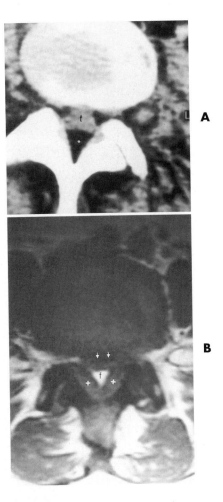

Fig. 16-37   Spinal stenosis. **A,** Axial CT with compression of the thecal sac *(t)* by extradural fat *(asterisk).* **B,** Spinal stenosis secondary to hypertrophy of the ligamentum flavum. Axial T1WI demonstrates massively enlarged ligamentum flavum *(+).* One can also appreciate the posterior epidural fat *(f)* and the posterior margin of the disk *(arrows)* both compressing the thecal sac.

The width of the lateral recess in the lumbar region is measured from the posterior aspect of the vertebral body to the most anterior aspect of the superior articular facet. Width of 2 mm or less is considered stenotic. The nerve root buds out of the thecal sac to course in the lateral recess, then under the pedicle and out the neural foramen. Hypertrophy of the superior articular facet is the most common cause of narrowing of the lateral recess, although abnormalities of any components of the lateral recess may also compress the nerve.

Stenosis of the lumbar neural foramen can also occur. Normally the neural foramen is oval, with constriction in its inferior portion, and is bordered anteriorly by the vertebral body and disk, superiorly and inferiorly by the pedicles, and posteriorly by the pars interarticularis. Sagittal MR is the best modality to view the foramen (Fig. 16-38). The nerve and blood vessels usually lie in the superior portion of the foramen, which is normally filled with fat. The nerve may be compressed here by osteophyte or disk, or from spondylolisthesis. You should carefully evaluate the sagittal relationship between the nerve and components of the foramen to detect subtle forms of compression that may not be apparent on axial images. MR tends to overestimate the degree of spinal stenosis compared with myelography and myelo-CT.

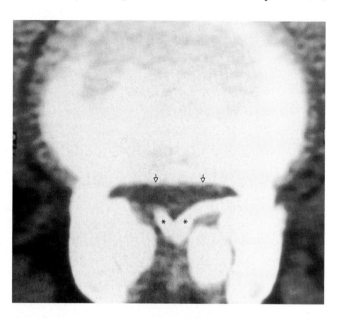

Fig. 16-39   Spinal stenosis. On this axial CT, the spinal canal is dramatically narrowed. Note the position of the lamina and the posterior margin of the vertebral body. Between the lamina *(asterisks)* and the posterior margin of the vertebral body *(arrows)* is a disk that is bulging and its lateral margins can be identified. We cannot find the exact location of the thecal sac in this stenotic canal to label it.

This is probably related to susceptibility effects, CSF motion, and truncation artifact.

Spinal stenosis can occur in children and adolescents with achondroplasia, mucopolysaccharidoses, congenital lipomas, and with acquired precipitating lesions such as an acute disk herniation in combination with preexisting idiopathic spinal stenosis (Fig. 16-39).

A lumbar laminectomy results in partial or complete removal of the lamina, the spinous process, the ligamentum flavum, and some of the contents of the patient's wallet. The extent of the procedure is determined by the disease and the surgical approach. On CT, loss of the lamina and absence of the ligamentum flavum indicate previous lumbar surgery. Postoperatively, on MR intermediate or high intensity on T2WI is observed in the region of the surgery. Mass effect (from the normal postoperative swelling, hemorrhage, and scar formation) can simulate preoperative disk herniation in size and signal intensity. This gradually resolves during a period of up to 6 months. Surgical disruption of the annulus appears as a line of high intensity on T2WI. Scar tissue can be seen in both asymptomatic and symptomatic patients. Enhancement in the postoperative patient is dynamic. There is normally enhancement of the facet joint, paraspinal muscles, previously compressed nerve roots (which may enhance proximally up to the conus), the postdiskectomy disk space, and vertebral end-plates. This enhancement is common and can persist for months or even longer. Siz-

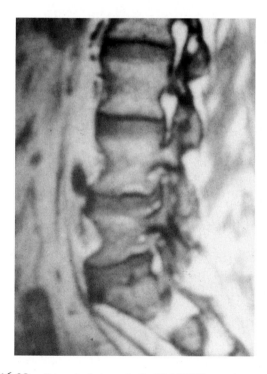

Fig. 16-38   Foraminal stenosis. Sagittal T1WI reveals narrowing of the L4-5 neural foramen. There is loss of the normal fat as well as decreased total neural foramen area. Similar changes, but to a lesser degree, are observed at L5-S1. Compare these changes to normal neural foramina at L3-4 or L2-3. The sagittal view, in the lumbar spine, is an excellent plane to image these changes.

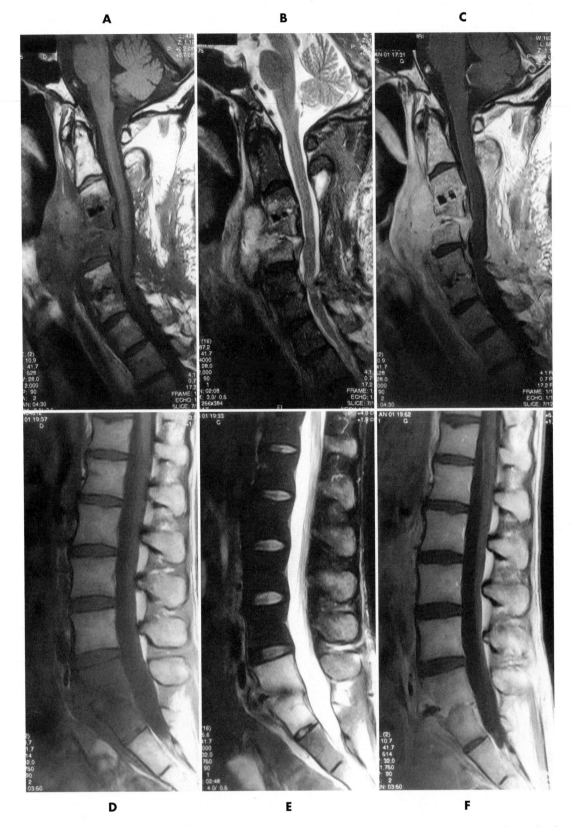

Fig. 16-40 Postoperative diskitis. **A,** Sagittal T1WI shows loss of disk space, hypointensity of the marrow, collapse, kyphosis, epidural compression, and a small (by Shaq's standards) anterior epidural mass. **B,** High signal in the disk and the adjacent marrow as well as the epidural and prevertebral mass is evident on this sagittal T2WI. **C,** After contrast, one completes the picture with enhancing disk material, endplates, epidural phlegmon, and prevertebral abscess. **D, E,** and **F,** Remarkable: The findings on the sagittal T1WI **(D),** T2WI **(E),** and enhanced T1WI **(F)** of the lumbar spine are identical to those of the cervical spine case in this patient with postoperative lumbar spine diskitis. Same disease, different location.

able scarring may be identified in more than 40% of patients postoperatively, and these persons may be asymptomatic.

Postoperative Diskitis

The classic MR findings of postoperative diskitis are decreased signal intensity within the disk and adjacent vertebral body marrow on T1WI; increased signal on T2WI in the disk and adjacent marrow, often with obliteration of the intranuclear cleft; and enhancement of the disk and end-plate (Fig. 16-40). A homogeneous pattern of enhancement can be identified as a horizontal band on either side of the disk space. Asymptomatic patients after diskectomy may have some of these findings. They do not even have to be uniformly present in patients with confirmed infections.

The bottom line is that the MR in the postoperative patient can be erroneously suggestive of residual diskitis, particularly within the first 6 months, even in patients who are asymptomatic. A little knowledge can be dangerous in this case; however, thorough appreciation of the normal postoperative MR findings can soothe your favorite neurosurgeon's or orthopedic surgeon's gastric mucosa (unless of course he or she operated on the wrong level, or you missed the incidental conus tumor).

Enhancement is not very specific in the postoperative patient to rule in or to rule out diskitis.

Dural ectasia   The phenomenon of dural ectasia is defined as enlargement of the dural sac and root sleeves anywhere along the spinal column but most often occurring in the lumbar and sacral regions. This results in scalloping of the posterior vertebral bodies, spinal canal dilatation with widening of the interpediculate distance and neural foramina, and thinning of the cortex of the pedicles and laminae. Anterior and posterior meningocele can also be seen in dural ectasia (Fig. 16-41). It is common in Marfan syndrome. It is also reported in neurofibromatosis, Ehlers-Danlos syndrome, and ankylosing spondylitis.

Myelopathy from degenerative disease   Cervical spondylosis compresses the spinal cord as well as its arterial and venous blood supply. Cervical myelopathy associated with high intensity on T2WI, extending over several vertebral body segments, has been reported in cases of cervical spondylosis in conjunction with instability on flexion extension films. Following successful stabilization and decompression, the high intensity can resolve suggesting an edematous etiology for the abnormality. Orthopedic conditions thought to have a correlation with spinal cord high signal intensity on T2WI include cervical disk herniation, ossification of the pos-

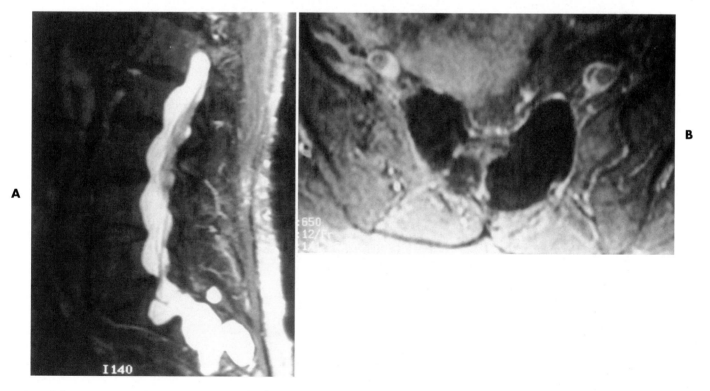

Fig. 16-41   Dural ectasia. **A,** Posterior scalloping and large sacral root cysts are present on the sagittal T2WI of this patient with Marfanoid patient with neurofibromatosis and ankylosing spondylitis. **B,** Post contrast T1WI shows the gross impression and remodeling of the sacrum.

terior longitudinal ligament, cervical spondylosis, atlantoaxial instability, vertebral body tumor, and ossification of the ligamentum flavum.

POSTOPERATIVE SPINE

Failed Back Surgery Syndrome (FBSS) (the Surgeon's Worst Nightmare)

A large problem confronting the clinician (and secondarily the radiologist) is recurrent or residual low back pain in the patient after lumbar disk surgery. This condition has a reported incidence of 5% to 40%, and the syndrome has been termed the "failed back" or the "failed back surgery" syndrome. The common causes of this condition are listed in Box 16-3.

Immediately following successful low back surgery imaging reveals mass effect on the anterior spinal canal usually greater than what was there preoperatively. This diminishes after the first week and its size does not correlate with outcome. There can also be posterior compression of the dural tube secondary to placement of an absorbable knitted fabric for hemostasis (Surgicel [Johnson & Johnson Medical, Arlington, TX, USA]), which ap-

---

Box 16-3   Causes of Failed Back Syndrome

Arachnoiditis
Central stenosis, foraminal stenosis
Conus tumor
Epidural fibrosis
Immediate postoperative complications including infection, hematoma, or surgical trauma to roots
Insufficient decompression of roots by residual soft tissue or bone
Mechanical instability
Pseudoarthrosis
Residual or recurrent disk
Spondylolisthesis
Surgery at wrong level

---

pears like a folded sponge surrounded by fluid. The MR appearance should not concern you unless the patient has significant referable clinical signs and symptoms.

All patients have varying degrees of scar tissue at 4 months. However, scar tissue cannot necessarily be implicated as an etiology of postoperative back pain be-

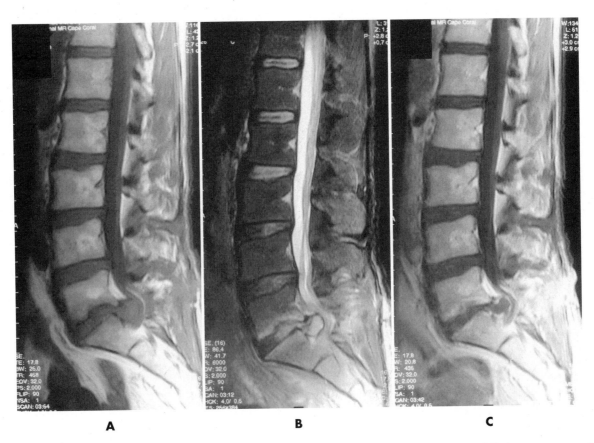

A   **B**   **C**

Fig. 16-42   Postoperative failed back. Sagittal T1WI (**A**), sagittal T2WI (**B**), and enhanced sagittal T1WI (**C**) show a recurrent herniated disk at L5–S1 and the spinous process defect from the laminectomy. Note that the disk does not enhance in **C**, but there is minimal peripheral granulation tissue.

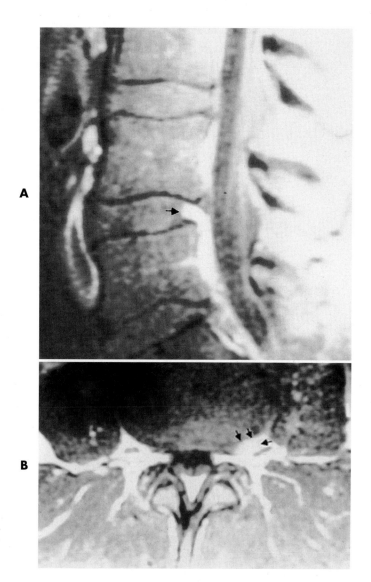

should be performed with fat saturation, because fat and enhancement are both hyperintense on T1WI without fat suppression. Conspicuity between scar (which enhances) and fat would thus be normally lacking. High dose contrast (0.3 mmol/kg) has been demonstrated experimentally to increase conspicuity of disk recurrent disk fragments although in walkie-talkie patients the added enhancement of scar did not provide additional diagnostic benefit and may indeed obscure recurrent disk.

There may be immediate enhancement around a herniated disk (Fig. 16-43), and fragmented disks can produce enhancement similar to scar. If scanning is delayed more than 20 minutes, disk may appear to enhance with an appearance not unlike scar. Enhancement also enables detection of the nerve root (unenhanced) surrounded by enhancing scar (Fig. 16-44).

Nerve roots have been noted to enhance up to 8 months postoperatively. These roots were nearly always

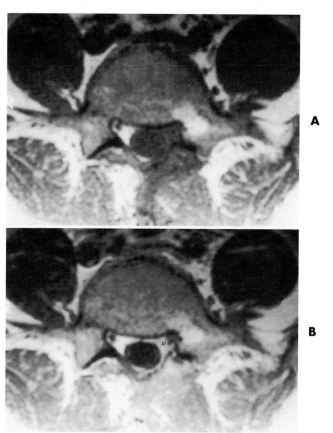

Fig. 16-43   Enhancement around an acute disk herniation. **A,** Sagittal T1WI shows enhancement *(arrow)* in an acutely herniated disk. **B,** Axial T1WI demonstrating the enhancing left lateral disk *(arrows)*.

cause everyone gets it and only some have chronic pain. In the failed back, it is critical to look carefully for other causes of pain including infection, residual or recurrent disk, or instability.

The diagnosis of scar versus disk is extremely important in this situation. Surgery is not indicated for scar (epidural fibrosis) but would be beneficial if disk can be diagnosed as the cause of the radiculopathy. Both may produce mass effect, although epidural fibrosis may cause traction of the dural tube. Nerve root displacement by a mass lesion is almost always associated with a recurrent herniated disk. Contrast is necessary in this situation. After injection, immediate scanning of scar demonstrates diffuse enhancement on T1WI whereas disk usually does not enhance (Fig. 16-42). Enhancement

Fig. 16-44   Scar around nerve root. **A,** On this axial unenhanced T1WI you can appreciate a mass in the left lateral recess obliterating the normal epidural fat. There is also evidence of a left-sided laminectomy. The nerve root is poorly visualized within this tissue. The question is, is the disk obliterating the lateral recess or is the nerve root wrapped in scar? **B,** Following contrast you can appreciate that the nerve root *(open arrow)* is completely surrounded by enhancing scar tissue. Enhancement is noted in the posterior scar as well.

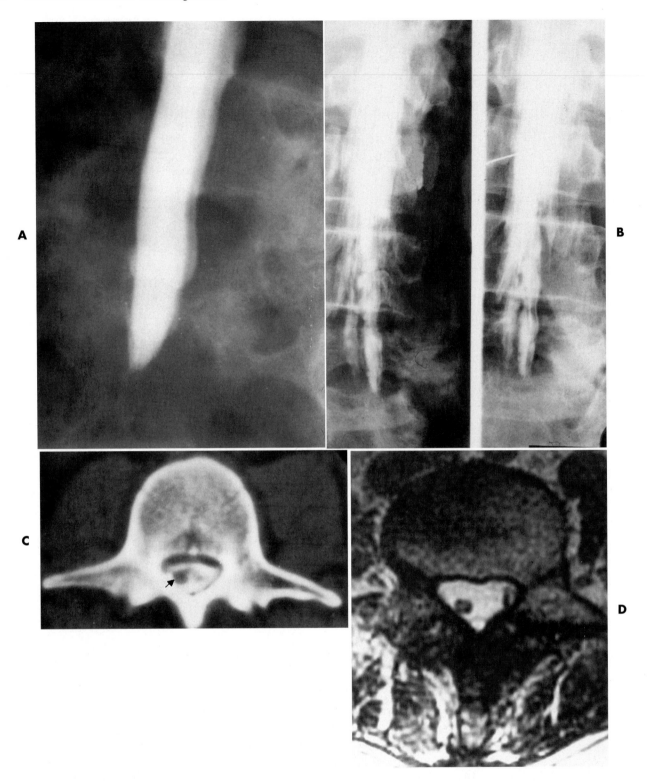

Fig. 16-45 Arachnoiditis. **A,** Myelogram of arachnoiditis. Note absence of root sleeves and the inability to define individual roots. **B,** Another example of arachnoiditis. Filling of the thecal sac is irregular, and the lumbar nerve roots appear thickened. **C,** Severe arachnoiditis. Postmyelogram CT in another patient demonstrates clumping of nerve roots *(arrow)* in this patient with severe arachnoiditis. **D,** T2WI shows a curious clump of adhered nerve roots within the right side of the thecal sac.

those compressed preoperatively suggesting ongoing repair and regeneration associated with an impaired blood-nerve barrier. Enhancement extends cephalad toward the conus. Relating the symptoms to root enhancement is controversial (both in the literature and in the court). In addition, this phenomenon occurs in 5% of symptomatic patients without surgery. An alternative explanation regarding lumbar root enhancement is that it results from obstruction of small radicular veins within the endoneurium of the nerve root related to nerve root compression. It may be the radicular veins (intravascular enhancement) and NOT roots that enhance. It may occur either physiologically or pathologically and may not be specific. Sorry for all the equivocation.

Arachnoiditis

Arachnoiditis, once a very common condition after contrast myelography, is an inflammatory disorder of the spinal leptomeninges particularly affecting the nerve roots resulting in intradural adhesions. It was particularly associated with the combination of hemorrhage from myelography/surgery and retained iophendylate (Pantopaque) (about 20% of cases). Nonionic contrast agents have markedly decreased the incidence of arachnoiditis after myelography, but it still occurs. Causes of arachnoiditis include infection (i.e., tuberculous or pyogenic meningitis), subarachnoid hemorrhage from any source (i.e., surgery [alone around 4%], trauma, arteriovenous malformation, or aneurysm), and inflammatory diseases. Remember that on good fast spin echo images in the lumbar spine you should be able to distinguish the anterior and posterior spinal roots until they leave thecal sac. In the lumbar region, arachnoiditis has a variable appearance, with loss of the ability to distinguish the roots in the thecal sac and obliteration of the root sleeves (mild) best visualized on axial images. With increasing severity there is loss of the morphology of the thecal sac, adhesion of the nerve roots to the dural tube ("empty sac") or clumping together of the nerve roots, leading to an appearance of a "pseudofilum" (Fig. 16-45). Arachnoiditis may or may not enhance (not very helpful), and the diagnosis is best made on the basis of the morphology of the roots and sac. Arachnoiditis has been cited as a cause in up to 16% of cases of failed back syndrome. It can be responsible for the development of arachnoid cysts particularly in the thoracic region.

Tuberculous arachnoiditis is somewhat different from other forms and involves the spinal cord, meninges, and nerve roots. On MR, there is loss of distinct margins of the cord and enhancement of the leptomeninges. Enhancing nodules have also been reported. The combination of leptomeningeal thickening, nodules of the spinal cord and roots, and spinal cord involvement should suggest tuberculous arachnoiditis (although other

Box 16-4   Diffuse Root Thickening
Arachnoiditis
Carcinomatous meningitis
Chronic inflammatory demyelinating polyradiculoneuropathy
CMV radiculitis
Guillain Barré
Hypertrophic interstitial polyneuritis (Dejerine-Sottas syndrome)
Lymphoma
Neurofibroma
Sarcoid
Spinal arteriovenous malformation

diseases such as sarcoid and metastatic disease could produce a similar picture). The differential diagnosis of nodular or diffuse root thickening is given in Box 16-4.

Occasionally, the dura can be torn at the time of surgery (by the Greek surgeon Euripides), with leakage of CSF from the wound (postoperatively) or with the formation of an organized CSF collection (pseudomeningocele), which can subsequently enlarge. This collection may need to be repaired. The differential diagnosis, particularly in the early postoperative period in the patient with pain and fever, is abscess, which might demonstrate significant peripheral enhancement.

We do not know anyone who won a Nobel Prize for making a major contribution to degenerative spine diseases. However, in practice this problem will occupy more of your time than you can imagine. Here the intellectual challenges are inversely proportional to wampum potential. Unfortunately, if you have ever had back pain, you would wish more Nobel Prize winners would lend their efforts to study the back rather than *Drosophila*.

SUGGESTED READINGS

Awwad EE, Martin DS, Smith KR, et al: MR imaging of lumbar juxtaarticular cysts, *J Comput Assist Tomogr* 14:415-417, 1990.

Awwad EE and Smith KR, Jr: MRI of marked dural sac compression by surgicel in the immediately postoperative period after uncomplicated lumbar laminectomy, *J Comput Assist Tomog* 23(6):969-975, 1999.

Bahk YW, Lee JM: Measure-set computed tomographic analysis of internal architectures of lumbar disk: clinical and histologic studies, *Invest Radiol* 23:17-23, 1988.

Beers GJ, Carter AP, McNary WF: Vertical foramina in the lumbosacral region: CT appearance, *AJNR* 5:617-619, 1984.

Berns DH, Ross JS, Kormos D, et al: The spinal vacuum phenomenon: evaluation by gradient echo MR imaging, *J Comput Assist Tomogr* 15:233-236, 1991.

Brown TR, Quinn SF, D'Agostino AN: Deposition of calcium pyrophosphate dihydrate crystals in the ligamentum flavum: evaluation with MR imaging and CT, *Radiology* 178:871-873, 1991.

Dorwart RH, Vogler JB III, Helms CA: Spinal stenosis, *Radiol Clin North Am* 21:301-321, 1983. 587-592, 1984.

Fitt GJ and Stevens JM: Postoperative arachnoiditis diagnosed by high resolution fast spin-echo MRI of the lumbar spine, *Neuroradiology* 37(2):139-145, 1995.

Flannigan BD, Lufkin RB, McGlade C, et al: MR imaging of the cervical spine: neurovascular anatomy, *AJNR* 8:27-32, 1987.

Fletcher G, Haughton VM, Ho K, et al: Age-related changes in the cervical facet joints: studies with cryomicrotomy, MR, and CT, *AJNR* 11:27-30, 1990.

Fox MW, Onofrio BM, Kilgore JE, et al: Neurological complications of ankylosing spondylitis, *J Neurosurg* 78(6):871-878, 1993.

Frymoyer JW: Back pain and sciatica, *N Engl J Med* 318:291-300, 1988.

Gallucci M, Bozzao A, et al: Does postcontrast MR enhancement in lumbar disk herniation have prognostic value? *J Comput Assist Tomogr* 19(1):34-38, 1995.

Gorey MT, Hyman RA, Black KS, et al: Lumbar synovial cysts eroding bone, *AJNR* 13:161-163, 1992.

Grenier N, Greselle J, Douws C, et al: MR imaging of foraminal and extraforaminal lumbar disk herniations, *J Comput Assist Tomogr* 14:243-249, 1990.

Grenier N, Grossman RI, Schiebler ML, et al: Degenerative lumbar disk disease: pitfalls and usefulness of MR imaging in detection of vacuum phenomenon, *Radiology* 164:861-865, 1987.

Grenier N, Kressel HY, Schiebler ML, et al: Normal and degenerative posterior spinal structures: MR imaging, *Radiology* 165:517-525, 1987.

Hajek PC, Baker LL, Goobar JE, et al: Focal fat deposition in axial bone marrow: MR characteristics, *Radiology* 162:245-249, 1987.

Hasso AN, McKinney JM, Killeen J, et al: Computed tomography of children an adolescents with suspected spinal stenosis, *J Comput Assist Tomogr* 11:609-611, 1987.

Haughton VM: MR imaging of the spine, *Radiology* 166:297-301, 1988.

Hoddick WK, Helms CA: Bony spinal canal changes that differentiate conjoined nerve roots from herniated nucleus pulposus, *Radiology* 154:119-120, 1985.

Hwang GJ, Suh JS, Na JB, et al: Contrast enhancement pattern and frequency of previously unoperated lumbar discs on MRI, *J Magnetic Res Imaging* 7(3):575-578, 1997.

Jackson DE, Atlas SW, Mani JR, et al: Intraspinal synovial cysts: MR imaging, *Radiology* 170:527-530, 1989.

Jinkins JR, Osborn AG, et al: Spinal nerve enhancement with Gd-DTPA: MR correlation with the postoperative lumbosacral spine, *AJNR* 14(2):383-394, 1993.

Kader DF, Wardlaw D, Smith FW, et al: Correlation between the MRI changes in the lumbar multifidus muscles and leg pain, *Clin Radiol* 55(2):145-149, 2000.

Ketonen L, Gyldensted C: Lumbar disk disease evaluated by myelography and postmyelography spinal computed tomography, *Neuroradiology* 28:144-149, 1986.

Kostelic JK, Haughton VM, Sether LA: Lumbar spinal nerves in the neural foramen: MR appearance, *Radiology* 178:837-839, 1991.

Lane JI, Koeller KK, Atkinson JL, et al: Enhanced lumbar nerve roots in the spine without prior surgery: radiculitis or radicular veins? *AJNR* 15(7):1317-1325, 1994.

Lee T, Chacha PB, Khoo J, et al: Ossification of posterior longitudinal ligament of the cervical spine in non-Japanese Asians, *Surg Neurol* 35:40-44, 1991.

Masaryk TJ, Ross JS, Modic MT, et al: High-resolution MR imaging of sequestered lumbar intervertebral disks, *AJNR* 9:351-358, 1988.

Modic MT, Herfkens RJ: Intervertebral disk: normal age-related changes in MR signal intensity, *Radiology* 177:332-334, 1990.

Modic MT, Masaryk T, Boumphrey F, et al: Lumbar herniated disk disease and canal stenosis: prospective evaluation by surface coil MR, CT, and myelography, *AJNR* 7:709-717, 1986.

Modic MT, Masaryk TJ, Ross JS, et al: Cervical radiculopathy: value of oblique MR imaging, *Radiology* 163:227-231, 1987.

Modic MT, Masaryk TJ, Ross JS, et al: Imaging of degenerative disk disease, *Radiology* 168:177-186, 1988.

Modic MT, Steinberg PM, Ross JS, et al: Degenerative disk disease: assessment of changes in vertebral body marrow with MR imaging, *Radiology* 166:193-199, 1988.

Modic MT, Ross JS, et al: Contrast-enhanced MR imaging in acute lumbar radiculopathy: a pilot study of the natural history [see comments], *Radiology* 195(2):429-435, 1995.

Morgan S and Saifuddin A: MRI of the lumbar intervertebral disc, *Clin Radiol* 54(11):703-723, 1999.

Murayama S, Numaguchi Y, Robinson AE: The diagnosis of herniated intervertebral disks with MR imaging: a comparison of gradient-refocused-echo and spin-echo pulse sequences, *AJNR* 11:17-22, 1990.

Nguyen C, An H, Ho KC, et al: Utility of high-dose contrast enhancement for detecting recurrent herniated intervertebral disks, *AJNR* 15(7):1291-1297, 1994.

Nowicki BH, Yu S, Reinartz J, et al: Effect of axial loading on neural foramina and nerve roots in the lumbar spine, *Radiology* 176:433-437, 1990.

Pate D, Goobar J, Resnick D, et al: Traction osteophytes of the lumbar spine: radiographic-pathologic correlation, *Radiology* 166:843-846, 1988.

Patel SC, Sanders WP: Synovial cyst of the cervical spine: case report and review of the literature, *AJNR* 9:602-603, 1988.

Penning L, Wilmink JT, Woerden V, et al: CT myelographic findings in degenerative disorders of the cervical spine: clinical significance, *AJNR* 7:119-127, 1986.

Prakash SG, Chandy MJ, Abraham J: Stenosis of the axis and cervical myelopathy, *J Neurosurg* 76:296-297, 1992.

Quaghebeur G, Jeffree M: Synovial cyst of the high cervical spine causing myelopathy, *AJNR* 13:981-982, 1992.

Ratliff J and Voorhies R: Increased MRI signal intensity in association with myelopathy and cervical instability: case report and review of the literature, *Surg Neurol* 53(1):8-13, 2000.

Remedios D, Natali C, Saifuddin A, et al: Case report: MRI of vertebral osteitis in early ankylosing spondylitis, *Clin Radiol* 53(7):534-536, 1998.

Reul J, Gievers B, Weis J, et al: Assessment of the narrow cervical spinal canal: a prospective comparison of MRI, myelography and CT-myelography, *Neuroradiology* 37(3):187-191, 1995.

Ricca GF, Robertson JT, Hines RS: Nerve root compression by herniated intradiskal gas, *J Neurosurg* 72:282-284, 1990.

Ricci C, Cova M, Kang YS, et al: Normal age-related patterns of cellular and fatty bone marrow distribution in the axial skeleton: MR imaging study, *Radiology* 177:83-88, 1990.

Roberts N, Gratin C, Whitehouse GH, et al: MRI analysis of lumbar intervertebral disc height in young and older populations, *J Magnetic Res Imaging* 7(5):880-886, 1997.

Robertson R, Maier S, Mulkern RV, et al: MR line-scan diffusion imaging of the spinal cord in children, *AJNR* 21(7):1344-1348, 2000.

Ross JS, Delamarter R, Hueftle MG, et al: Gadolinium-DTPA-enhanced MR imaging of the postoperative lumbar spine: time course and mechanism of enhancement, *AJNR* 10:37-46, 1989.

Ross JS, Masaryk TJ, Modic MT, et al: Lumbar spine: postoperative assessment with surface-coil MR imaging, *Radiology* 164:851-860, 1987.

Ross JS, Masaryk TJ, Modic MT: Postoperative cervical spine: MR assessment, *J Comput Assist Tomogr* 11:955-962, 1987.

Ross JS, Masaryk TJ, Schrader M, et al: MR imaging of the postoperative lumbar spine: assessment with gadopentetate dimeglumine, *AJNR* 11:771-776, 1990.

Ross JS, Perez-Reyes N, Masaryk TJ, et al: Thoracic disk herniation: MR imaging, *Radiology* 165:511-515, 1987.

Ross JS, Ruggieri PM, Tkach JA, et al: Gd-DTPA-enhanced 3D MR imaging of cervical degenerative disk disease: initial experience, *AJNR* 13:127-136, 1992.

Rothman SLG, Glenn WV: CT multiplanar reconstruction in 253 cases of lumbar spondylolysis, *AJNR* 5:81-90, 1984.

Russel EJ, D'Angele CM, Zimmerman RD, et al: Cervical disk herniation: CT demonstration after contrast enhancement, *Radiology* 152:703-712, 1984.

Russel EJ: Cervical disk disease, *Radiology* 177:313-325, 1990.

Saifuddin A and Burnett SJ: The value of lumbar spine MRI in the assessment of the pars interarticularis, *Clin Radiol* 52(9):666-671, 1997.

Sartoris DJ, Moskowitz PS, Kaufman RA, et al: Childhood diskitis: computed tomographic findings, *Radiology* 149:701-707, 1991.

Sato R, Takahashi M, Yamashita Y, et al: Calcium crystal deposition in cervical ligamentum flavum: CT and MR findings, *J Comput Assist Tomogr* 16:352-355, 1992.

Schellinger D, Manz HJ, Vidic B, et al: Disk fragment migration, *Radiology* 175:831-836, 1990.

Sether LA, Yu S, Haughton VM, et al: Intervertebral disk: normal age-related changes in MR intensity, *Radiology* 177:385-388, 1990.

Silbergleit R, Gebarski SS, Brunberg JA, et al: Lumbar synovial cysts: correlation of myelographic, CT, MR, and pathologic findings, *AJNR* 11:777-779, 1990.

Silverman CS, Lenchik L, Shimkin PM, et al: The value of MR in differentiating subligamentous from supraligamentous lumbar disk herniations [see comments], *AJNR* 16(3):571-579, 1995.

Solsberg MD, Lemaire C, Resch L, et al: High-resolution MR imaging of the cadaveric human spinal cord: normal anatomy, *AJNR* 11:3-7, 1990.

Taylor JR, McCormick CC: Lumbar facet joint fat pads: their normal anatomy and their appearance when enlarged, *Neuroradiology* 33:38-42, 1991.

Tyrrell PN, Davies AM, Evans N, et al: Signal changes in the intervertebral discs on MRI of the thoracolumbar spine in ankylosing spondylitis, *Clin Radiol* 50(6):377-383, 1995.

Udeshi UL and Reeves D: Routine thin slice MRI effectively demonstrates the lumbar pars interarticularis, *Clin Radiol* 54(9):615-659, 1999.

Weinreb JC: MR imaging of bone marrow: a map could help, *Radiology* 177:23-24, 1990.

Williams DM, Gabrielsen TO, Latack JT, et al: Ossification in the cephalic attachment of the ligamentum flavum, *Radiology* 150:423-426, 1984.

Wilmink JT: CT morphology of intrathecal lumbosacral nerve-root compression, *AJNR* 10:233-248, 1989.

Wilmink JT and Hofman PA: MRI of the postoperative lumbar spine: triple-dose gadodiamide and fat suppression [published erratum appears in *Neuroradiology* 1997 Nov;39(11):820], *Neuroradiology* 39(8):589-592, 1997.

Wilson DA, Prince JR: MR imaging determination of the location of the normal conus medullaris throughout childhood, *AJNR* 10:259-262, 1989.

Xu G, Haughton V, Carrera GF: Lumbar facet joint capsule: appearance at MR imaging and CT, *Radiology* 177:415-420, 1990.

Yamashita Y, Takahashi M, Matsuno Y, et al: Spinal cord compression due to ossification of ligaments: MR imaging, *Radiology* 175:843-848, 1990.

Yousem DM, Schnall MD: MR examination for spinal cord compression: impact of multicoil system on length of study, *J Comput Assist Tomogr* 15:598-604, 1991.

Yu S, Haughton VM, Sether LA, et al: Criteria for classifying normal and degenerated lumbar intervertebral disks, *Radiology* 170:523-526, 1989.

CHAPTER 17

Nondegenerative Diseases of the Spine

Infectious and Inflammatory Diseases

This chapter begins with infectious and noninfectious inflammatory diseases of the spine and spinal coverings. Cystic lesions of the cord followed by neoplastic diseases involving the spine and cord comprise the next two sections of this chapter. The last sections concern vascular diseases of the cord and spinal cord trauma. We have chosen this approach because it is disease oriented and in most settings the clinical findings generate the imaging algorithm. These diseases actually stimulate more intellectual discussion than questions such as, "Is it a small herniation or a focal bulge?" In fact, the diseases affecting the spine give the authors Lhermitte's shivers thinking about them. So, let us decompress the spine.

Diskitis and Osteomyelitis

Pyogenic disk space infections are usually the result of a blood-borne agent, particularly from the lung or urinary tract. The pathogen lodges in the region of the endplate and destroys the disk space and the adjacent vertebral bodies. The disk space infection may be acute, in which case pain is invariably present, or it may be more chronic. The symptoms start with focal back pain and progress to radicular, meningeal, and spinal cord involvement as the disease advances. Clinical settings include those cases in which there is a recent history of spine surgery or hematogenous dissemination from another infectious site. The lumbar spine is most frequently involved. The most common organism is *Staphylococcus;* other common causes include *Streptococcus, Pep-*

tostreptococcus, Escherichia coli, and *Proteus.* The sedimentation rate is elevated and there is a leukocytosis in most cases of disk space infection.

Although gallium radionuclide imaging is highly sensitive to inflammation, magnetic resonance imaging (MR) is the most specific method for cost-effective diagnosis. Gallium can also be quite sensitive to demonstrating that antibiotic therapy is effective by showing a decrease in radionuclide uptake. Conventional spin echo images reveal the disk space to be of low signal intensity on T1-weighted images (T1WI) and high signal intensity on T2-weighted images (T2WI) as a result of the associated edema (Fig. 17-1). The disk space, adjacent vertebral bodies (particularly at the end-plates), and, if present, the epidural and/or paravertebral soft tissues enhance. There is usually evidence of new bone formation as well as irregularity of the end-plate or bony sclerosis (best seen on computed tomography CT). Look carefully for epidural or paravertebral abscess.

Vertebral osteomyelitis usually occurs in the setting of disk space infection; however, osteomyelitis can occur without disk space infection from hematogenous dissemination directly to the vertebral body. The signal changes are similar to disk space infection. A three-phase technetium bone scan can differentiate cases of cellulitis from osteomyelitis based upon the combination of increased blood flow and persistent osseous uptake on delayed images in osteomyelitis. This exam may not be specific so that if there is a question of degenerative disease versus infection, a gallium scan or indium 111–labeled leukocyte scan may suggest an infectious process by demonstrating increased uptake and correlating it with the positive bone scan.

It is not uncommon to have spinal cord symptoms/signs without epidural compression in cases of pyogenic disk space infection or vertebral osteomyelitis. In this case, the cause is vasculitis of the medullary arteries and/or veins.

Renal Spondyloarthropathy

Patients undergoing dialysis can have changes in their spine (usually in the cervical region), which superficially may resemble infection (renal spondyloarthropathy). There is destruction of the disk space and adjacent vertebral bodies; however, the signal intensity on T2WI is usually low rather than high as in infection. Furthermore, there is no clinical evidence of infection. Amyloid deposition has been implicated as a possible cause.

Granulomatous Infections

The most common granulomatous infections of the spine are brucellosis, tuberculosis, and fungal infections (blastomycosis, cryptococcosis, and coccidioidomyco-

sis). Brucellosis is diagnosed by positive blood culture or serologic studies. Culture from biopsy is not definitive and usually contains nonspecific inflammatory changes. Brucellosis has a predilection for the lower lumbar spine generally, with less destruction of the vertebral body and disk space. Paravertebral mass and spinal deformity are rare.

Tuberculosis most often affects the lower thoracic spine (Pott disease, or tuberculous spondylitis), is indolent, and is frequently associated with epidural disease, particularly paravertebral, or subligamentous abscess, or abscess of the psoas muscle. Vertebral body destruction with relative sparing of the disk space occurs late in the disease (Fig. 17-2). Because of the infection, a gibbus deformity may develop. The posterior elements may be involved, and the infection can spread along the anterior longitudinal ligament and involve multiple levels. The disk can be of normal intensity on noncontrast MR but usually enhances. Spinal deformity is common. Approximately 50% of patients have obvious pulmonary disease. The diagnosis of tuberculosis requires isolation of the bacillus, characteristic histopathologic changes, and/or response to antibiotic therapy. Table 17-1 contrasts the features of bacterial infection, tuberculosis (TB), and neoplasm.

TB or not TB, phthisis the question—
Consumption be done about it?

Epidural Abscess

Epidural abscesses are the result of either direct extension of vertebral osteomyelitis or hematogenous dissemination from an infectious source. *Staphylococcus aureus* is the most common pathogen (45%), with the remainder being gram-negative rods, anaerobes, mycobacteria, and fungi. Rarely is the abscess caused by an epidural injection except in July when the new house officers begin. Patients are septic, with histories of intravenous drug abuse, immunosuppression, urinary tract infections, and cardiac infections; these patients present with tenderness over the spine, back pain, and progressive neurologic impairment. There is an association with blunt spine trauma with hematoma formation and secondary infection. The abscess is usually located in the dorsal epidural space, probably because of the close approximation of the ventral dura and the posterior longitudinal ligament, limiting anterior spread of the abscess. Incidentally, this is also why epidural hematoma is posterior.

MR is the modality of choice for imaging epidural abscesses (Fig. 17-3). The epidural mass has low signal intensity compared with normal spinal cord on T1WI and has high signal on T2WI. There are three patterns of enhancement: (1) homogeneous enhancement, representing diffuse inflamed tissue with microabscesses (phleg-

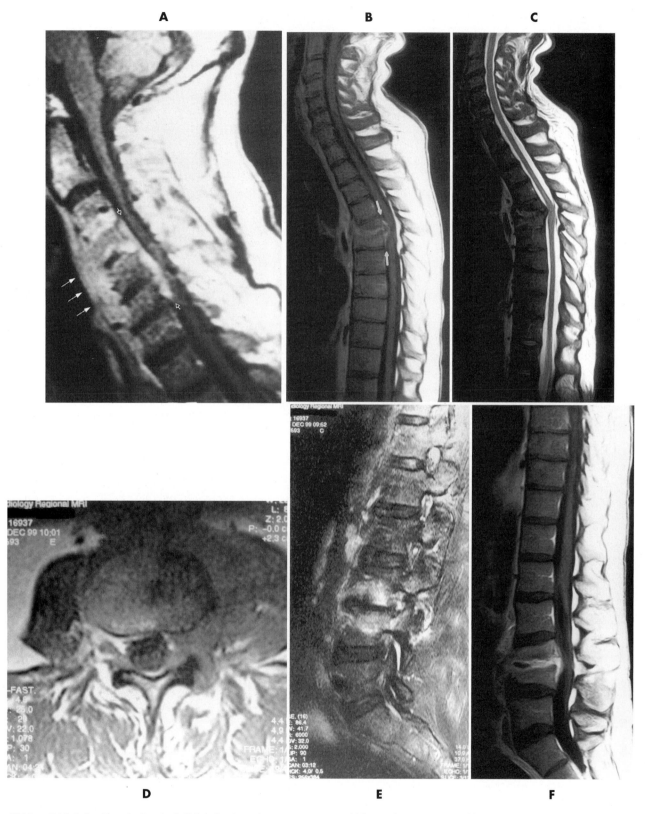

A   **B**   **C**

D   **E**   **F**

Fig. 17-1   Disk infection. **A,** Cervical disk infection after surgery. Sagittal T1W1 shows a prevertebral enhancing mass *(arrows)* and intraspinal enhancing epidural infection *(open arrows)* compressing the cord. Multiple disk spaces enhance after surgery at those levels. **B,** Sagittal T1WI shows a thoracic disk infection with compression of the spinal cord by associated epidural hematoma *(arrows).* The T2WI **(C)** shows the cord draped over the diseased segment. **D,** A lumbar study shows a left paraspinal mass extending into the foramen. **E,** The sagittal T2WI to the left reveals high signal in the endplates on either side of the diseased disk. **F,** Note the marked enhancement of the disk at L3-4 with a small epidural component.

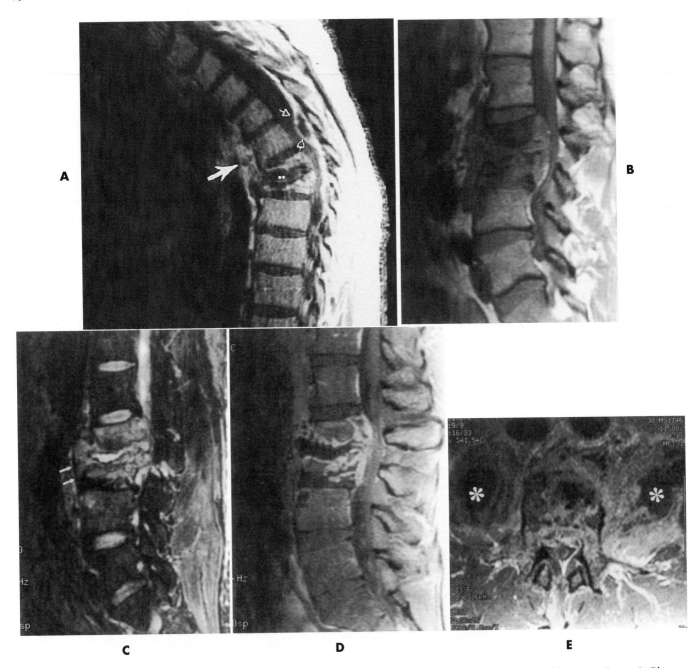

Fig. 17-2   Tuberculous osteomyelitis. **A,** T1 enhanced sagittal shows spread along the anterior longitudinal ligament *(arrow).* Observe the intraspinal abscess *(open arrows).* **B,** Another case with diskitis and osteomyelitis. T1 sagittal reveals anterior prespinal mass and thecal sac compression by an anterior epidural mass. **C,** Off midline sagittal T2WI nicely illustrates the bright disk and dark anterior ligament *(arrrows)* confining the infection. **D,** Note the bone necrosis on postcontrast scans. **E,** Psoas abscesses *(snowflakes)* are present bilaterally.

monous granulation tissue); (2) peripheral enhancement consistent with frank abscess including a necrotic center; and (3) a combination of tissue enhancement and frank abscess. Pattern (1) may be difficult to discern in the lumbar spine without the use of fat saturation techniques to distinguish between enhancement and epidural fat, which can be diffusely infiltrated by the inflammatory process. Epidural abscess produces symp-

toms by sheer mass effect and/or septic thrombophlebitis with cord edema and infarction. Think about spinal cord infarction secondary to thrombophlebitis in the setting of epidural abscess and high signal on T2WI in the cord. Meningitis (with increased intensity of the CSF on T1WI and enhancement of the CSF and nerve roots) can occasionally be identified along with the epidural abscess.

Table 17-1 Salient features of bacterial infection, TB, and neoplasm

Condition	Disk space	Paraspinous mass	Posterior elements	Spread
Bacterial infection	Always involved early on	May or may not be present	Very uncommon	Contiguous
TB	Occurs in the course of the disease	Usually large mass	Yes	May have skip areas
Neoplasm	Very rare	Yes	Yes	Noncontiguous

Subdural empyema has a similar presentation to epidural abscess, although it is much rarer in occurrence. Additionally there are iatrogenic causes including lumbar puncture, anesthesia, and diskography. Discrimination between the subdural and epidural compartments is usually difficult on MR.

Meningeal Sequelae

Infections of the meninges are discussed in Chapter 6. The sequela of bacterial meningitis may be arachnoiditis, which at times is associated with syringomyelia

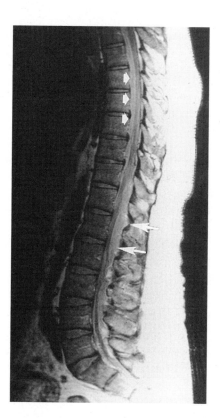

Fig. 17-3 Epidural abscess. Enhanced T1WI shows an anterior *(fat arrows)* and posterior *(arrows)* epidural collection. Observe the enhancement demarcating the lower lesion.

(see Cystic Lesions section in this chapter). In addition, cysticercosis can cause arachnoiditis (and rarely subarachnoid and spinal cord cysts). Pachymeningitis (thickened dura mater) has many causes (Box 17-1).

Clinically, meningeal infection may lead to symptoms of myelopathy and/or radiculopathy, which can progress to paralysis. These symptoms are related to compression of nerve roots and spinal cord by thickened dura. Infarction and cord cavitation are late sequelae of lepto or pachymeningitis. MR reveals poor definition of the cord or subarachnoid space on T1WI and diffuse thick enhancement of the leptomeninges.

Sarcoidosis

Only 6% to 8% of patients with neurosarcoidosis have spinal cord lesions with the most common location being the cervical region. Sarcoidosis can manifest as nodules on the surface of the cord, which can appear similar to tumor nodules and can be associated with cord enlargement. Rarely, sarcoid nodules may be on individual nerve roots. As in the brain, intramedullary lesions result from infiltration of the Virchow-Robin spaces (Fig. 17-4). Intramedullary sarcoidosis can present as a diffuse inflammatory lesion or as a discrete mass.

The lesions demonstrate high intensity on T2WI with diffuse leptomeningeal enhancement and/or nodular enhancement.

Box 17-1 Causes of Pachymeningitis

Fungus
Hemorrhage
Idiopathic
Leptomeningeal metastasis
Mucopolysaccharidosis
Rheumatoid granulation
Sarcoid
Syphilis
Tuberculosis

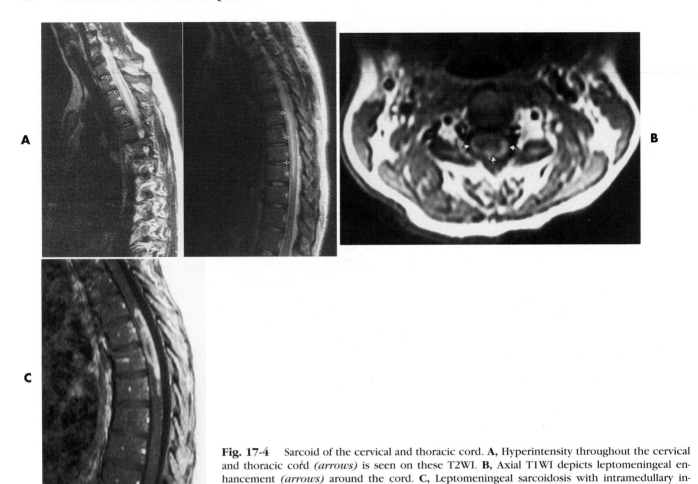

Fig. 17-4 Sarcoid of the cervical and thoracic cord. **A,** Hyperintensity throughout the cervical and thoracic cord *(arrows)* is seen on these T2WI. **B,** Axial T1WI depicts leptomeningeal enhancement *(arrows)* around the cord. **C,** Leptomeningeal sarcoidosis with intramedullary involvement is demonstrated on this postcontrast T1WI.

Intramedullary Lesions in Acquired Immunodeficiency Syndrome (AIDS)

A variety of conditions affect the cord in patients with acquired immunodeficiency syndrome (AIDS); these are listed in Box 17-2 (Fig. 17-5). Vacuolar myelopathy, identified in patients with AIDS, is defined as vacuolation in the spinal white matter associated with lipid-laden macrophages typically involving the dorsal columns and

Box 17-2 Intramedullary Lesions in AIDS

Cytomegalovirus infection
Herpes simplex virus infection
Herpes zoster virus infection
Non-Hodgkin's lymphoma
Subacute necrotizing myelopathy
Syphilis
Toxoplasmosis
Tuberculosis
Vacuolar myelopathy

lateral corticospinal tracts, although it may occur anywhere. Degeneration of the cortical spinal tract has also been reported, especially in children. Its incidence has been reported to be between 3% to 55%. The etiology is unknown but may be related to either primary or indirect effects of HIV, secondary infectious agents, nutritional deficiencies or toxic effects of drugs. The vertebral marrow can also be affected by these conditions (see Fig. 17-5E). High intensity on T2WI is seen in a spinal cord that may be normal or small in size. Nothing is specific about their MR appearance to separate them from other non-AIDS intramedullary lesions.

Transverse Myelitis and Multiple Sclerosis

Transverse myelitis is an inflammatory condition of the spinal cord associated with rapidly progressive neurologic dysfunction. The term either indicates bilateral dysfunction of the spinal cord or partial unilateral abnormality. Diseases causing this condition include acute disseminated encephalomyelitis (see Chapter 7—White Matter Diseases), multiple sclerosis, connective tissue diseases (lupus, rheumatoid arthritis, and Sjögren dis-

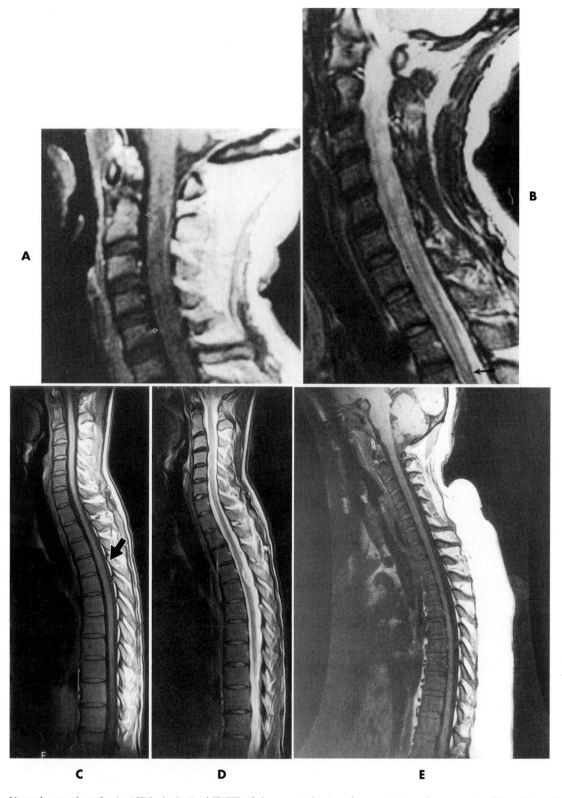

Fig. 17-5 Vacuolar myelopathy in AIDS. **A,** Sagittal T1WI of the cervical spine demonstrates enlargement and low intensity *(open arrows)* in the spinal cord. **B,** Diffuse high intensity in the cervical cord *(open arrows),* which ends in the thoracic region *(arrow)* can be appreciated on the T2WI. Herpes Zoster infection. **C,** Note the low intensity focus in the back of the cord on this sagittal T1WI. This is typical of Zoster as it grows along the dorsal roots. **D,** It is hyperintense on T2WI, yet the cord is not particularly expanded. The low signal of the marrow (less intense than the disks on the T1WI) should suggest the patient is immunocompromised. The diagnosis was herpes zoster myelitis. **E,** Marrow signal is often low on T1WI in patients who are HIV positive on the basis of nutritional, constitutional, and hematologic causes.

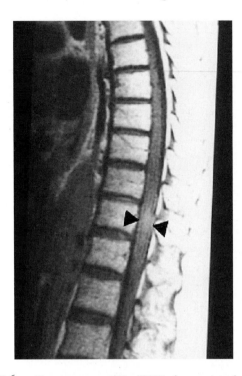

Fig. 17-6. Transverse myelitis. T1WI shows an enlarged enhancing cord at T11 *(arrowheads)*. Multiple sclerosis had been previously diagnosed in this patient.

ease), sarcoidosis, vascular malformations, vasculitides, and idiopathic. The spinal cord is focally enlarged with high signal on T2WI, and may enhance (Fig. 17-6).

Some authors believe that there is a distinct entity termed idiopathic acute transverse myelitis. The clinical course occurs over days to weeks. Pathology reveals demyelination, perivascular lymphocytic infiltrates, and necrosis. The lesion extends over multiple spinal cord segments and involved the entire cross section of the spinal cord. There is high intensity on T2WI with variable enhancement patterns (nodular, meningeal). In some cases, the cauda equina was observed to enhance suggesting a possible relationship with Guillain-Barré syndrome. It has been hypothesized that this is a result of a small vessel vasculopathy (perhaps immunologically mediated), either arterial or venous, affecting gray matter as well as white matter (Fig. 17-7).

Multiple sclerosis can affect the spinal cord and produce myelopathic signs and symptoms. It can be confined solely to the spinal cord (5% to 24% of cases), which may account for the "negative" brain MR findings in patients with definite disease. Multiple sclerosis lesions are isointense or of low intensity on T1WI and high

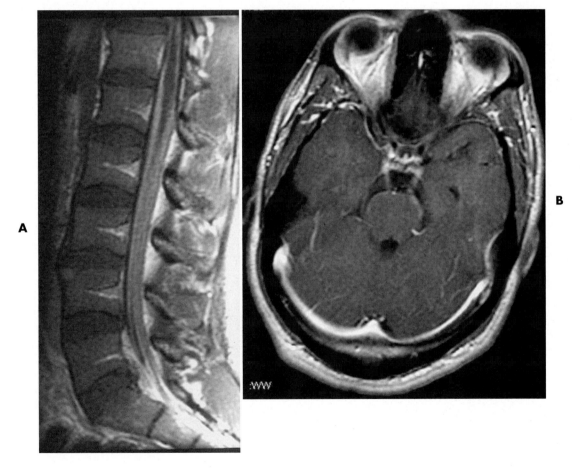

Fig. 17-7. Guillain Barre. **A,** Guillain Barre radiculitis is one potential source of a diffusely enchancing cauda equina, with or without enlarged nerve roots. **B,** In this case, the meningeal irritation was also evident intracranially with enhancing cranial nerves III and/or IV.

signal on T2WI. Sixty percent of the spinal cord lesions occur in the cervical region. The typical MS spinal cord lesion does not involve the entire cross-sectional area, is peripherally located, does not respect gray/white boundaries, and is less than 2 vertebral body segments in length (90% of the time). The cord is usually normal in size with enlargement seen in 6% to 14% of cases (Fig. 17-8). The majority of lesions are patchy in location, and demonstrate enhancement if the patient is referred for prob-

lems related to new spinal cord signs/symptoms. Spinal cord parenchymal loss, especially in the cervical region, can be detected over the course of the disease. Lesions in the spinal cord account for less than 20% of total disease burden. Nevertheless, a strategically placed lesion can profoundly affect disability. One other point—MS is a common disease, and it has not read the literature, so beware of unusual presentations particularly in young patients.

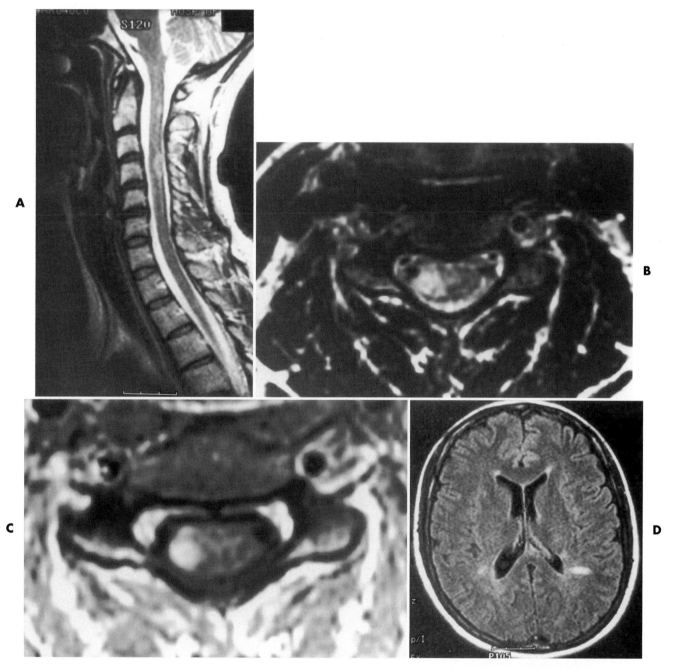

Fig. 17-8   Multiple sclerosis on parade. **A,** Multiple high signal intensity foci are depicted on this sagittal T2WI through the cervical cord. The absence of cord expansion places the lesion in the nonacute demyelination category. **B,** An axial T2WI through the cervical cord shows focal involvement of the right side of the cord. **C,** The plaque enhances. **D,** The next study should be the brain FLAIR sequence and voilà, the one can see Dawson's fingers at play—multiple periventricular plaques.

It is useful to image the brain if questions are raised concerning the cause of the transverse myelitis, because asymptomatic high signal abnormalities in young adult brains help favor multiple sclerosis as the cause of the transverse myelitis. Try the sagittal FLAIR and look at the callosal septal interface.

Lupus Myelitis

This is a recognized complication of systemic lupus erythematosus presenting as transverse myelitis with back pain, paraparesis or quadriparesis, and sensory loss. The spinal cord may be enlarged with high intensity on T2WI involving 4 to 5 vertebral body segments (larger than MS) of the cord (Fig. 17-9). Contrast enhancement can be detected in about 50% of cases. Etiology of the lesion is vacuolar degeneration from an autoimmune process or ischemia.

Subacute Combined Degeneration (SCD)

SCD, a complication of cobalamin (B12) deficiency, causes a myelopathy affecting the cervical and upper thoracic spinal cord, but it can also produce lesions in the optic tracts, brain, and peripheral nerves. Clinical find-

ings include paresthesias of the hands and feet, loss of position and vibratory sensation, sensory ataxia, spasticity, and lower extremity weakness. Pernicious anemia, the inability to absorb B12 due to inactivation of intrinsic factor (secreted by gastric parietal cells), is the most frequent cause of B12 deficiency in the United States. It is an immune-mediated process that results in loss of gastric parietal cells and leads to achlorhydria, atrophic gastritis, and decreased levels of intrinsic factor. The B12 intrinsic factor complex binds to the mucosa of the terminal ileum, where B12 is absorbed so that diseases that affect the terminal ileum such as regional enteritis or tropical sprue can produce B12 deficiency. Pathologically, demyelination and axonal loss in the posterior and lateral spinal cord columns is seen.

Box 17-3 provides the differential diagnosis of degenerative lesions involving the posterior columns. On T2WI, high intensity is observed longitudinally in the posterior columns (Fig. 17-10). Following treatment this can regress and disappear if caught early enough, however, if undetected permanent axonal loss and gliosis results. The bone marrow can also be low intensity on T1WI and T2WI associated with enhancement indicating benign hyperplasia of the hematopoietic marrow (secondary to the pernicious anemia).

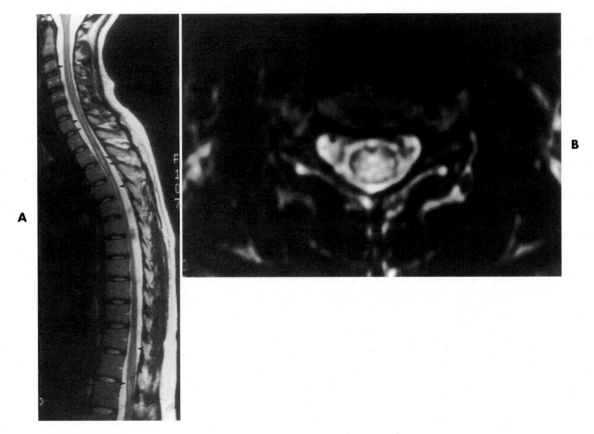

Fig. 17-9 Lupus myelitis. **A,** As opposed to multiple sclerosis, this case of lupus myelitis involves multiple disk levels (*arrowheads*) and the entity favors the central aspect of the cord (**B**).

Box 17-3 Conditions Associated with Degeneration of the Posterior Columns of the Spinal Cord

Carcinomatous radiculopathy
Charcot-Marie-Tooth disease
Cobalamin (B12) deficiency
Folic acid deficiency
Friedreich's ataxia
Joseph disease
Multiple sclerosis
Spinal trauma or tumor
Tabes dorsalis (syphilis)
Toxins
    Clioquinol (SMON)
    Organophosphorous
    Thallium
    Vincristine
Vacuolar myelopathy

RADIATION-INDUCED CHANGES

Spinal radiation converts normal bone marrow to fatty marrow (Fig. 17-11). This is manifested on MR by diffuse high signal on T1WI in the vertebral bodies and lower intensity on conventional T2WI. If the cord is high signal on T2WI, it may be the result of radiation myelitis or

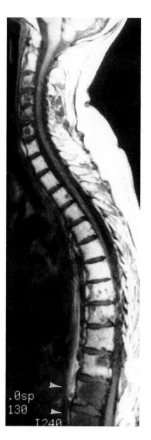

Fig. 17-11   Radiation changes to spine. Note the bright signal intensity of the marrow ALMOST throughout the entire spine. Unfortunately, the T12 and L1 vertebrae *(arrowheads)* bucked the trend. They had resistant metastatic small cell carcinoma in them. The cervical region shows changes of treated carcinoma. At least the cord looked good.

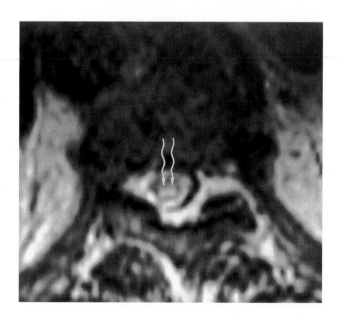

Fig. 17-10   Subacute combined degeneration. The two high signal intensity areas *(squiggly arrows)* in the posterior portion of the cord represent the dorsal columns (fasciculus gracilis and cuneatus). This is classic for B12 deficiency and subacute combined degeneration.

residual tumor, if the reason for the initial therapy was a cord tumor. Cord atrophy is another manifestation of radiation therapy. Box 17-4 provides a list of conditions that produce increased or decreased marrow signal on T1WI.

ADULT TETHERED CORD

Symptoms of adult tethered cord have been associated with a precipitating traumatic event. This is seen in young women more often than in men and is accompanied by diffuse back and perianal pain, leg weakness, and urinary tract dysfunction. The symptoms may occur in conjunction with pregnancy, childbirth, and pelvic examination. Imaging reveals the tip of the conus medullaris to be below L2, which is considered the lower limit of normal. The filum is thickened (>2 mm); however, it is difficult to distinguish between a thickened filum and a low-lying conus. The conus may be tethered by spina bifida occulta and/or an intradural lipoma, and posteriorly displaced by fat, glial cells, and collagen. Cutaneous stigmata of dysraphism including hairy patch, sinus tract, or subcutaneous lipoma are common.

> There once was a tethered cord from Long Island
> That eventually destroyed all of the myelin;
> The surgeon said with a grin as she bovied the skin
> "I'll need asylum after cutting the filum."

CYSTIC LESIONS

Arachnoid Cyst

Arachnoid cysts occur on a congenital basis or result from trauma or inflammation. On CT myelography, you can see an extraaxial mass, which may compress the cord. The cyst may or may not fill with contrast. On MR focal impression on the cord can be seen with intensity similar to that of cerebrospinal fluid (CSF) without enhancement (Fig. 17-12). Carefully scrutinize the smoothness of the cord, any indentation suggests the presence of arachnoid cyst. These cysts can be under pressure and produce symptoms by spinal cord compression.

Tarlov's Cyst

Cystic dilatation of the sacral root pouches (Tarlov's cysts named after Isadore) can be large and may be as-

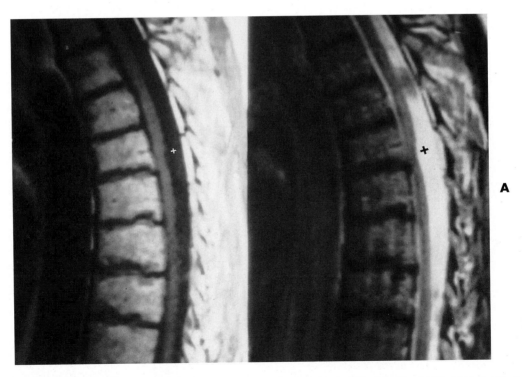

Fig. 17-12 Arachnoid cyst. **A,** Sagittal T1WI *(left)* and T2WI *(right)* demonstrate a CSF collection *(+)* behind the thoracic spinal cord. The spinal cord is pushed anteriorly by this posterior CSF-containing mass. This arachnoid cyst has produced spinal cord atrophy and compression.

Illustration continued on following page

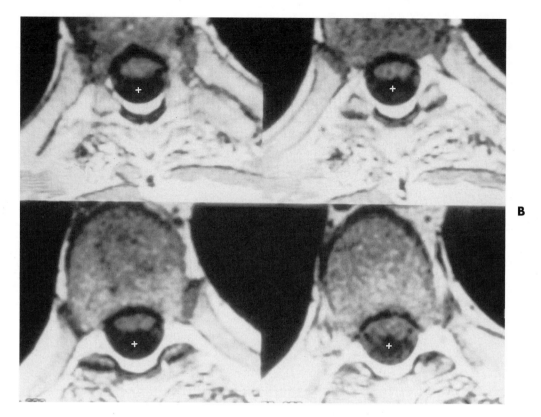

B

Fig. 17-12 *Continued.* **B,** Axial images through the region of the arachnoid cyst *(+)* demonstrate posterior compression and mild atrophic change in the spinal cord.

sociated with bone erosion. These are caused by a ball-valve phenomenon at the ostium of the nerve root sheath with CSF flowing into the cyst with arterial pulsation. After instillation of subarachnoid contrast these cysts fill and are routinely visualized during myelographic CT (Fig. 17-13). These may or may not be symptomatic (rare cause of sciatica); only the patient's disability board knows for sure. The differential diagnosis includes meningocele, arachnoid cyst, neurofibroma, and dural ectasia.

Epidermoid Cyst

Epidermoid cysts represent less than 1% of intraspinal tumors, with a higher incidence in children. They are usually extramedullary but rarely can be intramedullary, and can be congenital or acquired. Congenital epidermoids result from displaced ectoderm inclusions occurring early in fetal life perhaps from faulty closure of the neural tube. The acquired cysts result from lumbar puncture with inclusion of skin tissue in the spine. On MR, a discrete mass, which has a variable signal intensity depending on the cyst contents, is present (Fig. 17-14). The lesion can calcify and rarely can be associated with peripheral enhancement. Inclusion of endoderm results in an enterogenous cyst that is lined by mucin-secreting cells, which can produce contents with similar intensity (high

signal on T1WI and T2WI) to mucoceles. These can be associated with developmental defects in the skin and vertebral bodies, and with fistulous communications to cysts in the mediastinum, thorax, or abdomen. Other cysts include dermoid cysts (which contain fatty elements) and ependymal cysts (which follow CSF intensity).

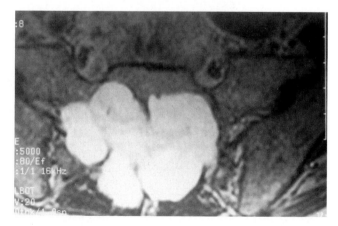

Fig. 17-13 Humongous sacral root cysts. There is very little spinal canal left on this T2WI because of the confluent sacral root cysts in this patient with Marfan syndrome (see Fig. 16-41 also).

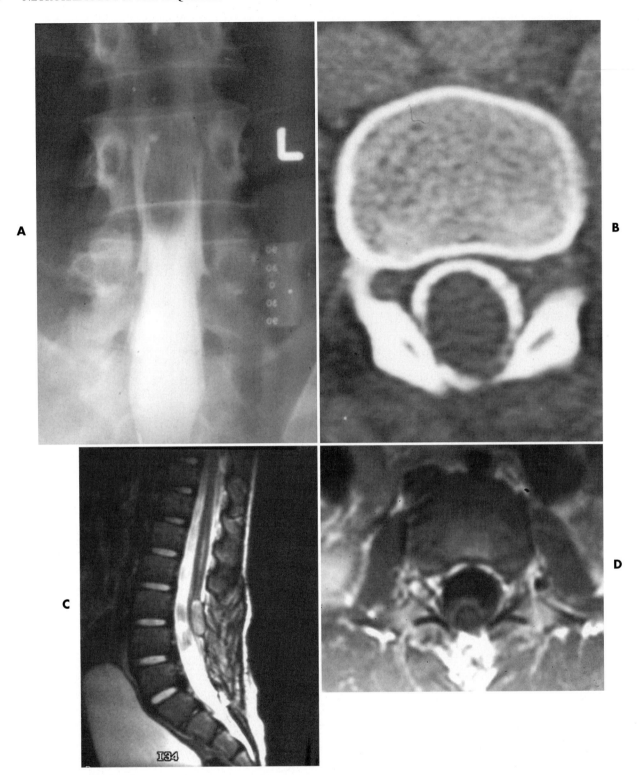

Fig. 17-14 Lumbar epidermoid. **A,** Lumbar myelogram mass in the L3 region. The mass is delineated by contrast. **B,** CT following the myelogram reveals what appears to be a cystic lesion surrounded by contrast. **C,** T2 weighted sagittal MR with the epidermoid (high intensity) easily seen. **D,** Axial T1 enhanced image reveals a rim of enhancement surrounding the lesion.

Syringomyelia (Syringohydromyelia)

This topic is controversial and even confusing—different names for the same condition and a host of theo-

ries to explain the creation—some might think you need to be a brain surgeon or worse, a basic scientist, to understand what syrinxes are and how they grow. Recall, you are reading the Requisites, and that means the nuts and bolts for all of us tire-kicker, low IQ radiologists. So

Box 17-5   Lesions Associated with Hydromyelia

Basliar invagination
Chiari malformations
Disatematomyelia
Klippel-Feil syndrome
Paget's disease
Spinal dysraphism
Tethered cord syndrome

relax, here is the pablum. First morsal—syrinxes are well demarcated spinal cavities containing fluid similar to CSF.

In the fetus and in newborns the central canal (in the central spinal cord gray matter) contains a small amount of CSF and is lined by ependymal cells. You should also know that the central canal extends from the obex of the fourth ventricle to the filum terminale. In the region of the conus medullaris the canal expands as a fusiform terminal ventricle, the ventriculus terminalis (fifth ventricle), which completely obliterates by about 40 years

of age. There are probably variations in the patency of the central canal with maturation. States that alter the flow of CSF (Chiari malformations, arachnoid cysts, and adhesions) and/or that produce abnormal CSF pressure ultimately result in transmission of the fluid pressure into what is left of the central canal. How precisely this occurs is open to much speculation but you can imagine higher CSF pressure transmitted along the perivascular spaces and into the interstitial spaces toward the central canal. This dilates the central canal remnant, and depending on where it is patent, is associated with the development of varieties of syringomyelia.

There are three types of syringomyelia. The first is a central canal syrinx that communicates with the fourth ventricle and is associated with hydrocephalus. These are produced by obstruction of CSF circulation distal to the outlets of the fourth ventricle. The second occurs in a region of the central canal that is dilated but does not communicate with the fourth ventricle. Here we are thinking (we know, do not think just list—Box 17-5) about Chiari I malformations, extramedullary intradural tumors, arachnoid cysts/arachnoiditis, cervical spinal stenosis, basilar invagination, and so on (Fig. 17-15). The

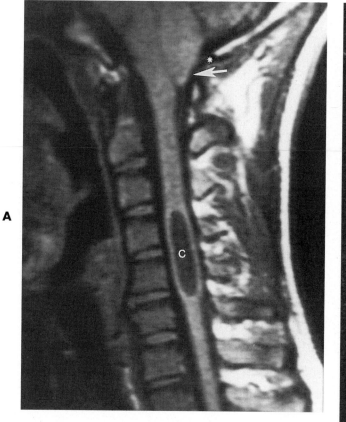

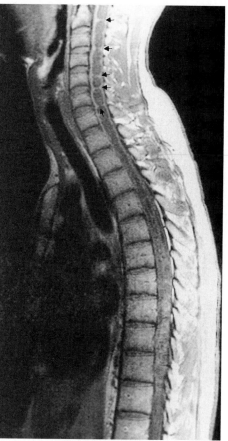

Fig. 17-15   **A,** Chiari I malformation with hydromyelia. Sagittal T1WI has tonsils *(arrow)* below the foramen magnum (*) and has a hydromyelic cyst *(c)*. **B,** Glial adhesions in a syrinx. Glial adhesions *(arrows)* are identified on this sagittal T1WI of a large syrinx. This linked-sausage appearance is classic in syringohydromyelia.

Box 17-6   Lesions Associated with Syringomyelia

Arachnoid cysts
Arachnoiditis
Cord infarction
Meningioma
Myelitis
Neurofibroma
Pott's disease
Spinal cord neoplasms: ependymoma, astrocytoma, hemangioblastoma
Spondylotic compression
Trauma
Vertebral body tumors

first and second cases have also been termed hydromyelia. There may also be cases of asymptomatic localized dilatation of the central canal without any predisposing factors such as Chiari malformation (there are exceptions to any theory).

The third differs from the first two in that it is centered in the spinal cord parenchyma and not centered in the central canal (Box 17-6). These are found in watershed regions of the spinal cord and associated with direct spinal cord injury such as trauma or infarction.

There has recently been described a situation where alterations of CSF flow are recognized before syringomyelia occurs. The spinal cord becomes edematous, appears enlarged with high intensity on T2WI. This has been termed a presyrinx. This condition appears reversible if the condition producing the altered CSF pressure is treated.

To add further confusion to the story the general terms *syrinx* or *syringohydromyelia* have been advocated to lump all the conditions together.

Rarely an eccentric syrinx can be identified. This can be confused with arachnoid cyst. One wonders if at least a few of the arachnoid cysts noted with syringomyelia may actually be eccentric syrinxes. An evaginated syrinx has been termed an exosyrinx (Fig. 17-16).

Posttraumatic myelomalacia is a lesion with cord cavitation, associated with significant spinal cord trauma in-

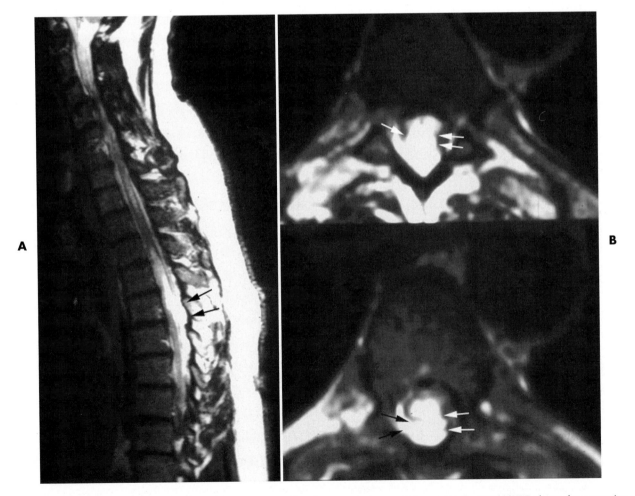

Fig. 17-16   Exosyrinx. **A,** Sagittal T2WI with syrinx protruding from posterior cord *(arrows)*. **B,** Axial T2WI show the posterior extent of the syrinx beyond the confines of the spinal cord *(arrows)*.

cluding hemorrhage or infarction. Altered CSF dynamics from adhesions may predispose to development of syrinx formation in this myelomalacic cavity. The question for radiologists in this setting is to determine if there is cystic or noncystic myelopathy. The former is a treatable cause of myelopathy. Although not perfect, cystic myelomalacia should follow CSF intensity on all pulse sequences whereas noncystic or microcysticmyelomalacia is high signal on proton density-weighted images (PDWI) and T2WI. The reality is that PDWI may not be totally reliable particularly if the fluid in the cyst is not subject to the same pulsations as CSF or has slightly elevated protein content. We normally now image using fast spin echo T2WI without PDWI which is another problem. You can also try intraoperative ultrasound, but that has low RVU's/minute. Our best buy recommendation—use the T1WI to distinguish cystic and noncystic myelomalacia—they are cost effective and liberate you from spending hours in the OR with your surgical colleagues. Let them do the ultrasound while you coil your next aneurysm.

NEOPLASTIC DISEASES

Intramedullary Lesions

MR has had a great impact on the diagnosis of neoplastic diseases of the cord. Neoplasms have three general characteristics: (1) they tend to enlarge the cord either focally or diffusely, (2) on PDWI and T2WI they produce high signal intensity, and (3) they enhance (Fig. 17-17). Tumors involving the cord may be primary, such as astrocytoma or ependymoma, or metastatic. It is virtually impossible to separate ependymoma from astrocytoma. Symptoms include pain, weakness, and muscle atrophy. Box 17-7 provides the differential diagnosis of the enlarged spinal cord. This is an essential diagnosis to know—memorize it! You must appreciate, however, that not all enlarged cords are neoplasms. As can be appreciated from this box, inflammatory and demyelinating diseases may enlarge the spinal cord. Especially in young patients with acute or subacute myelopathic symptoms, you should not glibly suggest that an enlarged spinal cord with high signal in it represents a tumor. Rather, think about the case, get an MR of the brain, and assess whether there are additional lesions. In this patient population, corroborative findings might favor a demyelinating process, such as multiple sclerosis, over a spinal cord tumor.

Let us now consider individual neoplastic lesions of the cord that are uncommon, representing 4% to 10% of all central nervous system tumors. We should point out that although certain trends may exist with respect to particular lesions, the specific diagnosis with MR in many situations is not usually possible. One final word here.

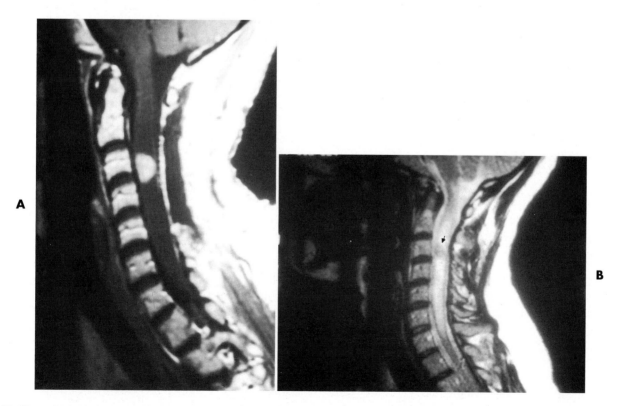

Fig. 17-17 Intramedullary breast metastasis. **A,** Sagittal T1WI demonstrates an enhancing intramedullary breast metastasis. Metastases generally evoke considerable edema and mass effect. **B,** T2WI also shows the extent of the edema, which involves the entire cervical cord. The metastatic nodule is identified *(arrow)*.

Box 17-7   Spinal Cord Enlargement

DEMYELINATING DISEASES

Acute disseminated encephalomyelitis
Multiple sclerosis
Other
Transverse myelitis

INFECTIONS

Cord swelling from extramedullary infectious process
    such as meningitis, producing vascular compromise
AIDS (see Box 17-2)

TUMOR

Metastases to cord
Primary spinal cord tumor

INFLAMMATION

Sarcoid
Systemic lupus erythematosus

SYRINGOHYDROMYELIA

**CAUSES OF SUBACUTE NECROTIZING MYELOPATHY
(SEE BOX 17-11)**

VASCULAR LESIONS

Acute infarction
Arteriovenous malformation
Cavernous angioma
Hemorrhage
Venous hypertension (Foix-Alajouanine syndrome)

The most important aspect of the radiologic workup is to identify that the cord is abnormal. As we just stated it is extremely difficult if not impossible to distinguish between astrocytoma and ependymoma—no kidding!

Cysts associated with neoplasia Just to confuse the reader further neoplasms of the spinal cord commonly have cysts associated with them. These cysts have been termed tumoral (or intratumoral) and nontumoral (reactive) (Fig. 17-18). Cysts rostral or caudal to the solid portion of the tumor (nontumoral) are secondary to dilatation of the central canal. They do not enhance, are not echogenic on intraoperative ultrasound, do not have septations, and usually disappear after resection of the solid lesion. Allegedly, fluid produced by the tumors dilates the central canal producing the cyst. Tumoral cysts (more common in astrocytoma) occur within the tumor and may show peripheral enhancement.

Astrocytoma These neoplasms make up approximately 40% of spinal tumors and usually occur in the children (most common intramedullary tumor), and adults in their third to fifth decade of life (with a mean age of 29 years). Males are affected more than females.

The thoracic cord is most commonly involved followed by the cervical region. The tumors are hypercellular, generally large without obvious margins, and involve the full diameter of the cord, but are more eccentric than ependymomas. The presentation is of pain and paresthesias followed by motor signs. In children, these lesions behave as grade 1 pilocystic astrocytomas with a good prognosis. Adults have a worse outcome related to the infiltrative nature of the lesion. Astrocytomas are graded I to IV with I being the pilocytic astrocytoma, II the low grade or fibrillary astrocytoma, III the anaplastic astrocytoma, and IV the glioblastoma multiforme. Most of the spinal cord astrocytomas are low grade with less than 2% being glioblastomas.

These tumors may produce mild scoliosis, widen the interpediculate distance, and vertebral scalloping but less than ependymomas. They are iso to low intensity on T1WI and high intensity on T2WI. The average length of involvement is 7 body segments. They may have an associated cystic component (usually tumoral with small irregular or eccentric morphology), which may be appreciated on T1WI as hypointensity (this is a generalization and may not always hold true, as with other generalizations on intensity) (Fig. 17-19). Hemorrhage is uncommon. Syrinx is common in the pilocytic variety. Enhancement is the general rule, although it may be uneven compared with the intense enhancement of ependymoma. Malignant potential is generally less than that of brain astrocytomas. Exophytic components are sometimes present. The size of the tumor does not necessarily reflect its malignant potential (repeatedly we see that size is overrated). These tumors are associated with neurofibroma type 1 (NF1), infiltrating and not generally resectable.

Ependymoma Ependymomas are generally more focal (involving an average of 3.6 vertebral body segments), although they can be extensive (reported to involve 15 vertebral body segments), and as they arise from ependymal cells from the central canal, they tend to occupy the central portion of the cord. They account for 50% to 60% of spinal cord tumors in the third to fifth decade of life (most common intramedullary neoplasm in adults), and may be associated with neurofibromatosis type 2. Although unencapsulated, these glial neoplasms are well circumscribed, noninfiltrating, histologically benign with slow growth and, in certain circumstances, are totally resectable. They most commonly involve the cervical spinal cord (44%), with extension into the upper thoracic spinal cord in an additional 23%. Twenty-six percent are located in the thoracic cord alone. Symptoms are generally mild, delaying diagnosis, with back or neck pain the most common complaint followed by sensory deficits and motor weakness, and bowel and bladder dysfunction. The 5 year survival is over 80%. Metastatic spread to extraspinal

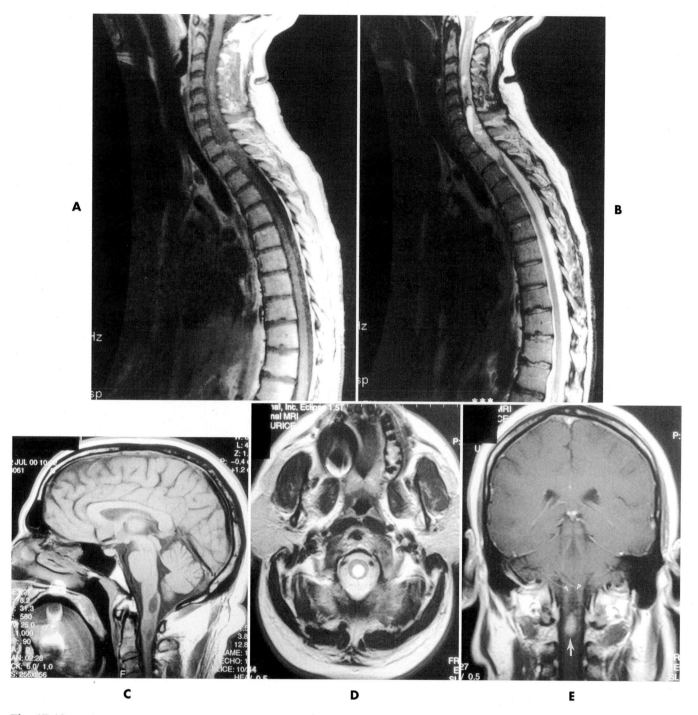

Fig. 17-18   Neoplastic cysts gallery. **A,** The tumoral cyst is not as evident on the sagittal T1WI as it is on the T2WI (**B**) where a fluid-fluid level *(arrowheads)* in the cervical spine is seen. **C,** In this case the cyst above the tumor is reactive and nonneoplastic. It is bright on T2WI axial imaging (**D**), but (**E**) it does not enhance *(arrowheads)* on the postcontrast study. As one would expect, the tumor does enhance *(arrows).*

sites include the retroperitoneum and lymph nodes. Ependymomas outside the CNS (broad ligament and sacrococcygeal region) have a strong association with spina bifida occulta.

They appear iso to hypointense with respect to the cord on T1WI and may have a multinodular high signal picture on T2WI that occupies the whole width of the cord. Commonly there is edema surrounding the tumor. Ependymomas have a propensity to hemorrhage, with hypointense rims ("cap sign") on T2WI, that histopathologically represent residual hemosiderin from hemorrhage. They can be the cause of subarachnoid hemor-

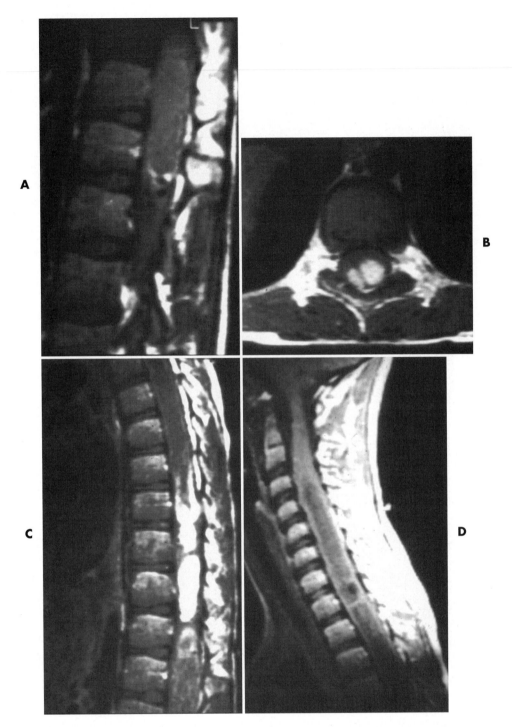

Fig. 17-19   Astrocytoma of thoracic spinal cord. **A,** Sagittal T1WI. **B,** Postcontrast axial T1WI reveals homogeneous enhancement in the tumor. **C,** Sagittal postcontrast T1WI. **D,** Observe the extensive reactive cysts in the cervical region above the tumor.

rhage. Hemosiderosis has also been reported to result from ependymoma. Enhancement is common, and the tumor may have sharply defined, intensely enhancing margins. They may be associated with extensive cyst formation (in up to 84% of ependymomas—mostly nontumoral cysts but tumoral cysts may also occur), which does not usually enhance. Other associated radiographic

findings include scoliosis, canal widening with vertebral body scalloping, pedicle erosion, or laminar thinning (Fig. 17-20).

Ependymoma is the most common primary spinal cord tumor of the lower spinal cord, conus medullaris and filum terminale (6.5% of spinal ependymomas), and often produces a lobulated mass. Thus, these neo-

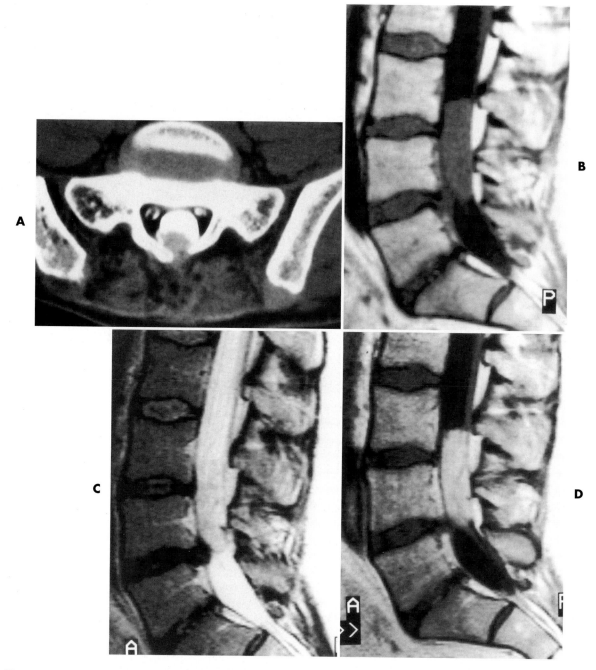

Fig. 17-20   Gallery of ependymoma. **A**, CT with intrathecal contrast outlining mass. **B**, Sagittal T1WI shows a mass filling the thecal sac in the mid lumbar region. **C**, It is very bright on the T2WI and could easily be overlooked without (**D**). **D**, the enhanced scan.

Illustration continued on following page

plasms can be both intramedullary and extramedullary intradural.

Myxopapillary ependymoma (13% of all spinal ependymomas) affects the filum with extension into the conus and in the subcutaneous sacrococcygeal region. The mean age on diagnosis is 35 and the lesion is more common in males. The presentation is of low back pain, leg pain, lower extremity weakness, and bladder dysfunction. These lesions are multilobulated, usually encapsu-

lated, mucin containing tumors that may hemorrhage and calcify. On MR they are usually isointense on T1WI, high intensity on T2WI, and enhance (see Fig. 17-20 E and F) However, as a result of calcification or hemorrhage they may be high intensity on T1 and T2WI.

Hemangioblastoma   Hemangioblastomas are vascular lesions that may involve the cervical and thoracic spinal cord. They are the third most common intramedullary spinal neoplasm (1% to 7% of all spinal cord

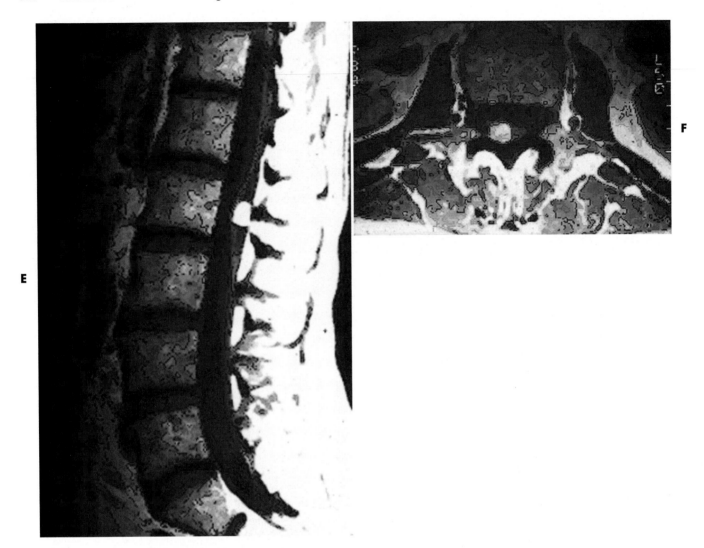

Fig. 17-20 *Continued.* **E,** This is a myxopapillary ependymoma of the lumbar region that is exophytic off the filum terminale. Its intrathecal location is better appreciated on the axial enhanced scan (**F**).

neoplasms). The tumor is composed of a dense network of capillary and sinus channels. They diffusely widen the spinal cord and may have both a cystic and solid component, with the solid component enhancing intensely. These tumors are associated with considerable edema (Fig. 17-21). Hemangioblastoma may be solid in 25% of cases.

Hemorrhagic components may be seen in the tumor nodule. There may be multiple lesions (20% of the time) in the spine and they may be eccentric, at times appearing extramedullary, or pial based, and they can occur on the nerve roots. With this presentation, the question of dropped hemangioblastoma from a cerebellar lesion versus primary spinal cord or nerve root lesions is always raised. Spinal angiography shows dilated arteries, a tumor stain, and draining vein. On MR, flow voids can be identified at times within the tumor and promi-

nent posterior draining veins can also be seen. They are variable intensity on T1WI and high intensity on T2WI with prominent flow voids. Edema can be noted surrounding the lesions. Avid homogeneous enhancement is visualized in the solid portion of the tumor.

Spinal cord hemangioblastomas may be an isolated lesion (80%), but one third of cases are associated with von Hippel-Lindau disease and are multiple (see Chapter 9). Von Hippel-Lindau disease has been isolated to chromosome 3.

Ganglioglioma/Gangliocytoma The terms ganglioglioma and gangliocytoma are frequently used synonymously. For the stickler ganglioglioma are derived from neurons or ganglion cells and gangliocytomas are derived from Schwann cells. Most important for radiologists is that they look the same, behave then same, and are treated the same. These are rare tumors (1.1% of all spinal

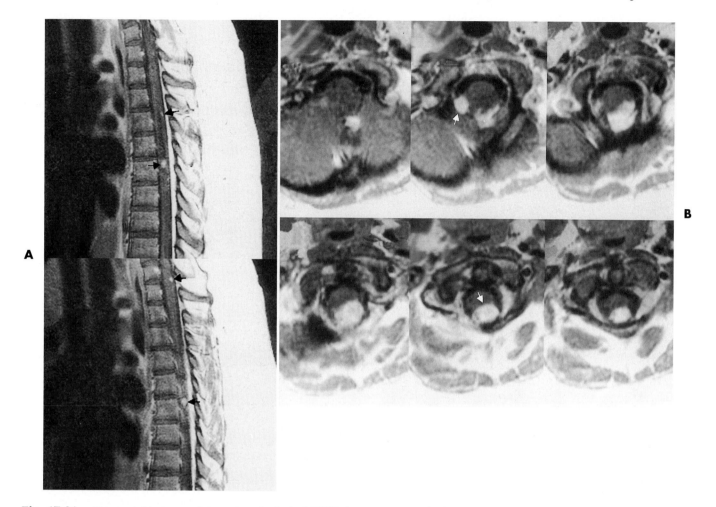

Fig. 17-21   Hemangioblastoma of the spine. **A,** Sagittal T1WI demonstrates multiple enhancing nodules *(arrows)* along the thoracic spinal cord. The cord is enlarged and there is low intensity centrally. **B,** Axial T1WI at the cervicomedullary junction shows enhancement of multiple masses *(arrows)* representing other hemangioblastomas in this region. Note that in this case the lesions are solid.

cord neoplasms), most frequent in children and young adults (average age of 12), consisting of neoplastic large mature neurons or ganglion cells and neoplastic glial cells. These lesions are slow growing, relatively benign neoplasms with the majority occurring in the cervical cord and less commonly involving the thoracic cord, conus, or entire spinal cord. Findings in this tumor include involvement consisting of long segments of tumor (commonly extending to over 8 vertebral body segments) associated with scoliosis and bony remodeling, mixed signal on T1WI and high intensity on T2WI, prominent tumoral cysts, patchy enhancement that extends to the pial surface without central enhancement (15% of cases demonstrate no enhancement), lack of edema, hemosiderin, or calcification, and an average patient age of 12 years. Gross resection of the tumor is recommended.

Intradural metastatic disease   Metastases can deposit on the dura, pia-arachnoid region, and rarely in the cord itself (Fig. 17-22). The incidence of leptomeningeal and intramedullary metastases (up to 3% of patients with metastatic disease) is increasing as patients with cancer live longer. Patients may have nonspecific symptoms (headache, back pain) or focal neurologic symptoms. Intramedullary lesions result from tumor growth along the Virchow-Robin spaces because of CSF spread. Spinal cord metastases may also occur as a result of hematogenous dissemination. Intramedullary metastases enlarge the cord, are associated with edema, and enhance (see Fig. 17-17). The most common location is the cervical cord followed by the thoracic region. They are usually solitary lesions involving 2 to 3 vertebral body segments. Box 17-8 lists lesions that commonly metastasize to the spinal cord or its coverings.

Intraspinal metastases are usually low intensity on T1WI and high intensity on T2WI (prominent edema surrounding the tumor nodule) with avid homogeneous enhancement of the tumor nodule.

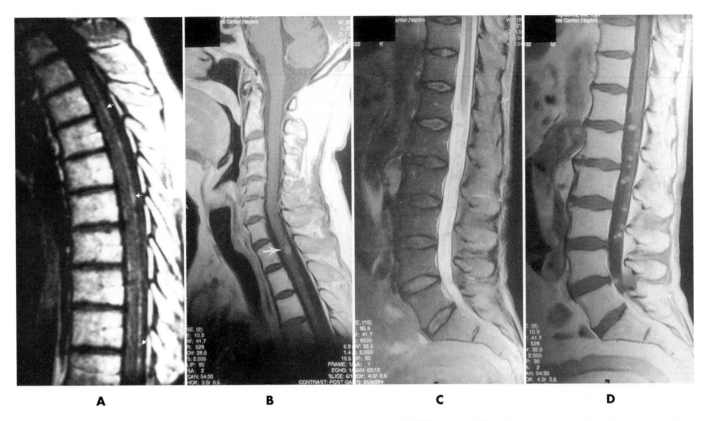

Fig. 17-22   **A,** Subarachnoid seeding from metastatic melanoma. Enhanced T1WI shows diffuse linear and nodular enhancement *(arrows)* on posterior and anterior surface of the spinal cord. **B,** This man with lung cancer had an intramedullary metastasis *(arrow)* in the thoracic cord, but he also had subarachnoid spread seen by the second year fellow (a vanishing breed) on the T2WI **(C)** and by the second year resident on the post contrast T1WI **(D).**

Box 17-8   Lesions that Commonly Metastasize to the Spinal Cord or Leptomeninges

CHILDREN

Chord plexus tumors
Ependymoma
Glioblastoma
Leukemia
Lymphoma
Neuroblastoma
Pineal region tumors (e.g., germinoma, pineoblastoma)
Primitive neuroectodermal tumor
Retinoblastoma

ADULTS

Glioblastoma multiforme
Hemangioblastoma
Lymphoma leukemia
Melanoma (primary or metastasis)
Metastases from lung, breast, renal, and gastric carcinomas
Oligodendroglioma

CSF spread of tumor in the leptomeninges may be diagnosed either by MR or by myelography combined with CT (myelo-CT). We prefer enhanced MR in the workup of leptomeningeal metastases; however, one additional benefit of myelography is the obtained CSF. Lumbar puncture in carcinomatous meningitis is abnormal, with positive cytology on serial punctures, in 90% of cases. MR reveals enhancement of the metastatic nodules, producing an irregular cord margin rather than its usual smooth contour. The entire subarachnoid space can enhance (sugar-coated appearance), and tumor nodules can be seen on nerve roots or in the cauda equina (Christmas balls). Pial metastases reveal linear enhancement on the surface of the cord (Fig. 17-22A); however, this can be observed in nonmalignant disease including sarcoidosis and infection. The CSF on T1WI can be more intense than normal and the conspicuity between CSF and cord may be diminished. Cerebral MR is necessary in this situation because leptomeningeal metastases may be the result of CSF seeding from brain parenchymal metastases.

Parameningeal masses are a preferred presentation for leukemia (termed chloromas), which can grow through the intervertebral foramina, a mode of spread also noted in both Hodgkin and non-Hodgkin lymphoma. CNS lymphoma rarely occurs as an intramedullary lesion (3%).

Extramedullary Intradural Lesions

Meningioma *Meningiomas* are well-circumscribed, globular lesions with a female predominance and constitute about 25% of spinal canal neoplasms. They are usually located in the thoracic region (approximately 80%) but can occur in any location throughout the spine. They may coexist with neurofibromas or neurofibromatosis type 2. The vast majority are extramedullary intradural but in rare cases they can be both intra and extradural or purely extradural (higher tendency to be malignant).

These tumors are isointense to slightly hypointense on T1WI and may have a heterogeneous texture. Most of the time these typical intradural extramedullary lesions are obvious on nonenhanced images (Fig. 17-23).

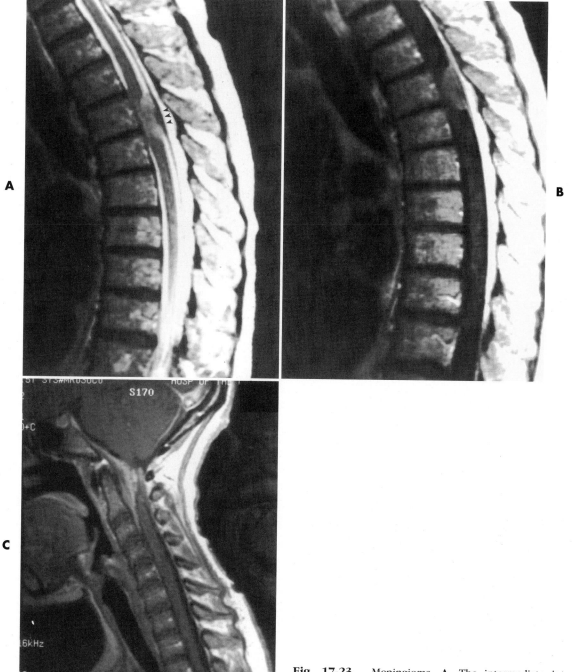

Fig. 17-23 Meningioma. **A,** The intermediate intensity intradural extramedullary mass has a meniscus sign seen on the T2WI. Note the dural thickening *(arrowheads).* **B,** The lesion faintly enhances. **C,** This cervicomedullary meningioma exhibits more of an en plaque configuration to the enhancement.

Meningiomas enhance and may show a dural tail. On T2WI they are iso to slightly high intensity with respect to the spinal cord and are usually well demarcated by the bright CSF. They shove the spinal cord to the opposite side and enlarge the CSF above and below the tumor on the ipsilateral side.

They originate from the denticulate ligament, are usually subdural in location, and may compress the cord but do not invade it. Meningiomas may demonstrate calcification and may widen the neural foramen, but far less often than schwannomas. Other characteristics that distinguish meningiomas from nerve sheath tumors include: (a) their position, with meningiomas posterolateral and nerve sheath tumors anterior; (b) there is a tendency for multiplicity of nerve sheath tumors; and (c) nerve sheath tumors may have low intensity central regions on postgadolinium T1WI and T2WI (see following section).

Nerve sheath tumors: schwannoma and neurofibroma Two types of benign nerve sheath tumors can be distinguished histopathologically: the schwannoma and the neurofibroma. Schwannomas (also termed neurinoma or neurilemoma) are encapsulated masses arising from a focal point. They are frequently associated with hemorrhage, intrinsic vascular changes (such as thrombosis or sinusoidal dilatation), cysts, and fatty degeneration. Neurofibromas consist of diffuse proliferation of Schwann cells and are well circumscribed but not encapsulated. Collagen is a conspicuous element in the neurofibroma as opposed to the schwannoma. Unlike schwannoma, they demonstrate little proclivity toward hemorrhage, vascular change, or fatty degeneration. In patients with NF1, all spinal nerve root tumors are neurofibromas; however, neurofibromas can occur in patients without NF1. In patients with neurofibromatosis type 2, almost all spinal nerve root tumors are schwannomas or mixed tumors rather than neurofibromas. In the spine, solitary lesions are usually schwannomas. In spinal neurofibromatosis, there is also a higher incidence of schwannomas than neurofibromas. In dumbbell lesions with both intraforaminal and extraforaminal components, schwannomas are seen as solitary lesions whereas neurofibromas are often multiple and occur with neurofibromatosis. One issue is that not every dumbbell shaped spinal tumor is of neurogenic origin. Indeed, any mass in the spinal canal can assume a dumbbell shape. Benign lesions tend to have regular margins and enlarge the intervertebral foramina in contrast to malignant lesions with irregular margins. Schwannomas occur more commonly in the sensory root. A young patient with a neurofibroma is likely to have NF1, whereas the patient with a schwannoma may have neurofibromatosis type 2 or neither type 1 nor 2.

Schwannomas are composed of Antoni tissue type A and type B. The type B tissue is responsible for the cystic changes sometimes noted within the mass. Schwannomas may occur in a purely intradural location (two thirds of cases), be partially intradural and extradural (one sixth), or purely extradural (one sixth). Neural foramina are enlarged, and tumor transgressing the foramen can be noted. These lesions may be multiple in neurofibromatosis and may undergo malignant degeneration.

It is impossible to separate schwannoma from neurofibroma by imaging (but Table 17-2 attempts to compare these entities), and thus they are clumped together. They are usually isointense on T1WI and are hyperintense on T2WI. They also enhance. Areas that are isointense or of high intensity on T1WI and low signal on PDWI and T2WI have been associated with hemorrhage (Fig. 17-24). A low intensity area ("dot") has been seen on postcontrast T1WI and thought to increase specificity for the diagnosis of neurofibroma/neurilemmoma. The substrate of this nonenhancing area includes calcification, old hemorrhage, fibrosis, foam cells, microcysts, edema, (we know—who cares?) These benign tumors (both schwannoma and neurofibroma) are slow growing and tend to erode bone, particularly if they are dumbbell shaped. (The authors have observed many other dumbbells, not all of them lesions.) Calcification is rare

---

Table 17-2 Schwannoma versus neurofibroma*

Schwannoma (aka neurinoma/neuilemoma)	Neurofibroma
Encapsulated mass arises from a focal point on sensory root	Diffuse proliferation of Schwann's cells, well circumscribed but not encapsulated
Hemorrhage	No hemorrhage, vascular changes, or fatty degeneration
Intrinsic vascular changes (thrombosis; sinusoidal dilatation)	Spinal nerve root tumors in NF1
Cysts	Can also be seen in patients without NF1
Fatty degeneration	
Spinal nerve root tumors in NF2	Spinal nerve root tumors in NF1
Solitary lesions	Solitary or multiple
Noninfiltrative	Can be plexiform and infiltrative

*This table is not worth much because they cannot be distinguished readily by radiologists.

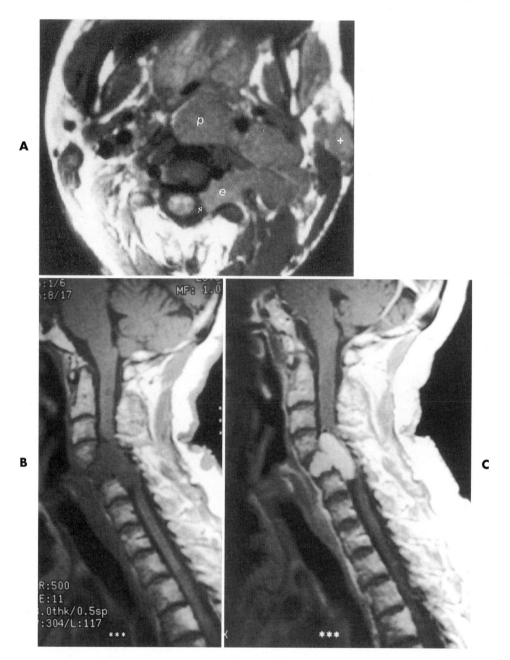

Fig. 17-24   Neurogenic tumor parade of champions. **A,** Dumbbell neurofibroma. Axial T1WI in a patient with neurofibromatosis delineates the intradural portion of the neurofibroma *(arrow)* and the extradural intraforaminal tumor *(e)*. Anteriorly there is a large plexiform neurofibroma *(p)*, and a subcutaneous neurofibroma *(+)*. Asymmetry can be seen in the muscles of the neck. **B,** Sagittal T1WIs on this case before **(B)** and after **(C)** contrast show an extra-axial, markedly enhancing mass associated with a slight reversed gibbus deformity.

Illustration continued on following page

compared with meningioma. Careful evaluation of the sagittal image reveals expansion of the neural foramen. Other findings that are associated with neurofibromatosis and that occasionally can be confused with nerve tumors are enlarged neural foramina and vertebral scalloping secondary to dural ectasia, lateral meningocele, or an arachnoid cyst. Lesions having a diffuse multi-nodular appearance have been termed plexiform neurofibro-

mas, being either schwannomas or neurofibromas, and are usually associated with neurofibromatosis.

Hereditary motor and sensory neuropathies (HMSN)   This is a group of diseases, in some cases, associated with hypertrophic peripheral and cranial nerves. We have excluded HMSN 2 and 4 because of the lack of imaging findings—we think. These diseases are characterized by concentric proliferation of Schwann

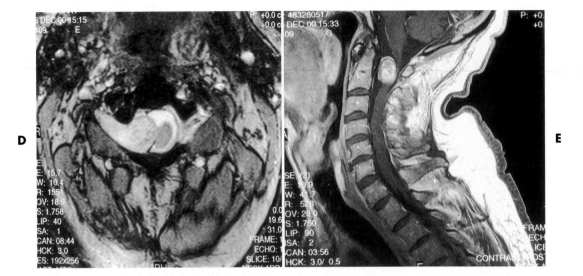

Fig. 17-24 *Continued.* **D,** Another schwannoma at the C2 level is both compressing the cord and expanding the neural foramen with a spectrum of intensities. It has a lamellated appearance to its enhancement (**E**).

cells, interspersed with collagen, in response to multiple episodes of demyelination and remyelination. This process results in an "onion bulb" appearance to the nerve. Cases present with a variety of signs and symptoms depending on the particular disease. On MR, enlargement and, at times, enhancement of the nerve roots can be seen. We have placed our discussion in this location because they are in the radiological differential diagnosis of neurofibromatosis.

Charcot-Marie-Tooth disease (CMT or HMSN 1) is usually an autosomal dominant disease that presents with slowly progressive distal atrophy (common peroneal muscular atrophy) and weakness in conjunction with pes cavus and scoliosis. The posterior columns, optic, and acoustic nerves may be involved. CMT is commonly misdiagnosed as a primary orthopedic problem.

Dejerine-Sottas disease (HMSN III) is an autosomal recessive condition with slowly progressive motor and sensory loss and ataxia. Scoliosis and pes cavus are frequent. There are enlarged peripheral and cranial nerves with hypomyelination. Imaging findings included enlarged nerves best demarcated on T2WI with variable enhancement (Fig 17-25).

Chronic inflammatory demyelinating polyradiculoneuropathy (CIDP) is an acquired disorder characterized by the slow onset of proximal weakness, paresthesias, and numbness. Cranial and peripheral nerves may be enlarged and can enhance. CIPD is often associated with lesions in the brain that appear similar to those of multiple sclerosis. Knowledge of these entity will score extra brownie points at rounds.

Lastly, you should appreciate that paraneoplastic syndromes have been reported to enlarged nerves cranial and peripheral nerves produced by a microvasculitis with associated with inflammatory changes.

Lipoma   Lipomas are usually seen in the first three decades of life and are most common in the thoracic region but can be seen throughout the spine. In the lumbar region, they are associated with myelodysplasia or the tethered cord (see Chapter 9). They are commonly identified in the filum terminale (1.5% to 5% prevalence). Lipomas may be intradural (60% of cases) or extradural (40%). Imaging characteristics include low density on CT or high signal on T1WI, and lower signal on standard T2WI (not fast spin-echo images). With fat suppression, they appear dark. These lesions can be extensive and compress the spinal cord. Lipomas could be confused superficially with hemorrhage, but signal intensity is suppressed with fat-suppression techniques whereas hemorrhage remains high signal. Chemical shift artifact can be identified along the frequency-encoding axis (Fig. 17-26). The differential diagnosis of fat-like lesions is provided in Box 17-9.

If you observe fat in a sacrococcygeal mass, consider the diagnosis of teratoma. There is a female predominance and a high incidence (as high as 60%) of malignant transformation, especially in male patients. There is also a high association of other anomalies, including anorectal ones. Lesions present as a large expansile mass, with fatty, cystic, and solid components, and may even be hemorrhagic. Elevated levels of α-fetoprotein are associated with the tumor. Teratomas may also occur within the spinal cord (see Fig. 17-26).

Extradural Neoplastic and Nonneoplastic Lesions

The vertebral bodies are the most frequent site of metastatic disease to the spine. Contrary to previous notions, the vast majority of metastases begin in the verte-

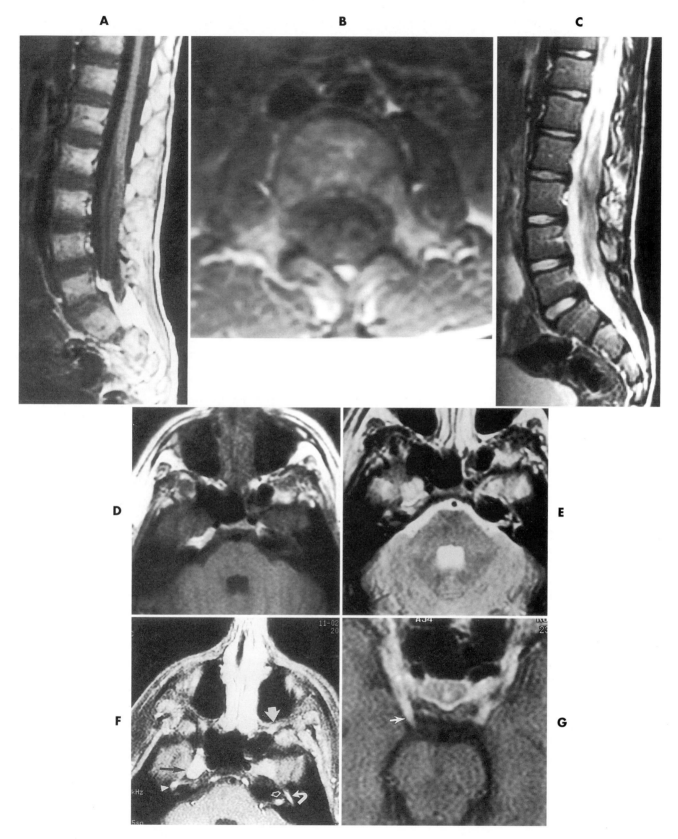

Fig. 17-25   **A to C,** Dejerine Sottas. Markedly thickened lumbar nerve roots are present in this patient with HMSN-3. The roots did not enhance. **D** and **E,** T1 and T2WI of enlarged cranial nerves at skull base. (Difficult to see without contrast F and G.) **F** and **G,** Enhanced T1WI. Enhancing and enlarged 3rd division of trigeminal *(arrow)* and greater superficial petrosal nerve *(arrowheads)* left VII *(curved arrows),* VIII nerve *(open arrow),* pterygopalatine ganglia *(fat arrow).* **G,** Enlarged enhancing right 3rd nerve *(arrow).*

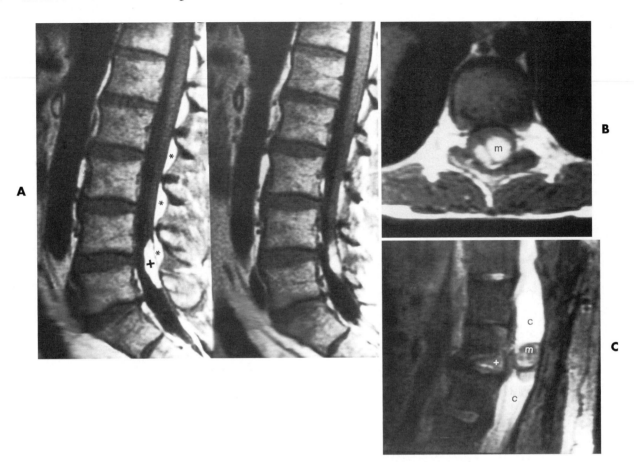

Fig. 17-26   Fatty intraspinal masses. **A,** Extramedullary lipoma *(+)* with a tethered cord is seen on this sagittal T1WI. You can appreciate the normal epidural fat *(∗)*. **B,** Axial T1WI of a patient with an *intramedullary* fatty mass *(m)* shows high intensity and septations. **C,** Sagittal T2WI of the same patient as in **B** shows a vertebral anomaly *(+)* at the level of the mass. Note that the mass has cystic *(c)* and fatty *(m)* components. This combination of findings suggests a teratoma.

bral body and subsequently grow into the region of the pedicle and posterior elements. The normal high intensity on T1WI from fatty marrow is replaced by lower signal intensity from tumor cells and associated increased water content (Fig. 17-27). Later there is destruction of the bony trabeculae, usually without periosteal response. MR is thus more sensitive in most cases at diagnosing metastatic disease than plain films or CT. On conventional T2WI the tumor-replaced marrow appears as high

Box 17-9 Differential Diagnosis of Fat-like Lesions

Epidural lipomatosis˚
Melanoma
Neurenteric cysts
Pantopaque˚
Rupture dermoid˚
Subacute hemorrhage
Teratoma˚

˚Suppress with fat saturation

signal intensity compared with the normal fatty marrow, which is of lower signal intensity. Common cancers associated with spinal metastasis include breast, prostate, lung, and kidney. Other lesions include Ewing sarcoma (which usually is seen in the sacrum and lumbar spine in the first three decades of life), neuroblastoma, melanoma, lymphoma, leukemia, multiple myeloma, and sarcoma. Pelvic lesions metastasize through the epidural plexus of veins (Batson's plexus) to the thoracolumbar bodies. Lymphoma rarely can present as an epidural mass without bone involvement.

On plain films most metastases are osteolytic or a combination of osteolytic and osteoblastic. Particular metastases associated with osteoblastic changes include prostate, breast, carcinoid, ovarian, and transitional cell carcinoma, and lymphoma. These lesions are not bright on T2WI but are still hypointense on T1WI. There appear to be two distinct patterns of breast metastases excluding patients with extensive diffuse metastases. Those patients with the presence of positive tumor estrogen or progesterone receptors develop osseous but not brain metastases. Patients with negative receptors tend to have brain and not osseous metastases.

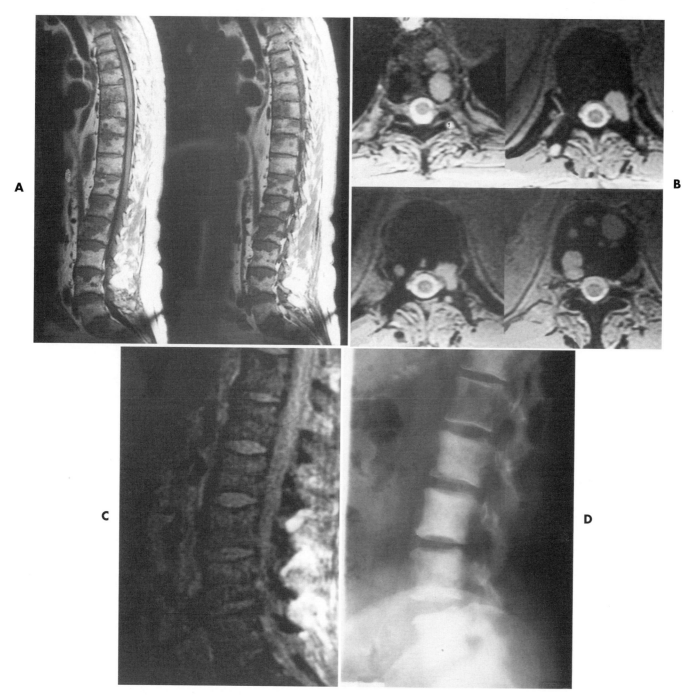

Fig. 17-27   Metastatic lesions. **A,** Note the low intensity lesions outlined by residual fat in the vertebral bodies on this sagittal T1WI in a patient with breast metastases. **B,** (Same patient as **A.**) Axial T2WI of one vertebra reveals multiple high intensity metastases in the vertebral body and pedicles. **C,** No, this is not a poorly photographed image. Rather, it is, believe it or not, a T1WI in another patient with diffuse osteoblastic breast metastases. Note that the disks are of higher intensity than the vertebral bodies. This is a tip-off that something is not kosher. Another observation is that the CSF is higher in intensity than normal. This was due to the high protein content caused by leptomeningeal seeding. **D,** Lateral spine radiograph confirms the osteoblastic metastases.

Osteoporosis

Osteoporosis is characterized by decreased bone mass. It is associated with compression fractures that are spontaneous or associated with minimal trauma (Fig.

17-28). These are usually located in the midthoracic and in the lower thoracic high lumbar regions. Osteoporosis is the most common cause of compression fractures and is particularly observed in elderly women.

Osteoporotic vertebral compression fractures have a reduction in vertebral height of more than 15%. Their

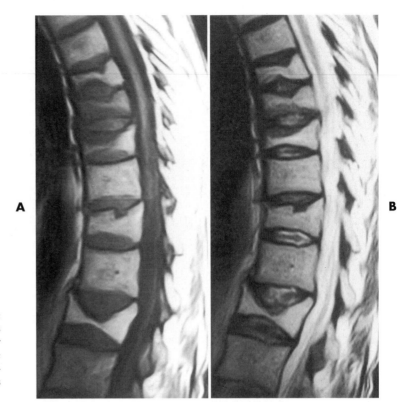

Fig. 17-28 Osteoporotic compression fractures: Note that the normal signal intensity of the bone marrow is preserved on the T1WI (**A**) and FSE T2WI. **B,** The linear striations of the upper vertebrae also are more indicative of benign compression fractures as opposed to neoplastic ones. There is no bone destruction or soft tissue mass associated with these fractures.

prevalence in women over 50 has been estimated to be 26%. It is difficult to distinguish between acute osteoporotic vertebral collapse and acute collapse from metastatic disease. Both may be associated with pain, and compress the spinal canal. The pain from an acute fracture usually lasts 4 to 6 weeks and is associated with exquisite pain at the fracture site. The spinal cord may be compressed in these fractures.

Table 17-3 provides CT criteria that have been reported to be useful in the separation of benign versus malignant acute compression fracture. The presence of all bone fragments from the original cortex (puzzle sign) is both very constant and quite specific for benign disease. It is interesting that sclerosis, marked comminution of cancellous bone of the vertebral body, Schmorl's

nodes, or fracture of a pedicle have low specificity for separating benign from malignant disease.

On MR, both may have low signal on T1WI and high signal on T2WI, and enhance. Both could involve multiple vertebral bodies and be associated with soft-tissue masses. Paraspinal mass is more likely to be metastatic disease. If the fracture has normal-appearing marrow signal on all pulse sequences, it is benign. Diffuse replacement of the entire vertebral body strongly suggests malignant disease. Cortical destruction, abnormal signal throughout vertebral bodies that are not compressed, and involvement of the posterior elements all suggest malignant disease. In the presence of other metastatic lesions in the spine, the collapsed vertebra most likely results from metastatic disease. Recently, diffusion

Table 17-3 CT features of benign and malignant acute compression fractures	
Benign	**Malignant**
Cortical fractures of the vertebral body without cortical bone destruction (puzzle sign)	Destruction of the anterolateral or posterior cortical bone of the vertebral body
Retropulsion of a bone fragment of the posterior cortex of the vertebral body into the spinal canal	Destruction of the cancellous bone of the vertebral body
Fracture lines within the cancellous bone of the vertebral body	Destruction of the vertebral pedicle
Thin diffuse paraspinal soft tissue mass	Focal paraspinal soft tissue mass
Intravertebral vacuum phenomenon	Epidural mass

Table 17-4   MR features of benign and malignant acute compression fractures

Benign	Malignant
Low intensity T1-acutely but returns to normal signal over 4–6 weeks	Low intensity T1—only returns to normal signal following radiation or at heaven's gate
High intensity T1-chronically	
Stripes of dark and bright on T1WI	Complete replacement of vertebral body with low intensity on T1WI
Enhances post gadolinium (not helpful)	Enhances post gadolinium (not helpful)
Smaller paraspinal soft tissue mass	Larger paraspinal soft tissue mass
Posterior elements less commonly affected	Posterior elements more commonly involved
ADC negative	ADC positive when there is cellular packing of the marrow
Usually not associated with an epidural mass	Epidural mass common
Overall mass of body diminished	Overall mass of body increased

weighted imaging has been applied in an attempt to distinguish benign from malignant. Compression fractures that are high intensity on diffusion weighted images (compared to normal bone marrow) were considered to be malignant whereas lesions with low intensity on diffusion were benign or traumatic. However, the results at this time are controversial and the methodology has not been generally implemented.

In the case of a single collapsed vertebral body in a patient with or without metastatic disease, a repeat image in 4 to 6 weeks is recommended. In this interval benign collapse progresses to isointensity on T1WI and T2WI, with decreased enhancement, whereas metastatic disease remains stable or progresses in size without a change in intensity. Although this waiting may be viewed as a cop-out, many times it is not possible to distinguish between acute, nontraumatic benign and metastatic vertebral body collapse. Naturally, the patient will have a full workup for occult malignancy, including bone scan to determine whether there are other lesions. The MR features are enumerated in Table 17-4. However, bone biopsy is the only definitive test for distinguishing benign versus malignant disease.

The list of diseases that can produce vertebral compression includes metastases, osteomyelitis, congenitally deficient vertebral endplates, benign and malignant primary vertebral neoplasms, osteomalacia, osteitis cystica of hyperparathyroidism, hemochromatosis, myeloproliferative disorders, and trauma.

Neural crest tumors Tumors of neural crest origin occur in infancy and arise from the sympathetic plexus. These include neuroblastoma (patients <5 years old), ganglioneuroblastoma (5 to 8 years old), and ganglioneuroma (5 to 8 years old) (Fig. 17-29). Calcification occurs in 30% of cases, and hemorrhage has been reported. These paravertebral masses, which usually occur in the thoracic region, can extend through the neural foramina to compress the thecal sac. They all enhance.

Melanoma Primary melanoma rarely can occur in the spinal cord or on spinal nerve roots. These may arise from melanocytes or Schwann cells, which share both, arise from the neural crest. If melanotic, this tumor can be high intensity on T1WI and low intensity on T2WI.

Hemangioma Hemangiomas are common benign lesions of the vertebral body and are most often incidental findings. They are composed of fully developed adult blood vessels. More than half of solitary hemangiomas occur in the spine and they have been found in approximately 12% of spines at autopsy. Multiple hemangiomas can occur in about a third of cases. There is a

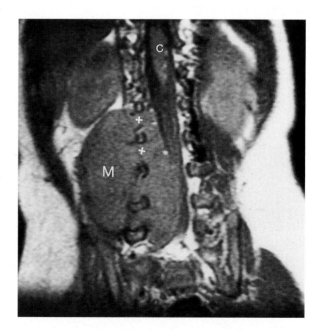

Fig. 17-29   Neuroblastoma. This paraspinal tumor mass *(M)* has spread through the neural foramen *(+)* into the epidural region and is compressing the nerve roots. Conus is identified *(c)*. The origin of this tumor may have been the sympathetic nervous plexus around the organ of Zuckerkandl (look it up!).

2:1 female/male predominance, with most lesions found in the lower thoracic and lumbar vertebrae. These lesions can be round or can be extensive, replacing the entire vertebral body with extension into the pedicles, arches, and spinous processes. The cortical margins are usually distinct, yet vertebral bodies with hemangiomas can have compression fractures or epidural extension and compromise the spinal canal or neural foramen. They have a striated appearance on plain films. The vertical striations represent vascular channels interspersed with thickened trabeculae. MR reveals high signal intensity on T1WI and T2WI because of their fat and water content (Fig. 17-30). With extraosseous extension, the signal intensity of the exophytic portion of the lesion may be dark on T1WI and high on T2WI. Problems occur when these lesions expand and compress the spinal cord or when they become hypervascular and produce venous hypertension. On spinal angiography, these lesions are vascular. On CT thick trabeculae with a salt-and-pepper picture are seen (boring analogy—if radiologists had more creativity, they would be cooks). Most

hemangiomas are asymptomatic; however, pain is associated with growth (especially in women during pregnancy) or compression fracture. Rarely, they can produce myelopathy from cord compression. The differential diagnosis is focal fatty marrow replacement. This can be distinguished on standard T2WI by noting decreased intensity of the focal fatty lesion and high signal in the nonfat containing regions of the hemangioma. If fast spin-echo imaging is used, then the fat and hemangioma are both bright on the T2WI, so that fat saturation should be used.

Chordoma Chordomas are a slow-growing, locally invasive neoplasm derived from remnants of the notochord, with approximately 50% originating in the sacral region and 15% affecting the spine (particularly the cervical region). In the spine, tumor mass is associated with lytic lesions of the bone, at times with a sclerotic rim and calcification. There is a spectrum of intensity patterns with some lesions demonstrating high signal on T1WI and T2WI. These lesions may involve the disk space and multiple vertebral bodies. In the differential

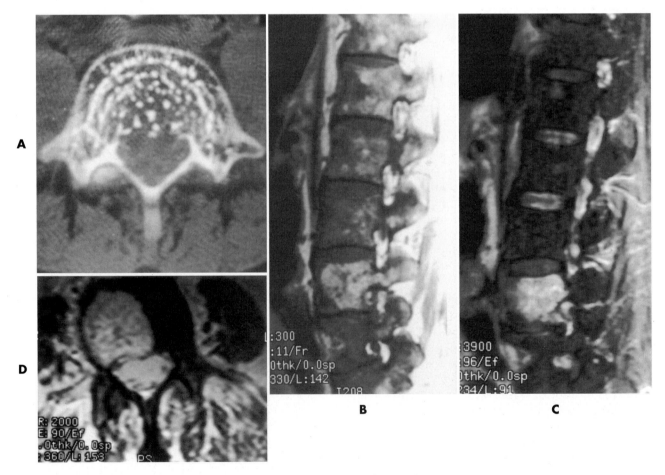

Fig. 17-30   A, Hemangioma. Unenhanced CT shows the characteristic polka-dot vertebra caused by vertical trabecular striations, with low density areas and high density spicules in this hemangioma. **B,** Parasagittal T1WI shows a high intensity bony mass in the vertebral body. **C,** The lesion is also bright on T2WI. Observe that the hemangioma extends to the pedicle. **D,** Note how closely the appearance on the axial T2WI mirrors that of the CT in (**A**).

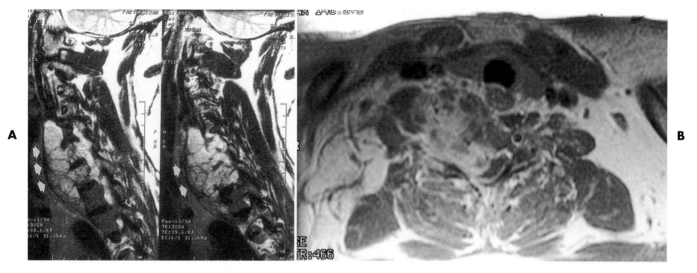

Fig. 17-31   Chordoma. **A,** This cervical spine mass displaces the longus colli musculature *(arrows)* anteriorly. It is very bright on T2WI, a feature that is characteristic of this tumor. **B,** The lesion erodes the lateral aspect of the vertebral body and extends to the right neural foramen. Chordomas can masquerade as herniated disks, schwannomas, and ependymomas.

diagnosis think about chordoma in bizarre cervical lesions that resemble large herniated disks, schwannoma, or unusual osteomyelitis (Fig. 17-31).

Chondrosarcoma   Chondrosarcoma may also occur in the spine and is associated with destruction of bone in the body or posterior elements. The hallmark of this lesion is chondroid calcification, which is much better detected on CT or plain film.

Aneurysmal bone cyst, giant cell tumor, osteoblastoma, and osteoid osteoma   Benign bony tumors of the spine include aneurysmal bone cyst, giant cell tumor, osteoblastoma, and osteoid osteoma and are best imaged on CT and plain films. These lesions have some characteristics that may help distinguish them. Osteoblastoma

(>1.5 cm) is larger than osteoid osteoma (<1.5 cm) and is much more common in the spine. Both have a propensity for the posterior elements or transverse process, have a lytic and/or calcific nidus surrounded by a sclerotic rim, and are associated with pain, which in the case of osteoid osteoma is classically described as nocturnal and relievable by aspirin (Fig. 17-32). Giant cell tumors are lytic lesions found commonly in the sacrum and vertebral bodies. Aneurysmal bone cysts are usually circumscribed multiloculated lytic lesions, occasionally containing hemorrhage (with fluid levels) and involving the posterior elements, particularly the lamina.

Eosinophilic granuloma   Eosinophilic granuloma affects children and predominantly involves the vertebral body. It is a rapidly growing tumor, producing bone loss and vertebral collapse associated with normal vertebral disk spaces (vertebra plana Box 17-10) (Fig. 17-33).

There may be associated soft-tissue extension from the vertebral body posteriorly into the vertebral canal or anteriorly. MR shows a collapsed vertebral body with heterogeneous intensity on T1WI. A bullet-shaped vertebral body in Hurler (mucopolysaccharidosis I) and Morquio (mucopolysaccharidosis IV) diseases may simulate vertebra plana of eosinophilic granuloma.

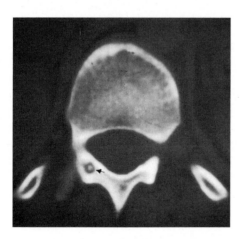

Fig. 17-32   Osteoid osteoma. There is a circumscribed lytic region in the right lamina on this CT with bone windows. In the central portion of the hypodense region *(arrow)* is a punctate area of high density. This is another classic!

Box 17-10   **Causes of Vertebral Plana**
Eosinophic granuloma
Fracture, osteogenesis imperfecta
Osteoporosis
Steroids
Tumors (leukemia, myeloma)

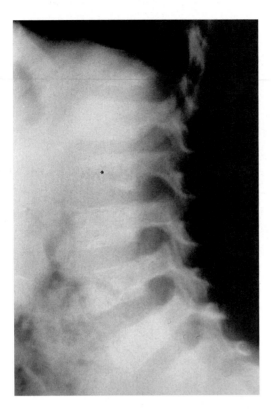

Fig. 17-33 Eosinophilic granuloma of the spine. Lateral spine film demonstrates vertebra plana *(asterisk)*. This is characteristic of eosinophilic granuloma involving the spine.

Osteochrondroma These lesions usually arise from the posterior elements and commonly involve the thoracic or lumbar vertebrae. They are commonly found in teenagers where they grow and occasionally cause neurologic symptoms. On MR these lesions are heterogeneous having high intensity on T2WI (from the cartilaginous portion of the lesion) and low intensity on all pulse sequences from the ossified part of the tumor.

Paget disease Paget disease commonly involves the spine and produces enlargement of all the vertebral elements. It usually demonstrates thickened bone cortex (distinguishing it from fibrous dysplasia), and sclerosis (late phase), with low intensity on T1WI and T2WI. Involvement is associated with back and neck pain and neurologic dysfunction associated with facet arthropathy, lateral recess syndrome, and central spinal stenosis. It is difficult at times to distinguish from osteoblastic metastatic disease. There is the possibility of malignant transformation to osteogenic sarcoma in approximately 10% of cases. The appearance of osteogenic sarcoma is variable, depending on whether the lesion is lytic, blastic, or mixed. Osteoid matrix or calcification appears as a signal void on all MR pulse sequences.

Multiple myeloma In multiple myeloma three patterns of marrow involvement have been observed on sagittal MR. The most common type reveals focal lesions with low intensity on T1WI and high intensity on T2WI. Rarely, lesions may be hyperintense on T1WI, probably because of hemorrhage within the myeloma foci. A second pattern consists of a variegated (inhomogeneous) appearance with tiny foci of hypointensity on T1WI and hyperintensity on T2WI. The third diffuse pattern represents total marrow involvement so that on T1WI the disks are hyperintense to the replaced fatty marrow. The diffuse and variegated appearance on T1WI can be confused with inhomogeneous distribution of fat in older patients. Both these lesion patterns enhance, which distinguishes them from inhomogeneous marrow. The focal lesion pattern also enhances. Vertebral compression may occur without the marrow being diffusely abnormal on MR. Vertebral compression fractures occur in 50% to 70% of patients and spinal cord compression in 10% to 15% of these cases, however, it appears that no correlation exists between the preexistence of focal vertebral marrow changes and the subsequent development of vertebral fractures.

MR patterns of diffuse and focal disease appear to correlate with more abnormal values of serum hemoglobin and the percentage of bone marrow plasmacytosis. Both symptomatic and asymptomatic patients may reveal these patterns early in the course of the disease.

A solitary plasmacytoma may be indistinguishable from a lytic metastasis and is a harbinger of multiple myeloma (Fig. 17-34). Plain films and CT demonstrate purely lytic lesions or diffuse osteopenia. It is unusual for myeloma to involve the pedicles. Consider myeloma in a patient with diffuse osteopenia and compression fractures (particularly male patients). On CT, destruction of cortical bone is much less common in myeloma than metastatic disease whereas cancellous vertebral body destruction occurs in both metastatic and myelomatous lesions. Rarely, less than 1% of cases can involve the leptomeninges with enhancement of the nerve roots. Remember that myeloma is one of the diseases that may be difficult to detect with bone scans.

Vertebroplasty This technique has been used to treat both benign osteoporotic and malignant vertebral body collapse as well as benign tumors such as hemangiomas of the vertebral body. The procedure involves injection of bone cement into the affected vertebral body. The methodology is beyond the price of this text. The procedure is useful in ameliorating pain resulting from vertebral body collapse. Complications result from leakage of cement into veins resulting in compression of the spinal cord or nerves or pulmonary embolism. Patients at the highest risk for complications are those with metastatic disease owing to destruction of the posterior cortex. Increased activity on bone scan in a vertebral compression fracture has been suggested to be predictive of a favorable outcome after vertebroplasty.

Epidural lipomatosis Epidural lipomatosis can occur from a number of different causes including obesity,

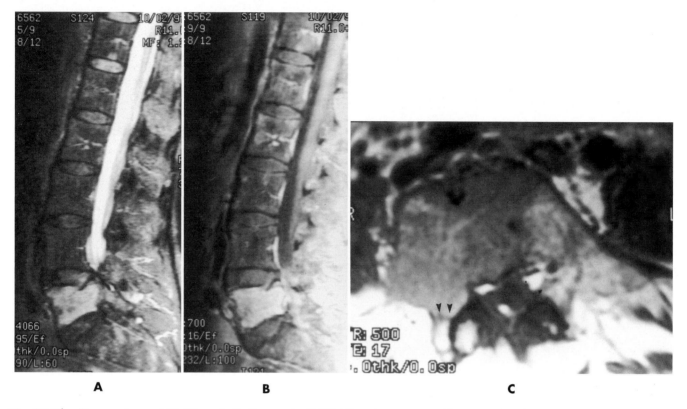

Fig. 17-34   Plasmacytoma of L5. The only finding on the T2WI (**A**) and postcontrast T1WI (**B**) that would suggest multiple myeloma and a plasmacytoma in this case is the low intensity marrow signal of the uninvolved vertebral bodies on the enhanced study (**B**). This could easily be a metastasis. (**C**) The lesion *(arrowheads)* spares the pedicle.

steroids (usually after prolonged use of oral steroids), and Cushing's syndrome. The fatty tissue is seen posteriorly and can produce significant cord compression. This is an obvious diagnosis on T1W1.

VASCULAR LESIONS

Infarction

Spinal cord ischemia and infarction can occur at any location in the cord but has a propensity for the upper thoracic or thoracolumbar regions because of the tenuous blood supply. The clinical presentation includes profound impairment of bowel and bladder function, loss of perineal sensation, and moderate impairment of sensory and motor function of the lower extremities. Ischemia to the conus may result from poor collateral supply after occlusion of the dominant blood supply (artery of Adamkiewicz). Rarely posterior spinal artery infarcts can be seen (think about vasculitis here).

In patients with the acute onset of symptoms referable to the spinal cord, conus medullaris, or cauda equina, and with what appears to be an enlarged cord or tumorlike conus on MR, think spinal cord infarction (Fig. 17-35). Infarction can be the result of problems as-

sociated with the descending aorta, such as atheroma, aortic surgery, and dissecting aneurysm. Other causes include vertebral occlusion or dissection, arteritis, vascular malformations, pregnancy, hypotension, sickle cell anemia, caisson disease, tuberculosis, meningitis, arachnoiditis, vascular malformation, diabetes, degenerative disease of the spine, and disk herniation with spinal artery injury or perhaps fibrocartilaginous emboli.

On MR high signal on T2WI is noted in the cord, which is usually enlarged, whereas enhancement may or may not be present. Occasionally, vertebral body high signal intensity on T2WI can be identified and is most likely the result of concomitant infarction (see Fig. 17-35B). Seeing high intensity in a vertebra in association with an acute nontraumatic myelopathy should strongly suggest spinal cord infarction. Careful attention should be paid to the aorta for aortic dissection or aneurysms as a cause.

Arteriovenous Malformations

There are a variety of classifications for spinal vascular malformations (Fig. 17-36). We present a simple one (sticking with our philosophy that if you wanted sophistication you would be reading the original manuscripts rather than Bob and Dave's simple book—from

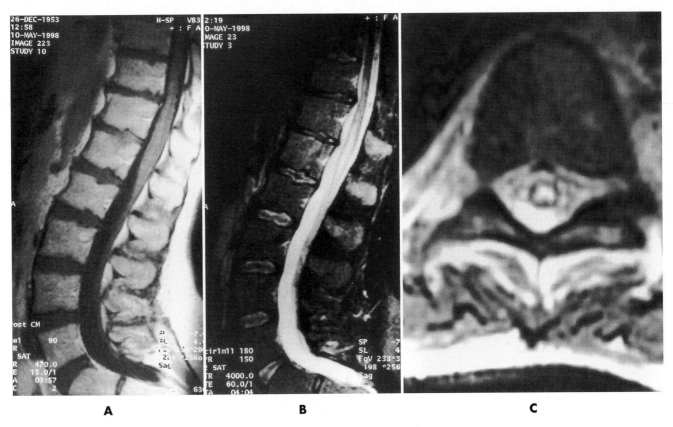

Fig. 17-35   Cord infarct. **A,** Swelling of the conus medullaris is present on this T1WI. **(B)** The signal intensity of the swollen cord is abnormally bright on the T2WI. Note the high intensity in the vertebral body, possibly from a bone infarct. **C,** Central cord high signal intensity is characteristic of a cord infarct. Sparing posteriorly is the norm.

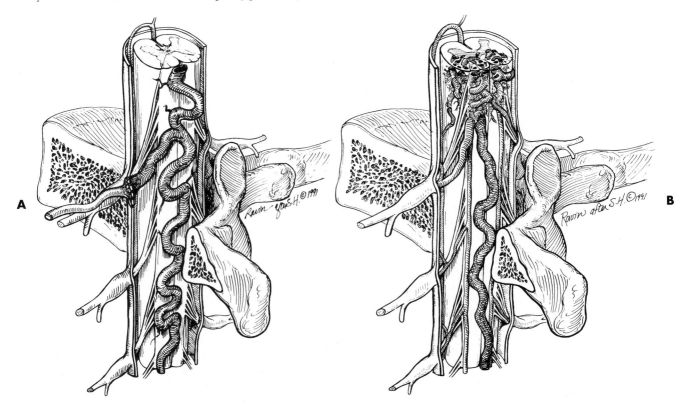

Fig. 17-36   Cord arteriovenous malformations (AVMs). **A,** Posterolateral view of the spinal cord with part of the lamina and dura removed. The fistula site of this type I spinal AVM is located in the proximal nerve root sleeve. Surgical ligation of the fistula interrupts the direct flow of arterial blood into the coronal venous plexus. Stripping the dilated venous network is unnecessary and can even produce neurologic morbidity. **B,** Type II or intramedullary spinal AVM. It has multiple arterial feeders from both the anterior and posterior spinal arteries. The nidus is located within the spinal cord and drains into a dilated venous plexus.

Illustration continued on following page

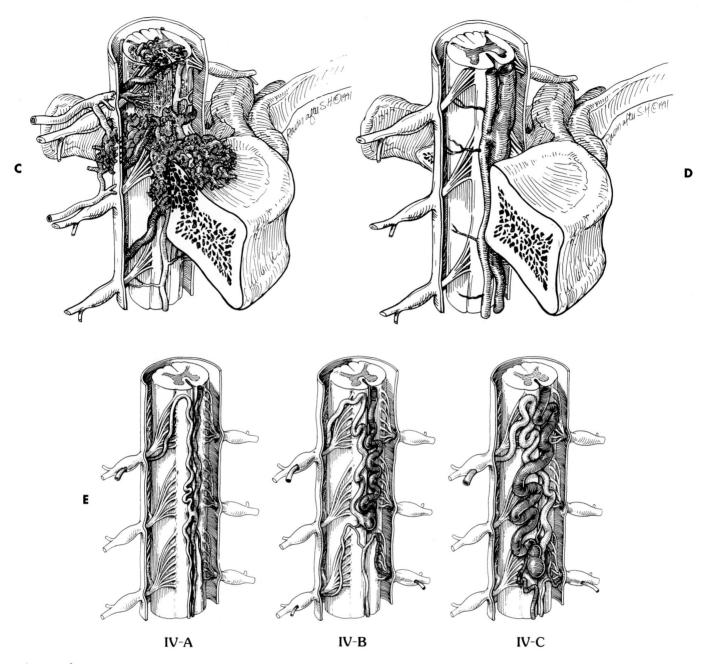

C   D

E

IV-A   IV-B   IV-C

Fig. 17-36 *Continued.* **C,** Juvenile AVM (type III) involving the spinal cord, vertebral body, and extraspinal structures. These lesions usually become symptomatic during childhood or early adulthood. Even with treatment the prognosis is poor. **D,** Type IV AVM. **E,** The three categories of type IV spinal cord AVMs. In all three types the nidus is intradural and located on the ventral or lateral surface of the spinal cord. Type IV-A AVMs have a small fistula, while type IV-C AVMs are formed by a large arterial feeder and a massively dilated venous system. Venous aneurysms are often associated with these lesions. (A, B, D, and E from Barrow Neurological Institute. C modified from Spetzler RF, Zabramski JM, Flom RA: Management of juvenile spinal AVMs by embolization and operative excision: Case Report, *J Neurosurg* 70:628-632, 1989.)

simple authors to simple readers). These may be separated into spinal dural arteriovenous fistula (malformation) (SDAVF or Type I AVMs), spinal cord arteriovenous malformations (SCAVM) also known as Type II and III (Juvenile) AVMs, and spinal cord arteriovenous fistula (SCAVF) also known as Type IV AVMs (Fig. 17-37). Table 17-5 summarizes the clinical differences between SDAVF and SCAVM. Treatment of spinal AVMs is dependent on

many factors, including age, AVM type, and neurologic condition, and consists of embolization, surgery, or a combination of the two. Blood supply to the malformation is very important in determining whether to proceed with embolization of the malformation or to perform surgery.

Spinal Dural arteriovenous fistula (SDAVF)   SDAVF is the most common spinal vascular malformation hav-

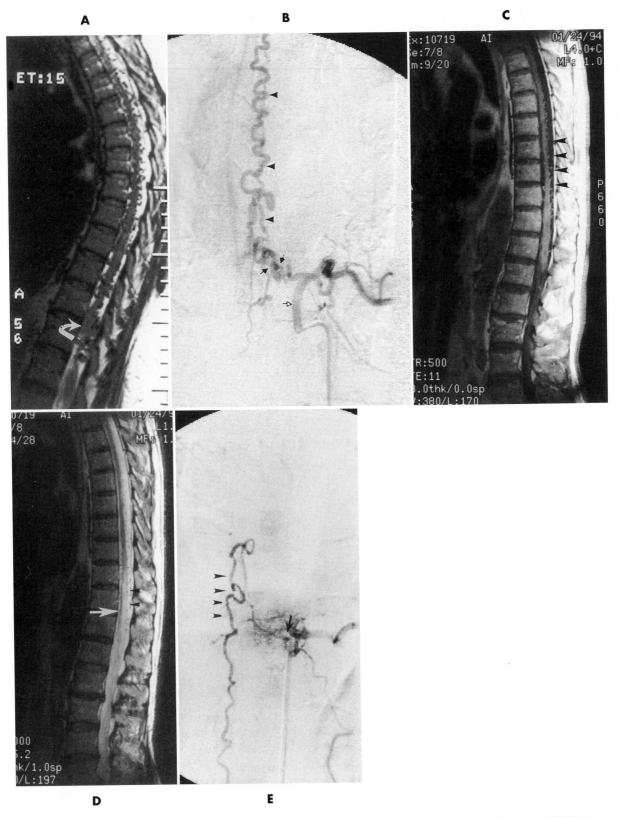

Fig. 17-37 Spinal vascular malformations. **A,** Note the numerous flow voids around the spinal cord on this sagittal T2WI. Lower down the cord is actually compressed by a varicose vein *(white curved arrow).* **B,** Spinal arteriogram. AP projection with injection of T10 intercostal artery *(open arrow)* reveals the dural malformation *(arrows)* and the veins draining the malformation *(arrowheads).* **C,** A post-contrast scan in a different patient shows enhancing vessels along the posterior margin of the cord and ever so slight enhancement of the conus. **D,** High signal in the cord *(arrowheads)* on T2WI is very characteristic of symptomatic Foix Alajouanine. Peripheral hypointensity *(arrow)* is present as well. **E,** The dural fistula *(black arrow)* is demonstrated on the intercostals artery injection with opacification of the draining vein *(arrowheads).*

Table 17-5 Summarizes the clinical differences between SDAVF and SCAVM

	SDAVF	SCAVM
Age	5–6th decade	3rd decade
M:F	>5:1	1:1.1
Onset	Insidious	Acute
Hemorrhage	Very rare	>50%

ing a nidus on the nerve root sleeve. This AVM, which is most frequently found on the dorsal aspect of the lower thoracic cord or conus medullaris sometimes has the eponym *Foix-Alajouanine syndrome* attached to it when myelopathy is present. In about 85% of cases a single radicular artery with systemic pressure is identified draining into spinal pial veins (low pressure). However, there are cases with many arterial feeders originating from either a single or multiple levels that may be either unilateral or bilateral. The systemic pressure in the spinal veins initially dilates these vessels with subsequent kinking and poor venous drainage. This results in venous hypertension defined histopathologically by stasis, edema, ischemia, and leading to infarction of the spinal cord. A large varix can be mistaken for a mass lesion. The veins may also appear serpentine.

Usually the anterior spinal artery does not arise at the same level as the SDAVF. If it does then an endovascular approach is contraindicated and surgical treatment is required. If the malformation is supplied by other vessels, embolization with permanent occlusive agents appears to be the procedure of choice (particularly if the neurointerventionalist is a member of the radiology department). Spinal angiography requires careful attention to all possible vascular pathways that may supply the malformation. You should inject all the standard vessels including intercostal, vertebral, costocervical, thyrocervical, and subclavian arteries. The blood supply, however, may arrive through vessels distant from the malformation including the iliac arteries, hypogastric arteries, and sacral arteries.

Complaints begin with an insidious onset of lower extremity weakness or sensory changes, associated with nonradiating pain starting in the caudal spinal segments and progressing superiorly. There is a propensity for these to occur in men in their fifth or sixth decade of life. These lesions are difficult to detect, and patients may have persistent neurologic sequelae if the lesions go unrecognized, although partial recovery is possible. This clinical presentation can sometimes be mistaken for degenerative disk disease. CSF protein can be increased mistakenly leading to the thought of a spinal cord tumor. Careful evaluation of the MR at this point can separate neoplasm (except perhaps in hemangioblastoma) from

dural AVM if prominent vessels are detected. Such vessels can be subtle. Spinal angiography is suggested in equivocal cases rather than going to myelography and CT. Spinal angiography is also necessary when the MR is unequivocal to define all of the feeders to the malformation.

Indeed, there can be a very significant delay between presentation and diagno$i$. Although 40% of patients may have lower extremity paresis at presentation up to 90% of patients may have it by the time diagnosis is made. This is even worse for bowel/bladder/and most importantly sexual function.

The MR findings are key. The spinal cord may be of normal size or enlarged with intramedullary high intensity seen on T2WI. Associated with this are usually (but NOT always) prominent vessels on the posterior aspect of the spinal cord. Look carefully for subtle bumps along the surface of the spinal cord, which is normally perfectly smooth. Obviously, these vessels enhance, however, in the outpatient HMO driven setting of "efficient" imaging the technologist may just get a history of lower back pain and default to the lumbar disk protocol. The first evidence that you may have missed the lesion is in the summons requesting the patient's records. The spinal cord itself, in addition to the veins, may or may not enhance.

Another finding recently recognized is the presence of peripheral hypointensity on T2WI, which in combination with high intensity within the cord should increase the specificity for the diagnosis of venous hypertension. This is thought to represent pial capillaries containing deoxyhemoglobin secondary to venous hypertension (see Fig. 17-37D).

SDAVF has also been associated with the syndrome of subacute necrotizing myelopathy, which involves progressive myelopathy in combination with necrosis of the spinal cord. Box 17-11 lists diseases that may manifest this syndrome. The bottom line is to consider the diagnosis of SDAVF in ALL patients with progressive myelopathic signs or symptoms and positive MR findings.

Occasionally, intracranial dural arteriovenous malformations (fistula) may have intraspinal drainage (<5%). The arterial supply is from meningeal branches of the external carotid artery or the vertebral artery. These usually involve the medulla or cervical spine and may present acutely with hemorrhage, quadriparesis, or medullary dysfunction. High intensity on T2WI in the medulla and/or cervical spine associated with peripheral cord or medullary hypointensity should suggest this possible diagnosis with rapid angiographic confirmation and endovascular treatment.

Spinal cord arteriovenous malformation (SCAVM) Spinal cord AVMs (Type II) are intramedullary lesions fed by branches of the anterior or posterior spinal arteries, into a nidus and then into spinal veins. These are true arteriovenous malformations just like the brain with similar angioarchitecture. These lesions are associated with spinal artery aneurysms. Acute symptoms are caused by intramedullary hemorrhage. Unlike SDAVF, there is no sexual preference and progressive myelopathy is less common. Juvenile AVMs (Type III) are rare lesions with extensive lesions with intramedullary, extramedullary, and extraspinal components. They occur early in life and tend to have a poor prognosis.

Spinal cord arteriovenous fistula (SCAVF) SCAVF (Type IV AVMs) are intradural extramedullary arteriovenous fistulas (without an intervening capillary network) located on the pial surface. They are seen ventrally or laterally involving the anterior and posterior spinal arteries with a single arteriovenous communication. Clinical presentations can vary from progressive myelopathy to hemorrhage including subarachnoid hemorrhage (up to 30%). Venous aneurysm can be seen with this malformation (see Fig. 17-37A).

When malformations produce increased venous pressure they can produce a subarachnoid hemorrhage. If the venous drainage is intracranial (particularly with SCAVF), patients may present with intracranial subarachnoid hemorrhage. The differential diagnosis of subarachnoid hemorrhage and hematomyelia is provided in Box 17-12.

Recently, MR angiography has been advocated to detect and characterize spinal vascular malformations. A variety of techniques have been suggested and to date reports have been limited. Phase contrast (2D and 3D) methods have been used with encoding for slow flow to emphasize slow venous flow (V_{enc} = 25 cm/sec).

Cavernous Angioma

Cavernous angiomas of the spinal cord are uncommon intramedullary vascular lesions. They appear similar to those in the brain, which are common. The age of

---

Box 17-12   Spinal Subarachnoid Hemorrhage and Hematomyelia

SCAVM
Cavernous angioma
Spinal cord tumor
Coarctation of the aorta
Spinal artery aneurysm
Spinal venous aneurysm
Vasculitis
Coagulation disorders/anticoagulation
Trauma

---

presentation is 30 to 50 with a 1:4 male to female ratio. These lesions usually occur in the cervical or thoracic region and may be familial.

MR is the imaging study of choice, with the malformation appearing round with regions of high signal intensity (methemoglobin) on T1WI and T2WI surrounded by low signal intensity on T2WI (hemosiderin) (Fig. 17-38). There is minimal mass effect or edema unless there has been recent hemorrhage. These lesions can enhance. Hematomyelia can be seen within the lesion. The clinical course is progressive, with Brown-Séquard syn-

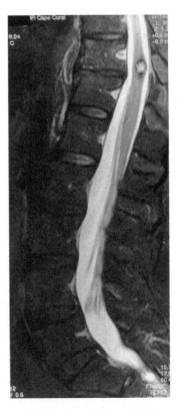

Fig. 17-38   Cavernoma of cord: Low signal intensity marks the hemosiderin stain from this cavernous malformation of the thoracic spinal cord.

drome (hemiparaplegia, ipsilateral loss of proprioceptive sensation, hyperesthesia, and contralateral loss of pain and temperature—this saves you a trip to your friendly neurology text) being the most common presentation, although acute neurologic deficits and pain from hemorrhage have been reported. Myelography may be normal or may reveal atrophy or cord expansion. Angiography is usually negative in these cases, although late venous pooling or abnormal draining veins may be found. Calcification has been reported, and cavernous lesions enhance.

Venous malformations occur in the cord and rarely may hemorrhage.

Siderosis Recurrent hemorrhage from spinal vascular malformations or hemorrhagic tumors such as ependymoma or hemangioblastoma, is associated with hemosiderin deposition throughout the leptomeninges and with hemosiderosis (see Chapter 4) of the central nervous system.

Transdural spinal cord herniation This is a rare bird (but, unlike the dodo, it does presently exist). It occurs spontaneously, posttraumatically, or may be a postoperative complication usually becoming symptomatic 1 to several years following the event. Clinical presentation includes myelopathy, radiculopathy, sensory symptoms, or Brown-Sequard syndrome. Herniation secondary to previous spine surgery is quite understandable particularly if the dura had been opened or torn. Here the cord herniates posteriorly through the defect. Trauma can also tear the dura and the arachnoid. Evidence of a nuclear trail sign (sclerotic changes in the vertebral endplate or disk representing the path of a previously herniated nuclear disk fragment) is commonly seen and probably is associated with traumatic disk herniation. In those cases without surgery or trauma, a congenital dural defect has been implicated. MR demonstrates the cord to be small, rotated and displaced with dilated CSF space (which can be confused with an arachnoid cyst) opposite to the herniation (Fig. 17-39). High signal intensity on T2WI may be seen with the cord. Surgery is usually beneficial.

SPINAL TRAUMA

In acute spinal injury CT is the best method for detecting bone fragments or compromise of the canal. The reader should appreciate some problems associated with CT. These include the following: (1) increases in intervertebral distances are not as evident on CT as on plain films; (2) subluxation, dislocation, and abnormal angulation are more difficult to recognize on axial images; (3) fractures oriented in the axial plane may be completely missed on CT; and (4) partial volume averaging may mask or mimic fractures. CT aids in visualizing C-1, C-2, C-6, and C-7 vertebrae, which are difficult to visualize in many cases on plain films (particularly at our institution). The swimmer's view is useful for alignment but is of little value in detecting C6 and C7 fractures. CT is an important adjunct to plain films at these levels. It is time to donate your tomography unit to the third world as 3D reconstructions using multidector CT is now state-of-the-

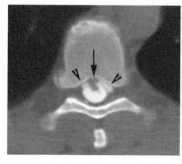
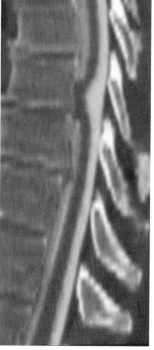

Fig. 17-39 Transdural spinal cord herniation. Post myelogram C. **A,** Axial image. Arrowheads reveal tear in dura with pseudomenigocele. Arrow show the transdural herniation. **B,** Reconstructed sagittal showing the herniated spinal cord.

art. Spiral CT has been reported to detect about 10% of cervicothoracic junction fractures occult by conventional radiography, however, most of the fractures detected were not clinically significant. These images assess the cause and degree of cervical subluxation and are the gold standard for atlantooccipital dislocations, subluxations of the vertebral bodies, and fractures of the lateral masses, articular processes, vertebral bodies, and dens.

MR is the only technique that can reliably reveal intrinsic injury to the cord and ligaments. In acute spinal cord injury abnormalities include intramedullary hemorrhage, which may be petechial or diffuse, and swelling, both of which can be appreciated on MR. In severe spinal cord trauma, lacerations and spinal cord transections (also seen in fetal hyperextension, breech delivery, flexion-hyperextension injury in children, and direct crush injuries) are present. MR can also visualize subluxations and vertebral body fractures, soft-tissue injuries such as ligamentous tears, hematomas around these tears, and traumatic disk herniations (see Fig. 17-39).

Carefully assess the prevertebral region for the presence of swelling and/or hemorrhage. Hematomas here result from adjacent soft-tissue injury or fractures involving the anterior vertebral column. The upper limit of prevertebral soft tissue at C3 level is 4 mm.

The radiologist must determine the extent of cord injury, cord compression and/or canal stenosis, as well as search for unexpected diseases such as odontoid fracture, and detect the sequelae of trauma such as atrophy of the cord or cystic changes.

Patients with acute spinal cord injury and normal MR findings have the best prognosis, whereas patients with hemorrhage and/or low or high signal intensity on T1WI and high signal on T2WI have the poorest prognosis. Enhancement has been observed at about 2 weeks after injury with a duration of between 2 to 3 months. It has been reported to represent early necrosis, absorption, and reorganization of the spinal cord, and may be an early indicator of damage. Cases with isointensity on T1WI and high signal on T2WI have some potential for reversible change and improved outcome. High intensity on T2WI in the dorsal column rostral to the main site of injury in a chronic injury likely represents Wallerian degeneration.

The pathologic consequences of significant spinal cord trauma (Fig. 17-40) may be (1) atrophy, (2) myelomalacia, (3) posttraumatic syrinx, (4) arachnoid cyst, and (5) arachnoiditis. The first two situations may not be amenable to treatment and are rather easy to recognize in most circumstances.

The onset of symptoms in a posttraumatic syrinx is extremely variable and not necessarily related to the extent of the lesion, so that MR is appropriate in following up all patients with spinal cord injury, even those who are relatively asymptomatic. MR displays a cystic lesion in the cord that grows over time. Identification is important because this is a treatable cause of deterioration after spinal cord injury. Intrinsic damage to the cord associated with dynamic changes in CSF pressure, and arachnoiditis, are factors implicated in development of posttraumatic syrinx.

Whiplash injury (personal experience) This results from a hyperextension and subsequent hyperflexion injury. One of the authors was sitting in the back of a smelly Philadelphia taxi cab, minding his own business while breathing through his mouth, when a falafel truck rear-ended the taxi. The falafel guy ran out of his car claiming that he did not do anything, but humus and babaganush flowed in the street. The author had 6 weeks of weird nonradicular, frequently intense upper extremity pains, at times associated with signs (like temperature and color changes in the digits of his hands) reminiscent of reflex sympathetic dystrophy (probably the result of microhemorrhages in the sympathetic nerves). Other symptoms frequently reported in the "whiplash syndrome" include headache, neck pain, pain in the interscapular region, paresthesias, vertigo, and general tiredness. Flexion and extension views occasionally show a kyphotic angle, a result of muscle spasm. Some investigators believe that the facet joints are the source of the pain secondary to occult fracture, capsular ruptures, and intraarticular hemorrhage.

MR, as it usually is in these cases, was normal but was reassuring. Most reports indicate that MR is not justified in these cases (except in physicians and HMO executives). The problem for the patient is that the symptoms are very troublesome and the MR offers little insight into the lesion. So remember the next time you think the patient is a turkey, MR is no electron microscope.

Ligamentous injuries MR is the method of choice for imaging ligamentous injury to the spine. The fibrous nature of the spinal ligaments results in their normal hypointensity on all MR pulse sequences. They should have well demarcated margins throughout their course. Tears or partial tears resulting in edema are best visualized on short inversion recovery (STIR) images (and almost as well on fat suppressed T2WI) as high intensity. The sagittal plane depicts injury to the anterior and posterior longitudinal ligaments, the ligamentum flavum, and the interspinous ligaments. Ligamentous injury is often associated with traumatic disk herniation.

Cervical Nerve Root Avulsion

Cervical nerve root avulsions are the result of traction injuries on the upper extremities that tear the roots from the spinal cord (Fig. 17-41). The roots are absent on the ipsilateral side and the cord is pulled to the contralateral side. Pseudomeningoceles are associated with this injury. They result from tears of the arachnoid and dura and can

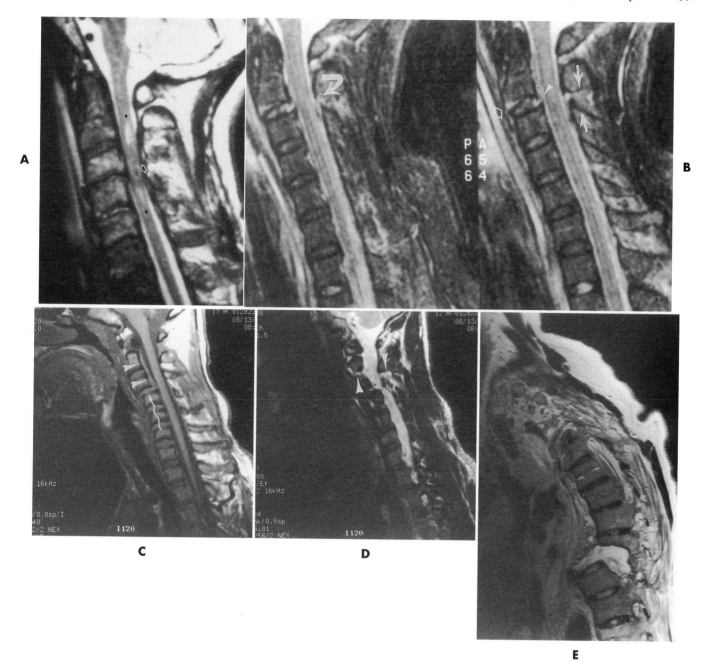

Fig. 17-40 Spinal trauma. **A,** Cervical spinal cord trauma. Cord is swollen with a hemorrhage *(open arrow)* at the level of the C3 vertebral body. Also observe the disk compressing the spinal cord at C3–C4. Edema is seen above and below this injury *(arrows)*. **B,** This sagittal T2WI set shows a rent in the spinal-laminar ligaments *(curved arrow)* and interspinous ligaments *(straight arrows)* as well as the posterior longitudinal ligament *(arrowhead)*. The plane of damage crosses the endplate to affect the anterior longitudinal ligament *(open arrow)*. Three column disease is DEFINITELY unstable. **C,** Subluxation of C3 on C4 *(squiggly arrow)* suggests a ligamentous injury. Also observe the epidural hematoma *(arrowheads)*. **D,** There is high signal intensity in the posterior ligaments *(arrowheads)*. **E,** What can we say besides "Ooooh Baby. That's a bad one!"

be identified on MR or CT myelography. After healing, some pseudomeningoceles may not communicate with the subarachnoid space and can present as epidural mass lesions. Focal displacement of epidural fat can confirm the location of the lesion and rule out posttraumatic arachnoid cyst.

Spine Fractures and Dislocations

It is important to appreciate the definition of clinical stability and instability. This turns out to be a controversial topic. (What isn't? Answer: motherhood, apple

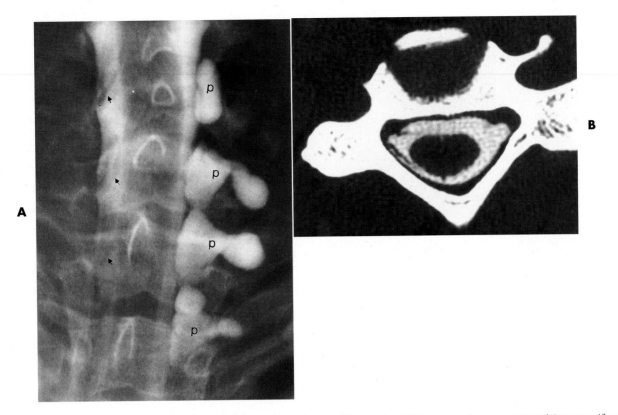

Fig. 17-41   Cervical root avulsion. **A,** Cervical root avulsion. Myelogram illustrates multiple cervical nerve root avulsions manifested by multiple pseudomeningoceles *(p)* from the torn arachnoid and dura. Ipsilateral nerve roots are not seen, having been torn and retracted. Contralateral nerve roots *(arrows)* can be identified. This is a classic! **B,** Note the absence of anterior and posterior roots on the left side with an incipient pseudomeningocele from the empty root sleeve.

pie, higher reimbursements??) We shall provide the classification scheme for the blue-collar radiologists. There is a method to our simplicity—as classification schemes become more complex they provide less utility and tend not to be implemented. In the cervical and thoracic spine, the concept of stability has lead to several classification schemes. Stability has been defined as the capacity of the spine under physiologic loads to limit displacement so as not to compromise or damage the spinal cord and nerve roots. Stability also denotes prevention of deformity or pain secondary to anatomical changes. Conversely, clinical instability may be defined as greater than normal range of motion within a spinal segment so as to assume a risk of neurologic injury. In the cervical spine clinical instability has been defined as anterior translation of greater than 3.5 mm and vertebral body angulation of greater than 11 degrees compared with the bodies above and below on standard lateral radiographs. Bones and ligaments are responsible for spinal cord stability. The implication of clinical instability is that surgical intervention is necessary to stabilize the spine.

Classification scheme and definitions   The spinal column can be divided into three columns. The anterior column is composed of the anterior longitudinal ligament, the anterior annulus, and the anterior portion of the vertebral body. The middle column delineated by the posterior longitudinal ligament, the posterior portion of the annulus, and the posterior aspect of the vertebral body and disk. The posterior column contains the neural arch, facet joints and capsules, ligamentum flavum, and all other posterior spinal ligaments. The middle column is critical as instability occurs when two of the three columns are injured (Fig. 17-42). Compression fractures result in anterior column injury (usually stable) whereas burst fractures affect the anterior and middle columns (unstable). Flexion-distraction injuries affect the middle and posterior columns and fracture-dislocation injuries result in a three column injury. Think about this as the inverse Chinese restaurant problem—the more columns the worse the injury.

Hyperflexion is a forward rotation and/or translation of a vertebra with both distraction of the posterior column and compression of the anterior column. Hyperextension injuries involve posterior rotation/translation.

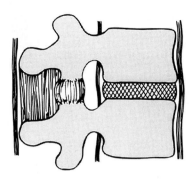

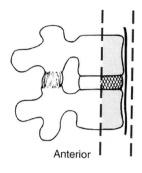

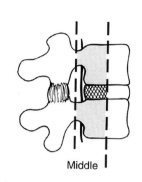

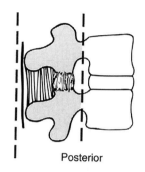

Anterior   Middle   Posterior

Fig. 17-42 The three-column classification model of the spine proposed by Denis represented an advance in thinking about spinal injuries over the previous two-column model. The concept of the middle column composed of the posterior longitudinal ligament, the posterior aspect of the annulus fibrosis and the posterior portion of the vertebral body and disk were added. (From Garfin SR, et al: Thoracic and upper lumbar spine injuries. In Browner BD, Jupiter JB, Levine AM, et al (eds): *Skeletal Trauma: Fracture, Dislocations, Ligamentous Injuries*, vol 1, ed 2. Philadelphia, WB Saunders, 1998, p 967.)

Here the anterior and middle columns bear the brunt of the injury (anterior longitudinal ligament, disc and posterior longitudinal ligament). "Sprains" are minor tears of the supraspinous, interspinous, and facet capsules from flexion-distraction injuries, which can result in anterior subluxation. Anterior subluxation is seen on lateral radiographs as a hyperkyphotic angulation of the cervical spine with widening of the distance between the spinous processes and interlaminar space when compared to other levels (fanning). Other findings include narrowing of the anterior disc space with widening of its posterior aspect with or without anterior translation of the involved vertebral body, widening of the space between the subluxed vertebral body and the superior articular facet of the lower vertebral body, and subluxation of the facet joints. Flexion-extension views can best demonstrate this injury. There are a range of ligamentous injuries from facet subluxations to perched facets to bilateral facet dislocations. Specific injuries to the cervical spine are discussed in the following paragraphs.

At present, good spine films and CT supplemented by MR are the most complete methods for evaluating spine fractures. MR with STIR imaging is most useful for associated ligamentous and spinal cord injury.

Cervical spine injury following blunt trauma has been reported to be low in patients who meet the following criteria: (1) no midline tenderness; (2) no focal neurologic deficit; (3) normal alertness; (4) no intoxication; (5) no painful, distracting injury. Patients who meet these clinical criteria do not need to be imaged. Table 17-6 lists spine injuries that are considered to be stable and unstable.

Atlantooccipital Dislocation

Atlantooccipital dislocation is customarily considered a fatal injury, although there are many case reports of survival. Severe injuries include pontomedullary junction laceration, contusion or laceration of the inferior medulla and spinal cord, injury to the midbrain, subarachnoid hemorrhage, subdural hemorrhage, and vascular dissection. The incidence is increased in children predominantly because of their small occipital condyles and horizontal plane of the atlantooccipital joints. The high-velocity shearing forces are directed to the face or posterior of the skull. Atlantooccipital dislocation can be associated with severe hyperextension, type I odontoid fracture (see Odontoid Fracture subsection), loss of the normal relationship of the occipital condyles to C1, and retropharyngeal swelling (greater than 10 mm at C2) (prevertebral hematoma) (Fig. 17-43). Longitudinal distraction, anterior or posterior dislocation of the occiput

Table 17-6   Stability of cervical spin fractures*

Stable	Unstable
Anterior subluxation	Atlantooccipital subluxation/dislocation
Burst fracture, lower cervical vertebrae	Bilateral C1-2 dislocation
Pillar fracture	Bilateral facet, laminae, or pedicle fractures and/or dislocation
Posterior neural arch fracture, atlas	Extension teardrop fracture (stable in flexion, unstable in extension)
Unilateral facet dislocation	Flexion teardrop fracture
Spinous process fracture	Hangman's fracture
Clay-shoveler's fracture	Hyperextension fracture–dislocation
Transverse process fracture	Type II odontoid fracture
Compression fracture of <25% of vertebral body height	Jefferson fracture
Anterior wedge fracture	
Isolated avulsion without ligamentous tear	
Type I odontoid fracture	
End plate fracture	
Osteophyte fracture (not including corner or teardrop fracture)	
Trabecular bone injury	

*Beware; patients and their lawyers are not as magnanimous as the authors.

relative to the atlas, is observed as a result of tearing of the tectoral membrane and alar ligaments and is seen as increased distance between the basion and dens (greater than 12 mm). CT can detect basion and condylar frac-

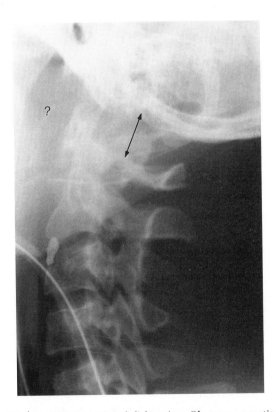

Fig. 17-43   Atlantooccipital dislocation. Observe separation between the occiput and the atlas *(arrows)* on this lateral spine film. Swelling is noted in the anterior neck *(?).*

tures with coronal and axial reformatted images showing widening between the lateral masses of C1 and the occipital condyles. MR with T2WI and STIR images reveal prevertebral soft tissue injury, ligamentous tears, epidural hematoma, spinal cord and brain stem injury.

In children, this diagnosis can be problematic because of variable bone ossification in the craniocervical junction, especially in the dens where the basion-dens interval is reported to be unreliable under the age of 13.

Figure 17-44 shows the three types of occipital condyle fractures.

Atlantoaxial Distraction

This injury is also the result of severe extension. There is disruption of the articular capsules, alar ligaments, transverse ligament, and tectorial membrane between C1 and C2. Occasionally, there is a type I dens fracture. There is obvious widening of the space between C1 and C2. Look for prevertebral swelling on plain films and CT. On MR, edema can be identified on STIR or T2WI in the prevertebral, interspinous, and nuchal ligaments. Other reported findings may be facet widening, epidural hematoma and increased intensity in the spinal cord.

Atlantoaxial Rotation

Atlantoaxial rotation results in torticollis, so that the atlas is rotated and dislocated from the articular processes of the axis. Head rotation does not correct what appears to be an asymmetric odontoid with respect to the lateral masses, nor does the spinous process of C1 move. To evaluate this you should perform the CT with

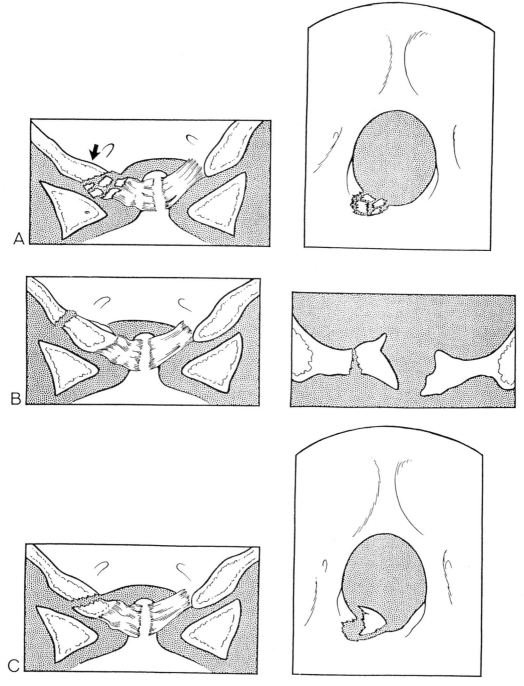

Fig. 17-44   The classification of Anderson and Montesano describes three basic types of occipital condyle fractures. The first (**A**) is an impaction-type fracture, which is usually the result of an asymmetrical axial load to the head; it may be associated with other lateral mass fractures in the upper cervical spine. The next type (**B**) is a basilar skull—type occipital condyle fracture, which may be the result of a distraction force applied through the alar and apical ligament complex.. (Redrawn from Anderson P, Montesano P: Morphology and treatment of occipital condyle fractures. *Spine* 13:731, 1988) **C,** Type III—avulsion-type occipital condyle fracture.

head turned to the left, right and in the neutral position to reveal the lack of correction.

Jefferson's fractures are breaks in the ring of the atlas that were classically described as having four sites (junctions of the anterior and posterior arches with the lat-eral masses, which are where the bone is thinnest) although there are many variations in the number of fractures. They are caused by compressive forces. Tears of the transverse ligament are associated with Jefferson's fracture.

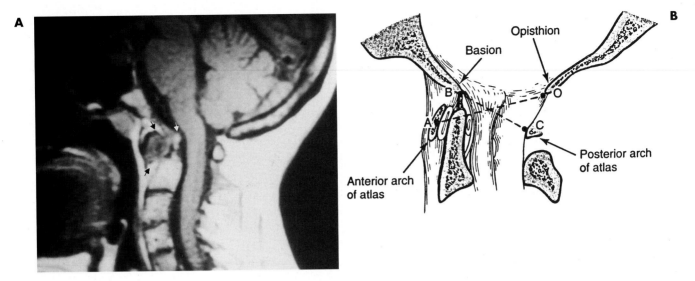

Fig. 17-45   Atlantoaxial dislocation. **A,** Sagittal T1WI in a patient with rheumatoid arthritis depicts pannus formation *(black arrows).* There is penciling of the odontoid process *(white arrow)* and dislocation between the anterior arch of C1, which is poorly visualized, and the odontoid process. **B,** Powers' ratio. If BC:OA is greater than 1, and anterior occipitoatlantal dislocation exists. Ratios less than 1 are normal except in posterior dislocations, associated fractures of the odontoid process or ring of the atlas, and congenital anomalies of the foramen magnum. *Abbreviations:* B, basion; C, posterior arch of C1; O, opisthion; A, anterior arch of C1.

Atlantoaxial Dislocation

Atlantoaxial dislocation can be caused by trauma with associated fractures and rupture of the transverse ligament, or may be seen in nontraumatic situations associated with transverse ligament problems or odontoid process malformations (os odontoideum, ossiculum terminale or agenesis of the odontoid base, apical segment, or the entire base) (Fig. 17-45). Other nontraumatic causes include infections such as tonsillitis and pharyngitis (Grisels syndrome—rotatory subluxation secondary to adjacent inflammatory mass), Downs syndrome (trisomy 21), Marfans syndrome, neurofibromatosis, ankylosing spondylitis, rheumatoid arthritis, and bone tumors. This injury can be fatal or totally asymptomatic.

Odontoid Fracture

Odontoid fractures have been divided into oblique fractures through the upper portion of the dens (type I), a transverse fracture through the junction of the dens with the body of the axis (type II) (unstable), and a fracture extending into the cancellous portion of the body of the axis (type III) (Fig. 17-46).

Fat C2 sign   On a lateral plain spine film obliquely oriented fractures of body of C2 appear as though C2 is larger in its anteroposterior dimension ("fat" C2 sign). This is the result of isolated hyperflexion or hyperextension or a combination of the two involving the vertebral body of C2. The oblique nature of the fracture is due to additional rotational forces. This fracture may result from a complex fracture of the body of C2, a low

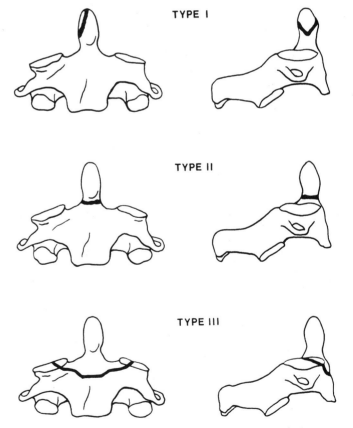

Fig. 17-46   Classification of odontoid fractures. This diagram illustrates the nomenclature associated with the three types of odontoid fractures. (From Modic M, Masaryk T, Ross J: *Magnetic resonance imaging of the spine,* ed. 1, Chicago, 1988, Year Book Medical Publishers.)

dens fracture (type III), or an atypical traumatic spondylolisthesis. It is associated with ligamentous injury and is potentially unstable.

Hangman's Fracture

Hangman's fractures result from hyperextension of the neck and are fracture dislocations of C2. The spectrum of traumatic spondylolisthesis is seen in Figure 17-47. When both pedicles are fractured, there is anterior subluxation of the body of C2 on C3 whereas the posterior ring does not move, being fixed by the inferior articular processes. (Fig. 17-47A).

Os odontoideum Os odontoideum is a round smooth bony ossicle that is seen proximal to the base of the dens. Its position is variable either in the position of the odontoid process (orthotopic) or at the foramen magnum near the base of the occiput (dystopic). On lateral radiographs there is commonly a smoothly marginated bone ossicle, separated by a zone of radiolucency, above the superior facets of axis (Fig. 17-48). This etiology of the os is controversial. Originally thought to be a congenital or developmental anomaly it is now thought to be the result of an acquired or posttraumatic cause. There is an association, albeit infrequent, with Klippel-Feil syndrome, myelodysplasia, Morquio's syndrome, Down's syndrome, spondyloepiphyseal dysplasia.

The os is embedded within the transverse atlantoaxial ligament, and is associated with atlantoaxial instability, translating over the axis and at times producing spinal cord compression. This usually requires surgical correction most of the time by posterior atlantoaxial fusion. The issue for radiologists is the differentiation of the os from a type I or type II odontoid fractures. Fractures do not have smooth corticate margins, rather they have sharp radiolucent margins.

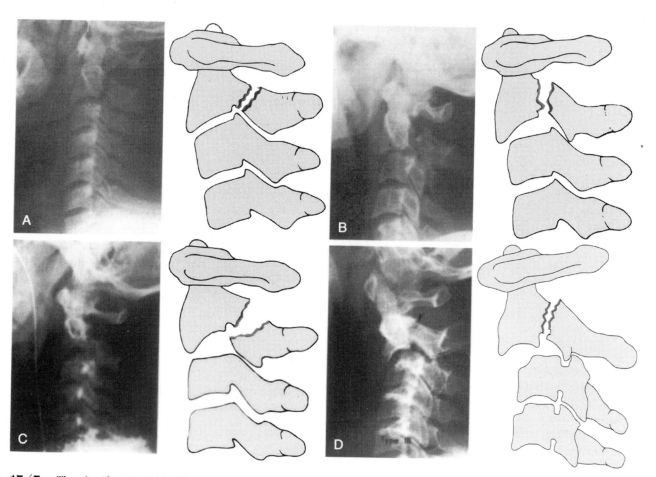

Fig. 17-47   The classification devised by Levine and Edwards for traumatic spondylolisthesis of the axis accounts for the majority of fractures of this type. **A,** The most commom pattern is type I, which is characterized radiographically by a fracture through the neural arch with minimal translation (<3 mm) and minimal angulation. Not pictured in the classification is the later addition of type IA, which has also been called atypical hangman's fracture. **B,** Type II fractures have significant angulation (>3 degrees) and translation (>3 mm) and are much more unstable than type I fractures. **C,** Type IIA fractures are identified radiographically by an oblique fracture line with minimal translation but significant angulation. **D,** Type III axial fractures combine bilateral facet dislocation between C2 and C3 with a fracture of the neural arch of the axis. (A-C, from Levine et al: *J Bone Joint Surg Am* 67: 217-226, 1985; D from Levine: Orthop Clin North Am 17:42, 1986.)

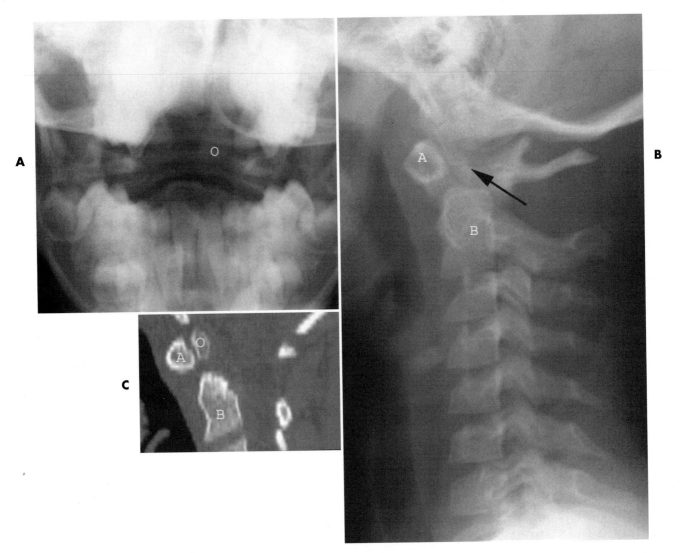

Fig. 17-48   Nice Oses. **A,** Open mouth view of os (o). **B,** Lateral view of spine. Anterior arch of C1 (**A**), odontoid (**B**), arrow points to os. **C,** CT with bone windows of os (o), anterior arch (**A**) and odontoid (**B**).

Compression Fractures

A classification of compression fractures (defined by an intact posterior wall—middle column) has been proposed. Compression fractures classified as type A involve both end-plates, without or with a fracture a coronal fracture through the body. Type B is the most common and is a fracture through the superior end-plate. Type C is a fracture through the inferior end-plate. Type D is a buckling fracture of the anterior cortex with both end-plates intact (Fig. 17-49).

Thoracolumbar Fractures

One classification scheme divides these fractures into 3 categories. Type A have vertebral body compression caused by axial load with or without an element of flex-ion but without disruption of soft tissues in the transverse plane. Type B injuries involve both the anterior and posterior elements with distortion concomitant with soft-tissue disruption in the transverse plane. Type C injuries are Type B injuries superimposed with a rotational component. These injuries may be further subdivided but that elaborate subdivision is beyond the scope of us dilettantes so you get a break.

Burst Fracture

In the thoracolumbar region, significant axial forces can produce comminuted or burst fractures of the vertebral body, with elements compromising the spinal canal with neurologic deficits. Anterior wedge fractures, when associated with disruption of the posterior elements (key), are usually accompanied by neurologic

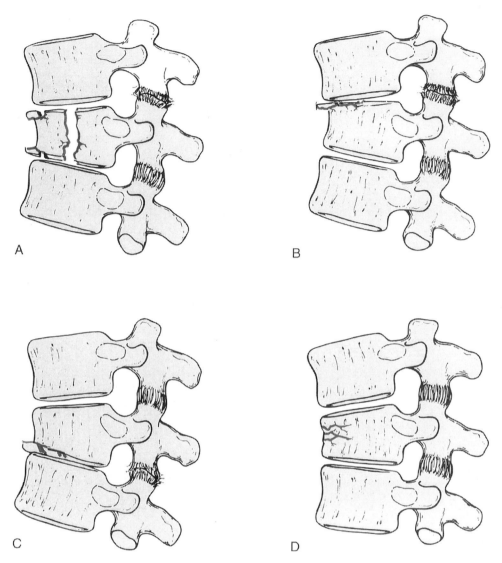

Fig. 17-49   Although it has not been as widely used as the classification of burst fractures, Denis proposed a classification of compression fractures. The critical feature of all four types is that the posterior wall of the vertebral body is intact with the fracture line either involving the end plates of the anterior portion of the body. **A,** Theses fractures may involve both end plates, with or without a coronal plane fracture. **B,** The most common type involves f ractures of the superior end plate alone. **C,** However, isolated fracture of the inferior end plated can occur. **D,** The final pattern is a buckling fracture of the anterior cortex with both end plates intact. This type must be carefully differentiated from a minimally displace flexion-distraction injury. (From Garfin SR, et al: Thoracic and upper lumbar spine injuries. In Browner BD, Jupiter JB, Levine AM, et al (eds), *Skeletal Trauma: Fracture, Dislocations, Ligamentous Injuries,* vol 1, ed 2. Philadelphia, WB Saunders, 1998, p 968.)

problems. These may also be classified into five types. Type A involves comminution of both end-plates as well as the pedicles and posterior elements, and represent about 40% of all burst fractures. It is the result of axial loading and there is minimal kyphosis. Type B involves the superior end-plate and upper portion of the vertebral body with retropulsion of the posterior superior corner of the vertebral body into the spinal canal. It results from axial loading and flexion and are present in 40% of cases. Type C fractures involve the inferior portion of the vertebral body and end-plate with retropulsion of the posterior inferior corner of the body into the canal.

These fractures are very uncommon and are the result of flexion compression injury. Type D fracture is a type A fracture with rotation best appreciated on AP film. Type E is a lateral burst fracture that results from a combination of axial loading and lateral bending best again seen on AP films (Fig. 17-50).

Chance Fracture

Lap seat belt injuries are associated with horizontal fractures of L2 or L3 and are termed Chance fractures (Fig. 17-51). There are several variations of this fracture,

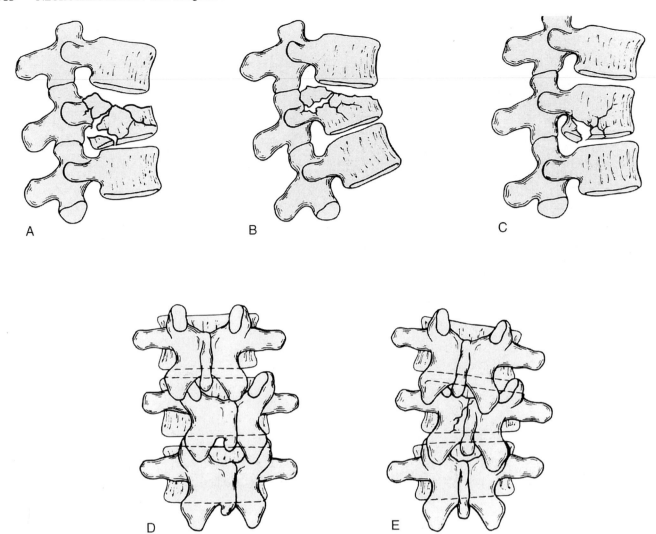

Fig. 17-50 The Denis classification of burst fractures is used to describe the majority of injuries of this type and is helpful in subdividing the injuries according to different treatment pattern. The common element is disruption of the posterior wall of the vertebral body in all cases. **(A)** The type A fracture is predominantly an axial loading injury with minimal kyphosis. A comminution of both end plates occurs, and there may also be fractures in the posterior elements. **(B)** Type B fractures tend to have more kyphosis and sparing of the posterior elements. Comminution of the superior end plates and upper portion of the vertebral body occur, with retropulsion of the posterosuperior portion into the canal. The first two types represent 80% to 90% of all burst fractures. **(C)** Type C fractures involve the inferior portion of the vertebral body and end plate with retropulsion of the posterior inferior corner of the body into the canal. These are extremely uncommon. **(D)** The type D fracture is a combination of a type A fracture with rotation, which is best appreciated on an anteroposterior radiograph. This type must be carefully differentiated from a shear injury. **(E)** Type E is a lateral burst fracture that results from a combination of axial loading and lateral bending and is again best appreciated on AP x-ray. (From Garfin SR, et al: Thoracic and upper lumbar spine injuries. In Browner BD, Jupiter JB, Levine AM, et al (eds): *Skeletal Trauma: Fracture, Dislocations, Ligamentous Injuries,* vol 1, ed 2. Philadelphia, WB Saunders, 1992, p 975.)

which can involve the body and posterior elements of a single vertebra or two levels.

Insufficiency Fractures of the Sacrum

These result from the inability of bone to withstand stress and are seen after radiation therapy or secondary to postmenopausal or steroid-induced osteoporosis. In addition to the sacrum, they can occur in the lower ex-

tremities, ilium, and pubis. The major finding is linear sclerosis running vertically (parallel to the sacroiliac joints) in the sacral alae, usually at the first through third sacral segments. Radionuclide bone scans reveal increased uptake ("Honda" sign). Their appearance can be mistaken for metastatic disease.

We have now finished the scientific portion of the text. Unfortunately you may become an expert on all the previous material and still not be able to hit the side of

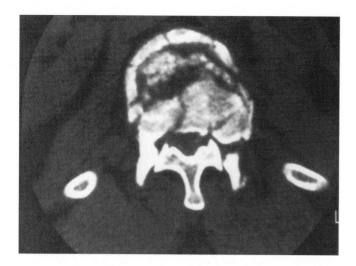

Fig. 17-51   Chance fracture. Note the comminuted nature of this L1 vertebral body fracture in a lawyer with a lap seat belt injury who had just settled a large malpractice suit and purchased his first Ferrari—oh well, he took his chances. Spinal canal diameter is compromised.

the barn. The last chapter is concerned with the art of the specialty, which will make you an M.V.P. (most valuable practitioner).

SUGGESTED READINGS

Afshani E, Kuhn JP: Common causes of low back pain in children, *Radiographics* 11:269-291, 1991.

Algra PR, Bloem JL, Tissing H, et al: Detection of vertebral metastases: comparison between MR imaging and bone scintigraphy, *Radiographics* 11:219-232, 1991.

Anson JA, Spetzler RF: Classification of spinal arteriovenous malformations and implications for treatment, *BNQI* 8, 1992.

Atlas SW, Regenbogen V, Rogers LF, et al: The radiographic characterization of burst fractures of the spine, *AJNR* 7:675-682, 1986.

Awad IA, Barnett GH: Neurological deterioration in a patient with a spinal arteriovenous malformation following lumbar puncture, *J Neurosurg* 72:650-653, 1990.

Azn R, Thijssen H, Merx JL, et al: The absent cervical pedicle syndrome, *Neuroradiology* 29:69-72, 1987.

Baker LL, Goodman SB, Perkash I, et al: Benign versus pathologic compression fractures of vertebral bodies: assessment with conventional spin-echo, chemical-shift, and STIR MR imaging, *Radiology* 174:485-502, 1990.

Barakos JA, Mark AS, Dillon WP, et al: MR imaging of acute transverse myelitis and AIDS myelopathy, *J Comput Assist Tomogr* 14:45-50, 1990.

Barnsley L, Lord SM, Wallace BJ, et al: The prevalence of chronic cervical zygapophysial joint pain after whiplash, *Spine* 20(1):20-25; discussion 26, 1995.

Barnwell SL, Dowd CF, Davis RL, et al: Cryptic vascular malformations of the spinal cord: diagnosis by magnetic resonance imaging and outcome of surgery, *J Neurosurg* 72:403-407, 1990.

Bartels RH, Jong TR, Grotenhuis JA: Spinal subdural abscess: case report, *J Neurosurg* 76:307-311, 1992.

Baur A, Huber A, Ertl-Wagner B, et al: Diagnostic value of increased diffusion weighting of a steady-state free precession sequence for differentiating acute benign osteoporotic fractures from pathologic vertebral compression fractures, *AJNR* 22(2):366-372, 2001.

Baur A, Stabler A, Bruning R, et al: Diffusion-weighted MR imaging of bone marrow: differentiation of benign versus pathologic compression fractures, *Radiology* 207(2):349-356, 1998.

Biondi A, Merland JJ, Hodes JE, et al: Aneurysms of spinal arteries associated with intramedullary arteriovenous malformations. I. Angiographic and clinical aspects, *AJNR* 13:913-922, 1992.

Biondi A, Merland JJ, Hodes JE, et al: Aneurysms of spinal arteries associated with intramedullary arteriovenous malformations. II. Results of AVM endovascular treatment and hemodynamic considerations, *AJNR* 13:923-931, 1992.

Blews DE, Wang H, Kumar AJ, et al: Intradural spinal metastases in pediatric patients with primary intracranial neoplasms: Gd-DtPA enhanced MR vs. CT myelography, *J Comput Assist Tomogr* 14:730-735, 1990.

Bluemke DA, Wang H: Primary spinal cord lymphoma: MR appearance, *J Comput Assist Tomogr* 14:812-814, 1990.

Blumenkopf B, Bennett WF: Delayed presentation of posttraumatic cervical disk herniation, *AJNR* 7:722-724, 1986.

Bobman SA, Atlas SW, Listerud J, et al: Postoperative lumbar spine: contrast-enhanced chemical shift MR imaging, *Radiology* 179:557-562, 1991.

Castillo M, Malko JA, Hoffman JC: The bright intervertebral disk: an indirect sign of abnormal spinal bone marrow on T1-weighted MR images, *AJNR* 11:23-26, 1990.

Castillo M and Mukherji SK: MRI of enlarged dorsal ganglia, lumbar nerve roots, and cranial nerves in polyradiculoneuropathies, *Neuroradiology* 38(6): 516-520, 1996.

Castillo M, Arbelaez A, Smith JK, et al: Diffusion-weighted MR imaging offers no advantage over routine noncontrast MR imaging in the detection of vertebral metastases, *AJNR* 21(5):948-953, 2000.

Criscuolo GR, Oldfield EH, Doppman JL: Reversible acute and subacute myelopathy in patients with dural arteriovenous fistulas, *J Neurosurg* 70:354-359, 1989.

Davis SJ, Teresi LM, Bradley WG, et al: Cervical spine hyperextension injuries: MR findings, *Radiology* 180:245-251, 1991.

Deliganis A, Baxter A, Hanson JA, et al: Radiologic spectrum of craniocervical distraction injuries, *Radiographics* 20:237S-250, 2000.

Demachi H, Takashima T, Kadoya M, et al: MR imaging of spinal neurinomas with pathological correlation, *J Comput Assist Tomogr* 14:250-254, 1990.

Dickinson LD, Farhat SM: Eosinophilic granuloma of the cervical spine: a case report and review of the literature, *Surg Neurol* 35:57-63, 1991.

Digman KE, Partington CR, Graves VB: MR imaging of spinal pachymeningitis, *J Comput Assist Tomogr* 14:988-990, 1990.

Djindjian M, Nguyen J, Gaston A, et al: Multiple vertebral hemangiomas with neurological signs: case report, *J Neurosurg* 76:1025-1028, 1992.

Duprez TP, Gille M, Vande Berg BC, et al: MRI of the spine in cobalamin deficiency: the value of examining both spinal cord and bone marrow, *Neuroradiology* 38(6):511-515, 1996.

Elksnis SM, Hogg JP, Cunningham ME: MR imaging of spontaneous spinal cord infarction, *J Comput Assist Tomogr* 15:228-232, 1991.

Fischbein NJ, Dillon WP, Cobbs C, et al: The "presyrinx" state: a reversible myelopathic condition that may precede syringomyelia [see comments], *AJNR* 20(1):7-20, 1999.

Flanders AE, Schaefer DM, Doan HT, et al: Acute cervical spine trauma: correlation of MR imaging findings with degree of neurologic deficit, *Radiology* 177:25-33, 1990.

Fontaine S, Melanson D, Cosgrove R, et al: Cavernous hemangiomas of the spinal cord: MR imaging, *Radiology* 166:839-841, 1988.

Gaensler EHL, Jackson DE, Halbach VV: Arteriovenous fistulas of the cervicomedullary junction as a cause of myelopathy: radiographic findings in two cases, *AJNR* 11:518-521, 1990.

Gebarski SS, Maynard FW, Gabrielson TO, et al: Posttraumatic progressive myelopathy, *Radiology* 157:379-385, 1985.

Gilsanz V, Gibbens DT, Roe TF, et al: Vertebral bone density in children: effect of puberty, *Radiology* 166:847-850, 1988.

Goldberg AL, Baron B, Daffner RH: Clinical images: atlantooccipital dislocation—MR demonstration of cord damage, *J Comput Assist Tomogr* 15:174-178, 1991.

Gomori JM, Grossman RI, Golberg HI, et al: Occult cerebral vascular malformations: high-field MR imaging, *Radiology* 158:707-713, 1986.

Gouliamos AD, Kontogiannis DS, Androulidakis J, et al: Spinal neurilemmomas and neurofibromas: central dot sign in postgadolinium MRI, *J Comput Assist Tomogr* 17(3):446-468, 1993.

Guerra J, Garfin SR, Resnick D: Vertebral burst fractures: CT analysis of the retropulsed fragment, *Radiology* 153:769-772, 1984.

Hackney DB: Denominators of spinal cord injury, *Radiology* 177:18-20, 1990.

Halliday AL, Sobel RA, Martuza RL: Benign spinal nerve sheath tumors: their occurrence sporadically and in neurofibromatosis types 1 and 2, *J Neurosurg* 74:248-253, 1991.

Hanakita J, Suwa H, Nagayasu S, et al: Capillary hemangioma in the cauda equina: neuroradiological findings, *Neuroradiology* 33:458-461, 1991.

Hanigan WC, Asner NG, Elwood PW: Magnetic resonance imaging and the nonoperative treatment of spinal epidural abscess, *Surg Neurol* 34:408-413, 1990.

Hashimoto T, Mitomo M, Hirabuki N, et al: Nerve root avulsion of birth palsy: comparison of myelography with CT myelography and somatosensory evoked potential, *Radiology* 178:841-845, 1991.

Hayes CW, Conway WF, Walsh JW, et al: Seat belt injuries: radiologic findings and clinical correlation, *RadioGraphics* 11:23-36 , 1991.

Heinz R, Curnes J, Friedman A, et al: Exophytic syrinx, an extreme form of syringomyelia: CT, myelographic, and MR imaging features, *Radiology* 183(1):243-246, 1992.

Hoffman JR, Mower WR, Wolfson AB, et al: Validity of a set of clinical criteria to rule out injury to the cervical spine in patients with blunt trauma. National Emergency X-Radiography Utilization Study Group [see comments], *New Engl J Med* 343(2):94-99, 2000.

Isoda H, Takahashi M, Mochizuki T, et al: MRI of dumbbell-shaped spinal tumors, *J Comput Assist Tomogr* 20(4):573-582, 1996.

Jack CR, Kokmen E, Onofrio BM: Spontaneous decompression of syringomyelia: magnetic resonance imaging findings, *J Neurosurg* 74:283-286, 1991.

Jelly L, Evans D, Easty MJ, et al: Radiography versus spiral CT in the evaluation of cervicothoracic junction injuries in polytrauma patients who have undergone intubation, *Radiographics* 20:251S-259, 2000.

Jinkins JR, Bashir R, Al-Mefty O, et al: Cystic necrosis of the spinal cord in compressive cervical myelopathy: demonstration by lopamidol CT-myelography, *AJNR* 7:693-701, 1986.

Jinkins JR and Sener RN: Idiopathic localized hydromyelia: dilatation of the central canal of the spinal cord of probable congenital origin, *J Comput Assist Tomogr* 23(3):351-353, 1999.

Jones DN, Knox AM, Sage MR: Traumatic avulsion fracture of the occipital condyles and clivus with associated unilateral atlantooccipital distraction, *AJNR* 11:1181-1183, 1990.

Kapeller P, Fazekas F, Krametter D, et al: Pyogenic infectious spondylitis: clinical, laboratory and MRI features, *Eur Neurol* 38(2):94-98, 1997.

Kaplan P, Resnick D, Murphey M, et al: Destructive noninfectious spondyloarthropathy in hemodialysis patients: a report of four cases, *Radiology* 162:241-244, 1987.

Kendall BE, Logue V: Spinal epidural angiomatous malformations draining into intrathecal veins, *Neuroradiology* 13:181-189, 1977.

Kesterson L, Benzel E, Orrison W, et al: Evaluation and treatment of atlas burst fractures (Jefferson fractures), *J Neurosurg* 75:213-220, 1991.

Kim RC: Necrotizing myelopathy, *AJNR* 12:1084-1086, 1992, *AJR* 158, 1992.

Klein SL, Sanford RA, Muhlbauer MS: Pediatric spinal epidural metastases, *J Neurosurg* 74:70-75, 1991.

Knudsen LL, Voldby B, Stagarrd M: Computed tomographic myelography in spinal subdural empyema, *Neuroradiology* 29:99, 1987.

Koeller K, Rosenblum R, Morrison AL, et al: Neoplasms of the spinal cord and filum terminale: radiologic-pathologic correlation *Radiographics* 20(6):1721-1749, 2000.

Kraus GE, Bucholz RD, Weber TR: Spinal cord arteriovenous malformation with an associated lymphatic anomaly, *J Neurosurg* 73:768-773, 1990.

Kulkarni MV, McArdle CB, Kopanicky D, et al: Acute spinal cord injury: MR imaging at 1.5T, *Radiology* 164:837-843, 1987.

Laredo J, Assouline E, Gelbert F, et al: Vertebral hemangiomas: fat content as a sign of aggressiveness, *Radiology* 177:467-472, 1990.

Laredo J, Reizine D, Bard M, et al: Vertebral hemangiomas: radiologic evaluation, *Radiology* 161:183-189, 1986.

Laredo JD, Lakhdari K, Bellaiche L, et al: Acute vertebral collapse: CT findings in benign and malignant nontraumatic cases, *Radiology* 194(1):41-48, 1995.

Larsson EM, Desai P, Hardin CW, et al: Venous infarction of the spinal cord resulting from dural arteriovenous fistula: MR imaging findings, *AJNR* 12:739-743, 1991.

Lecouvet F, Vande Berg B, Michaux L, et al: Development of vertebral fractures in patients with multiple myeloma: does MRI enable recognition of vertebrae that will collapse? *J Comput Assist Tomogr* 22(3):430-436, 1998.

Lee C, Woodring JH, Goldstein SJ, et al: Evaluation of traumatic atlantooccipital dislocations, *AJNR* 8:19-26, 1987.

Lee C, Woodring JH: Unstable Jefferson variant atlas fractures: an unrecognized cervical injury, *AJNR* 12:1105-1110, 1992; *AJR* 158, 1992.

Lim V, Sobel DF, Zyroff J: Spinal cord pial metastases: MR imaging with gadopentetate dimeglumine, *AJNR* 11:975-982, 1990; *AJR* 155:1077-1084, 1990.

Lin-Greenberg A, Cholankeril J: Vertebral arch destruction in tuberculosis: CT features, *J Comput Assist Tomogr* 14:300-302, 1990.

Maki DD and Grossman RI: Patterns of disease spread in metastatic breast carcinoma: influence of estrogen and progesterone receptor status, *AJNR* 21(6):1064-6, 2000.

Masaryk TJ, Ross JS, Modic MT, et al: Radiculomeningeal vascular malformations of the spine: MR imaging, *Radiology* 168: 845-849, 1987.

Mascalchi M, Bianchi MC, Quilici N, et al: MR angiography of spinal vascular malformations, *AJNR* 16(2):289-297, 1995.

McCarthy JT, Dahlberg PJ, Kriegshauser JS, et al: Erosive spondyloarthropathy in long-term dialysis patients: relationship to severe hyperparathyroidism, *Mayo Clin Proc* 63:446-452, 1988.

McCormick PC, Torres R, Post KD, et al: Intramedullary ependymoma of the spinal cord, *J Neurosurg* 72:523-532, 1990.

Melhem ER, Wang H: Intramedullary spinal cord tuberculoma in a patient with AIDS, *AJNR* 13:986-988, 1992.

Mendelsohn DB, Zollars L, Weatherall PT, et al: MR of cord transection, *J Comput Assist Tomogr* 14:909-911, 1990.

Meyer JE, Lepke RA, Lindfors KK, et al: Chordomas: their CT appearance in the cervical, thoracic and lumbar spine, *Radiology* 1 53:693-696, 1984.

Mikulis DJ, Ogilvy CS, McKee A, et al: Spinal cord infarction and fibrocartilaginous emboli, *AJNR* 13:155-160, 1992.

Mirich DR, Kucharczyk W, Keller AM, et al: Subacute necrotizing myelopathy: MR imaging in four pathologically proved cases, *AJNR* 12:1077-1083, 1991.

Mirvis SE, Geisler FH, Jelinek JJ, et al: Acute cervical spine trauma: evaluation with 1.5-T MR imaging, *Radiology* 166: 807-816, 1988.

Modic MT, Feiglin DH, Piraino DW, et al: Vertebral osteomyelitis: assessment using MR, *Radiology* 157:157-166, 1985.

Nowicki BH, Haughton VM: Neural foraminal ligaments of the lumbar spine: appearance at CT and MR imaging, *Radiology* 183:257-264, 1992.

Oner F, van Gils A, Dhert WJ, et al: MRI findings of thoracolumbar spine fractures: a categorization based on MRI examinations of 100 fractures, *Skeletal Radiol* 28(8):433-443, 1999.

Parizel PM, Baleriaux D, Rodesch G, et al: Gd-DTPA-enhanced MR imaging of spinal tumors, *AJNR* 10:249-258, 1989.

Patel U, Pinto RS, Miller DC, et al: MR of spinal cord ganglioglioma [see comments], *AJNR* 19(5):879-887, 1998.

Paulsen RD, Call GA, Murtagh FR, et al: Prevalence and percutaneous drainage of cysts of the sacral nerve root sheath (Tarlov cysts), *AJNR* 15(2):293-297; discussion 298-299, 1994.

Pech P, Kilgore DP, Pojunas KW, et al: Cervical spinal fractures: CT detection, *Radiology* 157:117-120, 1985.

Pellei D: The fat C2 sign, *Radiology* 217(2):359-360, 2000.

Pope TL, Wang G, Whitehill R: Discogenic vertebral sclerosis: a potential mimic of disc space infection or metastatic disease, *Orthopedics* 13:1389-1397, 1990.

Post MJD, Sze G, Quencer RM, et al: Gadolinium-enhanced MR in spinal infection, *J Comput Assist Tomogr* 14:721-729, 1990.

Price AC, Allen JH, Eggers FM, et al: Intervertebral disk-space infection: CT changes, *Radiology* 149:725-729, 1983.

Provenzale JM, Barboriak DP, Gaensler EH, et al: Lupus-related myelitis: serial MR findings, *AJNR* 15(10):1911-1917, 1994.

Pryce AP, Wiender SN: Syringomyelia associated with Paget disease of the skull, *AJR* 155:881-882, 1990.

Puljic S, Schechter MM: Multiple spinal canal meningiomas, *AJNR* 1:325-327, 1980.

Quint DJ, Levy R, Krauss JC, et al: MR of myelomatous meningitis, *AJNR* 16(6):1316-1317, 1995.

Raghavan N, Barkovich AJ, Edwards M, et al: MR imaging in the tethered spinal cord syndrome, *AJNR* 10:27-36, 1989.

Ragland RL, Abdelwahab IF, Braffman B, et al: Posterior spinal tuberculosis: a case report, *AJNR* 11:612-613, 1990.

Ravin B, Loevner LA, Bank W, et al: MR findings in subacute combined degeneration of the spinal cord: a case of reversible cervical myelopathy, *AJR* 174(3):863-865, 2000.

Robertson DP, Kirkpatrick JP, Harper RL, et al: Spinal intramedullary ependymal cyst, *J Neurosurg* 75:312-316, 1991.

Ronnen HR, de Korte PJ, et al: Acute whiplash injury: is there a role for MR imaging?—a prospective study of 100 patients, *Radiology* 201(1):93-96, 1996.

Russo CP, Katz DS, et al: Gangliocytoma of the cervicothoracic spinal cord, *AJNR* 16(4 Suppl):889-891, 1995.

Santosh CG, Bell JE, et al: Spinal tract pathology in AIDS: postmortem MRI correlation with neuropathology, *Neuroradiology* 37(2):134-138, 1995.

Sartoris DJ, Clopton P, Nemcek A, et al: Vertebral-body collapse in focal and diffuse disease: patterns of pathologic processes, *Radiology* 160:479-483, 1986.

Sartoris DJ, Resnick D, Guerra J: Vertebral venous channels: CT appearance and differential considerations, *Radiology* 155:745-749, 1985.

Satran R: Spinal cord infarction, *Curr Concepts Cerebrovasc Dis Stroke* 22:13-17, 1987.

Scott EW, Haid RW, Peace D: Type I fractures of the odontoid process: implications for atlanto-occipital instability, *J Neurosurg* 72:488-492, 1990.

Sharif HS, Clark DC, Aabed MY, et al: Granulomatous spinal infections: MR imaging, *Radiology* 177:101-107, 1990.

Shimada K, T Tokioka: Sequential MRI studies in patients with cervical cord injury but without bony injury, *Paraplegia* 33(10):573-578, 1995.

Shuman WP, Rogers JV, Sickler ME, et al: Thoracolumbar burst fractures: CT dimensions of the spinal canal relative to postsurgical improvement, *AJNR* 6:337-341, 1985.

Silbergeld DL, Laohaprasit V, Grady MS, et al: Two cases of fatal atlantoaxial distraction injury without fracture or rotation, *Surg Neurol* 35:54-56, 1991.

Silverstein AM, Quint DJ, McKeever PE: Intradural paraganglioma of the thoracic spine, *AJNR* 11:614-616, 1990.

Stern Y, Spiegelman R, Sadeh M: Spinal intradural arachnoid cysts, *Neurochirurgia* 34:127-130, 1991.

Sze G, Stimac GK, Bartlett C, et al: Multicenter study of gadopentetate dimeglumine as an MR contrast agent: evaluation in patients with spinal tumors, *AJNR* 11:967-974, 1990.

Tartaglino LM, Croul SE, et al: Idiopathic acute transverse myelitis: MR imaging findings, *Radiology* 201(3):661-669, 1996.

Tator CH, Fehlings MG: Review of the secondary injury theory of acute spinal cord trauma with emphasis on vascular mechanisms, *J Neurosurg* 75:15-26, 1991.

Thomeier WC, Brown DC, Mirvis SE: The laterally tilted dens: a sign of subtle odontoid fracture on plain radiography, *AJNR* 11:605-608, 1990.

Thruss A, Enzmann D: MR imaging of infectious spondylitis, *AJNR* 11:1171-1180, 1990.

Timms SR, Cure JK, Kurent JE, et al: Subacute combined degeneration of the spinal cord: MR findings, *AJNR* 14(5):1224-1227, 1993.

Van Lom KJ, Kellerhouse LE, Pathria MN, et al: Infection versus tumor in the spine: criteria for distinction with CT, *Radiology* 166:851-855, 1988.

Voyvodic F, Dolinis J, Moore VM, et al: MRI of car occupants with whiplash injury, *Neuroradiology* 39(1):35-40, 1997.

Watters MR, Stears JC, Osborn AG, et al: Transdural spinal cord herniation: imaging and clinical spectra [see comments], *AJNR* 19(7):1337-1344, 1998.

Waubant E, Manelfe C, Bonafe A, et al: MRI of intramedullary sarcoidosis: follow-up of a case, *Neuroradiology* 39(5):357-360, 1997.

White P, Seymour R, Powell N, et al: MRI assessment of the pre-vertebral soft tissues in acute cervical spine trauma, *Br J Radiol* 72(860):818-823, 1999.

Wiener MD, Boyko OB, Friedman HS, et al: False-positive spinal MR findings for subarachnoid spread of primary CNS tumor in postoperative pediatric patients, *AJNR* 11:1100-1103, 1990.

Williams MP, Olliff JFC, Rowley MR: CT and MR findings in parameningeal leukaemic masses, *J Comput Assist Tomogr* 14:736-742, 1990.

Yuh WTC, Marsh EE, Wang AK, et al: MR imaging of spinal cord and vertebral body infarction, *AJNR* 13:145-154, 1992.

Zager EL, Ojemann RG, Poletti CE: Acute presentations of syringomyelia, *J Neurosurg* 72:133-138, 1990.

Zlatkin MB, Lander PH, Hadjipavlou AG, et al: Paget disease of the spine: CT with clinical correlation, *Radiology* 160:155-159, 1986.

Zweig G, Russell EJ: Radiation myelopathy of the cervical spinal cord: MR findings, *AJNR* 11:1188-1190, 1990.

Zwimpfer TJ, Bernstein M: Spinal cord concussion, *J Neurosurg* 72:894-900, 1990.

CHAPTER 18

Approach and Pitfalls in Neuroimaging

READING "FOOLOSOPHY," OR "A RADIOLOGIST AND HIS MONEY ARE SOON PARTED"

If you have read the preceding chapters with due diligence, we can assume that you have the knowledge base for grandilloquating and titubating on the various entities that frequent the neuroradiologic realm. Etiologies, pathogeneses, complications, and clinical manifestations of many of the disorders of the central nervous system and head and neck should be firmly entrenched in your hippocampus. However, that is only half the task in radiology. The first step is to "make the finding." The next step is integrating the clinical information with the radiologic findings. We hope to present to the reader in this chapter the "Search Engine" for identification and

understanding the findings. The most important part of reading films in any branch of radiology is (1) the detection of abnormalities and (2) the classification of lesions into various differential diagnoses. It is easy to teach you the facts about diseases. Our goal in this chapter is to train you to have "good eyes." We always teach our fellows "you see what you know." The Sylvan Learning Center for wayward, obtuse neuroradiologists (SLCWON) says, "reading is fun-damental." The ultimate compliment for the radiologist is that "She is brilliant AND she has great eyes." Of course such a compliment may transcend the radiology application.

From a medicolegal standpoint, radiologists are easy prey. The answer (the evidence) is always on the film, PACS, or magnetic tape and does not go away. As we move down the road towards greater and greater softcopy reading, imaging data will be stored on computers for longer and longer periods in excellent condition. No longer will water stains and browning of the silver or blurred copy films help to obscure findings from old studies retrieved for malpractice suits. Lesions invisible on today's study will be readily detected through a 20/20 "retrospectoscope" on a review 6 years from now. Radiologists cannot retreat behind the usual clinical dodges of "That murmur was not present 3 months ago," or "The patient did not have a foot drop when I examined him," or, "That is a new rash." The good, the bad, and the ugly of radiology is that the answer is always on the images. The combination of the prior studies and follow-up films are a powerful and sometimes embarrassing force. With that continuum it is easy to identify our mistakes in a court of law.

Why do we bring up all of this fatalistic medicolegal mumbo-jumbo? We want to impress on you the need for an organized, thorough review of **all** images of a study. Many radiologists have picked up parotid masses, posterior triangle lymphadenopathy, cervical syringohydromyelic cavities, nasopharyngeal carcinomas, C1-2 dislocations, and cervical vascular disease, on sagittal "scout" images. For all of us potential defendants, do not neglect to look consistently at all images of all scans. And learn from your mistakes. To err is human, but it feels divine if presented as a learning tool. Nothing is more constructive (and instructive) than a missed case. How do you think we became so brilliant? Lots of mistakes made!! Keep track of your misses so you will be sure to look at that part of the image in the future. Enough nagging, more teaching!

Reading a CT

The approach to reading a case varies according to the clinical indication for the study and personal habits. As long as the modus operandi is consistent, thorough, and organized, the film will be read appropriately. We will provide one technique with a generic example of a commonly scribbled CT request: "Emergency room study: rule out bleed." Sometimes you do not even get that much information—it may be totally nonspecific, misleading, or illegible! (What do you expect?) What is the context of the "rule-out bleed" study? Is it in the setting of a stroke, trauma, or worst headache of one's life? An ounce of clinical information is worth a pound of radiologist banal statements (BS) in the report (and since "rule out bleed" is not even a reimbursable ICD-9 code, you may not even get paid for your meaningless read).

Start by taking the central to peripheral approach, looking at each image from first slice to last individually. Your first "gestalt" of a CT is based on an analysis of the ventricles and basal cisterns. Because CT is increasingly being relegated to the role of the emergency room study for trauma or acute neurologic deficits, the first thing to assess is whether there is mass effect or subarachnoid hemorrhage. If present, to what degree? Are the ventricles shifted from their normal position, and are the cisterns or sulci effaced by mass effect? Be careful, subtle sulcal effacement may be the only clue to a mass lesion or early stroke. Is herniation (e.g., subfalcian, uncal, transtentorial, upward) present, detectable by shift of the lateral ventricles, dilatation of the temporal horn, compression of ambient cisterns, or fourth ventricular displacement? If so, call someone before dictating the case. Are all the basal cisterns effaced and the ventricles small, suggestive of diffuse cerebral swelling? Call 911. Are the ventricles, and in particular the temporal horns enlarged, suggestive of hydrocephalus, or are they appropriate for the patient's age and clinical status? A 70-year-old book editor with small ventricles should put your hair on end for masses. Asymmetry of the ventricles is not uncommon, but it should heighten the suspicion of a unilateral obstructive mass or septation at the foramen of Monroe. If there is hydrocephalus, is it communicating or noncommunicating? Look carefully at the density of the basal cisterns. Is blood present? Is there blood in the interhemispheric fissure, ventricles, or sylvian fissure?

By the analysis of the ventricles and cisterns, you should have determined whether a surgical emergency is present. Has an aneurysm bled? Does the patient need to be shunted? Is there brain swelling requiring steroids and diuretics or surgical decompression? Is there potential herniation from a mass that needs to be removed emergently? Are you going to be up all night doing an angiogram and/or postoperative imaging?

Here is a commonly overlooked emergency—the cerebellar infarct. This "mass" may be obscured by beam-hardening artifact but it can be lethal. In a short time, the infarcted tissue, in the closed space of the posterior fossa, may quickly obstruct the fourth ventricle leading to acute hydrocephalus, or cause tonsillar herniation. Always identify the fourth ventricle, determine its midline position, and search for density differences in the parenchyma around it.

Next on the agenda is looking at the periphery of the brain for extraaxial collections. Again, CT is commonly used now in the setting of acute head trauma, and a subdural or epidural hematoma is a major source of morbidity. You may already have a suspicion that the patient may have mass effect on the basis of effacement of sulci, midline shift, buckling of the gray-white matter interface, or compression of ventricles. Now search for that mass, most commonly an extraaxial collection, in the case of a CT after closed head injury. Bilateral extracerebral collections may not cause ventricular shift. Beware, mon frere. The isodense subdural hematoma may be very subtle if you do not notice that the white matter is not approaching the periphery of the brain and there is absence of normal sulcation. Pay particular attention to the scans with intermediate windows that are more sensitive to subtle density differences and less susceptible to volume averaging of cortex.

On the peripheral pass through the brain you may detect soft-tissue scalp swelling, which hints to the site of the head trauma. Pay particular attention to the underlying brain as well as to the contrecoup direction. You may detect a skull fracture (if you look at the bone window settings) and should be wary about epidural hematomas over the temporal lobes or near venous sinuses. Foreign bodies or scalp lacerations may hint at the nature of the injury.

Next, begin to look at the brain parenchyma itself. An initial run-through from central to peripheral will identify any obvious areas of density differences suggestive of hemorrhage or necrosis. In the setting of trauma petechial hemorrhages that are rather subtle on CT may be the only evidence of a shearing injury. Check the gray-white junction and the splenium for white matter tears. Mass effect may be present without gross density changes because of the microscopic nature of this process. Another setting where hemorrhage is common is with hypertensive crises. Hypertensive bleeds occur most commonly in deep gray matter structures near the ventricles, so start there. Work outward to detect cortical hemorrhages from infarcts or contusions. Again, you may be directed to look at a particular site on the basis of analysis of the ventricular displacement, scalp findings or peripheral collections. Do not expect clinical information to guide you since the ER docs are often as aphasic on request slips as the GCS-3 patient. Sulcal effacement, a pet finding of one of the authors, may clue you in here as well.

Now it is time to look for subtle areas of distorted architecture or density differences. To be frank, clinicians know whether a patient has had a stroke. They do not need a neuroradiologist to tell them that, but **it is important** to let them know whether the stroke is hemorrhagic or is causing mass effect, shift, or herniation. Does it involve more than a third of the MCA distribution, leading to greater risk of thrombolytic therapy? Look for those subtle areas of lower density to suggest edema from a stroke, nonhemorrhagic shearing injuries, demyelination, or early neoplasms. But more important, make sure you look for subtle hemorrhage, because that also figures prominently in therapeutic decision-making as to whether to anticoagulate. You should not feel too bad if you miss a stroke on an early CT, because this is often a clinical diagnosis. But you probably will feel horrible if you miss the hemorrhage associated with that stroke, the clinicians heparinize or tPA the patient, and the dude herniates and subsequently dies from a massive bleed. Bad miss, Saddam. You should feel equally glum about overlooking subarachnoid hemorrhage, a life-threatening mass, or an extraaxial collection that demands treatment. The lawyers are sure to gain as they put you in pain, and drive you insane, create an asset drain, and mess with your brain.

When looking at the parenchyma it is important to know the vascular anatomy and the common sites for various pathologic entities. Look for clots in the middle cerebral artery and for strokes in the MCA distribution around the insula and temporal lobe and in deep gray matter structures. Check the watershed areas for strokes caused by hypotension or hypoxia. In hypertensive patients or ones with atherosclerosis, be sure to check for lacunar infarctions in the capsules and the lentiform nuclei. In trauma, carefully evaluate the temporal tips, subfrontal regions, and occipital lobes where coup-contrecoup injuries occur. For posterior fossa lesions check the fourth ventricle to see which way it is pushed; look at the contralateral cerebellar hemisphere. Check the temporal lobes in any patient with a fever and a change in mental status; herpes resides there (. . . and down there too, but that is a different herpes virus).

Finally it is time to make a last survey of the rest of the scan for abnormalities. Once again, check the age of the patient. Are the sulci and ventricles appropriately sized for age? When too big, this may indicate acquired immunodeficiency syndrome (AIDS) or Alzheimer disease. It also occasionally tells you whether the patients are substance abusers. If too small, check for that isodense subdural or diffuse cerebral swelling. Is sinusitis present? Is there a nasopharyngeal or airway mass present? Are the globes normal, and are there orbital masses? Do you detect papilledema, seen as reversed cupping of the optic nerve head insertion into the globe? If so, check again for causes of increased intracranial pressure. Check the scans with bone windows. Are any skull base foramina enlarged or eroded? Are fractures present? Sinusitis, mastoiditis, otitis media in a search for a source of fever? TMJ disease in a patient with headaches? Always check the scout topogram; you will be surprised how often you will pick up cervical spine injuries, spondylosis, bone metastases, basilar invagination, platybasia, myeloma, an enlarged sella, and other conditions on the basis of the scout view. These findings may not be readily apparent on the axial images.

Here is an alternative approach regarding the request slip. Blot out the clinical history and view the scan in a vacuum. What is your overall impression of the case? Be an umpire; call it as you see it—blind. Commit. *Then* factor in the clinical history. Now you are ready for *the show.*

Reading an MR

Magnetic resonance (MR) imaging is a lot harder to read than CT, because you are bombarded by information, all of it potentially useful to the analysis of the case. Complex cases have simple, easy to understand, but often wrong diagnoses. It is much harder to give a blueprint for how to read MR than CT because of the different pulse sequences, planes, and scan parameters available. CT is to MR as checkers is to chess. Here is a brief summary of one approach.

Use the same routine: start from central to peripheral. The first image to look at is the sagittal midline image on the scout T1WI. If that scan is hard to recognize, then it is likely that a mass displaces the midline, but the mass will be better seen on axial scans. On the midline image start from bottom to top and identify the cervical spine, nasopharynx, clivus, cerebellar tonsils, fourth ventricle, vermis, brain stem, basilar artery, cerebral aqueduct, sella, pituitary, optic chiasm, third ventricle, corpus callosum, pericallosal arteries, cingulate gyrus, cerebral cortex, sagittal sinus, and the partridge in the pear tree. Are any of these structures displaced upward or downward, not present at all, or of abnormal signal intensity? From the midline go to the more peripheral images and make sure you search for extraaxial collections, the carotid and vertebral arteries, al Quaeda operatives, and abnormal signal intensity (usually high) to suggest hemorrhage. Again, check the temporal tips and the temporal lobes for hemorrhage or sulcal distortion, particularly in the setting of trauma.

Remember that the sagittal image is usually the only one that also gives you a peek at the cervical spine and neck, because most axial scans start at the foramen magnum and go up. This is your only chance for that outstanding edge of the film neck call that elevates you over the less proficient radiologists who bought less profound and more expensive books than this one. The sagittal scans have more information that can potentiate a lawsuit. Is a Chiari malformation present? Is there a syrinx in the cervical spinal cord? Are there herniated cervical disks? Is posterior triangle lymphadenopathy present? Is a parotid, submandibular gland, lingual, pharyngeal, or laryngeal mass present? Are the orbits normal?

The next sequence performed is usually a T2-weighted one, be it a FLAIR or fast spin echo T2WI. Just as with axial CT, follow the path from central to peripheral, to central, to peripheral again until you are dazed, nystagmoid, and vertiginous. As you analyze the ventricles and cisterns for displacements, the subdural and epidural spaces for collections, the deep gray matter structures for signal intensity abnormalities, and the peripheral cortex for subtleties of intensity differences and mass effect, recall how easy things seemed during your medicine internship. Remember, reading the cases is like doing an arteriotomy—if at first you don't succeed, just keep stabbing at it. Eventually you'll hit on *something*.

Check out the sulcal pattern and size with relation to patient age, and check the bone marrow and base of skull for masses. The FLAIR/T2WI is the most sensitive (but often least specific) sequence you perform. FLAIR scans will lull you into a state of complacency as the contrast of edema from normal tissue is so exquisite. But BEWARE! Posterior fossa signal intensity abnormalities are not as contrasty on FLAIR and you should use the T2WI to double-check this vital real estate. Remember also that as cystic and encephalomalacic areas approach water content, they will be hypointense on FLAIR scans and may be less conspicuous. Do not drop your guard if that FLAIR crutch seems normal at first glance. Do not be a neurologist reading the scans! Pay attention or the game may be lost right here.

If you still perform proton density weighted scans, analyze the signal intensity of the lesion on the first and second echoes to see how it changes from short to long TE. This may add specificity to the analysis of the composition of the lesion (lacunes versus Virchow-Robin spaces, CSF versus epidermoid). Remember that with FLAIR and T2WI you are basically looking only at T2 characteristics of a lesion—you have lost the marginal contribution of hydrogen density by dropping a PDWI.

You may next view diffusion-weighted images (DWI).

There are potential pitfalls here as well. Not everything that is bright on DWI is an infarct because of the inherent T2-weighting of these studies. One should be cognizant of the concept of T2 shine-through. Therefore, if you do not have the capability of performing (or do not routinely construct) apparent diffusion coefficient (ADC) maps to determine if the bright areas on DWI are from cytotoxic edema (decreased ADC) or from a T2 effect (increased ADC), you must hedge your bets, or spend the money to purchase the software. Remember also that some entities cause decreased ADC but are not strokes—pyogenic abscesses, some tumors, herpes, some demyelinating lesions, and so on. Therefore, one must look at the distribution of the lesion. Remember that the evaluation of stroke may not end at a negative DWI scan. In centers with active stroke intervention programs you may be required to perform a perfusion scan to demonstrate the ischemic penumbra. In some settings this will lead to medical therapy designed to optimize cerebral blood flow (hypertensive, hypervolemic therapy) or thrombolysis. The brain tissue may not be infarcted (DWI negative) yet, but leave the patient alone and in 2 hours it will be. We good doctors would like to prevent that!

Often there is an enhanced scan to review. By this time the PDWI/FLAIR/T2WI/DWI will have been assessed and a mass may be suspected on the basis of morphologic criteria and/or a signal intensity abnormality; however, numerous lesions are apparent only on enhanced scans. The first place to start is simple: are there any intraparenchymal bright areas on the enhanced image that were not present on the precontrast study? If you have not performed a pregadolinium axial T1W scan (and most centers are dropping these in the interest of throughput), you must rely on your sagittal T1WI to determine this. In the event of a particularly vexing case, before bringing the patient back to your imaging center for pregadolinium scans, reformat your sagittals into the axial plane and see if you can make the call. For this reason you may perform high quality (5-mm interleaved ear to ear) sagittal T1WI—it is your one shot for pregadolinium T1WI evaluation. Next, look at the periphery. Is there abnormal enhancement of the meninges, dura, cisterns, exiting nerves, ependyma, or extraaxial fluid collections? Do the arteries enhance? (They should not on non–flow-compensated images because of fast flow so maybe they are not arteries or there is slow flow in them.) Finally, look at the areas that *normally* enhance to determine whether there are nonenhancing abnormalities. Do the adenohypophysis and pituitary stalk enhance uniformly? Do the venous sinuses enhance? Choroid? Area postrema (oh make me puke!)?

Return once again to that sagittal sequence and assess the precontrast signal intensity of any lesion you have identified subsequently. Retrace the hidden areas of the spine, neck, and midline structures.

While this approach may seem frightening,
Soon you'll be fast as lightning,
Your senses will be heightening,
And your differentials will be tightening.

A resident reading this chapter
Thought, "I wonder what the authors are after"
I know how to read 'em
I don't have to heed them
The lawyers could hardly contain their laughter
(As they hung him from the rafter)

HOW TO INTERPRET AN IMAGE

Knowledge of the implications of signal intensity and density changes in normal and abnormal tissue, together with a lesion's morphology, location, and clinical presentation, enables accurate diagnosis. At no extra cost we have included tables of useful radiologic gamuts in Appendix A after this chapter. Tear them out or tear them up, use them as you wish, but they may be helpful to intimidate your colleagues on the plane to the board examinations.

Detection of lesions begins with a knowledge of normal anatomy and its variants. It is only through reviewing numerous cases day after day that one obtains a mental image of the normal anatomy from which deviations can be readily identified. This is the source of the speed of the readings made by the codgey old professors of neuroradiology—they have burned a CD template into their brain of the pattern recognition for normality. Thus,

they can scan an image at light speed and still detect the subtlest abnormalities. One colleague of ours was known to chat with the resident as he continuously motored through the 50 board alternator, making the findings without having to remove his foot from the pedal control. Of course he is now on the West Coast, sipping Starbucks coffee, doing the same thing, and striking gold in Silicon Valley. But he too once had to slog through the numerous, boring normal scans of the brain and spine, to imprint that template of normality. The trainees who view the most cases will be served well in this regard— they will have the easiest time detecting lesions.

Let us start with the complicated modality—MR. MR lends itself to image analysis from several perspectives. These are based on intensity, morphology, and location. We believe that you can evaluate a lesion with very little knowledge—how do you think we got this far? Liken yourself to a stock market technical analyst. Note the trends. You really do not have to know that much about the company (pathology) if you just follow the basics and avoid Arthur Anderson analyses.

The first question is the intensity of the lesion on conventional pulse sequences: (1) T1WI, (2) PDWI, (3) T2WI, (4) FLAIR, (5) DWI, and (6) gradient echo scans. Remember that the B zero images from a diffusion-weighted scan are a poor man's gradient echo scan in just 40 to 50 seconds—film them and use them. Table 18-1 provides useful information concerning the characterization of lesion types with intensity information. Unfortunately, all too often MR lacks specificity, because most lesions are dark on T1WI and bright on T2WI. There is presently no signal *intensity* pattern hallmark

---

Table 18-1   Signal intensity characteristics of tissue on T1WI and T2WI

High intensity on T1WI	Low intensity on T1WI	High intensity on T2WI (hyperintense)	Low intensity on T2WI (hypointense)
High protein	Water (CSF, edema)	Water (CSF, edema)	High protein
Subacute hemorrhage (methemoglobin)	Acute hemorrhage (deoxyhemoglobin)		Acute hemorrhage (deoxyhemoglobin)
Gadolinium	Chronic hemorrhage (hemosiderin)		Chronic hemorrhage (hemosiderin)
Other paramagnetics (manganese, calcium, melanin)	Diamagnetic effects (calcification, air)		Early subacute hemorrhage (intracellular methemoglobin)
Blood flow (flow-related enhancement or even-echo rephasing)	Fast flow		Other paramagnetics (melanin, calcium)
Fat	Very viscous protein		Diamagnetics (calcification, air)
Cholesterol/cholesterin	Susceptibility artifact		High concentrations of gadolinium
	Low protein		Fast flow
			Fat (non-fast spin echo)
			Metal
			Susceptibility artifact

that clearly distinguishes, say, multiple sclerosis plaques from infarction or tumor. If a lesion decreases in intensity as the T2 weighting increases, you are more likely to be dealing with a lesion that has susceptibility effects. Gradient echo scanning emphasizes susceptibility differences and flow. Therefore, lesions that are hypointense on pulse sequences emphasizing T2 information appear significantly more hypointense on gradient echo scans if magnetic susceptibility is present.

The morphology of the lesion is important in its categorization. Several criteria are critical here: mass effect, atrophy, texture, edema pattern, extent of lesion, nature (solid versus cystic), number (single or multiple), distribution (e.g., along vascular supplies, Virchow-Robin spaces, cranial nerves, meninges, white matter tracts) involvement of one or both hemispheres, and enhancement characteristics. The presence or absence of mass effect is usually obvious. Lesions possessing mass effect are usually "active," whereas those, which do not, may be either old or very new. Examples of the former include a tumor or new stroke, whereas the latter would include an old stroke or old traumatic injury to the brain. Mass effect can be subtle, with slight effacement of sulci; however, such changes are highly significant with respect to arriving at the correct diagnosis. Careful observation is necessary. Absence of mass effect does not necessarily indicate benignity; rather, such lesions may be early in their evolution. The presence of focal atrophy (tissue loss) signifies past insult to the brain. Although the brain parenchyma decreases with age normally, focal loss of parenchyma is significant. Furthermore, global atrophic changes exceeding those for age suggest other processes such as steroid use, neurodegenerative disorders, human immunodeficiency virus (HIV) infection, and authors of second editions of books, to name a few.

Certain lesions have rather characteristic textures. For instance, oligodendrogliomas have a rather heterogeneous texture whereas lymphomas are more homogeneous. If edema is associated with a lesion, there is clearly an irritative element involved. The converse of this is not true; that is, if there is no edema, there is nothing harmful. Lesions without edema can be virulent: cortical metastases, gliomatosis cerebri, Creutzfeldt-Jakob disease, and HIV infection. The extent of the lesion also gives some clues to the diagnosis. In general, a lesion spanning both hemispheres is most likely tumor, because edema does not usually cross the connecting white matter tracts. Generally, lesions that are aggressive are poorly marginated and infiltrative. Again, the converse is not true. Many lesions have cystic components or are themselves cystic yet span the spectrum of aggressiveness. These include colloid cysts, craniopharyngioma, cystic astrocytoma, or necrotic glioblastomas. FLAIR images can distinguish CSF containing structures (hypointense) from more complex cystic lesions, the latter being high signal intensity with contents that have complex constituents including high levels of protein. Multiplicity of lesions changes the radiologic diagnostic gamut (e.g., metastatic lesions, multiple strokes, multicentric tumor, neurofibromas, and multiple sclerosis).

Enhancement is very important. It establishes that the lesion has an abnormal blood-brain barrier. It does not, however, indicate whether a lesion is benign malignant, nor does it demarcate the border of the lesion. It is instrumental in increasing our sensitivity to detecting abnormalities, particularly extraaxial and cortical neoplasms. We err on the side of giving contrast because it improves our sensitivity and specificity and enables us to read faster with more conviction.

Finally, location (just as in real estate) is of critical importance in making the correct diagnosis. Is the lesion intraaxial, extraaxial, or both? Obviously, extraaxial lesions suggest a different differential diagnosis from those that are purely intraaxial. Multiplanar images help resolve this question. Certain lesions have a propensity for specific locations; for example, herpes simplex affects the temporal lobe, oligodendroglioma the frontotemporal lobe, and juvenile pilocytic astrocytomas the posterior fossa and suprasellar region. Does the lesion involve the cortex, white matter, or both? This provides the initial diagnostic algorithm. If the lesion is predominantly in the white matter we might consider multiple sclerosis whereas if it affects both white and gray matter it may suggest a stroke. In the latter instance the lesion should follow a vascular distribution (but sometimes lesions do not read our book).

The interpretation of CT overlaps that of MR with respect to location, morphology, presentation, and enhancement features. The exception to this rule is that vessels enhance on CT, whereas, if there is fast flow, they do not enhance on MR. For your limbic pleasure, consider the density characteristics of lesions on CT in Table 18-2.

REVIEW OF BRAIN NEOPLASMS

To repeat for a third time in this book (Murphy's law: that which is repeated most will be the first forgotten), the most fundamental question that neuroradiologists

Table 18-2 Density characteristics of lesions on CT

Hypodense	Isodense	Hyperdense
Water (CSF, edema)	Intermediate protein	High protein (hemorrhage)
Fat	Normal brain	Calcium
Air		Metal
Low protein		Iodine
		Pantopaque

must ask themselves when faced with an intracranial or intraspinal mass is, "Is the lesion intraaxial or extraaxial?" This assumes you have correctly answered the question, "Is there a mass present (*cherchez la lésion*)?" Happily, most extraaxial nonosseous masses are benign and are limited to a few entities (meningiomas, schwannomas, epidermoids, arachnoid cysts, dural metastases, and subarachnoid seedings) that can usually be parceled out based on enhancement characteristics and morphology. For the purposes of this discussion intraventricular lesions are considered extraaxial lesions.

It is dangerous to make general statements about specific lesions. In this chapter, entitled "Approach and Pitfalls in Neuroimaging," we indulge in making broad statements about common entities to provide algorithms for the mundane lesion analysis. This buys you an admission ticket to the ballpark, and we hope you will hit some home runs after reading this chapter. But beware of the "pitfalls"—you still may strike out at the plate. By reading the whole book, we are sure you will be an all-star, and perhaps be elected to Cooperstown.

> The authors thought that a metaphor
> Would make reading less of a chore
> They went for broke
> With every joke
> But the text still was a bore!
> (Quoth the Raven, nevermore!)

Extraaxial Brain Neoplasms

Neuroradiologists ascertain whether a mass is intraaxial or extraaxial by several criteria. Extraaxial lesions tend to push the intraaxial structures rather than infiltrate them. Therefore, one sees buckling of gray and white matter around the extraaxial mass. Extraaxial masses tend to have flat, broad bases along the skull or spinal canal. On MR one often sees a "cleft" of (1) low-intensity dura being draped around the mass, (2) cortical vessels being displaced inwardly by the mass, and/or (3) CSF trapped around a mass. Occasionally, particularly in the spinal canal, you will see a meniscus of CSF above and/or below the extraaxial mass. Ipsilateral CSF expansion with contralateral compression of the CSF is the hallmark of intradural extraaxial lesions. The degree of edema (relative to the size of the mass) is less with extraaxial masses than intraaxial ones. Cerebral extraaxial masses tend to be supplied by external carotid artery branches, although occasionally, they parasitize pial vessels. Of extraaxial masses, meningiomas classically demonstrate dural tails in which enhancement is seen to extend in a triangular fashion along the dura, "tailing off" away from the mass. This is not specific for meningiomas, however.

In contrast to extraaxial lesions, intraaxial lesions tend to infiltrate the white matter and expand the superficial brain tissue. They blur the distinction between white and gray matter. They tend to have tongues of tissue that extend deeply in the white matter and may cross the midline through the white matter tracts of the commissures and corpus callosum. Internal carotid artery branches generally supply cerebral intraaxial masses.

Often, because of partial volume effects and the way extraaxial lesions may invaginate into the surrounding CNS tissue, it may not be possible to determine whether a lesion is intraaxial or extraaxial on the basis of a single plane. This underscores the tremendous advantage of MR for evaluating intracranial or intraspinal lesions: its multiplanar capability. In addition, the improved soft-tissue discrimination of MR may help to differentiate the signal intensity of extraaxial neoplasm, dura, vessels, gray matter, and white matter.

Having identified an extraaxial lesion, the next step in limiting the differential diagnosis lies in determining whether the lesion is benign or malignant. As stated previously, the common benign extraaxial masses of the central nervous system are meningiomas and schwannomas. Less common benign extraaxial lesions include lipomas, arachnoid cysts, epidermoids, and dermoids. The latter four do not enhance; meningiomas and schwannomas enhance. See, ain't that easy as Pi (3.141592)?

Malignant extraaxial neoplasms How is an extraaxial mass identified as benign or malignant? The majority of malignant extraaxial masses are due to metastatic bone disease. Although meningiomas may demonstrate some reactivity of the bone in a sclerotic (or, less commonly, lytic) pattern, the bone changes with malignancies tend to be much more destructive, aggressive, and infiltrative. Extraosseous soft tissue in the scalp is more common with metastatic bone disease, although it may occur with meningiomas. Sometimes patients are referred to the neuroradiologist on the basis of abnormalities on bone scans where multiple lesions are identified. Multiplicity favors metastatic disease. If only the inner table of the skull is involved and a dural mass is present, favor meningioma. Bone metastases usually involve both tables.

The other malignant extraaxial masses include the axes of evil; subarachnoid drop metastases (readily distinguishable from osseous metastases by the absence of bone lesions); dural metastases; and lymphoma (not readily distinguishable from anything as it can involve the subarachnoid space, epidural space, bone, dura, or parenchyma). These malignant extraaxial lesions have a higher rate of eliciting vasogenic edema in the subjacent brain, but remember because meningiomas (and sarcoid) are so much more common, they should also be included the differential diagnosis. Lymphoma and sarcoid are good diagnoses to blurt out when you have run out of things to say in conferences, at the boards, or on a blind date. They enhance—the conversation.

Benign extraaxial neoplasms You should be able to readily diagnose most of the *unusual* benign extraaxial masses on the basis of their signal intensity and/or CT density. Arachnoid cysts have density and intensity characteristics identical to that of CSF and do not enhance. Lipomas and dermoids have fat density and intensity and do not generally enhance. Chemical shift artifacts may suggest the presence of fat. Epidermoids follow CSF intensity, for the most part being low on T1WI, bright on T2WI, and low density on CT; however, the FLAIR and DWI scans will eliminate any confusion as they are bright as a light on these sequence. For those in underdeveloped MR regions who are PDWI retainers, epidermoids are also usually brighter than CSF. Looking at the T1WI, you may be able to distinguish an epidermoid as a "cystic" lesion as opposed to schwannomas and meningiomas, which are usually soft-tissue masses. The T2WI is often bright in all lesions.

MENINGIOMAS VERSUS SCHWANNOMAS   After eliminating the unusual nonenhancing extraaxial lesions, it then comes down to a differential diagnosis between meningiomas and schwannomas. What distinguishes these two benign extraaxial masses? CT may be useful. Generally, on unenhanced examinations meningiomas are slightly hyperdense as compared with schwannomas, which are isodense or hypodense. The presence of calcification on CT favors a meningioma. Cystic degeneration favors schwannomas, whereas fatty degeneration favors meningioma, although both can occur in either lesion. Hemorrhagic conversion favors a schwannoma.

On MR, the presence of a dural tail, vascular flow voids within and around the mass, and a broad dural base should lead you to favor meningioma. Obviously, lesions that are located in areas unlikely to have nerves spanning the extraaxial space are more likely to be meningiomas. Because the most common locations of meningiomas are at the sphenoid wing, parasagittally, over the convexities, and along the planum sphenoidale, the diagnosis is clear and the possibility of schwannoma is not even entertained. It is only within the spine, around the foramen magnum, ovale, and rotundum, intraorbitally, in the cerebellopontine angle, along the cavernous sinus, and in a suprasellar location that a differential diagnosis of schwannoma and meningioma is debated. Widening of a neural foramen, an orbital fissure, or a porus acousticus might favor a schwannoma. Schwannomas are more oblong or dumbbell shaped, you dumbbell, and they are usually brighter on T2WI.

An important caveat: anytime you say meningioma, we can say sarcoid, plasmacytoma, lymphoma, or dural met (as we reside in the ivory tower). You say tomato, we say. . . .

Intraventricular Neoplasms

The differential diagnosis of intraventricular lesions resides in a combination of the evaluation of the patient's age and the location of the lesion. In the pediatric age group, a lesion in the region of the trigone of the lateral ventricle is a choroid plexus papilloma until proved otherwise. The presence of calcification and/or hemorrhage within the lesion with intense enhancement will clinch the diagnosis. Meningiomas in children present near the trigone also. If the lesion is in the fourth ventricle or body of the lateral ventricle, consider ependymomas and medulloblastomas.

In an adult, the intraventricular masses to consider include meningiomas, oligodendrogliomas, intraventricular neurocytomas, colloid cysts, ependymomas, subependymal giant cell tumors, and ependymal cysts. Meningiomas occur near the glomus of the choroid plexus in the lateral ventricles. In the young adult an enhancing mass at the foramen of Monro may be a subependymal giant cell astrocytoma (check for stigmata of tuberous sclerosis); in older patients, think neurocytoma, glioblastoma multiforme, metastases, or lymphoma. If a mass at the foramen of Monro does not enhance, consider a low-grade glioma or colloid cyst if the patient is less than 30 years old, and a subependymoma if older than 30 years.

Intraventricular neurocytomas can occur anywhere but favor the septum pellucidum, temporal and frontal horns. Colloid cysts occur at the foramen of Monro. Colloid cysts, ependymal cysts, and epidermoids do not enhance; meningiomas do. Occasionally, a choroid plexus papilloma occurs in an adult; when present, it generally involves the fourth ventricle.

Pineal Region Neoplasms

Specific regions of the brain have more limited differential diagnoses than other areas, including the pineal and the suprasellar cistern regions. As stated in Chapter 3, pineal region tumors can best be differentiated on the basis of serology and the sex of the patient. The germinoma–germ cell lines of pineal region tumors are very uncommon in female patients. Therefore, if you encounter a pineal region tumor in a female patient, it is usually a pineocytoma, pineoblastoma, or tectal glioma mimicking a pineal region lesion. Just in case, look for the presence of fat and/or cystic areas to ensure that it is not a rare teratoma in a female patient. On the other hand, in a male patient favor the germ cell series, and if the lesion is hyperdense on unenhanced CT without evidence of fat or cystic areas, favor germinoma. Otherwise, the differential diagnosis is a toss-up between germinomas, pineocytomas, pineoblastomas, and gliomas. If you need to, punt the case to serology—most germ cell line tumors have a serologic marker (HCG, alpha-fetoprotein) that will suggest the correct diagnosis. Saved by the blood.

Suprasellar Neoplasms

In the suprasellar cistern, the differential diagnosis of masses includes vascular lesions, such as aneurysms, as well as congenital and neoplastic diseases. MR is preferable to CT in evaluating these lesions because it identifies aneurysms nicely with flow voids and/or flow-related artifacts.

A mnemonic for suprasellar masses is SATCHMOE. This mnemonic is an abbreviation for *s*uprasellar extension of pituitary adenomas and *s*arcoid, *a*neurysms and astrocytomas, *t*uberculum sellae meningiomas and tuberculosis, *c*raniopharyngiomas—Rathke cysts and choristomas, *h*ypothalamic gliomas and histiocytosis X, *m*etastatic lesions and myeloblastomas, *o*ptic nerve gliomas and optic neuritis, and *e*pidermoid-dermoid-teratomas and Erdheim-Chester disease. As stated previously, an aneurysm is easily separated from other lesions on MR owing to flow voids, pulsation artifacts, and signal intensity. The presence of high signal intensity in a suprasellar mass on a T1WI should suggest the diagnosis of a craniopharyngioma, Rathke cyst, hemorrhagic pituitary adenoma, lipoma, or teratoma. Think NF-1. The presence of a chemical shift artifact suggestive of fat in the teratoma or dermoid lesion mitigates against a craniopharyngioma or Rathke cyst, where the high signal intensity is thought to be due to either hemorrhage or hyperproteinaceous secretions. The distinction between optic chiasm gliomas and hypothalamic gliomas is moot because, often, these lesions encompass both regions. The presence of bony reaction along the planum sphenoidale or tuberculum sellae and the intensity characteristics will suggest the diagnosis of meningioma. Often on MR, evaluation of lesions in the suprasellar cistern the pituitary gland is separable from the lesion. This obviously is not possible with a pituitary adenoma. The presence of sellar expansion and the position of the diaphragma sellae (elevated with pituitary lesions and depressed with suprasellar lesions) also indicates the diagnosis of suprasellar extension of a pituitary adenoma.

Intraaxial Brain Neoplasms

The majority of intraaxial neoplasms in the brain result from "gliomas" (usually astrocytomas) and metastases. When faced with a single tumor in the brain, the numbers suggest that it is nearly a toss-up between primary astrocytomas and single metastases for the most common intraaxial lesion in the adult. To distinguish between a primary versus a metastatic lesion in the brain, enhanced MR is recommended. MR often shows a well-defined, enhancing, circumscribed mass within the brain, usually with surrounding edema (unless in the cortex) with metastatic disease. The edema associated with a metastasis may be impressive for the size of the enhancing mass. When you identify multiple enhancing lesions in the adult brain, you are most likely dealing with metastases.

As opposed to metastases, astrocytomas generally tend to be more infiltrative, less well defined, and less avidly enhancing. They are less likely to be multiple, although occasionally multifocal glioblastomas and hemangioblastomas may occur in multiple areas. If the lesion does not enhance, the patient has a chance. Eliminate the possibility of metastatic disease and move to the next paragraph.

Arriving at a limited differential diagnosis for gliomas ultimately may be purely mental gymnastics. Often, despite what a radiologist may say, a piece of tissue is required before treatment is instituted. For all the neuroradiologist's ruminations about whether the lesion is a medulloblastoma versus an ependymoma, the neurosurgeon may simply shrug his or her shoulders, hone the scalpel, lop it out and leave it to the pathologist and his myriad of new-fangled immunohistochemical stains to sort out. Nonetheless, it is fun to play the game of trying to predict histology on the basis of neuroimaging findings. Sort of like playing Clue—Colonel Mustard in the study with an oligodendroglioma.

Adult intraaxial neoplasms The very first thing to do in evaluating an intraaxial mass in the brain is to check the film for the patient's age. The set of tumors seen in children is different from that seen in adults, with only moderate overlap. In an adult astrocytomas are the most common neoplasms. There is a good correlation between higher grade of tumor and increasing age. A patient's advanced age (the reader's frame of reference is probably different from the emeritus professor's), the presence of necrosis, hemorrhage (best seen on gradient echo scans), enhancement, and high tumoral blood volume on perfusion imaging (corresponding to endothelial proliferation on histopathologic examination) suggest a diagnosis of malignant astrocytomas. The more choline, the more likely the higher grade.

In adults with an intraparenchymal mass look for the internal architecture of the lesion. A hyperdense non-hemorrhagic intraaxial tumor on unenhanced CT should suggest lymphoma or a "blastoma" (primitive neuroectodermal tumor). Hemorrhage should give you pause. Are you sure it is a tumor and not a hematoma from a vascular lesion, amyloid angiopathy, or hypertension? If there is a solid enhancing nodule nearby, then the gamut of a hemorrhagic tumor should be entertained and would include metastases (e.g., melanoma, choriocarcinoma, renal cell carcinoma, thyroid) or a high-grade malignancy, usually glioblastoma multiforme. When a calcified intraparenchymal mass is encountered, the differential diagnosis should include astrocytomas, oligodendrogliomas, and the rare intraparenchymal ependymoma. Cystic masses include gangliogliomas and pilocytic astrocytomas. A mass in the posterior fossa in the adult is most likely a metastasis; one with increased vascularity, a mural nodule, and/or cyst formation is usually a hemangioblastoma.

Pediatric intraaxial neoplasms As stated previously, the lesions in children tend to be different from those in adults. Posterior fossa masses predominate in the pediatric age group. The differential diagnosis often reduces to a choice of ependymoma, medulloblastoma (primitive neuroectodermal tumor), and pilocytic astrocytomas. Astrocytomas are usually identified in the cerebellar hemispheres and most often are cystic with an associated well-defined, enhancing nodule. In this regard they simulate the adult hemangioblastoma. Medulloblastomas, choroid plexus papillomas, and ependymomas may arise within the fourth ventricle in children and may be distinguished by the presence of calcification within the ependymoma and lack thereof in the medulloblastoma on unenhanced CT. In addition, ependymomas and choroid plexus tumors have a propensity for extending out the foramina of Magendie (medially) and Luschka (laterally), whereas medulloblastomas generally compress the fourth ventricle, arising from the medullary velum of the cerebellum. Choroid plexus tumors are more vascular (have more flow voids on MR) and enhance more dramatically than ependymomas. Fourth ventricular choroid plexus papillomas are more often seen in older patients; ones in the lateral ventricles favor children.

Brain stem gliomas occur more frequently in children. Usually, they are identified because of the distorted morphology; the density of these tumors (usually fibrillary astrocytomas) may mimic normal tissue. They infrequently enhance, and when they do it is spotty at best. What is in the differential diagnosis? Worldwide, tuberculosis is a common brain stem lesion, distinguished by greater enhancement and associated leptomeningeal disease. Rhombencephalitis. Listeria monocytogenes may simulate an infiltrative brain stem mass and is a bugger of a bug to try to grow in culture. Shake some ampicillin at it, though, and it will go away. Lymphomas may occur in the brain stem. Hopefully, they will be hyperdense on CT, to make that diagnosis. Demyelinating (multiple sclerosis, acute disseminated encephalomyelitis, central pontine myelinolysis) and vascular disorders may affect the brain stem; the presentations for these lesions (more abrupt in onset and usually not seen in children) should allow differentiation from an astrocytoma.

In the supratentorial space, gangliogliomas, low-grade astrocytomas, and cortical neuroblastomas predominate in children. These lesions may be identical in appearance, and unless you see cystic areas suggesting gangliogliomas, arriving at a specific diagnosis is very difficult. In children, think ET: PNET (primitive neuroectodermal tumor), DNET (dysembryoplastic neuroepithelial tumors).

NONNEOPLASTIC BRAIN LESIONS

Infarcts

The previous discussion assumes that a lesion is identified as neoplastic. In the adult, the major differential diagnosis of a lesion that has mass effect but is nonneoplastic is an infarct. As opposed to neoplastic lesions, infarcts follow a vascular distribution, may involve the gray matter preferentially, and generally are wedge shaped and wider at the cortical surface. Infarcts almost always present with an acute ictus and within a week or two lose mass effect and swelling, whereas neoplasms and untreated infections progress. Persistence of mass effect beyond 4 weeks strongly favors a nonischemic cause.

The diagnosis of acute infarction is no longer the "stroke of genius" thanks to diffusion weighted scanning. It is incredibly rare for a new completed infarct to be dark on DWI. Bank on this one. The specificity may be a little more shaky.

Difficulty arises when venous infarcts or peripheral septic emboli do not appear to be within an arterial distribution and do not obey the anterior, middle, and posterior cerebral artery territories. Depending upon which vein/sinus is occluded, one may see deep gray (internal cerebral vein, straight sinus), temporal lobe (transverse sinus, middle cerebral veins, vein of Labbé), or parasagittal (superior sagittal sinus) lesions. Venous infarcts on the whole are hemorrhagic, and often a thrombosed sinus and/or cortical vein are seen in association. Diffusion weighted scans are usually bright but there may be an element of reversibility with venous ischemia.

In young patients with strokes, think about predisposing conditions such as dissections (check your "voids"), hypercoaguable states (antiphospholipid antibody syndrome), MELAS, and vasculitis (the protection for dissection was a stent for the rent but infection at the insertion left correction uncertain).

Infections

Septic emboli may be located in subsegmental distributions of major vessels, usually the middle cerebral artery. Once again, they may induce a large amount of vasogenic edema because of the infection and they generally arise at the corticomedullary junction, with extension to the gray matter. These lesions are generally multiple, and the differential diagnosis usually includes metastases. Patients with valve lesions who self-medicate (e.g., shoot up), are the typical hosts.

When septic emboli induce abscess formation, the differentiation with a neoplasm becomes much more difficult. Do not read the scans in outer space. History is the best discriminator here. Let us assume you read in a vacuum. The classic description of abscess walls as thin and regular, with nodularity (if present) on the inner border, is a generalization that does not hold true in many cases. Abscesses induce a large amount of vasogenic edema. On unenhanced T1WI, a hyperintense rim around an abscess may be seen. As opposed to pyogenic abscess capsules, the capsule of a neoplasm or atypical (e.g., fungal) abscess is generally thicker and has nodularity along its outer aspects. The thinner wall of an abscess cavity is usually closer to the ventricle as the vascular supply is decreased.

This is not necessarily true with neoplasms. If meningeal enhancement associated with a ring-enhancing lesion is seen, consider the diagnosis of an inflammatory lesion to be much more likely because it is rarer for neoplasms to extend through the brain substance to the meninges. The DWI scan might suggest an abscess if the central necrotic area lights up—this does not happen with tumor necrosis. But it is inconstant in abscesses. Therefore good if positive, not much help if negative. Like a spouse.

The distinction between encephalitis and infarct is generally made on DWI, or barring the availability of this sequence in your armamentarium, clinical grounds. Encephalitis usually does not have a chronic course; this distinguishes it from a neoplasm. Encephalitides generally do not respect vascular distributions; however, with herpes virus infection, they may be localized to particular lobes of the brain. Herpes preferentially affects the gray matter and white matter of the temporal lobes and frontal lobes, and may be a unilateral process. In this case it may resemble an infarct; however, the vascular distribution of the middle cerebral artery is usually broached and there is sparing of the basal ganglia that would not be seen with a large embolus in the proximal middle cerebral artery. Some cases of herpes encephalitis are bright on DWI. Fever, bilaterality, confusion, and a rapidly progressive course over a few days distinguish herpes from tumors. In distinguishing a neoplasm from herpes, involvement of the basal ganglia or sparing of the gray matter implies a neoplasm. But don't burn your bridges until you come to them—first check the LP results on the electronic patient record.

The other viral encephalitides, including HIV infection and cytomegalovirus infection, may cause focal high signal intensity abnormalities in the white matter that resemble those of ischemic small vessel white matter disease. Once again, the differential diagnosis is generally made on clinical grounds, with the viral infections occurring in a younger age population and white matter ischemia in an older population. These entities do not usually enhance whereas multiple sclerosis might (see Demyelinating Disorders subsection).

Metabolic Disorders

Metabolic disorders of the brain can cause signal intensity abnormalities in the basal ganglia and deep gray matter structures as well as within the white matter. As opposed to neoplastic, vascular, or infectious causes, the metabolic diseases generally are bilateral and symmetric processes. Often they do not incite much edema or mass effect. Leave these diagnoses to serology, spectroscopy, and the fleas—they only deserve 4 sentences.

Demyelinating Disorders

What matters is white matter or your wit dithers (delta MS), mouth mutters (dysphasia), and might whithers (paresis). When one or more lesions are present in the white matter in the brain of an adult, the differential diagnosis may be extensive. Because multiple sclerosis (MS) is most often a clinical diagnosis and also the most common demyelinating disorder in adults, the neuroradiologist does not lose face if he or she recommends clinical correlation in the presence of areas of demyelination in the brain.

Because MS is a polyphasic disease, the presence of areas of abnormal intensity in the white matter that do and do not show enhancement suggests that the lesions are spaced out in time. Therefore, if you identify multiple white matter lesions in the brain, usually without mass effect, some of which enhance and some of which do not enhance, the likelihood of MS is increased. Ask for a history of optic neuritis and you may have your final clue (Professor Plum with the candlestick in the bedroom). It should be noted, however, that other polyphasic disorders such as Lyme disease, sarcoidosis, and vasculitides can appear in a similar manner.

The most common question you will be asked is, "Is it MS or is it ischemic white matter?" Patients with MS tend to be young adults as opposed to patients with ischemic white matter disease. Coincidence of basal ganglionic disease implicates a vascular etiology. Concomitant gray matter lesions in conjunction with white matter abnormalities are unusual in MS, and occur in only 5% of cases. In a similar vein (no pun intended) vasculitis typically has both white matter and gray matter involvement, although isolated gray or white matter disease is possible. Gray and white matter involvement is also seen with some infectious disorders including toxoplasmosis and some viral encephalitides.

The typical differential diagnosis of monophasic white matter lesions includes acute disseminated encephalomyelitis or posttraumatic white matter shearing injuries. Shearing injuries to the white matter may have hemorrhage associated with them best seen on gradient echo images. When hemorrhage is present in white matter lesions, search for a history of trauma. Also think amyloid. Usually in the chronic phase, hemosiderin is seen. Typically, posttraumatic injuries, migrainous white matter lesions, progressive multifocal leukoencephalopathy, and dilated Virchow-Robin spaces do not enhance. Acute disseminated encephalomyelitis, on the other hand, may enhance.

In relatively young patients with white matter disease and stroke think of cerebral autosomal dominant arteriopathy with subcortical infarcts and leukoencephalopathy (CADASIL). Diagnose that and you'll be in the Bush cabinet!

As opposed to demyelinating disorders, the dysmyelinating, peroxisomal, and metabolic disorders are spotted zebras and tend to be bilateral, symmetric, and more diffuse (bizarre). They are typically seen in a pediatric or at risk population. When diffuse white matter disease is associated with macrocephaly, Alexander and Canavan diseases should be suggested. If the white matter abnormality has an occipital predominance and has an enhancing advancing border, adrenal leukodystrophy is the usual diagnosis. It is left to serologic and enzymatic analysis to diagnose the most common dysmyelinating disorder, metachromatic leukodystrophy, as well as the lipodystrophies, mucopolysaccharidoses, and other leukodystrophies. The corollary to Murphy's law: the more obscure the entity, the more likely it is to occur on the day you are on service . . . with everyone else at the ASNR in Hawaii.

Hematomas

Let us say you find a hematoma in the frontal lobe. *Qu'est-ce que c'est?* History sometimes suggests a traumatic hematoma, but make sure the trauma preceded the ictus. Is the bleed the cause of the trauma (uh oh you've got to do an arteriorgram!) or did the trauma cause the bleed (shooo—you're in the clear). Mass effect out of proportion to the amount of hemorrhage, incomplete hemosiderin rings, persistent mass effect, and bizarre intensity progression strongly suggest a tumor. An enhancing nodule would seal the diagnosis. Subarachnoid hemorrhage associated with a hematoma might point to an aneurysm. Enlarged serpentine arteries and veins are seen with arteriovenous malformations, but beware, they may be transiently inapparent because of compression by the hematoma. Make sure the clinicians check the patient's blood pressure to exclude a hypertensive hemorrhage—basal ganglionic hemorrhages are common in patients with hypertension. Finally, advanced age and multiplicity suggest amyloid angiopathy. Siderosis may accompany this diagnosis. Tiny dots of parenchymal hemosiderin staining may also be found with amyloid angiopathy, but you must exclude etiologies such as micro-bleeds from hypertensive crises, radiation-induced telangiectasias, diffuse axonal injuries, or tiny cavernomas.

Fibroosseous Lesions

Just as you probably would not buy a used car from either of these authors be careful about believing too much in our discourses on fibroosseous bone lesions. The category of disease here includes fibrous dysplasia, nonossifying fibroma, osteoblastomas, giant cell tumors, ossifying fibroma, and malignant fibrous histiocytoma (MFH).

The soft tissue fibrous lesions are easier to deal with. MFH is the most common soft-tissue sarcoma in adults, accounting for 20% to 30% of all soft tissue malignancies. Peak age is in the 40s. Fortunately for us neuroradiologists, more than 75% occur in the extremities, with just 5% in the head and neck. Suffice it to say that these lesions may have a variety of histologic subtypes (storiform pleomor-

phic the most common, myxoid, giant cell, inflammatory, and angiomatoid) almost all of which show mixed to low signal intensity on T2WI, low density on CT, and necrosis. Calcification occurs in about 10% of cases.

Aggressive fibromatosis can infiltrate the neck and becomes particularly troublesome when it infiltrates the retropharyngeal space or the brachial plexus. Expect this lesion to obliterate fat planes, be low on T1WI and bright (though not excessively) on T2WI, and enhance markedly. Fibromyxomas are better defined lesions, strongly enhance, and may have hypointense fibrous septae.

Central cementing (non) ossifying fibromas of the maxilla are large, rounded odontogenic tumors of the maxillary alveolar ridge, maxillary sinus and hard palate. The tumors may be sparsely or heavily calcified. Ossifying fibromyxoid tumors are relatively dark on T2WI.

Some authors believe that in many cases fibrous dysplasia and ossifying fibroma of the facial bones are indistinguishable radiographically. Both are ground-glassy and expand bony medullary spaces. No good or reliable imaging findings correlate with histology, so several authors have proposed the term "benign fibroosseous lesion." We are not above taking a pawn in these cases and using this hedge (nor mixing our metaphors).

Fluid-fluid levels used to be the hallmark of aneurysmal bone cysts. Unfortunately, recent reports have included fluid levels in cases of telangiectatic osteosarcoma, chondroblastoma, giant cell tumor of bone, fibrous dysplasia, simple bone cyst, recurrent malignant fibrous histiocytoma of bone, soft-tissue hemangiomata, and synovial sarcomas.

SPINAL LESIONS

The earlier treatise on intracranial extraaxial lesions applies to the spinal canal as well. With regard to intramedullary lesions of the spine, the presence of multiplicity should suggest the diagnosis of a demyelinating disease, sarcoid, hemangioblastomas, neurofibromas, etc. These lesions may or may not enhance.

With a single intramedullary lesion, neoplasms should be first on your mind. It has been said in the past that nearly all the neoplasms of the spinal cord enhance. The enhancement is generally focal and nodular rather than limited and streaky as seen in the demyelinating and inflammatory disorders; however, occasionally, unusual spinal lesions such as herpes zoster, acute disseminated encephalomyelitis, collagen vascular disease, or tuberculosis simulate a neoplasm. Remember to scan the brain for associated lesions in MS. Cord neoplasm usually span many segments before they present clinically. Transverse myelitis may cross a few segments, but an MS plaque will involve just 1–2 levels.

It is not uncommon to see high T2WI signal intensity in the spinal cord opposite an area of disk herniation or severe spinal stenosis. This posttraumatic injury to the spinal cord does not enhance and is rarely associated with an element of hemorrhage that can be detected on gradient echo scans. Most believe it is a result of venous ischemia or subclinical stretching from trauma.

In patients with high intensity cords on T2WI be sure to scrutinize the enhanced sequence for evidence of serpentine veins on the posterior surface of the cord. Because a dural vascular malformation in the proper clinical setting (Foix-Alajouanine syndrome) may simulate a neoplasm, this may be your only chance to spare the patient a cord biopsy. Be vigilant.

Guess what? Only broad generalizations can be made

in trying to determine the histology of an intramedullary glioma, but you might as well take the plunge. More focal hemorrhagic lesions tend to be ependymomas, whereas diffuse infiltrated masses are typically astrocytomas. Hemangioblastomas are vascular and may have flow voids within them.

GRAND FINALE

There are always exceptions to our rules except this rule. Be careful (Table 18-3). It is a jungle out there, with herds of "zebras" and hungry lawyers stalking in

Table 18-3 Overrated signs in neuroradiology

Name of sign	Presumed significance	Pitfall
Delta sign (nonenhancing central area in sagittal sinus) on CT	Thrombosis of sagittal sinus	Routinely seen in normal patients
Hyperdense clot (hyperdensity in MCA vessel) on CT	Clot in vessel	Vessels are nearly always brighter than surrounding areas on 3rd generation or newer CT scanners
Insular ribbon sign (loss of density of cortex in insula) on CT	Sign of MCA infarct	Rarely seen
Murphy's tit (nubbin at apex of aneurysm)	Site of aneurysmal bleed	Too infrequently seen
Chiari I malformation (tonsils below foramen magnum)	Congenital anomaly	Too frequently seen
Partially empty sella (increased CSF in sella)	?	If you **don't** see it, it may be abnormal (that's how often we see it)
Stalk deviation (stalk pushed off midline)	Adenoma may be on opposite side, pushing stalk over	Seen in 3% of normal patients
Hippocampal-choroidal fissure dilatation	Suggestive of Alzheimer disease	Requires unusual plane of section to see reproducibly, found in department chairpersons
Hyperdense falx or tent (greater than brain density) on CT	Interhemispheric subdural hematoma	Falx and tentorium are naturally dense, often calcify
Dural tail sign	Sign of meningioma	Seen in any lesion involving the dura. The authors are keen observers of this sign.
Periventricular hyperintensity	Has been used to classify multiple sclerosis, age-related "ischemic" lesions in Alzheimer disease and depression	Universally seen. Only non-radiologists would use this "Simple Simon" approach
Bright CSF on FLAIR	Indicative of subarachnoid disease	Basal cisterns often normally bright. Anesthesia with use of 100% O_2 turns CSF bright. Nonspecific. Patients with renal failure after gad will have bright CSF on FLAIR and T1-weighted scans
Aqueductal flow void accentuation	Indicates normal-pressure hydrocephalus	Nonspecific. Correlates poorly with shunt success. Technique-dependent. Still looking for our first case of true NPH
CSF dimple-cleft sign	Cortical dysplasia	Still waiting to see first case
Books by other authors	Prettier, more expensive	Have you laughed once reading *their* books?

CSF, cerebrospinal fluid; MCA, middle cerebral artery.

Table 18-4 Overrated techniques

Name of technique	Presumed benefit	Pitfall
MRA		
Cervical	Evaluation for stenosis or occlusion	Overestimates degree of stenosis; poor for "string sign near occlusions"
Intracranial	Aneurysms, AVMs, stenosis	All over- and under-called depending on sequence, observers, scanners
Gadolinium enhanced	Origins from aorta; less artifact	Venous contamination; low volume evaluated; low resolution
Spinal	AVMs of spine	Technically limited; takes too long
MR venography	Venous or sinus thrombosis	Often equivocal; dependent on plane of imaging and stage of thrombosis; poor for cortical vein evaluation
DWI (that is diffusion-weighted imaging, not driving while intoxicated)	Specific for strokes	Also positive with some abscesses, demyelination; other lesions T2 shine-through obscures results; hemorrhage may limit application
Perfusion-weighted imaging	Ischemic penumbra	Does not take into account collateral flow, tandem lesions, bilateral disease; no universal postprocessing paradigm; not validated, single use (dynamic)
3DFT gradient echo of spine	Thin sections to assess foraminal disease	W-a-a-a-y overestimates disease; susceptibility artifact, post-op; unable to evaluate signal abnormality in cord
CT "stroke windows"	Supposed to show low-density strokes better	Never mind—send to DWI (above); irreproducible
CSF pulsation studies	To show effect of tonsils on CSF blood flow at cervicomedullary junction; evaluation for fibromyalgia/chronic fatigue syndrome	No one knows what normal looks like; high rate of positive Munchausen
Magnetic resonance spectroscopy (MRS)	Increased specificity in multiple diseases	If you need this to help you, go back to page 1; everything except Canavan has low NAA, high choline
Functional MRI	Localizes eloquent cortex	Movement degrades images; neovascularity of tumor, AVMs shift venous drainage; left-handed, right-handed, mixed-handed?; statistics are fraught with capacity for devious manipulation (there are liars, damned liars, and statisticians); it ain't electrophysiology; Penfield would plotz if he had to use this
Postgadolinium magnetization transfer imaging	Shows more "enhancing" lesions in brain	False-positives; many of these lesions are bright before gadolinium; increases the TE, decreases the available number of slices; decreases revenue of high-dose gadolinium pharmacy companies, need pre-gad scans, takes longer

the bushes. Do not subscribe to the notion, "The less I commit to a specific diagnoses, the less likely I am to be wrong." Get out there and be a "player." If you know everything in this book, we still invite you to apply for a staff position. We in academia are in desperate need for expanding staff due to the differential remuneration between academic and private practice salaries. By the time this second edition comes out we may be at retirement age, but cannot, due to poor reimbursement and low royalties. Unfortunately, we invested our royalties in ENRON, Global Crossing, and Al Quaida futures. Our children are still on ADC (aid to dependent co-authors).

We made it again, but this may be our last performance! Hold the calls for encores.

Thank you, thank you, thank you. We wish you well, *chers étudiants*. Live, learn, love, and leave a legacy.

APPENDIX: IMPORTANT DIAGNOSTIC GAMUTS

I. Morphology, density, intensity
 A. Calcified lesions
  1. Basal ganglia calcification
   a. Addison disease
   b. AIDS
   c. Carbon monoxide poisoning
   d. Cockayne syndrome
   e. Cysticerosis

f. Fahr disease
g. Hallervorden-Spatz
h. Hyperparathyroidism
i. Hypothyroidism
j. Hypoparathyroidism
k. Hypoxia
l. Idiopathic causes
m. Lead toxicity
n. Leigh disease
o. Methotrexate or radiation therapy
p. Neurofibromatosis
q. Normal (senescent)
r. Pseudohypoparathyroidism
s. Pseudopseudohypoparathyroidism
t. Sturge-Weber
u. TORCH infections
v. Tuberous sclerosis
w. Vitamin D intoxication

2. Calcified intraparenchymal lesions
    a. Arteriovenous malformations, occult cerebrovascular malformations, and aneurysms
    b. Cysticercosis, hydatid, sparganosis
    c. Cytomegalovirus infection
    d. Ependymoma
    e. Mucinous adenocarcinoma
    f. Oligodendroglioma
    g. Osteogenic sarcoma
    h. Sturge-Weber vascular abnormality
    i. Toxoplasmosis
    j. Tuberculomas
    k. Tubers, subependymal nodules

3. Calcified lesions of suprasellar region
    a. Aneurysms
    b. Chrondrosarcoma
    c. Chordoma
    d. Congenital lipoma
    e. Craniopharyngioma
    f. Germ cell tumor/Teratoma/Germinoma
    g. Meningioma
    h. Occult cerebrovascular malformations (OCVM)

4. Calcified lesion: pineal region
    a. Embryonal cell carcinoma
    b. Germinoma
    c. Pineal gland
    d. Pineocytoma/pineoblastoma
    e. Teratoma

5. Intraventricular calcified masses
    a. Astrocytoma
    b. Choroid plexus papilloma/carcinoma
    c. Ependymomas
    d. Meningioma
    e. Neurocytoma
    f. Oligodendrogliomas
    g. Xanthogranuloma

B. Cerebellar degeneration
    1. Alcohol abuse
    2. Ara-C therapy
    3. Ataxia telangiectasia
    4. Cerebellar infarction
    5. Gerstmann—Sträussler—Scheinker syndrome
    6. Hereditary disorders (Friedrich disease, olivopontocerebellar degeneration)
    7. Minamata disease (mercury poisoning)
    8. Paraneoplastic cause
    9. Phenytoin, phenobarbital
    10. Radiation therapy

C. Dense temporal bones
    1. Chronic osteitis
    2. Engelmann disease
    3. Fibrous dysplasia/fibroosseous lesions (what do you expect from 2 neuroradiologists)
    4. Meningioma
    5. Osteopetrosis
    6. Otosclerosis (late stage)
    7. Paget disease
    8. Radiation

D. Fat-containing lesions
    1. Dermoid
    2. Lipoma/lipomatosis
    3. Meningioma (fatty degeneration)
    4. Pantopaque
    5. Paté de Foie Gras embolus
    6. Silicone implants
    7. Teratoma

E. Gyriform Calcification
    1. Cortical tubers
    2. Infarction with laminar necrosis
    3. Meningoencephalitis
    4. Radiation therapy/chemotherapy
    5. Sturge-Weber

F. Hemorrhagic Neoplasms
    1. Hemorrhagic metastases
        a. Breast cancer
        b. Choriocarcinoma
        c. Lung cancer
        d. Melanoma
        e. Neuroblastoma
        f. Renal cell carcinoma
        g. Retinoblastoma
        h. Thyroid cancer
    2. Hemorrhagic primary tumors
        a. Acoustic schwannoma
        b. Choroid plexus carcinoma
        c. Craniopharyngioma
        d. Ependymoma
        e. High grade tumor
        f. Oligodendroglioma
        g. Primitive neuroectodermal tumor

(PNET)/Dysembryoplastic neuroectodermal tumor (DNET)

   h. Pituitary adenoma

G. Hyperdense *noncalcified* lesions on unenhanced CT

1. Blood in vessels (thrombosis, elevated hematocrit)
2. Colloid cyst
3. Germinoma
4. Gliadel wafers
5. Hemorrhage/Clot
6. Iodinated contrast
7. Iron-containing lesion (old hemorrhage/cavernomas/bullets)
8. Lymphoma
9. Medulloblastoma
10. Melanin
11. Meningioma
12. Pantopaque
13. Rathke cysts

H. Hyperintense basal ganglia on T1WI

1. AIDS
2. Carbon monoxide poisoning
3. Cockayne disease
4. Hallervorden-Spatz disease
5. Hemorrhage
6. Hepatic encephalopathy (manganese?)
7. Hyperalimentation (manganese?)
8. Hyperparathyroidism
9. Idiopathic calcification (Fahr disease)
10. Lead poisoning
11. Neurofibromatosis
12. Pseudohypoparathyroidism, pseudopseudo-hypoparathyroidism, hypoparathyroidism, hypervitaminosis D

I. Intracranial cysts

1. Arachnoid cyst
2. Cava interpositum and vergae
3. Colloid cyst
4. Cysticercosis
5. Cyst of cavum septum pellucidum
6. Dandy-Walker
7. Dermoid cyst
8. Ependymal cyst
9. Epidermoid cyst
10. Hydatid disease (*Echinococcus* infection)
11. Intratumoral cyst
12. Pineal cyst
13. Porencephaly
14. Rathke's cyst

J. Megalencephaly

1. Achondroplasia
2. Acromegaly
3. Alexander disease
4. Beckwith-Weidemann syndrome

5. Canavan disease
6. External hydrocephalus
7. Familial idiopathic
8. Hunter and Hurler syndromes
9. Hydrocephalus
10. Klippel—Trenaunay—Weber syndrome
11. Marfan
12. Neurofibromatosis
13. Proteus syndrome
14. Soto syndrome
15. Tay-Sachs disease
16. Tuberous sclerosis

K. Ring-enhancing lesions

1. Abscess
2. Infarcts
3. Metastases
4. Multiple sclerosis plaques
5. Primary neoplasm (high grade astrocytoma, lymphoma)
6. Radiation necrosis
7. Resolving hematomas

L. Tumor versus infarct

1. Clinical presentation
2. Concurrent basal ganglia lesion
3. Cortical ribbon sign (loss of insular cortex)
4. Decreasing mass size with time
5. Dense vessel on CT*
6. Diffusion—weighted scan (ADC) positive
7. Vascular distribution
8. Vascular occlusion on MRA

II. Location

A. Causes of dilated Virchow-Robin spaces

1. Amyloid angiopathy
2. Cryptococcosis
3. Meningioangiomatosis
4. Meningiomelanomatosis
5. Mucopolysaccharidoses (Hunter, Hurler).
6. Normal variation
7. Sarcoidosis
8. Sturge-Weber
9. Tuberculosis
10. Cerebrotendinous xanthomatosis

B. Cavernous sinus masses

1. Chondrosarcoma
2. Chordoma
3. Infection
4. Inflammatory lesions (Tolosa-Hunt syndrome)
5. Lymphoma
6. Meningioma
7. Metastasis
8. Pituitary adenoma
9. Schwannoma
10. Vascular lesions (ectatic carotid, aneurysms, thrombosis, fistulas, occult cerebrovascular malformations)

C. Cerebellopontine angle lesions
1. Aneurysms
2. Arachnoid cyst
3. Chondrosarcoma, chordoma, cordovas
4. Cysticercosis
5. Ependymoma, medulloblastoma
6. Epidermoid-dermoid
7. Exophytic gliomas
8. 5th/7th nerve schwannoma
9. Glomus tumor
10. Lipoma
11. Meningioma
12. Metastases
13. Vestibular schwannoma
D. Clivus masses
1. Chondroid tumors
2. Chordoma
3. Meningioma
4. Metastases
5. Nasopharyngeal carcinoma
6. Plasmacytoma
E. Cranial nerve lesions
1. Actinomycoses
2. Charcot-Marie-Tooth
3. Chronic inflammatory demyelinating polyradiculoneuropathy (CIDP)
4. Dejerine-Sottas
5. Guillain-Barré
6. Hemangioma
7. Lyme disease
8. Lymphoma
9. Multiple sclerosis
10. Perineural malignant spread
11. Sarcoid
12. Subarachnoid seeding
13. Schwannoma/neurofibroma
14. Viral inflammation
F. Enlarged neural foramen
1. Arachnoid cyst
2. Chordoma
3. Congenital absence of pedicle
4. Dural ectasia (Neurofibromatosis)
5. Intraspinal neoplasm
6. Meningioma
7. Metastasis to pedicle
8. Perineural cyst (e.g., Tarlov cyst)
9. Pseudomeningocele (e.g., avulsed nerve root, Marfan, Ehlers-Danlos, ankylosing spondylitis)
10. Schwannoma/neurofibroma
G. Exits from pterygopalatine fossa
1. Foramen rotundum
2. Greater and lesser palatine canals
3. Inferior orbital fissure
4. Pterygomaxillary fissure
5. Sphenopalatine foramen
6. Vidian (pterygoid) canal
H. External auditory canal masses
1. Basal cell carcinoma
2. Branchial cleft abnormality
3. Ceruminoma
4. Epidermoids
5. Exostosis, osteoma
6. Hemangioma
7. Keratosis obturans
8. Langerhans cell histiocytosis
9. Malignant external otitis
10. Melanoma
11. Papilloma
12. Polyp
13. Squamous cell carcinoma
I. Hyperdense disk
1. Ankylosing spondylitis
2. Calcium pyrophosphate deposition disease
3. Diffuse idopathic skeletal hyperostosis (DISH)
4. Degenerative joint disease (DJD)
5. Gout
6. Hemochromatosis
7. Hyperparathyroidism
8. Ochronosis
9. Sequella of infection
10. Spinal fusion (bone graft)
11. Wilson disease
J. Hypoglossal canal lesions
1. Chondroid lesion
2. Chordoma
3. Meningioma
4. Metastasis
5. Perineural spread of tumor
6. Persistent hypoglossal artery
7. Schwannoma
K. Intracanalicular lesions
1. Acoustic schwannoma (90%)
2. Facial nerve schwannoma
3. Hemangioma
4. Infection or inflammation (sarcoidosis, Lyme disease, tuberculosis, Bell's palsy)
5. Labyrinthine artery of anterior inferior cerebellar artery
6. Meningioma
7. Siderosis
8. Subarachnoid seeding
L. Intraventricular masses
1. Arteriovenous malformations
2. Astrocytomas
3. Capillary hemangiomas
4. Central neurocytoma (Oligodendroglioma)
5. Choroid plexus papillomas/carcinomas
6. Colloid cyst
7. Craniopharyngioma

8. Cysticercosis
9. Ependymal cyst
10. Ependymomas/subependymoma
11. Epidermoid/Dermoid
12. Hamartomas
13. Meningiomas
14. Metastases
15. PNET
16. Xanthogranuloma

M. Jugular foramen masses
1. Chondroid and chordoma lesions
2. Expanded jugular bulb
3. Glomus jugulare
4. Lymph node metastatic disease
5. Meningioma
6. Metastasis
7. Nasopharyngeal carcinoma
8. Schwannoma

N. Lesions associated with agenesis of corpus callosum
1. Chiari malformations
2. Dandy-Walker syndrome
3. Encephaloceles
4. Holoprosencephaly
5. Isolated
6. Lipoma
7. Trisomy 13, 15, 18

O. Lesions with decreased ADC, positive DWI scans
1. Carmofur leukoencephalopathy. (Carmofur is an antitumor drug that exerts a defect and gradual conversion into 5-fluorouracil. The degradation product has toxic effects on the myelin, which causes myelin edema)
2. Creutzfeldt-Jakob disease
3. Diffuse axonal injury
4. Encephalitis (HSV)
5. Empyemas
6. Hypoxic ischemic encephalopathy.
7. Infarction,
8. Multiple sclerosis
9. Phenylketonuria
10. Status epilepticus
11. Transneuronal degeneration secondary to striadal infarction
12. Venous infarction,
13. Wallerian degeneration

P. Location of encephaloceles
1. Foraminal (i.e., enlargement of skull base foramen)
2. Frontoethmoidal
3. Nasoethmoidal
4. Nasofrontal
5. Occipital
6. Parietal
7. Sphenoidal
8. Transsphenoidal

Q. Petrous apex masses
1. Cholesterol granulomas
2. Chondroid lesions
3. Epidermoids
4. 5th nerve schwannomas
5. Langerhans Cell Histiocytosis
6. Meningioma
7. Metastases
8. Mucoceles
9. Petrous carotid aneurysm

R. Pituitary masses
1. Abscess
2. Choristoma
3. Granuloma
4. Infarct-apoplexy
5. Intrasellar craniopharyngioma
6. Lymphocytic infundibular adenohypophysitis
7. Metastasis
8. Pituitary adenoma
9. Pituitary hyperplasia (puberty, pregnancy, nelson syndrome, hypothyroidism)
10. Rathke cleft cyst

S. Pituitary stalk-enhancing lesions
1. Craniopharyngioma
2. Erdheim-Chester
3. Germinoma
4. Hypothalamic glioma
5. Langerhans' cell histiocytosis
6. Lymphoma, leukemia
7. Metastases
8. Sarcoidosis
9. TB

T. Prepontine lesions
1. Arachnoid cysts
2. Basilar artery aneurysms
3. Chondroma/Chondrosarcoma
4. Chordoma
5. Dermoids, epidermoids
6. Exophytic brain stem gliomas
7. Meningioma
8. Metastases
9. Schwannoma

U. PRES (Posterior reversible encephalopathy syndrome)
1. ARA-A/ARA-C
2. Cis-platinum
3. Cyclosporine
4. DMSO
5. Eclampsia/Pre-eclampsia
6. FK 506 (Tacrolimus)

7. Hypertension
8. SLE, cryoglobulinema, hemolytic uremia syndrome

V. Primary central nervous system tumors with propensity for subarachnoid seeding
1. Choroid plexus papilloma/carcinoma
2. Ependymoblastoma
3. Germinoma
4. Glioblastoma multiforme
5. Medulloblastoma
6. Oligodendroglioma
7. Pineoblastoma
8. Retinoblastoma

W. Spinal lesions
1. Extradural spinal masses
   a. Arteriovenous malformations
   b. Disk herniations
   c. Extramedullary hematopoesis
   d. Fat/lipoma
   e. Hematoma
   f. Infections
   g. Metastases and primary bone tumors lymphoma
   h. Neurenteric cyst
   i. Neuroblastoma
   j. Osteophytes, hypertrophy of ligamentum flavum, synovial cysts
   k. Sacrococcygeal teratoma
   l. Schwannoma
   m. Trauma and fractures
2. Intradural extramedullary lesions
   a Arachnoid cyst
   b. Arteriovenous malformations
   c. Cysticercosis
   d. Ependymoma
   e. Intradural disk
   f. Lipoma
   g. Lymphoma
   h. Meningiomas
   i. Neurofibromas
   j. Paraganglioma
   k. Sarcoid
   l. Siderosis
   m. Subarachnoid space seeding
3. Intramedullary spinal lesions
   a. Astrocytoma
   b. Contusion
   c. Demyelination (Transverse myelitis, mul-

tiple sclerosis, acute disseminated encephalomyelitis, Devic syndrome)
   d. Ependymoma
   e. Ganglioglioma
   f. Hemangioblastoma
   g. Infection (toxoplasmosis, herpes zoster, herpes simplex, other)
   h. Intramedullary metastases
   i. Lymphoma
   j. Myelitis
   k. Schwannoma
   l. Syringohydromyelia
   m. Vacuolar myelopathy in AIDS
   n. Vascular lesions
   o. Venous hypertension

X. Suprasellar masses
1. Aneurysm
2. Arachnoid cyst
3. Chordoma
4. Craniopharyngioma-Rathke's cyst
5. Cysticercosis, hydatid cyst
6. Epidermoid
7. Germ cell tumors
8. Hypothalamic-chiasmatic glioma
9. Hypothalamic hamartomas
10. Lipoma
11. Lymphoma
12. Meningioma
13. Metastasis
14. Occult cerebrovascular malformations
15. Sarcoid and other granulomatous diseases
16. Suprasellar extension of pituitary mass

Y. Vascular intratympanic masses
1. Aberrant carotid or aneurysm
2. Arteriovenous malformation
3. Cholesteatoma
4. Chronic inflammation
5. Glomus jugulare
6. Glomus tympanicum
7. Hemangioma
8. High, dehiscent jugular bulb
9. Persistent stapedial artery

Z. Endings to book
1. So long
2. Farewell
3. Auf wiedersehen
4. Good night
5. See you in another 8 years

Index

Note: Page numbers followed by f refer to figures; page numbers followed by t refer to tables; and page numbers followed by b refer to boxes.

Note: Page numbers followed by f refer to figures; page numbers followed by t refer to tables; and page numbers followed by b refer to boxes.

Note: Page numbers followed by f refer to figures; page numbers followed by t refer to tables; and page numbers followed by b refer to boxes.

Note: Page numbers followed by f refer to figures; page numbers followed by t refer to tables; and page numbers followed by b refer to boxes.

Note: Page numbers followed by f refer to figures; page numbers followed by t refer to tables; and page numbers followed by b refer to boxes.

Note: Page numbers followed by f refer to figures; page numbers followed by t refer to tables; and page numbers followed by b refer to boxes.

Note: Page numbers followed by f refer to figures; page numbers followed by t refer to tables; and page numbers followed by b refer to boxes.

Note: Page numbers followed by f refer to figures; page numbers followed by t refer to tables; and page numbers followed by b refer to boxes.

Note: Page numbers followed by f refer to figures; page numbers followed by t refer to tables; and page numbers followed by b refer to boxes.

Note: Page numbers followed by f refer to figures; page numbers followed by t refer to tables; and page numbers followed by b refer to boxes.

Note: Page numbers followed by f refer to figures; page numbers followed by t refer to tables; and page numbers followed by b refer to boxes.

Note: Page numbers followed by f refer to figures; page numbers followed by t refer to tables; and page numbers followed by b refer to boxes.

Note: Page numbers followed by f refer to figures; page numbers followed by t refer to tables; and page numbers followed by b refer to boxes.

Note: Page numbers followed by f refer to figures; page numbers followed by t refer to tables; and page numbers followed by b refer to boxes.

Note: Page numbers followed by f refer to figures; page numbers followed by t refer to tables; and page numbers followed by b refer to boxes.

Note: Page numbers followed by f refer to figures; page numbers followed by t refer to tables; and page numbers followed by b refer to boxes.

Note: Page numbers followed by f refer to figures; page numbers followed by t refer to tables; and page numbers followed by b refer to boxes.

Note: Page numbers followed by f refer to figures; page numbers followed by t refer to tables; and page numbers followed by b refer to boxes.

Note: Page numbers followed by f refer to figures; page numbers followed by t refer to tables; and page numbers followed by b refer to boxes.

Note: Page numbers followed by f refer to figures; page numbers followed by t refer to tables; and page numbers followed by b refer to boxes.

Note: Page numbers followed by f refer to figures; page numbers followed by t refer to tables; and page numbers followed by b refer to boxes.

Note: Page numbers followed by f refer to figures; page numbers followed by t refer to tables; and page numbers followed by b refer to boxes.

Note: Page numbers followed by f refer to figures; page numbers followed by t refer to tables; and page numbers followed by b refer to boxes.

Note: Page numbers followed by f refer to figures; page numbers followed by t refer to tables; and page numbers followed by b refer to boxes.

Note: Page numbers followed by f refer to figures; page numbers followed by t refer to tables; and page numbers followed by b refer to boxes.

Note: Page numbers followed by f refer to figures; page numbers followed by t refer to tables; and page numbers followed by b refer to boxes.

Note: Page numbers followed by f refer to figures; page numbers followed by t refer to tables; and page numbers followed by b refer to boxes.

Note: Page numbers followed by f refer to figures; page numbers followed by t refer to tables; and page numbers followed by b refer to boxes.

Note: Page numbers followed by f refer to figures; page numbers followed by t refer to tables; and page numbers followed by b refer to boxes.

Spinal cord—cont'd
  sarcoidosis of, 799, 800f
  subacute combined degeneration of, 804, 805b, 805f
  syringohydromyelia of, 465-466
  tethered, 463-464, 464f, 805-806
  transdural herniation of, 837, 837f
  transverse myelitis of, 800, 802-804, 802f, 804f
  tumoral cysts of, 812, 813f
  vascular lesions of, 831-837, 832f-834f, 835b, 835t, 836b, 836f, 837f
Spinal nerves
  anatomy of, 752-753, 752f, 753f
  cervical, 753
    avulsion of, 838-839, 840f
  conjoined, 752-753
Spindle cell sarcoma, 677-678
Spine, 751-791. *See also* Spinal cord; Vertebrae.
  anatomy of, 752-757, 752f-756f
  aneurysmal bone cyst of, 829
  arachnoid cyst of, 806, 806f-807f
  burst fracture of, 846-847, 848f
  central canal of, 809
  cervical
    atlantoaxial dislocation at, 844, 844f
    atlantoaxial distraction at, 842
    atlantoaxial rotation at, 842-843
    atlantooccipital dislocation at, 841-842, 842f
    congenital anomalies of, 459
    hangman's fracture of, 845, 845f, 846f
    myelography of, 29f, 30
    odontoid fracture at, 844-845, 844f
    on contrast CT, 762
    on plain films, 762-763, 763f
    stability/instability of, 840-841, 842t
    trauma to, 838-839, 839f, 840f, 841, 842t
  chondrosarcoma of, 829
  chordoma of, 828-829, 829f
  columns of, 840, 841f
  compression fracture of, 825-827, 826f, 826t, 827t
    classification of, 846, 847f
    on CT, 826, 826t
    on MR, 826-827, 826f, 827t
  congenital anomalies of, 459-466. *See also specific anomalies.*
  cystic lesions of, 806-811, 806f-810f
  degenerative diseases of, 765-788. *See also specific diseases.*
  diffuse idiopathic skeletal hyperostosis of, 781-782, 782f
  eosinophilic granuloma of, 829, 830f
  fatty masses of, 822, 824b, 824f
  formation of, 411-413, 413t
  fracture of, 825-827, 826f, 826t, 827t
    Chance, 847-848, 849f
    classification of, 846, 847f
    thoracolumbar, 846-847, 848f
  giant cell tumor of, 829
  granulomatous infection of, 796, 798f, 799t
  hemangioma of, 827-828, 8282f
  inflammatory diseases of, 795-805, 799t. *See also specific diseases.*
  instability of, 839-841, 841f, 842t
  lipoma of, 822, 824b, 824f
  lipomatosis of, 830-831
  lumbar
    Chance fracture of, 847-848, 849f

Spine—cont'd
    on plain films, 754f, 763
    schwannoma of, 758f
  marrow of, 765
    changes in, 805, 805f, 806b
  meningioma of, 819-820, 819f
  metastatic disease of, 822, 824, 825f
  multiple myeloma of, 830, 831f
  neoplastic diseases of, 799t, 811-831
    extradural, 822, 824-825, 825f
    extramedullary, 819-822, 820t, 821f-824f, 824b
    intramedullary, 811-818, 811f, 812b, 813f-818f, 818f, 864-865
  neural crest tumors of, 827, 827f
  normal, 763, 765, 765f
  on CT, 761-762, 762f
  on CT myelography, 759, 759f
  on diskography, 762
  on MR, 8-9, 9f, 757-759, 758f, 760f, 763, 765, 765f
  on myelography, 759-761, 759f, 760f
  on plain films, 762-763, 763f
  osteoblastoma of, 829
  osteochondroma of, 830
  osteoid osteoma of, 829, 829f
  Paget disease of, 830, 831f
  postoperative, 788-791. *See also* Failed back surgery syndrome.
  radiation-induced changes in, 805, 805f
  sacral, fracture of, 848-489
  stability of, 839-841, 841f, 842t
  stenosis of, 784-785, 784f, 785f, 787
  Tarlov's cyst of, 806-807, 807f
  terminology for, 751-752
  thoracic, on plain films, 763
  thoracolumbar, fracture of, 846-847, 848f
  trauma to, 837-849, 839f-842f, 842t, 843f-849f
    ligamentous injury with, 838
    on CT, 837-838
    on MR, 838
    pathologic consequences of, 838, 839f
    terminology for, 840-841
    whiplash, 838
  venous plexus of, 765, 765f
Spinocerebellar tract, 48f, 49f, 51f
Spinothalamic tract, 42f-49f, 61-64, 62f-63f
Splenium, 39f, 51, 70f
  lymphoma of, 146f, 147f
Spondylitis, tuberculous, 796
Spondylolisthesis, 763, 764f, 782-783
Spondylolysis, 763, 764f, 782-783
Spondylosis deformans, 774-775, 776f
Spongiform degeneration, 361-362, 364f
Squamous cell carcinoma
  external auditory canal, 569, 570f
  laryngeal. *See* Larynx, squamous cell carcinoma of.
  lip, 662
  masticator space, 702f, 720
  nasopalatine nerves in, 665
  oral cavity, 662-665, 664b, 664f, 691
  oropharyngeal. *See* Oropharynx, squamous cell carcinoma of.
  palatine tonsil, 657-658, 658f
  paranasal sinus, 634, 634f
  parotid gland, 711, 711f
  sinonasal, 634, 634f
  tonsil, 657-658, 658f

Note: Page numbers followed by f refer to figures; page numbers followed by t refer to tables; and page numbers followed by b refer to boxes.

Note: Page numbers followed by f refer to figures; page numbers followed by t refer to tables; and page numbers followed by b refer to boxes.

Note: Page numbers followed by f refer to figures; page numbers followed by t refer to tables; and page numbers followed by b refer to boxes.

Note: Page numbers followed by f refer to figures; page numbers followed by t refer to tables; and page numbers followed by b refer to boxes.

Note: Page numbers followed by f refer to figures; page numbers followed by t refer to tables; and page numbers followed by b refer to boxes.

Note: Page numbers followed by f refer to figures; page numbers followed by t refer to tables; and page numbers followed by b refer to boxes.